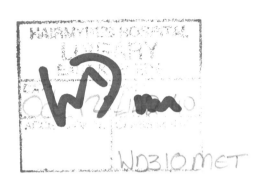

Food Allergy

We dedicate this edition to our wives and children who have supported and encouraged (and tolerated) our career interests; and to the many dedicated investigators who are helping those with adverse reactions to foods and additives.

Food Allergy

Adverse Reactions to Foods and Food Additives

Dean D. Metcalfe, MD

Chief, Laboratory of Allergic Diseases
National Institute of Allergy and Infectious Diseases
National Institutes of Health
Bethesda, Maryland, USA

Hugh A. Sampson, MD

Professor of Pediatrics and Immunobiology
Dean for Translational Biomedical Sciences
Chief of Pediatric Allergy and Immunology
Mount Sinai School of Medicine
New York, New York, USA

Ronald A. Simon, MD

Head, Division of Allergy, Asthma, and Immunology
Adjunct Member, Department of Molecular and Experimental Medicine
The Scripps Research Institute
La Jolla, California, USA

FOURTH EDITION

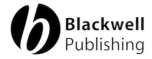

Blackwell
Publishing

First published 2008

1 2008

Library of Congress Cataloging-in-Publication Data

Food allergy : adverse reactions to foods and food additives/edited by
Dean D. Metcalfe, Hugh A. Sampson, Ronald A. Simon. — 4th ed.
    p.; cm.
  Includes bibliographical references and index.
  ISBN: 978-1-4051-5129-0 (alk. paper)
  1. Food allergy. 2. Food additives—Health aspects. I. Metcalfe, Dean D.
II. Sampson, Hugh A. III. Simon, Ronald A.
  [DNLM: 1. Food Hypersensitivity. 2. Food Additives—adverse
effects. WD 310 F68567 2008]
RC596.F6543 2008
616.97′5dc—22

                    2007036832

A catalogue record for this title is available from the British Library

Set in 9/12 Meridien by Charon Tec Ltd (A Macmillan Company), Chennai, India
Printed and bound in Singapore by Fabulous Printers Pte Ltd

Commissioning Editor: Alison Brown
Editorial Assistant: Jenny Seward
Development Editor: Elisabeth Dodds
Production Controller: Debbie Wyer

For further information on Blackwell Publishing, visit our website:
http://www.blackwellpublishing.com

The publisher's policy is to use permanent paper from mills that operate a sustainable
forestry policy, and which has been manufactured from pulp processed using acid-free
and elementary chlorine-free practices. Furthermore, the publisher ensures that the text
paper and cover board used have met acceptable environmental accreditation standards.

Contents

List of Contributors

Shradha Agarwal, MD

The Jeffrey Modell Division of Clinical Immunology
Mount Sinai School of Medicine
New York, New York, USA

Staffan Ahlstedt, PhD

Phadia AB, Uppsala, Sweden; and
National Institute of Environmental Medicine
Center of Allergy Research
Karolinska Institute
Stockholm, Sweden

Matthew Aresery, MD

Allergy and Asthma Associates of Maine
Portland, Maine, USA

James D. Astwood, PhD

V.P. Nutrition, Scientific and Regulatory Affairs
ConAgra Foods
Omaha, Nebraska, USA

James L. Baldwin, MD

Associate Professor
Division of Allergy and Immunology
University of Michigan Medical School
Ann Arbor, Michigan, USA

Gary A. Bannon, PhD

Lead, Protein and Molecular Sciences
Regulatory Product Characterization Organization
Monsanto
St Louis, Missouri, USA

M. Cecilia Berin, PhD

Assistant Professor of Pediatrics
Jaffe Food Allergy Institute
Mount Sinai School of Medicine
New York, New York, USA

Kirsten Beyer, MD

Klinik fuer Paediatrie m.S. Pneumologieund
Immunologie
Berlin, Germany

Carsten Bindslev-Jensen, MD, PhD, DMSc

Professor and Head
Allergy Center and Department of Dermatology
Odense University Hospital
Odense, Denmark

Stephan C. Bischoff, MD

Professor of Medicine
Director, Department of Nutritional Medicine and Immunology
University of Hohenheim
Stuttgart, Germany

Bengt Björkstén, MD, PhD

Emeritus Professor of Paediatrics and Allergy
Prevention
The National Institute of Environmental Medicine/IMM
Division of Physiology
Karolinska Institute
Stockholm, Sweden

S. Allan Bock, MD

National Jewish Medical Research Center; and
Clinical Professor
University of Colorado Health Sciences Center
Denver, Colorado, USA

John V. Bosso, MD

Chief, Allergy and Immunology
Nyack Hospital
New York Presbyterian Healthcare System
West Nyack, New York, USA

Heimo Breiteneder, PhD

Associate Professor
Department of Pathophysiology
Medical University of Vienna
Vienna, Austria

A. Wesley Burks, MD

Professor of Pediatric
Chief, Division of Allergy and Immunology
Duke University Medical Center
Durham, North Carolina, USA

Robert K. Bush, MD

Department of Medicine, Allergy, and
Immunology
University of Wisconsin-Madison
Madison, Wisconsin, USA

André Cartier, MD

Service de Pneumologie
Hôpital du Sacré-Coeur de Montréal
Montréal, Québec, Canada

Soheil Chegini, MD

Assistant Professor of Medicine & Pediatrics
Penn State Hershey Medical Center
Hershey, Pennsylvania, USA

Leslie G. Cleland, MD, FRACP

Rheumatology Unit
Royal Adelaide Hospital
Adelaide, Australia

Lourdes B. de Asis, MD, MPH

Assistant Clinical Professor
Department of Medicine
Division of Allergy and Immunology
Albert Einstein College of Medicine
Bronx, New York, USA

Raymond C. Dobert, PhD

Lead, Oilseeds Regulatory Affairs
Monsanto
St. Louis, Missouri, USA

George Du Toit, PhD

Consultant in Paediatric Allergy
Evelina Children's Hospital
Guy's and St Thomas' NHS Foundation Trust
Kings College London
London, UK

Philippe A. Eigenmann, MD

Head, Pediatric Allergy
Hôpital des Enfants
Geneva, Switzerland

John M. Fahrenholz, MD

Division of Allergy, Pulmonary and Critical
Care Medicine
Vanderbilt University Medical Center
Nashville, Tennessee, USA

David M. Fleischer, MD

Assistant Professor
Division of Pediatric Allergy/Immunology
National Jewish Medical and Research Center; and
Department of Pediatrics
University of Colorado Health Sciences Center
Denver, Colorado, USA

James P. Franciosi, MD, MS

Fellow-Physician
The Children's Hospital of Philadelphia
Division of Gastroenterology, Hepatology
and Nutrition
University of Pennsylvania School of Medicine
Philadelphia, Pennsylvania, USA

Roy L. Fuchs

Director, Regulatory Sciences and Regulatory Affairs
Monsanto
St. Louis, Missouri, USA

Matthew Greenhawt, MD

Division of Allergy and Immunology
University of Michigan Medical School
Ann Arbor, Michigan, USA

Marion Groetch, MS, RD, CDN

Mount Sinai School of Medicine
The Elliot and Roslyn Jaffe Food Allergy Institute
Department of Pediatrics
Division of Allergy and Immunology
New York, New York, USA

Ralf G. Heine, MD, FRACP

Paediatric Gastroenterologist and Allergist
Department of Allergy and Immunology
Royal Children's Hospital
Melbourne, Australia

David J. Hill, MD

Senior Consultant Allergist
Murdoch Children's Research Institute
Royal Children's Hospital
Melbourne, Australia

Clifford S. Hosking, MD, FRACP, FRCPA

Emeritus Immunologist
Department of Allergy
Royal Children's Hospital
Melbourne, Australia

Jonathan O'B. Hourihane, DM, FRCPCH

Professor of Paediatrics and Child Health
Clinical Investigations Unit
Cork University Hospital
Wilton, Cork, Ireland

John M. James, MD

Colorado Allergy and Asthma Centers, P.C.
Fort Collins, Colorado, USA

Stacie M. Jones, MD

Associate Professor of Pediatrics
Chief, Division of Allergy and Immunology
University of Arkansas for Medical Sciences and
Arkansas Children's Hospital
Little Rock, Arkansas, USA

Robert W. Keeton, MD
Division of Allergy and Immunology
University of Michigan Medical School
Ann Arbor, Michigan, USA

Anita Kober, PhD
Phadia AB
Uppsala, Sweden

Hirsh D. Komarow, MD
Staff Clinician
Laboratory of Allergic Diseases
National Institute of Allergy and Infectious Diseases
National Institutes of Health
Bethesda, Maryland, USA

Gideon Lack
Professor of Paediatric Allergy/Head of Paediatric
Allergy Service
King's College London
Guy's and St Thomas' NHS Foundation Trust
London, UK

Samuel B. Lehrer, PhD
Professor of Medicine
Tulane University
New Orleans, Louisiana, USA

Donald Y.M. Leung, MD
Division of Pediatric Allergy-Immunology
National Jewish Medical and Research Center; and
Department of Pediatrics
University of Colorado Health Sciences Center
Denver, Colorado, USA

Xiu-Min Li, MD
Associate Professor of Pediatrics
Pediatric Allergy and Immunology
The Mount Sinai School of Medicine
New York, New York, USA

Chris A. Liacouras, MD
Professor of Pediatrics
The Children's Hospital of Philadelphia
Division of Gastroenterology and Nutrition
University of Pennsylvania School of Medicine
Philadelphia, Pennsylvania, USA

Jonathan E. Markowitz, MD, MSCE
Attending Pediatric Gastroenterologist
Children's Center for Digestive Health
Greenville Hospital System University Medical
Center; and
Associate Professor of Pediatrics
University of South Carolina School of Medicine
Greenville, South Carolina, USA

Lloyd Mayer, MD
Professor of Medicine and Immunobiology
Chief, The Jeffrey Modell Division of Clinical Immunology
Mount Sinai School of Medicine
New York, New York, USA

E. N. Clare Mills, PhD
Institute of Food Research
Norwich Research Park
Colney, Norwich, UK

Michelle M. Montalbano, MD
Department of Allergy / Immunology
The Doctors Clinic
Bremerton, Washington, USA

Anne Muñoz-Furlong
Founder & CEO
The Food Allergy & Anaphylaxis Network
Fairfax, Virginia, USA

Joseph A. Murray, MD
Division of Gastroenterology and Hepatology
Mayo Clinic
Rochester, Minnesota, USA

Jennifer A. Namazy, MD
Division of Allergy, Asthma, and Immunology
Scripps Clinic and Research Foundation
La Jolla, California, USA

Bodo Niggemann, MD
Department of Pediatric Pneumology and Immunology
University Children's Hospital Charité
Berlin, Germany

Julie A. Nordlee, MS
Department of Food Science and Technology
Food Allergy Research and Resource Program
University of Nebraska – Lincoln
Lincoln, Nebraska, USA

Anna Nowak-Wegrzyn, MD
Assistant Professor of Pediatrics
Mount Sinai School of Medicine
The Elliot and Roslyn Jaffe Food Allergy Institute
Department of Pediatrics
Division of Allergy and Immunology
New York, New York, USA

Miae Oh
Fellow, Pediatric Allergy and Immunology
The Mount Sinai School of Medicine
New York, New York, USA

Morten Osterballe, MD
Department of Dermatology
Odense University Hospital
Odense, Denmark

Alberto Rubio-Tapia, MD
Division of Gastroenterology and Hepatology
Mayo Clinic
Rochester, Minnesota, USA

Gernot Sellge, MD, PhD
Unité de Pathogénie Microbienne Moléculaire
Institut Pasteur
INSERM
Paris, France

Scott H. Sicherer, MD
Associate Professor of Pediatrics
The Elliot and Roslyn Jaffe Food Allergy Institute
Department of Pediatrics
Division of Allergy and Immunology
Mount Sinai School of Medicine
New York, New York, USA

Maxcie Sikora, MD
Tulane University Health Sciences Center
New Orleans, Louisiana, USA

Andrew M. Singer, MD
Division of Allergy and Immunology
University of Michigan Medical School
Ann Arbor, Michigan, USA

Keegan M. Smith, MD
Division of Allergy, Pulmonary and Critical
Care Medicine
Vanderbilt University Medical Center
Nashville, Tennessee, USA

Lars Söderström, BSc
Phadia AB
Uppsala, Sweden

Lisa K. Stamp, FRACP, PhD
Department of Medicine
University of Otago
Christchurch, New Zealand

Donald D. Stevenson, MD
Senior Consultant
Division of Allergy, Asthma, and Immunology
Scripps Clinic
Adjunct Member, Dept of Molecular and Experimental Medicine
The Scripps Research Institute
La Jolla, California, USA

Steve L. Taylor, PhD
Professor of Food Science and Technology
Director, Food Allergy Research & Resource Program
University of Nebraska
Lincoln, Nebraska, USA

Ashraf Uzzaman, MD
Clinical Fellow, Mast Cell Biology Section
Laboratory of Allergic Diseases
National Institute of Allergy and Infectious Diseases
National Institutes of Health
Bethesda, Maryland, USA

Julie Wang, MD
Assistant Professor of Pediatrics
Mount Sinai School of Medicine
The Elliot and Roslyn Jaffe Food Allergy Institute
Department of Pediatrics
Division of Allergy and Immunology
New York, New York, USA

Richard W. Weber, MD
Professor of Medicine
National Jewish Medical & Research Center
University of Colorado Health Sciences Center
Denver, Colorado, USA

Laurianne Wild, MD
Tulane University Health Sciences Center
New Orleans, Louisiana, USA

Adam N. Williams, MD
Clinical Fellow, Division of Allergy, Asthma, and Immunology
Scripps Clinic and Green Hospital
La Jolla, California, USA

Katharine M. Woessner, MD
Member, Division of Allergy, Asthma, and Immunology
Scripps Clinic and Green Hospital
La Jolla, California, USA

Robert A. Wood, MD
Professor of Pediatrics and International Health
Department of Pediatrics
Division of Allergy and Immunology
Johns Hopkins University School of Medicine
Baltimore, Maryland, USA

Preface

It is the privilege of the editors to present the fourth edition of Food Allergy: Adverse Reactions to Foods and Food Additives. As in the first three editions, we have attempted to create a book that in one volume would cover pediatric and adult adverse reactions to foods and food additives, stress efforts to place adverse reactions to foods and food additives on a sound scientific basis, select authors to present subjects on the basis of their acknowledged expertise and reputation, and reference each contribution thoroughly. The growth in knowledge in this area continues to be gratifying, and is reflected in the increased length of this edition. Again this book is directed toward clinicians, nutritionists, and scientists interested in food reactions, but we also hope that others interested in such reactions will find the book to be a valuable resource.

The chapters cover basic and clinical perspectives of adverse reactions to food antigens; adverse reactions to food additives; and contemporary topics. The number of chapters addressing these areas has been increased from 29 chapters in the first edition, 38 chapters in the second edition, and 42 chapters in the third edition, to 47 chapters in the fourth edition. Basic science begins with overview chapters on immunology of particular relevance to the gastrointestinal tract as a target organ in allergic reactions and the properties that govern reactions initiated at this site. Included are chapters relating to biotechnology and to thresholds or reactivity. This is followed by chapters reviewing the clinical science of adverse reactions to food antigens from the oral allergy syndrome to anaphylaxis. The section on diagnosis of adverse reactions to foods constitutes a review of the approaches available for diagnosis; and their strengths and weaknesses. Adverse reactions to food additives include chapters addressing specific clinical reactions and reactions to specific agents. The final section on contemporary topics includes discussions of the pharmacologic properties of food, the history and prevention of food allergy, diets and nutrition, neurologic reactions to foods and food additives, psychological considerations and adverse reactions to seafood toxins.

Each of the chapters in this book is capable of standing alone, but when placed together they present a mosaic of the current ideas and research on adverse reactions to foods and food additives. Overlap is unavoidable but, we hope, is held to a minimum. Ideas of one author may sometimes differ from those of another, but in general there is remarkable agreement from chapter to chapter. We, the editors, thus present the fourth edition of a book that we believe represents a fair, balanced, and defensible review of adverse reactions of foods and food additives.

Dean D. Metcalfe
Hugh A. Sampson
Ronald A. Simon

Abbreviations

AA	Arachidonic acid	CCD	Cross-reactive carbohydrate determinants
AAF	Amino acid-based formula	CCP	Cyclic citrullinated peptide
AAP	American Association of Pediatrics	CDC	Centers for Disease Control and Prevention
ACCD	1-Aminocyclopropane-1-carboxylic acid deaminase	CFA	Chemotactic factor of anaphylaxis
		CFR	Code of Federal Regulations
ACD	Allergic contact dermatitis	CGRP	Calcitonin gene-related peptide
AD	Atopic dermatitis	CIU	Chronic idiopathic urticaria
ADA	Americans with Disabilities Act	CIUA	Chronic idiopathic urticaria/angioedema
AE	Atopic eczema	CLA	Cutaneous lymphocyte-associated antigen
AEC	Absolute eosinophil count	CLSI	Clinical and Laboratory Standards Institute
AERD	Aspirin exacerbated respiratory disease	CM	Cow's milk
AFP	Antifreeze protein	CMA	Cow's milk allergy
AGA	Anti-gliadin antibodies	CMF	Cow's milk formula
AI	Adequate intake	CMP	Cow's milk protein
ALA	Alimentary toxic aleukia	CMV	Cucumber mosaic virus
ALDH	Aldehyde dehydrogenase	CNS	Central nervous system
ALS	Advanced Life Support	COX	Cyclo-oxygense
ALSPAC	Avon Longitudinal Study of Parents and Children	CRH	Corticotropin-releasing hormone
		CRP	C-reactive protein
AMDR	Acceptable Macronutrient Distribution Ranges	CRS	Chinese restaurant syndrome
		CSPI	Center for Science in the Public Interest
AMP	Almond major protein	CSR	Class-switch recombination
APC	Antigen-presenting cell	CTL	Cytotoxic T-lymphocyte
APT	Atopy patch test	CTX	Ciguatoxins
ASCA	Anti-Saccharomyces cerevisiae	CU	Cholinergic urticaria
ASHMI	Anti-asthma Herbal Medicine Intervention	DAO	Diamine oxidase
ASP	Amnesic shellfish poisoning	DBPC	Double-blind, placebo-controlled
AZA	Azaspiracid	DBPCFC	Double-blind, placebo-controlled food challenge
AZP	Azaspiracid shellfish poisoning		
BAL	Bronchoalveolar lavage	DC	Dendritic cell
BAT	Basophil activation test	DHA	Docosahexaenoic acid
BCR	B-cell receptor	DMARD	Disease modifying anti-rheumatic agent
BER	Bioenergy regulatory	DoH	Department of Health
BFD	Bioelectric functions diagnosis	DRI	Dietary reference intakes
BHA	Butylated hydroxyanisole	DSP	Diarrhetic shellfish poisoning
BHR	Basophil histamine release	DTH	Delayed-type hypersensitivity
BHT	Butylated hydroxytoluene	DTT	Dithiothreitol
BLG	β-lactoglobulin	DTX	Dinophysistoxins
BMI	Body mass index	EAR	Estimate average requirement
BN	Brown–Norway	EAV	Electroacupuncture according to Voll
BP	Blood pressure	ECP	Eosinophil cationic protein
BPRS	Brief Psychiatric Rating Scale	EDN	Eosinophil-derived neurotoxin
BTX	Brevetoxins	EDS	Electrodermal screening
CAS	Chemical Abstract Society		

EE	Eosinophilic esophagitis	HBGF	Heparin-binding growth factors
EEG	Electroencephalogram	HCN	Hydrogen cyanide
EER	Estimated energy requirement	HE	Hen's egg
EFA	Essential fatty acid	HEL	Hen's egg lysozyme
EFSA	European Food Safety Authority	HEV	High endothelial venules
EGID	Eosinophil-associated gastrointestinal disorders	HKE	Heat-killed *Esherichia coli*
EIA	Enzyme immunoassay	HKL	Heat-killed *Listeria monocytogene*
ELISA	Enzyme-linked immunosorbent assays	HKLM	Heat-killed *Listeria monocytogenes*
EMA	Anti-endomysial	HLA	Human leukocyte antigen
EMT	Emergency Medical Technical	HMW	High molecular weight
EoE	Eosinophilic esophagitis	HNL	Human neutrophil lipocalin
EoG	Eosinophilic gastroenteritis	HPF	High-powered field
EoP	Eosinophilic proctocolitis	HPLC	High-performance liquid chromatography
EPA	Eicosapentaneoic acid	HPP	Hydrolyzed plant protein
EPO	Eosinophilic peroxidase	HRFs	Histamine releasing factors
EPSPS	Enzyme 5-enolpyruvylshikimate-3-phosphate synthase	HRP	Horseradish peroxidase
		HSP	Hydrolyzed soy protein
EPX	Eosinophil protein X	HVP	Hydrolyzed vegetable protein
ESR	Erythrocyte sedimentation rate	IAAs	Indispensable amino acids
FAAN	Food Allergy & Anaphylaxis Network	ICD	Irritant contact dermatitis
FAE	Follicle-associated epithelium	IDECs	Inflammatory dendritic epidermal cells
FAFD	Food-additive-free diet	IEC	Intestinal epithelial cells
FALCPA	Food Allergen Labeling and Consumer Protection Act	IEI	Idiopathic environmental intolerances
		IgA	Immunoglobulin A
FAO	Food and Agricultural Organization	IgE	Immunoglobulin E
FASEB	Federation of American Societies for Experimental Biology	IgG	Immunoglobulin G
		IgM	Immunoglobulin M
FDA	Food and Drug Administration	ISB	Isosulfan blue
FDDPU	Food-dependent delayed pressure urticaria	ISS	Immunostimulatory sequences
		IST	Intradermal skin test
FDEIA	Food-dependent exercise-induced anaphylaxis	ITAM	Immunoreceptor tyrosine-based activation motif
FEC	Food-and-exercise challenge	ITIM	Immunoreceptor tyrosine-based inhibitory motif
FEIA	Fluorescent-enzyme immunoassay	IUIS	International Union of Immunological Societies
FFQs	Food Frequency Questionnaires	JECFA	Expert Committee on Food Additives
FFSPTs	Fresh food skin prick tests	KA	Kainic acid
FPIES	Food protein-induced enterocolitis syndrome	KGF	Keratinocyte growth factor
FSIS	Food Safety Inspection Service	KLH	Key-hole limpet hemocyanin
GALT	Gut-associated lymphoid tissue	LA	Linoleic acid
GBM	Glomerular basement membrane	LCPUFA	Long-chain polyunsaturated fatty acids
GER	Gastroesophageal reflux	LCs	Langerhans cells
GERD	Gastroesophageal reflux disease	LFI	Lateral flow immunochromatographic
GFD	Gluten-free diet	LGG	Lactobacillus rhamnosus GG
GH	Growth hormone	LLDC	Langerhans-like dendritic cell
GHRH	Growth hormone releasing hormone	LMW	Low molecular weight
GI	Gastrointestinal	LOAELs	Lowest observed adverse effect level
GINI	German Infant Nutritional Interventional	LOX	Lipoxygenase
GOX	Glyphosate oxidoreductase	LP	Lamina propria
GrA	Granzymes A	LPL	LP lymphocytes
GRAS	Generally recognized as safe	LPS	Lipopolysaccharide
GrB	Granzymes B	LRTIs	Lower respiratory tract infections
GRS	Generally regarded as safe	LSD	Lysergic acid diethylamide
GSH	Glutathione	LT	Leukotrienes
GVHD	Graft-versus-host disease	LTP	Lipid-transfer protein
HACCP	Hazard analysis and critical control point	MALDI	Matrix-assisted laser desorption/ionization
HAQ	Health Assessment Questionnaire		

MALT	Mucosa-associated lymphoid tissue	PMN	Polymorphonuclear leukocytes
MAO	Monoamine oxidase	PPA	Positive predictive accuracy
MAPK	Mitogen-activated protein kinase	PPI	Protein phosphatase inhibition
MAS	Multicenter Allergy Study	PPs	Peyer's patches
MBP	Major basic protein	PPT	PP-derived T-cells
MC	Mast cell	PPV	Positive predictive value
MCS	Multiple chemical sensitivity	PR	Pathogenesis-related
MED	Minimal eliciting dose	PSP	Paralytic shellfish poisoning
MFA	Multiple food allergies	PST	Prick skin test
MHC	Major histocompatibility complex	PTX	Pectenotoxins
MIP	Macrophage inflammatory protein-1	PUFA	Polyunsaturated fatty acids
MMP	Matrix metalloproteinase	PUVA	Psoralen + ultraviolet A radiation
MMPI	Minnesota Multiphasic Personality Inventory	RADS	Reactive airways dysfunction syndrome
MMR	Measles–mumps–rubella	RAST	Radioallergosorbent test
MPO	Myeloperoxidase	RBA	Receptor-binding assay
MSG	Monosodium glutamate	RBL	Basophilic leukemia
MTX	Maitotoxins	RDA	Recommended dietary allowances
MUFA	Monounsaturated fatty acids	RDBPC	Randomized double–blind, placebo-controlled
MWL	Mushroom worker's lung	RF	Rheumatoid factor
NADPH	Nicotinamide dinucleotide phosphate	RIA	Radioimmunoassay
NASN	National Association of School Nurses	ROS	Reactive oxygen species
NCHS	National Center for Health Statistics	SBPC	Single-blinded placebo-controlled
NDGA	Nordihydroguaiaretic acid	SC	Secretory component
NIAID	National Institute of Allergy and Infectious Diseases	SCF	Stem cell factor
NIOSHA	National Institute for Occupational Safety and Health	SCIT	Subcutaneous immunotherapy
		SCN	Soybean cyst nematode
NK	Natural killer	SFAP	School Food Allergy Program
NLEA	National Labeling and Education Act	SGF	Simulated gastric fluid
NOEL	No observable effect level	SHM	Somatic hyper mutation
NPA	Negative predictive accuracy	SIF	Simulated intestinal fluid
NPIFR	Nasal peak inspiratory flow	SIgA	Secretory IgA
NPV	Negative predictive values	SIgM	Secretory IgM
NSAID	Non-steroidal anti-inflammatory drugs	SIT	Specific immunotherapy
NSBR	Non-specific bronchial responsiveness	SLIT	Sublingual immunotherapy
NSP	Neurotoxic shellfish poisoning	SPECT	Single photon emission computed tomography
OAS	Oral allergy syndrome	SPT	Skin prick test
ODN	Oligodeoxynucleotides	STX	Saxitoxins
OFC	Oral food challenge	SVR	Sequential vascular response
OPRA	Occupational Physicians Reporting Activity	TCM	Traditional Chinese medicine
OT	Oral tolerance	TCR	T-cell receptor
OVA	Ovalbumin	TLP	Thaumatin-like protein
PAF	Platelet-activating factor	TLR	Toll-like receptor
PAMP	Pathogen-associated molecular pattern	TNF	Tumor necrosis factor
PBB	Polybrominated biphenyls	TPA	Tetradecanoylphorbol-13-acetate
PBMC	Peripheral blood mononuclear cell	TSA	Transportation Security Administration
PBT	Peripheral blood T-cells	TTG	Tissue transglutaminase
PCB	Polychlorinated biphenyls	TTX	Tetrodotoxin
PEF	Peak expiratory flow	UGI	Upper GI
PEFR	Peak expiratory flow rate	UL	Upper intake level
PFS	Pollen–food syndrome	USDA	United States Department of Agriculture
PFT	Pulmonary function testing	VAR	Voice-activated audiotape recording
PHA	Phytohemagglutinin	VIP	Vasoactive intestinal peptide
PK	Prausnitz-Küstner	WHO	World Health Organization
PKC	Protein kinase C	YTX	Yessotoxin

PART 1

Adverse Reactions to Food Antigens: Basic Science

CHAPTER 1

Mucosal Immunity

Shradha Agarwal and Lloyd Mayer

KEY CONCEPTS

- The gastrointestinal tract is the largest lymphoid organ in the body. The mucosal immune system is unique in its ability to suppress responses against commensal flora and dietary antigens.

- The mucosal immune system is characterized by unique cell populations (intra-epithelial lymphocytes, lamina propria lymphocytes) and antigen-presenting cells (epithelial cells, tolerized macrophages, and dendritic cells) that contribute to the overall non-responsive state.

- Numerous chemical (extremes of pH, proteases, bile acids) and physical (tight junctions, epithelial membranes, mucus, trefoil factors) barriers reduce antigen access to the underlying mucosal immune system (non-immune exclusion).

- The one positive aspect of mucosal immunity, secretory IgA, serves as a protective barrier against infection by preventing attachment of bacteria and viruses to the underlying epithelium (immune exclusion).

- Oral tolerance is the active non-response to antigen administered via the oral route. Factors affecting the induction of oral tolerance to antigens include: the age and genetics of the host; the nature, form, and dose of the antigen; and the state of the mucosal barrier.

Introduction

An allergic response is thought to be an aberrant, misguided, systemic immune response to an otherwise harmless antigen. An allergic response to a food antigen then can be thought of as an aberrant mucosal immune response. The magnitude of this reaction is multiplied several fold when one looks at this response in the context of normal mucosal immune responses; that is, responses that are suppressed or downregulated. The current view of mucosal immunity is that it is the antithesis of a typical systemic immune response. In the relatively antigen pristine environment of the systemic immune system, foreign proteins, carbohydrates, or even lipids are viewed as potential pathogens. A coordinated reaction seeks to decipher, localize, and subsequently rid the host of the foreign invader. The micro- and macroenvironment of the gastrointestinal (GI) tract is quite different, with continuous exposure to commensal bacteria in the mouth, stomach, and colon and dietary substances (proteins, carbohydrates, and lipids) that if injected subcutaneously would surely elicit a systemic response. The complex mucosal barrier consists of the mucosa, epithelial cells, tight junctions, and the lamina propria (LP) containing Peyer's patches (PP), lymphocytes, antigen-presenting

macrophages, dendritic cells (DCs), and T-cells with receptors for MHC class I- and II-mediated antigen presentation. Those cells exist in an acidic environment replete with digestive enzymes. Failure to maintain this barrier may result in food allergies. Recent studies in murine models demonstrated that anti-ulcer therapy with H2-receptor blockers or proton pump inhibitors may promote the development of IgE antibodies toward digestion-labile dietary compounds, implying that acidity may play a role in the prevention of allergies and in promoting tolerance [1]. Pathways have been established in the mucosa to allow such non-harmful antigens/organisms to be tolerated [2,3]. In fact, it is believed that the failure to tolerate commensals and food antigens is at the heart of a variety of intestinal disorders (e.g. celiac disease and gluten [4,5], inflammatory bowel disease and normal commensals [6–8]). Thus, it makes sense that some defect in mucosal immunity predisposes a person to food allergy. This chapter will lay the groundwork for the understanding of mucosal immunity. The subsequent chapters will focus on the specific pathology seen when the normal immunoregulatory pathways involved in this system are altered.

Mucosal immunity is associated with suppression: the phenomena of controlled inflammation and oral tolerance

As stated in the introduction, the hallmark of mucosal immunity is suppression. Two-linked phenomena symbolize

---

Food Allergy: Adverse Reactions to Foods and Food Additives, 4th edition.
Edited by Dean D. Metcalfe, Hugh A. Sampson, and Ronald A. Simon.
© 2008 Blackwell Publishing, ISBN: 978-1-4501-5129-0.

this state: controlled/physiologic inflammation and tolerance. The mechanisms governing these phenomena are not completely understood, as the dissection of factors governing mucosal immunoregulation is still evolving. It has become quite evident that the systems involved are complex and that the rules governing systemic immunity frequently do not apply in the mucosa. There is unique compartmentalization, cell types, and routes of antigen trafficking which come together to produce the immunosuppressed state.

Controlled/physiologic inflammation (Fig. 1.1)

The anatomy of the mucosal immune system underscores its unique aspects. There is a single layer of columnar epithelium that separates a lumen replete with dietary, bacterial, and viral antigens from the lymphocyte-rich environment of the underlying loose connective tissue stroma called the lamina propria (LP). Histochemical staining of this region reveals an abundance of plasma cells, T-cells, B-cells, macrophages, and DCs [3,9–11]. The difference between the LP and a peripheral lymph node is that there is no clear-cut organization in the LP and the cells in the LP are virtually all activated memory cells. While the cells remain activated, they do not cause destruction of the tissue or severe inflammation. The cells appear to reach a stage of activation but never make it beyond that stage. This phenomenon has been called controlled/physiologic inflammation. The entry and activation of the cells into the LP is antigen driven. Germ-free mice have few cells in the LP. However, within hours to days following colonization with normal intestinal flora (no pathogens) there is a massive influx of cells [12–15]. Despite the persistence of an antigen drive (luminal bacteria), the cells fail to develop into aggressive, inflammation producing lymphocytes and macrophages. Interestingly, many groups have noted that cells activated in the systemic

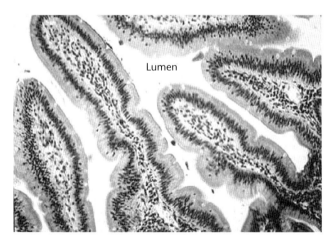

Lumen

Figure 1.1 Hematoxylin and eosin stain of a section of normal small intestine (20×). Depicted is the villi lined with normal absorptive epithelium. The loose connective tissue stroma (LP) is filled with lymphocytes, macrophages, and DCs. This appearance has been termed controlled or physiologic inflammation.

immune system tend to migrate to the gut. It has been postulated that this occurs due to the likelihood of re-exposure to a specific antigen at a mucosal rather than a systemic site. Activated T-cells and B-cells express the mucosal integrin $\alpha_4\beta_7$ which recognizes its ligand, MadCAM [12–19], on high endothelial venules (HEV) in the LP. They exit the venules into the stroma and remain activated in the tissue. Bacteria or their products play a role in this persistent state of activation. Conventional ovalbumin–T-cell receptor (OVA-TCR) transgenic mice have activated T-cells in the LP even in the absence of antigen (OVA) while OVA-TCR transgenic mice crossed on to a RAG-2 deficient background fail to have activated T-cells in the LP [20]. In the former case, the endogenous TCR can rearrange or associate with the transgenic TCR generating receptors that recognize luminal bacteria. This tells us that the drive to recognize bacteria is quite strong. In the latter case the only TCR expressed is that which recognizes OVA and even in the presence of bacteria no activation occurs. If OVA is administered orally to such mice, activated T-cells do appear in the LP. So antigen drive is clearly the important mediator. The failure to produce pathology despite the activated state of the lymphocytes is the consequence of suppressor mechanisms in play. Whether this involves regulatory cells, cytokines, or other, as yet undefined, processes is currently being pursued. It may reflect a combination of events. It is well known that LP lymphocytes (LPLs) respond poorly when activated via the TCR [21,22]. They fail to proliferate although they still produce cytokines. This phenomenon may also contribute to controlled inflammation (i.e. cell populations cannot expand, but the cells can be activated). In the OVA-TCR transgenic mouse mentioned above, OVA feeding results in the influx of cells however, no inflammation is seen even when the antigen is expressed on the overlying epithelium [23]. Conventional cytolytic T-cells (class I restricted) are not easily identified in the mucosa and macrophages respond poorly to bacterial products such as lipopolysaccharide (LPS) because they downregulate a critical component of the LPS receptor, CD14, which associates with Toll-like receptor-4 (TLR-4) and MD2 [24]. Studies examining cellular mechanisms regulating mononuclear cell recruitment to inflamed and non-inflamed intestinal mucosa demonstrate that intestinal macrophages express chemokine receptors but do not migrate to the ligands. In contrast, autologous blood monocytes expressing the same receptors do migrate to the ligands and chemokines derived from LP extracellular matrix [25]. These findings imply that monocytes are necessary in maintaining the macrophage population in non-inflamed mucosa and are the source of macrophages in inflamed mucosa. The inability of intestinal macrophages to participate in receptor-mediated chemotaxis suggests dysregulation in signal transduction, possibly a defect in the signal transduction pathway leading to nuclear factor-κB activation (P.D. Smith, manuscript in preparation). All of these observations support the existence of control mechanisms that tightly regulate mucosal immune responses.

Clearly, there are situations where the inflammatory reaction is intense, such as infectious diseases or ischemia. However, even in the setting of an invasive pathogen such as *Shigella* or *Salmonella*, the inflammatory response is limited and restoration of the mucosal barrier following eradication of the pathogen is quickly followed by a return to the controlled state. Suppressor mechanisms are thought to be a key component of this process as well.

Oral tolerance (Fig. 1.2)

Perhaps the best-recognized phenomenon associated with mucosal immunity and equated with suppression is oral tolerance [27–32]. Oral tolerance can be defined as the active, antigen-specific non-response to antigens administered orally. Many factors play a role in tolerance induction and it may be that there are multiple forms of tolerance elicited by these different factors. The concept of oral tolerance arose from the recognition that we do not frequently generate immune responses to foods we eat, despite the fact that they can be quite foreign to the host. Disruption in oral tolerance results in food allergies and food intolerances such as celiac disease. Part of the explanation for this observation is trivial, relating to the properties of digestion. These processes take large macromolecules and, through aggressive proteolysis, carbohydrate, and lipid degradation, render potentially immunogenic substances, non-immunogenic. In the case of proteins, digestive enzymes break down large polypeptides into non-immunogenic di- and tri-peptides, too small to bind to major histocompatibility complex (MHC) molecules. However, several groups have reported that upward of 2% of dietary proteins enter the draining enteric vasculature intact [33]. Two percent is not a trivial amount, given the fact that Americans eat 40–120 g of protein in the form of beef, chicken, or fish.

The key question then is this: How do we regulate the response to antigens that have bypassed complete digestion? The answer is oral tolerance. Its mechanisms are complex (Table 1.1) and depend on age, genetics, nature of the antigen, form of the antigen, dose of the antigen, and the state of the mucosal barrier.

Several groups have noted that oral tolerance is difficult to achieve in neonates [34]. This may relate to the rather

Table 1.1 Factors affecting the induction of oral tolerance

Age of host (reduced tolerance in the neonate)
Genetics of the host
Nature of the antigen (protein $\ggg$ carbohydrate $\ggggg$ lipid)
Form of the antigen (soluble $>$ particulate)
Dose of the antigen (low dose $\rightarrow$ regulatory T-cells: high dose $\rightarrow$ clonal deletion or anergy)
State of the barrier (decreased barrier $\rightarrow$ decreased tolerance)

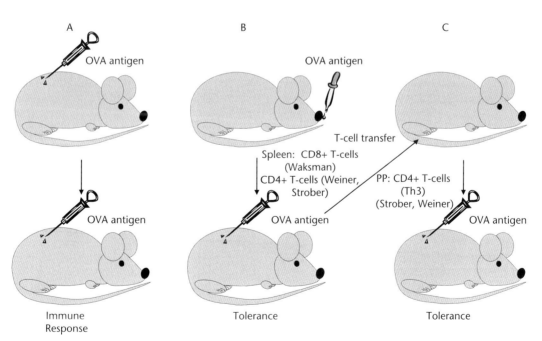

Figure 1.2 Comparison of immune responses elicited by changing the route of administration of the soluble protein antigen OVA. Panel A represents the outcome of systemic immunization. Mice generate both T-cell and antibody responses. Panel B: If mice are fed OVA initially, systemic immunization fails to generate a T- or B-cell response. Panel C: When T-cells transferred from mice initially fed OVA antigen to naïve mice, systemic immunization fails to generate a T- or B-cell response. Tolerance is an active process since it can be transferred by either PP CD4+ T-cells or splenic CD8+ T-cells. These latter findings suggest that there are multiple mechanisms involved in tolerance induction. (Adapted from Chehade and Mayer [26], with permission from the American Academy of Allergy, Asthma and Immunology.)

permeable barrier that exists in the newborn or the immaturity of the mucosal immune system. Within 3 weeks of age (in mice), oral tolerance can be induced, and many previous antibody responses to food antigens are suppressed. The limited diet in the newborn may serve to protect the infant from generating a vigorous response to food antigens.

The next factor involved in tolerance induction is the genetics of the host. Lamont and co-workers [35] published a report detailing tolerance induction in various mouse strains using the same protocol. Balb/c mice tolerize easily while others failed to tolerize at all. Furthermore, some of the failures to tolerize were antigen specific; upon oral feeding, a mouse could be rendered tolerant to one antigen but not another. This finding suggested that the nature and form of the antigen play a significant role in tolerance induction. Protein antigens are the most tolerogenic while carbohydrate and lipids are much less effective in inducing tolerance [36]. The form of the antigen is also critical; for example, a protein given in soluble form (e.g. OVA) is quite tolerogenic whereas, once aggregated, it loses its potential to induce tolerance. The mechanisms underlying these observations have not been completely defined but appear to reflect the nature of the antigen-presenting cell (APC) and the way in which the antigen traffics to the underlying mucosal lymphoid tissue. Insolubility or aggregation may also render a luminal antigen incapable of being sampled [3]. In this setting, non-immune exclusion of the antigen would lead to ignorance from lack of exposure of the mucosa-associated lymphoid tissue (MALT) to the antigen in question. Lastly, prior sensitization to an antigen through extraintestinal routes affects the development of a hypersensitivity response. Sensitization to peanut protein was demonstrated by application of skin preparations containing peanut oil to inflamed skin in children [37]. Similar results were obtained by Hsieh's group in epicutaneous sensitized mice to the egg protein OVA [38].

The dose of antigen administered is also critical to the form of oral tolerance generated. In mouse models, low doses of antigen appear to activate regulatory/suppressor T-cells [39,40]. There are an increasing number of such cells identified, of both CD4 and CD8 lineages. Th3 cells were the initial regulatory/suppressor cells described in oral tolerance [40–42]. These cells appear to be activated in the PP and secrete transforming growth factor-β (TGF-β). This cytokine plays a dual role in mucosal immunity; it is a potent suppressor of T- and B-cell responses while promoting the production of IgA (it is the IgA switch factor) [34,43–45]. TGF-β is the most potent immunosuppressive cytokine defined and its activities are broad and non-specific. A recent investigation of the adaptive immune response to cholera toxin B subunit and macrophage-activating lipopeptide-2 in mouse models lacking the TGF-βR in B-cells (TGFβRII-B) demonstrated undetectable levels of antigen-specific IgA-secreting cells, serum IgA, and

secretory IgA (SIgA) [46]. These results demonstrate the critical role of TGF-βR in antigen-driven stimulation of SIgA responses *in vivo*. The production of TGF-β by Th3 cells elicited by low-dose antigen administration helps explain an associated phenomenon of oral tolerance, bystander suppression. As mentioned earlier, oral tolerance is antigen specific, but if a second antigen is co-administered systemically with the tolerogen, suppression of T- and B-cell responses to that antigen will occur as well. The participation of other regulatory T-cells in oral tolerance is less well defined. Tr1 cells produce interleukin (IL)-10 and appear to be involved in the suppression of graft-versus-host disease (GVHD) and colitis in mouse models, but their activation during oral antigen administration has not been as clearcut [47–49]. Frossard *et al.* demonstrated increased antigen induced IL-10 producing cells in PP from tolerant mice after β-lactoglobulin feeding but not in anaphylactic mice, suggesting that reduced IL-10 production in PPs may support food allergies [50]. There is some evidence for the activation of CD4+CD25+ regulatory T-cells during oral tolerance induction protocols but the nature of their role in the process is still under investigation [51–54]. Experiments in transgenic mice expressing TCRs for OVA demonstrated increased numbers of CD4+CD25+ T-cells expressing cytotoxic T-lymphocyte antigen 4 (CTLA-4) and cytokines TGF-β and IL-10 following OVA feeding. Adoptive transfer of CD4+CD25+ cells from the fed mice suppressed *in vivo* delayed-type hypersensitivity responses in recipient mice [55]. Furthermore, tolerance studies done in mice depleted of CD25+ T-cells along with TGF-β neutralization failed in the induction of oral tolerance by high and low doses of oral OVA suggesting that CD4+CD25+ T-cells and TGF-β together are involved in the induction of oral tolerance, partly through the regulation of expansion of antigen-specific CD4+ T-cells [56]. Markers such as glucocorticoid-induced TNF receptor and transcription factor FoxP3, whose genetic deficiency results in an autoimmune and inflammatory syndrome, have been shown to be expressed by CD4+CD25+ Tregs [57,58]. Lastly, early studies suggested that antigen-specific CD8+ T-cells were involved in tolerance induction since transfer of splenic CD8+ T-cells following feeding of protein antigens could transfer the tolerant state to naïve mice [59–62]. Like the various forms of tolerance described, it is likely that the distinct regulatory T-cells defined might work alone depending on the nature of the tolerogen or in concert to orchestrate the suppression associated with oral tolerance and more globally to mucosal immunity.

Higher doses of antigen lead to a different response, either the induction of anergy or clonal deletion [63]. In this setting, tolerance is not infectious and transfer of T-cells from such tolerized animals does not lead to the transfer of tolerance. Clonal deletion via FAS-mediated apoptosis [64] may be a common mechanism given the enormous antigen load in the GI tract.

The last factor affecting tolerance induction is the state of the barrier. This was alluded to earlier in the discussion relating to the failure to generate tolerance in the neonate since intestinal permeability is greater. However, several states of barrier dysfunction are associated with aggressive inflammation and a lack of tolerance. Increased permeability throughout the intestine has been shown in animal models of anaphylaxis where antigens are able to pass through paracellular spaces by the disruption of tight junctions [65–67]. It is speculated that barrier disruption leads to altered pathways of antigen uptake and failure of conventional mucosal sampling and regulatory pathways. For example, treatment of mice with interferon-γ (IFN-γ) can disrupt the mucosal barrier. These mice fail to develop tolerance to OVA feeding [68,69]. IFN-γ disrupts the inter-epithelial tight junctions allowing for paracellular access by fed antigens. IFN-γ influences many different cell types so mucosal barrier disruption may be only one of several defects induced by such treatment. N-cadherin dominant negative mice develop mucosal inflammation (loss of controlled inflammation) [70]. N-cadherin is a component of the epithelial cell barrier. These mice are immunologically intact yet failed to suppress inflammation, possibly because of the enormous antigenic exposure produced by a leaky barrier. Although no oral tolerance studies have been performed in these animals, the concept that controlled inflammation and oral tolerance are linked phenomena suggest that defects in tolerance would exist here as well.

Do these phenomena relate to food allergy? There is no clear answer yet. No studies of oral tolerance to protein antigens have been performed in food-allergic individuals, and data conflict in studies on the integrity of the mucosal barrier in children with various GI diseases [71–75]. The studies required to answer this question are reasonably straightforward and the answer is critically important for our understanding of food allergy. Oral tolerance has been demonstrated in humans although its efficacy is limited. One clear difference between humans and mice is that tolerance is induced for T-cells but not for B-cells [76,77]. This difference may have relevance in human antibody-mediated diseases.

The nature of antibody responses in the gut-associated lymphoid tissue

IgE is largely the antibody responsible for food allergy. In genetically pre-disposed individuals an environment favoring IgE production in response to an allergen is established. The generation of T-cell responses promoting a B-cell class switch to IgE has been described (i.e. Th2 lymphocytes secreting IL-4). The next question, therefore, is whether such an environment exists in the gut-associated lymphoid tissue (GALT), and what types of antibody responses predominate in this system.

The production of a unique antibody isotype-SIgA was the first difference noted between systemic and mucosal immunity. In fact, given the surface area of the GI tract (the size of one tennis court), the cell density and the overwhelming number of plasma cells within the GALT, IgA produced by the mucosal immune system far exceeds the quantity of any other antibody in the body. SIgA is a dimeric form of IgA produced in the LP and transported into the lumen by a specialized pathway through the intestinal epithelium (Figs 1.1–1.3) [78]. SIgA is also unique in that it is anti-inflammatory in nature. It does not bind classical complement components but rather binds to luminal

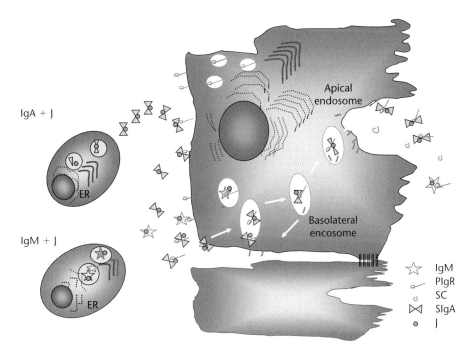

IgA + J

IgM + J

Apical endosome

Basolateral encosome

ER

☆ IgM
↙ PIgR
↺ SC
⋈ SIgA
● J

Figure 1.3 Depiction of the transport of SIgA and SIgM. Plasma cells produce monomeric IgA or IgM that polymerizes after binding to J chain. Polymeric immunoglobulins are secreted into the LP and taken up by the PIgR or SC produced by IECs and expressed on the basolateral surface. Bound SIgA or SIgM are internalized and transcytosed in vesicles across the epithelium and releases with SC into the intestinal lumen. SC protects the SIg from degradation once in the lumen.

antigens, preventing their attachment to the epithelium or promoting agglutination and subsequent removal of the antigen in the mucus layer overlying the epithelium. These latter two events reflect "immune exclusion," as opposed to the non-specific mechanisms of exclusion alluded to earlier (the epithelium, the mucus barrier, proteolytic digestion, etc.). SIgA has one additional unique aspect – its ability to bind to an epithelial cell-derived glycoprotein called secretory component (SC), the receptor for polymeric Ig receptor (pIgR) [79–82]. SC serves two functions: it promotes the transcytosis of SIgA from the LP through the epithelium into the lumen, and, once in the lumen, it protects the antibody against proteolytic degradation. This role is critically important, because the enzymes used for protein digestion are equally effective at degrading antibody molecules. For example, pepsin and papain in the stomach digest IgG into F(ab)$'_2$ and Fab fragments. Further protection against trypsin and chymotrypsin in the lumen allows SIgA to exist in a rather hostile environment.

IgM is another antibody capable of binding SC (pIgR). Like IgA, IgM uses J chain produced by plasma cells to form polymers; in the case of IgM, a pentamer. SC binds to the Fc portions of the antibody formed by the polymerization. The ability of IgM to bind SC may be important in patients with IgA deficiency. Although not directly proven, secretory IgM (SIgM) may compensate for the absence of IgA in the lumen.

What about other Ig isotypes? The focus for years in mucosal immunity was SIgA. It was estimated that upward of 95% of antibody produced at mucosal surfaces was IgA. Initial reports ignored the fact that IgG was present not only in the LP, but also in secretions [83,84]. These latter observations were attributed to leakage across the barrier from plasma IgG. However, recent attention has focused on the potential role of the neonatal Fc receptor, FcR_N, which might serve as a bidirectional transporter of IgG [85,86]. The FcR_N is expressed early on, possibly as a mechanism to take up maternal IgG in breast milk. Its expression was thought to be downregulated after weaning, but recent studies suggest that it may still be expressed in adult lung, kidney, and possibly gut epithelium. As suggested above, there are new data indicating that it might serve to transport IgG both to and from the lumen. In a series of inflammatory diseases of the bowel, marked increases in IgG in the LP and lumen have been observed [87].

We are left then with IgE. Given the modest amounts present in the serum, it has been even more difficult to detect IgE in mucosal tissues or secretions. However, there have not been many studies attempting to do so. Mucosal mast cells are well described in the gut tissue. The IgE Fc receptor, FcεRI, is present and mast cell degranulation is reported (although not necessarily IgE related). FcεRI is not expressed by the intestinal epithelium so it is unlikely that this molecule would serve a transport function. CD23 (FcεRII), however, has been described on gut epithelial cells,

and one model has suggested that it may play a role in facilitated antigen uptake and consequent mast cell degranulation [88,89]. In this setting, degranulation is associated with fluid and electrolyte loss into the luminal side of the epithelium, an event clearly associated with an allergic reaction in the lung and gut. Thus, the initial concept that IgA was the be-all and end-all in the gut may be shortsighted and roles for other isotypes in health and disease require further study.

The anatomy of the gut-associated lymphoid tissue: antigen trafficking patterns (Fig. 1.4)

The final piece of the puzzle is probably the most critical for regulating mucosal immune responses, the cells involved in antigen uptake and presentation. As alluded to earlier, antigens in the GI tract are treated very differently than in the systemic immune system. There are additional hurdles to jump. Enzymes, detergents (bile salts), extremes of pH can alter the nature of the antigen before it comes into contact with the GALT. If the antigen survives this onslaught, it has to deal with a thick mucous barrier, a dense epithelial membrane, and intercellular tight junctions. Mucin produced by goblet cells and trefoil factors produced by epithelial cells provide a viscous barrier to antigen passage. However, despite these obstacles, antigens manage to find their way across the epithelium and immune responses are elicited.

Probably the best defined pathway of antigen traffic is in the GI tract through the specialized epithelium overlying the organized lymphoid tissue of the GALT; the PP. This specialized epithelium has been called follicle-associated epithelium (FAE) or microfold cell (M-cell). The M-cell is unique in contrast to the adjacent absorptive epithelium. It has few microvilli, a limited mucin overlayer, a thin elongated cytoplasm and a shape that forms a pocket around subepithelial lymphocytes, macrophages, and DCs. The initial description of the M-cell not only documented its unique structure, but also its ability to take up large particulate antigens from the lumen into the subepithelial space [90–93]. M-cells contain few lysosomes so little or no processing of antigen can occur [94]. M-cells protrude into the lumen, pushed up by the underlying PP. This provides a larger area for contact with luminal contents. The surface of the M-cell is special in that it expresses a number of lectin-like molecules which help promote binding to specific pathogens. For example, poliovirus binds to the M-cell surface via a series of glycoconjugate interactions [95]. Interestingly, antigens that bind to the M-cell and get transported to the underlying PP generally elicit a positive (SIgA) response. Successful oral vaccines bind to the M-cell and not to the epithelium. Thus, this part of the GALT appears to be critical for the positive aspects of mucosal immunity.

The M-cell is a conduit to the PP. Antigens transcytosed across the M-cell and into the subepithelial pocket are

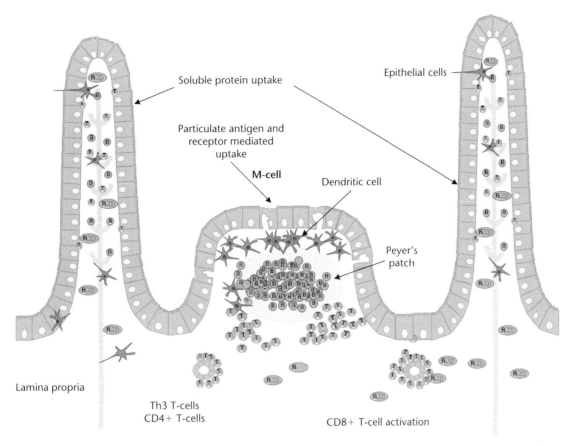

Figure 1.4 Sites of antigen uptake in the gut. Antigen taken up by M-cells travel to the underlying PP where Th3 (TGF-β secreting) T-cells are activated and isotype switching to IgA occurs (B-cells). This pathway favors particulate or aggregated antigen. Antigen taken up by intestinal epithelial cells (IECs) may activate CD8+ T-cells which suppress local (and possibly systemic – tolerance) responses. This pathway favors soluble antigen.

taken up by macrophages/DCs and carried into the PP. Once in the patch, TGF-β-secreting T-cells promote B-cell isotype switching to IgA [45]. These cells leave the patch and migrate to the mesenteric lymph node and eventually to other mucosal sites where they undergo terminal maturation to dimeric IgA producing plasma cells. In relation to food allergy and tolerance mechanisms, Frossard *et al.* compared antigen-specific IgA-secreting cells in PP from mice sensitized to β-lactoglobulin resulting in anaphylaxis versus tolerant mice. Tolerant mice were found to have higher numbers of β-lactoglobulin-specific IgA-secreting cells in PPs in addition to higher fecal β-lactoglobulin-specific IgA titers compared to anaphylactic mice. The increase in antigen-specific SIgA is induced by IL-10 and TGF-β production by T-cells from PPs [96].

Several groups have suggested that M-cells are involved in tolerance induction as well. The same TGF-β producing cells activated in the PP that promote IgA switching also suppress IgG and IgM production and T-cell proliferation. These are the Th3 cells described initially by Weiner's group [39]. There are some problems with this scenario however. First, M-cells are more limited in their distribution, so that

antigen sampling by these cells may be modest in the context of the whole gut. Second, M-cells are rather inefficient at taking up soluble proteins. As stated earlier, soluble proteins are the best tolerogens. These two factors together suggest that sites other than PPs are important for tolerance induction. Recent studies have attempted to clearly define the role of M-cells and the PP in tolerance induction. Work initially performed by Kerneis *et al.* documented the requirement of PP for M-cell development [97]. The induction of M-cell differentiation was dependent on direct contact between the epithelium and PP lymphocytes (B-cells).

In the absence of PP there are no M-cells. In B-cell deficient animals (where there are no PP), M-cells have not been identified [98]. Several groups looked at tolerance induction in manipulated animals to assess the need for M-cells in this process. In most cases, there appeared to be a direct correlation between the presence of PP and tolerance; however, each manipulation (LTβ–/–, LTβR–/–, treatment with LTβ-Fc fusion protein *in utero*) [99–101] is associated with abnormalities in systemic immunity as well (e.g. no spleen, altered mesenteric LNs, etc.) so interpretation of these data is clouded. Furthermore, compared to mice with intact PPs, PP deficient mice were found to have the same frequencies of APCs in secondary lymphoid organs after oral administration of soluble antigen [102].

More recent data demonstrate that tolerance can occur in the absence of M-cells and PPs. Kraus *et al.* created a mouse model of surgically isolated small bowel loops (fully vascularized with intact lymphatic drainage) that either contained or were deficient in M-cells and PPs. They were able to generate comparable tolerance to OVA peptides in the presence or absence of PPs. These data strongly support the concept that cells other than M-cells are involved in tolerance induction [103].

DCs play an important role in the tolerance and immunity of the gut. They function as APCs, help in maintaining gut integrity through expression of tight junction proteins, and orchestrate Th1 and Th2 responses. DCs continuously migrate within lymphoid tissues even in the absence of inflammation and present self-antigens, likely from dying apoptotic cells, to maintain self-tolerance [104]. DCs process internalized antigens slower than macrophages, allowing adequate accumulation, processing, and eventually presentation of antigens [105]. They have been found within the LP and their presence is dependent on chemokine receptor CX3CR1 to form transepithelial dendrites which allows for direct sampling of antigen in the lumen [106,107]. Studies are ongoing to determine the chemokines responsible for migration of DCs to the LP. However, what has been found is that epithelial cell-expressed CCL25, the ligand for CCR9 and CCR10, may be a DC chemokine in the small bowel, and CCL28, ligand for CCR3 and CCR10, may be a DC chemokine in the colon [108–110]. DCs in the LP were found to take up the majority of orally administered protein, suggesting they may be tolerogenic [111]. Mowat, Viney and colleagues expanded DCs in the LP by treating mice with Flt-3 ligand. The increase in gut DCs directly correlated with enhanced tolerance [112]. The continuous sampling and migration by DCs is thought to be responsible for T-cell tolerance to food antigens [113]. Several studies have examined the pathways by which DCs maybe tolerogenic including their maturation status at the time of antigen presentation to T-cells; downregulation of costimulatory molecules CD80 and CD86, production of suppressive cytokines IL-10, TGF-β and IFN-α, and interaction with costimulatory molecules CD200 [107,114,115]. Man *et al.* examined DC–T-cell cross-talk in relation to IgE-mediated allergic reactions to food, specifically investigating T-cell-mediated apoptosis of myeloid DCs from spleen and PPs of mice with cow's milk allergy. DCs from mice with milk allergy exhibited reduced apoptosis compared to DCs from control non-allergic donors. This suggests that dysregulation of DCs, systemic and gut derived, influences the development of food allergy and is necessary for controlling immune responses [116].

The other cell type potentially involved in antigen sampling is the absorptive epithelium. These cells not only take

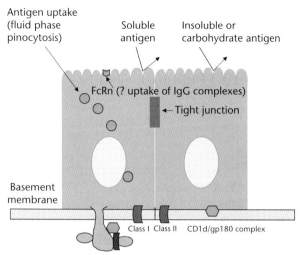

Figure 1.5 Antigen uptake by IECs. Soluble proteins are taken up by fluid phase endocytosis and pursue a transcellular pathway (endolysosomal pathway). Particulate and carbohydrate antigens are either not taken up or taken up with slower kinetics. Paracellular transport is blocked by the presence of tight junctions. In the case of antigen presentation by the IEC, a complex of a non-classical class I molecule (CD1d) and a CD8 ligand, gp180, is recognized by a subpopulation of T-cells in the LP (possibly intra-epithelial space as well). The interaction of IEC with the LPL occurs by foot processes extruded by the IEC into the LP through fenestrations in the basement membrane. Antigens can also be selectively taken up by a series of Fc receptors expressed by IEC (neonatal FcεR for IgG or CD23 for IgE). The consequences of such uptake may affect responses to food antigens (food allergy).

up soluble proteins, but also expresses MHC class I, II, as well as non-classical class I molecules to serve as restriction elements for local T-cell populations (Fig. 1.5). Indeed, a number of groups have documented the capacity of intestinal epithelial cells (IECs) to serve as APCs to both CD4+ and CD8+ T-cells [117–124]. In man, *in vitro* studies have suggested that normal IECs used as APCs selectively activate CD8+ suppressor T-cells [122]. Activation of such cells could be involved in controlled inflammation and possibly oral tolerance. Epithelial cells could interact with intra-epithelial lymphocytes (IELs) (CD8+ in the small intestine) or LPLs. The studies by Kraus *et al.* alluded to above (loop model) strongly support a role of IECs in tolerance induction. However, a role for IECs in the regulation of mucosal immunity is best demonstrated in studies of inflammatory bowel disease. In *in vitro* co-culture experiments, IECs from patients with inflammatory bowel disease stimulated CD4+ T-cells rather than suppressive CD8+ cells activated by normal enterocytes [125]. Furthermore, Kraus *et al.* demonstrated that oral antigen administration does not result in tolerance in patients with inflammatory bowel disease but rather results in active immunity [77].

Once again how does this fit into the process of food allergy? Do allergens traffic differently in predisposed individuals? Is there a Th2 dominant environment in the

GALT of food-allergic patients? As mentioned earlier, IECs do express CD23 induced by IL-4 so there is a potential pathway for allergen/IgE complexes to enter from the lumen. However, these are secondary events. The real key is how the initial IgE is produced and what pathways are involved in its dominance. The answers to these questions will provide major insights into the pathogenesis of food allergy.

References

1 Untersmayr E, Bakos N, Scholl I, *et al*. Anti-ulcer drugs promote IgE formation toward dietary antigens in adult patients. *Faseb J* 2005;19:656–8.

2 Kiyono H. Mucosal immune system: close encounter in the uncharted world of immunology. *Ophthalmologica* 2001;215:22–32.

3 Mayer L, Sperber K, Chan L, *et al*. Oral tolerance to protein antigens. *Allergy* 2001;56:12–15.

4 Farrell RJ, Kelly CP. Celiac sprue. *N Engl J Med* 2002;346:180–8.

5 Freeman H, Lemoyne M, Pare P. Coeliac disease. *Best Pract Res Clin Gastroenterol* 2002;16:37–49.

6 Farrell RJ, LaMont JT. Microbial factors in inflammatory bowel disease. *Gastroenterol Clin North Am* 2002;31:41–62.

7 Basset C, Holton J. Inflammatory bowel disease: Is the intestine a Trojan horse? *Sci Prog* 2002;85:33–56.

8 Prantera C, Scribano ML. Crohn's disease: the case for bacteria. *Ital J Gastroenterol Hepatol* 1999;31:244–6.

9 Geboes K. From inflammation to lesion. *Acta Gastroenterol Belg* 1994;57:273–84.

10 Sartor RB. Current concepts of the etiology and pathogenesis of ulcerative colitis and Crohn's disease. *Gastroenterol Clin North Am* 1995;24:475–507.

11 Mayer L. Mucosal immunity and gastrointestinal antigen processing. *J Pediatr Gastroenterol Nutr* 2000;30:S4–12.

12 Anderson JC. The response of gut-associated lymphoid tissue in gnotobiotic piglets to the presence of bacterial antigen in the alimentary tract. *J Anat* 1977;124:555–62.

13 Ishikawa K, Satoh Y, Tanaka H, Ono K. Influence of conventionalization on small-intestinal mucosa of germ-free Wistar rats: quantitative light microscopic observations. *Acta Anat (Basel)* 1986;127:296–302.

14 Cebra JJ, Periwal SB, Lee G, *et al*. Development and maintenance of the gut-associated lymphoid tissue (GALT): the roles of enteric bacteria and viruses. *Dev Immunol* 1998;6:13–18.

15 Rothkotter HJ, Ulbrich H, Pabst R. The postnatal development of gut lamina propria lymphocytes: number, proliferation, and T and B cell subsets in conventional and germ-free pigs. *Pediatr Res* 1991;29:237–42.

16 Hamann A, Andrew DP, Jablonski-Westrich D, *et al*. Role of alpha 4-integrins in lymphocyte homing to mucosal tissues in vivo. *J Immunol* 1994;152:3282–93.

17 Shyjan AM, Bertagnolli M, Kenney CJ, Briskin MJ. Human mucosal addressin cell adhesion molecule-1 (MAdCAM-1) demonstrates structural and functional similarities to the alpha

18 De Keyser F, Elewaut D, De Wever N, *et al*. The gut associated addressins: lymphocyte homing in the gut. *Baillieres Clin Rheumatol* 1996;10:25–39.

19 Viney JL, Jones S, Chiu HH, *et al*. Mucosal addressin cell adhesion molecule-1: a structural and functional analysis demarcates the integrin binding motif. *J Immunol* 1996;157:2488–97.

20 Saparov A, Kraus LA, Cong Y, *et al*. Memory/effector T cells in TCR transgenic mice develop via recognition of enteric antigens by a second, endogenous TCR. *Int Immunol* 1999;11:1253–64.

21 Qiao L, Schurmann G, Betzler M, Meuer SC. Activation and signaling status of human lamina propria T lymphocytes. *Gastroenterology* 1991;101:1529–36.

22 De Maria R, Fais S, Silvestri M, *et al*. Continuous *in vivo* activation and transient hyporesponsiveness to TcR/CD3 triggering of human gut lamina propria lymphocytes. *Eur J Immunol* 1993;23:3104–8.

23 Vezys V, Olson S, Lefrancois L. Expression of intestine-specific antigen reveals novel pathways of CD8 T cell tolerance induction. *Immunity* 2000;12:505–14.

24 Smith PD, Smythies LE, Mosteller-Barnum M, *et al*. Intestinal macrophages lack CD14 and CD89 and consequently are down-regulated for LPS- and IgA-mediated activities. *J Immunol* 2001;167:2651–6.

25 Smythies LE, Maheshwari A, Clements R, *et al*. Mucosal IL-8 and TGF-beta recruit blood monocytes: evidence for cross-talk between the lamina propria stroma and myeloid cells. *J Leukoc Biol* 2006;80:492–9.

26 Chehade M, Mayer L. Oral tolerance and its relation to food hypersensitivities. *J Allergy Clin Immunol* 2005;115:3–12; quiz 13.

27 Xiao BG, Link H. Mucosal tolerance: a two-edged sword to prevent and treat autoimmune diseases. *Clin Immunol Immunopathol* 1997;85:119–28.

28 Whitacre CC, Gienapp IE, Meyer A, *et al*. Treatment of autoimmune disease by oral tolerance to autoantigens. *Clin Immunol Immunopathol* 1996;80:S31–9.

29 Weiner HL, Mayer LF. Oral tolerance: mechanisms and applications. Introduction. *Ann NY Acad Sci* 1996;778:xiii–xviii.

30 Titus RG, Chiller JM. Orally induced tolerance. Definition at the cellular level. *Int Arch Allergy Appl Immunol* 1981;65:323–38.

31 Strober W, Kelsall B, Marth T. Oral tolerance. *J Clin Immunol* 1998;18:1–30.

32 MacDonald TT. T cell immunity to oral allergens. *Curr Opin Immunol* 1998;10:620–7.

33 Webb Jr KE. Amino acid and peptide absorption from the gastrointestinal tract. *Fed Proc* 1986;45:2268–71.

34 Strobel S. Neonatal oral tolerance. *Ann NY Acad Sci* 1996;778:88–102.

35 Lamont AG, Mowat AM, Browning MJ, Parrott DM. Genetic control of oral tolerance to ovalbumin in mice. *Immunology* 1988;63:737–9.

36 Garside P, Mowat AM. Mechanisms of oral tolerance. *Crit Rev Immunol* 1997;17:119–37.

37 Lack G, Fox D, Northstone K, Golding J. Factors associated with the development of peanut allergy in childhood. *N Engl J Med* 2003;348:977–85.

38 Hsieh KY, Tsai CC, Wu CH, Lin RH. Epicutaneous exposure to protein antigen and food allergy. *Clin Exp Allergy* 2003;33:1067–75.

39 Friedman A, Weiner HL. Induction of anergy or active suppression following oral tolerance is determined by antigen dosage. *Proc Natl Acad Sci USA* 1994;91:6688–92.

40 Hafler DA, Kent SC, Pietrusewicz MJ, *et al.* Oral administration of myelin induces antigen-specific TGF-beta 1 secreting T cells in patients with multiple sclerosis. *Ann NY Acad Sci* 1997;835:120–31.

41 Fukaura H, Kent SC, Pietrusewicz MJ, *et al.* Induction of circulating myelin basic protein and proteolipid protein- specific transforming growth factor-beta1-secreting Th3 T cells by oral administration of myelin in multiple sclerosis patients. *J Clin Invest* 1996;98:70–7.

42 Inobe J, Slavin AJ, Komagata Y, *et al.* IL-4 is a differentiation factor for transforming growth factor-beta secreting Th3 cells and oral administration of IL-4 enhances oral tolerance in experimental allergic encephalomyelitis. *Eur J Immunol* 1998;28:2780–90.

43 Kunimoto DY, Ritzel M, Tsang M. The roles of IL-4, TGF-beta and LPS in IgA switching. *Eur Cytokine Netw* 1992;3:407–15.

44 Kim PH, Kagnoff MF. Transforming growth factor beta 1 increases IgA isotype switching at the clonal level. *J Immunol* 1990;145:3773–8.

45 Coffman RL, Lebman DA, Shrader B. Transforming growth factor beta specifically enhances IgA production by lipopolysaccharide-stimulated murine B lymphocytes. *J Exp Med* 1989;170:1039–44.

46 Borsutzky S, Cazac BB, Roes J, Guzman CA. TGF-beta receptor signaling is critical for mucosal IgA responses. *J Immunol* 2004;173:3305–9.

47 Groux H, O'Garra A, Bigler M, *et al.* A CD4+ T-cell subset inhibits antigen-specific T-cell responses and prevents colitis. *Nature* 1997;389:737–42.

48 Levings MK, Roncarolo MG. T-regulatory 1 cells: a novel subset of CD4 T cells with immunoregulatory properties. *J Allergy Clin Immunol* 2000;106:S109–12.

49 Roncarolo MG, Bacchetta R, Bordignon C, *et al.* Type 1 T regulatory cells. *Immunol Rev* 2001;182:68–79.

50 Frossard CP, Tropia L, Hauser C, Eigenmann PA. Lymphocytes in Peyer patches regulate clinical tolerance in a murine model of food allergy. *J Allergy Clin Immunol* 2004;113:958–64.

51 Sakaguchi S, Toda M, Asano M, *et al.* T cell-mediated maintenance of natural self-tolerance: its breakdown as a possible cause of various autoimmune diseases. *J Autoimmun* 1996;9:211–20.

52 Sakaguchi S, Sakaguchi N, Shimizu J, *et al.* Immunologic tolerance maintained by CD25+ CD4+ regulatory T cells: their common role in controlling autoimmunity, tumor immunity, and transplantation tolerance. *Immunol Rev* 2001;182:18–32.

53 Shevach EM, Thornton A, Suri-Payer E. T lymphocyte-mediated control of autoimmunity. *Novartis Found Symp* 1998;215:200–11; discussion 211–30.

54 Nakamura K, Kitani A, Strober W. Cell contact-dependent immunosuppression by CD4(+)CD25(+) regulatory T cells is mediated by cell surface-bound transforming growth factor beta. *J Exp Med* 2001;194:629–44.

55 Zhang X, Izikson L, Liu L, Weiner HL. Activation of CD25(+)CD4(+) regulatory T cells by oral antigen administration. *J Immunol* 2001;167:4245–53.

56 Chung Y, Lee SH, Kim DH, Kang CY. Complementary role of CD4+CD25+ regulatory T cells and TGF-beta in oral tolerance. *J Leukoc Biol* 2005;77:906–13.

57 Hori S, Nomura T, Sakaguchi S. Control of regulatory T cell development by the transcription factor Foxp3. *Science* 2003; 299:1057–61.

58 McHugh RS, Shevach EM. The role of suppressor T cells in regulation of immune responses. *J Allergy Clin Immunol* 2002;110:693–702.

59 Mowat AM, Lamont AG, Strobel S, Mackenzie S. The role of antigen processing and suppressor T cells in immune responses to dietary proteins in mice. *Adv Exp Med Biol* 1987:709–20.

60 Mowat AM, Lamont AG, Parrott DM. Suppressor T cells, antigen-presenting cells and the role of I-J restriction in oral tolerance to ovalbumin. *Immunology* 1988;64:141–5.

61 Mowat AM. Depletion of suppressor T cells by 2'-deoxyguanosine abrogates tolerance in mice fed ovalbumin and permits the induction of intestinal delayed-type hypersensitivity. *Immunology* 1986;58:179–84.

62 Mowat AM. The role of antigen recognition and suppressor cells in mice with oral tolerance to ovalbumin. *Immunology* 1985;56:253–60.

63 Whitacre CC, Gienapp IE, Orosz CG, Bitar DM. Oral tolerance in experimental autoimmune encephalomyelitis. III. Evidence for clonal anergy. *J Immunol* 1991;147:2155–63.

64 Chen Y, Inobe J, Marks R, *et al.* Peripheral deletion of antigen-reactive T cells in oral tolerance. *Nature* 1995;376:177–80.

65 Brandt EB, Strait RT, Hershko D, *et al.* Mast cells are required for experimental oral allergen-induced diarrhea. *J Clin Invest* 2003;112:1666–77.

66 Li XM, Schofield BH, Huang CK, *et al.* A murine model of IgE-mediated cow's milk hypersensitivity. *J Allergy Clin Immunol* 1999;103:206–14.

67 Berin MC, Kiliaan AJ, Yang PC, *et al.* The influence of mast cells on pathways of transepithelial antigen transport in rat intestine. *J Immunol* 1998;161:2561–6.

68 Madara JL, Stafford J. Interferon-gamma directly affects barrier function of cultured intestinal epithelial monolayers. *J Clin Invest* 1989;83:724–7.

69 Zhang ZY, Michael JG. Orally inducible immune unresponsiveness is abrogated by IFN-gamma treatment. *J Immunol* 1990;144:4163–5.

70 Hermiston ML, Gordon JI. Inflammatory bowel disease and adenomas in mice expressing a dominant negative N-cadherin. *Science* 1995;270:1203–7.

71 Jakobsson I. Intestinal permeability in children of different ages and with different gastrointestinal diseases. *Pediatr Allergy Immunol* 1993;4:33–9.

72 Troncone R, Caputo N, Florio G, Finelli E. Increased intestinal sugar permeability after challenge in children with cow's milk allergy or intolerance. *Allergy* 1994;49:142–6.

73 Laudat A, Arnaud P, Napoly A, Brion F. The intestinal permeability test applied to the diagnosis of food allergy in paediatrics. *West Indian Med J* 1994;43:87–8.

74 Ahmed T, Fuchs GJ. Gastrointestinal allergy to food: a review. *J Diarrhoeal Dis Res* 1997;15:211–23.

75 Kalach N, Rocchiccioli F, de Boissieu D, *et al*. Intestinal permeability in children: variation with age and reliability in the diagnosis of cow's milk allergy. *Acta Paediatr* 2001;90:499–504.

76 Husby S, Mestecky J, Moldoveanu Z, *et al*. Oral tolerance in humans. T cell but not B cell tolerance after antigen feeding. *J Immunol* 1994;152:4663–70.

77 Kraus TA, Toy L, Chan L, *et al*. Failure to induce oral tolerance to a soluble protein in patients with inflammatory bowel disease. *Gastroenterology* 2004;126:1771–8.

78 Kagnoff MF. Immunology of the intestinal tract. *Gastroenterology* 1993;105:1275–80.

79 Brandtzaeg P, Valnes K, Scott H, *et al*. The human gastrointestinal secretory immune system in health and disease. *Scand J Gastroenterol Suppl* 1985;114:17–38.

80 Mostov KE, Kraehenbuhl JP, Blobel G. Receptor-mediated transcellular transport of immunoglobulin: synthesis of secretory component as multiple and larger transmembrane forms. *Proc Natl Acad Sci USA* 1980;77:7257–61.

81 Mostov KE, Blobel G. Transcellular transport of polymeric immunoglobulin by secretory component: a model system for studying intracellular protein sorting. *Ann NY Acad Sci* 1983;409:441–51.

82 Mostov KE, Friedlander M, Blobel G. Structure and function of the receptor for polymeric immunoglobulins. *Biochem Soc Symp* 1986;51:113–15.

83 Raux M, Finkielsztejn L, Salmon-Ceron D, *et al*. IgG subclass distribution in serum and various mucosal fluids of HIV type 1-infected subjects. *AIDS Res Hum Retroviruses* 2000;16:583–94.

84 Schneider T, Zippel T, Schmidt W, *et al*. Increased immunoglobulin G production by short term cultured duodenal biopsy samples from HIV infected patients. *Gut* 1998;42:357–61.

85 Israel EJ, Taylor S, Wu Z, *et al*. Expression of the neonatal Fc receptor, FcRn, on human intestinal epithelial cells. *Immunology* 1997;92:69–74.

86 Dickinson BL, Badizadegan K, Wu Z, *et al*. Bidirectional FcRn-dependent IgG transport in a polarized human intestinal epithelial cell line. *J Clin Invest* 1999;104:903–11.

87 MacDermott RP, Nash GS, Bertovich MJ, *et al*. Alterations of IgM, IgG, and IgA synthesis and secretion by peripheral blood and intestinal mononuclear cells from patients with ulcerative colitis and Crohn's disease. *Gastroenterology* 1981;81:844–52.

88 Berin MC, Kiliaan AJ, Yang PC, *et al*. Rapid transepithelial antigen transport in rat jejunum: impact of sensitisation and the hypersensitivity reaction. *Gastroenterology* 1997;113:856–64.

89 Berin MC, Yang PC, Ciok L, *et al*. Role for IL-4 in macromolecular transport across human intestinal epithelium. *Am J Physiol* 1999;276:C1046–52.

90 Bhalla DK, Owen RL. Migration of B and T lymphocytes to M cells in Peyer's patch follicle epithelium: an autoradiographic and immunocytochemical study in mice. *Cell Immunol* 1983;81:105–17.

91 Kraehenbuhl JP, Pringault E, Neutra MR. Review article: intestinal epithelia and barrier functions. *Aliment Pharmacol Ther* 1997;11:3–8; discussion 8–9.

92 Neutra MR. Current concepts in mucosal immunity. V. Role of M cells in transepithelial transport of antigens and pathogens to the mucosal immune system. *Am J Physiol* 1998;274:G785–91.

93 Owen RL. Sequential uptake of horseradish peroxidase by lymphoid follicle epithelium of Peyer's patches in the normal unobstructed mouse intestine: an ultrastructural study. *Gastroenterology* 1977;72:440–51.

94 Allan CH, Mendrick DL, Trier JS. Rat intestinal M cells contain acidic endosomal–lysosomal compartments and express class II major histocompatibility complex determinants. *Gastroenterology* 1993;104:698–708.

95 Sicinski P, Rowinski J, Warchol JB, *et al*. Poliovirus type 1 enters the human host through intestinal M cells. *Gastroenterology* 1990;98:56–8.

96 Frossard CP, Hauser C, Eigenmann PA. Antigen-specific secretory IgA antibodies in the gut are decreased in a mouse model of food allergy. *J Allergy Clin Immunol* 2004;114:377–82.

97 Kerneis S, Bogdanova A, Kraehenbuhl JP, Pringault E. Conversion by Peyer's patch lymphocytes of human enterocytes into M cells that transport bacteria. *Science* 1997;277:949–52.

98 Gonnella PA, Waldner HP, Weiner HL. B cell-deficient (mu MT) mice have alterations in the cytokine microenvironment of the gut-associated lymphoid tissue (GALT) and a defect in the low dose mechanism of oral tolerance. *J Immunol* 2001;166:4456–64.

99 Fujihashi K, Dohi T, Rennert PD, *et al*. Peyer's patches are required for oral tolerance to proteins. *Proc Natl Acad Sci USA* 2001;98:3310–15.

100 Spahn TW, Fontana A, Faria AM, *et al*. Induction of oral tolerance to cellular immune responses in the absence of Peyer's patches. *Eur J Immunol* 2001;31:1278–87.

101 Spahn TW, Weiner HL, Rennert PD, *et al*. Mesenteric lymph nodes are critical for the induction of high-dose oral tolerance in the absence of Peyer's patches. *Eur J Immunol* 2002;32:1109–13.

102 Kunkel D, Kirchhoff D, Nishikawa S, *et al*. Visualization of peptide presentation following oral application of antigen in normal and Peyer's patches-deficient mice. *Eur J Immunol* 2003;33:1292–301.

103 Kraus TA, Brimnes J, Muong C, *et al*. Induction of mucosal tolerance in Peyer's patch-deficient, ligated small bowel loops. *J Clin Invest* 2005;115:2234–43.

104 Steinman RM, Hawiger D, Nussenzweig MC. Tolerogenic dendritic cells. *Annu Rev Immunol* 2003;21:685–711.

105 Delamarre L, Pack M, Chang H, *et al*. Differential lysosomal proteolysis in antigen-presenting cells determines antigen fate. *Science* 2005;307:1630–4.

106 Niess JH, Brand S, Gu X, *et al*. CX3CR1-mediated dendritic cell access to the intestinal lumen and bacterial clearance. *Science* 2005;307:254–8.

107 Niess JH, Reinecker HC. Lamina propria dendritic cells in the physiology and pathology of the gastrointestinal tract. *Curr Opin Gastroenterol* 2005;21:687–91.

108 Kunkel EJ, Campbell DJ, Butcher EC. Chemokines in lymphocyte trafficking and intestinal immunity. *Microcirculation* 2003;10:313–23.

109 Zhao X, Sato A, Dela Cruz CS, *et al*. CCL9 is secreted by the follicle-associated epithelium and recruits dome region Peyer's patch CD11b+ dendritic cells. *J Immunol* 2003;171:2797–803.

110 Caux C, Vanbervliet B, Massacrier C, *et al*. Regulation of dendritic cell recruitment by chemokines. *Transplantation* 2002;73:S7–11.

111 Chirdo FG, Millington OR, Beacock-Sharp H, Mowat AM. Immunomodulatory dendritic cells in intestinal lamina propria. *Eur J Immunol* 2005;35:1831–40.

112 Viney JL, Mowat AM, O'Malley JM, *et al*. Expanding dendritic cells *in vivo* enhances the induction of oral tolerance. *J Immunol* 1998;160:5815–25.

113 Mowat AM, Donachie AM, Parker LA, *et al*. The role of dendritic cells in regulating mucosal immunity and tolerance. *Novartis Found Symp* 2003;252:291–302; discussion 302–5.

114 Gorczynski RM, Lee L, Boudakov I. Augmented induction of CD4+CD25+ Treg using monoclonal antibodies to CD200R. *Transplantation* 2005;79:488–91.

115 Yamagiwa S, Gray JD, Hashimoto S, Horwitz DA. A role for TGF-beta in the generation and expansion of CD4+CD25+ regulatory T cells from human peripheral blood. *J Immunol* 2001;166:7282–9.

116 Man AL, Bertelli E, Regoli M, *et al*. Antigen-specific T cell-mediated apoptosis of dendritic cells is impaired in a mouse model of food allergy. *J Allergy Clin Immunol* 2004;113:965–72.

117 Bland PW. Antigen presentation by gut epithelial cells: secretion by rat enterocytes of a factor with IL-1-like activity. *Adv Exp Med Biol* 1987:219–25.

118 Bland PW, Kambarage DM. Antigen handling by the epithelium and lamina propria macrophages. *Gastroenterol Clin North Am* 1991;20:577–96.

119 Hershberg RM, Framson PE, Cho DH, *et al*. Intestinal epithelial cells use two distinct pathways for HLA class II antigen processing. *J Clin Invest* 1997;100:204–15.

120 Hershberg RM, Cho DH, Youakim A, *et al*. Highly polarized HLA class II antigen processing and presentation by human intestinal epithelial cells. *J Clin Invest* 1998;102:792–803.

121 Hershberg RM, Mayer LF. Antigen processing and presentation by intestinal epithelial cells – polarity and complexity. *Immunol Today* 2000;21:123–8.

122 Mayer L, Shlien R. Evidence for function of Ia molecules on gut epithelial cells in man. *J Exp Med* 1987;166:1471–83.

123 Mayer L. The role of the epithelium in mucosal immunity. *Res Immunol* 1997;148:498–504.

124 Kaiserlian D, Vidal K, Revillard JP. Murine enterocytes can present soluble antigen to specific class II-restricted CD4+ T cells. *Eur J Immunol* 1989;19:1513–16.

125 Mayer L, Eisenhardt D. Lack of induction of suppressor T cells by intestinal epithelial cells from patients with inflammatory bowel disease. *J Clin Invest* 1990;86:1255–60.

CHAPTER 2

The Immunological Basis of IgE-Mediated Reactions

Gernot Sellge and Stephan C. Bischoff

KEY CONCEPTS

- Sensitization to food allergens can occur via the gastrointestinal tract (true food allergens) or via the pulmonary route (cross-reactive aeroallergens).

- Food allergens enter the mucosal barrier and can be transported throughout the body in an immunologically intact form.

- A dysregulated immune response to food allergens, consisting of a strong Th2 and IgE response and a low regulatory T-cell and IgG/IgA response, leads to allergic disease.

- Genetic and environmental (hygiene hypothesis) factors influence the individual immune reactions to food allergens.

- Cross-linking of IgE on tissue mast cells triggers the release of pro-inflammatory mediators and initiates the acute-phase reaction and the recruitment of eosinophils, basophils, and lymphocytes.

Introduction

Food allergy defined as immune-mediated food intolerance can be divided into "IgE-mediated" disorders (immediate-type gastrointestinal hypersensitivity, oral allergy syndrome, acute urticaria and angioedema, allergic rhinitis, acute bronchospasm, anaphylaxis) and "non-IgE-mediated" (dietary protein-induced enterocolitis and proctitis, celiac disease, and dermatitis herpetiformis). This classification has been extended by supposing a third subgroup of "mixed IgE- and non-IgE-mediated" disorders such as allergic eosinophilic esophagitis and gastroenteritis, atopic dermatitis, and allergic asthma [1,2].

In this chapter, the underlying immune mechanism of IgE-mediated allergic reactions with a particular focus on food allergy will be discussed. The development of food allergy is a multi-step process, requiring repetitive challenges with a particular food antigen, in contrast to non-immune-mediated reactions which can cause symptoms even after a single food exposure. The disease is preceded by a sensitization phase without symptoms, in which allergen-specific T- and B-cells are primed and IgE is produced. Recurrent

Food Allergy: Adverse Reactions to Foods and Food Additives, 4th edition.
Edited by Dean D. Metcalfe, Hugh A. Sampson, and Ronald A. Simon.
© 2008 Blackwell Publishing, ISBN: 978-1-4501-5129-0.

allergen challenge of sensitized individuals results in IgE cross-linking bound on tissue mast cells that subsequently release their pro-inflammatory mediators.

Route of sensitization

Food allergy might result from sensitization to ingested food proteins or to aeroallergens through the respiratory route. Several pollen allergens can confer cross-reactivity to homologous proteins in plant foods. It has been suggested that oral sensitization only occurs when allergens are highly resistant to digestion in the gastrointestinal tract, while pollen food cross-reactive proteins are labile [2]. The route of sensitization might therefore influence the allergenic pattern on a molecular level and influence the clinical manifestation after challenge. This relationship has been confirmed in a recent multi-center study across Europe [3]. In the Netherlands, Austria, and northern Italy apple allergy is mild (>90% present exclusively oral symptoms) and precedes birch pollen allergy. The apple allergy arises as a result of the cross-reactivity between the birch pollen allergen Bet v 1 and the apple allergen Mal d 1. In Spain, exposure to birch pollen is virtually absent and the main apple allergen is Mal d 3. The authors suggested that apple allergy in Spain is a result of a primary sensitization to peach and its major allergen Pru p 3, which is cross-reactive to Mal d 3. Both proteins belong to the non-specific lipid transfer proteins, which are resistant to proteolysis. Consequently, about 35% of the Spanish patients have systemic reactions after double-blind, placebo-controlled food challenges with apple [3].

Allergen uptake in the intestine

The intestinal mucosa is constantly challenged with food and the commensal flora, which may be harmful after uncontrolled uptake. Therefore, innate and adoptive mechanisms have been developed to control the immune balance to food and commensals and to fend off pathogens [1,4,5]. Gastric acid, mucus, an intact epithelial layer, digestive enzymes, and the intestinal peristaltic are unspecific factors forming the "non-immunological" barrier [6]. The immunological defense mechanisms include innate (antimicrobial peptides, immune cells expressing pattern recognition molecules, etc.) and adaptive mechanisms (lymphocytes, IgA) [4]. Despite this tight mucosal barrier, macromolecules and intact bacteria can pass through or can be even actively taken up by the intestinal epithelium. Macromolecular uptake can be beneficial in delivering essential growth factors and in sampling the antigenic milieu of the gastrointestinal tract in order to enable the induction of immune tolerance to environmental antigens [6,7].

Breakdown of the intestinal barrier is associated with the development of food allergy. Neutralization of gastric acid results in increased mucosal transport of ingested proteins and sensitization to allergens [8]. Intestinal permeability is increased in patients suffering from food allergy [9]. Interestingly, one study showed that intestinal permeability is increased in patients with bronchial asthma, supporting the hypothesis that a general defect of the mucosal system may facilitate the development of allergic diseases [10]. Further evidence that a barrier dysfunction is a risk factor for developing food allergy comes from the notion that early introduction of solid food in babies (immature barrier) [11] and IgA deficiency or retarded IgA development in infants [12] is associated with a higher risk of atopy.

Many food allergens are fairly stable to heat, acid, and proteases making them resistant to digestion, a critical role allowing them to get in contact with the intestinal immune system. It has been demonstrated that ingested food proteins can be transported throughout the body in an immunologically intact form [2,13]. This might explain why symptoms of food allergies are not restricted to the gastrointestinal tract, but very often cause additionally or even exclusively extra-intestinal symptoms. Considering that the intestine is an immunologically privileged site, it is not surprising that hyperresponsive reactions to food allergens occur in some patients only outside the gastrointestinal system, independent from the site of initial antigen uptake.

T-cell response in IgE-mediated allergy

A hallmark of IgE-mediated allergic disorders is the generation of allergen-specific CD4+ Th2 lymphocytes. These cells produce a characteristic Th2-cytokine profile consisting of IL-4, IL-5, IL-9, and IL-13. IL-4 and IL-13 induce IgE class-switching in B-cells, IL-4 and IL-9 are important growth and activation factors for mast cells, and IL-5 promotes eosinophil development and recruitment. IL-13 additionally triggers mucus secretion in the lung and provokes airway hypersensitivity [14,15]. In the 1990s, allergic sensitization to harmless environmental proteins (allergens) was attributed to a dysregulation of the Th1/Th2 balance. However, the simple dichotomy of the Th1/Th2 system has been challenged by the discovery of a plethora of new T-cell subsets, including Th17 cells [16], non-classical T-cells such as NKT [17] and γδ T-cells, different subsets of CD8+ T-cells (Tc1 and Tc2), and, most importantly, regulatory T (Treg) cells [14,18,19]. The actual concept states that allergies and also autoimmune diseases result from a dysbalance between a protective Treg response and a disease inducing effector Th2 (in the case of allergy) or Th1/Th17 response (in the case of autoimmune diseases; recent observations suggest that Th17 cells are the main effectors) [16]. However, it is clear that different effector T-cell subsets have counter-regulatory functions, which also play a role in the immune-regulatory network [14,18,19].

Several subtypes of Treg cells have been described, which also have some overlapping phenotypes. Naturally occurring CD4+CD25+FoxP3+ Treg cells are distinguished from antigen-driven IL-10 (Tr1) and TGF-β (Th3)-secreting CD4+ Treg cells. The former subset originates from the thymus and acts by cell–cell contact in an antigen-independent manner. Tr1 and Th3 cells originate in the periphery and operate by the production of the anti-inflammatory cytokines IL-10 and TGF-β via an antigen-driven mechanism [14,18]. However, inducible and naturally occurring Treg cells share a functional relationship. The modulatory functions of Treg cells have also been attributed to the production of IL-10 and TGF-β and can eventually be induced in the periphery. Antigen-specific Treg cells may also function through cell–cell contact independently of IL-10 and TGF-β. It has been suggested that IL-10 producing T cells might not be exclusively generated from naïve CD4+, but also from Th1 or Th2 cells that have undergone chronic stimulation, resulting in the disappearance of effector cytokines [18].

Evidence that both subtypes of Treg cells play a major role in the prevention of allergen sensitization and modulation of disease activity comes from human and animal studies [18]. The function of Treg cells are impaired or dysregulated in allergic patients [20]. It is noteworthy to mention that a large number of healthy individuals are sensitized to allergens. However, these persons likely mount a balanced immune response, consisting of allergen-specific

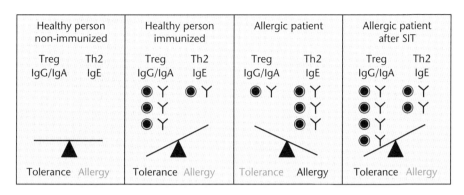

Figure 2.1 Immune response to allergens in healthy and allergic individuals.

Tr1 cells and high levels of protective antigen-specific IgG4 and IgA (Fig. 2.1) [19,20]. Treg cells modulate different cells and effector functions, which are associated with allergic diseases. They downregulate Th2 cell activation, stimulate IgG4 (indirectly induced by IL-10) and IgA (induced by TGF-β) class-switch in B-cells [18], and might inhibit mast cell and eosinophil functions through the production of IL-10 and TGF-β [21,22]. Further evidence for the importance of Treg cells in the prevention of allergy arises from the finding that successful specific immunotherapy (SIT) is associated with a decrease in allergen-specific Th2 cell responses and the induction of allergen-induced Tr1 and TH3 cells (Fig. 2.1) [23,24].

B-cell response in IgE-mediated allergy

Antigen-specific IgE produced by B-cells is essential for type I allergic reactions. Apart from its pathological function in allergies, antigen-specific IgE is an important component of protective immunity against helminths [25].

IgE class-switch recombination (CSR) is strongly dependent on antigen-specific Th2 cells [26], although some evidence exists that other cells, including mast cells, basophils, and eosinophils, can provide the required signals [27,28]. Naïve B-cells capture their specific antigen (allergen) by the B-cell receptor (BCR), process it, and present it in the context of MCH class II to Th2 cells. This interaction illustrates why B- and T-cell epitopes are frequently found in the same protein. Th2 cells provide the major signals responsible for the IgE CSR; IL-4 and IL-13, as well as CD40L on T-cells, which binds CD40 on B-cells. The activation of the transcription factors STAT6 (induced by IL-4 and IL-13) and NF-κB (induced by CD40) in the B-cells promotes the CSR to IgE [26]. Given the potent, and potentially life-threatening effects of allergen-specific IgE, the class-switch is tightly controlled by several antagonizing signals, such as cytokines (IFN-γ, IL-21, TGF-β), B-cell surface receptors (CTLA4, CD45, BCR, CD23), and transcription factors (BCL6, ID2) [26]. Activated B-cells subsequently expand and are subjected to affinity maturation by somatic hyper mutation (SHM). However, there is less evidence for mutational maturation of antigen selection by IgE compared to IgG, although the existence of high-affinity IgE antibodies has convincingly been demonstrated [29]. CSR and SHM take place in secondary lymphoid organs, from which the cells migrate to mucosal effectors sites and undergo terminal differentiation to plasma cells [4]. However, it is becoming increasingly apparent that CSR and SHM may also occur at mucosal sites of allergic patients [30,31].

Secreted antibodies provide humoral immunity against pathogens, but persistent production of specific IgE is also a hallmark of type I allergies. IgE plasma level is the lowest (<100 μg/l in normal adults) and the biological half-life is the shortest (~12 hours in the serum [32] and ~14 days in the skin [33]) of all immunoglobulin classes. Elevated titers of antigen-specific IgE are found in allergic patients and after helminth infections, even in the absence of antigen for several years [25,34]. This conclusion is consistent with clinical experience, since patients can develop recurrent allergic symptoms despite long-term allergen avoidance. Stable maintenance of B-cell memory can be divided into two broad categories: long-lived plasma cells and memory B-cells. Three competing concepts, which are not mutually exclusive, might explain humoral memory. First, short-lived plasma cells (which do not divide) are constantly generated from memory B-cells, a process that might be driven by persisting antigen. Second, long-lived plasma cells with a defined half-life of several weeks develop from cytokine-receptor or Toll-like receptor (TLR) activated memory B-cells. Third, memory arises from long-lived plasma cells that survive in appropriate survival niches, which are located in the bone marrow and possibly in secondary lymphoid organs and inflamed tissue [35]. Whether IgE is predominately produced within or outside mucosal sites is a matter of debate [35,36]. The fact that allergen-specific IgE production can be transferred by bone marrow transplantation argues that bone marrow-derived IgE might contribute to the sensitization of effector cells at mucosal surfaces [37]. The persistence of allergen-specific IgE even under immunosuppressive therapy suggests that long-lived plasma cells (possibly located in the bone marrow) contribute substantially to IgE-mediated allergy, because long-lived plasma cells are resistant to immunosuppression [35].

Allergen-specific IgG and IgA

Allergen-specific IgG1, IgG4, and IgA are frequently detectable in allergic and non-allergic individuals. It has been proposed that these immunoglobulin subclasses might prevent allergic reactions and that the ratio of antigen-specific IgE and antigen-specific IgG determines the severity of an allergic reaction following allergen exposure (Fig. 2.1) [14,19,38]. Evidence for the protective effect of allergen-specific IgG arises from SIT studies. Although specific IgE levels not always decrease after successful SIT [39], several studies show that allergen-specific IgG1 and, in particular, IgG4 levels increase [40–42], most likely as a result of the change in the T cell profile (Fig. 2.1).

Allergen-specific IgG may compete with IgE for the binding of allergens and inhibit, therefore, high-affinity Fc receptor (FcεRI) cross-linking [14,43–45]. Furthermore, allergen-specific IgG (in particular IgG1) may co-aggregate FcγRIIB with FcεRI. FcγRIIB contains an intra-cytoplasmatic immunoreceptor tyrosine-based inhibitory motif (ITIM) and has been reported to inhibit IgE-induced mast cell and basophil activation [43,46]. Its inhibitory function in allergy has been demonstrated by studies using knock-out mice [47]. Co-cross-linking of FcγRIIB and FcεRI might also be exploited for the engineering of safe therapeutic agents for SIT that maintain all B- and T-cell epitopes. A human IgG1 Fc fragment fused to the cat allergen Fel d 1 was reported to inhibit Fel d 1-induced activation of human mast cells and basophils sensitized with serum from patients allergic to Fel d 1; and also Fel d 1-induced anaphylaxis in human FcεRIα transgenic mice [48]. However, the relationship between the efficacy of SIT and the induction of allergen-specific IgG has also been questioned, because some studies failed to observe a correlation [45,49]. These conflicting data might be explained by the fact that allergen-specific IgG can also have immune-enhancing effects. For example, IgG can stimulate immune and inflammatory cells such as mast cells and eosinophils through binding to Fcγ receptors (Table 2.1) [50,51]. Allergen-specific IgG may enhance allergic reactions by the formation of larger allergen aggregates (super-cross-linking) [52] or by activating complement (IgG1–3, not IgG4). Furthermore, the binding of certain IgG to allergens can enhance IgE affinity, which may be due to changes of the three-dimensional allergen structure [53]. However, IgG4 seems to be of particular importance to prevent allergic reactions. It binds only with low affinity to Fcγ receptors and does not activate complement. Furthermore, it has been shown very recently that IgG4 antibodies are dynamic molecules

Table 2.1 Fc receptors on mast cells, eosinophils, and basophils

Receptor (CD)	Chains	Binding affinity	Ligands	Expression MC, E, B	Other cells
FcγRI (CD64)	α, γ	Ig1: 10^8 M^{-1}	(1) IgG1 = IgG3, (2) IgG4, (3) IgG2	MC, E[1]	M, N[1], DC
FcγRII-A (CD32)	α	Ig1: 2×10^6 M^{-1}	(1) IgG1, (2) IgG2[2] = IgG3, (3) IgG4	MC, E, B[3]	M, N, LC, P
FcγRII-B (CD32)	α[4]	Ig1: 2×10^6 M^{-1}	(1) IgG1 = IgG3, (2) IgG4, (3) IgG2	MC, E, B[3]	M, N, B
FcγRIII (CD16)	α, β, γ	Ig1: 5×10^5 M^{-1}	(1) IgG1 = IgG3, (2) IgG4, (3) IgG2	E	M, N, B
FcαRI (CD89)	α, γ	IgA1, IgA2: 10^7 M^{-1}	IgA1 = IgA2	E	M, N
FcεRI	α, β, γ	IgE: 10^{10} M^{-1}	IgE	MC, B, E[1,5]	M[5], DC[5], LC[5]
FcεRII (CD23)	Single	IgE: 10^8 M^{-1}	IgE, others[6]	E	B, T, M, LC, P

MC, mast cells; E, eosinophils; B, basophils; M, monocytes; N, neutrophils; B, B-cells; T, T-cells; DC, dendritic cells; LC, Langerhans' cells; P, platelets.
[1] Inducible.
[2] Only some allotypes of FcγRII-A bind IgG2.
[3] CD32 expression has been shown, but to date it is not clear whether FcγRII-A or FcγRII-B is expressed.
[4] Contains an ITIM motif (inhibitory).
[5] β chain is not expressed.
[6] See text (IgE receptors). Modified from Janeway CA *et al.* [55].

that exchange Fab arms by swapping a heavy chain and attached light chain (half-molecule) with a heavy-light chain pair from another molecule, which results in bispecific antibodies. IgG4 molecules thereby lose their ability to cross-link antigen and to form immune complexes under most conditions. This mechanism might provide the basis for the anti-inflammatory activity attributed to IgG4 [53b].

Obviously, the clinical consequences of an allergen exposure are influenced by several factors: (i) allergen structure, (ii) dose and duration of exposure, (iii) epitope specificity and affinity of the antibodies, (iv) absolute and relative amounts of immunoglobulin subclasses, (v) expression profiles of Fc receptors on effector cells, (vi) composition and activation status of immune cells in the exposed tissue, and (vii) profile of allergen-specific effector T cells [14,54]. This demonstrates that monitoring of SIT by measurement of antigen-specific immunoglobulins can be sometimes misleading and that complex biological systems are required to analyze the immunological effects of SIT.

Genes and environment

It is generally acknowledged that risk factors for the development of allergic diseases include genetic and environmental factors, but certainly also individual factors such as psychological conditions.

Sibling and family studies have revealed that the genetic background affects the risk of developing allergy. These observations can be related to several gene polymorphisms. Not surprisingly, many of these genes encode for key factors of Th2-type and IgE-related immune reactions, such as FcεRI β chain, IL-4R, IL-13, and STAT6 [56,57]. Interestingly, also genes for innate immune receptors, such as CD14 and NOD1, might be associated with allergy [58,59]. These analyses suggest that the threshold of the immune system to environmental stimuli is controlled by natural genetic variation and gene–environment interaction.

Prevalence of allergic disorders is considerably lower in developing countries and in rural area in comparison to urban areas within one country. Furthermore, the number of allergic patients has strongly increased within the last decades, further arguing that environmental factors are substantially responsible for atopy [60,61]. However, there is little consistent evidence to suggest that obvious risk factors, such as increased exposure to indoor allergens, pollution, or changes in diet and breast-feeding, could account for the rise in allergic diseases. Another category of environmental factors that show overwhelming inverse association with atopy are infections, vaccinations, absence of antibiotic treatment, traditional farming environments, older siblings, day care attendance, and pet ownership [60–62]. These findings lead to the "hygiene hypothesis" which proposes that reduced exposure to particular microbiological stimuli [63], which decrease with improved living standards and higher personal hygiene, might result in an increased risk of developing allergy. Indeed, perinatal treatment (mothers prenatal and infants 6-month postnatal) with the probiotic *Lacobacillus GG* strain significantly reduced the development of allergies up to the age of 4 years [64]. Although the "hygiene hypothesis" is widely accepted, the underlying mechanisms are controversial. In particular, the molecular link between environmental stimuli and immune hyper-responsiveness is far from being understood. It has been suggested that a chronic stimulation of the immune system by microbes creates a kind of immunotolerant environment. This concept is attractive, since it would also explain the known relation between increased hygiene standards, decline in infection rates, and increase in autoimmune diseases [65]. Tolerance induction might involve both the innate and the adaptive immune systems. Animal studies show protective effects of certain TLR ligands in allergen-induced inflammation [60]. Furthermore, microbial components such as CpG-containing immunostimulatory DNA, a TLR9 agonist, or the bacterial cell wall component monophosphoryl lipid A have been used successfully as adjuvants in clinical studies for SIT. These compounds considerably improve immunological surrogate markers and clinical outcome [66,67]. Chronic infections might induce Treg cells which provide non-specific bystander suppression [61]. Moreover, it has been suggested that cross-reactive IgE and IgG-binding structures exist in allergens and parasite antigens [61]. Interestingly, parasite-specific IgG4 antibodies can inhibit IgE-mediated degranulation of effector cells isolated from allergic patients, suggesting that chronic parasite infections induce allergen-cross-reactive "blocking antibodies" [68].

Innate immune recognition of allergens

The concept that the driving force for the induction of an adaptive immune response is the innate immune recognition system in dendritic cells and other immune cells has been generally accepted [69]. In light of this model, it is interesting to note that certain allergens contain immune stimulatory properties that target the innate immune system. For example, pollens contain intrinsic NAPDH oxidase activity, generating reactive oxygen species (ROS) [70] and/or bioactive lipids (phytoprostanes) [71]. These pollen intrinsic bioactivities have been shown to instruct a Th2 cell polarization. Furthermore, the pollen NADPH-induced ROS vigorously augments specific IgE production and allergic airway inflammation induced by the major pollen antigens in mice [70]. Several allergens have enzymatic functions, frequently protease activities that facilitate transepithelial allergen delivery and spreading, but also activation of epithelial cells via protease-activated receptors, resulting in the production of pro-inflammatory cytokines [15]. Most interestingly, a recent study reports that the major peanut allergen Ara h 1 is recognized by DC-SIGN, a C-type lectin acting as a pathogen recognition molecule. Ara h 1 challenged dendritic cells primed a Th2-skewed T-cell response [72]. Ara h 1 is an N-glycan that shares structural similarities to N-glycans from *Schistosoma mansoni* egg antigens, that are well studied Th2 PAMPs (pathogen-associated molecular pattern). These data suggest that at least some allergens provoke allergies by a two-signal strategy, in which signal 1 is the innate response and signal 2 the adaptive response.

Allergic inflammation

Once an individual is sensitized and allergen-specific IgE has been formed, recurrent antigen exposure readily induces the manifestations of atopic disease. The response has been categorized into three phases: (i) acute or immediate-phase reaction, (ii) late-phase reaction, and (iii) chronic allergic inflammation (Fig. 2.2).

An acute reaction occurs when the allergen, after crossing the mucosa, binds to antigen-specific IgE on the surface of mast cells and eventually basophils. This induces cross-linking of FcεRI resulting in the release of pro-inflammatory mediators, such as histamine, eicosanoids, and cytokines. Clinical signs of the acute response (weal and flare) develop within seconds to minutes. A particular characteristic of intestinal food allergy might be a delayed "acute reaction" because of the passage time of dietary antigens through the esophagus and the stomach. The immediate reaction may be followed by a late-phase reaction starting after 4–48 hours. Mast cell-derived mediators induce expression of adhesion molecules on endothelial cells, which bind its ligand on the surface of eosinophils, basophils, Th2 cells, and NKT cells [17,73]. This leads to the preferential extravasations of these cells through vessel walls into sites of inflammation. Their recruitment to the target organ depends on the production of a number of chemokines [74]. Within the tissue, infiltrating cells are further activated by the inflammatory environment and allergens via antigen-specific recognition (IgE on basophils and MHC class II-dependent antigen presentation to Th2 cells). Late-phase reactions may be developed independent of IgE. It has been reported that birch pollen-related food allergen that lost capacity to bind to IgE because of cooking, but retained their T-cell stimulatory potency, does not induce an acute-phase reaction such as the oral allergy syndrome; but can still induce a late-phase response like atopic eczema [73]. Repeated allergen exposure may lead to a chronic inflammatory response causing persistent infiltration of mast cells, eosinophils, basophils, and lymphocytes and subsequent chronic structural changes of the tissue, such as mucus cell and smooth muscle hypertrophy, fibrosis, and organ dysfunction. The specific clinical features of each of the different phases vary according to the anatomical site affected (Fig. 2.2).

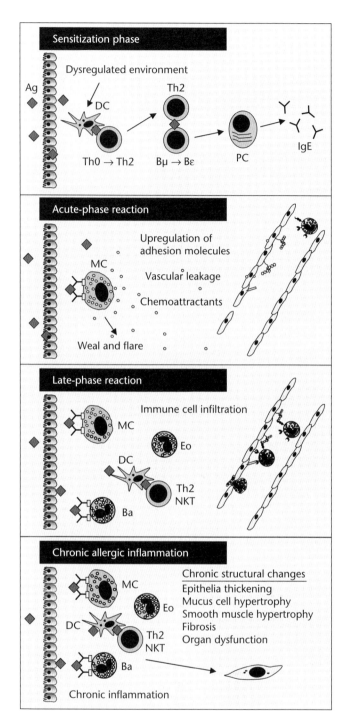

Figure 2.2 Phases of allergic disease. For details see text. Ag, antigen; DC, dendritic cell; Th0, naïve CD4+ lymphocyte. Th2, Th2 lymphocyte; Bμ, naïve B-cell; Bε, primed B-cell after IgE class-switch; PC, plasma cell; MC, mast cell; Eo, eosinophil; Ba, basophil; NKT, NKT cell.

IgE receptors

Most of the IgE is bound to its FcεRI expressed on mast cells, basophils, monocytes, dendritic cells, Langerhans cells, eosinophils, and platelets (Table 2.1). Monomeric IgE binds to FcεRI with high affinity and has a very slow dissociation rate (half-life of about 20 hours). The FcεRI is composed of an IgE-binding α chain, a tertaspanning transmembrane β chain, and a homodimeric disulfide-linked γ chain. The β chain, which is only expressed in mast cells and basophils, functions as an amplifier and in its absence the receptor initiates only weak signals. Cross-linking of FcεRI initiates signaling mediated through the immunoreceptor tyrosine-based activation motif (ITAM) encoded in the cytoplasmic tails of the β and γ chains. For a detailed description of the signaling events via FcεRI, the reader is referred to some recent and comprehensive reviews [46,75–77]. In brief, downstream signaling results in intracellular Ca++ release and activation of PKC (protein kinase C), MAPK (mitogen-activated protein kinase) pathways, NF-κB (nuclear factor-kappaB), PI3K (phosphoinositide-3 kinase), and PLA$_2$ (phospholipase A$_2$). In mast cells and basophils these events result in degranulation, generation of arachidonic acid metabolites, and enhanced expression of genes encoding for pro-inflammatory cytokines and chemokines. IgE binding in the absence of antigen increases receptor expression, induces anti-apoptotic signals, and triggers low-level cytokine production in mast cells [78,79]. The downstream signaling induced by monomeric IgE binding remains elusive. In antigen-presenting cells, FcεRI has been shown to facilitate antigen presentation by IgE-dependent capture of antigens [36,80].

The low-affinity IgE receptor (FcεRII/CD23) is not a member of the Ig superfamily. CD23 is a type II integral membrane protein with a C-lectin domain at the distal *C*-terminal end of the extracellular sequence. The lectin domain contains the binding sites for all known ligands of CD23 including IgE, complement receptors CR2, CR3, and CR4 (also termed CD21, CD18-CD11b, CD18-CD11c, respectively), and vitronectin. CD23 facilitates antigen presentation of B-cells and acts as a negative feedback regulator of the IgE class-switch. In enterocytes, CD23 facilitates the bidirectional transport of IgE–antigen complexes and thus may participate in antigen sampling from the intestinal lumen [36].

Mast cells

Mast cells are widely distributed throughout the body, frequently found around blood vessels, attached to nerves and at mucosal surfaces. Bone marrow-derived mast cell progenitors migrate via the peripheral blood into the tissue, where they undergo final maturation under the influence of local microenvironmental factors. Stem cell factor (SCF), produced either in a soluble or membrane-bound form by fibroblasts, endothelial cells, and stromal cells, is the essential factor for both mast cell maturation and survival of mature mast cells [81]. The importance of SCF and its receptor KIT is stressed by the fact that KIT-deficient mice basically lack mast cells. Mature mast cells are long-living cells that maintain the capability to grow. In particular IL-4, but also IL-3

and IL-9, induces proliferation of tissue mast cells in an SCF-dependent manner [82–84].

Human mast cells are commonly classified according to their protease content and related ultrastructural signatures of their granules. Mast cells containing only tryptase (MC$_T$) predominate in the lung and intestinal mucosa. Tryptase and chymase positive mast cells (MC$_{TC}$) are mainly located in the skin and the intestinal submucosa. It has been suggested that these subtypes can be further classified according to their responsiveness to certain IgE-independent agonists. This heterogeneity might reflect that mast cells exhibit differences in biochemical and functional properties, depending on the anatomical site in which the cells reside; and/or the biological process, in which they participate [76].

Mast cells exert their biological functions mainly by the release of humoral mediators. Mast cell, as well as eosinophil and basophil, mediators can be categorized into three groups: (i) preformed secretory granule-associated mediators, (ii) *de novo* synthesized eicosanoid metabolites, and (iii) cytokines and chemokines which are mainly *de novo* synthesized but are also sometimes found to be stored within secretory granules (Table 2.1). Secretory granule-associated mediators of mast cells are mainly histamine, proteases, and proteoglycans. Histamine exerts its wide-ranging biological activities via binding to four histamine receptors (H1–4). With regard to allergic inflammation, the H1-receptor seems to be of particular importance. Its activation affects the function of blood vessels (dilation and increased permeability), smooth muscles (contraction), epithelial cells (mucus production), and Th2 lymphocytes (recruitment) [85]. Mast cell proteases can cleave several host proteins, including protease activating receptors, and have been linked to immune as well as non-immune functions of mast cells, such as tissue repair and fibrinolysis [86]. Very recently, two exiting studies showed that mast cell-derived proteases cleave endogenous (endothelin-1, induced by bacterial infection) and exogenous (snake and honeybee venoms) toxins and subsequently limit pathology [87,88]. Moreover, mast cell proteases mediate cleavage of allergens. This might be an important negative feedback loop terminating or weakening allergic inflammation [89]. The main mast cell-produced metabolites of arachidonic acid (and their prominent function) are PGD$_2$ (smooth muscle contraction, chemoattractant for eosinophils, and Th2 cells), LTC$_4$ (increase of vascular permeability, mucus production, and smooth muscle contraction), and LTB$_4$ (chemoattractant for neutrophils, eosinophils, and CD8+ T-cells) [90]. A significant amount of cytokines and chemokines are produced by mast cells. Among them, IL-3, IL-5, and IL-13 seem to be specifically important in allergic reactions [91]. They mediate basophil (IL-3), and eosinophil recruitment (IL-5), IgE class-switching, mucus production, and airway hyperreactivity (all IL-13). Although detectable in rodent mast cells [92], human mast cells produce no or only small amounts of IL-4 [27,91].

Table 2.2 Mediators of mast cells, eosinophils, and basophils

Mast cells

Granule-associated	Histamine, tryptase, chymase, carboxypeptidase A, heparine, chondroitinsulfate E, many acid hydrolases, catepsin G
De novo synthesized	LTC$_4$, LTB$_4$, PGD$_2$, PAF
Cytokines/chemokines	IL-1β, IL-3, IL-5, IL-6, IL-8, IL-9, IL-10, IL-11, IL-13, IL-16, IL-18, IL-25, TNF-α, TGF-β, GM-CSF, MIP-1α, bFGF, VPF/VEGF, and others

Eosinophils

Granule-associated	ECP, EDN (formerly called EPX), MBP, EPO, CLC
De novo synthesized	LTC$_4$, LTB$_4$, PAF, PGE$_1$/E$_2$, thromboxane B$_2$, oxygen metabolites (H$_2$O$_2$, O$_2^-$)
Cytokines/chemokines	IL-2, IL-3, IL-4, IL-5, IL-6, IL-8, IL-10, IL-12, IL-13, IL-16, IL-18, TNF-α, TGF-α, TGF-β, GM-CSF, RANTES, MIP-1α, MCP-1, eotaxin-1, VPF/VEGF, PDGF-B

Basophils

Granule-associated	Histamine, chondroitin sulfate A, neutral protease with bradykinin-generating activity, β-glucoronidase, elastase, cathepsin G-like enzyme, MBP, CLC, granzyme B (induced by IL-3)
De novo synthesized	LTC$_4$
Cytokines/chemokines	IL-4, IL-13, MIP-1α

Cross-linking of the FcϵRI is the most potent trigger to activate mast cells for the release of all three classes of mediators. Degranulation and eicosanoid production occur within minutes. Cytokines, if not stored within the granules, are mainly transcriptionally regulated and produced within 2–6 hours [91]. IL-3, IL-4, and IL-5 enhance FcϵRI-mediated reactions [83,91,93], ensuring an autocrine and paracrine positive feedback loop, because the main producers of these cytokines are mast cells (IL-3, IL-5) and, after recruitment, basophils (IL-4), eosinophils (IL-3, IL-5), and Th2 cells (IL-4, IL-5) (Table 2.2). IL-4 induces IL-5 production by mast cells even in the absence of IgE-cross-linking [93]. On the other hand, the central modulatory cytokines of Treg cells, IL-10 and TGF-β, have been shown to induce apoptosis in mast cells (TGF-β) and decrease FcϵRI-induced mediator production (IL-10 and TGF-β) [21,22]. Several IgE-independent mast cell triggers have been described. SCF, complement factors (C5a), neuropeptides (substance P), adenosine, IgG-cross-linking of FcγRI, and several TLR ligands stimulate mast cell effector functions, but are substantially less effective than FcϵRI-mediated signals [50,94].

Considering the multiple biological effects of mast cell mediators, one can propose several possible functions of mast cells *in vivo*. A mouse mast cell "knock-in" model has considerably contributed to the understanding of the role of mast cells in several pathologies. Apart from allergies, recent studies point out that mast cells are important effector cells in immune complex-induced autoimmune models (mediated via Fcγ on mast cells) [95] and confer protection against acute bacterial infections [94,96,97]. Using this mast cell knock-in model, it has been shown that mast cells contribute to all stages of immunopathology in allergic asthma, which are the immediate-phase, late-phase, and chronic allergic

reactions. Mast cell effector functions were mainly, but not exclusively, dependent on FcϵRI/FcγRIII expression [98].

An exiting new field of mast cell research concerns the questions whether and how mast cells contribute to the instruction of the adaptive immune response? Several lines of evidence now indicate that mast cells deliver signals important for dendritic cell activation and T-/B-cell priming, such as cytokines (e.g. TNF-α) and co-stimulatory molecules (CD40L, OX40 ligand). *In vivo*, delayed-type hypersensitivity responses may be decreased in the absence of mast cells, although data are conflicting [99]. However, recent studies suggest that mast cells mediate regulatory functions [100,101]. In an allograft model, mast cells were absolutely essential in Treg cell-dependent peripheral tolerance. IL-9 represented the functional link through which Treg recruited and activated mast cells to mediate regional immune suppression [101]. However, it remains elusive as to whether mast cells play a role (either activating or tolerizing) during the sensitization phase of allergies.

Despite the new enthusiasm about the multiple functions of mast cells in immune diseases and immune regulation, one should consider that most of the data derived from the murine system, in particular with regard to mast cell functions, may not always reflect the human situation [102].

Basophils

Basophils have often been considered as the circulating progenitor of tissue mast cells, because of their similar morphology and staining characteristics due to the basophilic granule contents; and their overlapping functional properties. It is now generally accepted that mast cells and basophils originate from separate lineages [103,104]. Basophils fully mature within the bone marrow and are subsequently released to the peripheral blood, where they form the smallest population of leukocytes (0.5–1% of total leukocytes, considerably increased in allergic patients). IL-3 is the most important basophil growth factor, but other growth factors such as IL-5, GM-CSF, NGF, and TGF-β have been identified [103]. Basophils enter the tissue at sites of inflammation, being directed by adhesion molecules and chemoattractants [74,105]. This array of growth factors and chemoattractants largely overlap with the factors promoting eosinophil development and recruitment. This may explain the combined involvement of both cell types in many diseases. In contrast to mast cells, both basophils and eosinophils are short-living cells, surviving in the tissue only for several days [103,106]. Basophils have been detected particularly in allergic late-phase reactions within the skin and the lung [107]; whereas their involvement in gastrointestinal pathologies is largely unknown.

Similar to mast cells, basophils release large amounts of histamine and LTC4, but no PGD_2, which is specifically mast cell-derived. Basophils are a major source of IL-4 and IL-13 [108,109] that can be released upon IgE-dependent and IgE-independent stimulation. On a per cell basis, activated basophils produce more IL-4 and IL-13 than any other cell type. Basophils produced a much more limited cytokine profile than mast cells and eosinophils (Table 2.1). However, the specific expression of IL-4, which is hardly produced by mast cells and eosinophils, suggests a particular role for basophils in the antigen-specific priming of Th2 cells [110].

After cross-linking of FcεRI, the release of histamine and eicosanoid is nearly complete by 20 minutes, whereas IL-4 and IL-13 production follows a time course with a maximal response after 4 and 20 hours, respectively. Small amounts of IL-4 ($<10\,pg/10^6$ basophils) become detectable within 5–10 minutes after stimulation, suggesting that preformed IL-4 is released [106]. IgE-independent secretagogues are the anaphylatoxins C3a and C5a, platelet-activating factor (PAF), eosinophil-derived major basic protein (MBP), cytokines (IL-3, IL-5, GM-CSF), and chemokines (MCP-1, -3, eotaxin, RANTES, MIP-1α, IL-8). Of particular interest is the observation that IL-3, IL-5, and GM-CSF only induce small amounts of mediator release, but substantially enhance the effects of almost all IgE-dependent and IgE-independent agonists. The latter seems to be of greater importance; particularly in the allergic late-phase reaction characterized by enhanced cytokine production, and has been named "basophil priming." Similar observations could be made for other inflammatory cells such as eosinophils, suggesting a rather general way of inflammatory cell regulation [103,106,111].

A growing body of evidence suggests that basophils are involved in the defense against helminth infections [112]. However, basophil *in vivo* studies are limited, because a basophil-deficient mouse strain does not exist. Mukai *et al.* recently demonstrated a series of elegant transfer studies, that basophils, in the absence of T-cells and reacting mast cells, induce an IgE-dependent delayed-onset allergic inflammation, whereas mast cells were necessary for the immediate-phase response [113].

Eosinophils

Eosinophils fully maturate within the bone marrow, from which they enter the bloodstream. IL-3, IL-5, and GM-CSF are particularly effective in regulating eosinophil growth and maturation. Of these three, IL-5 is the most specific and potent. Eosinophils normally account for only 1–3% of peripheral blood leukocytes and, under physiological conditions, their presence in tissue is primarily limited to the gastrointestinal mucosa which forms the largest eosinophil reservoir of the body. In the course of several diseases, including allergy, eosinophilic gastroenteritis, and helminth infection, eosinophils can selectively accumulate in the peripheral blood or any tissue [28,114]. Recruitment of eosinophils depends on the production of a number of chemokines (e.g. RANTES and the eotaxins). Only IL-5 and the eotaxins selectively regulate eosinophil trafficking [28,74]. Anti-IL-5 treatment reduced tissue eosinophilia in asthma patients by 55%, however, without affecting symptoms [115].

Eosinophils secrete an array of cytotoxic granule cationic proteins that are present in large quantities in the cells: eosinophil cationic protein (ECP), eosinophil-derived neurotoxin (EDN), major basic protein (MBP), and eosinophilic peroxidase (EPO). The enzymatic activities and several functions of these proteins have been defined and have been recently reviewed in detail [28,116]. Apart from their toxic effects and antiviral activity, these proteins activate mast cells (EPO, MBP) and suppress T-cell proliferation (ECP) and immunoglobulin synthesis (ECP). Eosinophils produce several eicosanoid metabolites, oxygen radicals, and multiple cytokines/chemokines [28] (Table 2.1).

C5a, C3a, and PAF cause degranulation in eosinophils, whereas other stimuli, such as the cytokines IL-3, IL-5, and GM-CSF, have a weak or no direct effect. However, this set of cytokines "prime" eosinophils for enhanced mediator release to other stimuli, including otherwise ineffective agonists [117]. Interestingly, PAF produced by eosinophils has been considered as an autocrine secretagogue [118]. Furthermore, chemokines, such as the CCR3 ligands MCP-3, MCP-4, RANTES, and eotaxin, induce degranulation in eosinophils [119]. Eosinophils express FcαRI, FcγRII, and FcγRI (inducible, Table 2.2) and secretory IgA and IgG are strong signals for degranulation [51,120,121] mediating for example antibody (or complement)-dependent cellular toxity against helminthes. The role of the FcεRI on the eosinophil is still a matter of controversy [122]. Eosinophil activation by cytokines and immunoglobulins is critically dependent on β2-integrins, especially on Mac-1 binding to ICAM-1 [123], suggesting that their activity is silenced in the bloodstream.

There is strong evidence that eosinophils play a considerable role in the defense against helminthes. This is supported by findings in both humans and animal models [28,124]. Recently, two eosinophil-deficient mouse models have been developed. In both strains, eosinophils substantially impact on experimental allergic asthma, but apart from this common finding, they give divergent results. While the *PHIL* mice are completely protected from developing airway hyperresponsiveness and show partial protection from airway mucous metaplasia, the Δdbl GATA mice lack improvement of these parameters, and rather show attenuation of airway remodeling. However, airway remodeling has not been investigated in the PHIL mice [125,126].

Conclusion

The allergen-specific Th2 and B-cell priming, the function of IgE and FcεRI, and the biology of allergic effector cells have been intensively studied during the last few decades. The current advances in understanding these fundamental immunological mechanisms lead to the design of new treatment approaches, of which some have reached the level of clinical trails or approval [14,115,127]. We are only beginning to understand the regulatory network of the immune system, in particular the function of Treg cells and "blocking" allergen-specific antibodies. Therefore, we still need to learn how we can direct the immune system toward a tolerizing response to introduce more rational and safer vaccine strategies [14]. The link between environmental stimuli and allergy remains poorly understood and requires further investigation.

A specific problem concerning food allergy lies in the fact that the general pathophysiological concepts of allergy have mainly been developed in model systems of non-food-related atopy. This applies also to this chapter, which reviews in large part data generated in studies of non-food allergy. This is further reflected by the fact that new drugs are often designed for the treatment of asthma, rhinoconjunctivitis, atopic dermatitis, or insect allergy, but rarely for food allergy. The pathophysiology and the clinical management of food allergy might be considered more complex in comparison to other allergic disorders, in particular, as the gastrointestinal tract is difficult to access for investigation and the symptoms are often variable and unspecific. Therefore, a better understanding of the specific immunopathology of food allergy and an improvement in the diagnostic approach are necessary to provide improved treatment options.

Acknowledgment

We thank Thomas Kufer for critical reading.

References

1 Bischoff S, Crowe SE. Gastrointestinal food allergy: new insights into pathophysiology and clinical perspectives. *Gastroenterology* 2005;128:1089–113.

2 Sampson HA. Update on food allergy. *J Allergy Clin Immunol* 2004;113:805–19.

3 Fernandez-Rivas M, Bolhaar S, Gonzalez-Mancebo E, *et al*. Apple allergy across Europe: how allergen sensitization profiles determine the clinical expression of allergies to plant foods. *J Allergy Clin Immunol* 2006;118:481–8.

4 Brandtzaeg P, Johansen FE. Mucosal B cells: phenotypic characteristics, transcriptional regulation, and homing properties. *Immunol Rev* 2005;206:32–63.

5 Sansonetti PJ. War and peace at mucosal surfaces. *Nat Rev Immunol* 2004;4:953–64.

6 Sanderson IR, Walker WA. Uptake and transport of macromolecules by the intestine: possible role in clinical disorders (an update). *Gastroenterology* 1993;104:622–39.

7 Niedergang F, Kweon MN. New trends in antigen uptake in the gut mucosa. *Trends Microbiol* 2005;13:485–90.

8 Untersmayr E, Jensen-Jarolim E. The effect of gastric digestion on food allergy. *Curr Opin Allergy Clin Immunol* 2006;6:214–19.

9 Ventura MT, Polimeno L, Amoruso AC, *et al*. Intestinal permeability in patients with adverse reactions to food. *Dig Liver Dis* 2006;38:732–6.

10 Benard A, Desreumeaux P, Huglo D, *et al*. Increased intestinal permeability in bronchial asthma. *J Allergy Clin Immunol* 1996;97:1173–8.

11 Zeiger RS, Heller S, Mellon MH, *et al*. Effect of combined maternal and infant food-allergen avoidance on development of atopy in early infancy: a randomized study. *J Allergy Clin Immunol* 1989;84:72–89.

12 Taylor B, Norman AP, Orgel HA, *et al*. Transient IgA deficiency and pathogenesis of infantile atopy. *Lancet* 1973;2:111–13.

13 Husby S, Foged N, Host A, Svehag SE. Passage of dietary antigens into the blood of children with coeliac disease. Quantification and size distribution of absorbed antigens. *Gut* 1987;28:1062–72.

14 Larche M, Akdis CA, Valenta R. Immunological mechanisms of allergen-specific immunotherapy. *Nat Rev Immunol* 2006;6:761–71.

15 Akdis CA. Allergy and hypersensitivity mechanisms of allergic disease. *Curr Opin Immunol* 2006;18:718–26.

16 Veldhoen M, Stockinger B. TGFbeta1, a "Jack of all trades": the link with pro-inflammatory IL-17-producing T cells. *Trends Immunol* 2006;27:358–61.

17 Umetsu DT, Dekruyff RH. A role for natural killer T cells in asthma. *Nat Rev Immunol* 2006;6:953–8.

18 Hawrylowicz CM, O'Garra A. Potential role of interleukin-10-secreting regulatory T cells in allergy and asthma. *Nat Rev Immunol* 2005;5:271–83.

19 Akdis M. Healthy immune response to allergens: T regulatory cells and more. *Curr Opin Immunol* 2006;18:738–44.

20 Akdis M, Verhagen J, Taylor A, *et al*. Immune responses in healthy and allergic individuals are characterized by a fine balance between allergen-specific T regulatory 1 and T helper 2 cells. *J Exp Med* 2004;199:1567–75.

21 Royer B, Varadaradjalou S, Saas P, *et al*. Inhibition of IgE-induced activation of human mast cells by IL-10. *Clin Exp Allergy* 2001;31:694–704.

22 Gebhardt T, Lorentz A, Detmer F, *et al*. Growth, phenotype, and function of human intestinal mast cells are tightly regulated by transforming growth factor beta1. *Gut* 2005;54:928–34.

23 Jutel M, Akdis M, Budak F, *et al*. IL-10 and TGF-beta cooperate in the regulatory T cell response to mucosal allergens in normal immunity and specific immunotherapy. *Eur J Immunol* 2003;33:1205–14.

24 Akdis CA, Blesken T, Akdis M, *et al*. Role of interleukin 10 in specific immunotherapy. *J Clin Invest* 1998 ;102:98–106.

25 Mitre E, Nutman TB. IgE memory: persistence of antigen-specific IgE responses years after treatment of human filarial infections. *J Allergy Clin Immunol* 2006;117:939–45.

26 Geha RS, Jabara HH, Brodeur SR. The regulation of immunoglobulin E class-switch recombination. *Nat Rev Immunol* 2003;3:721–32.

27 Pawankar R, Okuda M, Yssel H, *et al*. Nasal mast cells in perennial allergic rhinitics exhibit increased expression of the Fc epsilonRI, CD40L, IL-4, and IL-13, and can induce IgE synthesis in B cells. *J Clin Invest* 1997;99:1492–9.

28 Rothenberg ME, Hogan SP. The eosinophil. *Annu Rev Immunol* 2006;24:147–74.

29 Dahlke I, Nott DJ, Ruhno J, *et al*. Antigen selection in the IgE response of allergic and nonallergic individuals. *J Allergy Clin Immunol* 2006;117:1477–83.

30 Takhar P, Smurthwaite L, Coker HA, *et al*. Allergen drives class switching to IgE in the nasal mucosa in allergic rhinitis. *J Immunol* 2005;174:5024–32.

31 Coker HA, Durham SR, Gould HJ. Local somatic hypermutation and class switch recombination in the nasal mucosa of allergic rhinitis patients. *J Immunol* 2003;171:5602–10.

32 Vieira P, Rajewsky K. The half-lives of serum immunoglobulins in adult mice. *Eur J Immunol* 1988;18:313–16.

33 Tada T, Okumura K, Platteau B, *et al*. Half-lives of two types of rat homocytotropic antibodies in circulation and in the skin. *Int Arch Allergy Appl Immunol* 1975;48:116–31.

34 Golden DB, Kagey-Sobotka A, Norman PS, *et al*. Outcomes of allergy to insect stings in children, with and without venom immunotherapy. *N Engl J Med* 2004;351:668–74.

35 Radbruch A, Muehlinghaus G, Luger EO, *et al*. Competence and competition: the challenge of becoming a long-lived plasma cell. *Nat Rev Immunol* 2006;6:741- 50.

36 Gould HJ, Sutton BJ, Beavil AJ, *et al*. The biology of IGE and the basis of allergic disease. *Annu Rev Immunol* 2003;21:579–628.

37 Hallstrand TS, Sprenger JD, Agosti JM, *et al*. Long-term acquisition of allergen-specific IgE and asthma following allogeneic bone marrow transplantation from allergic donors. *Blood* 2004; 104:3086–90.

38 Crameri R, Rhyner C. Novel vaccines and adjuvants for allergen-specific immunotherapy. *Curr Opin Immunol* 2006;18:761–8.

39 van RR, Van Leeuwen WA, Dieges PH, *et al*. Measurement of IgE antibodies against purified grass pollen allergens (Lol p 1, 2, 3 and 5) during immunotherapy. *Clin Exp Allergy* 1997;27:68–74.

40 Reisinger J, Horak F, Pauli G, *et al*. Allergen-specific nasal IgG antibodies induced by vaccination with genetically modified allergens are associated with reduced nasal allergen sensitivity. *J Allergy Clin Immunol* 2005;116:347–54.

41 Niederberger V, Horak F, Vrtala S, *et al*. Vaccination with genetically engineered allergens prevents progression of allergic disease. *Proc Natl Acad Sci USA* 2004;101:14677–82.

42 Jutel M, Jaeger L, Suck R, *et al*. Allergen-specific immunotherapy with recombinant grass pollen allergens. *J Allergy Clin Immunol* 2005;116:608–13.

43 Strait RT, Morris SC, Finkelman FD. IgG-blocking antibodies inhibit IgE-mediated anaphylaxis *in vivo* through both antigen interception and Fc gamma RIIb cross-linking. *J Clin Invest* 2006;116:833–41.

44 Ejrnaes AM, Svenson M, Lund G, *et al*. Inhibition of rBet v 1-induced basophil histamine release with specific immunotherapy -induced serum immunoglobulin G: no evidence that FcgammaRIIB signalling is important. *Clin Exp Allergy* 2006; 36:73–82.

45 Flicker S, Valenta R. Renaissance of the blocking antibody concept in type I allergy. *Int Arch Allergy Immunol* 2003;132:13–24.

46 Bruhns P, Fremont S, Daeron M. Regulation of allergy by Fc receptors. *Curr Opin Immunol* 2005;17:662–9.

47 Watanabe T, Okano M, Hattori H, *et al*. Roles of FcgammaRIIB in nasal eosinophilia and IgE production in murine allergic rhinitis. *Am J Respir Crit Care Med* 2004;169:105–12.

48 Zhu D, Kepley CL, Zhang K, *et al*. A chimeric human–cat fusion protein blocks cat-induced allergy. *Nat Med* 2005;11:446–9.

49 Djurup R, Malling HJ. High IgG4 antibody level is associated with failure of immunotherapy with inhalant allergens. *Clin Allergy* 1987;17:459–68.

50 Okayama Y, Kirshenbaum AS, Metcalfe DD. Expression of a functional high-affinity IgG receptor, Fc gamma RI, on human mast cells: up-regulation by IFN-gamma. *J Immunol* 2000;164:4332–9.

51 Zhu X, Hamann KJ, Munoz NM, *et al*. Intracellular expression of Fc gamma RIII (CD16) and its mobilization by chemoattractants in human eosinophils. *J Immunol* 1998;161:2574–9.

52 Sellge G, Laffer S, Mierke C, *et al*. Development of an *in vitro* system for the study of allergens and allergen-specific immunoglobulin E and immunoglobulin G: Fcepsilon receptor I supercross-linking is a possible new mechanism of immunoglobulin G-dependent enhancement of type I allergic reactions. *Clin Exp Allergy* 2005;35:774–81.

53 Denepoux S, Eibensteiner PB, Steinberger P, *et al*. Molecular characterization of human IgG monoclonal antibodies specific

for the major birch pollen allergen Bet v 1. Anti-allergen IgG can enhance the anaphylactic reaction. *FEBS Lett* 2000;465:39–46.

53b van der Neut Kolfschoten M, Schuurman J, Losen M, Bleeker WK, Martinez-Martinez P, Vermeulen E, den Bleker TH, Wiegman L, Vink T, Aarden LA, De Baets MH, van de Winkel JG, Aalberse RC, Parren PW. Anti-inflammatory activity of human IgG4 antibodies by dynamic Fab arm exchange. Science 2007; 317:1554–7.

54 Nimmerjahn F, Ravetch JV. Divergent immunoglobulin g subclass activity through selective Fc receptor binding. *Science* 2005;310:1510–12.

55 Janeway CA, Travers P, Walport M, Shlomchik M. *Immunobiology: the Immune System in Health and Disease*, 5th edn. New York: Garland Publishing, a member of the Taylor & Francis Group, 2001.

56 Barnes KC. Genetic epidemiology of health disparities in allergy and clinical immunology. *J Allergy Clin Immunol* 2006; 117:243–54.

57 Vercelli D. Genetic polymorphism in allergy and asthma. *Curr Opin Immunol* 2003;15:609–13.

58 Vercelli D, Baldini M, Stern D, *et al.* CD14: a bridge between innate immunity and adaptive IgE responses. *J Endotoxin Res* 2001;7:45–8.

59 Eder W, Klimecki W, Yu L, *et al.* Association between exposure to farming, allergies and genetic variation in CARD4/NOD1. *Allergy* 2006;61:1117–24.

60 Vercelli D. Mechanisms of the hygiene hypothesis – molecular and otherwise. *Curr Opin Immunol* 2006;18:733–7.

61 Yazdanbakhsh M, Kremsner PG, van RR. Allergy, parasites, and the hygiene hypothesis. *Science* 2002;296:490–4.

62 de MG, Janssen NA, Brunekreef B. Early childhood environment related to microbial exposure and the occurrence of atopic disease at school age. *Allergy* 2005;60:619–25.

63 Mazmanian SK, Liu CH, Tzianabos AO, Kasper DL. An immunomodulatory molecule of symbiotic bacteria directs maturation of the host immune system. *Cell* 2005;122:107–18.

64 Kalliomaki M, Salminen S, Poussa T, *et al.* Probiotics and prevention of atopic disease: 4-year follow-up of a randomised placebo-controlled trial. *Lancet* 2003;361:1869–71.

65 Bach JF. Infections and autoimmune diseases. *J Autoimmun* 2005;25:74–80.

66 Simons FE, Shikishima Y, Van NG, *et al.* Selective immune redirection in humans with ragweed allergy by injecting Amb a 1 linked to immunostimulatory DNA. *J Allergy Clin Immunol* 2004;113:1144–51.

67 von BV, Hermes A, von BR, *et al.* Allergoid-specific T-cell reaction as a measure of the immunological response to specific immunotherapy (SIT) with a Th1-adjuvanted allergy vaccine. *J Investig Allergol Clin Immunol* 2005;15:234–41.

68 Hussain R, Poindexter RW, Ottesen EA. Control of allergic reactivity in human filariasis. Predominant localization of blocking antibody to the IgG4 subclass. *J Immunol* 1992;148:2731–7.

69 Sansonetti PJ. The innate signaling of dangers and the dangers of innate signaling. *Nat Immunol* 2006;7:1237–42.

70 Boldogh I, Bacsi A, Choudhury BK, *et al.* ROS generated by pollen NADPH oxidase provide a signal that augments antigen-induced allergic airway inflammation. *J Clin Invest* 2005;115:2169–79.

71 Traidl-Hoffmann C, Mariani V, Hochrein H, *et al.* Pollen-associated phytoprostanes inhibit dendritic cell interleukin-12 production and augment T helper type 2 cell polarization. *J Exp Med* 2005;201:627–36.

72 Shreffler WG, Castro RR, Kucuk ZY, *et al.* The major glycoprotein allergen from Arachis hypogaea, Ara h 1, is a ligand of dendritic cell-specific ICAM-grabbing nonintegrin and acts as a Th2 adjuvant *in vitro. J Immunol* 2006;177:3677–85.

73 Bohle B, Zwolfer B, Heratizadeh A, *et al.* Cooking birch pollen-related food: divergent consequences for IgE- and T cell-mediated reactivity *in vitro* and *in vivo. J Allergy Clin Immunol* 2006;118:242–9.

74 Bochner BS, Schleimer RP. Mast cells, basophils, and eosinophils: distinct but overlapping pathways for recruitment. *Immunol Rev* 2001;179:5–15.

75 Blank U, Rivera J. The ins and outs of IgE-dependent mast-cell exocytosis. *Trends Immunol* 2004;25:266–73.

76 Galli SJ, Kalesnikoff J, Grimbaldeston MA, *et al.* Mast cells as "tunable" effector and immunoregulatory cells: recent advances. *Annu Rev Immunol* 2005;23:749–86.

77 Gilfillan AM, Tkaczyk C. Integrated signalling pathways for mast-cell activation. *Nat Rev Immunol* 2006;6:218–30.

78 Matsuda K, Piliponsky AM, Iikura M, *et al.* Monomeric IgE enhances human mast cell chemokine production: IL-4 augments and dexamethasone suppresses the response. *J Allergy Clin Immunol* 2005;116:1357–63.

79 Kalesnikoff J, Huber M, Lam V, *et al.* Monomeric IgE stimulates signaling pathways in mast cells that lead to cytokine production and cell survival. *Immunity* 2001;14:801–11.

80 Maurer D, Ebner C, Reininger B, *et al.* The high affinity IgE receptor (Fc epsilon RI) mediates IgE-dependent allergen presentation. *J Immunol* 1995;154:6285–90.

81 Bischoff SC, Sellge G. Mast cell hyperplasia: role of cytokines. *Int Arch Allergy Immunol* 2002;127:118–22.

82 Bischoff SC, Sellge G, Lorentz A, *et al.* IL-4 enhances proliferation and mediator release in mature human mast cells. *Proc Natl Acad Sci USA* 1999;96:8080–5.

83 Gebhardt T, Sellge G, Lorentz A, *et al.* Cultured human intestinal mast cells express functional IL-3 receptors and respond to IL-3 by enhancing growth and IgE receptor-dependent mediator release. *Eur J Immunol* 2002;32:2308–16.

84 Matsuzawa S, Sakashita K, Kinoshita T, *et al.* IL-9 enhances the growth of human mast cell progenitors under stimulation with stem cell factor. *J Immunol* 2003;170:3461–7.

85 Bryce PJ, Mathias CB, Harrison KL, *et al.* The H1 histamine receptor regulates allergic lung responses. *J Clin Invest* 2006;116:1624–32.

86 Valent P, Sillaber C, Baghestanian M, *et al.* What have mast cells to do with edema formation, the consecutive repair and fibrinolysis? *Int Arch Allergy Immunol* 1998;115:2–8.

87 Maurer M, Wedemeyer J, Metz M, *et al*. Mast cells promote homeostasis by limiting endothelin-1-induced toxicity. *Nature* 2004;432:512–16.

88 Metz M, Piliponsky AM, Chen CC, *et al*. Mast cells can enhance resistance to snake and honeybee venoms. *Science* 2006;313:526–30.

89 Rauter I, Krauth MT, Flicker S, *et al*. Allergen cleavage by effector cell-derived proteases regulates allergic inflammation. *FASEB J* 2006;20:967–9.

90 Ott VL, Cambier JC, Kappler J, *et al*. Mast cell-dependent migration of effector CD8+ T cells through production of leukotriene B4. *Nat Immunol* 2003;4:974–81.

91 Lorentz A, Schwengberg S, Sellge G, *et al*. Human intestinal mast cells are capable of producing different cytokine profiles: role of IgE receptor cross-linking and IL-4. *J Immunol* 2000;164:43–8.

92 Plaut M, Pierce JH, Watson CJ, *et al*. Mast cell lines produce lymphokines in response to cross-linkage of Fc epsilon RI or to calcium ionophores. *Nature* 1989;339:64–7.

93 Ochi H, De Jesus NH, Hsieh FH, *et al*. IL-4 and -5 prime human mast cells for different profiles of IgE-dependent cytokine production. *Proc Natl Acad Sci USA* 2000;97:10509–13.

94 Dawicki W, Marshall JS. New and emerging roles for mast cells in host defence. *Curr Opin Immunol* 2006;19:31–8.

95 Benoist C, Mathis D. Mast cells in autoimmune disease. *Nature* 2002;420:875–8.

96 Malaviya R, Ikeda T, Ross E, Abraham SN. Mast cell modulation of neutrophil influx and bacterial clearance at sites of infection through TNF-alpha. *Nature* 1996;381:77–80.

97 Echtenacher B, Mannel DN, Hultner L. 1996. Critical protective role of mast cells in a model of acute septic peritonitis. *Nature* 381:75–77.

98 Yu M, Tsai M, Tam SY, *et al*. Mast cells can promote the development of multiple features of chronic asthma in mice. *J Clin Invest* 2006;116:1633–41.

99 Galli SJ, Nakae S, Tsai M. Mast cells in the development of adaptive immune responses. *Nat Immunol* 2005;6:135–42.

100 Depinay N, Hacini F, Beghdadi W, *et al*. Mast cell-dependent down-regulation of antigen-specific immune responses by mosquito bites. *J Immunol* 2006;176:4141–6.

101 Lu LF, Lind EF, Gondek DC, *et al*. Mast cells are essential intermediaries in regulatory T-cell tolerance. *Nature* 2006;442:997–1002.

102 Bischoff SC. Role of mast cells in allergic and non-allergic immune responses: a comparison of human and murine data. *Nat Rev Immunol* 2007;7:93–104.

103 Falcone FH, Haas H, Gibbs BF. The human basophil: a new appreciation of its role in immune responses. *Blood* 2000;96:4028–38.

104 Arinobu Y, Iwasaki H, Gurish MF, *et al*. Developmental checkpoints of the basophil/mast cell lineages in adult murine hematopoiesis. *Proc Natl Acad Sci USA* 2005;102:18105–10.

105 Lim LH, Burdick MM, Hudson SA, *et al*. Stimulation of human endothelium with IL-3 induces selective basophil accumulation *in vitro*. *J Immunol* 2006;176:5346–53.

106 Schroeder JT, MacGlashan Jr, DW, Lichtenstein LM. Human basophils: mediator release and cytokine production. *Adv Immunol* 2001;77:93–122.

107 Macfarlane AJ, Kon OM, Smith SJ, *et al*. Basophils, eosinophils, and mast cells in atopic and nonatopic asthma and in late-phase allergic reactions in the lung and skin. *J Allergy Clin Immunol* 2000;105:99–107.

108 Brunner T, Heusser CH, Dahinden CA. Human peripheral blood basophils primed by interleukin 3 (IL-3) produce IL-4 in response to immunoglobulin E receptor stimulation. *J Exp Med* 1993;177:605–11.

109 Devouassoux G, Foster B, Scott LM, *et al*. Frequency and characterization of antigen-specific IL-4- and IL-13-producing basophils and T cells in peripheral blood of healthy and asthmatic subjects. *J Allergy Clin Immunol* 1999;104:811–19.

110 Oh K, Shen T, Le GG, Min B. Induction of Th2 type immunity in a mouse system reveals a novel immunoregulatory role of basophils. *Blood* 2007;109:2921–7.

111 Bischoff SC, de Weck AL, Dahinden CA. Interleukin 3 and granulocyte/macrophage-colony-stimulating factor render human basophils responsive to low concentrations of complement component C3a. *Proc Natl Acad Sci USA* 1990;87:6813–17.

112 Mitre E, Nutman TB. Basophils, basophilia and helminth infections. *Chem Immunol Allergy* 2006;90:141–56.

113 Mukai K, Matsuoka K, Taya C, *et al*. Basophils play a critical role in the development of IgE-mediated chronic allergic inflammation independently of T cells and mast cells. *Immunity* 2005;23:191–202.

114 Kato M, Kephart GM, Morikawa A, Gleich GJ. Eosinophil infiltration and degranulation in normal human tissues: evidence for eosinophil degranulation in normal gastrointestinal tract. *Int Arch Allergy Immunol* 2001;125:55–8.

115 Leckie MJ, ten BA, Khan J, *et al*. Effects of an interleukin-5 blocking monoclonal antibody on eosinophils, airway hyper-responsiveness, and the late asthmatic response. *Lancet* 2000;356:2144–8.

116 Moqbel R, Lacy P. Exocytotic events in eosinophils and mast cells. *Clin Exp Allergy* 1999;29:1017–22.

117 Gleich GJ. Mechanisms of eosinophil-associated inflammation. *J Allergy Clin Immunol* 2000;105:651–63.

118 Bartemes KR, McKinney S, Gleich GJ, Kita H. Endogenous platelet-activating factor is critically involved in effector functions of eosinophils stimulated with IL-5 or IgG. *J Immunol* 1999;162:2982–9.

119 Fujisawa T, Kato Y, Nagase H, *et al*. Chemokines induce eosinophil degranulation through CCR-3. *J Allergy Clin Immunol* 2000;106:507–13.

120 Abu-Ghazaleh RI, Fujisawa T, Mestecky J, *et al*. IgA-induced eosinophil degranulation. *J Immunol* 1989;142:2393–400.

121 Egesten A, Calafat J, Janssen H, *et al*. Granules of human eosinophilic leucocytes and their mobilization. *Clin Exp Allergy* 2001;31:1173–88.

122 Kita H, Kaneko M, Bartemes KR, *et al*. Does IgE bind to and activate eosinophils from patients with allergy? *J Immunol* 1999;162:6901–11.

123 Horie S, Kita H. CD11b/CD18 (Mac-1) is required for degranulation of human eosinophils induced by human recombinant granulocyte-macrophage colony-stimulating factor and platelet-activating factor. *J Immunol* 1994;152:5457–67.

124 Rothenberg ME, Mishra A, Brandt EB, Hogan SP. Gastrointestinal eosinophils. *Immunol Rev* 2001;179:139–55.

125 Humbles AA, Lloyd CM, McMillan SJ, *et al*. A critical role for eosinophils in allergic airways remodeling. *Science* 2004; 305:1776–9.

126 Lee JJ, Dimina D, Macias MP, *et al*. Defining a link with asthma in mice congenitally deficient in eosinophils. *Science* 2004;305:1773–6.

127 Busse W, Corren J, Lanier BQ, *et al*. Omalizumab, anti-IgE recombinant humanized monoclonal antibody, for the treatment of severe allergic asthma. *J Allergy Clin Immunol* 2001;108:184–90.

CHAPTER 3

The Immunologic Basis of Non-IgE-Mediated Reactions

Ashraf Uzzaman and Hirsh D. Komarow

KEY CONCEPTS

- Genetic, environmental, and developmental factors as well as antigenic properties of food proteins influence the development of non-IgE-mediated food allergy.

- The mucosal barrier in concert with the innate and adaptive arms of the immune system comprises the primary defense of the gastrointestinal tract against luminal antigens.

- The uptake and transport of luminal antigens is facilitated by intestinal epithelial cells, microfold cells, and dendritic cells.

- Food antigens are presented to T-cells in association with MHC class II molecules.

- Oral tolerance is a physiologic, active non-response to an encountered antigen and a failure of its induction leads to immunologic reactions to foods.

Introduction

The first authentic report of food hypersensitivity, over 2300 years ago, is attributed to Hippocrates for his findings that there exist individual differences in reactions to milk ingestion [1,2]. Quantitatively, food proteins account for one of the largest antigenic challenges confronting the human immune system [3]. Nonetheless, only a small number of foods instigate the majority of abnormal immune responses.

Abnormal responses to foods may be classified as toxic, such as to food contaminants, which are not dependent on individual susceptibility; and non-toxic, which are dependent on individual susceptibility. Non-toxic responses may be separated into non-immune mediated, such as food intolerance to lactose, and immune mediated, such as food allergy. The mechanisms of immune-mediated adverse reactions may be further divided into IgE-mediated or immediate-in-time and non-IgE-mediated or delayed-in-time responses [4,5]. Consistent with the global increase in the prevalence of atopic diseases, there has been a significant rise in both IgE and non-IgE-mediated food allergies [6,7].

This chapter provides a comprehensive overview of the immunologic basis of non-IgE-mediated, as well as mixed IgE-mediated mechanisms of food allergy. We elaborate on factors affecting the development of food allergy; the immunologic anatomy and defense mechanisms of the gut which avert the development of food allergy; the processing of enteral food antigens and their presentation to immune competent cells of the gastrointestinal tract; and the effector cells and inflammatory mediators critical to the propagation and consequences of abnormal reactions to foods.

Development of food allergy

Genetic, environmental, and developmental factors, as well as a number of antigenic characteristics of food proteins, appear to influence the onset of food allergy. Genetic factors, such as a family history of atopic disease [8] and genetic polymorphisms [9], have been implicated. Early infectious exposure [10,11], rural upbringing with exposure to animals [12], and commensal [13] and pathogenic microorganisms within the GI tract are environmental factors that have been correlated with reduced atopic sensitization. Developmental factors, which include immaturity of the gut mucosa and the gut immune system, as seen among infants and children, may contribute to the development of food allergy. In addition, a number of antigenic characteristics of food proteins also impact the occurrence of food allergy.

The genetic basis of IgE-mediated food allergies have been more thoroughly characterized [14–19] than for non-IgE-mediated food allergies [20,21]. Studies of familial clustering, twin studies, and isolation of genetic polymorphisms

Food Allergy: Adverse Reactions to Foods and Food Additives, 4th edition.
Edited by Dean D. Metcalfe, Hugh A. Sampson, and Ronald A. Simon.
© 2008 Blackwell Publishing, ISBN: 978-1-4501-5129-0.

illustrate the genetic influences on non-IgE-mediated diseases. For example, celiac disease (CD), a prototypical non-IgE-mediated food allergy, shows familial clustering [22,23] and a high concordance rate of approximately 75% among monozygotic twins [24,25]. This disease has also been shown to be associated with two conventional DQ molecules, HLA-DQ2 and HLA-DQ8 [20,26,27]. Moreover, studies showing the genetic contribution of the HLA region on the familial clustering of CD suggest that HLA haplotypes are an important genetic background to the development of CD. However, additional susceptibility factors need to be identified [27]. Genetic associations with disease have also been made in eosinophilic esophagitis where familial clustering occurs, and observation of a single nucleotide polymorphism in the human eotaxin-3-gene has been made [28]. The genetic basis of food allergy, however, remains unclear [29].

A number of environmental factors appear to influence the development of allergy [30]. Studies show that improved social conditions may lead to a more "sanitary" living environment which may increase the risk for developing allergies, including food allergy [31]. A dominant role of early environmental exposures in the development of immune tolerance has also been reported. For instance, a farm upbringing, particularly with exposure to animals and livestock, has been shown to be relatively protective against the development of allergies [32]. This concept is often referred to as the "hygiene hypothesis" and is supported by a recent study which documented a decreased prevalence of allergic sensitization in children growing up on farms compared to their counterparts residing in the same geographic regions [33]. The inheritance of primary eosinophilic disorders appears to be multi-factorial, with an interplay between genetic and environmental factors where a majority of individuals are atopic [9]. Moreover, individuals demonstrate symptomatic improvement when the offending food allergen is eliminated from their diet [34].

Both commensal and pathogenic microorganisms in the gut appear to stimulate local B-cells and T-cells to induce normal development of the GI mucosal immune system. Animals reared in a germ-free environment have an underdeveloped GI mucosal immune system [13,35]. Toll-like receptors (TLRs) and secretion of chemokines, such as CCL20, IL-8, and MIP3α, which are involved in luminal bacterial recognition, appear to be critical for the development of the innate as well as the adaptive arm of the mucosal immune system [36,37]. It has been proposed that disturbances in the gut flora, along with disruption of the gut barrier and breakdown of innate mucosal immunity caused by enteral pathogenic microorganisms, may contribute to the development of allergies. Further, microorganisms play a role in the pathogenesis of reflux esophagitis [38], gastritis and gastric ulcers [39], and infectious diarrheas [40], which are characterized by disruptions of the gut barrier resulting in irregularities in permeability and antigen transport across the GI epithelium, perhaps fostering the development of food allergy.

The prevalence of food allergy is higher among infants and in children who are less than 3 years of age [41]. In infants, the relative immaturity of the GI mucosal immune system and mucosal barrier functions may be responsible for the increased prevalence [1]. The mucosal immune system immaturity is characterized by low basal acid output in the stomach, relative low levels of proteolytic activity, and immaturity of the barrier function. These conditions result in decreased luminal breakdown of antigen which leads to increased antigen absorption, as well as absorption of large antigenic molecules that interact with the mucosal immune system and predispose to food allergy [30].

Antigenic characteristics of food proteins may contribute to specific food allergies [42]. Physical characteristics of food proteins, such as size of the antigen, relative abundance [43] and resistance to acidic and enzymatic denaturation and digestion [44], their immunogenicity and the method by which they are presented to T-cells, are key determinants of their antigenic potential [45]. Food proteins that are allergenic also tend to be resistant to processing and heating and to acidic degradation and digestion within the GI tract [46].

Gut anatomy

The primary anatomical constituents which relate to immunologic responses in the GI tract include mucus, the glycocalyx, microvilli, the epithelial layer, the lamina propria, the muscularis mucosa, and gut-associated lymphoid tissue (GALT) (Fig. 3.1). The mucus layer is composed of mucin, free protein, dialyzable salts and is 95% water. It forms an adherent mucus gel layer over epithelial cells and creates a near-neutral pH at the epithelial surface, which is resistant to acidic and proteolytic digestion, thereby protecting the underlying mucosa [47]. Internal to the mucus layer is the cell surface coat, the glycocalyx, which is composed primarily of carbohydrates and contains various enzymes such as enteropeptidases, dipeptidases, and disaccharidases; and non-enzymatic proteins that are essential for terminal digestion of food and absorption of nutrients [48,49]. Luminal to the epithelial cells and beneath the glycocalyx are dense microvilli, which increase the absorptive surface area [50]. The epithelial layer is singular and composed of columnar cells, and together with the luminal mucus, functions as the primary separation between the mucosal immune system and the microbiota and enteral food antigens [51]. The epithelium also contains mucus goblet cells, undifferentiated crypt epithelial cells, and intra-epithelial lymphocytes, each of which performs a unique and integrated function (Fig. 3.1(a)). The intestinal epithelial cells (IECs) are bound by tight junctions at their apical surfaces, which function as a selective barrier to prevent the absorption of harmful

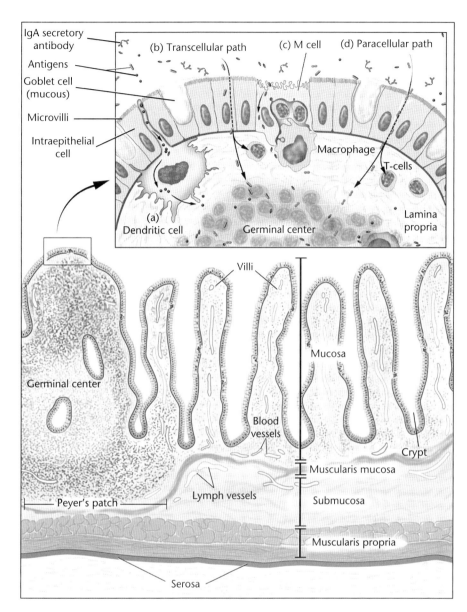

Figure 3.1 Ultrastructure of the GI wall illustrating some of its physical characteristics which comprises the intrinsic factors of the defense mechanisms. (Inset) Pathways of antigen uptake in the gut: (a) dendritic cells extend foot processes to sample luminal antigens; (b) antigen uptake across the apical surface of the IECs; (c) uptake of antigens by M cells, which subsequently deliver them to the germinal centers; and (d) uptake of antigen via the tight junctions of the IECs.

viruses, bacteria, and antigens, while allowing the transport of essential nutrients [52]. The lamina propria is a connective and supportive tissue layer between the basement membrane upon which the epithelium rests and the underlying muscularis mucosa. The lamina propria contains significant numbers of adaptive and innate immunocompetent cells: dendritic cells, T-cells (predominantly CD4+ and TCRαβ+ cells), plasma cells (mostly IgA producing), eosinophils, macrophages, and mast cells [53].

The mucosal immune system of the GI tract which resides within the mucosal layer is considered to be the largest immunologic organ in the body [51]. Humans have a well-developed gut immune system by 19 weeks' gestation, similar to most lymphoid tissues. The GALT is larger in children than in adults, and consists of lymphoid follicles and lymphoid cells. The lymphoid follicles are distributed

within the wall of the GI tract as Peyer's patches and also as solitary lymphoid follicles in the small intestine [54,55]. Lymphoid cells are present diffusely within the epithelium as intra-epithelial lymphocytes, within the lamina propria, and in the Peyer's patches [56]. Peyer's patches serve as antigen sampling sites for the gut immune system [57]. Each Peyer's patch consists of many follicles, and each follicle is made up of a central germinal center. The germinal center develops after antigenic exposure at birth [58] and is composed of B-lymphocytes and surrounded by a number of T-lymphocytes [59]. Overlying the follicle is a dome region consisting of the follicle-associated epithelium (Fig. 3.1) which contains the specialized microfold cells (M cells) [60,61]. M cells are derived from IECs and have microfolds on their luminal surface unlike epithelial cells which possess microvilli [62]. The M cells facilitate the uptake of antigens from the gut lumen and present them to dendritic cells and macrophages which are contained beneath the follicle-associated epithelium. In the small intestine, other lymphoid tissues aggregates have also been described, which include isolated mucosal lymphoid follicles and submucosal lymphoid aggregations that are thought to be solitary Peyer's patch follicles [55]. The appendix is a prominent constituent of the GALT. It is organized into a large number of repeating lymphoid follicles which are morphologically similar to those present in the Peyer's patches [63].

Within the colon, lymphoid follicles may be present as lymphoglandular complexes, which are organized lymphoid structures [64] and appear to be intimately associated with the luminal epithelium. The complexes are located at points of defects in the muscularis mucosa and consist of compact spherical aggregates of lymphocytes situated below the muscularis mucosa. These complexes are also in continuity with a less clearly circumscribed collection of lymphocytes located within the colonic lamina propria. Individual lymphoid follicles may be found within the colonic submucosa and lamina propria, and are most common in the rectum [56]. The cell types present in these lymphoglandular complexes, such as dendritic cells, T- and B-lymphocytes, macrophages, and epithelial cells, have ultrastructural characteristics similar to M cells and appear to be similar to cells that exist in the lymphoepithelial complexes of the small intestine [64].

Defense mechanisms

The GI epithelium functions, in essence, as a gatekeeper, allowing the passage of essential nutrients necessary for growth and development, while maintaining an effective barrier against antigenic food proteins, and commensal and pathogenic microorganisms. The mucosal barrier in conjunction with the innate and adaptive immune systems comprises the primary host defense of the GI tract. The innate immune system provides protection by barrier mechanisms, while the adaptive immune system prevents indiscriminate immune responses to innocuous antigens [65].

An abnormal immune response may be observed when there are perturbations in these defense mechanisms, which in certain disease processes may be triggered by small amounts of residual, non-degraded dietary enteral proteins [66]. The GI defense system may also be divided into extrinsic factors, which are features that restrict the quantity of antigen that is able to reach the epithelial surface, and intrinsic factors, which are characteristics of the physical barriers of the GI wall. The extrinsic and intrinsic factors appear to act synergistically to limit the absorption of food antigens.

The extrinsic factors consist of proteolysis of food proteins, GI acidity, mucin production, peristalsis, and secretory IgA. The stomach produces proteolytic enzymes, such as pepsin

and papain, while the small intestine harbors trypsin, chymotrypsin, and the pancreatic proteases that lead to protein denaturation and degradation which alters the epitopes necessary for immunologic recognition [42,44]. A number of diseases and the effects of some medications lead to reduced gastric acidity, which may promote increased antigen absorption [67]. Patients with cystic fibrosis are deficient in pancreatic enzymes, which may lead to increased antigen absorption [68]. Mucus produced by goblet cells coats the epithelial surface and acts as a physical barrier, while its viscous nature in unison with the peristaltic activity of the gut impedes the access of food antigens. Peristaltic waves results in mixing of mucus with food antigens, which limits the interaction with the absorptive epithelial surface and subsequent uptake [69]. Large intestine peristaltic waves are fewer and less vigorous compared to the small intestine, which promotes the absorption of food antigens [70]. Secretory antibodies provide the immunologic barrier within the gut lumen. Breast milk, especially colostrum, appears to provide, as well as enhance, secretory IgA production, a majority of which remains within the gut lumen [71]. Luminal IgA binds to food antigens which hastens their transport within the GI tract [72]. IgA may also act as a cell surface receptor and attach to food antigens, which facilitates their transport into epithelial cells where such antigens are digested within the phagolysosomes [73,74].

The intrinsic barrier consists of the microvillus and IECs with their tight junctions, intracellular organelles, and proteolytic enzymes. Food antigen must maneuver across the components of the extrinsic barrier prior to coming in contact with the intrinsic barrier. The abundant microvilli, which cover the epithelial cell surface, constitute a significant barrier due to their size, close apposition to each other [75], and their negative charge [76]. The IECs appear to be more than just passive barriers to the luminal contents, given the presence of a selectively permeable membrane at the base of the microvilli [77]. The IECs are hyperpolarized and joined together by tight junctions which further augment barrier function [78]. Food proteins are ultimately endocytosed into vesicles where they are acidified and degraded by proteases and delivered to lysosomes where most antigens are eventually destroyed.

Oral tolerance

Immune responses against foods may lead to decreased absorption of food constituents and essential nutrients. Abnormal responses to foods may result in intestinal pathology, as exemplified by CD and other food-sensitive enteropathies. Under physiologic conditions, when a novel antigen is ingested, IgA antibodies are secreted in the mucosa, which is followed by a systemic humoral and/or a cell-mediated immune response. Subsequently, a systemic and local immune hyporesponsiveness may develop which prevents a deleterious immune response with subsequent encounter of the specific antigen. This is referred to as oral tolerance [79].

Although the mechanisms of oral tolerance have been primarily elucidated in animal models [80,81], there does exist clinical and experimental evidence of oral tolerance in humans [82]. Studies have suggested that at least two mechanisms are responsible for the development of oral tolerance: induction of clonal anergy (or deletion) of antigen-specific T-cells, and stimulation of regulatory T-cells (Treg) which mediate active suppression of the immune response to food antigens. Clonal anergy results from a lack of co-stimulatory molecules on the antigen-presenting cells, namely CD80 and CD86, or interaction with inhibitory co-stimulatory molecules, such as CD152 or cytotoxic T-lymphocyte-associated antigen-4 (CTLA4) and PD-1 [83–87]. Clonal anergy is an outcome of the activation of apoptotic pathways which permanently remove antigen-specific T-cells [88]. Further, a single high dose of food antigen is more likely to induce tolerance by clonal anergy whereas repeated intake of low doses may stimulate Treg cell activity [89–91]. Stimulation of Treg cells is the other mechanism by which oral tolerance may be induced. However, recent studies show that clonal anergy and active regulation by Treg cells are not necessarily distinct aspects of T-cell function [86]. Current research suggests that Treg cells are more likely to be CD4+ cells than the earlier believed CD8+ T-cells. Several subsets of CD4+ Treg cells have been identified, which include TGF-β producing Th3 cells, IL-10 producing Tr1 and CD4+CD25+ Treg cells [86]. Th3 cells are formed in the GALT and appear to be pivotal in the mediation of tolerance to dietary antigens which are ingested in low doses, and inhibit the activation of all lymphocytes in close proximity. This is often referred to as bystander tolerance. Th3 cells then migrate to lymphoid organs where they suppress immune responses by hindering the generation of effector cells, and to target organs where they suppress disease by releasing antigen non-specific cytokines [92]. Studies have shown that compared to normal individuals, children suffering from food allergies, immediate as well as delayed, may have reduced numbers of Th3 cells in their duodenal mucosa, which supports the finding that TGF-β is an important regulator of intestinal immunity in humans [93]. Antigen and naïve T-cell interactions lead to a preferential induction of Treg cells which secrete downregulatory cytokines such as IL-10, TGF-β, and IL-4. IL-10 appears to downregulate inflammatory cytokines such as IL-1α, IL-6, and TNF-α, which are secreted by gut wall macrophages upon interacting with luminal bacteria [94]. Thymus dependent CD4+CD25+ Treg cells have been shown in experimental studies to prevent colitis, possibly relating to increased levels of TGF-β [95]. Oral tolerance once induced suppresses T-cell allergic responses, the basis of most non-IgE-mediated food-allergic diseases. A breakdown of oral tolerance may lead to CD and cow's milk-protein allergy in which aberrant CD4+ T-cell responses to gliadin and milk-protein antigens, respectively, lead to mucosal injury [96].

Antigen transport

Nutrients and antigens from enteral food are primarily absorbed by IECs across their apical surface or through their tight junctions or by M cells. IECs absorb antigens in a fluid phase as well as soluble antigens, whereas M cells primarily deliver samples of large particulate antigens to the lymphoid tissues via an active vesicular transport [97,98]. Studies have suggested that this membrane traffic is charge dependent, as is seen in polarized epithelial cells [99]. The M cells have a limited number of cytoplasmic lysosomes, which makes intracellular processing of antigenic foods unlikely. The large particulate antigens which are absorbed across M cells are more likely to be of bacterial and viral origin [100].

Antigens are transported at the apical surface via the transcellular pathway or through the tight junctions by means of the paracellular pathway. Across the apical surface, antigens are transported in membrane-bound vesicles by pinocytosis (Fig. 3.1) [76]. The tight junctions, under physiologic conditions, make paracellular transport of antigens and other macromolecules almost unachievable. The tight junctions appear to be dynamic structures. Activation of certain transport systems embedded within the apical membrane of the IEC may lead to transient and reversible increases in permeability. For example, activation of the Na+ coupled transport of glucose and amino acids dilates tight junctions and allows for increased absorption of food antigens [101,102]. Similarly, TNF-α, IFN-γ, IL-4, and IL-13 increase epithelial permeability, but TGF-β appears to enhance barrier functions [103–106].

Antigen processing and presentation

The uptake, processing, and presentation of food antigens to naïve T-cells are necessary for the mounting of an immune response by immune competent cells of the GI tract. The uptake of antigens peaks during the neonatal period and decreases as the gut matures. In the adult GI tract, minute quantities of ingested food antigens may be absorbed and transported to the portal venous and systemic circulations in immunologically intact forms [107]. Subsequent to uptake, the processing of antigenic food proteins by IECs is achieved by proteolysis within endosomes. The antigens may then be presented to T-cells by eosinophils and mast cells, the non-professional antigen-presenting cells, which express class II MHC molecules on their cell surface when activated; and dendritic cells, macrophages, and B-cells, the professional antigen-presenting cells that constitutively express class II MHC molecules. However, IECs appear to be the only non-professional antigen-presenting cells that constitutively express MHC class II molecules on their surface [108]. The antigen may be taken up by the antigen-presenting cells by endocytosis, which is non-specific and less efficient than by receptor-mediated methods which appear to be more efficient [109]. Only professional antigen-presenting cells with the following three key characteristics are able to activate normally naïve T-cells to become memory and effector cells [110]. First, there must be expression of surface glycoproteins, which are products of class II MHC molecules. Second, absorption of antigens must occur by either receptor-mediated or fluid-phase endocytosis. Finally, there must be processing of the absorbed antigens within intracytoplasmic organelles, forming a complex with products of class II MHC molecules and presenting them to T-cells.

In addition to their role in barrier function and as non-professional antigen-presenting cells, IECs may also play a role in the regulation of regional immunologic function. These cells absorb and process antigens and may present them directly to T-cells in an MHC-dependent manner [111]. The IECs express class II MHC molecules, mostly on their basolateral surface, where they interact with lymphocytes in the intra-epithelial spaces and in the lamina propria. The expression of MHC molecules appears to be enhanced during gut inflammation [112]. Absorbed luminal antigens may be processed by dissimilar proteolytic enzymes contained in different phagolysosomes that generate a diversity of antigenic epitopes which ultimately interact with T-cells [113]. An antigen absorbed at the apical surface usually may not elicit an immune response, but may if it is absorbed at the basolateral surface [114]. In contrast to professional antigen-presenting cells, IECs may selectively activate CD8+ suppressor T-cells which enhance the suppression of the gut immune response [115]. This process appears to be regulated by the non-classical MHC class I molecule CD1d and an IEC membrane glycoprotein, the CD8 ligand gp180 [116–118]. The precise mechanisms implicated and the roles played in downregulating the mucosal immune responses, however, remain to be characterized.

Dendritic cells are derived from circulating monocytes, which originate from bone-marrow-derived myeloid precursors [119,120]. Dendritic cells are specialized for the uptake, processing, transport, and presentation of antigens, as well as the priming of naïve T-cells. During differentiation, dendritic cells upregulate expression of MHC class II molecules which increases their antigen-presenting efficiency. They also alter their expression of chemokine receptors and production of cytokines which are vital to T-cell differentiation [121,122]. Microbes within the intestinal lumen also appear to stimulate dendritic cells to secrete immunostimulatory cytokines, including IL-12, which upregulate the expression of MHC class II molecules, as well as produce co-stimulatory molecules [121]. Within gut lymphoid follicles, dendritic cells may be classified as follicular and non-follicular cells. Follicular dendritic cells express antigens,

which are vital for the maintenance of memory B-cells. The non-follicular dendritic cells are preferentially localized within the dome regions of Peyer's patches, the lamina propria, in T-cell zones and in certain other parts of the GALT.

The uptake of antigens by dendritic cells may be achieved by macropinocytosis or by receptor-dependent mechanisms [123,124]. Dendritic cells may also send foot processes between IECs [125] or they may become lodged between adjacent IECs and endocytose luminal antigens before migrating to the lamina propria [126]. Subsequently, they reach secondary lymphoid organs, such as mesenteric lymph nodes, where they may interact with and activate naïve T-cells [127]. Occasionally, antigens may reach dendritic cells within secondary lymphoid organs by direct dissemination through draining gastrointestinal lymphatics or bloodstream.

T-cells

The production of food-antigen-specific IgE antibodies is facilitated by cytokines produced by T-cells, such as IL-4 and IL-13. Non-IgE-mediated food allergies result in part from an imbalance between inflammatory cytokines secreted by T-cells such as, IFN-γ, TNF-α, and IL-15 and regulatory cytokines such as IL-10 [128,129].

Antigenic stimulation of naïve T-cells leads to priming, followed by proliferation into memory T-cells and subsequent entrance into the circulation. From the vasculature, memory T-cells may return to the GI tract to function as effector cells in disease pathogenesis. Increased expression of $\alpha 4\beta 7$ on memory T-cell subsets correlates with enhanced recruitment into Peyer's patches. Naïve T-cells which are $\alpha 4\beta 7$low and the subset of memory T-cells which are $\alpha 4\beta 7$high are equally well recruited to Peyer's patches. However, the subset of memory T-cells which are $\alpha 4\beta 7$low are excluded [130]. The specific ligand for $\alpha 4\beta 7$ on vascular endothelial cells within the high endothelial venules is mucosal addressin-cell adhesion molecule-1 (MAdCAM-1), which facilitates the migration of T-cells. Stimulation of peripheral T-cells by β lactoglobulin present in cow's milk results in the selective increased expression of $\alpha 4\beta 7$, which suggests that allergen exposure enhances the migration of memory T-cells [131]. Patients with subclinical CD have increased numbers of T-cells within the gut mucosa which proliferate further when the individual becomes symptomatic [132,133].

CD is characterized by the presence of gluten-specific CD4+ T-cells in the lamina propria and increased numbers of intra-epithelial lymphocytes of the TCR$\alpha\beta$+ CD8+CD4− and TCR$\gamma\delta$+ CD8−CD4− lineage [134]. Cytokines secreted by CD4+ cells, intra-epithelial lymphocytes, and IECs are the primary effectors of mucosal injury in CD. Gluten-activated mucosal CD4+ cells secrete IFN-γ, which together with TNF-α secreted by macrophages, leads to increased permeability and direct cytotoxic effect on the small IECs [135,136]. Activated stromal cells within the lamina propria are induced by TNF-α to produce keratinocyte growth factor (KGF), an epithelial mitogen, which stimulates small intestinal epithelial cell proliferation and results in crypt cell hyperplasia [137]. IECs, dendritic cells, and macrophages produce IL-15, which is upregulated within the lamina propria and the intestinal epithelium during active disease and plays a critical role in the pathogenesis of CD [138]. Gliadin may act independently or in consort with IL-15 on IECs to activate them and induce the expression of the non-conventional HLA I molecule, MHC class I chain A related molecule (MICA). Expression of MICA leads to direct cytotoxicity of IECs in an antigen non-specific manner [139]. IL-15 may also upregulate the expression of NKG2D, the natural killer receptor which is normally expressed on most NK cells as well as on CD8+ TCRαβ+ and TCRγδ+ cells [140–142]. MICA serves as a ligand for the activating natural killer cell receptor, NKG2D, which may result in lymphocyte-mediated cytotoxicity of IECs and in villus atrophy and small intestinal mucosal injury [143]. However, T-cell mechanisms which mediate injury and exert their damaging effects on the mucosa are yet to be completely understood.

In a subset of individuals, the underlying mechanism of cow's milk allergy may be non-IgE mediated. Persons with cow's milk allergy, in contrast to individuals with CD, usually do not develop villous atrophy nor an increased mononuclear cell infiltrate within the lamina propria. However, TCRγδ+ CD8−CD4− cells may occur as the majority of intra-epithelial lymphocytes, which suggests that a cytokine imbalance leads to the disease phenotype [144]. CD is primarily Th1 biased, whereas cow's milk-protein allergy in individuals with an atopic predisposition appears to be predominantly Th2 biased. This is evidenced by a high production of IL-4, IL-5, and IL-13 and a low production of IFN-γ [145,146]. However, non-atopic individuals may exhibit a Th0-like cytokine phenotype [147]. A recent study has demonstrated differences in an immune activation profile between individuals with non-IgE-mediated cow's milk allergy and CD. The group with cow's milk allergy demonstrated an upregulation of CCR4 and IL-6mRNA and downregulation of IL-18 and IL-2mRNA within the gut mucosal tissue, suggesting a Th2-biased immune response. In contrast, individuals with CD showed upregulation of IFN-γ and downregulation of IL-12p35, IL-12p40, and IL-18-specific mRNA [148].

Eosinophils

Eosinophils play an important role in the pathogenesis of allergic disorders in the lung, skin, and gut [149]. Mixed IgE and non-IgE food-allergic reactions are the basis of eosinophil-associated gastrointestinal disorders (EGID) [1,9]. Individuals with EGID are often allergic to multiple foods,

have an eosinophil-rich infiltrate within the wall of the esophagus, stomach and small and large intestines [150], an elevated serum IgE in a majority and peripheral eosinophilia in a few [151,152].

Numerous inflammatory mediators have been implicated in the recruitment of eosinophils to tissues. Of these, eotaxin, which is constitutively expressed by the GI epithelium, and IL-5 appear to be relatively specific eosinophil chemoattractants [153]. Eotaxin appears to modulate the recruitment of eosinophils by selectively binding and signaling through the chemokine receptor, CCR3, found primarily on eosinophils [154]. Eotaxin also appears to facilitate the movement of eosinophils from blood vessels to the gut tissue, which is dependent on the interaction of α4β7 present on eosinophils with MAdCAM-1 [155]. In a physiologic state, eosinophils exist in small numbers within the GI wall and the presence of relatively large numbers denotes an underlying disease process. However, the esophageal wall lacks eosinophils and their presence indicates a pathologic course [156]. IL-5 has also been shown to be involved in eosinophil differentiation, proliferation, survival, recruitment, and trafficking within the GI tract and has been implicated as the principal modulator of gut inflammation in EGID [157].

A step-wise interaction between endothelial cells of the blood vessels and eosinophils promotes their migration to the mucosal tissues. The rolling of an eosinophil over the endothelial cell surface is assisted primarily by P-selectin, the adhesion molecule present on endothelial cells [158]. Rolling is followed by adherence facilitated by adhesion molecules of the integrin family [159]. Within the mucosal tissues, eosinophil survival is cytokine dependent, where GM-CSF increases the survival of tissue eosinophils and IL-12 appears to increase apoptosis [160].

Studies have demonstrated that in addition to eosinophils, the cellular component of the inflammatory infiltrate in EGID also consists of increased numbers of activated CD4+ T-cells and mast cells [161]. Monocytes and neutrophils are other cell types that are associated with the disease [162]. Eosinophils propagate disease pathogenesis and may instigate mucosal injury by release of inflammatory mediators, eosinophilic cytotoxic granule proteins, cytokines, and reactive oxygen intermediates. Cytokines, immunoglobulins, and complement components may activate eosinophils to generate numerous inflammatory mediators, such as IL-1, IL-3, IL-4, IL-5, IL-13, GM-CSF, TNF-α, MIP 1α, and vascular endothelial cell growth factor. This suggests that eosinophils may modulate the many features of the immune response [163]. Furthermore, epithelial growth, fibrosis, and tissue remodeling may be influenced by eosinophil-derived TGF-β and the eosinophilic cytotoxic granule proteins including eosinophilic cationic protein [164], major basic protein [165], and eosinophil peroxidase [166]. The eosinophilic cationic protein may insert pores into the IEC membrane, which leads to the entry of other toxic

Table 3.1 An overview of immune mechanisms and symptoms of non-IgE-mediated and mixed food allergies

Disease	Immune mechanism	Symptoms
Food-protein-induced enterocolitis	Cell mediated	Profuse vomiting, diarrhea (±microscopic blood), severe symptoms may lead to lethargy, dehydration, and shock
Food-protein-induced proctocolitis	Cell mediated	Gradual onset bleeding progressing to streaks of blood, infant typically thriving and usually well
Food-protein-induced enteropathy (gluten-sensitive enteropathy)	Cell mediated	Dyspepsia, reflux, diarrhea, abdominal distension, flatulence, failure to thrive, other symptoms depend on extraintestinal manifestations
Allergic eosinophilic esophagitis	Cell mediated and/or IgE mediated	Difficulty in feeding, failure to thrive, gastroesophageal reflux, vomiting, epigastric pain, dysphagia and food impaction
Allergic eosinophilic gastroenteritis	Cell mediated and/or IgE mediated	Recurrent abdominal pain and vomiting, failure to thrive, peripheral blood eosinophilia (50%).

molecules [167]. Major basic protein induces smooth muscle reactivity and may initiate degranulation of mast cells and basophils [168].

Respiratory burst enzyme pathways in eosinophils generate superoxide that may cause mucosal damage [169]. Eosinophil peroxidase generates toxic hydrogen peroxide and halic acids which may trigger further injury [170]. Neutrophils also generate lipid mediators, such as LTC4, LTD4, and LTE4 which lead to increased vascular permeability, mucin secretion, and smooth muscle contraction [171]. Moreover, the extent of GI wall eosinophil infiltration and the quantity of eosinophilic cytotoxic proteins correlate with disease severity [172,173].

Table 3.1 lists diseases with non-IgE and mixed immune-mediated mechanisms and a summary of their clinical features [174–178].

Food-protein-induced enterocolitis and proctocolitis

Food-protein-induced enterocolitis and proctocolitis occur predominantly in infants with food allergies and are characterized by severe small and large intestine mucosal injury. The common dietary culprits implicated in the pathogenesis of food-allergic reactions in infants are cow's milk and soybean. Cereal grains (rice, oat, barley), fish, poultry, and vegetables are infrequent offenders [179]. The diagnosis is chiefly made by clinical symptoms and challenge testing, but may also be supported by resolution of symptoms after dietary elimination of the perpetrator protein. Typical symptoms consist of vomiting and diarrhea with presence of blood, leukocytes, eosinophils, and increased carbohydrate content in the stool [180]. Histologic studies of endoscopic biopsy specimens in symptomatic patients reveal nonspecific markers of inflammation, which include prominent eosinophilia and plasma cells, crypt abscesses, and mild villous injury. A few infants may also show evidence of gastritis and esophagitis [181].

Celiac disease

CD is often categorized as an autoimmune disorder affecting the small intestines, induced by the intake of gluten in wheat and analogous proteins present in barley and rye. CD is closely associated with genes that code HLA-II antigens, mainly of DQ2 and DQ8 classes [182,183]. CD may manifest early in life following the introduction of gluten in the diet or may develop later in life. The clinical manifestations include abdominal pain with distension, dyspepsia, presence of gastroesophageal reflux disease (GERD), recurrent episodes of altered bowel habits (diarrhea and/or constipation), weight loss, bone disease, anemia, and weakness. Symptoms tend to remit upon strict compliance to a gluten-free diet. The demonstration of circulatory IgA antibodies to transglutaminase (tTG-IgA) is supportive of the diagnosis. Histologic examination of endoscopic samples is confirmatory [184]. However, patchy involvement of the mucosa may lead to a false-negative diagnosis. Histologic changes within the mucosa include villus atrophy/flattening, crypt hyperplasia, thickening of the epithelial basement membrane, and reduced numbers of goblet cells. Evidence of mucosal inflammation is manifested by an increase in intra-epithelial lymphocytes and an influx of immune cells within the small intestinal lamina propria, and loss of basal nuclear orientation as well as change of the IECs to a cuboidal morphology.

Allergic eosinophilic esophagitis and gastroenteritis

Primary eosinophilic gastrointestinal disorders include eosinophilic esophagitis, gastritis, gastroenteritis, enteritis, and eosinophilic colitis. These diseases are occurring with increasing frequency and are mediated by mixed immune mechanisms [185]. They are characterized by an eosinophil-rich infiltrate within the gut wall in the absence of other causes of gut wall eosinophilia such as drug reactions, parasitic infections, and malignancy. The constellation of
```
```

symptoms includes abdominal pain, dysphagia, vomiting, diarrhea, gastric dysmotility, irritability, and failure to thrive [186]. The diagnosis of primary eosinophilic gastrointestinal disorders is contingent upon the histologic assessment of endoscopic biopsy samples with vigilant consideration of the quantity, location, and characteristics of the eosinophilic infiltration [9].

Conclusions

We have reviewed non-IgE-mediated mechanisms of food allergy. We have detailed the barrier functions of the gut; the processing, absorption, and presentation of antigens to the immune competent cells; the mounting of a response; and the inflammatory changes and mucosal damage as propagated by infiltrating cells within the gut mucosa. It is apparent that non-IgE-mediated gastrointestinal allergic diseases may be associated with gastrointestinal epithelial barrier dysfunction. However, it is not clear if barrier dysfunction is an outcome, or a contributing factor to development of food allergies. Intertwined in the disease pathogenesis are roles of T-cells which are pivotal to the induction of oral tolerance as well as the propagation of disease, and eosinophils which are central in the pathogenesis and modulation of eosinophilic gastrointestinal disorders. An appreciation of the immune mechanisms involved in food hypersensitivities and its associated diseases, and the counseling of genetically susceptible individuals will facilitate the development of new and novel approaches to treating patients with these diseases.

References

1 Sampson HA. Food allergy. Part 1. Immunopathogenesis and clinical disorders. *J Allergy Clin Immunol* 1999;103:717–28.

2 Hippocrates. *The Medical Works of Hippocrates*. Oxford Press, Oxford 1950.

3 Buckley RH, Metcalfe D. Food allergy. *JAMA* 1982;248: 2627–31.

4 Johansson SG, Hourihane JO, Bousquet J, *et al*. A revised nomenclature for allergy. An EAACI position statement from the EAACI nomenclature task force. *Allergy* 2001;56:813–24.

5 Johansson SG, Bieber T, Dahl R, *et al*. Revised nomenclature for allergy for global use: report of the Nomenclature Review Committee of the World Allergy Organization, October 2003. *J Allergy Clin Immunol* 2004;113:832–6.

6 Grundy J, Matthews S, Bateman B, *et al*. Rising prevalence of allergy to peanut in children: data from 2 sequential cohorts. *J Allergy Clin Immunol* 2002;110:784–9.

7 Cherian S, Smith NM, Forbes DA. Rapidly increasing prevalence of eosinophilic esophagitis in Western Australia. *Arch Dis Child* 2006;91:1000–4.

8 Murch SH. The immunologic basis for intestinal food allergy. *Curr Opin Gastroenterol* 2000;16:552–7.

9 Rothenberg ME. Eosinophilic gastrointestinal disorders (EGID). *J Allergy Clin Immunol* 2004;113:11–28; quiz 9.

10 Rook GA, Stanford JL. Give us this day our daily germs. *Immunol Today* 1998;19:113–6.

11 Schiffrin EJ, Blum S. Interactions between the microbiota and the intestinal mucosa. *Eur J Clin Nutr* 2002;56:S60–4.

12 Dimich-Ward H, Chow Y, Chung J, Trask C. Contact with livestock – a protective effect against allergies and asthma? *Clin Exp Allergy* 2006;36:1122–9.

13 Cebra JJ. Influences of microbiota on intestinal immune system development. *Am J Clin Nutr* 1999;69:1046S–51S.

14 Sicherer SH, Furlong TJ, Maes HH, *et al*. Genetics of peanut allergy: a twin study. *J Allergy Clin Immunol* 2000; 106:53–6.

15 Kalogeromitros DC, Makris MP, Gregoriou SG, *et al*. Grape anaphylaxis: a study of 11 adult onset cases. *Allergy Asthma Proc* 2005;26:53–8.

16 Blanco C, Sanchez-Garcia F, Torres-Galvan MJ, *et al*. Genetic basis of the latex–fruit syndrome: association with HLA class II alleles in a Spanish population. *J Allergy Clin Immunol* 2004;114:1070–6.

17 Liu X, Beaty TH, Deindl P, *et al*. Associations between total serum IgE levels and the 6 potentially functional variants within the genes IL4, IL13, and IL4RA in German children: the German Multicenter Atopy Study. *J Allergy Clin Immunol* 2003;112:382–8.

18 Liu X, Beaty TH, Deindl P, *et al*. Associations between specific serum IgE response and 6 variants within the genes IL4, IL13, and IL4RA in German children: the German Multicenter Atopy Study. *J Allergy Clin Immunol* 2004; 113:489–95.

19 Matsuo H, Kohno K, Morita E. Molecular cloning, recombinant expression and IgE-binding epitope of omega-5 gliadin, a major allergen in wheat-dependent exercise-induced anaphylaxis. *FEBS J* 2005;272:4431–8.

20 Tollefsen S, Arentz-Hansen H, Fleckenstein B, *et al*. HLA-DQ2 and -DQ8 signatures of gluten T cell epitopes in celiac disease. *J Clin Invest* 2006;116:2226–36.

21 Blanchard C, Wang N, Rothenberg ME. Eosinophilic esophagitis: pathogenesis, genetics, and therapy. *J Allergy Clin Immunol* 2006;118:1054–9.

22 Risch N. Assessing the role of HLA-linked and unlinked determinants of disease. *Am J Hum Genet* 1987;40:1–14.

23 Macdonald WC, Dobbins III WO, Rubin CE. Studies of the familial nature of celiac sprue using biopsy of the small intestine. *N Engl J Med* 1965;272:448–56.

24 Greco L, Romino R, Coto I, *et al*. The first large population based twin study of coeliac disease. *Gut* 2002;50:624–8.

25 Bardella MT, Fredella C, Prampolini L, *et al*. Gluten sensitivity in monozygous twins: a long-term follow-up of five pairs. *Am J Gastroenterol* 2000;95:1503–5.

26 Periolo N, Chernavsky AC. Coeliac disease. *Autoimmun Rev* 2006;5:202–8.

27 Petronzelli F, Bonamico M, Ferrante P, *et al*. Genetic contribution of the HLA region to the familial clustering of coeliac disease. *Ann Hum Genet* 1997;61:307–17.

28 Blanchard C, Wang N, Stringer KF, *et al*. Eotaxin-3 and a uniquely conserved gene-expression profile in eosinophilic esophagitis. *J Clin Invest* 2006;116:536–47.

29 Bjorksten B. Genetic and environmental risk factors for the development of food allergy. *Curr Opin Allergy Clin Immunol* 2005;5:249–53.

30 Kaczmarski M, Kurzatkowska B. The contribution of some environmental factors to the development of cow's milk and gluten intolerance in children. *Rocz Akad Med Bialymst* 1988;33–34:151–65.

31 von Mutius E, Weiland SK, Fritzsch C, *et al.* Increasing prevalence of hay fever and atopy among children in Leipzig, East Germany. *Lancet* 1998;351:862–6.

32 Ege MJ, Bieli C, Frei R, *et al.* Prenatal farm exposure is related to the expression of receptors of the innate immunity and to atopic sensitization in school-age children. *J Allergy Clin Immunol* 2006;117:817–23.

33 Alfven T, Braun-Fahrlander C, Brunekreef B, *et al.* Allergic diseases and atopic sensitization in children related to farming and anthroposophic lifestyle – the PARSIFAL Study; 2006.

34 Markowitz JE, Spergel JM, Ruchelli E, Liacouras CA. Elemental diet is an effective treatment for eosinophilic esophagitis in children and adolescents. *Am J Gastroenterol* 2003;98:777–82.

35 MacPherson GG, Liu LM. Dendritic cells and Langerhans cells in the uptake of mucosal antigens. *Curr Top Microbiol Immunol* 1999;236:33–53.

36 Kelly D, Conway S. Bacterial modulation of mucosal innate immunity. *Mol Immunol* 2005;42:895–901.

37 Abreu MT, Fukata M, Arditi M. TLR signaling in the gut in health and disease. *J Immunol* 2005;174:4453–60.

38 Nordenstedt H, Nilsson M, Johnsen R, *et al.* Helicobacter pylori infection and gastroesophageal reflux in a population-based study (The HUNT Study). *Helicobacter* 2007;12:16–22.

39 Figura N, Perrone A, Gennari C, *et al.* CagA-positive *Helicobacter pylori* infection may increase the risk of food allergy development. *J Physiol Pharmacol* 1999;50:827–31.

40. Zuckerman MJ, Watts MT, Bhatt BD, Ho H. Intestinal permeability to [51Cr]EDTA in infectious diarrhea. *Dig Dis Sci* 1993; 38:1651–7.

41 Bock SA. Prospective appraisal of complaints of adverse reactions to foods in children during the first 3 years of life. *Pediatrics* 1987;79:683–8.

42 Bannon GA. What makes a food protein an allergen? *Curr Allergy Asthma Rep* 2004;4:43–6.

43 Metcalfe DD, Astwood JD, Townsend R, *et al.* Assessment of the allergenic potential of foods derived from genetically engineered crop plants. *Crit Rev Food Sci Nutr* 1996;36:S165–86.

44 Untersmayr E, Jensen-Jarolim E. The effect of gastric digestion on food allergy. *Curr Opin Allergy Clin Immunol* 2006;6:214–9.

45 Sen M, Kopper R, Pons L, *et al.* Protein structure plays a critical role in peanut allergen stability and may determine immunodominant IgE-binding epitopes. *J Immunol* 2002;169: 882–7.

46 Astwood JD, Leach JN, Fuchs RL. Stability of food allergens to digestion *in vitro*. *Nat Biotechnol* 1996;14:1269–73.

47 Allen A, Flemstrom G. Gastroduodenal mucus bicarbonate barrier: protection against acid and pepsin. *Am J Physiol Cell Physiol* 2005;288:C1–19.

48 Poley JR. Loss of the glycocalyx of enterocytes in small intestine: a feature detected by scanning electron microscopy in children with gastrointestinal intolerance to dietary protein. *J Pediatr Gastroenterol Nutr* 1988;7:386–94.

49 Ito S. Structure and function of the glycocalyx. *Fed Proc* 1969; 28:12–25.

50 Danielsen EM, Hansen GH. Lipid raft organization and function in brush borders of epithelial cells. *Mol Membr Biol* 2006;23:71–9.

51 Chehade M, Mayer L. Oral tolerance and its relation to food hypersensitivities. *J Allergy Clin Immunol* 2005;115:3–12; quiz 3.

52 Guttman JA, Li Y, Wickham ME, *et al.* Attaching and effacing pathogen-induced tight junction disruption *in vivo*. *Cell Microbiol* 2006;8:634–45.

53 MacDonald TT. The mucosal immune system. *Parasite Immunol* 2003;25:235–46.

54 Lugering A, Kucharzik T. Induction of intestinal lymphoid tissue: the role of cryptopatches. *Ann NY Acad Sci* 2006;1072:210–7.

55 Moghaddami M, Cummins A, Mayrhofer G. Lymphocyte-filled villi: comparison with other lymphoid aggregations in the mucosa of the human small intestine. *Gastroenterology* 1998;115:1414–25.

56 Langman JM, Rowland R. The number and distribution of lymphoid follicles in the human large intestine. *J Anat* 1986;149:189–94.

57 Van Kruiningen HJ, West AB, Freda BJ, Holmes KA. Distribution of Peyer's patches in the distal ileum. *Inflamm Bowel Dis* 2002;8:180–5.

58 Bridges RA, Condie RM, Zak SJ, Good RA. The morphologic basis of antibody formation development during the neonatal period. *J Lab Clin Med* 1959:331–57.

59 Strobel S. Mechanisms of mucosal immunology and gastrointestinal damage. *Pediatr Allergy Immunol* 1993;4:25–32.

60 Spahn TW, Kucharzik T. Modulating the intestinal immune system: the role of lymphotoxin and GALT organs. *Gut* 2004; 53:456–65.

61 Fujimura Y, Kihara T, Ohtani K, *et al.* Distribution of microfold cells (M cells) in human follicle-associated epithelium. *Gastroenterol Jpn* 1990;25:130.

62 Owen RL, Jones AL. Epithelial cell specialization within human Peyer's patches: an ultrastructural study of intestinal lymphoid follicles. *Gastroenterology* 1974;66:189–203.

63 Bockman DE. Functional histology of appendix. *Arch Histol Jpn* 1983;46:271–92.

64 O'Leary AD, Sweeney EC. Lymphoglandular complexes of the colon: structure and distribution. *Histopathology* 1986;10: 267–83.

65 Seibold F. Food-induced immune responses as origin of bowel disease? *Digestion* 2005;71:251–60.

66 Mahe S, Messing B, Thuillier F, Tome D. Digestion of bovine milk proteins in patients with a high jejunostomy. *Am J Clin Nutr* 1991;54:534–8.

67 Untersmayr E, Bakos N, Scholl I, *et al.* Anti-ulcer drugs promote IgE formation toward dietary antigens in adult patients. *FASEB J* 2005;19:656–8.

68 Walker WA, Wu M, Isselbacher KJ, Bloch KJ. Intestinal uptake of macromolecules. IV. The effect of pancreatic duct ligation on

the breakdown of antigen and antigen-antibody complexes on the intestinal surface. *Gastroenterology* 1975;69:1223–9.

69 Reinhardt MC. Macromolecular absorption of food antigens in health and disease. *Ann Allergy* 1984;53:597–601.

70 Walker WA, Bloch KJ. Gastrointestinal transport of macromolecules in the pathogenesis of food allergy. *Ann Allergy* 1983;51:240–5.

71 Roberts SA, Freed DL. Neonatal IgA secretion enhanced by breast feeding. *Lancet* 1977;2:1131.

72 Levinsky RJ. Factors influencing intestinal uptake of food antigens. *Proc Nutr Soc* 1985;44:81–6.

73 Matthews DM. Absorption of amino acids and peptides from the intestine. *Clin Endocrinol Metab* 1974;3:3–16.

74 Kraehenbuhl JP, Neutra MR. Molecular and cellular basis of immune protection of mucosal surfaces. *Physiol Rev* 1992;72: 853–79.

75 Phillips AD, France NE, Walker-Smith JA. The structure of the enterocyte in relation to its position on the villus in childhood: an electron microscopical study. *Histopathology* 1979;3:117–30.

76 Snoeck V, Goddeeris B, Cox E. The role of enterocytes in the intestinal barrier function and antigen uptake. *Microbes Infect* 2005;7:997–1004.

77 Schindler J, Nothwang HG. Aqueous polymer two-phase systems: effective tools for plasma membrane proteomics. *Proteomics* 2006;6:5409–17.

78 Massey-Harroche D. Epithelial cell polarity as reflected in enterocytes. *Microsc Res Tech* 2000;49:353–62.

79 Ko J, Mayer L. Oral tolerance: lessons on treatment of food allergy. *Eur J Gastroenterol Hepatol* 2005;17:1299–303.

80 Strobel S, Ferguson A. Modulation of intestinal and systemic immune responses to a fed protein antigen, in mice. *Gut* 1986; 27:829–37.

81 Strobel S, Ferguson A. Immune responses to fed protein antigens in mice. 3. Systemic tolerance or priming is related to age at which antigen is first encountered. *Pediatr Res* 1984;18: 588–94.

82 Korenblat PE, Rothberg RM, Minden P, Farr RS. Immune responses of human adults after oral and parenteral exposure to bovine serum albumin. *J Allergy* 1968;41:226–35.

83 Nakada M, Nishizaki K, Yoshino T, *et al.* CD80 (B7-1) and CD86 (B7-2) antigens on house dust mite-specific T cells in atopic disease function through T–T cell interactions. *J Allergy Clin Immunol* 1999;104:222–7.

84 Teft WA, Kirchhof MG, Madrenas J. A molecular perspective of CTLA-4 function. *Annu Rev Immunol* 2006;24:65–97.

85 Greenwald RJ, Freeman GJ, Sharpe AH. The B7 family revisited. *Annu Rev Immunol* 2005;23:515–48.

86 von Boehmer H. Mechanisms of suppression by suppressor T cells. *Nat Immunol* 2005;6:338–44.

87 Leibson PJ. The regulation of lymphocyte activation by inhibitory receptors. *Curr Opin Immunol* 2004;16:328–36.

88 van Parijs L, Perez VL, Abbas AK. Mechanisms of peripheral T cell tolerance. *Novartis Found Symp* 1998;215:5–14; discussion 20, 33–40.

89 Friedman A, Weiner HL. Induction of anergy or active suppression following oral tolerance is determined by antigen dosage. *Proc Natl Acad Sci USA* 1994;91:6688–92.

90 Melamed D, Friedman A. Direct evidence for anergy in T lymphocytes tolerized by oral administration of ovalbumin. *Eur J Immunol* 1993;23:935–42.

91 Melamed D, Friedman A. *In vivo* tolerization of Th1 lymphocytes following a single feeding with ovalbumin: anergy in the absence of suppression. *Eur J Immunol* 1994;24:1974–81.

92 Faria AM, Weiner HL. Oral tolerance. *Immunol Rev* 2005;206: 232–59.

93 Perez-Machado MA, Ashwood P, Thomson MA, *et al.* Reduced transforming growth factor-beta1-producing T cells in the duodenal mucosa of children with food allergy. *Eur J Immunol* 2003;33:2307–15.

94 Fiorentino DF, Zlotnik A, Mosmann TR, *et al.* IL-10 inhibits cytokine production by activated macrophages. *J Immunol* 1991;147:3815–22.

95 Duchmann R, Zeitz M. T regulatory cell suppression of colitis: the role of TGF-beta. *Gut* 2006;55:604–6.

96 Kagnoff MF. Celiac disease: pathogenesis of a model immunogenetic disease. *J Clin Invest* 2007;117:41–9.

97 Wolf JL, Bye WA. The membranous epithelial (M) cell and the mucosal immune system. *Annu Rev Med* 1984;35:95–112.

98 Neutra MR, Pringault E, Kraehenbuhl JP. Antigen sampling across epithelial barriers and induction of mucosal immune responses. *Annu Rev Immunol* 1996;14:275–300.

99 Neutra MR. M cells in antigen sampling in mucosal tissues. *Curr Top Microbiol Immunol* 1999;236:17–32.

100 Niedergang F, Kweon MN. New trends in antigen uptake in the gut mucosa. *Trends Microbiol* 2005;13:485–90.

101 Pappenheimer JR, Volpp K. Transmucosal impedance of small intestine: correlation with transport of sugars and amino acids. *Am J Physiol* 1992;263:C480–93.

102 Madara JL, Pappenheimer JR. Structural basis for physiological regulation of paracellular pathways in intestinal epithelia. *J Membr Biol* 1987;100:149–64.

103 Planchon SM, Martins CA, Guerrant RL, Roche JK. Regulation of intestinal epithelial barrier function by TGF-beta 1. Evidence for its role in abrogating the effect of a T cell cytokine. *J Immunol* 1994;153:5730–9.

104 Resta-Lenert S, Barrett KE. Probiotics and commensals reverse TNF-alpha- and IFN-gamma-induced dysfunction in human intestinal epithelial cells. *Gastroenterology* 2006;130:731–46.

105 Colgan SP, Resnick MB, Parkos CA, *et al.* IL-4 directly modulates function of a model human intestinal epithelium. *J Immunol* 1994;153:2122–9.

106 Madden KB, Whitman L, Sullivan C, *et al.* Role of STAT6 and mast cells in IL-4- and IL-13-induced alterations in murine intestinal epithelial cell function. *J Immunol* 2002;169:4417–22.

107 Husby S, Jensenius JC, Svehag SE. Passage of undegraded dietary antigen into the blood of healthy adults. Quantification, estimation of size distribution, and relation of uptake to levels of specific antibodies. *Scand J Immunol* 1985;22:83–92.

108 Scott H, Solheim BG, Brandtzaeg P, Thorsby E. HLA-DR-like antigens in the epithelium of the human small intestine. *Scand J Immunol* 1980;12:77–82.

109 Bajtay Z, Csomor E, Sandor N, Erdei A. Expression and role of Fc- and complement-receptors on human dendritic cells. *Immunol Lett* 2006;104:46–52.

110 Brandtzaeg P. Nature and function of gastrointestinal antigen-presenting cells. *Allergy* 2001;56:16–20.

111 Hershberg RM, Framson PE, Cho DH, *et al*. Intestinal epithelial cells use two distinct pathways for HLA class II antigen processing. *J Clin Invest* 1997;100:204–15.

112 Mayer L, Eisenhardt D, Salomon P, *et al*. Expression of class II molecules on intestinal epithelial cells in humans. Differences between normal and inflammatory bowel disease. *Gastroenterology* 1991;100:3–12.

113 Hershberg RM, Cho DH, Youakim A, *et al*. Highly polarized HLA class II antigen processing and presentation by human intestinal epithelial cells. *J Clin Invest* 1998;102:792–803.

114 Hershberg RM, Mayer LF. Antigen processing and presentation by intestinal epithelial cells – polarity and complexity. *Immunol Today* 2000;21:123–8.

115 Mayer L, Shlien R. Evidence for function of Ia molecules on gut epithelial cells in man. *J Exp Med* 1987;166:1471–83.

116 Panja A, Blumberg RS, Balk SP, Mayer L. CD1d is involved in T cell-intestinal epithelial cell interactions. *J Exp Med* 1993; 178:1115–9.

117 Campbell NA, Park MS, Toy LS, *et al*. A non-class I MHC intestinal epithelial surface glycoprotein, gp180, binds to CD8. *Clin Immunol* 2002;102:267–74.

118 Yio XY, Mayer L. Characterization of a 180-kDa intestinal epithelial cell membrane glycoprotein, gp180. A candidate molecule mediating t cell-epithelial cell interactions. *J Biol Chem* 1997;272:12786–92.

119 Banchereau J, Steinman RM. Dendritic cells and the control of immunity. *Nature* 1998;392:245–52.

120 Tacke F, Randolph GJ. Migratory fate and differentiation of blood monocyte subsets. *Immunobiology* 2006;211:609–18.

121 Thoma-Uszynski S, Kiertscher SM, Ochoa MT, *et al*. Activation of toll-like receptor 2 on human dendritic cells triggers induction of IL-12, but not IL-10. *J Immunol* 2000;165:3804–10.

122 Wu L, Dakic A. Development of dendritic cell system. *Cell Mol Immunol* 2004;1:112–8.

123 Inaba K, Inaba M, Naito M, Steinman RM. Dendritic cell progenitors phagocytose particulates, including bacillus Calmette-Guerin organisms, and sensitize mice to mycobacterial antigens *in vivo*. *J Exp Med* 1993;178:479–88.

124 Jiang W, Swiggard WJ, Heufler C, *et al*. The receptor DEC-205 expressed by dendritic cells and thymic epithelial cells is involved in antigen processing. *Nature* 1995;375:151–5.

125 Niess JH, Brand S, Gu X, *et al*. CX3CR1-mediated dendritic cell access to the intestinal lumen and bacterial clearance. *Science* 2005;307:254–8.

126 Rescigno M, Urbano M, Valzasina B, *et al*. Dendritic cells express tight junction proteins and penetrate gut epithelial monolayers to sample bacteria. *Nat Immunol* 2001;2:361–7.

127 Chirdo FG, Millington OR, Beacock-Sharp H, Mowat AM. Immunomodulatory dendritic cells in intestinal lamina propria. *Eur J Immunol* 2005;35:1831–40.

128 Eigenmann PA, Frossard CP. The T lymphocyte in food-allergy disorders. *Curr Opin Allergy Clin Immunol* 2003;3:199–203.

129 Guandalini S, Gokhale R. Update on immunologic basis of celiac disease. *Curr Opin Gastroenterol* 2002;18:95–100.

130 Williams MB, Butcher EC. Homing of naive and memory T lymphocyte subsets to Peyer's patches, lymph nodes, and spleen. *J Immunol* 1997;159:1746–52.

131 Eigenmann PA, Tropia L, Hauser C. The mucosal adhesion receptor alpha4beta7 integrin is selectively increased in lymphocytes stimulated with beta-lactoglobulin in children allergic to cow's milk. *J Allergy Clin Immunol* 1999;103:931–6.

132 Veres G, Helin T, Arato A, *et al*. Increased expression of intercellular adhesion molecule-1 and mucosal adhesion molecule alpha4beta7 integrin in small intestinal mucosa of adult patients with food allergy. *Clin Immunol* 2001;99:353–9.

133 Vandezande LM, Wallaert B, Desreumaux P, *et al*. Interleukin-5 immunoreactivity and mRNA expression in gut mucosa from patients with food allergy. *Clin Exp Allergy* 1999;29:652–9.

134 Lopez-Botet M, Llano M, Navarro F, Bellon T. NK cell recognition of non-classical HLA class I molecules. *Semin Immunol* 2000;12:109–19.

135 Madara JL, Stafford J. Interferon-gamma directly affects barrier function of cultured intestinal epithelial monolayers. *J Clin Invest* 1989;83:724–7.

136 Deem RL, Shanahan F, Targan SR. Triggered human mucosal T cells release tumour necrosis factor-alpha and interferon-gamma which kill human colonic epithelial cells. *Clin Exp Immunol* 1991;83:79–84.

137 Bajaj-Elliott M, Poulsom R, Pender SL, *et al*. Interactions between stromal cell-derived keratinocyte growth factor and epithelial transforming growth factor in immune-mediated crypt cell hyperplasia. *J Clin Invest* 1998;102:1473–80.

138 Mention JJ, Ben Ahmed M, Begue B, *et al*. Interleukin 15: a key to disrupted intraepithelial lymphocyte homeostasis and lymphomagenesis in celiac disease. *Gastroenterology* 2003; 125:730–45.

139 Hue S, Mention JJ, Monteiro RC, *et al*. A direct role for NKG2D/MICA interaction in villous atrophy during celiac disease. *Immunity* 2004;21:367–77.

140 Reinecker HC, MacDermott RP, Mirau S, *et al*. Intestinal epithelial cells both express and respond to interleukin 15. *Gastroenterology* 1996;111:1706–13.

141 Ebert EC. Interleukin 15 is a potent stimulant of intraepithelial lymphocytes. *Gastroenterology* 1998;115:1439–45.

142 Bauer S, Groh V, Wu J, *et al*. Activation of NK cells and T cells by NKG2D, a receptor for stress-inducible MICA. *Science* 1999;285:727–9.

143 Meresse B, Chen Z, Ciszewski C, *et al*. Coordinated induction by IL15 of a TCR-independent NKG2D signaling pathway converts CTL into lymphokine-activated killer cells in celiac disease. *Immunity* 2004;21:357–66.

144 Kokkonen J, Holm K, Karttunen TJ, Maki M. Children with untreated food allergy express a relative increment in the density of duodenal gammadelta+ T cells. *Scand J Gastroenterol* 2000;35:1137–42.

145 Nilsen EM, Lundin KE, Krajci P, *et al.* Gluten specific, HLA-DQ restricted T cells from coeliac mucosa produce cytokines with Th1 or Th0 profile dominated by interferon gamma. *Gut* 1995;37:766–76.

146 Schade RP, Van Ieperen-Van Dijk AG, Van Reijsen FC, *et al.* Differences in antigen-specific T-cell responses between infants with atopic dermatitis with and without cow's milk allergy: relevance of TH2 cytokines. *J Allergy Clin Immunol* 2000;106:1155–62.

147 Schade RP, Tiemessen MM, Knol EF, *et al.* The cow's milk protein-specific T cell response in infancy and childhood. *Clin Exp Allergy* 2003;33:725–30.

148 Paajanen L, Kokkonen J, Karttunen TJ, *et al.* Intestinal cytokine mRNA expression in delayed-type cow's milk allergy. *J Pediatr Gastroenterol Nutr* 2006;43:470–6.

149 Weller PF. The immunobiology of eosinophils. *N Engl J Med* 1991;324:1110–8.

150 Kelly KJ. Eosinophilic gastroenteritis. *J Pediatr Gastroenterol Nutr* 2000;30:S28–35.

151 Jaffe JS, Metcalfe DD. Cytokines and their role in the pathogenesis of severe food hypersensitivity reactions. *Ann Allergy* 1993;71:362–4.

152 Johnstone JM, Morson BC. Eosinophilic gastroenteritis. *Histopathology* 1978;2:335–48.

153 Rothenberg ME, Zimmermann N, Mishra A, *et al.* Chemokines and chemokine receptors: their role in allergic airway disease. *J Clin Immunol* 1999;19:250–65.

154 Xu B, Aoyama K, Takeuchi M, *et al.* Expression of cytokine mRNAs in mice cutaneously exposed to formaldehyde. *Immunol Lett* 2002;84:49–55.

155 Mishra A, Hogan SP, Brandt EB, *et al.* Enterocyte expression of the eotaxin and interleukin-5 transgenes induces compartmentalized dysregulation of eosinophil trafficking. *J Biol Chem* 2002;277:4406–12.

156 Fox VL, Nurko S, Furuta GT. Eosinophilic esophagitis: it's not just kid's stuff. *Gastrointest Endosc* 2002;56:260–70.

157 Hogan SP, Rothenberg ME. Review article: the eosinophil as a therapeutic target in gastrointestinal disease. *Aliment Pharmacol Ther* 2004;20:1231–40.

158 Symon FA, Walsh GM, Watson SR, Wardlaw AJ. Eosinophil adhesion to nasal polyp endothelium is P-selectin-dependent. *J Exp Med* 1994;180:371–6.

159 Wardlaw AJ, Walsh GM, Symon FA. Adhesion interactions involved in eosinophil migration through vascular endothelium. *Ann NY Acad Sci* 1996;796:124–37.

160 Rothenberg ME. Eosinophilia. *N Engl J Med* 1998;338:1592–600.

161 Hogan SP, Rothenberg ME. Eosinophil function in eosinophil-associated gastrointestinal disorders. *Curr Allergy Asthma Rep* 2006;6:65–71.

162 Hogan SP, Rothenberg ME, Forbes E, *et al.* Chemokines in eosinophil-associated gastrointestinal disorders. *Curr Allergy Asthma Rep* 2004;4:74–82.

163 Miike S, Kita H. Human eosinophils are activated by cysteine proteases and release inflammatory mediators. *J Allergy Clin Immunol* 2003;111:704–13.

164 Venge P, Bystrom J, Carlson M, *et al.* Eosinophil cationic protein (ECP): molecular and biological properties and the use of ECP as a marker of eosinophil activation in disease. *Clin Exp Allergy* 1999;29:1172–86.

165 Furuta GT, Nieuwenhuis EE, Karhausen J, *et al.* Eosinophils alter colonic epithelial barrier function: role for major basic protein. *Am J Physiol Gastrointest Liver Physiol* 2005;289:G890–7.

166 Wang J, Slungaard A. Role of eosinophil peroxidase in host defense and disease pathology. *Arch Biochem Biophys* 2006;445:256–60.

167 Young JD, Peterson CG, Venge P, Cohn ZA. Mechanism of membrane damage mediated by human eosinophil cationic protein. *Nature* 1986;321:613–6.

168 O'Donnell MC, Ackerman SJ, Gleich GJ, Thomas LL. Activation of basophil and mast cell histamine release by eosinophil granule major basic protein. *J Exp Med* 1983;157:1981–91.

169 Otamiri T, Sjodahl R. Oxygen radicals: their role in selected gastrointestinal disorders. *Dig Dis* 1991;9:133–41.

170 Spalteholz H, Panasenko OM, Arnhold J. Formation of reactive halide species by myeloperoxidase and eosinophil peroxidase. *Arch Biochem Biophys* 2006;445:225–34.

171 Nielsen OH, Ahnfelt-Ronne I, Elmgreen J. Abnormal metabolism of arachidonic acid in chronic inflammatory bowel disease: enhanced release of leucotriene B4 from activated neutrophils. *Gut* 1987;28:181–5.

172 Rothenberg ME, Mishra A, Brandt EB, Hogan SP. Gastrointestinal eosinophils. *Immunol Rev* 2001;179:139–55.

173 Talley NJ, Shorter RG, Phillips SF, Zinsmeister AR. Eosinophilic gastroenteritis: a clinicopathological study of patients with disease of the mucosa, muscle layer, and subserosal tissues. *Gut* 1990;31:54–8.

174 Powell GK. Milk- and soy-induced enterocolitis of infancy. Clinical features and standardization of challenge. *J Pediatr* 1978;93:553–60.

175 Lake AM. Food-induced eosinophilic proctocolitis. *J Pediatr Gastroenterol Nutr* 2000;30:S58–60.

176 Green PH, Jabri B. Celiac disease. *Annu Rev Med* 2006;57:207–21.

177 Walsh SV, Antonioli DA, Goldman H, *et al.* Allergic esophagitis in children: a clinicopathological entity. *Am J Surg Pathol* 1999;23:390–6.

178 Sampson HA. Food allergy. *J Allergy Clin Immunol* 2003;111:S540–7.

179 Nowak-Wegrzyn A, Sampson HA, Wood RA, Sicherer SH. Food protein-induced enterocolitis syndrome caused by solid food proteins. *Pediatrics* 2003;111:829–35.

180 Sicherer SH. Food protein-induced enterocolitis syndrome: clinical perspectives. *J Pediatr Gastroenterol Nutr* 2000;30:S45–9.

181 Odze RD, Wershil BK, Leichtner AM, Antonioli DA. Allergic colitis in infants. *J Pediatr* 1995;126:163–70.

182 Sollid LM, Jabri B. Is celiac disease an autoimmune disorder? *Curr Opin Immunol* 2005;17:595–600.

183 Stepniak D, Koning F. Celiac disease – sandwiched between innate and adaptive immunity. *Hum Immunol* 2006;67:460–8.

184 Rostom A, Dube C, Cranney A, *et al*. The diagnostic accuracy of serologic tests for celiac disease: a systematic review. *Gastroenterology* 2005;128:S38–46.

185 Furuta GT. Emerging questions regarding eosinophil's role in the esophago-gastrointestinal tract. *Curr Opin Gastroenterol* 2006;22:658–63.

186 Guajardo JR, Plotnick LM, Fende JM, *et al*. Eosinophil-associated gastrointestinal disorders: a world-wide-web based registry. *J Pediatr* 2002;141:576–81.

CHAPTER 4

Food Allergens: Molecular and Immunological Characteristics

Heimo Breiteneder and E.N. Clare Mills

KEY CONCEPTS

- Food allergens belong to a limited number of protein families with different molecular properties, which may mean routes of sensitization differ for different allergen families.

- Food allergens that sensitize via the gastrointestinal tract have molecular features that enhance stability to thermal and proteolytical denaturation.

- Two allergen families (caseins and cupins) thought to sensitize via the gastrointestinal tract retain their allergenicity even after digestion for reasons which are not understood.

- Plant food allergens related to pollen allergens generally have no stability-enhancing characteristics and only induce oral allergy syndrome (OAS) as a secondary reaction to primary sensitization to pollen.

Introduction

The post-genomic era, with its explosion of information about protein and genome sequences, is allowing us to study molecular relationships in new ways, and notably within the context of evolution. Allergenic proteins have not suddenly appeared on the protein landscape but are the result of a long chain of formative processes that resulted in the creation of protein architectures that are treated as allergenic by an atopic immune system. Allergens are restricted to a very small number of protein families which share characteristic three-dimensional structures or scaffolds, as has been shown for plant food [1] and pollen allergens [2]. For some of these protein scaffolds, their origins can be followed back today to even archaebacteria as has been done for the cupin superfamily [3]. Although most members of the prolamin superfamily seem to be restricted to the seeds of dicotyledonous plants [4], proteins related to 2S albumins have been identified in the spores of ostrich fern [5]. The common ancestors of ferns and angiosperms lived more than 300 million years ago. Some of the evolved structures have been proven so successful that they are conserved between plants and animals as is the case for thaumatin-like

proteins [6]. Consequently, allergenicity seems to be linked to certain structural features of molecules that are members of a limited number of protein families. In general, within a given protein family, those known to be allergens represent only a fraction of its members, which has been well demonstrated for the Bet v 1 family of proteins [7]. In addition to any intrinsic allergenicity of the protein scaffold, this also may relate to issues of exposure, with some forms not being found in edible tissues or transiently expressed during development such that levels in the exposing agent are low. The most important food allergen families will be discussed in this chapter.

Food allergen protein families

Based on their shared amino acid sequences and conserved three-dimensional structures, proteins can be classified into families using various bioinformatics tools which form the basis of several protein family databases, one of which is Pfam [8]. Over the past 10 years or so there has been an explosion in the numbers of well characterized allergens, which have been sequenced and are being collected into a number of databases to facilitate bioinformatic analysis [9]. We have undertaken this analysis for both plant [1] and animal food allergens [10] along with pollen allergens [2]. They show similar distributions with the majority of allergens in each group falling into just 3–12 families with a tail

---

Food Allergy: Adverse Reactions to Foods and Food Additives, 4th edition.
Edited by Dean D. Metcalfe, Hugh A. Sampson, and Ronald A. Simon.
© 2008 Blackwell Publishing, ISBN: 978-1-4501-5129-0.

of between 14 and 23 families comprising between 1 and 3 allergens each. With regards to food allergens, around 65% of those from plants belong to just four protein families, the prolamin, cupin, Bet v 1-like, and profilin families [1], supporting molecular and structural approaches to the classification of plant food allergens [4,11]. Similarly, animal food allergens can be classified into three main families, the tropomyosins, EF-hand proteins, and caseins [10]. Such patterns of behavior beg the question of why certain protein scaffolds dominate the landscape of allergen structures? Are there structural features that predispose certain proteins to becoming allergens? Certainly detailed analysis of the secondary structural elements in proteins has not shown any relationship with allergenicity [12], but protein structure–function relationships can be very subtle. Using the food allergen family classification, we will summarize the properties of known food allergens and discuss how their structures and properties might determine their allergenic potency.

Food allergens of animal origin (Table 4.1)

Tropomyosins

Tropomyosins are a family of closely related proteins present in muscle and non-muscle cells [13]. Together with actin and myosin, tropomyosins play a key regulatory role in muscle contraction. Tropomyosins contain 40 uninterrupted heptapeptide repeats and are two-stranded proteins that occur as α-helical coiled coils [14]. Tropomyosins form head-to-tail polymers along the length of an actin filament [15] and are the major allergens of two invertebrate groups, Crustacea and Mollusca, that are generally referred to as shellfish. Shrimp, crab, squid, and abalone are assumed to be largely responsible for seafood allergies. Tropomyosins were originally identified as major shrimp allergens by several laboratories [16–18] and today they are recognized as invertebrate pan-allergens [19]. The first two residues of the IgE-binding region (epitope) in the *C*-terminal portion of the protein appear to be crucial for IgE binding and is not found in vertebrate tropomyosin. As a consequence of the lack of homology in the IgE epitopes, there is no cross-reactivity of IgE from shellfish-allergic individuals to animal muscle tropomyosins. Allergenic tropomyosins are heat stable and cross-reactive between the various crustacean and mollusk species [20]. Extracts from boiled *Penaeus indicus* shrimp contained Pen i 1 with unaltered allergenicity [21]. Water-soluble shrimp allergens were also detected in the cooking water after boiling [22].

Parvalbumins

The second largest animal food allergen family are the parvalbumins. Abundant in the white muscle of many fish species, parvalbumins are characterized by the possession of a widely found calcium-binding domain which is known as the EF-hand [23]. The EF-hand is a motif that consists of a loop of 12 amino acid residues that is flanked on either side by a 12-residue α-helical domain. Parvalbumins comprise three such domains [24], two of which are able to bind calcium [25]. Parvalbumins are important for the relaxation of muscle fibers by binding free intracellular calcium [26]. The binding of the calcium ligands is necessary for the correct parvalbumin conformation, loss of calcium resulting in a large change in conformation with an associated loss of IgE-binding capacity [27,28]. Parvalbumins with bound calcium ions possess a remarkable stability to denaturation by heat [29]. The ability to act as major fish allergens is obviously linked to the stability of parvalbumins to heat, denaturing chemicals, and proteolytic enzymes [30]. Parvalbumins can be subdivided into two distinct evolutionary lineages, the α- and the β-parvalbumins, although their overall architectures are very similar. The β-parvalbumins are generally allergenic. Gad c 1, a codfish allergen, was the first allergenic fish parvalbumin that was purified and characterized [31,32]. Today, allergenic β-parvalbumins have been characterized from many different fish species and are considered as pan-allergens in fish [33]. The cross-reactivity of fish and frog muscle in fish-allergic individuals has been attributed to the structural similarities between their parvalbumins [34]. An α-parvalbumin of frog has also been described as allergenic [35].

Caseins

Structurally mobile proteins, they are found in mammalian milk at a concentration of around 15 mg/ml and are responsible for binding calcium through clusters of phosphoserine and/or phosphothreonine residues in α_{s1}-, α_{s2}-, and β-caseins although the α_{s2}-casein gene is not expressed in man. The casein polypeptides form a shell around amorphous calcium phosphate to form microstructures called nanoclusters allowing calcium levels in milk to exceed the solubility limit of calcium phosphate. The nanoclusters are assembled into the casein micelles found in milk which are in turn stabilized by κ-casein [36]. The α- and β-caseins are related to the secretory calcium-binding phosphoprotein family together with proteins involved in mineralization and salivary proteins whilst κ-caseins may be distantly related to fibrinogen γ-chain [37]. Caseins are a major food allergen involved in cow's milk allergy, which affects predominantly young children. Studies on the IgE cross-reactivity between different types of casein in a group of cow's milk-allergic infants found that 90% had serum IgE against α_{s2}-casein, 55% against α_{s1}-casein, whilst only 15% had IgE against β-casein [38]. This pattern of reactivity appears to be related to the degree of similarity between bovine and human casein with caseins least like human caseins being more reactive. Thus, bovine β-casein appears to be the least reactive and has the highest identity to human casein of 53% whilst bovine α_{s2}-caseins were the

Table 4.1 Food allergens of animal origin

Animal food allergen family	Function	Source	Allergen name	Sequence accession	Reference
Tropomyosin superfamily	Tropomyosins bind to actin in muscle increasing thin filament stability and rigidity. It may play an important role with troponin in controlling muscle contraction	Brown shrimp (*Farfantepenaeus aztecus*)	Pen a 1	AAZ76743	[16]
		Greasy backed shrimp (*Metapenaeus ensis*)	Met e 1	Q25456	[39]
		Black tiger shrimp (*Penaeus monodon*)	Pen m 1	Not known	[40]
		Indian prawn (*Fenneropenaeus indicus*)	Pen i 1	Peptides only	[16]
		Snail (*Helix aspersa*)	Hel as 1	O97192	[41]
		Squid (*Todarodes pacificus*)	Tod p 1	Peptides only	[42]
		Oyster (*Crassostrea gigas*)	Cra g 1 Cra g 2 Cra g 1.03	Q95WY0	[43]
		Crab (*Charybdis feriatus*)	Cha f 1	Q9N2R3	[44]
		Abalone (*Haliotis diversicolor*)	Hal d 1	Q9GZ71	[45]
Parvalbumin superfamily	Parvalbumins control the flow of calcium from troponin C back to membrane-bound pumps after a muscle contraction	Cod (*Gadus morhua*)	Gad c 1	Q90YK9, Q90YL0	[46]
		Carp (*Cyprinus carpio*)	Cyp c 1.01 Cyp c 1.02	Q8UUS3 Q8UUS2	[47]
		Salmon (*Salmo salar*)	Sal s 1.01 Sal s 1.02	Q91482 Q91483	[48]
		Tuna (*Thunnus tonggol*)	Thu o 1.01 Thu o 1.02	None	[49]
		Edible frog (*Rana esculenta*)	Ran e 1	Q8JIU2 P02627	[35]
			Ran e 2	Q8JIU1, P02617	
Caseins	Caseins form stable micellar calcium phosphate protein complexes in mammalian milks	Domestic cow (*Bos taurus*)	Bos d 8		[50]
			α_{s1n}	P02662	
			α_{s2}	P02663	
			β-casein	P02666	
			κ-casein	P02668	
		Goat (*Capra hircus*)	α_{s1n}	P18626	[51]
			α_{s2}	P33049	
			β-casein	P33048	
			κ-casein	P02670	
		Sheep (*Ovis aries*)	α_{s1n}	P04653	[52]
			α_{s2}	P04654	
			β-casein	P11839	
			κ-casein	P02669	

most reactive being least similar with only ~16% identity to the human homolog. There is considerable similarity in the caseins from different mammalian milks used for human consumption, which explains their IgE cross-reactivity. It has been observed that cow's milk-allergic patients generally react to goat's milk on oral challenge [51], whose caseins have sequence identities of over 90%. However, it appears that when this sequence identity drops to between 22% and 66%, as is the case between mare's and cow's milk caseins, it is associated with tolerance, since individuals with cow's milk can tolerate mare's milk [53] and do not show IgE cross-reactivity to milk proteins from species such as camels [54].

Minor families
Lipocalins
The lipocalins are a group of diverse proteins sharing about 20% sequence identity with conserved three-dimensional structures characterized by a central tunnel which can often accommodate a diversity of lipophilic ligands [55]. They are thought to function as carriers of odorants, steroids, lipids, and pheromones amongst others. The majority of lipocalin allergens are respiratory, having been identified as the major allergens in rodent urine, animal dander, and saliva as well as in insects such as cockroaches, although the only lipocalin which acts as a food allergen is the cow's milk allergen, β-lactoglobulin [56].

Lysozyme family
Lysozyme type C and α-lactalbumins belong to the glycoside hydrolase family 22 clan of the O-glycosyl hydrolase superfamily and have probably evolved from a common ancestral protein. However, they have distinctly different functions; α-lactalbumin is involved in lactose synthesis in milk, and lysozyme acts as a muramidase hydrolyzing peptidoglycans found in bacterial cell walls. Furthermore α-lactalbumin, unlike hen's egg lysozyme, binds calcium. Two food allergens belong to this clan, the minor hen's egg allergen, lysozyme (Gal d 4) and the minor cow's milk allergen, α-lactalbumin, these proteins share little sequence homology, but are superimposable three-dimensional structures [57].

Transferrin family
Transferrins are eukaryotic sulfur-rich iron-binding glycoproteins which function in vivo to control the level of free iron. Members of the family that have been identified as minor food allergens include milk lactotransferrin (lactoferrin) and hen egg white ovotransferrin [58,59].

Serpins
Serpins are a class of serine protease inhibitors and are found in all types of organisms with the exception of fungi and are involved in a variety of physiological processes. Many of the family members have lost their inhibitory activity [60]. Only one food allergen has been identified as belonging to this family, the hen's egg allergen ovalbumin [61].

Arginine kinases
Arginine kinases have been identified as allergens in invertebrates including food allergens such as in shrimp [40] and as cross-reactive allergens in the Indian meal moth and king prawn, lobster, and mussel [62]. This protein belongs to a family of structurally and functionally related ATP:guanido phosphotransferases that reversibly catalyze the transfer of phosphate between ATP and various phosphogens.

Ovomucoids
Kazal inhibitors which inhibit a number of serine proteases belong to a family of proteins that includes pancreatic secretory trypsin inhibitor, avian ovomucoid, and elastase inhibitor. These proteins contain between 1 and 7 Kazal-type inhibitor repeats [63]. Avian ovomucoids contain three Kazal-like inhibitory domains [64]. Chicken ovomucoid has been shown to be the dominant hen's egg white allergen Gal d 1 [61]. Gal d 1 comprises 186 amino acid residues that are arranged in three tandem domains (Gal d 1.1, Gal d 1.2, Gal d 1.3). Each domain contains three intradomain disulfide bonds. Gal d 1.1 and Gal d 1.2 contain two carbohydrate chains each, and about 50% of the Gal d 1.3 domains contain one carbohydrate chain which may act to stabilize the protein against proteolysis [65].

Food allergens of plant origin (Table 4.2)
The prolamin superfamily
The prolamin superfamily was initially defined by Kreis and co-workers [66] who observed that three groups of apparently unrelated seed proteins contained a conserved pattern of cysteine residues. These included two types of cereal seed proteins, namely the sulfur-rich prolamins and the α-amylase/trypsin inhibitors of monocotyledonous cereal seeds, together with the 2S storage albumins (Fig. 4.1(a)) found in a variety of dicotyledonous seeds including castor bean and oilseed rape. Subsequently other low molecular weight (LMW) allergenic proteins have been identified as belonging to this superfamily including soybean hydrophobic protein (Fig. 4.1(b)), non-specific lipid-transfer proteins (nsLTPs, Fig. 4.1(c)) and α-globulins. The conserved cysteine skeleton comprises a core of eight cysteine residues which includes a characteristic Cys–Cys and Cys–X–Cys motif (X representing any other residue). Two additional cysteine residues are found in the α-amylase/trypsin inhibitors. In the cereal seed storage prolamins the disulfide skeleton has been disrupted by the insertion of a repetitive domain comprising motifs rich in proline and glutamine. Whilst the way in which the disulfide connectivities formed by the cysteine residues are different in the different types of prolamin superfamily members, they share a common three-dimensional structure, examples of which are shown in Fig. 4.1. This figure illustrates the three-dimensional structures shared by these

Table 4.2 Food allergens of plant origin

Plant food allergen family	Function in plant	Botanical source	Allergen name	Sequence accession	Reference
Prolamin superfamily					
Prolamins	Seed storage protein		α- and γ-gliadin	BAA12318	[67–69]
				BAA11251	
			LMW glutenin	BAA23162	
Non-specific lipid-transfer proteins (nsLTPs)	Function uncertain; maybe involved in transport of suberin monomers	Apple (*Malus domestica*)	Mal d 3	Q9M5X7	[70]
		Apricot (*Prunus armeniaca*)	Pru ar 3	G7404406	[71]
		Cherry (*Prunus avium*)	Pru av 3	AAF26449	[72]
		Peach (*Prunus persica*)	Pru p 3 (originally Pru p 1)	P81402	[73]
		Garden plum (*Prunus domestica*)	Pru d 3	P82534	[74]
		Strawberry (*Fragaria ananassa*)	Fra a 3	Q4PLT5-9	[75]
				Q4PLU0	
		Orange (*Citrus sinensis*)	Cit s 3	P84161	[76]
		Grape (*Vitis vinifera*)	Vit v 1	P80274	[77]
		Chestnut (*Castanea sativa*)	Cas s 8	N-terminus only	[78]
		Walnut (*Juglans regia*)	Jug r 3	Not known	[79,80]
		Hazelnut (*Corylus avellana*)	Cor a 8	AF329829	[81]
		Asparagus (*Asparagus officinalis*)	Aspa o 1		[82]
		Lettuce (*Lactuca sativa*)	Lac s 1	N-terminus only	[83]
		Cabbage (*Brassica oleracea*)	Bra o 3	Q2A988	[84]
		Maize (*Zea mays*)	Zea m 14	P19656	[85]
α-amylase/trypsin inhibitors	Provide protection against degradative proteases and amylases produced by insect pests and pathogens	Barley (*Hordeum vulgaris*)	Hor v 1	CAA45085	[85,86]
		Rice (*Oryza sativa*)	Rag 1, 2 5, 5.b, 14, 14b, 16, 17	Q01881	[87–89]
				S59922	
				S59924	
				S59925	
				BAA01997	
				BAA01998	
				BAA01999	
				BAA02000	
2S albumins	Seed storage protein	Walnut (*Juglans regia*)	Jug r 1	JRU66866	[90]
		Almond (*Prunus dulcis*)		P82944	[91]
		Brazil nut (*Bertholletia excelsa*)	Ber e 1	CAA38362	[92]
		Cashew nut (*Anacardium occidentale*)	Ana o 3	Q8H2B8	[93]
		White mustard (*Sinapis alba*)	Sin a 1	P15322	[94]
		Black mustard (*Brassica juncea*)	Bra j 1	P80207	[95]

(Continued)

Table 4.2 (Continued)

Plant food allergen family	Function in plant	Botanical source	Allergen name	Sequence accession	Reference
		Chickpea (*Cicer arietinum*)	None	None	[96]
		Peanut (*Arachis hypogaea*)	Ara h 2	L77197	[97–99]
			Ara h 6	AF091737	
			Ara h 7	AF092846	
		Sesame (*Sesamum indicum*)	Ses i 1	AAD42943	[100]
			Ses i 2	Q9XHP1	[101]
		Sunflower (*Helianthus annuus*)	SFA-8		[102]
Bet v 1 superfamily		Apple (*Malus domestica*)	Mal d 1	P43211	[103]
		Pear (*Pyrus communis*)	Pyr c 1	O65200	[104]
		Cherry (*Prunus avium*)	Pru av 1 (originally Pru a 1)	O24248 Q6QHU3 Q6QHU2	[105]
		Strawberry (*Fragaria ananassa*)		AY679601	[106]
		Carrot (*Daucus carota*)	Dau c 1	O04298	[107]
		Celery root (*Apium graveolens*)	Api g 1	P49372 P92918	[108]
		Hazelnut (*Corylus avellana*)	Cor a 1.04	Q9FPK2,3,4 Q9SWR4	[109]
		Soy (*Glycine max*)	Gly m 4	P26987	[110]
Cupin superfamily 7S (vicilin like) Globulins	Seed storage protein	Peanut (*Arachis hypogaea*)	Conarachin, Ara h 1	L34402	[111]
		Soy (*Glycine max*)	β-conglycinin	αP13916 α′: P11827 β:P25974	[112]
		Buckwheat (*Fagopyrum esculentum*)	BWI-1c BWI-2 BWI-2b BWI-2c	Q6QJL1	[113]
		Almond (*Prunus dulcis*)	Conglutin Gamma	P82952	[91]
		Walnut (*Juglans regia*)	Jug r 2	AAB41308	[114]
		Hazelnut (*Corylus avellana*)	Cor a 11	Q8S4P9	[115]
		Cashew nut (*Anacardium occidentale*)	Ana o 1.0101	Q8L5L5	[116]
			1.0102	Q8L5L6	
		Sesame (*Sesamum indicum*)	Ses i 3	Q9AUD0	[101]

11S (legumin like) Globulins	Seed storage protein	Peanut (*Arachis hypogaea*)	Arachin Ara h 3 Ara h 4	AF093541 AF086821	[97,117]
		Soy (*Glycine max*)	Glycinin	Gy1 (A1aBx): P04776 Gy2 (A2B1a): P04405 Gy3 (AB): P11828 Gy4 (A4/5B3): P02858 Gy (A3B4): P04347	[118]
		Buckwheat (*Fagopyrum esculentum*)	BW24KD Fag e 1 FAGAG1 FA02 FA18	Q9XFM4 O23880 O23878	[113]
		Almond (*Prunus dulcis*)	Major almond protein, amandin, prunin	Q43607	[119,120]
		Cashew nut (*Anacardium occidentale*)	Ana o 2	Q8GZP6	[121]
		Brazil nut (*Bertholletia excelsa*)	Ber e 2, Excelsin	Q84ND2	[79]
Cysteine protease C 1 family	Cysteine proteases	Kiwi (*Actinidia deliciosa*)	Actinidin	Q43367	[122]
		Soy (*Glycine max*)	Gly m Bd 30K; P34; Gly m 1	P22895	[123]

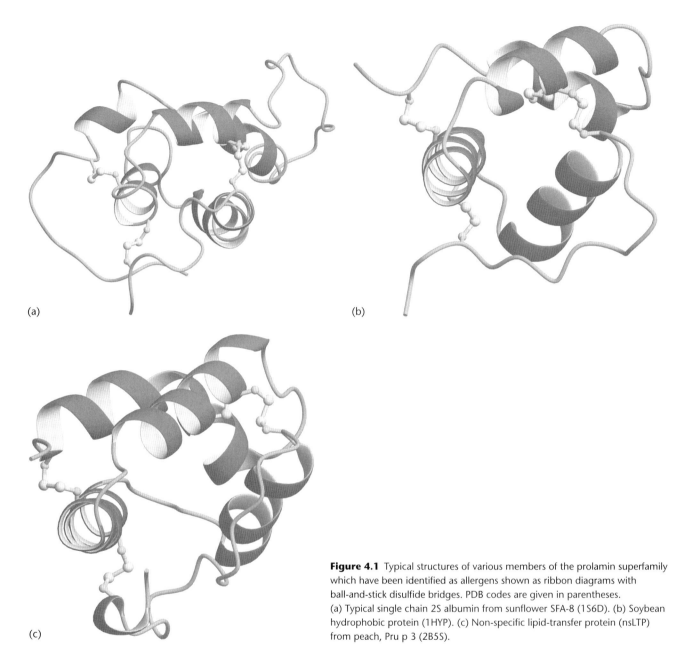

(a)

(b)

(c)

Figure 4.1 Typical structures of various members of the prolamin superfamily which have been identified as allergens shown as ribbon diagrams with ball-and-stick disulfide bridges. PDB codes are given in parentheses. (a) Typical single chain 2S albumin from sunflower SFA-8 (1S6D). (b) Soybean hydrophobic protein (1HYP). (c) Non-specific lipid-transfer protein (nsLTP) from peach, Pru p 3 (2B5S).

proteins, which consist of bundles of four α-helices stabilized by disulfide bonds which are arranged in such a way as to create a lipid-binding tunnel in the nsLTPs, which is collapsed in the 2S albumin structures. As yet no ancestral type has been identified, and consequently this scaffold appears to be found almost exclusively in flowering plants.

The lipid-binding tunnel of the nsLTPs shows considerable flexibility being able to accommodate a diverse range of lipophiles including prostaglandins [124] and up to two fatty acids lying side by side [125]. Apart from the seed storage prolamins, whose properties are dominated by the inserted repetitive domain, the physichochemical properties of prolamin superfamily members are dominated by their intramolecular disulfide bonds. Compact proteins, the disulfide

bonds in the prolamin superfamily members, are responsible for maintaining the three-dimensional structure even after heating, which is associated with retaining their allergenic properties after cooking [126]. Their structure and IgE-binding properties are only being altered if severe heating results in hydrolysis of these bonds [127]. These same structural attributes underlie their resistance to proteolysis, with several members, including the 2S albumins [128] and nsLTP allergens [129] being highly resistant to gastric and duodenal digestion. Any degradation that does occur appears to leave the major IgE-binding sites intact explaining the fact that simulated gastrointestinal digestion does not alter their ability to elicit skin reactions *in vivo*, as has been observed for the grape nsLTP [130].

Cereal prolamins

As a consequence of the inserted repetitive domain, the α-helical structure has been disrupted in the seed storage prolamins. Their properties are dominated by the repetitive domain which is thought to adopt an ensemble of unfolded and secondary structures comprising overlapping β-turns or poly-L-proline II structures which may form a loose spiral structure [131]. They comprise around half of the protein found in grain from the related cereals, wheat, barley, and rye, those from wheat being able to form large disulfide-linked polymers which comprise the viscoleastic protein fraction known as gluten. These proteins are characteristically insoluble in dilute salt solutions, either in the native state or after reduction of inter-chain disulfide bonds, being soluble instead in aqueous alcohols. In addition to their role in triggering celiac disease, several types of cereal storage prolamins have been identified as triggering IgE-mediated allergies including γ-, α-, and ω-5 gliadins [67,68,132] in addition to the polymeric HMW and LMW subunits of glutenin [69,133–135]. Cooking appears to affect allergenicity and one study suggested that baking may be essential for allergenicity of cereal prolamins [136].

Bifunctional inhibitors

The other group of prolamin superfamily allergens unique to cereals are the α-amylase/trypsin inhibitors which have been found to sensitize individuals via the lungs resulting in occupational allergies to wheat flour such as Baker's asthma or via the gastrointestinal tract for cereal-containing foods including wheat, barley, and rice. They were initially identified in extracts made with chloroform/water mixtures (and hence called CM proteins) but are also soluble in water, dilute saline, or alcohol/water mixtures. More detailed studies have revealed a range of monomeric, dimeric, and tetrameric forms, many of the subunits being glycosylated [137]. The individual subunits are either inactive or inhibitory to trypsin (and sometimes other proteinases), α-amylases from insects (including pests) or both enzymes (i.e. the inhibitors are bifunctional). The best characterized allergens are the α-amylase inhibitors of rice grain [87], although there is one report of a M_r ~15,000 subunit being involved in wheat allergy [138]. Allergens with M_r of 16,000 have also been characterized in corn and beer (originating from barley) which appear to belong to the α-amylase inhibitor family [85,86].

2S albumins

The 2S albumins are a major family of storage proteins [139] and appear to be restricted to seeds of dicotyledonous plants where they may accompany the cupin globulin seed storage proteins (see below). Most 2S albumins are synthesized as single chains of M_r 10,000–15,000 which, depending on the plant species, may be post-translationally processed to give small and large subunits that usually remain joined by disulfide bonds. In some plant species such as peanut and sunflower, the precursors are unprocessed and remain as a single polypeptide chain (Fig. 4.1(a)). 2S albumins can act as both occupational (sensitizing through inhalation of dusts) and food allergens, having been identified as the major allergenic components of many foods including the peanut allergens Ara h 2, 6, and 7 [97,98], oriental and yellow mustard allergens Bra j 1 and Sin a 1 [94,95], the walnut allergen Jug r 1 [90], Ses i 1 and 2 from sesame [100,101], Ber e 1 from Brazil nut [92], and 2S albumins from almond [91] and sunflower seeds [102]. There is also some evidence that the 2S albumins of soy [140] and chickpea [96] are also allergenic.

Non-specific lipid-transfer proteins

One of the most important groups of allergens to have been identified in the last decade are the nsLTPs which appear to be involved in severe allergies to fresh fruits such as peach in the south of Europe around the Mediterranean. They have been termed as "pan-allergens" [70] and are the most widely distributed type of prolamin being found in a variety of plant organs including seeds, fruits, and vegetative tissues. Thus, in addition to being identified in many different fruits and seeds, they have also been characterized in pollen of plant species such as olive and *Parietaria judaica* [141,142]. nsLTPs as major allergens have been identified in fruits such as Pru p 3 (Fig. 4.1(c)) in peach [143], Mal d 3 in apple [70], and Vit v 1 in grape [77]. Allergenic nsLTPs have also been characterized in vegetables such as asparagus [82], cereals such as maize [85], and in a number of nuts including hazelnut [144]. As their name implies, nsLTPs were originally defined on the basis of their ability *in vitro* to transfer a range of phospholipid types from liposomes to various types of membranes such as those from mitochondria. However, this is not their *in vivo* function and it is emerging that plants have used the nsLTP scaffold in a wide range of contexts. Those involved in food allergies are found in epidermal tissues. This observation, along with their lipid-binding characteristics, has led to the view that they play a role in transporting lipids involved in the synthesis of waxy cutin and suberin layers in outer plant tissues in seeds and pollen.

The cupin superfamily

The cupins are a functionally diverse protein superfamily which has probably evolved from a prokaryotic ancestor but has not found its way into the animal kingdom. They possess a characteristic β-barrel structure, the name "cupin" being derived from Latin for barrel [3]. This basic scaffold has been utilized in a diverse range of functions including sporulation proteins in fungi, sucrose-binding activities and enzymatic activities found in germins where manganese is bound in the center of the barrel. The cupin motif has been duplicated in flowering plants to give rise to the bi-cupin 7S and 11S globulin seed storage globulins, the three-dimensional structure of the 11S globulin of soy proglycinin is shown in Fig. 4.2(b). The 11S–12S globulins are found in the seeds of many monocotyledonous and dicotyledonous plants with homologs having been identified in gymnosperms (including conifers). They are sometimes termed legumins because they are particularly found in legume seeds and are oligomers of M_r ~300,000–450,000. Each oligomer consists of six subunits of M_r about 60,000, the products of a multigene family, non-covalently associated by intertwining α-helical regions. Each subunit is post-translationally processed to give rise to acidic (M_r about 40,000) and basic (M_r about 20,000) chains, linked by a single disulfide bond and rarely, if ever, glycosylated [145]. In contrast the 7S/8S globulins are usually trimeric proteins of M_r about 150,000–190,000, comprising subunit M_r ~40,000–80,000, but typically about

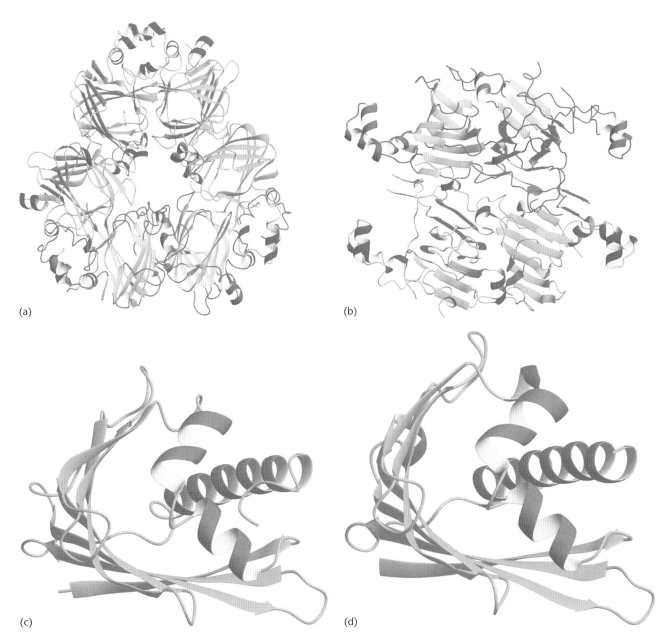

(a)

(b)

(c)

(d)

Figure 4.2 Typical structures of the cupin and Bet v 1 superfamily allergens shown as ribbon diagrams with ball-and-stick disulfides. PDB codes are given in parentheses. (a) Trimeric structure of soybean 7S globulin β-conglycinin comprising solely β-subunits (1UIJ). (b) Edge-on view of soybean 11S globulin showing the way in which individual subunits are stacked within the hexamer (2D5H). (c) Major birch pollen allergen Bet v 1 (1BV1). (d) Allergenic Bet v 1 homolog from celery root, Api g 1 (2BK0).

50,000. They are also termed vicilins since they are particularly found in the Viciae group of legumes. The subunits are again the products of a multigene family and also undergo proteolytic processing and glycosylation the extent of which varies depending on the plant species [145].

Major allergens include the 7S (Fig. 4.2(a)) and 11S globulins (Fig. 4.2(b)) of soybean [112,118,145], Ara h 1 and Ara h 3 of peanut [97,111,117], Ana c 1 and Ana c 2 of cashew nut [116,121], the 7S globulins Jug r 2 of walnut [114] and Len c 1 of lentil [147], and the 7S globulins of sesame [101] and hazelnut [144]. The 11S globulins have also been shown to be allergens in almond, also known as almond major protein (AMP) [148], and in hazelnut [149]. In general, these vicilin- and legumin-like seed globulins exhibit a high degree of thermostability, requiring temperatures in excess of 70°C for denaturation, and have a propensity to form large aggregates on heating which still retain, to a large degree, their native secondary structure [150–152]. At high protein concentrations these proteins can form heat-set gels [152].

Since the globulins are partially or fully insoluble between pH 3.5 and 6.5 it is likely that only limited solubilization of globulins would occur when they enter the stomach. However, the 7S globulins seem to be highly susceptible to pepsinolysis, although several LMW polypeptides seem to persist following digestion of the peanut 7S globulin allergen Ara h 1 [153,154], and there is evidence that they still possess IgE-binding sites following proteolysis [155]. Similarly *in vitro* simulated gastrointestinal digestion results in rapid and almost complete degradation of the protein to relatively small polypeptides although these retain their allergenic properties [156]. There are indications that the peptides do not remain monomeric but can assemble into larger structures and it may be that this propensity to aggregate is responsible for the protein retaining its allergenic properties even when hydrolyzed.

The Bet v 1 family

The association of plant food allergies with birch pollen allergy is the most frequently observed of the cross-reactivity syndromes [157]. The clinical symptoms of the birch pollen allergy-related OAS are caused by cross-reactive IgE between the major birch pollen allergen Bet v 1 (Fig. 4.2(c)) and its homologs in a wide range of fruits and vegetables, including apple [103], celery (Fig. 4.2(d)) [118], peanut [158], mung bean [159], sharon fruit [160], and even jackfruit [121]. Bet v 1 was the first allergen identified that possessed similarities to family 10 of the pathogenesis-related (PR) proteins [162,163]. As a possible biological function in plants, a general plant-steroid carrier function for Bet v 1 and related PR-10 proteins was suggested [164]. The known structures of Bet v 1 [164,165] and its homologs in cherry [166] and celery [167] illustrate the high identity of the molecular surfaces that are accessible to IgE and

thus offer a molecular explanation for the observed clinical cross-reactivities. A structural bioinformatic analysis of Bet v 1 and its homologous allergens from apple, soybean, and celery showed that conservation of three-dimensional structure plays an important role in conservation of IgE-binding epitopes and underlies the birch pollen – plant food syndrome [1]. There is evidence on the T-cell level that Bet v 1 is the relevant sensitizing agent [168]. It has been shown that a subpopulation of patients with birch pollen allergy and atopic dermatitis reacted with worsening of eczema after oral challenge with foods harboring Bet v 1 homologous proteins [169]. Bet v 1-specific T-cells could be found in the lesional skin of these patients [169]. T-cell cross-reactivity between Bet v 1 and related food allergens occurs independently of IgE cross-reactivity. Gastrointestinal or heat degradation destroyed the histamine releasing but not the T-cell activating properties of Bet v 1 homologous food allergens [170,171]. Thus, ingestion of cooked birch pollen allergy-related foods did not induce OAS but caused atopic eczema to worsen [171].

Minor families
Class I chitinases
Chitinases are enzymes that catalyze the hydrolysis of chitin polymers. Chitinases are members of the glycoside hydrolase families 18 or 19 [172]. Endochitinases from plants belong to 19 (also known as classes IA or I and IB or II) and are able to degrade chitin, a major structural component of the exoskeleton of insects and of the cell walls of many pathogenic fungi [173]. Class I chitinases contain an *N*-terminal so-called hevein domain with putative chitin-binding properties [174]. This hevein domain shares high sequence identity with the major *Hevea brasiliensis* latex allergen Hev b 6.02, hevein [175]. Class I chitinases from fruits such as avocado [176], banana [177], and chestnut [178] have been identified as major allergens that cross-react with Hev b 6.02. Pers a 1, an allergenic class I chitinase from avocado, was extensively degraded when subjected to simulated gastric fluid digestion. However, the resulting peptides, particularly those corresponding to the hevein-like domain, were clearly reactive both *in vitro* and *in vivo* [179]. The 43-residue polypeptide chain of hevein-like domains contains four disulfide bonds to which they owe their stability [180].

Cysteine protease superfamily
Cysteine proteases of the C1, or papain-like, family were originally characterized by having a cysteine residue as part of their catalytic site, which has now been extended to include conserved glutamine, cysteine, histidine, and asparagine residues [181]. Whilst sharing the fold of the C1 protease family, some members may have lost the capacity to act as proteases, a notable example being the soybean P34 protein in which a glycine has replaced the active site

cysteine residue [182]. Two major food allergens belong to this family, actinidin (Act c 1) from kiwi fruit [122] and an allergen involved in soybean-induced atopic dermatitis known as Gly m Bd 30K, Gly m 1, or P34 [123].

Profilins

Profilins from higher plants constitute a family of highly conserved proteins with sequence identities of at least 75% even between members of distantly related organisms [183]. Profilins are cytosolic proteins of 12–15 kDa in size that are found in all eukaryotic cells. Profilins bind to monomeric actin and a number of other proteins, thus regulating the actin polymerization and depolymerization during processes such as cell movement, cytokinesis, and signaling [184]. Originally, plant profilins were discovered as cross-reactive pollen allergens eliciting IgE responses in 10–20% of pollen-allergic patients. Later, they were also described as allergens in plant foods and *Hevea* latex [185]. Structures of three plant profilins have been elucidated so far, those from *Arabidopsis thaliana* pollen [186], birch pollen [187], and *Hevea brasiliensis* latex. Since profilin-specific IgE cross-reacts with homologs from virtually every plant source, sensitization to these allergens has been considered a risk factor for allergic reactions to multiple pollen sources [188] and for pollen-associated food allergy [189]. However, the clinical relevance of plant food profilin-specific IgE is still under debate [190]. Despite sequence identities of below 30%, plant profilin structures are highly similar to the structures of profilins from mammals, fungi, and amoeba. IgE directed to plant profilins weakly binds to the human homolog as well [191]. However, no profilins from sources other than plants have been shown to elicit allergic reactions.

Protease inhibitors and lectins

The Kunitz/bovine pancreatic trypsin inhibitor family is active against serine, thiol, aspartic, and subtilisin proteases. They are generally small (~50 residue) with three disulfide bonds constraining the proteins three-dimensional structure and belong to a superfamily of structurally related proteins, which share no sequence similarity and that includes such diverse proteins as interleukin-1 proteins, heparin-binding growth factors (HBGF), and histactophilin. In plants they probably play a role in defense against pests and pathogens. Minor allergens have been identified belonging to the Kunitz inhibitor family in soybean [192,193] and potato [194]. It is thought that their stability to processing and digestion is important for their allergenic activity. In addition to agglutinin, a lectin found in peanut has been identified as a minor allergen [193].

Thaumatin-like proteins

Thaumatin-like proteins (TLPs) derive their name from their sequence similarities to thaumatin, an intensely sweet tasting protein isolated from the fruits of the West African rain forest shrub *Thaumatococcus daniellii*. TLPs accumulate in plants in response to pathogen challenge and belong to the PR-5 family of proteins that also includes thaumatin and osmotin [195]. Recent phlyogenetic and structural studies revealed that PR-5 proteins constitute an ancient protein family that is conserved between plants, insects, and nematodes [6]. Several allergenic TLPs from fruits have been described. These include Mal d 2 from apple [196], Cap a 1 from bell pepper [197], Pru av 2 from sweet cherry [198,199], Act c 2 from kiwi [200], and an allergenic TLP from grape [77]. The conformation of TLPs is stabilized by eight disulfide bonds. This extensive disulfide cross-linking confers high stability to proteolysis to the TLP scaffold as has been shown for a zeamatin, a TLP from corn [201]. This is also the reason why the allergenic TLPs produced by grape berries persist during the entire vinification process and are among the major proteins present in wine [202].

What does this mean?

Many of the proteins that have been described as allergens in plant foods function as seed storage proteins, providing the nutrients for a developing plant, with the cow's milk caseins functioning in a similar fashion to provide essential nutrition to young mammals. This relationship may not be so surprising since these are the proteins predominantly found in nuts and seeds and as a consequence exposure in the human diet, especially to the abundant storage proteins, is considerable. Extent of exposure to a given protein probably plays a role in determining its allergenicity, with extensive exposure now thought to be important for tolerization, total exclusion precluding an individual from developing an allergy, with low levels of exposure possibly being more effective at sensitizing [203,204]. However, it is emerging that there is a complex dialog between different routes of exposure with evidence from animal models that cutaneous exposure may prevent oral tolerance developing [205].

There are a number of allergens which are less abundant in foods, notably the nsLTPs where the prolamin superfamily fold may play a role in potentiating the allergenicity of these proteins. Intriguingly many of the allergens that are less abundant in plant-derived foods have a role in plant protection. Others have alluded to the fact that many plant food allergens are involved in defense [206], with many of them being classified as pathogenesis-related proteins according to the criteria defined by van Loon and van Strien [207]. These include for example the PR-10 proteins from the Bet v 1 family of allergens, the PR-14 nsLTPs, whilst others, such as the cereal α-amylase inhibitors that have not been classified as PR proteins, are thought to have a protective function. In addition, certain minor animal food allergens also have an imputed protective function. Many PR proteins are resistant to the effects of extremes in pH and highly resistant to proteolysis, possibly to evade the degradative environment created by pests and pathogens infecting plant tissues [4].

It has been hypothesized that resistance to digestion is important in allowing sufficient immunologically active fragments to come into contact with the immune system, particularly with regards to sensitization via the gastro-intestinal tract. However, it is evident that some allergen families, notably the caseins and the cupins, are readily degraded in the gastrointestinal tract. Nevertheless, for the cupins at least, there is evidence that degradation does not affect the ability of these proteins to elicit histamine release *in vitro* [156], although the impact of digestion on the sensitization potential of these proteins is not clear. For animal allergens there may also be the need to consider the evolutionary distance from man, since animal food allergens, notably the tropomyosins, lie at the borders of self–non-self recognition. Thus, it may be that in addition to the routes and extent of exposure, the mechanisms whereby different scaffolds sensitize and elicit allergic reactions may differ. Such complex interacting factors underlie the reasons why we still do not understand why some food proteins, and not others, cause allergic reactions in man. Other factors, such as the role of food processing and modification of allergens, or adjuvant effects of other food components, may also play a role in stimulating IgE, rather than IgG responses to foods such as peanuts. Only an improved understanding of these factors and the mechanisms underlying the generation of aberrant IgE responses will enable us to understand what makes a protein become an allergen.

Acknowledgments

Author HB wishes to thank the Austrian Science Fund Grant SFB F1802 for support. ENC Mills was supported by the Competitive Strategic grant from BBSRC.

References

1 Jenkins JA, Griffiths-Jones S, Shewry PR, *et al*. Structural relatedness of plant food allergens with specific reference to cross-reactive allergens: an in silico analysis. *J Allergy Clin Immunol* 2005;115:163–70.

2 Radauer C, Breiteneder H. Pollen allergens are restricted to few protein families and show distinct patterns of species distribution. *J Allergy Clin Immunol* 2006;117:141–7.

3 Dunwell JM, Purvis A, Khuri S. Cupins: the most functionally diverse protein superfamily? *Phytochemistry* 2004;65:7–17.

4 Mills EN, Jenkins JA, Alcocer MJ, Shewry PR. Structural, biological, and evolutionary relationships of plant food allergens sensitizing via the gastrointestinal tract. *Crit Rev Food Sci Nutr* 2004;44:379–407.

5 Rodin J, Rask L. Characterization of matteuccin, the 2.2S storage protein of the ostrich fern. Evolutionary relationship to angiosperm seed storage proteins. *Eur J Biochem* 1990;28;192:101–7.

6 Shatters Jr RG, Boykin LM, Lapointe SL, *et al*. Phylogenetic and structural relationships of the PR5 gene family reveal an ancient multigene family conserved in plants and select animal taxa. *J Mol Evol* 2006;63:12–29.

7 Liscombe DK, MacLeod BP, Loukanina N, *et al*. Evidence for the monophyletic evolution of benzylisoquinoline alkaloid biosynthesis in angiosperms. *Phytochemistry* 2005;66:2501–20.

8 Bateman A, Coin L, Durbin R, *et al*. The Pfam protein families database. *Nucleic Acids Res* 2004;1:32(Database issue):D138–41.

9 Gendel SM, Jenkins JA. Allergen sequence databases. *Mol Nutr Food Res* 2006;50:633–7.

10 Jenkins JA, Breiteneder H, Mills EN. Evolutionary distance from human homologs reflects allergenicity of animal food proteins. DOI information: 10.1016/j.jaci.2007.08.019.

11 Breiteneder H, Radauer C. A classification of plant food allergens. *J Allergy Clin Immunol* 2004;113:821–30.

12 Aalberse RC. Structural biology of allergens. *J Allergy Clin Immunol* 2000;106:228–38.

13 MacLeod AR. Genetic origin of diversity of human cytoskeletal tropomyosins. *Bioessays* 1987;6:208–12.

14 Li Y, Mui S, Brown JH, *et al*. The crystal structure of the *C*-terminal fragment of striated-muscle alpha-tropomyosin reveals a key troponin T recognition site. *Proc Natl Acad Sci USA* 2002;99:7378–83.

15 Gunning PW, Schevzov G, Kee AJ, Hardeman EC. Tropomyosin isoforms: divining rods for actin cytoskeleton function. *Trends Cell Biol* 2005;15:333–41.

16 Shanti KN, Martin BM, Nagpal S, *et al*. Identification of tropomyosin as the major shrimp allergen and characterization of its IgE-binding epitopes. *J Immunol* 1993;151:5354–63.

17 Daul CB, Slattery M, Reese G, Lehrer SB. Identification of the major brown shrimp (*Penaeus aztecus*) allergen as the muscle protein tropomyosin. *Int Arch Allergy Immunol* 1994;105:49–55.

18 Leung PS, Chu KH, Chow WK, *et al*. Cloning, expression, and primary structure of Metapenaeus ensis tropomyosin, the major heat-stable shrimp allergen. *J Allergy Clin Immunol* 1994;94:882–90.

19 Reese G, Ayuso R, Lehrer SB. Tropomyosin: an invertebrate pan-allergen. *Int Arch Allergy Immunol* 1999;119:247–58.

20 Motoyama K, Ishizaki S, Nagashima Y, Shiomi K. Cephalopod tropomyosins: identification as major allergens and molecular cloning. *Food Chem Toxicol* 2006;44:1997–2002.

21 Naqpal S, Rajappa L, Metcalfe DD, Rao PV. Isolation and characterization of heat-stable allergens from shrimp (*Penaeus indicus*). *J Allergy Clin Immunol* 1989;83:26–36.

22 Lehrer SB, Ibanez MD, McCants ML, *et al*. Characterization of water-soluble shrimp allergens released during boiling. *J Allergy Clin Immunol* 1990;85:1005–13.

23 Lewit-Bentley A, Rety S. EF-hand calcium-binding proteins. *Curr Opin Struct Biol* 2000;10:637–43.

24 Ikura M. Calcium binding and conformational response in EF-hand proteins. *Trends Biochem Sci* 1996;21:14–17.

25 Declercq JP, Tinant B, Parello J, Rambaud J. Ionic interactions with parvalbumins. Crystal structure determination of pike

4.10 parvalbumin in four different ionic environments. *J Mol Biol* 1991;220:1017–39.

26 Pauls TL, Cox JA, Berchtold MW. The Ca2+(-)binding proteins parvalbumin and oncomodulin and their genes: new structural and functional findings. *Biochim Biophys Acta* 1996;1306:39–54.

27 Bugajska-Schretter A, Elfman L, Fuchs T, *et al.* Parvalbumin, a cross-reactive fish allergen, contains IgE-binding epitopes sensitive to periodate treatment and Ca2+ depletion. *J Allergy Clin Immunol* 1998;101:67–74.

28 Bugajska-Schretter A, Grote M, Vangelista L, *et al.* Purification, biochemical, and immunological characterisation of a major food allergen: different immunoglobulin E recognition of the apo- and calcium-bound forms of carp parvalbumin. *Gut* 2000;46:661–9.

29 Filimonov VV, Pfeil W, Tsalkova TN, Privalov PL. Thermodynamic investigations of proteins. IV. Calcium binding protein parvalbumin. *Biophys Chem* 1978;8:117–22.

30 Elsayed S, Aas K. Characterization of a major allergen (cod). Observations on effect of denaturation on the allergenic activity. *J Allergy* 1971;47:283–91.

31 Aas K, Jebsen JW. Studies of hypersensitivity to fish. Partial purification and crystallization of a major allergenic component of cod. *Int Arch Allergy Appl Immunol* 1967;32:1–20.

32 Elsayed S, Bennich H. The primary structure of allergen M from cod. *Scand J Immunol* 1975;4:203–8.

33 Bernhisel-Broadbent J, Scanlon SM, Sampson HA. Fish hypersensitivity. I. *In vitro* and oral challenge results in fish-allergic patients. *J Allergy Clin Immunol* 1992;89:730–7.

34 Hilger C, Thill L, Grigioni F, *et al.* IgE antibodies of fish allergic patients cross-react with frog parvalbumin. *Allergy* 2004; 59:653–60.

35 Hilger C, Grigioni F, Thill L, *et al.* Severe IgE-mediated anaphylaxis following consumption of fried frog legs: definition of alpha-parvalbumin as the allergen in cause. *Allergy* 2002;57:1053–8.

36 Tuinier R, de Kruif CG. Stability of casein micelles in milk. *J Chem Phys* 2002;117:1290–5.

37 Kawasaki K, Weiss KM. Mineralized tissue and vertebrate evolution: the secretory calcium-binding phosphoprotein gene cluster. *Proc Natl Acad Sci USA* 2003;100:4060–5.

38 Natale M, Bisson C, Monti G, *et al.* Cow's milk allergens identification by two-dimensional immunoblotting and mass spectrometry. *Mol Nutr Food Res* 2004;48:363–9.

39 Reese G, Tracey D, Daul CB, *et al.* IgE and monoclonal antibody reactivities to the major shrimp allergen Pen a 1 (tropomyosin) and vertebrate tropomyosins. *Adv Exp Med Biol* 1996;409:225–30.

40 Yu CJ, Lin YF, Chiang BL, Chow LP. Proteomics and immunological analysis of a novel shrimp allergen, Pen m 2. *J Immunol* 2003;170:445–53.

41 Asturias JA, Eraso E, Arilla MC, *et al.* Cloning, isolation, and IgE-binding properties of Helix aspersa (brown garden snail) tropomyosin. *Int Arch Allergy Immunol* 2002;128:90–6.

42 Miyazawa H, Fukamachi H, Inagaki Y, *et al.* Identification of the first major allergen of a squid (*Todarodes pacificus*). *J Allergy Clin Immunol* 1996;98:948–53.

43 Leung PS, Chu KH. cDNA cloning and molecular identification of the major oyster allergen from the Pacific oyster Crassostrea gigas. *Clin Exp Allergy* 2001;31:1287–94.

44 Leung PS, Chen YC, Gershwin ME, *et al.* Identification and molecular characterization of Charybdis feriatus tropomyosin, the major crab allergen. *J Allergy Clin Immunol* 1998;102:847–52.

45 Chu KH, Wong SH, Leung PS. Tropomyosin is the major mollusk allergen: reverse transcriptase polymerase chain reaction, Expression and IgE Reactivity. *Mar Biotechnol (NY)* 2000;2:499–509.

46 Van Do T, Hordvik I, Endresen C, *et al.* The major allergen (parvalbumin) of codfish is encoded by at least two isotypic genes: cDNA cloning, expression and antibody binding of the recombinant allergens. *Mol Immunol* 2003;39:595–602.

47 Swoboda I, Bugajska-Schretter A, Verdino P, *et al.* Recombinant carp parvalbumin, the major cross-reactive fish allergen: a tool for diagnosis and therapy of fish allergy. *J Immunol* 2002;168:4576–84.

48 Lindstrom CD, van Do T, Hordvik I, *et al.* Cloning of two distinct cDNAs encoding parvalbumin, the major allergen of Atlantic salmon (*Salmo salar*). *Scand J Immunol* 1996;44:335–44.

49 Shiomi K, Hamada Y, Sekiguchi K, *et al.* Two classes of allergens, parvalbumins and higher molecular weight substances, in Japanese eel and bigeye tuna. *Fish Sci* 1999;65:943–8.

50 Bernard H, Creminon C, Yvon M, *et al.* Specificity of the human IgE response to the different purified caseins in allergy to cow's milk proteins. *Int Arch Allergy Immunol* 1998;115:235–44.

51 Bellioni-Businco B, Paganelli R, Lucenti P, *et al.* Allergenicity of goat's milk in children with cow's milk allergy. *J Allergy Clin Immunol* 1999;103:1191–4.

52 Spuergin P, Walter M, Schiltz E, *et al.* Allergenicity of alpha-caseins from cow, sheep, and goat. *Allergy* 1997;52:293–8.

53 Businco L, Giampietro PG, Lucenti P, *et al.* Allergenicity of mare's milk in children with cow's milk allergy. *J Allergy Clin Immunol* 2000;105:1031–4.

54 Restani P, Gaiaschi A, Plebani A, *et al.* Cross-reactivity between milk proteins from different animal species. *Clin Exp Allergy* 1999;29:997–1004.

55 Flower DR. The lipocalin protein family: structure and function. *Biochem J* 1996;318:1–14.

56 Virtanen T. Lipocalin allergens. *Allergy* 2001;56:48–51.

57 Nitta K, Sugai S. The evolution of lysozyme and alpha-lactalbumin. *Eur J Biochem* 1989;182:111–8.

58 Aabin B, Poulsen LK, Ebbehoj K, *et al.* Identification of IgE-binding egg white proteins: comparison of results obtained by different methods. *Int Arch Allergy Immunol* 1996;109:50–7.

59 Holen E, Elsayed S. Characterization of four major allergens of hen egg-white by IEF/SDS-PAGE combined with electrophoretic transfer and IgE-immunoautoradiography. *Int Arch Allergy Appl Immunol* 1990;91:136–41.

60 van Gent D, Sharp P, Morgan K, Kalsheker N. Serpins: structure, function and molecular evolution. *Int J Biochem Cell Biol* 2003;35:1536–47.

61 Bernhisel-Broadbent J, Dintzis HM, Dintzis RZ, Sampson HA. Allergenicity and antigenicity of chicken egg ovomucoid (Gal d III)

compared with ovalbumin (Gal d I) in children with egg allergy and in mice. *J Allergy Clin Immunol* 1994;93:1047–59.

62 Binder M, Mahler V, Hayek B, *et al*. Molecular and immunological characterization of arginine kinase from the Indianmeal moth, Plodia interpunctella, a novel cross-reactive invertebrate pan-allergen. *J Immunol* 2001;167:5470–7.

63 Laskowski Jr M, Kato I, Ardelt W, *et al*. Ovomucoid third domains from 100 avian species: isolation, sequences, and hypervariability of enzyme-inhibitor contact residues. *Biochemistry* 1987;26:202–21.

64 Kato I, Schrode J, Kohr WJ, Laskowski Jr. M. Chicken ovomucoid: determination of its amino acid sequence, determination of the trypsin reactive site, and preparation of all three of its domains. *Biochemistry* 1987;26:193–201.

65 Cooke SK, Sampson HA. Allergenic properties of ovomucoid in man. *J Immunol* 1997;159:2026–32.

66 Kreis M, Forde BG, Rahman S, *et al*. Molecular evolution of the seed storage proteins of barley, rye and wheat. *J Mol Biol* 1985;183:499–502.

67 Palosuo K, Alenius H, Varjonen E, *et al*. A novel wheat gliadin as a cause of exercise-induced anaphylaxis. *J Allergy Clin Immunol* 1999;103:912–17.

68 Palosuo K, Varjonen E, Kekki OM, *et al*. Wheat omega-5 gliadin is a major allergen in children with immediate allergy to ingested wheat. *J Allergy Clin Immunol* 2001;108:634–8.

69 Maruyama N, Ichise K, Katsube T, *et al*. Identification of major wheat allergens by means of the Escherichia coli expression system. *Eur J Biochem* 1998;255:739–45.

70 Sanchez-Monge R, Lombardero M, Garcia-Selles FJ, *et al*. Lipid-transfer proteins are relevant allergens in fruit allergy. *J Allergy Clin Immunol* 1999;103:514–9.

71 Pastorello EA, D'Ambrosio FP, Pravettoni V, *et al*. Evidence for a lipid transfer protein as the major allergen of apricot. *J Allergy Clin Immunol* 2000;105:371–7.

72 Scheurer S, Pastorello EA, Wangorsch A, *et al*. Recombinant allergens Pru av 1 and Pru av 4 and a newly identified lipid transfer protein in the *in vitro* diagnosis of cherry allergy. *J Allergy Clin Immunol* 2001;107:724–31.

73 Pastorello EA, Farioli L, Pravettoni V, *et al*. The major allergen of peach (Prunus persica) is a lipid transfer protein. *J Allergy Clin Immunol* 1999;103:520–6.

74 Pastorello EA, Farioli L, Pravettoni V, *et al*. Characterization of the major allergen of plum as a lipid transfer protein. *J Chromatogr B Biomed Sci Appl* 2001;756:95–103.

75 Zuidmeer L, Salentijn E, Rivas MF, *et al*. The role of profilin and lipid transfer protein in strawberry allergy in the Mediterranean area. *Clin Exp Allergy* 2006;36:666–75.

76 Ahrazem O, Ibanez MD, Lopez-Torrejon G, *et al*. Orange germin-like glycoprotein Cit s 1: an equivocal allergen. *Int Arch Allergy Immunol* 2006;139:96–103.

77 Pastorello EA, Farioli L, Pravettoni V, *et al*. Identification of grape and wine allergens as an endochitinase 4, a lipid-transfer protein, and a thaumatin. *J Allergy Clin Immunol* 2003;111:350–9.

78 Sanchez-Monge R, Blanco C, Lopez-Torrejon G, *et al*. Differential allergen sensitization patterns in chestnut allergy with or without associated latex-fruit syndrome. *J Allergy Clin Immunol* 2006;118:705–10.

79 Asero R, Mistrello G, Roncarolo D, *et al*. Allergy to minor allergens of Brazil nut. *Allergy* 2002;57:1080–1.

80 Pastorello EA, Farioli L, Pravettoni V, *et al*. Lipid transfer protein and vicilin are important walnut allergens in patients not allergic to pollen. *J Allergy Clin Immunol* 2004;114:908–14.

81 Schocker F, Luttkopf D, Scheurer S, *et al*. Recombinant lipid transfer protein Cor a 8 from hazelnut: a new tool for *in vitro* diagnosis of potentially severe hazelnut allergy. *J Allergy Clin Immunol* 2004;113:141–7.

82 Diaz-Perales A, Tabar AI, Sanchez-Monge R, *et al*. Characterization of asparagus allergens: a relevant role of lipid transfer proteins. *J Allergy Clin Immunol* 2002;110:790–6.

83 San Miguel-Moncin M, Krail M, Scheurer S, *et al*. Lettuce anaphylaxis: identification of a lipid transfer protein as the major allergen. *Allergy* 2003;58:511–7.

84 Palacin A, Cumplido J, Figueroa J, *et al*. Cabbage lipid transfer protein Bra o 3 is a major allergen responsible for cross-reactivity between plant foods and pollens. *J Allergy Clin Immunol* 2006;117:1423–9.

85 Pastorello EA, Farioli L, Pravettoni V, *et al*. The maize major allergen, which is responsible for food-induced allergic reactions, is a lipid transfer protein. *J Allergy Clin Immunol* 2000;106:744–51.

86 Curioni A, Santucci B, Cristaudo A, *et al*. Urticaria from beer: an immediate hypersensitivity reaction due to a 10-kDa protein derived from barley. *Clin Exp Allergy* 1999;29:407–13.

87 Nakase M, Adachi T, Urisu A, *et al*. Rice (Oryza sativa L.) alpha amylase inhibitors of 14–16 kDa are potential allergens and products of a multi gene family. *J Agric Food Chem* 1996;44:2624–8.

88 Alvarez AM, Adachi T, Nakase M, *et al*. Classification of rice allergenic protein cDNAs belonging to the alpha-amylase/trypsin inhibitor gene family. *Biochim Biophys Acta* 1995;1251:201–4.

89 Izumi H, Adachi T, Fujii N, *et al*. Nucleotide sequence of a cDNA clone encoding a major allergenic protein in rice seeds. Homology of the deduced amino acid sequence with members of alpha-amylase/trypsin inhibitor family. *FEBS Lett* 1992;302:213–16.

90 Teuber SS, Dandekar AM, Peterson WR, Sellers CL. Cloning and sequencing of a gene encoding a 2S albumin seed storage protein precursor from English walnut (Juglans regia), a major food allergen. *J Allergy Clin Immunol* 1998;101:807–14.

91 Poltronieri P, Cappello MS, Dohmae N, *et al*. Identification and characterisation of the IgE-binding proteins 2S albumin and conglutin gamma in almond (Prunus dulcis) seeds. *Int Arch Allergy Immunol* 2002;128:97–104.

92 Pastorello EA, Farioli L, Pravettoni V, *et al*. Sensitization to the major allergen of Brazil nut is correlated with the clinical expression of allergy. *J Allergy Clin Immunol*. 1998;102:1021–7.

93 Robotham JM, Wang F, Seamon V, *et al*. Ana o 3, an important cashew nut (Anacardium occidentale L.) allergen of the 2S albumin family. *J Allergy Clin Immunol* 2005;115:1284–90.

94 Menendez-Arias L, Moneo I, Dominguez J, Rodriguez R. Primary structure of the major allergen of yellow mustard (Sinapis alba L.) seed, Sin a I. *Eur J Biochem* 1988;177:159–66.

95 Monsalve RI, Gonzalez de la Pena MA, Menendez-Arias L, et al. Characterization of a new oriental-mustard (Brassica juncea) allergen, Bra j IE: detection of an allergenic epitope. *Biochem J* 1993;293:625–32.

96 Vioque J, Sanchez-Vioque R, Clemente A, et al. Purification and partial characterization of chickpea 2S albumin. *J Agric Food Chem* 1999;47:1405–9.

97 Burks AW, Williams LW, Connaughton C, et al. Identification and characterization of a second major peanut allergen, Ara h II, with use of the sera of patients with atopic dermatitis and positive peanut challenge. *J Allergy Clin Immunol* 1992;90:962–9.

98 Kleber-Janke T, Crameri R, Appenzeller U, et al. Selective cloning of peanut allergens, including profilin and 2S albumins, by phage display technology. *Int Arch Allergy Immunol* 1999;119:265–74.

99 Stanley JS, King N, Burks AW, et al. Identification and mutational analysis of the immunodominant IgE binding epitopes of the major peanut allergen Ara h 2. *Arch Biochem Biophys* 1997;342:244–53.

100 Pastorello EA, Varin E, Farioli L, et al. The major allergen of sesame seeds (Sesamum indicum) is a 2S albumin. *J Chromatogr B Biomed Sci Appl* 2001;756:85–93.

101 Beyer K, Bardina L, Grishina G, Sampson HA. Identification of sesame seed allergens by 2-dimensional proteomics and Edman sequencing: seed storage proteins as common food allergens. *J Allergy Clin Immunol* 2002;110:154–9.

102 Kelly JD, Hlywka JJ, Hefle SL. Identification of sunflower seed IgE-binding proteins. *Int Arch Allergy Immunol* 2000;121:19–24.

103 Vanek-Krebitz M, Hoffmann-Sommergruber K, Laimer da Camara Machado M, et al. Cloning and sequencing of Mal d 1, the major allergen from apple (Malus domestica), and its immunological relationship to Bet v 1, the major birch pollen allergen. *Biochem Biophys Res Commun* 1995;214:538–51.

104 Karamloo F, Scheurer S, Wangorsch A, et al. Pyr c 1, the major allergen from pear (Pyrus communis), is a new member of the Bet v 1 allergen family. *J Chromatogr B Biomed Sci Appl* 2001;756:281–93.

105 Scheurer S, Metzner K, Haustein D, et al. Molecular cloning, expression and characterization of Pru a 1, the major cherry allergen. *Mol Immunol* 1997;34:619–29.

106 Karlsson AL, Alm R, Ekstrand B, et al. Bet v 1 homologues in strawberry identified as IgE-binding proteins and presumptive allergens. *Allergy* 2004;59:1277–84.

107 Hoffmann-Sommergruber K, O'Riordain G, Ahorn H, et al. Molecular characterization of Dau c 1, the Bet v 1 homologous protein from carrot and its cross-reactivity with Bet v 1 and Api g 1. *Clin Exp Allergy* 1999;29:840–7.

108 Breiteneder H, Hoffmann-Sommergruber K, O'Riordain G, et al. Molecular characterization of Api g 1, the major allergen of celery (Apium graveolens), and its immunological and structural relationships to a group of 17-kDa tree pollen allergens. *Eur J Biochem* 1995;233:484–9.

109 Luttkopf D, Muller U, Skov PS, et al. Comparison of four variants of a major allergen in hazelnut (Corylus avellana) Cor a 1.04 with the major hazel pollen allergen Cor a 1.01. *Mol Immunol* 2002;38:515–25.

110 Mittag D, Vieths S, Vogel L, et al. Soybean allergy in patients allergic to birch pollen: clinical investigation and molecular characterization of allergens. *J Allergy Clin Immunol* 2004;113:148–54.

111 Burks AW, Williams LW, Helm RM, et al. Identification of a major peanut allergen, Ara h I, in patients with atopic dermatitis and positive peanut challenges. *J Allergy Clin Immunol* 1991;88:172–9.

112 Ogawa T, Bando N, Tsuji H, et al. Alpha-subunit of beta-conglycinin, an allergenic protein recognized by IgE antibodies of soybean-sensitive patients with atopic dermatitis. *Biosci Biotechnol Biochem* 1995;59:831–3.

113 Kondo Y, Urisu A, Wada E, et al. [Allergen analysis of buckwheat by the immunoblotting method]. *Arerugi* 1993;42:142–8.

114 Teuber SS, Jarvis KC, Dandekar AM, et al. Identification and cloning of a complementary DNA encoding a vicilin-like proprotein, jug r 2, from English walnut kernel (Juglans regia), a major food allergen. *J Allergy Clin Immunol* 1999;104:1311–20.

115 Lauer I, Foetisch K, Kolarich D, et al. Hazelnut (Corylus avellana) vicilin Cor a 11: molecular characterization of a glycoprotein and its allergenic activity. *Biochem J* 2004;383:327–34.

116 Wang F, Robotham JM, Teuber SS, et al. Ana o 1, a cashew (Anacardium occidental) allergen of the vicilin seed storage protein family. *J Allergy Clin Immunol* 2002;110:160–6.

117 Rabjohn P, Helm EM, Stanley JS, et al. Molecular cloning and epitope analysis of the peanut allergen Ara h 3. *J Clin Invest* 1999;103:535–42.

118 Beardslee TA, Zeece MG, Sarath G, et al. Soybean glycinin G1 acidic chain shares IgE epitopes with peanut allergen Ara h 3. *Int Arch Allergy Immunol* 2000;123:299–307.

119 Garcia-Mas J, Messeguer R, Arus P, et al. Molecular characterization of cDNAs corresponding to genes expressed during almond (Prunusamygdalus Batsch) seed development. *Plant Mol Biol* 1995;27:205–10.

120 Roux KH, Teuber SS, Robotham JM, et al. Detection and stability of the major almond allergen in foods. *J Agric Food Chem* 2001;49:2131–6.

121 Wang F, Robotham JM, Teuber SS, et al. Ana o 2, a major cashew (Anacardium occidentale L.) nut allergen of the legumin family. *Int Arch Allergy Immunol* 2003;132:27–39.

122 Pastorello EA, Conti A, Pravettoni V, et al. Identification of actinidin as the major allergen of kiwi fruit. *J Allergy Clin Immunol* 1998;101:531–7.

123 Ogawa T, Tsuji H, Bando N, et al. Identification of the soybean allergenic protein, Gly m Bd 30K, with the soybean seed 34-kDa oil-body-associated protein. *Biosci Biotechnol Biochem* 1993;57:1030–3.

124 Tassin-Moindrot S, Caille A, Douliez JP, et al. The wide binding properties of a wheat nonspecific lipid transfer protein. Solution structure of a complex with prostaglandin B2. *Eur J Biochem* 2000;267:1117–24.

125 Douliez JP, Jegou S, Pato C, et al. Binding of two monoacylated lipid monomers by the barley lipid transfer protein,

LTP1, as viewed by fluorescence, isothermal titration calorimetry and molecular modelling. *Eur J Biochem* 2001;268: 384–8.

126 Pastorello EA, Pompei C, Pravettoni V, *et al*. Lipid-transfer protein is the major maize allergen maintaining IgE-binding activity after cooking at 100 degrees C, as demonstrated in anaphylactic patients and patients with positive double-blind, placebo-controlled food challenge results. *J Allergy Clin Immunol* 2003;112:775–83.

127 Sancho AI, Rigby NM, Zuidmeer L, *et al*. The effect of thermal processing on the IgE reactivity of the non-specific lipid transfer protein from apple, Mal d 3. *Allergy* 2005;60:1262–8.

128 Moreno FJ, Mellon FA, Wickham MS, *et al*. Stability of the major allergen Brazil nut 2S albumin (Ber e 1) to physiologically relevant *in vitro* gastrointestinal digestion. *FEBS J* 2005;272:341–52.

129 Asero R, Mistrello G, Roncarolo D, *et al*. Lipid transfer protein: a pan-allergen in plant-derived foods that is highly resistant to pepsin digestion. *Int Arch Allergy Immunol* 2000;122:20–32.

130 Vassilopoulou E, Rigby N, Moreno FJ, *et al*. Effect of *in vitro* gastric and duodenal digestion on the allergenicity of grape lipid transfer protein. *J Allergy Clin Immunol* 2006;118:473–80.

131 Shewry PR, Halford NG, Belton PS, Tatham AS. The structure and properties of gluten: an elastic protein from wheat grain. *Philos Trans Roy Soc Lond B Biol Sci* 2002;357:133–42.

132 Matsuo H, Morita E, Tatham AS, *et al*. Identification of the IgE-binding epitope in omega-5 gliadin, a major allergen in wheat-dependent exercise-induced anaphylaxis. *J Biol Chem* 2004;279:12135–40.

133 Watanabe M, Tanabe S, Suzuki T, *et al*. Primary structure of an allergenic peptide occurring in the chymotryptic hydrolysate of gluten. *Biosci Biotechnol Biochem* 1995;59:1596–7.

134 Tanabe S, Arai S, Yanagihara Y, *et al*. A major wheat allergen has a Gln-Gln-Gln-Pro-Pro motif identified as an IgE-binding epitope. *Biochem Biophys Res Commun* 1996;219:290–3.

135 Simonato B, Pasini G, Giannattasio M, *et al*. Food allergy to wheat products: the effect of bread baking and *in vitro* digestion on wheat allergenic proteins. A study with bread dough, crumb, and crust. *J Agric Food Chem* 2001;49:5668–73.

136 Simonato B, De Lazzari F, Pasini G, *et al*. IgE binding to soluble and insoluble wheat flour proteins in atopic and non-atopic patients suffering from gastrointestinal symptoms after wheat ingestion. *Clin Exp Allergy* 2001;31:1771–8.

137 Carbonero P, García-Olmedo F. *A Multigene Family of Trypsin/Alpha-Amylase Inhibitors from Cereals*. Dordrecht, The Netherlands: Kluwer Academic Publishers, 1999.

138 James JM, Sixbey JP, Helm RM, *et al*. Wheat alpha-amylase inhibitor: a second route of allergic sensitization. *J Allergy Clin Immunol* 1997;99:239–44.

139 Shewry PR, Pandya MJ. *The 2S Albumin Storage Proteins*. Dordrecht, The Netherlands: Kluwer Academic Publishers, 1999.

140 Shibasaki M, Suzuki S, Tajima S, *et al*. Allergenicity of major component proteins of soybean. *Int Arch Allergy Appl Immunol* 1980;61:441–8.

141 Duro G, Colombo P, Costa MA, *et al*. cDNA cloning, sequence analysis and allergological characterization of Par j 2.0101, a new major allergen of the Parietaria judaica pollen. *FEBS Lett* 1996;399:295–8.

142 Tejera ML, Villalba M, Batanero E, Rodriguez R. Identification, isolation, and characterization of Ole e 7, a new allergen of olive tree pollen. *J Allergy Clin Immunol* 1999;104:797–802.

143 Pastorello EA, Farioli L, Robino AM, *et al*. A lipid transfer protein involved in occupational sensitization to spelt. *J Allergy Clin Immunol* 2001;108:145–6.

144 Pastorello EA, Vieths S, Pravettoni V, *et al*. Identification of hazelnut major allergens in sensitive patients with positive double-blind, placebo-controlled food challenge results. *J Allergy Clin Immunol* 2002;109:563–70.

145 Mills ENC, Jenkins JA, Bannon GA. *Plant Seed Globulin Allergens*. Oxford: Blackwell Publishing, 2004.

146 Burks Jr AW, Brooks JR, Sampson HA. Allergenicity of major component proteins of soybean determined by enzyme-linked immunosorbent assay (ELISA) and immunoblotting in children with atopic dermatitis and positive soy challenges. *J Allergy Clin Immunol* 1988;81:1135–42.

147 Lopez-Torrejon G, Salcedo G, Martin-Esteban M, *et al*. Len c 1, a major allergen and vicilin from lentil seeds: protein isolation and cDNA cloning. *J Allergy Clin Immunol* 2003;112:1208–15.

148 Roux KH, Teuber SS, Sathe SK. Tree nut allergens. *Int Arch Allergy Immunol* 2003;131:234–44.

149 Beyer K, Grishina G, Bardina L, *et al*. Identification of an 11S globulin as a major hazelnut food allergen in hazelnut-induced systemic reactions. *J Allergy Clin Immunol* 2002;110:517–23.

150 Mills EN, Huang L, Noel TR, *et al*. Formation of thermally induced aggregates of the soya globulin beta-conglycinin. *Biochim Biophys Acta* 2001;1547:339–50.

151 Mills EN, Marigheto NA, Wellner N, *et al*. Thermally induced structural changes in glycinin, the 11S globulin of soya bean (*Glycine max*) – an *in situ* spectroscopic study. *Biochim Biophys Acta* 2003;1648:105–14.

152 Yamauchi F, Yamagishi T, Iwabuchi S. Molecular understanding of heat-induced phenomena of soybean protein. *Food Rev Intt* 1991;7:283–322.

153 Maleki SJ, Kopper RA, Shin DS, *et al*. Structure of the major peanut allergen Ara h 1 may protect IgE-binding epitopes from degradation. *J Immunol* 2000;164:5844–9.

154 Kopper RA, Odum NJ, Sen M, *et al*. Peanut protein allergens: gastric digestion is carried out exclusively by pepsin. *J Allergy Clin Immunol* 2004;114:614–8.

155 Shin DS, Compadre CM, Maleki SJ, *et al*. Biochemical and structural analysis of the IgE binding sites on ara h1, an abundant and highly allergenic peanut protein. *J Biol Chem* 1998;273:13753–9.

156 Eiwegger T, Rigby N, Mondoulet L, *et al*. Gastro-duodenal digestion products of the major peanut allergen Ara h 1 retain an allergenic potential. *Clin Exp Allergy* 2006;36:1281–8.

157 Vieths S, Scheurer S, Ballmer-Weber B. Current understanding of cross-reactivity of food allergens and pollen. *Ann NY Acad Sci* 2002;964:47–68.

158 Mittag D, Akkerdaas J, Ballmer-Weber BK, *et al.* Ara h 8, a Bet v 1-homologous allergen from peanut, is a major allergen in patients with combined birch pollen and peanut allergy. *J Allergy Clin Immunol* 2004;114:1410–17.

159 Mittag D, Vieths S, Vogel L, *et al.* Birch pollen-related food allergy to legumes: identification and characterization of the Bet v 1 homologue in mungbean (*Vigna radiata*), Vig r 1. *Clin Exp Allergy* 2005;35:1049–55.

160 Bolhaar ST, van Ree R, Ma Y, *et al.* Severe allergy to sharon fruit caused by birch pollen. *Int Arch Allergy Immunol* 2005;136:45–52.

161 Bolhaar ST, Ree R, Bruijnzeel-Koomen CA, *et al.* Allergy to jackfruit: a novel example of Bet v 1-related food allergy. *Allergy* 2004;59:1187–92.

162 Breiteneder H, Pettenburger K, Bito A, *et al.* The gene coding for the major birch pollen allergen Betv1, is highly homologous to a pea disease resistance response gene. *EMBO J* 1989;8:1935–8.

163 Hoffmann-Sommergruber K. Plant allergens and pathogenesis-related proteins. What do they have in common? *Int Arch Allergy Immunol* 2000;122:155–66.

164 Markovic-Housley Z, Degano M, Lamba D, *et al.* Crystal structure of a hypoallergenic isoform of the major birch pollen allergen Bet v 1 and its likely biological function as a plant steroid carrier. *J Mol Biol* 2003;325:123–33.

165 Gajhede M, Osmark P, Poulsen FM, *et al.* X-ray and NMR structure of Bet v 1, the origin of birch pollen allergy. *Nat Struct Biol* 1996;3:1040–5.

166 Neudecker P, Schweimer K, Nerkamp J, *et al.* Allergic cross-reactivity made visible: solution structure of the major cherry allergen Pru av 1. *J Biol Chem* 2001;276:22756–63.

167 Schirmer T, Hoffimann-Sommergrube K, Susani M, *et al.* Crystal structure of the major celery allergen Api g 1: molecular analysis of cross-reactivity. *J Mol Biol* 2005;351:1101–9.

168 Bohle B, Radakovics A, Jahn-Schmid B, *et al.* Bet v 1, the major birch pollen allergen, initiates sensitization to Api g 1, the major allergen in celery: evidence at the T cell level. *Eur J Immunol* 2003;33:3303–10.

169 Reekers R, Busche M, Wittmann M, *et al.* Birch pollen-related foods trigger atopic dermatitis in patients with specific cutaneous T-cell responses to birch pollen antigens. *J Allergy Clin Immunol* 1999;104:466–72.

170 Schimek EM, Zwolfer B, Briza P, *et al.* Gastrointestinal digestion of Bet v 1-homologous food allergens destroys their mediator-releasing, but not T cell-activating, capacity. *J Allergy Clin Immunol* 2005;116:1327–33.

171 Bohle B, Zwolfer B, Heratizadeh A, *et al.* Cooking birch pollen-related food: divergent consequences for IgE- and T cell-mediated reactivity *in vitro* and *in vivo*. *J Allergy Clin Immunol* 2006;118:242–9.

172 Henrissat B. A classification of glycosyl hydrolases based on amino acid sequence similarities. *Biochem J* 1991;280:309–16.

173 Kasprzewska A. Plant chitinases – regulation and function. *Cell Mol Biol Lett* 2003;8:809–24.

174 Beintema JJ. Structural features of plant chitinases and chitin-binding proteins. *FEBS Lett* 1994;350:159–63.

175 Salcedo G, Diaz-Perales A, Sanchez-Monge R. The role of plant panallergens in sensitization to natural rubber latex. *Curr Opin Allergy Clin Immunol* 2001;1:177–83.

176 Sowka S, Hsieh LS, Krebitz M, *et al.* Identification and cloning of prs a 1, a 32-kDa endochitinase and major allergen of avocado, and its expression in the yeast *Pichia pastoris*. *J Biol Chem* 199823;273:28091–7.

177 Sanchez-Monge R, Blanco C, Diaz-Perales A, *et al.* Isolation and characterization of major banana allergens: identification as fruit class I chitinases. *Clin Exp Allergy* 1999;29:673–80.

178 Diaz-Perales A, Collada C, Blanco C, *et al.* Class I chitinases with hevein-like domain, but not class II enzymes, are relevant chestnut and avocado allergens. *J Allergy Clin Immunol* 1998;102:127–33.

179 Diaz-Perales A, Blanco C, Sanchez-Monge R, *et al.* Analysis of avocado allergen (Prs a 1) IgE-binding peptides generated by simulated gastric fluid digestion. *J Allergy Clin Immunol* 2003;112:1002–7.

180 Breiteneder H, Mills EN. Molecular properties of food allergens. *J Allergy Clin Immunol* 2005;115:14–23; quiz 4.

181 Rawlings ND, Barrett AJ. Evolutionary families of peptidases. *Biochem J* 1993;290:205–18.

182 Kalinski A, Weisemann JM, Matthews BF, *et al.* Molecular cloning of a protein associated with soybean seed oil bodies that is similar to thiol proteases of the papain family. *J Biol Chem* 1990;265:13843–8.

183 Radauer C, Willerroider M, Fuchs H, *et al.* Cross-reactive and species-specific immunoglobulin E epitopes of plant profilins: an experimental and structure-based analysis. *Clin Exp Allergy* 2006;36:920–9.

184 Witke W. The role of profilin complexes in cell motility and other cellular processes. *Trends Cell Biol* 2004;14:461–9.

185 Radauer C, Hoffimann-Sommergrube K. *Profilins*. Oxford: Blackwell Publishing, 2004.

186 Thorn KS, Christensen HE, Shigeta R, *et al.* The crystal structure of a major allergen from plants. *Structure* 1997; 5:19–32.

187 Fedorov AA, Ball T, Mahoney NM, *et al.* The molecular basis for allergen cross-reactivity: crystal structure and IgE-epitope mapping of birch pollen profilin. *Structure* 1997;5:33–45.

188 Mari A. Multiple pollen sensitization: a molecular approach to the diagnosis. *Int Arch Allergy Immunol* 2001;125:57–65.

189 Asero R, Mistrello G, Roncarolo D, *et al.* Detection of clinical markers of sensitization to profilin in patients allergic to plant-derived foods. *J Allergy Clin Immunol* 2003;112:427–32.

190 Wensing M, Akkerdaas JH, van Leeuwen WA, *et al.* IgE to Bet v 1 and profilin: cross-reactivity patterns and clinical relevance. *J Allergy Clin Immunol* 2002;110:435–42.

191 Valenta R, Duchene M, Pettenburger K, *et al.* Identification of profilin as a novel pollen allergen; IgE autoreactivity in sensitized individuals. *Science* 1991;253:557–60.

192 Moroz LA, Yang WH. Kunitz soybean trypsin inhibitor: a specific allergen in food anaphylaxis. *N Engl J Med* 1980;302: 1126–8.

193 Burks AW, Cockrell G, Connaughton C, *et al.* Identification of peanut agglutinin and soybean trypsin inhibitor as minor legume allergens. *Int Arch Allergy Immunol* 1994;105:143–9.

194 Seppala U, Majamaa H, Turjanmaa K, *et al.* Identification of four novel potato (*Solanum tuberosum*) allergens belonging to the family of soybean trypsin inhibitors. *Allergy* 2001;56:619–26.

195 van Loon LC, Rep M, Pieterse CM. Significance of inducible defense-related proteins in infected plants. *Annu Rev Phytopathol* 2006;44:135–62.

196 Krebitz M, Wagner B, Ferreira F, *et al.* Plant-based heterologous expression of Mal d 2, a thaumatin-like protein and allergen of apple (*Malus domestica*), and its characterization as an antifungal protein. *J Mol Biol* 2003;329:721–30.

197 Fuchs HC, Hoffmann-Sommergrube K, Wagner B, *et al.* Heterologous expression in Nicotiana benthamiana of Cap a 1, a thaumatin-like protein and major allergen from bell pepper (*Capsicum annuum*). *J Allergy Clin Immunol* 2002;109(S):134–5.

198 Inschlag C, Hoffmann-Sommergruber K, O'Riordain G, *et al.* Biochemical characterization of Pru a 2, a 23-kD thaumatin-like protein representing a potential major allergen in cherry (*Prunus avium*). *Int Arch Allergy Immunol* 1998;116:22–8.

199 Fuchs HC, Bohle B, Dall'Antonia Y, *et al.* Natural and recombinant molecules of the cherry allergen Pru av 2 show diverse structural and B cell characteristics but similar T cell reactivity. *Clin Exp Allergy* 2006;36:359–68.

200 Gavrovic-Jankulovic M, cIrkovic T, Vuckovic O, *et al.* Isolation and biochemical characterization of a thaumatin-like kiwi allergen. *J Allergy Clin Immunol* 2002;110:805–10.

201 Roberts WK, Selitrennikoff CP. Zeamatin, an antifungal protein from maize with membrane-permeabilizing activity. *J Gen Microbiol* 1990;136:1771–8.

202 Flamini R, De Rosso M. Mass spectrometry in the analysis of grape and wine proteins. *Expert Rev Proteomics* 2006;3:321–31.

203 Lack G, Golding J. Peanut and nut allergy. Reduced exposure might increase allergic sensitisation. *BMJ* 1996;313:300.

204 Strid J, Thomson M, Hourihane J, *et al.* A novel model of sensitization and oral tolerance to peanut protein. *Immunology* 2004;113:293–303.

205 Strid J, Hourihane J, Kimber I, *et al.* Epicutaneous exposure to peanut protein prevents oral tolerance and enhances allergic sensitization. *Clin Exp Allergy* 2005;35:757–66.

206 Hoffmann-Sommergruber K. Pathogenesis-related (PR)-proteins identified as allergens. *Biochem Soc Trans* 2002;30:930–5.

207 Van Loon LC, Van Strien EA. The families of pathogenesis related proteins, their activities, and comparative analysis of PR-1-type proteins. *Physiol Mol Plant Pathol* 1999;5:85–97.

5

CHAPTER 5

Biotechnology and Genetic Engineering

Gary A. Bannon, James D. Astwood, Raymond C. Dobert, and Roy L. Fuchs

---

KEY CONCEPTS

- All agricultural biotechnology products are assessed for safety according to international guidelines to ensure the risk of allergy is appropriately addressed prior to their marketing, and that a consistent assessment approach is used around the world.

- The current allergy assessment process identifies the potential risks associated with the introduced protein as well as the overall allergenic risks associated with a transformed food crop.

- No single, predictive assay is capable of assessing the allergenic potential of all proteins introduced into food crops and, therefore, all aspects of the current safety assessment testing strategy need to be considered in a "weight of evidence" approach rather than relying too heavily on one test to determine protein safety.

- The protective value of current allergy testing approaches and future approaches that adopt sound risk assessment principles and new methods as they become validated, have in the past and will continue to provide robust assurances to risk managers and consumers alike for present and future biotech products.

Introduction

The population of the world is expected to increase by 2.5 billion people in the next 25 years. Food requirements for this growing population are expected to double by the year 2025. In contrast, there has been a decline in the annual rate of increase in cereal yield such that the annual rate of yield increase is below the rate of population increase [1]. In order to feed this growing population, crop yield will have to be increased and some of the increase in yield will be due to genetic engineering of foods. In addition, the incidence of food allergies appears to be on the rise, particularly in developed countries [2,3]. Genetic engineering of food crops should have little practical consequence for the occurrence, frequency, and natural history of food allergy if simple precautions are observed. Essential aspects of the health safety assessment for products derived from this technology are discussed in this chapter; and the accepted strategy for addressing any potential impact on food allergy will be reviewed in detail. It should be noted that no single, predictive assay appears to be capable of assessing the allergenic potential of all proteins introduced into food crops [4]. However, through the use of *in vivo* and *in vitro* immunological assays in combination with a comparative evaluation

relative to the characteristics of known food allergens, a sound scientific basis for allergenicity assessment has evolved. The biochemical properties of common food allergens have been described in this book and elsewhere [5,6]: allergens tend to be stable to proteolysis, tend to be abundant, tend to be resistant to heat (cooking or processing), and all have multiple IgE-binding epitopes. Thus, these factors have been used to discriminate potentially harmful allergens from safe proteins entering the food supply.

This chapter will briefly summarize the development and commercialization of food biotechnology products, the internationally recognized approach to food safety assessment for these foods, and will provide a comprehensive review of food allergy considerations in this context.

Plant biotechnology

Twenty years ago the improvement of crop productivity was a sophisticated process, albeit dependent on trial and error. Many years of meticulous observations were required to determine whether desired traits were stable in the new varieties and cultivars of food crops created by this process. Crop improvement and the science of plant breeding depended on existing intraspecies genetic variation of plants, interspecies introgression of traits from "wild" or taxonomically similar plants, and on the creation of new genetic variability by chemical or irradiation mutagenesis. While there are limitations to these approaches, crop scientists and geneticists were

Food Allergy: Adverse Reactions to Foods and Food Additives, 4th edition.
Edited by Dean D. Metcalfe, Hugh A. Sampson, and Ronald A. Simon.
© 2008 Blackwell Publishing, ISBN: 978-1-4501-5129-0.

nevertheless able to improve crop yield and food production per unit area of agricultural land several fold by creating new and more productive crops, and by improving agronomic practices.

With the advent of molecular biology and biotechnology it became possible not only to identify a desirable phenotypic trait but also to identify the precise genetic material responsible for that genetic trait. Recombinant DNA and plant transformation techniques have made it possible to alter the composition of individual plant components (lipids, carbohydrates, proteins) beyond what is easily possible through traditional breeding practices. Direct and stable gene transfer into plants was first reported in 1984 [7,8]. Since then, at least 88 different plant species and many economically important crops have been genetically engineered [9], usually via *Agrobacterium* [10,11] or particle gun technologies [12,13].

The thrust of most first-generation biotech crops has been to improve resistance to insect predation, increase resistance to pesticides for easier weed control, confer immunity to viral pathogens, and improve ripening characteristics of fresh fruits and vegetables. These crops are essentially unchanged from the non-transformed parental crops and have no significant changes in key nutrients. To a lesser extent, products with enhanced functional or nutritional properties have appeared as a result of intended alteration of specific metabolites such as oil (lipid) profiles, amino acid composition, and starch (carbohydrate) content. However, the majority of current products have had their biggest impact on agricultural practices of producers (i.e. by reducing pesticide use, improving soil conservation practices, and reducing energy inputs on farms). The availability of these so-called "agronomic" traits has driven the adoption of biotech crops since the introduction of the first product, Flavr Savr tomato, in 1994 (Fig. 5.1). Today, over 90% of the world-wide acreage of biotech crops are agronomic traits, as shown in Table 5.1 [14]. Of the principal food crops grown worldwide in 2006, biotech soybean occupies 58.6 million hectares and maize occupies 25.2 million hectares. Herbicide tolerance has consistently been the dominant trait planted in the field followed by insect resistance and then products containing both of these traits in a stacked combination. In 2006, herbicide tolerance deployed in soybean, maize, canola, cotton, and alfalfa occupied 69.9 million hectares (68%) of the global biotech 102 million hectares, with 19.0 million hectares (19%) planted to Bt crops and 13.1 million hectares (13%) to the stacked traits of Bt and herbicide tolerance. The accumulated hectarage from 1996 to 2006 exceeded half a billion hectares at 577 million hectares (1.4 billion acres), with an unprecedented 60-fold increase between 1996 and 2006, making biotech crops the fastest adopted crop technology in recent history [14]. Over the next 5–10 years it is expected that the proportion of food biotechnology products that have been developed for nutritional and functional benefits will increase significantly [15].

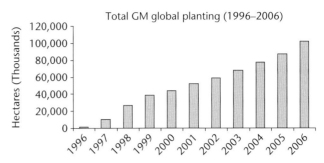

Figure 5.1 World-wide acreage of biotech crops since introduction in 1996. Based on data reported in Brooks and Barfoot [156] and James [14] and literature cited therein.

Below we describe the development of Roundup Ready soybeans to illustrate the application of agricultural biotechnology. We then briefly summarize the safety assessment procedures for food biotechnology illustrated by reference to the data developed for Roundup Ready soybeans. Following this general discussion, we provide a detailed account of current approaches and issues in allergy assessment for these products, also illustrated by the data developed for Roundup Ready soybeans.

Roundup Ready soybeans: a case study in food safety assessment

Soybean (*Glycine max*) ranks fifth in world production of major crops after wheat, maize, rice, and potato. In the United States, soybeans represent $5.6 billion in farm gate receipts [14,16]. Soybeans represent approximately one-third of all crops grown in the United States. The major food use of soybeans is the oil, whereas 96% of soybean meal is used for animal feed. Approximately 75% of vegetable food-grade oil used in foods such as shortenings, margarines, and salad/cooking oils is from soybeans. Soybean flour (meal) is used in foods such as soups, stews, beverages, desserts, bakery goods, cereals, and meat products and extenders [17]. Soybeans were the most common transgenic crop planted in 2006, representing 57% of the total acres planted with biotech traits, followed by maize (25%), cotton (13%), and canola (5%) [14]. The most common biotechnology trait was herbicide tolerance, followed by insect protection [14].

Development and benefits of Roundup Ready soybeans

The genetically engineered soybean line GTS 40-3-2 was developed to allow the use of glyphosate, the active ingredient in the wide-spectrum herbicide Roundup®, as a weed control option for soybean. This genetically engineered soybean line contains a glyphosate tolerant form of the plant enzyme 5-enolpyruvylshikimate-3-phosphate

Table 5.1 Current biotechnology food crops where FDA consultations have been completed through March 2007 (www.cfsan.fda.gov)

Crop	Introduced gene(s)	Source of gene(s)	Trait
Corn	Cry 3A	*Bacillus thuringiensis*	Resistance to corn rootworm
	cDHDPS	*Corynebacterium glutamicum*	Increase lysine level for use in animal feed
	Cry 3Bb1	*Bacillus thuringiensis*	Resistance to Colepteran insects, including corn root worm
	Cry34Ab1, Cry35Ab1/PAT	*Bacillus thuringiensis/Streptomyces iridochromogenes*	Resistance to Coleopteran insects/ tolerance to the herbicide glufosinate ammonium
	Cry 1F/PAT	*Bacillus thuringiensis/Streptomyces viridochromogenes*	Resistance to certain lepidopteran insects/ tolerance to the herbicide glufosinate
	EPSPS	*Agrobacterium*	Tolerance to the herbicide glyphosate
	Barnase	*Bacillus amyloliquefaciens*	Male sterility
	Modified EPSPS	Corn	Tolerance to the herbicide glyphosate
	Cry9C protein/PAT	*Bacillus thuringiensis/Streptomyces hygroscopicus*	Resistance to several lepidopteran insects/ tolerance to the herbicide glufosinate
	DAM/PAT	*Escherichia coli/Streptomyces viridochromogenes*	Male sterility/tolerance to glufosinate
	CrylAc	*Bacillus thuringiensis*	Resistance to European corn borer
	CrylAb/EPSPS	*Bacillus thuringiensis/ Agrobacterium*	Resistance to European corn borer; tolerance to the herbicide glyphosate
	CrylAb	*Bacillus thuringiensis*	Resistance to European corn borer
	Barnase/PAT	*Bacillus amyloliquefaciens/ Streptomyces hygroscopicus*	Male sterility/tolerance to glufosinate
	PAT	*Streptomyces hygroscopicus*	Tolerance to glufosinate
Canola	**Nitrilase**	*Klebsiella ozaenae*	Tolerance to the herbicide bromoxynil
	Phytase	*Aspergillus niger*	Degradation of phytate in animal feed
	Barnase/PAT	*Bacillus amyloliquefaciens/ Streptomyces hygroscopicus*	Male sterility/tolerance to glufosinate
	Barstar/PAT	*Bacillus amyloliquefaciens/ Streptomyces hygroscopicus*	Fertility restorer/tolerance to glufosinate
	PAT	*Streptomyces hygroscopicus*	Tolerance to glufosinate
	12:0 Acyl carrier protein thioesterase	*Umbellularia californica*	**High laurate canola oil**
	EPSPS/GOX	*Agrobacterium* sp. strain CP4, *Achromobacter*	Tolerance to the herbicide glyphosate
Soybean	PAT	*Streptomyces hygroscopicus*	Tolerance to glufosinate
	GmFad2-1 gene	Soybean	High oleic acid soybean oil
	EPSPS	*Agrobacterium* sp. strain CP4	Tolerance to the herbicide glyphosate
Cotton	Nitrilase/Cry1Ac protein	*Klebsiella pneumoniae/ Bacillus thuringiensis*	Tolerance to bromoxynil/resistance to certain lepidopteran insects
	Cry2ab; Cry1ac	*Bacillus thuringiensis*	Resistance to lepidopteran insects
	ALS	*Nicotiana tabacum*	Tolerance to the herbicide sulfonylurea
	EPSPS	*Agrobacterium* sp. strain CP4	Tolerance to the herbicide glyphosate
	Cry1F/PAT	*Bacillus thuringiensis/Streptomyces viridochromogenes*	Resistance to lepidopteran insects/ tolerance to the herbicide glufosinate ammonium
	VIP3A protein	*Bacillus thuringiensis*	Resistance to lepidopteran insects
	CrylAc protein	*Bacillus thuringiensis*	Resistance to cotton bollworm, pink bollworm, and tobacco budworm
	Nitrilase	*Klebsiella ozaenae*	Tolerance to the herbicide bromoxynil
Sugarbeet	EPSPS	*Agrobacterium* sp. strain CP4	Tolerance to the herbicide glyphosate
	PAT	*Streptomyces hygroscopicus*	Tolerance to glufosinate

(Continued)

Table 5.1 (*Continued*)

Crop	Introduced gene(s)	Source of gene(s)	Trait
Tomato	**CrylAc protein**	*Bacillus thuringiensis*	Resistance to certain lepidopteran insects
	S-adenosylmethionine hydrolase	*Escherichia coli* bacteriophage T3	Delayed fruit ripening due to reduced ethylene synthesis
	ACCS gene fragment	**Tomato**	Delayed ripening due to reduced ethylene synthesis
	PG	**Tomato**	Delayed softening due to reduced pectin degradation
	ACCD	Pseudomonas chloraphis	Delayed softening due to reduced ethylene synthesis
	PG antisense gene	**Tomato**	Delayed softening due to reduced pectin degradation
Potato	CrylIIA/PVY coat protein	*Bacillus thuringiensis*/PVY	Resistance to Colorado potato beetle and PVY
	CrylIIA/PLRV replicase	*Bacillus thuringiensis/ Potato Leafroll virus*	Resistance to Colorado potato beetle and PLRV
	CrylIIA	*Bacillus thuringiensis*	Resistance to Colorado potato beetle
Rice	PAT	*Streptomyces hygroscopicus*	Tolerance to glufosinate
Cantaloupe	S-adenosylmethionine hydrolase	*Escherichia coli* bacteriophage T3	Delayed fruit ripening due to reduced ethylene synthesis
Radicchio	Barnase/PAT	*Bacillus amyloliquefaciens/ Streptomyces hygroscopicus*	Male sterility/tolerance to glufosinate
Squash	Coat proteins from CMV, ZYMV, and WMV2	CMV, ZYMV, and WMV2	Resistance to the viruses CMV, ZYMV, and WMV2
	ZYMV and WMV2 coat proteins	ZYMV and WMV2	Resistance to the viruses ZYMV and WMV2
Papaya	**PRV coat protein**	PRSV	**Resistance to PRSV**
Flax	ALS (csr-1)	Arabidopsis	Tolerance to the herbicide sulfonylurea

ACCD, 1-aminocyclopropane-1-carboxylic acid deaminase; ALS, Acetolactate synthase; cDHDPS, Dihydrodipicolinate synthase; CMV, Cucumber mosaic virus; DAM, DNA adenine methylase; GOX, glyphosate oxidoreductase; PAT, Phosphinothricin acetyl transferase; PG, Polygalacturonase; PRSV, Papaya ringspot virus; PVY, Potato virus Y; WMV2, watermelon mosaic virus 2; ZYMV, zucchini yellow mosaic virus.

synthase (EPSPS) isolated from the common soil bacterium, *Agrobacterium tumefaciens* strain CP4 (CP4 EPSPS). The EPSPS enzyme is part of the shikimate pathway that is involved in the production of aromatic amino acids and other aromatic compounds in plants [18]. When conventional plants are treated with glyphosate, the plants cannot produce the aromatic amino acids needed to survive. GTS 40-3-2 was developed by introducing the CP4 EPSPS coding sequence into the soybean variety A5403, a commercial soybean variety of Asgrow Seed Company, using particle-acceleration (biolistic) transformation. A5403 is a maturity group V cultivar that combines consistently high-yield potential with resistance to races 3 and 4 of the soybean cyst nematode (SCN). It also possesses good standability, excellent seedling emergence, and tolerance to many leaf and stem diseases.

Weed control in soybeans represents a major financial and labor input by growers. Since soybeans are dicots, grassy weeds are controlled by one class of herbicides, and dicot (broadleaf) weeds are controlled by a second class of herbicides. Since soybeans are also broadleaf plants, their physiology and biochemistry are similar to broadleaf weeds. Therefore, in conventional soybeans, it is technically challenging to control both grassy and broadleaf weeds without harming the soybean plants themselves [16].

Glyphosate is used as a foliar-applied, non-selective herbicide and is effective against the majority of grasses and broadleaf weeds. Glyphosate has no pre-emergence or residual soil activity [18]. Furthermore, glyphosate is not prone to leaching, degrades rapidly in soil, and is essentially non-toxic to mammals, birds, and fish [19–21].

Roundup Ready soybeans offer growers an additional tool for improved weed control. Control of weeds in the soybean crop is essential, as weeds compete with the crop for sunlight, water, and nutrients. Failure to control weeds within the crop results in decreased yields and reduced crop quality. In addition, weeds reduce the efficiency of the mechanical harvest of the crop.

Roundup Ready soybeans have been produced commercially in the United States, Argentina, and Canada beginning in 1996 and provide the following environmental and economic benefits:

• Improved efficacy in weed control compared to herbicide programs used in conventional soybeans, as specific pre-emergent herbicides that are used as prevention are replaced by a broad-spectrum post-emergent herbicide that can be used on an "as needed" basis [22]. The introduction of Roundup Ready soybeans in the United States has resulted in a 12% reduction in the number of herbicide applications from 1996 to 1999, even though the total soybean acres increased by 18% [16]. The decrease in herbicide applications means that growers make fewer trips over the field to apply herbicides and translates into each of management.

• A reduction in herbicide costs for the farmer. It has been estimated that United States soybean growers spent $216 million less in 1999 for weed control (including a technology fee for Roundup Ready soybean), compared to 1995, the year before Roundup Ready soybeans were introduced [16].

• Less labor required due to the elimination of hand weeding and high-cost, early post-directed sprays, which require special equipment.

• High compatibility with integrated pest management and soil conservation techniques [23], resulting in a number of important environmental benefits including reduced soil erosion and improved water quality [24–26], improved soil structure with higher organic matter [27,28], improved wildlife habitat and improved carbon sequestration [29,30] and reduced CO_2 emissions [27,31].

Safety assessment of Roundup Ready soybeans
Safety assessment principles
In 1996, a joint report from an expert consultation sponsored by the World Health Organization (WHO) and the Food and Agricultural Organization (FAO) of the United Nations concluded that "biotechnology provides new and powerful tools for research and for accelerating the development of new and better foods" [32]. The FAO/WHO expert consultation also concluded that it is vitally important to develop and apply appropriate strategies and safety assessment criteria for food biotechnology to ensure the long-term safety and wholesomeness of the food supply.

Following these criteria, foods derived from biotechnology have been extensively assessed to assure they are as safe and nutritious as traditional foods. All foods, independent of whether they are derived from biotech crops or traditionally bred plants, must meet the same rigorous food safety standard. Numerous national and international organizations have considered the safety of foods derived

from biotech crops. They have concluded that the food safety considerations are basically of the same nature for food derived from biotech crops as for those foods derived using other methods like traditional breeding.

This concept of comparing the safety of the food from a biotech crop to that of a food with an established history of safe use is referred to as "substantial equivalence" [33,34]. The process of substantial equivalence involves comparing the characteristics, including the levels of key nutrients and other components, of the food derived from a biotech crop to the food derived from conventional plant breeding. When a food is shown to be substantially equivalent to a food with a history of safe use, then "the food is regarded to be as safe as its conventional counterpart" [32]. An FAO/WHO expert consultation in 1995 concluded "this approach provides equal or greater assurance of the safety of food derived from genetically modified organisms as compared to foods or food components derived by conventional methods" [32]. As a practical matter, this evaluation brings together an evaluation of the introduced proteins and accounts for unexpected effects due to the protein *per se*, or due to pleitropic effects created by gene insertion as assessed at the level of phenotype: the agronomic and compositional parameters of the biotech crop in comparison to traditional counterparts [35].

CP4 5-enolpyruvylshikimate-3-phosphate synthase protein safety
Usually when a gene is chosen for transformation into a crop, the encoded protein has been well characterized in terms of function (mechanism of action, evolutionary heritage, physicochemical properties, etc.). This information has been extensively evaluated during the development of biotech crops such as NewLeaf™ potato, [36] RoundupReady™ soybeans [37], and YieldGard™ corn [38]. An important consideration in protein safety is whether or not the protein can be established to have been used or eaten previously – is there a history of safe use?

The CP4 EPSP synthase protein produced in Roundup Ready soybeans is functionally similar to a diverse family of EPSPS proteins typically present in food and feed derived from plant and microbial sources [39]. The EPSPS proteins are required for the production of aromatic amino acids in plants and microbes. The enzymology and known function of EPSPS proteins generally, and CP4 EPSPS specifically, indicate that this class of enzymes perform a well-described and understood biochemical role in plants. From the perspective of safety, this characterization indicates that metabolic effects owing to the expression of the CP4 EPSPS gene are limited to conferring the Roundup Ready trait alone. Part of this evaluation includes the known structural relationship between CP4 EPSPS and other EPSPS proteins found in food as is demonstrated by comparison of the amino acid sequences with conserved identity of the active site residues, and the expected conserved three-dimensional structure based on similarity of the amino acid sequence. With respect to amino acid sequence, there is considerable divergence among known EPSPSs. For instance, the amino acid sequence of CP4 EPSPS is 41% identical at the amino acid level to *Bacillus subtilis* EPSPS, whereas the soybean EPSPS is 30% identical to *Bacillus subtilis* EPSPS. Thus, the divergence of the CP4 EPSPS amino acid sequence from typical food EPSPS sequences is on the same order as the divergence among food EPSPSs themselves [37].

The detailed enzymology [37] and subsequent biochemical composition evaluations [40,41] confirm and demonstrate that CP4 EPSPS, as expressed in line 40-3-2, has the predicted and expected metabolic effects on soybeans: the production of aromatic amino acids via the shikimic acid biosynthetic pathway.

Another aspect used for the assessment of potential toxic effects of proteins introduced into plants is to compare the amino acid sequence of the protein to known toxic proteins. Homologous proteins derived from a common ancestor have similar amino acid sequences, are structurally similar, and often share common function. Therefore, it is undesirable to introduce DNA that encodes for a protein that is homologous to a protein that is toxic to animals and people. Homology is determined by comparing the degree of amino acid similarity between proteins using published criteria [42]. The CP4 EPSPS protein does not show meaningful amino acid sequence similarity when compared to known protein toxins.

Lack of protein toxicity is confirmed by evaluating acute oral toxicity in mice or rats [43]. This study is typically a 2-week program in which the pure protein is fed to animals at doses that should be 100–1000 times higher than the highest anticipated exposure via consumption of the whole food product containing that protein. Table 5.2 summarizes the data from several acute oral toxicity studies. Although these studies were designed to obtain LD_{50}s, in fact no lethal dose has been achieved for these proteins [39,43–46]. For CP4 EPSPS, there were no treatment-related adverse effects in mice-administered CP4 EPSPS protein by oral gavage at dosages up to 572 mg/kg, the highest dose tested. This dose represents a significant (approximately 1300-fold) safety margin relative to the highest potential human consumption of CP4 EPSPS and assumes that the protein is expressed in multiple crops in addition to soybeans [39].

Phenotype evaluation (substantial equivalence)

Compositional analyses are a critical component of the safety assessment process that integrates with the evaluation of the trait (e.g. CP4 EPSP synthase) described above. Each of the measured parameters provides an assessment of the cumulative result of numerous biochemical pathways and hence provides an assessment of a wide range of metabolic pathways. Comparisons of various nutri-

Table 5.2 Summary of the data from standardized acute oral toxicity LD_{50} studies in mice. The no observable effect level (NOEL) was the highest dose tested for each protein. When accounting for the level of these proteins in the crops in which they are found (Table 5.1), these doses represent between 10^4 and 10^6 times the levels typically consumed as food

Protein	Crop	NOEL* (mg/kg)
Cry1Ac	Cotton, tomato	4200
Cry1Ab	Corn	4000
Cry2Aa	Cotton	3000
Cry2Ab	Corn, cotton	3700
Cry3A	Potato	5200
Cry3Bb1	Corn	3780
CP4 EPSPS	Soybean, cotton, canola, sugarbeet	572
NPTII	Cotton, potato, tomato	5000
GUS	Soybean, sugarbeet	100
GOX	Canola, cotton, corn, sugarbeet	100

*No observed effect level
Cry1Ac, Cry1Ab, Cry2Aa, Cry2Ab, Cry3A, Cry3Bb1 are all "crystal" proteins from *Bacillus thuringiensis*.
CP4 EPSPS, CP4 5-enolpyruvylshikimate-3-phosphate synthase; GOX, glyphosate oxidoreductase; GUS, β-glucuronidase; NPTII, neomycin phosphotransferase II.

ents and anti-nutrients are made to both a closely related traditional counterpart and the established published range for the specific component within that crop, to compare the observed levels to the natural variation of that component in current plant varieties. The composition of Roundup Ready soybeans has been thoroughly characterized and the results of these studies have been published [40,41]. Over 1400 individual analyses have been conducted and they establish that the composition of Roundup Ready soybeans is substantially equivalent to the non-transgenic parental soybean variety and other commercial soybean varieties. Table 5.3 summarizes the composition of Roundup Ready soybeans and traditional soybeans, which include:

- *Proximate analysis*: protein, fat, fibre, ash, carbohydrates, and moisture.
- *Anti-nutrients*: trypsin inhibitors, lectins, phytoestrogens (genistein and daidzein), stacchyose, raffinose, and phytate.
- *Fatty acid profile*: percentage of individual fatty acids.
- *Amino acid composition*: levels of individual amino acids.

In addition to a demonstration of substantially equivalent composition, further agronomic evaluation of the biotech crop is necessary to establish that there are no unexpected biological effects of the introduced trait. While compositional assessments provide good assurance that no untoward metabolic, nutritional, or anti-nutritional effects have occurred, an additional and very sensitive measure has been to compare a wide variety of biological characteristics at the whole plant level. The basic question asked is: Does the biotech crop fit within the usual definition of that crop? For example, do

Table 5.3 Summary of historical and literature ranges for the nutritional composition of Roundup Ready soybeans

Component	Historical Roundup Ready soybean range[a]	Literature soybean range[b]	Component	Historical Roundup Ready soybean range[a]	Literature soybean range[b]
Proximates (% dw)			Lysine	6.46–6.66	Not available
Moisture (% fw)	5.32–8.85	5.30–11 [47–49]	Methionine	1.36–1.46	Not available
Protein	37.0–45.0	36.9–46.4 [48]	Phenylalanine	4.89–5.04	Not available
Fat	13.27–23.31	13.2–22.5 [48,50]	Proline	5.20–5.27	Not available
Ash	4.45–5.87	4.29–5.88 [47]	Serine	5.76–6.08	Not available
Carbohydrates	27.6–40.74	29.3–41.3 [47]	Threonine	3.37–3.50	Not available
			Tryptophan	1.05–1.15	Not available
Fibre (% dw)			Tyrosine	3.50–3.66	Not available
Acid detergent fibre	9.76–12.46	Not available	Valine	4.50–4.66	Not available
Neutral detergent fibre	11.02–11.81	Not available	*Fatty Acids (% of total FA)[c]*		
Crude fibre	5.45–9.82	5.74–8.10 [47,53]	12:0 Lauric acid	<0.01% fw to 0.40	Not available
			14:0 Myristic acid	<0.01 fw to 0.17	Not available
Amino acid (g/100 g dw)			16:0 Palmitic acid	10.63–12.75	7–12 [54]
Alanine	1.48–1.88	1.49–1.87 [51,52]			9.63–13.09 [55]
Arginine	2.20–3.57	2.45–3.49 [51,52]	16:1 Palmitoleic acid	0.11–0.17	Not available
Aspartic acid	3.85–5.25	3.87–4.98 [51,52]	17:0 Heptadecanoic acid	0.10–0.17	0.11–0.14 [47]
Cystine	0.54–0.69	0.50–0.66 [47,53]	17:1 Heptadecenoic acid	<0.01% fw	Not available
Glutamic acid	6.00–8.34	6.10–8.72 [51,52]	18:0 Stearic acid	4.01–5.93	2–5.5 [54]
Glycine	1.48–1.90	1.60–2.02 [47,51,52]			2.69–4.40 [55]
Histidine	0.91–1.18	0.89–1.16 [1,51,52]	18:1 Oleic acid	15.56–32.52	20–50 [54]
Isoleucine	1.51–1.95	1.46–2.12 [51,52]			19.63–36.58 [55]
Leucine	2.60–3.37	2.71–3.37 [51,52]	18:2 Linoleic acid	42.41–54.48	35–60 [54]
Lysine	2.30–2.88	2.35–2.86 [51,52]			42.61–58.16 [55]
Methionine	0.50–0.62	0.49–0.66 [51,52]	18:3 Linolenic acid	4.99–10.37	2–13 [54]
Phenylalanine	1.64–2.20	1.70–2.19 [47,51,52]			5.66–8.58 [55]
Proline	1.76–2.30	1.88–2.61 [51,52]	20:0 Arachidic acid	0.30–0.51	0.31–0.43 [47]
Serine	1.80–2.60	1.81–2.32 [51,52]	20:1 Eicosenoic acid	0.14–0.28	0.14–0.26 [47]
Threonine	1.39–1.74	1.33–1.79 [51,52]	22:0 Behenic acid	0.49–0.62	0.46–0.59 [47]
Tryptophan	0.42–0.64	0.48–0.63 [47,53]	*Isoflavones (Total as aglycones)*		
Tyrosine	1.23–1.58	1.12–1.62 [51,52]	Daidzein (µg/g dw)	90.5–1260	161–1190 [47,53]
Valine	1.58–2.02	1.52–2.24 [51,52]	Genistein (µg/g dw)	106–1243	230–1380 [47,53]
Alanine	4.29–4.42	Not available	Glycitein (µg/g dw)	<10.8–184	Not available
Arginine	7.31–8.16	Not available	*Miscellaneous*		
Aspartic acid	11.46–11.98	Not available	Vitamin E mg/100g dw	1.85–4.26	1.95 [56]
Cystine	1.48–1.67	Not available	Trypsin inhibitor (TIU/mg DW)	35.5–59.5	26.4–93.2 [57]
Glutamic acid	18.53–19.02	Not available	Lectin (H.U./mg fw)	0.5–1.6	0.8–2.4 [47]
Glycine	4.34–4.41	Not available			
Histidine	2.66–2.72	Not available			
Isoleucine	4.29–4.43	Not available			
Leucine	7.63–7.87	Not available			

[a] Range of values from Roundup Ready soybean event: 40-3-2 [40,41].
[b] Commercial/non-transgenic control values: [1](40); [2](47); [3](48); [4](49); [5](50); [6](51); [7](41); [8](52); [9](53); [10](54): units in mg/100g edible portion); [11](55).
[c] "<0.01% fw" is below the lower limit of quantitation.

Roundup Ready soybeans still possess the expected plant performance of traditional soybeans? Agronomic and yield characteristics are very sensitive to untoward perturbations in metabolism and in genetic pleiotropy.

Wholesomeness (nutrition) of Roundup Ready soybeans

Farm animal nutrition studies have provided supplementary confirmation of the substantial equivalence and safety

in crop biotechnology. Currently there are many options for animal studies, the choice of which depends on the crop being engineered and its intended use. In over 65 farm animal studies completed to date, the factors evaluated include feed intake, body weight, carcass yield, feed conversion, milk yield, milk composition, digestibility, and nutrient composition of the resulting animal-derived foods [56].

A series of animal-feeding studies have been completed using diets incorporating raw or processed Roundup Ready soybeans. The animal-feeding studies included two separate 4-week studies in rats (one with unprocessed soybean meal and one with processed soybean meal), a 4-week dairy cow study, a 6-week chicken study, a 10-week catfish study, and a 5-day quail study. Animals were fed either raw soybean, unprocessed or processed soybean meal (dehulled, defatted, toasted). Included in these studies were control groups fed a non-modified parental soybean line from which both events were derived. Results from all groups were compared using conventional statistical methods to detect differences between groups in measured parameters.

All soybean samples tested provided similar growth and feed efficiency for rats, chickens, catfish, and quail [57]. Milk production, composition, and rumen fermentation parameters for dairy cows were also comparable across all groups [57]. Results for other parameters measured in each feeding study were also similar across all groups. When compared to the US population as a whole, the levels of soybean consumption (in mg/kg of body weight) in these animal-feeding studies were 100-fold or more higher than the average human daily consumption of soybean-derived foods in the United States. All these studies confirmed the food and feed safety and nutritional equivalence of diets from Roundup Ready soybeans.

General assessment strategy for food allergy

The consumer marketplace reflects widespread interest and concern about adverse reactions to certain foods and food additives. A consumer survey indicated 30% of the people interviewed reported that they or some family member had an allergy to a food product [58]. This survey also found that 22% avoided particular foods on the mere possibility that the food may contain an allergen. In reality, food-allergic reactions affect only about 6% of children and 4% of the adult population [59–61]. The most common food allergies known to affect children are IgE-mediated reactions to cow's milk, eggs, peanuts, soybeans, wheat, fish, and tree nuts. Approximately 80% of all reported food allergies in children are due to peanuts, milk, or eggs. While most childhood food allergies are outgrown, allergies to peanuts, tree nuts, and fish are rarely resolved in adulthood. In adults the most common food allergies are to peanuts, tree nuts, fish, and shellfish. The incidence of IgE-mediated reactions to specific food crops is increasing, particularly in developed countries, likely due to increased levels of protein consumption. Allergic reactions are typically elicited by a defined subset of proteins that are found in abundance in the food.

Identification and purification of allergens have been essential for the structural and immunological studies necessary to understand how these molecules stimulate IgE antibody formation [62]. In the past several years a number of allergens have been identified that stimulate IgE production and cause IgE-mediated disease in man. Significant information now exists on the identification and purification of allergens from a wide variety of sources, including foods, pollens, dust mites, animal dander, insects, and fungi [62]. However, despite increasing knowledge of the structure and amino acid sequences of the identified allergens, specific features associated with IgE antibody formation have not been fully determined [62].

Because potential allergens cannot at present be accurately identified based on a single characteristic, the allergy assessment testing strategy, as originally proposed by the US Food and Drug Administration (FDA) [63] and further modified by FAO/WHO scientific panels [64,65], proposes that all proteins introduced into crops be assessed for their similarity to a variety of structural and biochemical characteristics of known allergens. As the primary method of disease management for food-allergic people is avoidance, a core principle of these recommended strategies is to experimentally determine whether candidate proteins for genetic engineering into foods represent known food allergens currently. Prevention of unwanted exposures to food allergens is addressed by accurate labeling of food ingredients – labeling is seen as a central tool in food protection policy in the United States.

The current allergy assessment process is designed to identify the potential risks associated with the introduced protein as well as the overall allergenic risks associated with a transformed food crop. The current allergy assessment process follows recommendations made by Codex (www.codexalimentarius.net/web/index_en.jsp). Codex is an intergovernmental body representing 168 member states responsible for protecting the health of consumers and facilitating trade by setting international safety standards. The Codex recommendations for allergy assessment include evaluation of the introduced protein with respect to origin (from a known allergenic source or not), sequence homology to known allergens, stability in *in vitro* digestion assays, and when appropriate, IgE-binding capacity in *in vitro* and *in vivo* clinical tests.

Analyzing the sources of introduced genes

The source of the introduced gene is the first variable to consider in the allergy assessment process. If a gene transferred into a food crop is obtained from a source known to be allergenic, the assessment process calls for *in vitro* diagnostic tests to determine if the target protein binds IgE from patients allergic to the source of the protein. In addition, *in vivo* diagnostic tests such as skin prick tests and double-blind, placebo-controlled food challenges (DBPCFCs) may be required if the protein is to be introduced into a commodity crop. The USFDA recognizes this need and realizes that such risks to consumers can be avoided [63]. In addition to tests to determine potential allergenicity, the use of labels that clearly indicate the presence of ingredients that may cause harmful effects, such as allergies, gives consumers the opportunity to avoid these foods or food ingredients. For example, to assist people who suffer from celiac disease, the FDA has determined that products containing gluten should be identified as to the source – that is, wheat versus corn gluten (wheat gluten cannot be safely consumed by these patients, unlike corn gluten). In the case of food allergy, voluntary labeling already occurs for certain snack foods that do not ordinarily contain peanuts, but that may come into contact with peanuts during preparation. This type of labeling provides protection for peanut allergy sufferers and helps prevent accidental and unwanted exposure. The FDA has also stated that, if known allergens are genetically engineered into food crops, the resulting foods must be labeled disclosing the source of the introduced genes [63,66]. Moreover, proteins derived from known allergenic sources should be treated as allergens until demonstrated otherwise. The methodology to assess whether the transferred protein is allergenic is described below.

Different approaches can be taken to assess the potential allergenicity of a protein that originates from a non-allergenic source. As described below, a search for amino acid sequence homology of the introduced protein with all known allergens can be performed. In addition, the physicochemical properties of the introduced protein can be compared with the biochemical properties of known food allergens. From biochemical analysis of a limited number of allergens, certain characteristics shared by most but not necessarily all can be identified. For example, food allergens are typically relatively abundant in the food source, have multiple, linear IgE-binding epitopes, and are resistant to denaturation and digestion [67]. These characteristics are purported to be important to the allergenicity of a protein for various reasons. The observation that most food allergens are relatively abundant in the food source was explained by the idea that the immune system was more likely to encounter these proteins than one that was present as a small percentage of the total protein ingested. Resistance to denaturation and digestion of an allergen is thought to be an important characteristic because the longer a significant portion of the protein remains intact, the more likely it is to trigger an immune response. Finally, most food allergens have multiple, linear binding epitopes so that even when they are partially digested or denatured, they are still capable of interacting with IgE and causing an allergic reaction [68].

Amino acid sequence comparisons to known allergens

The proteins introduced into all genetically engineered plants that have been put into commerce in the United States have been screened by comparing their amino acid sequence to those of known allergens and gliadins as one of many assessments performed to evaluate product safety [4,69]. The purpose of bioinformatic analyses is to describe the biological and taxonomical relatedness of a query sequence to other functionally related proteins. In the context of allergy, the goal is to identify the level of amino acid

similarity and structural relatedness between a protein of interest and sequences from known allergens in order to determine whether the query protein is similar to known allergens or has the potential to cross-react with IgE directed against known allergens. Because candidate genes for transfer into commodity crops could be from a variety of sources, most allergen databases contain all known allergens including aeroallergens, food allergens, and proteins implicated in celiac disease. For example, the FARRP allergen database (www.allergenonline.com) contains all known allergen, gliadin, and glutenin protein sequences. The protein sequences in the FARRP allergen database were assembled and evaluated for evidence of allergenicity by an international panel of allergy experts, making this one of the more highly curated, publicly available allergen databases. High percentage matches between a query sequence and a sequence in the allergen database suggests that the query sequence could cross-react with IgE directed against that allergen. This is because homologous proteins share secondary structure and common three-dimensional folds [70] and are more likely to share allergenic cross-reactive conformational and linear epitopes than unrelated proteins; however, the degree of similarity between homologs varies widely and homologous allergens do not always share epitopes [71]. To distinguish among many matches, criteria can be used to judge the ranked scores produced by programs such as FASTA. For example, the Codex Alimentarius (www.codexalimentarius.net/web/index_en.jsp) recommended a percentage identity score of at least 35% matched amino acid residues of at least 80 residues as being the lowest identity criteria for proteins derived from biotechnology that could suggest IgE cross-reactivity with a known allergen. However, Aalberse [72] has noted that proteins sharing less than 50% identity across the full length of the protein sequence are unlikely to be cross-reactive, and immunological cross-reactivity may not occur unless the proteins share at least 70% identity. Recent published work has led to the harmonization of the methods used for bioinformatic searches and a better understanding of the data generated [73,74] from such studies.

An additional bioinformatics approach can be taken by searching for 100% identity matches along short sequences contained in the query sequence as they are compared to sequences in a database. These regions of short amino acid sequence homologies are intended to represent the smallest sequence that could function as an IgE-binding epitope [75]. If any exact matches between a known allergen and a transgenic sequence were found using this strategy, it could represent the most conservative approach to predicting potential for a peptide fragment to act as an allergen. Critical to this type of search algorithm is the selection of the overlapping sequence length (i.e. the sliding window). As the length of this window of overlapping amino acids to search with is shortened, the chance for random, false-positive matches becomes higher. Although different window lengths have been recommended, a length of eight amino acids has been shown to be informative without acquiring a majority of matches based on random chance [73,76,77].

There exist clear limits to the utility of performing sequence searches based on potential epitopes, with a major limitation being the lack of a comprehensive database of confirmed IgE-binding sequential epitopes for existing allergens. Development of this type of database represents a challenging task due to the fact that many allergens that bind IgE in patient sera and are known to cause clinical allergy symptoms do not have B- and T-cells epitopes described for them in the scientific literature [75]. At this time there is no database of epitope sequences which can fully describe epitopes for all of the known protein allergens. This makes assessments of biotechnology food protein sequences with an epitope database impractical at this time and is not recommended as a safety assessment strategy [73]. Thus, further research regarding epitope identity and sequence length is required in order to make short amino acid search strategies informative beyond the theoretical identity matching strategy currently available [73]. Moreover, it must also be noted that many IgE-binding epitopes are conformational in nature [75], not just a string of primary amino acid sequences. The analysis of conformational IgE epitopes is difficult and involves methods such as site-directed mutagenesis of the full length allergen, mimicking conformational IgE-binding sites by short phage displayed peptides, or even structural analysis of allergen immune complexes [78,79].

It should also be recognized that two IgE-binding epitopes on the same molecule are required to cross-link high-affinity IgE receptors on mast cells and induce an intracellular signal. If sufficient numbers of receptors are stimulated, the mast cell will degranulate, releasing histamine and leukotrienes. Therefore, a single match in this analysis may or may not be clinically significant and must be assessed by a second tier of studies such as *in vitro* and *in vivo* IgE assays discussed below.

Protein stability

One biophysical property shared by many but not all food allergens is resistance to degradation. That this biophysical aspect of some food proteins can be used to predict potential allergenicity is based on the premise that the longer significant portions of the protein remain intact, the more likely it is to trigger an immune response. There also appears to be a correlation between protein stability and allergenic potential [80], but this correlation is not absolute [81]. This property is not a predominant characteristic of aeroallergens, primarily because their route of sensitization is through the respiratory tract where they would not be expected to encounter the harsh conditions of the GI tract.

Initially, investigators [82,83] tested the correlation between protein stability and allergenicity by disrupting the secondary and tertiary structures of the major allergens from

milk and wheat and showed that the allergens were strikingly sensitive to pepsin digestion and lost their ability to elicit allergic reactions. Another food allergen, peanut allergen, Ara h 2, is stabilized by disulfide linkages that, when intact, protect a portion of the protein from degradation. Amino acid sequence analysis of the resistant protein fragments indicated that they contained most of the immunodominant IgE-binding eptiopes. These results provide a link between allergen structure and the most allergenic portions of the protein [84,85].

Models of digestion are commonly used to assess the stability of dietary proteins [86–88]. A digestion model using simulated gastric fluid (SGF) was adapted to evaluate the allergenic potential of dietary proteins [80]. In this model, stability to digestion by pepsin has been used as a criterion for distinguishing food allergens from safe, non-allergenic dietary proteins. Although these digestibility models are representative of human digestion, they are not designed to predict the $t_{1/2}$ of proteins *in vivo*, even though some investigators have attempted to measure protein half-life in this qualitative *in vitro* assay [89]. Thomas *et al.* [90] assessed changes to enzyme concentration, pH, protein purity, and method of detection in this SGF assay and proposed a standardized process so that results from different laboratories can be directly compared.

In addition to the SGF assay, simulated intestinal fluid (SIF) is also used for *in vitro* studies to assess the digestibility of food components [91]. SIF is an *in vitro* digestion model where proteins undergo digestion at neutral pH by a mixture of enzymes collectively known as pancreatin. However, the relationship between protein allergenicity and protein stability in the *in vitro* SIF study is limited because the protein has not been first exposed to the acidic, denaturing conditions of the stomach, as would be the case *in vivo* [92]. For this reason we recommend that the SGF and SIF assays be done sequentially to fully assess a protein's potential allergenicity.

In vitro immunoassays of allergenicity

In vitro assays such as radioallergosorbent tests (RAST) [93,94], enzyme-linked immunosorbent assays (ELISA) [95], or immunoblotting assays should be undertaken to determine if an allergen has been transferred to the target plant. These assays use IgE fractions of serum from appropriately sensitized individuals who are allergic to the food, from which the transferred gene was derived. Serum donors should meet clinically relevant criteria, including a convincing history or positive responses in DBPCFCs [93,96,97]. A recent FAO/WHO scientific panel [65] has recommended that in addition to using serum IgE from individuals who are allergic to the food from which the transferred gene was derived, the serum IgE from patients allergic to plants in the same botanical family also be used in these assays (targeted serum screening). However, the current Codex allergy assessment guidelines (www.codexalimentarius.net/web/index_en.jsp)

do not appear to support the recommendations for targeted serum screening because its usefulness had not been practically demonstrated [98]. Furthermore, the utility of serum screening in the absence of sufficient structural similarity between the protein of interest and a known allergen as recommended by Thomas *et al.* [73] (e.g. at a level of 35% over 80 or greater amino acids), has not been rigorously tested.

In vivo assays of allergenicity

For transgenic proteins from allergenic sources or with significant sequence homology with known allergens, further evaluation is required to determine if the introduced protein could precipitate IgE-mediated reactions. *In vivo* skin prick testing may be required for some proteins. Skin prick testing is an excellent negative predictor of allergenicity but is only 50–60% predictive if a positive result is obtained [99]. The best *in vivo* test of allergenicity is the DBPCFC. This procedure involves testing with sensitive and non-sensitive patients under controlled clinical conditions. Patients who are known to be allergic to proteins from the source would be tested directly for hypersensitivity to food containing the protein encoded by the gene from the allergenic source. The ethical considerations for this type of assessment would include factors such as the likelihood of inducing anaphylactic shock in test subjects, potential value to test subjects, availability of appropriate safety precautions, and approval of local institutional review boards. If sensitive patients underwent a reaction in these tests, food derived from crops containing the protein would require labeling. In practice, however, such a discovery has led to the discontinuation of product development for brazil-nut allergen containing soybeans.

Changes in endogenous allergens (substantial equivalence)

In the context of substantial equivalence, it is important to establish that the expression of new genes or effect due to the insertion of genes into plant genomes does not alter the levels of endogenous (existing) allergens in food crops. This is likely to be especially true for crops that are commonly allergenic, such as soybeans, wheat, rice, or tree nuts. From the perspective of human health risk, it is generally agreed that substantive change in the allergenicity of allergenic foods leading to increased incidence or severity of food allergy should be evaluated and considered in safety assessment [38]. To date, evaluations of endogenous allergens have typically been performed for crops that fall into the top eight "commonly" allergenic food groups. Experimentally, these evaluations involve *in vitro* IgE immunoassays by western blot, ELISA, ELISA inhibition, or a combination of these techniques. Examples utilizing each of these different techniques to determine the IgE-binding capacity of transgenic versus non-transgenic foods and biotech proteins have appeared in the literature [100–104]. All studies conducted

to date concluded that there were no meaningful differences between genetically modified and traditional food crops.

Allergy assessment summary: Roundup Ready soybeans

Source of CP4 EPSPS: The gene encoding CP4 EPSPS was isolated from the common soil bacterium *Agrobacterium tumefaciens* strain CP4. This enzyme is present in all plants, bacteria, and fungi. However, animals do not synthesize their own aromatic amino acids and therefore lack this enzyme. Because the aromatic amino acid biosynthetic pathway is not present in mammalian, avian, or aquatic life forms, glyphosate has little if any toxicity for these organisms. In addition, the EPSPS enzyme is normally present in food for human consumption derived from plant and microbial sources indicating that the protein has a long history of safe use.

Bioinformatic analysis of CP4 EPSPS: A search for amino acid sequence similarity between the CP4 EPSPS protein and known allergens was conducted according to the methods described in this chapter. The search revealed no significant amino acid sequence homologies with known allergens either by the FASTA alignment or the 8mer search. In addition, analysis of the amino acid sequence of the inserted CP4 EPSPS enzyme did not show homologies with known mammalian protein toxins and was not judged to have any potential for human toxicity.

In vitro digestibility of CP4 EPSPS: An *in vitro* pepsin digestion assay was performed using *E. coli* produced CP4 EPSPS that had previously been shown to be biochemically identical to that produced in plants. The intact CP4 EPSPS protein was digested rapidly and no stable fragments were detected after only 15 seconds exposure to the enzyme. These results indicate that the CP4 EPSPS protein is unlikely to be an allergen.

These data, taken together with the comprehensive characterization data for the CP4 EPSPS protein and very low expression level of the CP4 EPSPS gene (protein accumulates to less than 0.05% of total soybean meal protein), suggest that CP4 EPSPS is neither currently a known food allergen nor likely to become a food allergen as consumed in Roundup Ready soybeans.

Trends in the science of risk assessment

Animal models for predicting allergenicity

The potential for animal models to mimic the human disease process makes them an invaluable tool for potentially predicting allergenicity of nutritionally enhanced crops. Most of the allergy animal models developed to date have been designed to test reagents for immunotherapeutic treatment of allergic disease and to predict the potential allergenicity of proteins [105]. These two disparate goals, identifying effective treatment regimens and predicting potential human allergenicity, require many of the same variables to be considered in the development of an effective animal model. To date, animal models of food allergy developed to test immunotherapeutic reagents have seen some success [106–108]. On the other hand, animal models developed to predict allergenicity are not as prevalent [109,110] and are yet to be widely accepted.

There has been considerable interest in the development of animal models that would permit a more direct evaluation of the sensitizing potential of novel proteins. The development of a predictive animal model could help to address the third category of public health risk posed by introduction of GM proteins into food crops – that of a novel protein becoming an allergen. In this context, attention has focused on the production of IgE in response to the novel protein and a wide variety of organisms are being developed for this purpose including rodents [111–113], dogs [114], and swine [115]. Many variables are being tested in the development of each model organism including route of sensitization, dose, use of adjuvant, age of organism, diet, and genetics. Unfortunately, there are currently no validated models available for assessing the allergenic potential of specific proteins in naïve subjects. This is due in part to the extremely complex nature of the immune response to foods and proteins and also in part due to the fact that most animal models of food allergy were originally developed to understand the mechanisms of allergenicity rather than assessing the allergenic potential of novel proteins. The development of an animal model that can accurately predict human allergenicity would be an invaluable tool for assessing the allergenicity of nutritionally enhanced food crops. However, while some progress is being made in select models [116,117], there remains much work to be done before there is confidence that any one model will provide positive predictive value with regard to protein allergenicity in humans.

Refinements of *in vitro* pepsin digestion assay

As described above, the pepsin digestion assay can be a reasonable contributor to an overall allergy assessment of specific proteins. However, even more enlightening information may be obtained if the underlying structural basis for an allergen's ability to resist pepsin digestion was known. It is with this in mind that the sequence specificity of the pepsin substrate and the minimum peptide size required for eliciting the clinical symptoms of allergy are discussed.

Pepsin is an aspartic endopeptidase obtained from the gastric mucosa of vertebrates. However, all mammalian pepsins have similar specificities. Pepsin preferentially cleaves the peptide bond between any large hydrophobic residue (L, F, W, or Y) and most other hydrophobic or neutral residues except P [118]. In order to cleave the peptide bond between two hydrophobic residues, the active site groove of pepsin binds to a segment of the protein containing the sessile peptide bond and four amino acids on either side of the cleavage site. There have been a number of studies evaluating the efficiency of pepsin cleavage and the effect of various amino acids around the sessile peptide bond. To facilitate discussion, the positions have been assigned identification labels such that the amino acid (aa) residues located on the amino-terminal side of the sessile bond are labeled P_1, P_2, P_3, or P_4, and on the carboxyl-side labeled P_1'', P_2', etc. The bond between P_1 and P_1' is the sessile bond. The most efficiently cleaved peptides have aromatic or hydrophobic residues at both the P_1 and P_1' positions. The rate of pepsin cleavage is slowed if a proline is at amino acid position P_2' or if arginines are in the P_2, P_3, or P_4 positions [119,120].

The resistance of a protein to pepsin digestion raises the possibility that it will be taken up by antigen-processing cells at the mucosal surface of the small intestine and could sensitize susceptible individuals who have consumed the protein, leading to the production of antigen-specific IgE. In addition there is the possibility that a pepsin-resistant peptide could provoke an IgE-mediated allergic response in those who are already sensitized. IgE plays a pivotal role during the induction of an allergic response by triggering effecter cells such as the tissue mast cells (and possibly blood basophils) to release histamine, leukotrienes, and inflammatory proteases. This is accomplished when two or more IgE molecules are bound to a single peptide fragment while the antibody is bound to the high-affinity IgE receptors (FcεRI) on these effecter cells. Studies of rat basophilic leukemia (RBL) cells indicate that it probably requires the cross-linking of well over 1000 of the 200,000 or so FcεRI receptors on a single cell to cause degranulation of that cell [121]. IgE antibody cross-linking occurs through the binding of multivalent antigens by IgE molecules bound to the surface of mast cells. While various IgE–antigen binding arrangements are possible, only certain ones will lead to the productive signaling and degranulation of the mast cells [122,123]. The binding is only effective if it is maintained long enough (by a high-affinity interaction) and if the spatial relationship and rigidity of the antigen are sufficient to cross-link and induce intracellular signaling. Baird, Holowka and colleagues used haptens with linkers of various sizes to determine the effective spacing for degranulation and to study intracellular signaling. Results demonstrated that oligomerization of the FcεRI–IgE–antigen molecules was more effective at inducing degranulation. Further, minimum spatial distances were identified using the artificial hapten-spacer constructs indicating that while tight IgE binding can occur with bivalent haptens spanning 30 Å (angstroms), the RBL cells were not induced to degranulate. Bivalent haptens of ~50 Å were required to obtain modest degranulation while similar haptens spaced between 80 and 240 Å apart seemed to provide optimum degranulation [122,123]. These results may be used to provide guidance on the sizes of peptides that might be required to cause an allergic reaction upon challenge.

In order to evaluate the minimum peptide size that might effectively cross-link receptors on mast cells, the maximum overall spacing (length) may be calculated, but various assumptions must be made regarding epitope size and peptide conformation. The first assumption regards the size of a typical IgE-binding epitope observed in a food allergen. Most food allergen IgE-binding epitopes are reported to range in size from 6–15 amino acids in length [75]. Therefore the absolute minimum size of a peptide would have to be 12–30 amino acids long and contain two IgE-binding epitopes. However, this does not take into account the data of Kane et al. [124,125] that show the IgE-binding epitopes must be at least 80–240 Å apart to provide optimum degranulation. Assuming the two IgE-binding epitopes are separated by the minimum length of 80 Å and that the diameter size for an amino acid such as alanine is 5 Å, the minimum size for a peptide that would be expected to elicit the clinical symptoms of an allergic reaction would be 29 amino acids long or a peptide of about 3190 Da (29 aa $\times$ 110 average aa molecular weight). These calculations do not take into account the secondary structure of the peptide. For example, the peptide could be in an α-helical arrangement, a β-pleated sheet, or a random coil dependent on its amino acid sequence. Dependent on the secondary structure of the peptide, mast cell degranulation would only be possible if each end of the fragment represents a strong IgE-binding epitope and if the peptide is in a β-strand conformation. Based on this rationale it appears improbable that the presence of a protease-resistant fragment of <3 kDa in the in vitro pepsin digestion assay would have the ability to degranulate mast cells and therefore would not be likely to pose a risk to consumers.

While the discussion above is theoretical, there is recent evidence that pepsin-resistant allergen fragments produced in an in vitro pepsin digestion assay were >3 kDa and contained multiple IgE-binding epitopes. The major peanut allergen Ara h 2 is a 17-kDa protein that has eight cysteine residues that could form up to four disulfide bonds. Upon treatment with pepsin, a 10-kDa fragment was produced that was resistant to further enzymatic digestion. The resistant Ara h 2 peptide fragment contained intact IgE-binding epitopes and several potential enzyme cut sites that were protected from the enzyme by the compact structure of the protein. Amino acid sequence analysis of the resistant protein fragments indicates that they contained most of the immunodominant IgE-binding epitopes. These results provide a link between allergen structure and the immunodominant IgE-binding epitopes within a population of food-allergic individuals and lend additional biological relevance to the in vitro pepsin digestion assay [126].

The link between food allergenicity and protein stability appears to have been confirmed, at least for milk and wheat allergy. Buchanan and colleagues have shown that when stability of the major allergens from these foods is disrupted by reduction of disulfide bonds, the allergens were strikingly sensitive to pepsin digestion and lost their allergenicity as determined by their ability to provoke skin test and gastrointestinal symptoms in previously sensitized dogs [127,128]. Other food allergens will have to be tested in this same manner in order to determine if this is a general characteristic of food allergens.

In an attempt to assess the positive and negative predictive values (PPV and NPV, respectively) for the pepsin digestion assay in identifying potential food allergens, Bannon et al. [129] compared the stability of 20 known food allergens and 10 non-food allergens and calculated a PPV for these proteins of 0.95 and an NPV of 0.80. This analysis indicates that the pepsin digestion assay is a good positive and negative predictor of the potential of a protein to be an allergen. However, the results should be interpreted with some caution as food allergens associated with oral allergy syndrome (OAS) were not included in this analysis and only 30 proteins were tested in this manner. In any event, assay standardization and the study of many proteins (allergens and non-allergens) will inform the allergy assessment strategy with respect to the robustness and predictive power of this physicochemical property of proteins.

Proteomics and the allergy assessment strategy

Proteomics is a high-throughput technology platform that substantially increases the number of proteins that can be detected simultaneously. This type of approach has the potential to provide important quantitative information on multiple allergens that could aid in the allergy assessment process. However, there are key technical and data gaps that need to be addressed prior to this method being generally applied.

Generally speaking, proteomics relies on the ability to separate/fractionate complex protein mixtures and then to accurately annotate those proteins based on properties such as mass and amino acid sequence. Separation of complex protein mixtures is most often done using some variant of the classical two-dimensional polyacrylamide gel electrophoresis (2D-PAGE) method originally described by Laemmli [130]. Steady improvements to this methodology have evolved to include more precision in the isoelectric focusing with narrow range pH gradients [131], improved staining and detection protocols [132,133] and methods to quantitatively analyze proteins within a gel-based format [134]. Most of the problems with the 2-D gels stem from poor reproducibility due to methodological problems [135]. While the main strengths of 2-DE are good separation and visualization of complex samples, the resulting image and data analysis tend to introduce additional sources of variation. There have also been good advances in non-gel-based methods for protein fractionation, particularly in the area of affinity chromatography applications [136].

Once proteins have been adequately fractionated, identification of the proteins is typically performed using mass spectrometry. There are various types of mass spectrometers that can be used to identify proteins, including the basic matrix-assisted laser desorption/ionization (MALDI) systems that detect peptide masses; to complex multistage systems such as tandom time of flight (ToF–ToF) machines that in addition to mass detection are also able to detect structural features of the peptides (see review [137] for detailed comparisons of available mass spectrometers). Mass spectrometers differ in their mass accuracy, resolving power, sensitivity, and dynamic range; so choice of instrument is very dependent on the biological question being studied.

Although technology around protein fractionation and identification is continuing to improve, there continue to be challenges that must be resolved before it will become routinely acceptable to apply these technologies to determining the allergenicity of nutritionally enhanced food crops. The main technical challenges include technology variability (differences in platforms, methodology, sensitivity, reproducibility), data management (storage and visualization of complex gel images and MS spectra), and data analysis (incomplete databases of protein structure information, poor quality DNA sequence data, incomplete sequence annotation).

Another key challenge limiting the routine application of this technology to the allergy assessment process is the need to define the natural variability of allergen abundance in food crops with different genetic backgrounds and grown in different environments. Since protein abundance is a characteristic of known allergens, before informed decisions on whether a protein's abundance has significantly increased, we must first know the normal range of protein abundance that is seen in nature. Without this point of reference, it is impossible to interpret the effect of any changes that are detected in protein abundance. Another key point to keep in mind is that having the ability to detect a change, especially given the ongoing improvements in sensitivity of the equipment, does not immediately imply that the change will have any biological effect on allergenicity.

Removing allergens from foods

Genetic engineering can be used to reduce the levels of known allergens by post-transcriptional gene silencing using an RNA antisense approach, or to reduce their allergenicity by reducing disulfide bonds that are critical for allergenicity using thioredoxin, or by directly modifying the genes encoding the allergen(s).

The RNA antisense approach has been successfully applied to reduce the allergenic potential of rice. Most rice allergens have been found in the globulin fraction of rice seed [138–142]. The globulins and albumins have been estimated to comprise about 80–90% of the total protein in rice seeds. From this fraction a 16 kDa α-amylase/trypsin inhibitor-like protein was identified as the major allergen involved in hypersensitivity reactions to rice [138,139].

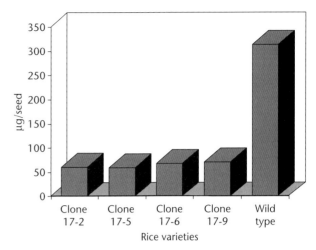

Figure 5.2 Suppression of a 16-kDa rice allergen using antisense technology. Rice allergen levels were quantified by ELISA from each genetically engineered rice variety (clones 17-2, 17-5, 17-6, and 17-9) and were compared with wild-type rice seeds. (From Matsuda T, Nakase M, Adachi T, *et al.* Allergenic proteins in rice: strategies for reduction and evaluation. Presented at the *Symposium of Food Allergies and Intolerances*, Bonn, Germany, May 10–13, 1995; permission from Matsuda.)

Using this antisense RNA approach, Nakamura and Matsuda [142] generated several rice lines that contained transgenes producing antisense RNA for the 16 kDa rice allergen. These authors successfully lowered the allergen content in rice by as much as 80% without a concomitant change in the amount of other major seed storage proteins (Fig. 5.2).

The concept of reducing disulfide bonds to reduce allergenicity has been tested on allergens in wheat and milk by Buchanan and colleagues and shown to significantly reduce the allergic symptoms elicited from sensitized dogs [127,128,143]. Briefly, the authors exposed either the purified allergens or an extract from the food source containing the allergens to thioredoxin purified from *E. coli* and then performed skin tests and monitored gastrointestinal symptoms in a sensitized dog model. Allergens that had their disulfide bonds reduced by thioredoxin showed greatly reduced skin reactions and gastrointestinal symptoms (Fig. 5.3). These results provide a critical proof of concept for this approach prior to constructing transgenic wheat lines that overproduce thioredoxin.

One of the more ambitious approaches to reducing allergenicity of food crops is by modification of the genes encoding the allergens so that they produce hypoallergenic forms of these proteins [144,145]. This approach is based on the observation that most food allergens have linear IgE-binding epitopes that can be readily defined using overlapping peptides representing the entire amino acid sequence of the allergen and serum IgE from a population of individuals with hypersensitivity reactions to the food in question [75]. Once the IgE-binding epitopes are determined,

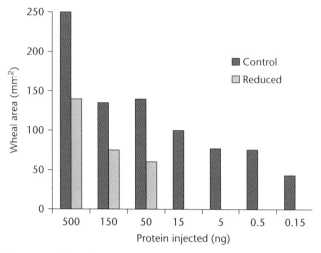

Figure 5.3 Thioredoxin mitigation of milk allergen reactivity in dogs sensitized to milk. Milk was incubated in physiological buffered saline containing 5 μl of 100 mmol/l dithiothreitol (DTT) and boiled for 5 minutes prior to skin testing in milk-allergic dogs. (Reproduced from de Val G. *et al.*, [128] with permission from Elsevier.)

critical amino acids can be identified that when changed to another amino acid result in loss of IgE binding to that epitope without modification of the function of that protein. Any changes that result in loss of IgE binding can then be introduced into the gene by site-directed mutagenesis.

Serum IgE from patients with documented peanut hypersensitivity and overlapping peptides were used to identify the IgE-binding epitopes of the major peanut allergens Ara h 1, Ara h 2, and Ara h 3. At least 23 different linear IgE-binding epitopes located throughout the length of the Ara h 1 molecule were identified [146]. In a similar fashion, 10 IgE-binding epitopes and 4 IgE-binding epitopes were identified in Ara h 2 and Ara h 3, respectively [147,148]. Mutational analysis of each of the IgE-binding epitopes revealed that single amino acid changes within these peptides had dramatic effects on IgE-binding characteristics. Substitution of a single amino acid led to loss of IgE binding [146,147,149]. Analysis of the type and position of amino acids within the IgE-binding epitopes that had this effect indicated that substitution of hydrophobic residues in the center of the epitopes was more likely to lead to loss of IgE binding [146]. Site-directed mutagenesis of the cDNA encoding each of these allergens was then used to change a single amino acid within each IgE-binding epitope. The hypoallergenic versions of these allergens were produced in *E. coli* and tested for their ability to bind IgE and to stimulate proliferation of T cells from peanut-allergic patients. The results of these studies indicated that it is possible to produce hypoallergenic forms of the peanut allergens that bind less allergen-specific IgE, interact with T cells from peanut-sensitive patients, and release significantly lower amounts of mediators from passively sensitized mast cells [150,151].

International consensus: a common strategy

The development of national and international regulations, guidelines, and policies to assess the safety of food products derived from genetically engineered plants has led to broad discussions and a general consensus on the types of information that are appropriate to assess the potential allergenicity of such foods. Gaining international consensus on allergy assessment is critical because many genetically engineered plant products are commodity products (e.g. corn, soybean, wheat) grown and traded globally. A consensus approach provides producers, regulators, and consumers with the assurance that the risk of allergy to these products is appropriately addressed prior to their marketing, and that a consistent assessment approach is used around the world.

Conclusion and future considerations

The allergy assessment testing strategy, as it is presently formulated, is a tiered, hazard identification approach that utilizes currently available scientific data regarding allergens and the allergic response. It is extremely important to emphasize that all aspects of the current safety assessment testing strategy need to be considered when assessing a novel protein, not just the results from a single arm of this strategy. While a hazard assessment approach has served the public interest well, it may not be adequate in the assessment of future products which may have proteins that may have unknown or unpredictable mechanisms of action or which may share one or more properties with food allergens while concomitantly providing significant nutritional and human health benefits. Considering the advances in the science of allergy assessment detailed in this chapter, the allergy assessment strategies proposed by Metcalfe *et al.* , and the most recent recommendations by the scientific advisory panel of the FAO/WHO we have described the current practices and issues in allergy assessment. This strategy takes advantage of the past assessments but by its tiered design attempts to place more importance on the "weight of evidence" from each test rather than relying too heavily on one test to determine whether a protein is likely to have allergenic potential.

We conclude that the current testing strategy will need to be integrated into a risk assessment model where risk is defined as a function of the level of the hazard and the level of exposure to the hazard. This strategy consists of four steps: hazard assessment, dose–response evaluation, exposure assessment, and risk characterization [152]. To apply risk assessment principles to the issue of the allergenicity of proteins and food biotechnology, new scientific data must be collected for each step in this process. This review of scientific progress on these issues indicates that this process of integration has already begun. For example, the issue of dose–response evaluation is beginning to be addressed by a variety of investigators exploring threshold doses for traditional allergenic foods in clinically allergic patients [153,154]. The issue of exposure assessment consists of three parts: the abundance of the protein in the food, the stability of the protein in the GI tract, and the amount of the GM crop consumed in the diet. We believe that the protective value of current testing approaches and future approaches that adopt sound risk assessment principles, have and will provide robust assurances to risk managers and consumers alike for present and future biotech products [155].

References

1 Somerville C, Briscoe J. Genetic engineering and water. *Science* 2001;292:2217.

2 Sicherer SH, Burks AW, Sampson HA. Clinical features of acute allergic reactions to peanut and tree nuts in children. *Pediatrics* 1998;102:e6.

3 Taylor SL, Lemanske Jr RF, Bush RK, Busse, WW. Chemistry of food allergens. Food allergy. In: Chandra RK (ed.) *Food allergy.* St John's Nutrition Research Education Foundation, 1987: 21–44.

4 Fuchs RL, Astwood JD. Allergenicity assessment of foods derived from genetically modified plants. *Food Tech* 1996;50:83–8.

5 Taylor SL. Chemistry and detection of food allergens. *Food Tech* 1992;46:146–52.

6 Stanley JS, Bannon GA. Biochemistry of food allergens. *Clin Rev Allergy Immunol* 1999;17:279–91.

7 Horsch RB, Fraley RT, Rogers SG, *et al.* Inheritance of functional foreign genes in plants. *Science* 1984;223:496–8.

8 De Block M, Herrera-Estrella L, Van Montagu M, *et al.* Expression of foreign genes in regenerated plants and their progeny. *EMBO J* 1984;3:1681–9.

9 Fiske HJ, Dandekar AM. The introduction and expression of transgenes in plants. *Sci Hort* 1993;55:5–36.

10 Van Larebeke N, Engler G, Holsters M, *et al.* Large plasmid in *Agrobacterium tumafaciens* is essential for crown gall inducing activity. *Nature* 1974;252:169.

11 Zambryski PC. Chronicles from the *Agrobacterium*-plant cell transfer story. *Annu Rev Plant Physiol Plant Mol Biol* 1992; 43:465–90.

12 Sanford JC, Klein TM, Wolf ED, Allen N. Delivery of substances into cells and tissues using a particle bombardment process. *J Part Sci Technol* 1987;5:27–37.

13 Sanford JC, Smith FD, Russell JA. Optimizing the biolistic process for different biological application. *Methods Enzymol* 1992;217:483–509.

14 James C. *Global Status of Commercialized Biotech/GM Crops.* ISAAA Brief No. 35. Ithaca, NY: ISAAA, 2006.

15 GAO Report on Biotechnology, 2002.

16 Carpenter J, Gianessi L. Herbicide use on roundup ready crops. *Science* 2000;287:803–4.

17 Liu K. *Soybeans: Chemistry, Technology and Utilization.* Chapman and Hall, 1997.

18 Steinrucken HC, Amrhein N. The herbicide glyphosate is a potent inhibitor of 5-enolpyruvyl-shikimate-3-phosphate synthase. *Biochem Biophys Res Commun* 2001;94:1207–12.

19 EPA. *Reregistration Eligibility Decision (RED): Glyphosate.* Office of Prevention, Pesticides and Toxic Substances, US Environmental Protection Agency, Washington, DC, 1993.

20 WHO. *Glyphosate.* World Health Organization (WHO), International Programme of Chemical Safety (IPCS), Geneva. Environmental Health Criteria No. 159, 1994.

21 Williams GM, Kroes R, Munro IC. Safety evaluation and risk assessment of the herbicide roundup and its active ingredient, glyphosate, for humans. *Regul Toxicol Pharmacol* 2000;31: 117–65.

22 Culpepper AS, York AC. Weed management in glyphosate-tolerant cotton. *J Cotton Sci.* 1998;2:174–85.

23 Keeling JW, Dotray PA, Osborn TS, Asher BS. Postemergence weed management with Roundup Ultra, Buctril and Staple in Texas High Plains cotton. *Proceedings of the Beltwide Cotton Conference,* 1998;1:861–2.

24 Baker JL, Laflen JM. Runoff losses of surface-applied herbicides as affected by wheel tracks and incorporation. *J Environ Qual* 1979;8:602–7.

25 Hebblethewaite JF. *The Contribution of No-Till to Sustainable and Environmentally Beneficial Crop Production: A Global Perspective.* West Lafayette, IN: Conservation Technology Information Center, 1995.

26 CTIC. *Crop Residue Management Survey.* West Lafayette, IN: Conservation Technology Information Center, 1998.

27 Kay BD. Soil quality: impact of tillage on the structure of tilth of soil. *Farming for a Better Environment.* Ankeny, IA: Soil and Water Conservation Society, 1995:7–9.

28 CTIC. *Top Ten Benefits.* West Lafayette, IN: Conservation Technology Information Center, 2000.

29 Reicosky DC. Impact of tillage on soil as a carbon sink. *Farming for a Better Environment.* Ankeny, IA: Soil and Water Conservation Society, 1995.

30 Reicosky DC, Lindstrom MJ. Impact of fall tillage on short-term carbon dioxide flux. In: Lal R, Kimble J, Levine E, Stewart BA (eds.) *Soils and Global Change.* Chelsea, MI: Lewis Publishers, 1995:177–87.

31 Kern JS, Johnson MG. Conservation tillage impacts on national soil and atmospheric carbon levels. *Soil Sci Soc Am J* 1993;57:200–10.

32 FAO/WHO. *Biotechnology and Food Safety.* Geneva: FAO/WHO, 1996:1–27.

33 FAO/WHO. *Strategies for Assessing the Safety of Foods Produced by Biotechnology.* Geneva: FAO/WHO, 1991: iii–59.

34 OECD. *Safety Evaluation of Foods Derived by Modern Biotechnology: Concepts and Principles.* Paris: Organization for Economic Cooperation and Development (OECD), 1993.

35 Astwood JD, Fuchs RL. Status and safety of biotech crops. In: Baker DR, Umetsu NK (eds.) *Agrochemical Discovery. Insect, Weed*

and Fungal Control. ACS Symposium Series 774. Washington, DC: American Chemical Society, 2001:152–64.

36 Lavrik PB, Bartnicki DE, Feldman J, *et al.* Safety assessment of potatoes resistant to colorado potato beetle. In: Engel KII, Takeoka GR, Teranishi R (eds.) *Genetically Modified Foods. Safety Issues.* ACS Symposium Series 605.Washington, DC: American Chemical Society, 1995:148–58.

37 Padgette SR, Re DB, Barry GF, *et al.* New weed control opportunities: development of soybeans with a Roundup Ready™ gene. In: Duke SO (ed.) *Herbicide-Resistant Crops. Agricultural, Environmental, Economic, Regulatory, and Technical Aspects.* CRC Lewis Publishers, 1996:53–84.

38 Sanders P, Lee TC, Groth ME, *et al.* Safety assessment of insect-protected corn. In: Thomas JA (ed.) *Biotechnology and Safety Assessment,* 2nd edn. Taylor & Francis, 1998:241–56.

39 Harrison LA, Bailey MR, Naylor MW, *et al.* The expressed protein in glyphosate-tolerant soybean, 5-enolpyruvylshikimate-3-phosphate synthase from *Agrobacterium* sp. strain CP4, is rapidly digested *in vitro* and is not toxic to acutely gavaged mice. *J Nutr* 1996;126:728–40.

40 Padgette SR, Taylor NB, Nida DL, *et al.* The composition of glyphosate-tolerant soybean seeds is equivalent to that of conventional soybeans. *J Nutr* 1996;126:702–16.

41 Taylor NB, Fuchs RL, MacDonald J, *et al.* Compositional analysis of glyphosate-tolerant soybeans treated with glyphosate. *J Agric Food Chem* 1999;47:4469–73.

42 Doolitltle RF. Searching through sequence databases. *Meth Enzymol* 1990;183:99–110.

43 McClintock JT, Schaffer CR, Sjoblad RD. A comparative review of the mammalian toxicity of *Bacillus thuringiensis*-based pesticides. *Pest Sci* 1995;45:95–105.

44 Fuchs RL, Ream JE, Hammond BG, *et al.* Safety assessment of the neomycin phosphotransferase II (NPTII) protein. *Bio/Technology* 1993;11:1543–7.

45 Gilissen LJ, Metz W, Stiekema W, Nap JP. Biosafety of *E. coli* beta-glucuronidase (GUS) in plants. *Transgenic Res* 1998;7:157–63.

46 Hammond BG, Fuchs RL. Safety evaluation for new varieties of food crops developed through biotechnology. In: Thomas JA (ed.) *Biotechnology and Safety Assessment.* Philadelphia, PA: Taylor & Francis, 1998:61–79.

47 Smith AK, Circle SJ. Chemical composition of the seed. In: Smith AK, Circle SJ (eds.) *Soybeans: Chemistry and Technology.* Westport, CT: Avi Publishing, 1972;1:61–92.

48 Perkins EG. Composition of soybeans and soybean products. In: Erickson DR (ed.) *Practical Handbook of Soybean Processing and Utilization.* Champaign, IL and St. Louis, MO: AOCS Press and United Soybean Board, 1995:9–28.

49 Wilcox JR. Breeding soybean for improved oil quantity and quality. In: Shible R (ed.) *World Soybean Research Conference III: Proceedings.* Boulder, CO: Westview Press, 1985:380–6.

50 Han Y, Parsons CM, Hymowitz T. Nutritional evaluation of soybeans varying in trypsin inhibitor content. *Poultry Sci* 1991;70:896–906.

51 Orthoefer FT. Processing and utilization. In: Norman AG (ed.) *Soybean Physiology, Agronomy, and Utilization.* New York: Academic Press, 1978:219–46.

52 Pryde EH. Composition of soybean oil. In: Erickson DR, Pryde EH, Brekke OL, Mounts, RTL, Falb, RA (eds.) *Handbook of Soy Oil Processing and Utilization.* St. Louis, MO and Champaign, IL: American Soybean Association and American Oil Chemists' Society, 1990.

53 Visentainer JV, Laguila JE, Matsushita M, *et al.* Fatty acid composition in several lines of soybean recommended for cultivation in Brazil. *Arg Biol Tecnol* 1991;34:1–6.

54 USDA Web Site. www.nal.usda.gov/fnic/cgi-bin/nut_search.pl?soybean. Subtopic: Soybeans, Mature Seeds, Raw 2001.

55 Kakade ML, Simons NR, Liener IE, Lambert JW. Biochemical and nutritional assessment of different lines of soybeans. *J Agric Food Chem* 1972;20:87–90.

56 Faust MA. New feeds from genetically modified plants: the US approach to safety for animals in the food chain. *Livest Prod Sci* 2002;74:239–54.

57 Hammond BG, Vicini JL, Hartnell GF, *et al.* The feeding value of soybeans fed to rats, chickens, catfish and dairy cattle is not altered by genetic incorporation of glyphosate tolerance. *J Nutr* 1996;126:717–27.

58 Sloan AE, Powers ME. A perspective on popular perceptions of adverse reactions to foods. *J Allergy Clin Immunol* 1986;78:127–33.

59 AAAAI. Overview of allergic disease. *The Allergy Report* 2000;1:1–3.

60 Sicherer SH, Sampson HA. Food allergy. *J Allergy Clin Immunol* 2006;117:S470–5.

61 Woods RK, Stoney RM, Raven J, *et al.* Reported adverse food reactions overestimate true food allergy in the community. *Eur J Clin Nutr* 2002;56:31–6.

62 Anderson JA, Sogn DD. *Adverse Reactions to Foods.* NIH Publication No. 84-2442, 1984;1–6.

63 US Food and Drug Administration, Department of Health and Human Services, Statement of policy: food derived from new plant varieties. *Fed Register* 1992;57:22984–3005.

64 FAO/WHO. Safety aspects of genetically modified foods of plant origin. *Report of a Joint FAO/WHO Expert Consultation on Allergenicity of Foods Derived from Biotechnology.* May 29–June 2, 2000. Geneva, Switzerland.

65 FAO/WHO. Evaluation of allergenicity of genetically modified foods. *Report of a Joint FAO/WHO Expert Consultation on Allergenicity of Foods Derived from Biotechnology.* January 22–25, 2001. Rome, Italy.

66 US Food and Drug Administration, Department of Health and Human Services. Secondary direct food additives permitted in food for human consumption; food additives permitted in feed and drinking water of animals; aminoglycoside 3′-phosphotransferase II. *Fed Register* 1994;59:26700–11.

67 Bannon, GA. What makes a food protein an allergen? *Curr Allergy Asthma Rep* 2004;4:43–6.

68 Burks W, Helm R, Stanley S, Bannon GA. Food allergens. *Curr Opin Allergy Clin Immunol* 2001;1:243–8.

69 Metcalfe DD, Astwood JD, Townsend R, *et al.* Assessment of the allergenic potential of foods derived from genetically engineered crop plants. *Crit Rev Food Sci Nutr* 1996;36:S165–86.

70 Pearson WR. Effective protein sequence comparison. *Meth Enzymol* 1996;266:227–58.

71 Astwood JD, Silvanovich A, Bannon, GA. Vicilins: a case study in allergen pedigrees. *J Allergy Clin Immunol* 2002;110:26–7.

72 Aalberse RC. Structural biology of allergens. *J Allergy Clin Immunol* 2000;106:228–38.

73 Thomas K, Bannon G, Hefle S, *et al.* In silico methods for evaluating human allergenicity to novel proteins. Bioinformatics Workshop Meeting Report, February 23–24, 2005. *Toxicol Sci* 2005;88:307–10.

74 Ladics GS, Bannon GA, Silvanovich A, Cressman, RF. Comparison of conventional FASTA identity searches with the 80 amino acid sliding window FASTA search for the elucidation of potential identities to known allergens. *Mol Nutr Food Res* 2007;51:985–998.

75 Bannon G, Ogawa T. Evaluation of available IgE-binding epitope data and its utility in bioinformatics. *Mol Nutr Food Res* 2006;50:638–44.

76 Hileman RE, Silvanovich A, Goodman RE, *et al.* Bioinformatic methods for allergenicity assessment using a comprehensive allergen database. *Int Archives Allergy Immunol* 2002;128:280–91.

77 Silvanovich A, Nemeth MA, Song P, *et al.* The value of short amino acid sequence matches for prediction of protein allergenicity. *Toxicol Sci* 2005;90:252–8.

78 Neudecker P, Lehmann K, Nerkamp J, *et al.* Mutational epitope analysis of Pru av 1 and Api g 1, the major allergens of cherry (*Prunus avium*) and celery (*Apium graveolens*): correlating IgE reactivity with three-dimensional structure. *Biochem J* 2003;376:97–107.

79 Mittag D, Batori V, Neudecker P, *et al.* A novel approach for investigation of specific and cross-reactive IgE epitopes on Bet v 1 and homologous food allergens in individual patients. *Mol Immunol* 2006;43:268–78.

80 Astwood JD, Leach JN, Fuchs RL. Stability of food allergens to digestion *in vitro*. *Nat Biotechnol* 1996;14:1269–73.

81 Fu T-J, Abbott UR, Hatzos C. Digestibility of food allergens and non-allergenic proteins in simulated gastric fluid and simulated intestinal fluid – a comparative study. *J Agric Food Chem* 2002;50:7154–60.

82 Buchanan BB, Adamidi C, Lozano RM, *et al.* Thioredoxin-linked mitigation of allergic responses to wheat. *Proc Natl Acad Sci USA* 1997;94:5372–7.

83 del Val G, Yee BC, Lozano RM, *et al.* Thioredoxin treatment increases digestibility and lowers allergenicity of milk. *J Allergy Clin Immunol* 1999;103:690–7.

84 Sen MM, Kopper R, Pons L, *et al.* Protein structure plays a critical role in peanut allergen stability and may determine immunodominant IgE-binding epitopes. *J Immunol* 2002; 169:882–7.

85 Lehmann K, Schweimer K, Reese G, *et al.* Structure and stability of 2S albumin-type peanut allergens: implications for the severity of peanut allergic reactions. *Biochem J* 2006;395:463–72.

86 Petschow BW, Talbott, RD. Reduction in virus-neutralizing activity of a bovine colostrum immunoglobulin concentrate by gastric acid and digestive enzymes. *J Pediatr Gastroenterol Nutr* 1994;19:228–35.

87 Silano M, De Vincenzi M. *In vitro* screening of food peptides toxic for coeliac and other gluten-sensitive patients: a review. *Toxicology* 1999;132:99–110.

88 Besler M, Steinhart H, Paschke A. Stability of food allergens and allergenicity of processed foods. *J Chromatogr B Biomed Sci Appl* 2001;756:207–28.

89 Herman RA, Woolhiser MM, Ladics GS, *et al.* Stability of a set of allergens and non-allergens in simulated gastric fluid. *Int J Food Sci Nutr* 2007;58:125–41.

90 Thomas K, Aalbers M, Bannon GA, *et al.* A multi-laboratory evaluation of a common *in vitro* pepsin digestion assay protocol used in assessing the safety of novel proteins. *Regul Toxicol Pharmacol* 2004;39:87–98.

91 Okunuki H, Techima R, Shigeta T, *et al.* Increased digestibility of two products in genetically modified food (CP4-EPSPS and Cry1Ab) after preheating. *J Food Hyg Soc Japan* 2002; 43:68–73.

92 Yagami T, Haishima Y, Nakamura A, *et al.* Digestibility of allergens extracted from natural rubber latex and vegetable foods. *J Allergy Clin Immunol* 2000;106:752–62.

93 Sampson HA, Albergo R. Comparison of results of skin test, RAST, and double blind, placebo-controlled food challenges in children with atopic dermatitis. *J Allergy Clin Immunol* 1984;74:26–33.

94 Yunginger JW, Adolphson CR. *Standardization of Allergens.* Washington, DC: American Society of Microbiology, 1992: 678–84.

95 Burks AW, Brooks JR, Sampson HA. Allergenicity of major component proteins of soybean determined by enzyme-linked immunosorbent assay (ELISA) and immunoblotting in children with atopic dermatitis and positive soy challenges. *J Allergy Clin Immunol* 1988;81:1135–42.

96 Sampson HA, Scanion, SM. Natural history of food hypersensitivity in children with atopic dermatitis. *J Pediatr* 1989;115:23–7.

97 Bock SA, Sampson HA, Atkins FM, *et al.* Double-blind, placebo-controlled food challenges (DBPCFC) as an office procedure. *J Allergy Clin Immunol* 1988;82:986–97.

98 Thomas K, Bannon G, Herouet-Guicheney C, *et al.* The utility of a global sera bank for use in evaluating human allergenicity to novel proteins. *Toxicol Sci* 2007;97:27–31.

99 Hill DJ, Hosking CS, Reyes-Benito V. Reducing the need for food allergen challenges in young children: a comparison of *in vitro* with *in vivo* tests. *Clin Exp Allergy* 2001;31:1031–5.

100 Kim SH, Kim HM, Ye YM, *et al.* Evaluating the allergic risk of genetically modified soybean. *Yonsei Med J* 2006;47:505–12.

101 Batista R, Nunes B, Carmo M, *et al.* Lack of detectable allergenicity of transgenic maize and soya samples. *J Allergy Clin Immunol* 2005;116:403–10.

102 Burks AW, Fuchs RL. Assessment of the endogenous allergens in glyphosate-tolerant and commercial soybean varieties. *J Allergy Clin Immunol* 1996;96:1008–10.

103 Park JH, Chung TC, Kim JH, *et al.* Comparison of allergens in genetically modified soybean with conventional soybean. *Yakhak Hoeji* 2001;45:293–301.

104 Hoff M, Son D-Y, Gubesch M, *et al.* Serum testing of genetically modified soybeans with special emphasis on potential allergenicity of the heterologous protein CP4 EPSPS. *Mol Nutr Food Res* 2007;51:946–955.

105 Knippels LM, van Wijk F, Penninks AH. Food allergy: What do we learn from animal models? *Curr Opin Allergy Clin Immunol* 2004;4:205–9.

106 Morafo V, Srivastava K, Huang CK, *et al.* Genetic susceptibility to food allergy is linked to differential TH2-TH1 responses in C3H/HeJ and BALB/c mice. *J Allergy Clin Immunol* 2003;111:1122–8.

107 Pons L, Ponnappan U, Hall RA, *et al.* Soy immunotherapy for peanut-allergic mice: modulation of the peanut-allergic response. *J Allergy Clin Immunol* 2004;114:915–21.

108 Srivastava KD, Kattan JD, Zou ZM, *et al.* The Chinese herbal medicine formula FAHF-2 completely blocks anaphylactic reactions in a murine model of peanut allergy. *J Allergy Clin Immunol* 2005;115:171–8.

109 Buchanan BB, Frick OL. The dog as a model for food allergy. *Ann NY Acad Sci* 2002;964:173–83.

110 Dearman RJ, Stone S, Caddick HT, *et al.* Evaluation of protein allergenic potential in mice: dose–response analyses. *Clin Exp Allergy* 2003;33:1586–94.

111 Li XM, Schofield BH, Huang CK, *et al.* A murine model of IgE-mediated cow's milk hypersensitivity. *J Allergy Clin Immunol* 1999;103:206–14.

112 Dearman RJ, Kimber I. Determination of protein allergenicity: studies in mice. *Toxicol Lett* 2001;120:181–6.

113 Akiyama H, Teshima R, Sakushima JI, *et al.* Examination of oral sensitization with ovalbumin in Brown Norway rats and three strains of mice. *Immunol Lett* 2001;78:1–5.

114 Frick OL. Food allergy in atopic dogs. *Adv Exp Med Biol* 1996;409:1–7.

115 Helm RM, Furuta GT, Stanley JS, *et al.* A neonatal swine model for peanut allergy. *J Allergy Clin Immunol* 2002;109:136–42.

116 Ermel RW, Kock M, Griffey SM, *et al.* The atopic dog: a model for food allergy. *Lab Anim Sci* 1997;47:40–9.

117 Li XM, Serebrisky D, Lee SY, *et al.* A murine model of peanut anaphylaxis: T- and B-cell responses to a major peanut allergen mimic human responses. *J Allergy Clin Immunol* 2000;106:150–8.

118 Voet D, Voet JG. *Biochemistry*, 2nd edn. New York: John Wiley & Sons Inc, 1995:112.

119 Shintani T, Nomura K, Ichishima E. Engineering of porcine pepsin. Alteration of S1 substrate specificity of pepsin to those of fungal aspartic proteinases by site-directed mutagenesis. *J Biol Chem* 1997;272:18855–61.

120 Dunn BM, Hung SH. The two sides of enzyme-substrate specificity: lessons from the aspartic proteinases. *Biochim Biophys Acta* 2000;1477:231–40.

121 Holowka D, Baird B. Antigen-mediated IGE receptor aggregation and signaling: a window on cell surface structure and dynamics. *Annu Rev Biophys Biomol Struct* 1996;25:79–112.

122 Schweitzer-Stenner R, Licht A, Pecht I. Dimerization kinetics of the IgE-class antibodies by divalent haptens. I. The Fab-hapten interactions. *Biophys J* 1992;63:551–62.

123 Schweitzer-Stenner R, Licht A, Pecht I. Dimerization kinetics of the IgE-class antibodies by divalent haptens. II. The interactions between intact IgE and haptens. *Biophys J* 1992;63:563–8.

124 Kane P, Erickson J, Fewtrell C, *et al.* Cross-linking of IgE-receptor complexes at the cell surface: synthesis and characterization of a long bivalent hapten that is capable of triggering mast cells and rat basophilic leukemia cells. *Mol Immunol* 1986;23:783–90.

125 Kane PM, Holowka D, Baird B. Cross-linking of IgE-receptor complexes by rigid bivalent antigens greater than 200 A in length triggers cellular degranulation. *J Cell Biol* 1988;107:969–80.

126 Sen MM, Kopper R, Pons L, *et al.* Protein structure plays a critical role in peanut allergen stability and may determine immunodominant IgE-binding epitopes. *J Immunol* 2002;169:882–7.

127 Buchanan B, Adamidi C, Lozano RM, *et al.* Thioredoxin-linked mitigation of allergic responses to wheat. *Proc Natl Acad Sci USA* 1997;94:5372–7.

128 de Val G, Yee BC, Lozano RM, *et al.* Thioredoxin treatment increases digestibility and lowers allergenicity of milk. *J Allergy Clin Immunol* 1999;103:690–7.

129 Bannon GA, Goodman RE, Leach JN, *et al.* Digestive stability in the context of assessing the potential allergenicity of food proteins. *Comments Toxicol* 2002;8:271–285.

130 Laemmli UK. Cleavage of structural proteins during the assembly of the head of bacteriophage T4. *Nature* 1970;227:680–5.

131 Hoving S, Gerrits B, *et al.* Preparative two-dimensional gel electrophoresis at alkaline pH using narrow range immobilized pH gradients. *Proteomics* 2002;2:127–34.

132 Unlu M, Morgan ME, *et al.* Difference gel electrophoresis: a single gel method for detecting changes in protein extracts. *Electrophoresis* 1997;18:2071–7.

133 Rabilloud T. Two-dimensional gel electrophoresis in proteomics: old, old fashioned but it still climbs up mountains. *Proteomics* 2002;2:3–10.

134 Tonge R, Shaw J, *et al.* Validation and development of fluorescence two-dimensional differential gel electrophoresis proteomics technology. *Proteomics* 2001;1:377–96.

135 Voss T, Haberl P. Observations on the reproducibility and matching efficiency of two-dimensional electrophoresis

gels: consequences for comprehensive data analysis. *Electrophoresis* 2000;21:3345–50.

136 Lee WC, Lee KH. Applications of affinity chromatography in proteomics. *Anal Biochem* 2004;324:1–10.

137 Domon B, Aebersold R. Challenges and opportunities in proteomics data analysis. *Mol Cell Proteomics* 2006;5:1921–6.

138 Shibasaki M, Suzuki S, Nemoto H, Kuroume T. Allergenicity and lymphocyte-stimulating property of rice protein. *J Allergy Clin Immunol* 1979;64:259–65.

139 Matsuda T, Sugiyama M, Nakamura R, Torii S. Purification and properties of an allergenic protein in rice grains. *Agric Biol Chem* 1988;52:1465–70.

140 Matsuda T, Nomura R, Sugiyama M, Nakamura R. Immunochemical studies on rice allergenic proteins. *Agric Biol Chem* 1991;55:509–13.

141 Nakase M, Alvarez AM, Adachi T, *et al.* Immunochemical and biochemical identification of the rice seed protein encoded by cDNA clone A3-12. *Biosci Biotechnol Biochem* 1996;60: 1031–42.

142 Nakamura R, Matsuda T. Rice allergenic protein and molecular-genetic approach for hypoallergenic rice. *Biosci Biotech Biochem* 1996;60:1215–21.

143 Buchanan BB, Schurmann P, Decottignies P, Lozano RM. Thioredoxin: a multifunctional regulatory protein with a bright future in technology and medicine. *Arch Biochem Biophys* 1994;314:257–60.

144 Bannon GA, Shin D, Maleki S, *et al.* Tertiary structure and biophysical properties of a major peanut allergen, implications for the production of a hypoallergenic protein. *Int Arch Allergy Immunol* 1999;118:315–16.

145 Burks AW, King N, Bannon GA. Modification of a major peanut allergen leads to loss of IgE binding. *Int Arch Allergy Immunol* 1999;118:313–14.

146 Burks AW, Shin D, Cockrell G, *et al.* Mapping and mutational analysis of the IgE-binding epitopes on Ara h 1, a legume vicilin protein and a major allergen in peanut hypersensitivity. *Eur J Biochem* 1997;245:334–9.

147 Stanley JS, King N, Burks AW, *et al.* Identification and mutational analysis of the immunodominant IgE binding epitopes of the major peanut allergen Ara h 2. *Arch Biochem Biophys* 1997;342:244–53.

148 Bannon GA, Cockrell G, Connaughton C, *et al.* Engineering, characterization and *in vitro* efficacy of the major peanut allergens for use in immunotherapy. *Int Arch Allergy Immunol* 2001;124:70–2.

149 Rabjohn P, Helm EM, Stanley JS, *et al.* Molecular cloning and epitope analysis of the peanut allergen Ara h 3. *J Clin Invest* 1999;103:535–42.

150 Rabjohn P, West CM, Connaughton C, *et al.* Modification of peanut allergen Ara h 3: effects on IgE binding and T cell stimulation. *Int Arch Allergy Immunol* 2002;128:15–23.

151 King N, Helm R, Stanley JS, *et al.* Allergenic characteristics of a modified peanut allergen. *Mol Nutr Food Res* 2005;49: 963–71.

152 Hodgson E, Levi PE. *A Textbook of Modern Toxicology*, 2nd edn. Stamford, CT: Appleton and Lange, 1997.

153 Taylor S, Hefle SL, Bindslev-Jensen C, *et al.* Factors affecting the determination of threshold doses for allergenic foods: How much is too much? *J Allergy Clin Immunol* 2002;109:24–30.

154 Taylor SL, Hefle SL, Bindslev-Jensen C, *et al.* A consensus protocol for the determination of the threshold doses for allergenic foods: How much is too much? *Clin Exp Allergy* 2004;34:689–95.

155 Bannon GA, Martino-Catt S. Application of current allergy assessment guidelines to next generation biotechnology derived crops. *J AOAC Int* 2007:90:1492–1499.

156 Brookes G, Barfoot P. *GM Crops: The First Ten Years – Global Socio-Economic and Environmental Impacts.* ISAAA Brief No. 36. Ithaca, NY: ISAAA, 2006.

CHAPTER 6

Food Allergen Thresholds of Reactivity*

Steve L. Taylor and Jonathan O'B. Hourihane

KEY CONCEPTS

- Threshold doses of food allergens do exist below which patients will not react adversely to residues of an allergenic food.

- Threshold doses vary considerably from one patient to another.

- Clinical determination of threshold doses is best done through double-blind, placebo-controlled food challenges.

- Knowledge of individual threshold doses can provide guidance to patients in the successful implementation of avoidance diets.

Until more innovative therapies are developed and implemented, food-allergic individuals must adhere to specific food avoidance diets. In general terms, allergists advise food-allergic patients to avoid completely the specific allergenic food(s) and all ingredients made from those food(s). The presumption is made that the threshold dose for the offending food is zero and thus complete avoidance is a necessity. From a practical perspective, this advice is probably prudent. Food-allergic individuals can react adversely to exposure to small quantities of the offending food [1,2], but it is now well documented that food-allergic individuals have threshold doses below which they will not experience adverse reactions [3,4]. Ultimately, that information could be helpful to allergic individuals, their physicians, the food industry, and governmental regulatory agencies in protecting the health of these consumers. However, the determination of individual threshold doses is not yet a common clinical procedure and no consensus exists on the establishment of regulatory threshold doses below which the vast majority of a population of patients allergic to a specific food, for example peanut, would not be expected to react.

Definition of threshold

A good discussion about the usefulness of threshold presupposes that there is a universally held definition for the term threshold. In much of the existing clinical literature, the threshold dose is operationally defined as the lowest dose capable of eliciting an allergic reaction. From the toxicology and risk assessment perspective, this dose would be known as the lowest observed adverse effect level (LOAEL) or the minimal eliciting dose (MED) [3]. However, from a risk assessment perspective, the threshold dose should actually be defined as the highest amount of the allergenic food which will not cause a reaction in individuals allergic to that food. This dose would be known as the no observed adverse effect level (NOAEL). Unfortunately, in much of the clinical literature on dose–response relationships for allergenic foods, the NOAEL is not clearly reported.

Clearly, NOAELs and LOAELs can be defined on either an individual basis or a population basis. For an individual, the NOAEL or LOAEL can be experimentally determined by challenge trials conducted in a clinical setting on a particular day. Individual NOAELs or LOAELs might vary from one day to another or from one season to another based on many factors that are not completely understood. Few studies have been done comparing individual NOAELs or LOAELs from one occasion to another, although it is well described that pediatric patients [5] and patients undergoing successful immunotherapy [6] can become more tolerant of an allergenic food. Certainly, considerable variation occurs in the NOAELs and LOAELs between individuals with a given food allergy. Individual NOAELs for peanut, for example, in controlled clinical challenges can range from low milligram levels to perhaps 10 g [7].

The population threshold can be defined as the largest amount of the allergenic food which will not cause a reaction

---

Food Allergy: Adverse Reactions to Foods and Food Additives, 4th edition.
Edited by Dean D. Metcalfe, Hugh A. Sampson, and Ronald A. Simon.
© 2008 Blackwell Publishing, ISBN: 978-1-4501-5129-0.

*This chapter is dedicated to the memory of Susan L. Hefle, Ph.D., who was originally invited to author this chapter and who provided inspiration to both of us over many years in debates and discussions about allergic reactions to foods and threshold doses.

when tested experimentally in a defined population of allergenic individuals. Of course, this definition presumes that a representative population can be identified and tested experimentally that would include some of the most highly sensitive (as defined by dose) individuals. Clinically that can be difficult, especially if some patients, such as those with histories of severe reactions, are excluded from the clinical threshold trial. The derivation of the population threshold can also be approached through modeling of the dose–response relationship [8]. In this approach, the individual thresholds of ideally a large number of patients are plotted and examined statistically. In this case, the threshold is defined as the amount of the allergenic food which will not cause a reaction in a specified proportion of an allergic population. These different definitions imply the use of different approaches to the determination of thresholds that would have different uses in advising patients, labeling of foods, and regulating the food industry.

Thresholds for sensitization versus elicitation

Allergic responses occur in two phases: sensitization and elicitation. Thresholds may apply to both phases [8]. In the sensitization phase, the susceptible individual develops allergen-specific IgE antibodies in response to allergen exposure. Because allergic reactions have not yet occurred, the level of exposure to the allergenic food can be quite high, for example feeding of milk-based formula to an infant. However, clinical experience suggests, but does not prove, that some infants are sensitized by exposure to much lower doses of the allergenic foods via breast milk where the level of the allergens is presumably restricted to the small amounts that can transfer from the mother's digestive tract to the breast milk [9]. Cutaneous exposure to food allergens has been implicated in sensitization in retrospective case control series [10] and animal studies have confirmed that this is possible, especially through inflamed skin [11,12]. Very little information is known about threshold doses for sensitization, and gathering clinical evidence about thresholds for sensitization is likely unethical.

Therefore, this chapter will be devoted to a discussion of the threshold dose for elicitation. The MED is the lowest amount of the allergenic food needed to elicit an allergic reaction in a previously sensitized individual. These food-allergic individuals are the ones who implement specific avoidance diets and must be reasonably protected by food industry practices and labeling standards.

Clinical determination of individual threshold doses

Double-blind, placebo-controlled food challenge (DBPCFC) remains the gold standard for diagnosis of food allergy [9,13]. The inclusion of extremely low doses of allergenic foods in challenges has been common in research practice for more than a decade [14]. Starting with lower doses means a longer challenge, as challenges must continue until the equivalent of a reasonable serving of the food has been consumed. While existing clinical data are somewhat limited, no correlation has yet been found between patients who react on challenge to very low doses and patients with histories of severe reactions. Indeed, severe reactions to the lowest doses used during the challenge have not been reported in any of the most cited studies and inclusion of low doses, for example 1 mg of peanut protein, is becoming the norm. It appears therefore that the inclusion of very low doses in DBPCFCs has further increased the safety of food challenges for research and clinical interests.

DBPCFCs that include low doses are now commonplace and most adhere to consensus protocols developed with input from stakeholders from the medical, industrial, and regulatory communities [15]. These challenges proceed in exactly the same fashion as "normal" food challenges. A major consideration has been how to set criteria for a definitive result. Subjective symptoms such as non-cooperation (in children particularly), abdominal pain, vomiting, or itch are easily elicited but are then difficult to quantify. Thresholds for subjective symptoms appear to be lower than for objective symptoms [16]. Comparison of apparently similar patients in similar or identical studies in different countries would be difficult if criteria for stopping a challenge were not standardized. It has been agreed that most low-dose challenges, especially in adults, should continue until objective signs are elicited, such as urticaria or angioedema. Subjective symptoms should be carefully recorded and more significant subjective symptoms such as abdominal pain in infants and children, in particular, are frequently considered as an adequate basis to stop the challenge trial [15]. However, as with other diagnostic food challenges, low-dose challenges should be stopped before more significant signs are elicited, such as wheeze. Put simply, low-dose challenge studies add up to three or four extra doses at the start of the challenge, but after the low doses have been safely consumed, there is nothing more complex about a low-dose challenge than there is for any other diagnostic food challenge.

There will always be concerns that volunteers for research studies are self-selected and that there are likely to be more sensitive subjects who do not wish to volunteer. Furthermore subjects who agree to undergo a challenge, whether clinically motivated or for research studies, must be in optimal health at the time of challenge, so the effects of asthma, reactivity to pollen, or use of medications such as ACE inhibitors are eliminated from the challenge in a way that they cannot be eliminated from exposures to allergens in the community [17]. Airway stability must be assessed before challenge by assessment of peak expiratory flow rate, FEV1 measurement, or formal spirometry. Regular medications that may affect elicitation of an allergic reaction during challenge, such as antihistamines, must be stopped appropriately before challenge [13,15].

The severity of previous reactions by history was not an exclusion criterion for the first threshold study of 14 peanut-allergic patients [14] and published data now exist on more than 70 low-dose peanut challenges in subjects including "severe reactors" [14,18,19]. Flinterman [16] reported low-dose challenges in a group of children with a spectrum of clinical reactivity so it appears, therefore, that within the constraints of research-motivated challenges in volunteers, both adult and children, that a spectrum of clinical reactivity has been fully represented in low-dose challenges to date.

The use of standardized protocols is critical for direct comparison of challenge studies, as the outcome of challenges can be affected by considerations such as use of different vehicles for challenges [20] or different types of allergen, for example pasteurized egg powder versus cooked egg, defatted peanut flour versus roasted peanut, etc. [3].

Repeated food challenge is often necessary in children to ascertain persistence or resolution of food allergy. Clinical experience in pediatric practice suggests that increasing amounts of allergen can be tolerated as oral tolerance is achieved, suggesting a change in individual threshold doses, but this has not been formally evaluated. Changes in thresholds over time have not been extensively investigated, with isolated reports suggesting there is no substantial change in adults [14,21].

Clinical correlates of thresholds of reactivity

Allergen-specific IgE levels in serum and skin prick test wheal size are now widely used in clinical practice to assess the progress of oral tolerance acquisition in pediatric patients and to determine appropriate times for confirmatory challenge trials [22,23]. Furthermore, a Dutch study [24] reported that nine subjects with the lowest eliciting dose of peanut (0.1–1.0 mg peanut flour) had a higher median peanut-specific IgE value (44 kU$_A$/l) than three subjects with a higher threshold (>10 mg, peanut-specific IgE values 4.7 kU$_A$/l, $p = 0.018$). Thus, some correlation seems to exist between the levels of allergen-specific IgE levels in serum and individual threshold doses. However, it has not been possible to strongly correlate serum allergen-specific IgE levels or skin prick test wheal sizes with the severity of both reported reactions, and more importantly, of future exposures, possibly because many other factors are in play in community exposures [17]. Studies designed to specifically examine low-dose reactivity, however, have begun to alter this perception. A British study has shown a moderate inverse correlation between peanut-specific IgE levels and challenge-induced reaction score, which is stronger in adults than in children [17]. Wensing et al. [25] reported that subjects who reported moderate to severe reactions during exposures to peanut in the community reacted (with mainly subjective symptoms) to significantly lower doses of peanut during low-dose DBPCFC than did subjects whose previous reactions had been mild ($p = 0.027$). In contrast, Hourihane et al. [18] found little correlation between "community" and "challenge" severity when an estimate of the dose of allergen was considered in the assessment of reaction severity. It appears possible that the inclusion of very low doses in challenges will improve the information that can be gathered from a challenge, and that the use of allergen-specific IgE levels could be developed for the prediction of the severity of reactions in challenges with peanut. This association remains to be demonstrated for other food allergens, and it is possible that the significance of allergen-specific IgE levels will remain confined to interpretation of low-dose challenge studies, rather than replacing them.

Minimal eliciting doses for specific foods

Oral challenges, often DBPCFCs, are often conducted as part of the clinical diagnostic procedure for patients suspected to have food allergy [9]. In the recommended clinical procedure, the initial dose for diagnostic challenges is described as less than that estimated by the patient to be required to produce symptoms [9]. Thus, considerable physician discretion and experience is involved in the selection of the initial dose in diagnostic DBPCFC. In routine clinical practice, challenge doses often start at 500 mg of the specific food [26], although lower initial doses are occasionally used when circumstances warrant. Sicherer et al. [26], in reporting on diagnostic DBPCFC experiences in 196 patients with 513 positive challenges, indicated that a large percentage of patients, ranging from 17% for fish to 55% for milk, reacted to the initial dose of the DBPCFC. While this approach is quite useful from a diagnostic perspective in clearly establishing the role of the specific food in the allergic reaction, it does not establish the individual NOAEL in patients reacting to the initial dose because doses well below 500 mg could provoke reactions in such patients. In fact, 11% of patients experienced severe reactions to the initial dose [26] perhaps suggesting that the initial dose was considerably higher than the patient's MED. Other clinical investigators have similarly reported severe reactions occurring to the initial dose in a diagnostic DBPCFC [27].

In their diagnostic experiences with DBPCFC, Sicherer et al. [26] reported that half or more of allergic individuals had MEDs of 600 mg or more, ranging up to 8 g [26]. Similar results were reported by Morisset et al. [7] in sharing clinical experiences with large numbers of patients involved in diagnostic DBPCFC and in results from several immunotherapy trials for peanut allergy [6,28,29]. Thus, the majority of food-allergic individuals are likely to experience reactions only when exposed to food that has been rather seriously contaminated or mislabeled.

Very importantly, some exceptionally sensitive patients exist. Individual patients with MEDs of 1 mg have been described for peanut and egg, with even occasional lower MEDs for milk in some infants [3]. The percentage of patients with individual MEDs that are well below (<100 mg) the typical initial dose used in diagnostic DBPCFC is unknown. The identification of such patients may be quite important, as these are predicted to be the individuals who would be at greatest risk from exposure to foods contaminated with trace levels of the offending food.

Clinical trials using low-dose challenges have been conducted on peanut [6,7,14,16,20,24,25,28–32], milk [7,32–35], egg [7,32,34,36], and hazelnut [37–39] for multiple purposes including diagnosis, the determination of thresholds, or the evaluation of various therapeutic treatments. Sufficient number of patients have been included in these various trials to perhaps allow the determination of a population-based threshold dose, although various factors, as discussed below, complicate the interpretation of the collective data [3]. Similar trials have been conducted on smaller groups of patients for soybeans [35,40], mustard [41,42], fish [43,44], and sesame seed [7], but the groups are too small to make population-based estimates. Table 6.1 provides a list of published studies where low-dose challenge studies have been conducted on one or more patients with peanut, egg, milk, hazelnut, soybean, fish, mustard, shrimp, or sesame seed allergy. From Table 6.1, individual MEDs appear to be quite variable, ranging from approximately 1 mg to as much as several grams.

The interpretation of these data to determine population-based thresholds is complicated by numerous factors. The use of a study population that is representative of the entire cross-section of individuals allergic to a particular food should be an essential feature in the determination of population-based thresholds. The compilations of diagnostic challenge experiences indicate that the majority of food-allergic patients have individual threshold doses above the typical 500 mg initial dose used in diagnostic challenges [7,26,27]. An examination of the studies reviewed in Table 6.1 indicates that low-dose challenge trials seem to include a preponderance of patients who have lower individual threshold doses. This observation is not surprising since the use of low doses in diagnostic challenges is typically predicated on the patient's historical accounts of reactions to ingestion of small amounts [9,26], but suggests that these individuals may not be representative of the entire population allergic to a particular food.

Other factors also lead to uncertainty in the establishment of population-based threshold using existing published data. In many cases, the LOAELs are reported but NOAELs are not or must be inferred. The doses are reported as discrete doses in some cases and cumulative doses in others. More importantly, the challenge materials are not consistent and need to be normalized to some factors such as protein, but the protein levels in the challenge materials are not given. For example, peanuts are approximately 25% protein while peanut flour

Table 6.1 Published studies on low-dose challenges

Reference	Number of patients	Range of MEDs[1]
Peanut		
May (1976) [32]	8	0.200–8.0
Atkins et al. (1985) [45]	3	0.500–50
Moneret-Vautrin et al. (1995) [34]	2	0.10–10
Oppenheimer et al. (1992) [28]	11	0.030–8.0
Hourihane et al. (1997) [14]	8	0.002–0.050
Nelson et al. (1997) [29]	12	0.016–2.8
Moneret-Vautrin et al. (1998) [31]	9	0.200–0.965
Wensing et al. (2002) [25]	26	0.0001–1.0[2]
Morisset et al. (2003) [7]	103	0.005–>7.11
Leung et al. (2003) [6]	23	0.001–2.0
Grimshaw et al. (2003) [20]	4	0.006–0.936
Lewis et al. (2005) [30]	40	0.001–3.936
Flinterman et al. (2006) [39]	23	0.100–>3.0
Peeters et al. (2007) [24]	26	0.012–4.412[2]
Cows' milk		
May (1976) [32]	1	2.0
Bernstein et al. (1982) [46]	2	14.1
Moneret-Vautrin et al. (1995) [34]	5	8.0–200
Fiocchi et al. (2003) [35]	12	0.012–0.180
Morisset et al. (2003) [7]	59	0.0001–0.200
Meglio et al. (2004) [33]	18	?–0.090[3]
Rolinck-Werninghaus et al. (2005) [47]	1	0.150
Egg		
May (1976) [32]	4	0.200–2.0
Atkins et al. (1985) [45]	1	50
Moneret-Vautrin et al. (1995) [34]	8	0.020–15
Morisset et al. (2003) [7]	125	0.002–>7.11
Rolinck-Werninghaus et al. (2005) [47]	2	0.013–0.200
Buchanan et al. (2007) [36]	6	0.018–1.01
Hazelnut		
Ispano et al. (1998) [38]	21	1.50–20[2]
Wensing et al. (2002) [37]	31	0.001–0.100[2]
Flinterman et al. (2006) [39]	12	0.100–>3.0[2]
Soybean		
Magnolfi et al. (1996) [40]	8	0.088–3.6
Fiocchi et al. (2003) [35]	18	0.012–0.180[4]
Mustard		
Rance et al. (2000) [41]	15	0.001–0.936
Figueroa et al. (2005) [42]	14	0.045–0.493
Fish		
Hansen and Bindslev-Jensen (1992) [43]	7	0.006–6.656
Helbling et al. (1999) [44]	6 (cod)	1.0–64
	5 (catfish)	0.25–64
	3 (snapper)	1.0–4.0
Sesame seed		
Morisset et al. (2003) [7]	12	0.030–?[5]
Shrimp		
Bernstein et al. (1982) [46]	1	14
Atkins et al. (1985) [45]	4	25–100

[1] MED: minimal eliciting dose (LOAEL) expressed in grams of the food as administered in the challenge trial (not normalized for protein content).
[2] Subjective symptoms as endpoint for some challenges in the group.
[3] Lowest doses of milk impossible to quantify (drop).
[4] Dose of soybean formula.
[5] Highest MED for sesame seed was not given.

is about 50% protein. In some studies, subjective responses, such as oral allergy syndrome, were used as the criterion for a positive response [25,38]. In other studies, LOAELs were reported on the basis of objective reactions [7,30].

A binomial probability approach has been considered as one way to estimate the population-based threshold [8]. In this approach, 29 patients allergic to a particular food are challenged in a low-dose manner to identify a dose below which none of the 29 patients experiences an adverse reaction. Binomial probability theory then allows the conclusion that there is 95% certainty that fewer than 10% of this food-allergic population will react to ingestion of this dose of the particular food [8]. Of course, the group of 29 subjects must be representative of the entire allergic population. Furthermore, this approach allows for the possibility that almost 10% of patients allergic to that food will react to ingestion of that dose and this possibility may be considered as too high. Modeling of collective data from several studies is probably the preferred approach to determine the population-based threshold, although the best statistical model to use remains to be determined [8].

Usefulness of individual thresholds for reactivity

Knowledge of an individual patient's threshold dose allows the allergist to provide the patient with more useful advice. While all food-allergic patients should employ avoidance diets, patients with comparatively low threshold doses are at greater risk because exposure to small residual amounts of allergenic foods is more likely to provoke an adverse reaction. These individuals must be extremely vigilant because shared utensils, cooking vessels, and frying oil might be expected to transfer milligram quantities of the allergenic food. Even kissing someone who has consumed the allergenic food may pose a risk [48,49].

Low-dose oral challenges allow determination of an individual's threshold dose for reactivity via ingestion. Anecdotally, food-allergic individuals have also reacted to exposure to very small quantities of allergenic foods through other routes such as skin contacts with food surfaces, inhalation of vapors from cooking of the food, and exposure to dust in airplane cabins [3,50,51]. Routes of exposure other than the oral route, for example inhalation or skin contact, may be comparatively more sensitive, although this has not been carefully studied. Thus, knowledge of the oral threshold dose may be of limited value in providing advice regarding other routes of exposure.

Infants and children are sometimes able to outgrow their food allergies apparently through the development of oral tolerance [5]. That is particularly true for milk, egg, soybean, and wheat allergies [5]. Although not carefully studied in a longitudinal manner, the individual thresholds of these children appear to increase until they can tolerate

typical servings of these foods. Thus, it is tempting to speculate that those individuals with very low individual threshold doses would be less likely to outgrow their food allergy or would require a longer time period for that to occur.

In at least one study [25], individuals with histories of severe food allergies had significantly lower individual threshold doses. Perhaps this observation should not be surprising, because exposure to small amounts of the allergenic food is likely to elicit reactions in such individuals and inadvertent exposure to large doses seems likely to provoke more serious manifestations. Because of their vulnerability to small doses of hidden allergens, individuals with comparatively low threshold doses should probably be among the patients who would benefit the most from carrying an emergency epinephrine kit. However, in other studies [18], the correlation between the severity of reactions suffered in the community and the severity of reactions elicited during low-dose challenges was poor. The doses involved in reactions occurring in the community are certainly not controlled and could affect attempts to make such correlations. Such observations do indicate the value of clinical conservatism in decisions about access to epinephrine.

Food industry and regulatory uses of threshold information

Unfortunately, scientific and regulatory consensus does not exist to allow the establishment of population-based threshold levels. Many reasons exist for the lack of consensus, but key issues are the lack of data due to the relatively low numbers of patients with known and published individual threshold doses, the lack of individual NOAELs even in cases where the individual LOAEL is published, uncertainties emanating from the possible exclusion of patients with histories of severe reactions from challenge trials, and uncertainties due to differences in clinical protocols for low-dose challenges.

Governmental regulatory agencies could make effective use of population-based thresholds. Regulatory agencies have the responsibility to assure the safety of the food supply in their country or region. Certainly, undeclared major allergens in packaged foods should be considered as a potential health hazard for consumers with that food allergy. Recalls of products from the marketplace are common in some countries (United States, Canada, and Australia) as a result of undeclared allergens. Currently, any level of an undeclared allergen can be the basis for a recall. With the establishment of population-based thresholds, enforcement could be focused on products with undeclared allergens at levels likely to exceed these thresholds.

The food industry has the responsibility for maintaining effective allergen control in their manufacturing facilities to assure the safety of food-allergic consumers. However, economic efficiencies mandate the use of shared equipment and shared facilities between more allergenic and less allergenic formulations. The establishment of population-based thresholds would allow the food industry to establish uniform and appropriate guidelines for evaluation of the effectiveness of their allergen control programs. Methods currently exist that allow the detection of residues of many commonly allergenic foods at ppm (μg per gram) levels [52]. The effectiveness of sanitation is often confirmed with these methods. However, the establishment of population-based thresholds would assure that these existing methods are sufficient to mitigate any possible hazards from allergen cross-contact.

The use of advisory labeling (e.g. "may contain peanut") has proliferated on packaged foods in recent years. Many foods have such labels even though allergen residues cannot be detected in those foods [53]. Food-allergic consumers should be advised to avoid products bearing such advisory statements but evidence indicates that these consumers are increasingly ignoring these statements [53]. These advisory labeling statements are voluntary and companies have widely differing criteria for the use of such statements on packages. The establishment of population-based thresholds could be used by regulatory agencies as the basis for criteria for the use of advisory labeling statements. Such action would likely curtail the rampant use of such labeling and improve the quality-of-life of consumers with restricted avoidance diets.

"Allergen-free" products are also appearing on the market in many countries. The use of such labeling is voluntary and not well regulated in most circumstances. While consumers probably believe that no residues of the allergenic food are present in such products, that belief is not documented in the case of most of these products. The establishment of population-based thresholds could provide the basis for "allergen-free" products. The use of gluten-free labeling on products for the benefit of patients with celiac disease is a good example of the use of such labeling and regulation. The regulatory standards for gluten-free products are variable around the world but range from <20 to <200 ppm gluten. Products containing <100 ppm gluten appear to be safe for the majority of celiac patients [54]. Thus, the establishment of a regulatory, population-based threshold based on clinical science has allowed the prudent development of a gluten-free market category that benefits these patients.

Conclusions

Diagnostic challenge procedures for food allergy could allow physicians to determine the individual threshold doses for patients. As it stands, most food-allergic patients do not know their individual threshold dose because few allergy clinics make this assessment. The knowledge of individual threshold doses would allow physicians to offer more complete advice to food-allergic patients in terms of their comparative vulnerability to hidden residues of allergenic foods. The clinical determination of large numbers of individual threshold doses would allow estimates of population-based thresholds using appropriate statistical modeling approaches. The food industry and regulatory agencies could also make effective use of information on population-based threshold doses to establish improved labeling regulations and practices and allergen control programs.

References

1 Gern JE, Yang E, Evrard HM, *et al*. Allergic reactions to milk-contaminated "non-dairy" products. *N Engl J Med* 1991;324:976–9.

2 Yman IM. Detection of inadequate labeling and contamination as causes of allergic reactions to foods. *Acta Aliment* 2004;33:347–57.

3 Taylor SL, Hefle SL, Bindslev-Jensen C, *et al*. Factors affecting the determination of threshold doses for allergenic foods: How much is too much? *J Allergy Clin Immunol* 2002;109:24–30.

4 Hefle SL, Taylor SL. How much food is too much? Threshold doses for allergenic foods. *Curr Allergy Asthma Reps* 2002;2:63–66.

5 Sampson HA. Epidemiology of food allergy. *Pediatr Allergy Immunol* 1996;7:42–50.

6 Leung DYM, Sampson HA, Yunginger JW, *et al*. Effect of anti-IgE therapy in patients with peanut allergy. *N Engl J Med* 2003;348:986–93.

7 Morisset M, Moneret-Vautrin DA, Kanny G, *et al*. Thresholds of clinical reactivity to milk, egg, peanut and sesame in immunoglobulin E-dependent allergies: evaluation by double-blind or single-blind placebo-controlled oral challenges. *Clin Exp Allergy* 2003;33:1046–51.

8 Crevel RWR, Briggs D, Hefle SL, *et al*. Hazard characterization in food allergen risk assessment: the application of statistical approaches and the use of clinical data. *Food Chem Toxicol* 2007;45:691–701.

9 Bock SA, Sampson HA, Atkins FM, *et al*. Double-blind, placebo-controlled challenge (DBPCFC) as an office procedure: a manual. *J Allergy Clin Immunol* 1988;82:986–97.

10 Lack G, Fox D, Northstone K, *et al*. Factors associated with the development of peanut allergy in childhood. *N Eng J Med* 2003;348:977–85.

11 Strid J, Hourihane J, Kimber I, *et al*. Disruption of the stratum corneum allows potent epicutaneous immunization with protein antigens resulting in a dominant systemic Th2 response. *Eur J Immunol* 2004;34:2100–9.

12 Adel-Patient K, Ah-Leung S, Bernard H, *et al*. Oral sensitization to peanut is highly enhanced by application of peanut extracts to intact skin, but is prevented when CpG and cholera toxin are added. *Int Arch Allergy Immunol* 2007;143:10–20.

13 Bindslev-Jensen C, Ballmer-Weber BK, Bengtsson U, *et al*. Standardization of food challenges in patients with immediate reactions to foods – position paper from the European Academy of Allergology and Clinical Immunology. *Allergy* 2004;59:690–7.

14 Hourihane J, Kilburn SA, Nordlee JA, *et al*. An evaluation of the sensitivity of subjects with peanut allergy to very low doses of peanut protein: a randomized, double-blind, placebo-controlled food challenge study. *J Allergy Clin Immunol* 1997;100:596–600.

15 Taylor SL, Hefle SL, Bindslev-Jensen C, *et al.* A consensus protocol for the determination of the threshold doses for allergenic foods: how much is too much? *Clin Exp Allergy* 2004;34:689–95.

16 Flinterman AE, Pasmans SG, Hoekstra MO, *et al.* Determination of no-observed-adverse-effect levels and eliciting doses in a representative group of peanut-sensitized children. *J Allergy Clin Immunol* 2006;117:448–54.

17 Hourihane JO'B, Knulst AC. Thresholds of allergenic proteins in foods. *Toxicol Appl Pharmacol* 2005;207:152–6.

18 Hourihane JO'B, Grimshaw KE, Lewis SA, *et al.* Does severity of low-dose, double-blind, placebo-controlled food challenges reflect severity of allergic reactions to peanut in the community? *Clin Exp Allergy* 2005;35:1227–33.

19 Nordlee JA, Hefle SL, Taylor SL, *et al.* Minimum elicitation dose determination using roasted peanut – low dose challenges. *J Allergy Clin Immunol* 2007;119:S158.

20 Grimshaw KEC, King RM, Nordlee JA, *et al.* Presentation of allergen in different food preparations affects the nature of the allergic reaction – a case series. *Clin Exp Allergy* 2003; 33:1581–5.

21 van der Zee JA, Wensing M, Penninks AH, *et al.* Threshold levels in peanut and hazelnut allergic patients do not change over time. *Proceedings of XXII Congress of European Academy of Allergology and Clinical Immunology*, Paris, 2003.

22 Sampson HA. Update on food allergy. *J Allergy Clin Immunol* 2004;113:805–19.

23 Roberts G, Lack G. Diagnosing peanut allergy with skin prick and specific IgE testing. *J Allergy Clin Immunol* 2005;115:1291–6.

24 Peeters KABM, Koppelman S, van Hoffen E, *et al.* Does skin prick test reactivity to purified allergens correlate with clinical severity of peanut allergy? *Clin Exp Allergy* 2007;37:108–15.

25 Wensing M, Penninks AH, Hefle SL, *et al.* The distribution of individual threshold doses eliciting allergic reactions in a population with peanut allergy. *J Allergy Clin Immunol* 2002;110:915–20.

26 Sicherer SH, Morrow EH, Sampson HA. Dose–response in double-blind, placebo-controlled oral food challenges in children with atopic dermatitis. *J Allergy Clin Immunol* 2000;105:582–6.

27 Perry TT, Matsu EC, Conover-Walker MK, *et al.* Risk of oral food challenges. *J Allergy Clin Immunol* 2004;114:1164–8.

28 Oppenheimer JJ, Nelson HS, Bock SA, *et al.* Treatment of peanut allergy with rush immunotherapy. *J Allergy Clin Immunol* 1992;90:256–62.

29 Nelson HS, Lahr J, Rule R, *et al.* Treatment of anaphylactic sensitivity to peanuts by immunotherapy with injections of aqueous peanut extract. *J Allergy Clin Immunol* 1997;99:744–51.

30 Lewis SA, Grimshaw KEC, Warner JO, *et al.* The promiscuity of immunoglobulin E binding to peanut allergens, as determined by Western blotting, correlates with the severity of clinical symptoms. *Clin Exp Allergy* 2005;35:767–73.

31 Moneret-Vautrin DA, Rance F, Kanny G, *et al.* Food allergy to peanuts in France – evaluation of 142 observations. *Clin Exp Allergy* 1998;28:1113–19.

32 May CD. Objective clinical and laboratory studies of immediate hypersensitivity reactions to foods in asthmatic children. *J Allergy Clin Immunol* 1976;58:500–15.

33 Meglio P, Bartone E. Plantamura M, *et al.* A protocol for oral desensitization in children with IgE-mediated cow's milk allergy. *Allergy* 2004;59:980–7.

34 Moneret-Vautrin DA, Fremont S, Kanny G, *et al.* The use of two multitests fx5 and fx10 in the diagnosis of food allergy in children: regarding 42 cases. *Allergie Immunologie* 1995;27:2–6.

35 Fiocchi A, Travaini M, D'Auria E, *et al.* Tolerance to a rice hydrolysate formula in children allergic to cow's milk and soy. *Clin Exp Allergy* 2003;33:1576–80.

36 Buchanan AD, Green TD, Jones SM, *et al.* Egg oral immunotherapy in nonanaphylactic children with egg allergy. *J Allergy Clin Immunol* 2007;119:199–205.

37 Wensing M, Penninks AH, Hefle SL, *et al.* The range of minimum provoking doses in hazelnut-allergic patients as determined by double-blind, placebo-controlled food challenges. *Clin Exp Allergy* 2002;32:1757–62.

38 Ispano M, Ansaloni R, Rotondo F, *et al.* Double blind placebo controlled food (DBPCFC) challenge in subjects believed to be allergic to hazelnut. *Abstract of the 7th International Symposium on Immunological, Chemical and Clinical Problems of Food Allergy*, Taormina, Italy, Munksgaard, Copenhagen, 1998:92.

39 Flinterman AE, Hoekstra MO, Meijer Y, *et al.* Clinical reactivity to hazelnut in children: association with sensitization to birch pollen or nuts? *J Allergy Clin Immunol* 2006;118:1186–9.

40 Magnolfi CF, Zani G, Lacava L, *et al.* Soy allergy in atopic children. *Ann Allergy Asthma Immunol* 1996; 77:197–201.

41 Rance F, Dutau G, Abbal M. Mustard allergy in children. *Allergy* 2000;55:496–500.

42 Figueroa J, Blanco C, Dumpierrez AG, *et al.* Mustard allergy confirmed by double-blind placebo-controlled food challenges: clinical features and cross-reactivity with mugwort pollen and plant-derived foods. *Allergy* 2005;60:48–55.

43 Hansen TK, Bindslev-Jensen C. Codfish allergy in adults – identification and diagnosis. *Allergy* 1992;47:610–17.

44 Helbling A, Haydel R, McCants ML, *et al.* Fish allergy: Is cross-reactivity among fish species relevant? Double-blind placebo-controlled food challenge studies in fish allergic adults. *Ann Allergy Asthma Immunol* 1999;83:517–23.

45 Atkins FM, Steinberg SS, Metcalfe DD. Evaluation of immediate adverse reactions to food in adult patients. II. A detailed analysis of reaction patterns during oral food challenge. *J Allergy Clin Immunol* 1985;75:356–63.

46 Bernstein M, Day JH, Welsh A. Double-blind food challenge in the diagnosis of food sensitivity in the adult. *J Allergy Clin Immunol* 1982;70:205–10.

47 Rolinck-Werninghaus C, Staden U, Mehl A, *et al.* Specific oral tolerance induction with food in children: transient or persistent effect on food allergy. *Allergy* 2005;60:1320–2.

48 Eriksson NE, Moller C, Werner S, *et al.* The hazards of kissing when you are food allergic. *J Invest Allergol Clin Immunol* 2003;13:149–54.

49 Hallett R, Haapanen LAD, Teuber SS. Food allergies and kissing. *N Engl J Med* 2002;346:1833–4.

50 Sicherer SH, Furlong TJ, DeSimone J, *et al.* Self-reported allergic reactions to peanut on commercial airlines. *J Allergy Clin Immunol* 1999;104:186–9.

51 Perry TT, Conover Walker MK, Pomes A, *et al.* Distribution of peanut allergen in the environment. *J Allergy Clin Immunol* 2004;113:973–6.

52 Koppelman SJ, Hefle SL (eds.). *Detecting Allergens in Food.* Cambridge, England: Woodhead Publishing Ltd, 2006:422 pp.

53 Hefle SL, Furlong TJ, Niemann L, *et al.* Consumer attitudes and risks associated with packaged foods having advisory labeling regarding the presence of peanuts. *J. Allergy Clin Immunol* 2007; 120:171–6.

54 Collin P, Thorell L, Kaukinen K, *et al.* The safe threshold for gluten contamination in gluten-free products. Can trace amounts be accepted in the treatment of coeliac disease? *Aliment Pharmacol Ther* 2004;19:1277–83.

7

CHAPTER 7

Development of Immunological Tolerance to Food Antigens

Bengt Björkstén

KEY CONCEPTS

- Oral tolerance to ingested antigens is an active immunological process, mediated through two primary effector mechanisms, low doses favoring the induction of regulatory T-cells, and high doses promoting antigen driven tolerance.

- Early T-cell responses are subject to a broad range of regulatory mechanisms which are dictated by the concentration, frequency, and route of allergen exposure as well as age and developmental status of the individual at the time of exposure.

- Genetic risk of allergy is associated with delayed postnatal maturation of immune regulation.

- Interaction with microbes, especially the normal gut microbiota, is the principal environmental signal for postnatal maturation of T-cell function. Oral tolerance, for example, does not develop in germ-free animals and they also have other signs of impaired immune regulation.

- Immunological interaction between the mother and her offspring, during gestation and through breast milk, may play a significant role in tolerance induction.

Introduction

The prevalence of allergic diseases has increased progressively since the 1960s, in particular in First World countries, and the rises appear to be continuing in many countries. The most prominent increases have occurred in allergy to inhaled antigens. However, there is evidence to suggest that at least some forms of food allergy are also increasing. The most notable example is peanut allergy, which was previously rare in many countries. The increase may be due to altered dietary habits in previously unexposed populations coupled with changes in processing procedures resulting in increased allergenicity of peanut antigens, but the issue remains unresolved.

This chapter focuses primarily on the underlying immunological mechanisms governing host responses to ingested antigens. The focus will initially be on what has been learned from basic studies in animal models, what has been deduced from extrapolation of these systems to immunocompetent human adults, and then what is known of the immunology underlying sensitization to dietary versus inhalant allergens during childhood.

Immunological tolerance to dietary antigens in experiment animals: the phenomenon of oral tolerance

The first formal description of experimental oral tolerance (OT) dates back to the work of H.G. Wells in 1911 [1]. His studies in the guinea pig involving repeated feeding of egg white protein (ovalbumin; OVA) are prototypical of several generations of subsequent laboratory research viz. repeated antigen feeding of immunologically naive animals elicited initial "hypersensitivity" responses which in some animals resulted in fatal anaphylaxis, but in the majority the symptomatology was transient and was followed by permanent unresponsiveness to the antigen. We now recognize the initial hypersensitivity manifestations as a hallmark of the "Th2 default" response of the mucosal immune system to a soluble protein antigen [2], and the ensuing state of (antigen specific) unresponsiveness as indicative of the subsequent onset of immunological tolerance (i.e. OT).

It is recognized that most aspects of the adaptive immune response may be experimentally downregulated by antigen feeding, in many cases via a single dose. The range of susceptible immunological phenomena include cellular immunity measured as delayed-type hypersensitivity (DTH [3–5]), contact sensitivity [6], cytotoxic CD8+ T-cell responses [7,8], production of cytokines [9], and antibody

Food Allergy: Adverse Reactions to Foods and Food Additives, 4th edition.
Edited by Dean D. Metcalfe, Hugh A. Sampson, and Ronald A. Simon.
© 2008 Blackwell Publishing, ISBN: 978-1-4501-5129-0.

secretion [10]. There is some evidence that local secretory IgA responses to the eliciting antigen may be preferentially "spared" in this tolerance induction process via generation of IgA T-helper cells in gut associated lymphoid tissues during tolerogenesis [11]. This may be part of a generalized mucosal protection process, since IgA antibodies would prevent antigen penetration through the gut wall and thus limit the scope for allergic sensitization.

Many host and environmental factors have been identified as partial determinants of susceptibility to OT induction. Prominent among host factors are hormonal balance [12], genetic background [13], and in particular postnatal age. A transient temporal window defining increasing susceptibility to sensitization to dietary antigens is operative in the mouse during the early postnatal period [14–16]. This seems to be due to poorly developed immune regulation, both at the levels of T-regulatory and antigen-presenting cells (APC) [17,18]. Host immune competence is a key feature underlying efficient OT, as demonstrated by the fact that administration of cytotoxic immunosuppressants seriously compromises the process [4].

Additional exogenous factors which interfere with OT induction include inflammatory adjuvants [19], low dose irradiation [3], and changes in host microbial flora [20,21].

The type and dose of antigen are also important factors in the induction of OT. While tolerance can be readily induced to all thymus-dependent soluble protein antigens, replicating and particulate antigens tend to induce active immunity. The inflammatory response elicited by replicating antigens bypasses OT mechanisms, and this can be mimicked with inert soluble protein antigen by coupling to adjuvants and/or microbial toxins [22,23]. The tolerogenic dose range for some antigens can also in some situations be within the immunogenic range for others, as shown in recent studies contrasting cow's milk whey proteins and OVA [18]. It is also noteworthy that while OT can be induced over a wide range of dosages and using varying feeding frequency regimes, continuous exposure leads to the most profound tolerance [24,25]. Furthermore, very low doses below the tolerogenic range can in some circumstances prime animals for subsequent immune responses [26].

Antigen presentation and processing in oral tolerance induction

Several pathways are operative in sampling and processing of ingested antigen, and it is possible that the particular pathway which is dominant within an individual immune response may ultimately determine the nature of ensuing immunity. There are three principal pathways for sampling of antigens from the luminal surface of the gut: between lining epithelial cells, through the epithelial cells themselves, or via M-cells with subsequent delivery into Peyer's patches (PP). In each situation, distinct populations of

potential APC will be encountered, and it is not clear what the contribution of each is in the OT process.

The full range of known professional APC have been identified throughout the gut wall and associated lymphoid tissues, comprising dendritic cells (DC), macrophages, and B-cells [27]. Many sites contain multiple APC populations. For example, at least three populations of DC with APC activity have been defined in PP [28–30], one of which has been proposed to selectively prime T-cells for IL-10 production [28].

Gut-derived DC are currently the focus of intense interest, as potential candidates for generation of the rate-limiting tolerogenic signal(s) in the OT process. In other organ systems, DC are recognized as the ultimate regulators of the immune response [17,31]. These cells are the most potent APC for activation of T-cells in primary immune responses, and they are increasingly being implicated in regulation of tolerance to self-antigens and to exogenous antigens. Administration of the growth factor Flt3L to mice markedly expands the numbers of DC in the intestine and associated lymphoid tissues, and at the same time increases susceptibility to OT induction [32].

An additional antigen presentation pathway which may also contribute to OT development involves the direct absorption into the circulation of breakdown products of ingested antigens (i.e. low molecular weight peptides) which are potentially tolerogenic [33,34].

Cellular mechanisms governing the induction and maintenance of oral tolerance

There are two primary effector mechanisms of OT. The first mechanism involves the induction of regulatory T-cells that mediate active suppression and the second is caused by clonal anergy. Low doses of antigen favor the generation of regulatory T-cell driven tolerance, whereas high doses of antigen promote antigen driven tolerance [35].

The initial evidence that OT is an active process came from studies involving adoptive transfer of OT to naive recipients via CD8+ splenocytes from tolerant donors [36]. However, this maneuver failed in many laboratories until careful studies revealed that several apparently distinct mechanisms are operative at the two extremes of the antigen exposure dose–response curve [35]. At one end of the spectrum, high-dose oral antigen exposure leads to functional elimination of antigen-specific T-cells via either deletion or anergy induction.

An alternative to deletion is T-cell anergy induction, in which antigen-response cells are functionally paralyzed. This also occurs in the high-dose range, most likely via aberrant antigen presentation by MHC class II-bearing APC which lack key costimulator molecules, such as CD80/CD86 [37]. These anergized cells do not apoptose and instead persist at the periphery. They presumably maintain their surface antigen receptors, but lose the capacity to clonally expand and secrete the full repertoire of cytokines following encounter with antigen. In particular, in some model systems cytokine secretion by anergized T-cells appears limited to IL-10. Consistent with the potential importance of this mechanism, evidence exists in some models of OT for the presence of tolerized T-cells whose ability to respond to antigen *in vivo* can be restored by exogenous IL-2 [38]. Further supporting evidence has been provided in transgenic mice [39].

In contrast, exposure of animals to low dose oral antigen is proposed to induce a form of "low zone tolerance" involving active antigen-specific suppression of immunity which can in some systems be adoptively transferred by CD8+ T-cells, and by CD4+ T-cells in others [40]. However, it should be noted that OT induction proceeds normally in CD8-knockout mice [7], suggesting that the role of these cells may be restricted to maintenance, rather than induction of OT. There is additional evidence to suggest that a subset of TcRγ/δ T-cells may also participate in the OT process [41].

Currently, much of the OT literature is focused on CD4+ T-regulatory cells and the cytokines they secrete. Two principal subtypes have been identified (i.e. Th3 cells which secrete TGFβ with or without IL-10 [42,43], and Tr1 cells which secrete IL-10 [42]). IL-4 has also been implicated in the OT inducing activity of Th3 cells; however, its role may be restricted to that of a non-essential growth factor [44] given that IL-4-knockout mice can still generate OT [45].

TGFβ has many roles in the control of epithelial growth and differentiation and in local control of secretory IgA production in the gut [46]. This may explain the selective preservation of secretory IgA antibody production during systemic OT induction [47]. Additionally, TGFβ has a number of potent immunosuppressive effects [46], including those targeted at APC functions. IL-10 is recognized as a powerful anti-inflammatory and immunomodulatory agent which plays a critical role in local homeostasis in the gastrointestinal mucosa, particularly via its damping effects on Th1 activity [27,48].

One interpretation of these findings is that many of the mechanisms defined experimentally may represent redundancies. However, it is more likely that each constitutes one component of a multi-layered integrated regulatory process, each of which is operative as dictated by prevailing conditions of antigen dosage and exposure frequency [18]. An intriguing additional possibility is that some of the T-regulatory populations may in fact be partially anergized T-cells, which despite functional downregulation have conserved their ability to secrete certain cytokines, such as IL-10 and TGFβ.

Oral tolerance in humans: How well do mouse models mimic the human situation?

As noted above, the baseline "default" response of laboratory mice appears biased toward a Th2-like cytokine profile, admixed with TGFβ production [2]. This Th2 default is also consistent with the pioneering studies of Wells in guinea pigs [1], wherein the first manifestations of immunological reactivity in a subset of his test animals during feeding was what we now recognize as anaphylaxis. However, this Th2 bias is clearly a transient state in most situations, given the fact that the hallmark of successfully induced OT is tolerance in the IgE antibody class.

Selective priming of T-cells in PP for production of IL-4 and TGFβ is a hallmark of this bias toward baseline Th2 in murine immune responses to oral antigen [49,50]. These cells migrate to peripheral sites and function as T-regulators to dampen Th1 immunity [51]. Such studies have not been performed in man. However, studies indicate that unlike the murine situation, the immunological milieu in human gut associated lymphoid structures such as PP is strongly Th1 biased [52], at least in adults. Thus, freshly isolated T-cells from the human gut lamina propria produce high levels of IFNγ relative to IL-4, IL-5, and IL-10 [53,54], and high levels of IL-12 production are observed in human PP [52,55]. This difference between mouse and humans may be a direct reflection of the markedly differing levels of microbial stimulation in humans versus specified pathogen-free mice housed under controlled conditions and fed exclusively sterilized food [52]. Under extreme conditions (i.e. in germ-free mice) OT does not even develop [20].

While these observations suggest significant differences between human immune responses to oral antigens and those seen in mice under experimental conditions, it is clear from several lines of evidence that the fundamental process of OT nevertheless occurs in man. Notably, feeding of keyhole limpet hemocyanin to immunologically naive volunteers selectively downregulated subsequent cellular immune responses to the antigen [56,57]. Furthermore, prospective studies have shown transient IgE antibody production to foods to be common during the first 2 years of life and then downregulated [58]. Also deliberate parenteral immunization of volunteers with the common dietary antigen bovine serum albumin elicited little or no antibody production [59]. Additionally, clinical trials aimed at amelioration of autoimmune disease by autoantigen feeding have provided varying levels of clinical effects [60], and have also provided evidence of the induction of Th3 responses in blood lymphocytes which are comparable to those reported in murine model [43].

Comparative studies on T-cell responses of PP-derived T-cells (PPT) versus peripheral blood T-cells (PBT) from normal subjects indicated consistent lymphoproliferation in PPT in response to the dietary antigen β-lactoglobulin (BLG), in contrast to low/non-responsiveness in PBT [55]. Moreover, the peripheral blood mononuclear cell responses were dominated by Th1 cytokines [55], mirroring the overall Th1-biased milieu of gut associated lymphoid tissues [49]. This apparent OT at the periphery with the concomitant presence of antigen-specific IFNγ-secreting T-cells in lymphoid compartments draining the intestinal mucosa, mimics precisely the situation reported for mice fed repeated doses of OVA [9], and may be indicative of the contribution of locally activated regulatory T-cells in the maintenance of systemic tolerance. It is clear that more fundamental studies are needed on human immune responses to dietary antigens, and in particular on the potential interactions between these and parallel responses to microbial stimuli provided by the local commensal flora.

Food allergy in humans: the clinical reality

Dietary antigen-induced enteropathies are believed to be central to the pathogenesis of a broad range of chronic inflammatory diseases in humans, including IgE-mediated food allergy, celiac disease, inflammatory bowel disease, and other enteropathies. The discussion below will focus on allergic-like manifestations of aberrant immunity to dietary antigens, in particular issues relating to the initiation of dietary allergies in early life. From a clinical point of view it is important to appreciate that similar clinical symptoms may be induced by immune reactions, various biochemical intolerances and toxic reactions. Thus, various food intolerances caused by non-immunologically mediated mechanisms are often erroneously called "food allergy". For example, the majority of adults in the world are lactose intolerant. Drinking milk may induce symptoms that may be interpreted as evidence of food allergy.

Allergy to food antigens in an infant is often the first manifestation of atopy and may be the forerunner of subsequently developing IgE-mediated allergy to inhalant allergens. IgE-mediated food allergy and atopic dermatitis in infancy may thus be the first steps in the "atopic march" [61–63]. In most instances, clinical tolerance to the food develops within the first 3 years of life; however, the atopic march continues with manifestations of allergic asthma and subsequently allergic rhinoconjunctivitis. The reasons for this switch from the gastrointestinal to the respiratory tract are unknown.

Clinical tolerance does not develop equally to all food allergens. For unknown reasons, IgE-mediated allergy to cow's milk and egg are uncommon after the age of 4 years, while allergy to soy protein tends to last for a longer time period, peanut allergy usually for many years, and celiac disease is regarded as a lifetime condition which will relapse at any age if the individual is exposed to gluten for some time.

The resolution of clinically manifest food allergy is accompanied by the development of tolerance to food antigens. This process has mostly been studied for allergens causing IgE-mediated reactions, while less is known regarding, for example, the kinetics of immune responses to antigens involved in the pathogenesis of celiac disease and other enteropathies. Prospective studies, in which immune responses to food antigens have been studied through the first several years of life, show that transient IgE antibody responses to, for example, egg and cow's milk are common

in healthy non-atopic infants [62]. In contrast, the IgE antibody responses are of higher magnitude and more prolonged in infants who develop food allergy and/or who will manifest respiratory allergy later during childhood. Indeed, high levels of IgE antibodies to egg or milk in an apparently healthy infant predict the appearance of respiratory allergy some years later [61–63].

Cellular mechanisms underlying control of T-cell immunity to dietary antigens in humans: lessons from studies on responses to aeroallergens

As noted above, studies on antibody production indicate that immune responses against environmental allergens are initiated very early in life in most individuals. These observations have prompted detailed investigations in many laboratories on the nature of underlying T-cell immunity during this life phase. The salient findings are reviewed below.

Firstly, it is clear that T-cells responsive to both dietary and inhalant allergens, as measured by lymphoproliferation and cytokine secretion, are present in cord blood from virtually all subjects [64–67]. Additionally, T-cell cloning and subsequent genotyping studies indicate that the responsive cells are of fetal origin and exhibit a Th2-polarized and/or Th0 cytokine profile [68]. It has been suggested [65,67] that these T-cells may have been primed by processed antigen crossing the placenta, perhaps bound to maternal IgG. Evidence showing the presence of detectable levels of allergen in complex with IgG antibodies in cord blood supports this suggestion [69]. However, it is also feasible that these T-cell responses may be directed against cross-reacting antigens or anti-idiotypic antibodies.

Secondly, it is evident that these early T-cell responses are subject to a variety of regulatory mechanisms postnatally, which are driven by direct exposure of the infant immune system to incoming environmental allergen. Given the experience from animal models, it is likely that a broad range of regulatory mechanisms will be involved, which are dictated by the concentration, frequency and route(s) of allergen exposure, the age and hence developmental status of the individual at the time of exposure, and potentially by allergen structure (e.g. susceptibility to proteolytic degradation). The relevant immunoregulatory mechanisms involved are likely to span the full range from classical low zone tolerance (essentially Th1/Th2 cross-regulation) through to high-zone tolerance phenomena (anergy and/or deletion via apoptosis), and will inevitably include important, but as yet uncharacterized contributions from recently described subsets of T-regulatory cells which appear to participate in a wide range of immunological control mechanisms.

Cross-sectional and prospective studies indicate that in atopic children, consolidation of Th2-polarized immunity against inhalant allergens is initiated in early infancy

[64,70,71] and may be completed by the end of the preschool years in children who develop clinically manifest allergy [72], or even earlier [64]. In contrast, in infants who develop allergic manifestations, low level Th1 responses are established [64]. Prospective studies from Estonia, with a low, and Sweden with a high prevalence of allergy, indicate that the regulatory mechanisms are established more rapidly and that also other mechanisms may be operative [64,73,74]. This is suggested by the observation that during the first 2 years of life, the incidence of positive skin prick tests was similar to that in recent studies from Western Europe, while at 5 years the prevalence was only 3%. At the same time the prevalence of circulating IgE antibodies to milk or egg increased to 36% and 47% to inhalant allergens. The discrepancy between positive skin prick tests and circulating IgE antibodies is interesting in a country with a low prevalence of atopic allergy, as well as Th1-dependent type I diabetes and a lifestyle similar to that prevailing in Scandinavia some 30–40 years ago. The findings may also suggest that clinical tolerance to a food does not exclude the presence of IgE antibodies and possibly other indicators of Th2 immunity. It is possible that a traditional lifestyle is associated with an early induction of a general regulation of T-cell immunity. This notion is supported by the close correlation globally between the prevalence of wheezing and type I diabetes [75].

In contrast to what appears to be positive selection for different forms of active T-cell immunity against inhalant allergens during infancy, the majority of subjects manifest active downregulation of T-cell responses to dietary allergens such as egg, as demonstrated by diminishing lymphoproliferative responses and by a progressive reduction in the number of egg-specific T-cell epitopes recognized *in vitro* [70,71]. This finding suggests the operation of control mechanisms akin to high-zone tolerance (anergy/deletion) in the mouse, although additional regulatory pathways may operate in parallel.

Microbial stimulation in the gastrointestinal tract as a potential modulator of human oral tolerance

Genetic risk for allergy is associated with delayed postnatal maturation of T-helper cell function [76]. Both the cloning frequency of CD4+ T-cells and the capacity of cloned CD4+ T-cells to secrete IFNγ and IL-4 were reduced in infants with positive atopic family history (AFH+) and the reduction was most marked in IFNγ, indicating an overall Th2 bias in T-cell function in this group [76]. Several groups have since reported similar findings in cord blood, both in countries with a high- and low-allergy prevalence [64,77–80]. It is recognized that T-cell function in fetal life is constitutively Th2 based, as part of a set of control mechanisms to limit potential damage to the placenta via toxic Th1 cytokines [81,82], and the more pronounced Th2 bias in AFH+ children may

reflect inappropriate persistence of one or more of these control mechanisms after birth [83].

It is also recognized that interaction with microbes, especially the normal microbial flora of the gastrointestinal tract, is the principal environmental signal for postnatal maturation of T-cell function (in particular the Th1 component) [84,85]. Recognition of these signals is mediated by a series of Toll-like receptors expressed on cells of the innate immune system, and other receptors such as CD14, and it is noteworthy that a polymorphism in the CD14 gene has been associated with high IgE levels [86].

International studies have drawn attention to the wide variations in allergy prevalence between different countries [87–89], and a variety of evidence suggests that these changes have been particularly pronounced over the last 30–40 years [90,91]. Variations in patterns of microbial colonization of the gastrointestinal tract, linked with lifestyle and/or geographic factors, may be important determinants of the heterogeneity in allergy prevalence throughout the world [84]. Ongoing cohort studies are focusing in detail on this complex question. These suggestions are supported by observations that germ-free mice do not develop tolerance in the absence of a gut flora [20,21] and by the demonstration of differences in the composition of the gut flora between infants living in countries with a high and a low prevalence of allergy [74,92] and between healthy and allergic infants [93–96]. Although all the studies confirm such differences, no particular protective or potentially harmful bacterial species can be identified so far. In the three prospective studies [94,96,97] and one cross-sectional study [93], the presence of bifidobacteria was associated with less allergy, while presence of *Clostridium difficile* has been linked to allergy. The administration of lactobacilli to mothers or their infants was recently reported to be associated with less atopic dermatitis during the first 2 years of life [96] but there was no reduction in respiratory allergies at 4 years of age [98].

Maternal influences

There is a close immunological interaction between the mother and her offspring, not only during pregnancy as already discussed, but also as long as the baby is breast-fed. Human milk contains numerous immunological components, including IgA and other antibodies, various chemokines [99] as well as cytokines, mainly with anti-inflammatory and IgA stimulatory properties, such as TGF-β, IL-8, and IL-10 [100]. It is well established that human milk often contains food antigens that may induce IgE antibody formation. Less is known regarding the immunological consequences of introducing foreign antigens while the infant is still breast-feeding. As indicated by studies of immunity to infectious agents, it is possible that this represents a mechanism by which immune responses are modulated [101]. In the early 1990s, there was a pronounced increase in the incidence of celiac disease among Swedish infants [102]. Prior to the increase in celiac disease, gluten was gradually introduced while the baby was still breast-fed. Then, gluten was avoided for the first 6 months. When the national recommendations were changed back to gradual introduction of gluten while the babies were still partly breast-fed, the incidence of celiac disease dropped rapidly.

Very recent studies with probiotics suggest that the maternal influences may be more pronounced in tolerance induction than previously appreciated. There are now at least three studies trying to prevent food allergy and infantile eczema with lactobacilli [96,103,104]. In the study with a negative outcome [104], the bacteria were given only to the babies, while in the two studies with some protective effect [96,98,103] they were also given to the mothers during the last month of gestation.

Concluding remarks

The development of immunological tolerance to food antigens is a complex process and depends on an intense interaction between the host and the environment, including microbial stimulation. It is intriguing that microbial stimulation, in particular via the gastrointestinal tract, has also been implicated as an etiological factor in respiratory allergic diseases. This suggests that microbial stimuli exert effects beyond the mucosal tissue microenvironments adjacent to sites of exposure, and presumably can influence systemic precursor compartments such as bone marrow and thymus. The underlying mechanism(s) are likely to include stimulation of functional maturation of cells within the innate and adaptive immune systems during the early postnatal period, a process which may ultimately determine the overall efficiency of immune/tolerance induction during early life, with major flow-on effects into adulthood. A full understanding of the underlying mechanisms may open new venues for the prevention by modification of the gut microflora, not only of food allergy, but also conceivably of respiratory allergies.

References

1 Wells HG, Osborne TB. The biological reactions of the vegetable proteins. I. Anaphylaxis. *J Infect Dis* 1911;8:66–124.

2 Weiner HL, Friedman A, Miller A, *et al*. Oral tolerance: immunologic mechanisms and treatment of animal and human organ-specific autoimmune diseases by oral administration of autoantigens. *Ann Rev Immunol* 1994;12:809–37.

3 Bruce MG, Strobel S, Hanson DG, Ferguson A. Irradiated mice lose the capacity to "process" fed antigen for systemic tolerance of delayed-type hypersensitivity. *Clin Exp Immunol* 1987;70:611–18.

4 Mowat AM, Strobel S, Drummond HE, Ferguson A. Immunological responses to fed protein antigens in mice. I. Reversal of oral tolerance to ovalbumin by cyclophosphamide. *Immunology* 1982;45:105–13.

5 Peng HJ, Turner MW, Strobel S. The kinetics of oral hyposensitization to a protein antigen are determined by immune status and the timing, dose and frequency of antigen administration. *Immunology* 1989;67:425–30.

6 Asherson GL, Zembala M, Perera MA, *et al*. Production of immunity and unresponsiveness in the mouse by feeding contact sensitizing agents and the role of suppressor cells in the peyer's patches, mesenteric lymph nodes and other lymphoid tissues. *Cell Immunol* 1977;33:145–55.

7 Garside P, Steel M, Liew FY, Mowat AM. CD4+ but not CD8+ T cells are required for the induction of oral tolerance. *Int Immunol* 1995;7:501–4.

8 Ke Y, Kapp JA. Oral antigen inhibits priming of CD8+ CTL, CD4+ T cells, and antibody responses while activating CD8+ suppressor T cells. *J Immunol* 1996;156:916–21.

9 Hoyne GF, Callow MG, Kuhlman J, Thomas WR. T-cell lymphokine response to orally administered antigens during priming and unresponsiveness. *Immunology* 1993;78:534–40.

10 Thompson HS, Staines NA. Could specific oral tolerance be a therapy for autoimmune disease? *Immunol Today* 1990;11:396–9.

11 Richman LK, Graeff AS, Yarchoan R, Strober W. Simultaneous induction of antigen-specific IgA helper T cells and IgG suppressor T cells in the murine Peyer's patch after protein feeding. *J Immunol* 1981;126:2079–83.

12 Mowat AM. Depletion of suppressor T cells by 2′-deoxyguanosine abrogates tolerance in mice fed ovalbumin and permits the induction of intestinal delayed-type hypersensitivity. *Immunology* 1986;58:179–84.

13 Holt PG, Britten D, Sedgwick JD. Suppression of IgE responses by antigen inhalation: studies on the role of genetic and environmental factors. *Immunology* 1987;60:97–102.

14 Strobel S, Ferguson A. Immune responses to fed protein antigens in mice. 3. Systemic tolerance or priming is related to age at which antigen is first encountered. *Pediatr Res* 1984;18:588–94.

15 Hanson DG. Ontogeny of orally induced tolerance to soluble proteins in mice. I. Priming and tolerance in newborns. *J Immunol* 1981;127:1518–24.

16 Miller A, Lider O, Abramsky O, Weiner HL. Orally administered myelin basic protein in neonates primes for immune responses and enhances experimental autoimmune encephalomyelitis in adult animals. *Eur J Immunol* 1994;24:1026–32.

17 Niess J, Reinecker H. Dendritic cells: the commanders-in-chief of mucosal immune defenses. *Curr Opin Gastroenterol* 2006;22:354–60.

18 Strobel S, Mowat AM. Immune responses to dietary antigens: oral tolerance. *Immunol Today* 1998;19:173–81.

19 Hornquist E, Grdic D, Mak T, Lycke N. CD8-deficient mice exhibit augmented mucosal immune responses and intact adjuvant effects to cholera toxin. *Immunology* 1996;87:220–9.

20 Moreau MC, Coste M, Gaboriau V, Dubuquoy C. Oral tolerance to ovalbumin in mice: effect of some parameters on the induction and persistence of the suppression of systemic IgE and IgG antibody responses. *Adv Exp Med Biol* 1995;371B:1229–34.

21 Sudo N, Sawamura S-A, Tanaka K, *et al*. The requirement of intestinal bacterial flora for the development of an IgE production

system fully susceptible to oral tolerance induction. *J Immunol* 1997;159:1739–45.

22 Maloy KJ, Donachie AM, Mowat AM. Induction of Th1 and Th2 CD4+ T cell responses by oral or parenteral immunization with ISCOMS. *Eur J Immunol* 1995;25:2835–41.

23 Pierre P, Denis O, Bazin H, *et al.* Modulation of oral tolerance to ovalbumin by cholera toxin and its B subunit. *Eur J Immunol* 1992;22:3179–82.

24 Melamed D, Fishman-Lovell J, Uni Z, *et al.* Peripheral tolerance of Th2 lymphocytes induced by continuous feeding of ovalbumin. *Int Immunol* 1996;8:717–24.

25 Melamed D, Friedman A. *In vivo* tolerization of Th1 lymphocytes following a single feeding with ovalbumin: anergy in the absence of suppression. *Eur J Immunol* 1994;24:1974–81.

26 Mowat AM. The regulation of immune responses to dietary protein antigens. *Immunol Today* 1987;8:93–8.

27 Faria AM, Weiner HL. Oral tolerance. *Immunol Rev* 2005; 206:232–59.

28 Iwasaki A, Kelsall BL. Freshly isolated Peyer's patch, but not spleen, dendritic cells produce interleukin 10 and induce the differentiation of T helper type 2 cells. *J Exp Med* 1999;190:229–39.

29 Iwaski A, Kelsall BL. Mucosal immunity and inflammation. I. Mucosal dendritic cells: their specialized role in initiating T cell responses. *Am J Physiol* 1999;276:G1074–8.

30 Strobel S, Mowat AM. Oral tolerance and allergic responses to food proteins. *Curr Opin Allergy Clin Immunol* 2006;6:207–13.

31 Akbari O, Umetsu DT. Role of regulatory dendritic cells in allergy and asthma. *Curr Opin Allergy Clin Immunol* 2004;4:533–8.

32 Viney JL, Mowat AM, O'Malley JM, Williamson E, Fanger NA. Expanding dendritic cells *in vivo* enhances the induction of oral tolerance. *J Immunol* 1998;160:5815–25.

33 Bruce MG, Ferguson A. The influence of intestinal processing on the immunogenicity and molecular size of absorbed, circulating ovalbumin in mice. *Immunology* 1986;59:295–300.

34 Webb KE. Amino acid and peptide absorption from the gastrointestinal tract. *Fed Proc* 1986;45:2268–71.

35 Friedman A, Weiner HL. Induction of anergy or active suppression following oral tolerance is determined by antigen dosage. *PNAS* 1994;91:6688–92.

36 Mowat AM. The role of antigen recognition and suppressor cells in mice with oral tolerance to ovalbumin. *Immunology* 1985;56:253–60.

37 Mueller DL, Jenkins MK, Schwartz RH. Clonal expansion versus functional clonal inactivation: a costimulatory signalling pathway determines the outcome of T cell antigen receptor occupancy. *Annu Rev Immunol* 1989;7:745–80.

38 Whitacre CC, Gienapp IE, Orosz CG, Bitar DM. Oral tolerance in experimental autoimmune encephalomyelitis. *J Immunol* 1991;147:2155–63.

39 Van Houten N, Blake SF. Direct measurement of anergy of antigen-specific T cells following oral tolerance induction. *J Immunol* 1996;157:1337–41.

40 Chen Y, Inobe J, Weiner HL. Induction of oral tolerance to myelin basic protein in CD8-depleted mice: both CD4+ and CD8+ cells mediate active suppression. *J Immunol* 1995;155:910–6.

41 Ke Y, Pearce K, Lake JP, *et al.* Gamma delta T lymphocytes regulate the induction and maintenance of oral tolerance. *J Immunol* 1997;158:3610–18.

42 Fowler E, Weiner HL. Oral tolerance: elucidation of mechanisms and application to treatment of autoimmune diseases. *Biopolymers* 1997;43:323–35.

43 Fukaura H, Kent SC, Pietrusewicz MJ, *et al.* Induction of circulating myelin basic protein and proteolipid protein-specific transforming growth factor-beta1-sectreting Th3 T cells by oral administration of myelin in multiple sclerosis patients. *J Clin Ivest* 1996;98:70–7.

44 Inobe J, Slavin AJ, Komagata Y, *et al.* IL-4 is a differentiation factor for transforming growth factor-beta secreting Th3 cells and oral administration of IL-4 enhances oral tolerance in experimental allergic encephalomyelitis. *Eur J Immunol* 1998;28:2780–90.

45 Garside P, Steel M, Worthey EA, *et al.* T helper 2 cells are subject to high dose oral tolerance and are not essential for its induction. *J Immunol* 1995;154:5649–55.

46 Faria AM, Weiner HL. Oral tolerance and TGF-beta-producing cells. *Inflamm Allergy Drug Targets* 2006;5:179–90.

47 Challacombe SJ, Tomasi TJ. Systemic tolerance and secretory immunity after oral immunization. *J Exp Med* 1980;152:1459–72.

48 Battaglia M, Gianfrani C, Gregori S, Roncarolo M. IL-10-producing T regulatory type 1 cells and oral tolerance. *Ann NY Acad Sci* 2004;1029:142–53.

49 Gonnella PA, Chen Y, Inobe J, *et al. In situ* immune response in gut-associated lymphoid tissue (GALT) following oral antigen in TCR-transgenic mice. *J Immunol* 1998;160:4708–18.

50 Santos LM, al-Sabbagh A, Londono A, Weiner HL. Oral tolerance to MBP induces regulatory TGFb secreting T cells in Peyer's patches of SJL mice. *Cell Immunol* 1994;157:439–47.

51 Khoury SJ, Hancock WW, Weiner HL. Oral tolerance to myelin basic protein and natural recovery from experimental autoimmune encephalomyelitis are associated with downregulation of inflammatory cytokines and differential upregulation of transforming growth factor β, interleukin-4, and prostaglandin E expression in the brain. *J Exp Med* 1992;176:1355–64.

52 MacDonald TT, Monteleone G. IL-12 and Th1 immune responses in human Peyer's patches. *Trends Immunol* 2001;22:224–47.

53 Carol M, Lambrechts A, Van Gossum A, *et al.* Spontaneous secretion of interferon gamma and interleukin 4 by human intraepithelial and lamina propria gut lymphocytes. *Gut* 1998;42:643–9.

54 Hauer AC, Breese EJ, Walker-Smith JA, MacDonald TT. The frequency of cells secreting interferon-gamma and interleukin-4, -5, and -10 in the blood and duodenal mucosa of children with cow's milk hypersensitivity. *Pediatr Res* 1997;42:629–38.

55 Nagata S, McKenzie C, Pender SLF, *et al.* Human Peyer's patch T cells are sensitized to dietary antigen and display a Th cell type 1 cytokine profile. *J Immunol* 2000;165:5315–21.

56 Husby S, Mestecky J, Moldoveanu Z, Elson CO. Oral tolerance in humans: T cell but not B cell tolerance to a soluble protein

antigen. In: Mestecky J (ed.) *Advances in Mucosal Immunology.* New York: Plenum Press, 1995:1225–8.

57 Husby S, Mestecky J, Moldoveanu Z, *et al.* Oral tolerance in humans: T cell but not B cell tolerance after antigen feeding. *J Immunol* 1994;152:4663–70.

58 Hattevig G, Kjellman B, Björkstén B. Appearance IgE antibodies to ingested and inhaled allergens during the first 12 years of life in atopic and non-atopic children. *Pediatr Allergy Immunol* 1993;4:182–6.

59 Kornblat PE, Rothberg RM, Minden P, Farr RS. Immune response of human adults after oral and parenteral exposure to bovine serum albumin. *J Allergy* 1968;41:226–35.

60 Faria AM, Weiner HL. Oral tolerance: therapeutic implications for autoimmune diseases. *Clin Dev Immunol* 2006;13:143–57.

61 Kulig M, Klettke U, Wahn V, *et al.* Development of seasonal allergic rhinitis during the first 7 years if life. *J Allergy Clin Immunol* 2000;106:832–9.

62 Sigurs N, Hattevig G, Kjellman B, *et al.* Appearance of atopic disease in relation to serum IgE antibodies in children followed up from birth for 4 to 15 years. J *Allergy Clin Immunol* 1994;94:757–63.

63 Van Asperen PP, Kemp AS, Mukhi A. Atopy in infancy predicts the severity of bronchial hyperresponsiveness in later childhood. *J Allergy Clin Immunol* 1990;85:790–5.

64 Böttcher MF, Jenmalm MC, Voor T, *et al.* Cytokine responses to allergens during the first 2 years of life in Estonian and Swedish children. *Clin Exp Allergy* 2006;36:619–28.

65 Holt PG, O'Keeffe PO, Holt BJ, *et al.* T-cell "priming" against environmental allergens in human neonates: sequential deletion of food antigen specificities during infancy with concomitant expansion of responses to ubiquitous inhalant allergens. *Pediatr Allergy Immunol* 1995;6:85–90.

66 Kondo N, Kobayashi Y, Shinoda S, *et al.* Cord blood lymphocyte responses to food antigens for the prediction of allergic disorders. *Arch Dis Child* 1992;67:1003–7.

67 Piastra M, Stabile A, Fioravanti G, *et al.* Cord blood mononuclear cell responsiveness to beta-lactoglobulin: T-cell activity in "atopy-prone" and "non-atopy-prone" newborns. *Int Arch Allergy Immunol* 1994;104:358–65.

68 Prescott SL, Macaubas C, Holt BJ, *et al.* Transplacental priming of the human immune system to environmental allergens: universal skewing of initial T-cell responses towards the Th-2 cytokine profile. *J Immunol* 1998;160:4730–7.

69 Casas R, Björkstén B. Detection of Fel d 1-IgG immune complexes in the cord blood and sera from allergic and non allergic mothers. *Pediatr Allergy Immunol* 2001;12:59–64.

70 Prescott SL, Macaubas C, Smallacombe T, *et al.* Development of allergen-specific T-cell memory in atopic and normal children. *Lancet* 1999;353:196–200.

71 Yabuhara A, Macaubas C, Prescott SL, *et al.* Th-2-polarised immunological memory to inhalant allergens in atopics is established during infancy and early childhood. *Clin Exp Allergy* 1997;27:1261–9.

72 Macaubas C, Sly PD, Burton P, *et al.* Regulation of Th-cell responses to inhalant allergen during early childhood. *Clin Exp Allergy* 1999;29:1223–31.

73 Julge K, Vasar M, Björkstén B. Development of allergy and IgE antibodies during the first five years of life in Estonian children. *Clin Exp Allergy* 2001;31:1854–61.

74 Sepp E, Naaber RP, Voor T, *et al.* Development of intestinal microflora during the first month of life in Estonian and Swedish infants. *J Microbiol Ecol Health* 2000;12:22–6.

75 Stene LC, Nafstad P. Relation between occurrence of type 1 diabetes and asthma. *Lancet* 2001;257:607–8.

76 Holt PG, Clough JB, Holt BJ, *et al.* Genetic "risk" for atopy is associated with delayed postnatal maturation of T-cell competence. *Clin Exp Allergy* 1992;22:1093–9.

77 Liao SY, Liao TN, Chiang BL, *et al.* Decreased production of IFN-γ and increased production of IL-6 by cord blood mononuclear cells of newborns with a high risk of allergy. *Clin Exp Allergy* 1996;26:397–405.

78 Martinez FD, Stern DA, Wright AL, *et al.* Association of interleukin-2 and interferon-γ production by blood mononuclear cells in infancy with parental allergy skin tests and with subsequent development of atopy. *J Allergy Clin Immunol* 1995;96:652–60.

79 Rinas U, Horneff G, Wahn V. Interferon-γ production by cord-blood mononuclear cells is reduced in newborns with a family history of atopic disease and is independent from cord blood IgE-levels. *Pediatr Allergy Immunol* 1993;4:60–4.

80 Tang MLK, Kemp AS, Thorburn J, Hill DJ. Reduced interferon-γ secretion in neonates and subsequent atopy. *Lancet* 1994;344:983–6.

81 Wegmann TG, Lin H, Guilbert L, Mosmann TR. Bidirectional cytokine interactions in the maternal–fetal relationship: Is successful pregnancy a Th2 phenomenon? *Immunol Today* 1993;14:353–6.

82 Zenclussen AC. Regulatory T cells in pregnancy. *Springer Semin Immunopathol* 2006;28:31–9.

83 Holt PG, Macaubas C. Development of long term tolerance versus sensitisation to environmental allergens during the perinatal period. *Curr Opin Immunol* 1997;9:782–7.

84 Björkstén B. Genetic and environmental risk factors for the development of food allergy. *Curr Opin Allergy Clin Immunol* 2005;5:249–53.

85 Demengeot J, Zelenay S, Moraes-Fontes MF, *et al.* Regulatory T cells in microbial infection. *Springer Semin Immunopathol* 2006;28:41–50.

86 Baldini M, Lohman IC, Halonen M, *et al.* A polymorphism in the 5′-flanking region of the CD14 gene is associated with circulating soluble CD14 levels with total serum IgE. *Am J Resp Cell Mol Biol* 1999;20:976–83.

87 Asher MI, Montefort S, Björkstén B, *et al.* Worldwide time trends in the prevalence of symptoms of asthma, allergic rhinoconjunctivitis, and eczema in childhood: ISAAC Phases One and Three repeat multicountry cross-sectional surveys. *Lancet* 2006;368:733–43.

88 European Community Respiratory Health Survey (ECRHS). Variation in the prevalence of respiratory symptoms, self-reported asthma attacks, and use of asthma medication in the

European Community Respiratory Health Survey (ECRHS). *Eur Resp J* 1996;9:687–95.

89 The International Study of Asthma and Allergies in Childhood (ISAAC) Steering Committee. Worldwide variations in the prevalence of symptoms of asthma, allergic rhinoconjunctivitis and atopic eczema. *Lancet* 1998;251:1225–32.

90 Bråbäck L, Hedberg A. Perinatal risk factors for atopic disease in conscripts. *Clin Exp Allergy* 1998;28:936–42.

91 Jögi R, Janson C, Björnsson E, *et al*. Atopy and allergic disorders among adults in Tartu, Estonia compared with Uppsala, Sweden. *Clin Exper Allergy* 1998;28:1072–80.

92 Sepp E, Julge K, Vasar M, *et al*. Intestinal microflora of Estonian and Swedish infants. *Acta Paediatr* 1997; 86:956–61.

93 Björkstén B, Naaber P, Sepp E, Mikelsaar M. The intestinal microflora in allergic Estonian and Swedish 2-year old children. *Clin Exp Allergy* 1999;29:342–6.

94 Björkstén B, Sepp E, Julge K, *et al*. Allergy development and the intestinal microflora during the first two years of life. *J Allergy Clin Immunol* 2001;108:516–20.

95 Böttcher M, Sandin A, Norin E, *et al*. Microflora associated characteristics in faeces from allergic and non-allergic children. *Clin Exp Allergy* 2000;30:590–6.

96 Kalliomaki M, Kirjavainen P, Eerola E, *et al*. Distinct patterns of neonatal gut microflora in infants developing or not developing atopy. *J Allergy Clin Immunol* 2001;107:129–34.

97 Sepp E, Julge K, Mikelsaar M, Björkstén B. Intestinal microbiota and immunoglobulin E responses in 5-year-old Estonian children. *Clin Exp Allergy* 2005;35:1141–6.

98 Kalliomaki M, Salminen S, Poussa T, *et al*. Probiotics and prevention of atopic disease: 4-year follow-up of a randomised placebo-controlled trial. *Lancet* 2003;361:1869–71.

99 Böttcher FM, Jenmalm MC, Björkstén B, Garofalo RP. Chemoattractant factors in breast milk of atopic and nonatopic mothers. *Pediatr Res* 2000;47:592–7.

100 Böttcher MF, Jenmalm MC, Garofalo RP, Björkstén B. Cytokines in breast milk from allergic and nonallergic mothers. *Pediatr Res* 2000;47:157–62.

101 de Martino M, Resti M, Appendino C, Vierucci A. Different degree of antibody response to hepatitis B virus vaccine in breast- and formula-fed infants born to HBsAg-positive mothers. *J Pediatr Gastroenterol Nutr* 1987;6:208–11.

102 Ivarsson A, Persson LA, Nystrom L, *et al*. Epidemic of coeliac disease in Swedish children. *Acta Paediatr* 2000;89:165–71.

103 Abrahamsson T, Jakobsson T, Fagerås Böttcher M, *et al*. Probiotics in prevention of IgE-associated eczema: a double blind randomised placebo-controlled trial. *J Allergy Clin Immunol* 2007;119:1174–80.

104 Taylor AL, Dunstan JA, Prescott SL. Probiotic supplementation for the first 6 months of life fails to reduce the risk of atopic dermatitis and increases the risk of allergen sensitization in high-risk children: a randomized controlled trial. *J Allergy Clin Immunol* 2007;119:184–91.

PART 2

Adverse Reactions to Food Antigens: Clinical Science

8

CHAPTER 8

The Spectrum of Allergic Reactions to Foods

Stacie M. Jones and A. Wesley Burks

KEY CONCEPTS

- Immunoglobulin E-mediated food allergy is the most common and well-recognized form of food hypersensitivity.
- Allergic reactions to food range from mild to life threatening.
- Risk factors for life-threatening anaphylaxis are important to recognize.
- Atopic dermatitis and asthma are allergic conditions in which hypersensitivity to a food(s) may play a role in disease activity.
- A subset of patients with eosinophilic gastrointestinal disorders may have food allergy-induced symptoms.

Introduction

An *adverse food reaction* is a general term that can be applied to a clinically abnormal response to an ingested food or food additive. Adverse food reactions are common and often assumed by patients to be allergic in nature. Food allergies are most prevalent during the first years of life, affecting about 6% of infants younger than 3 years [1–5]. About 2.5% of newborn infants have hypersensitivity reactions to cow's milk in the first year of life, with about 80% "outgrowing" the allergy by their fifth birthday [6]. Immunoglobulin E (IgE)-mediated reactions account for about 60% of milk-allergic reactions; about 25% of these infants retain their sensitivity into the second decade of life, and 35% go on to acquire other food allergies. About 1.5% of young children are allergic to eggs and 0.5% to peanuts. Some evidence suggests that the prevalence of peanut allergy has been increasing during the past two decades [7,8]. Children with atopic disorders tend to have a higher prevalence of food allergy; about 35% of children with moderate to severe atopic dermatitis (AD) have IgE-mediated food allergy [9], and about 6% of children with asthma have food-induced wheezing [10]. Adverse reactions to food additives also have been demonstrated to affect 0.5–1% of children [11–13]. Food allergy appears to be less common in adults, although

adequate epidemiologic studies are lacking. A survey in the United States indicated that peanut and tree nut allergies together affect 1.1% of American adults [7]. Overall, it is estimated that about 2% of adults in the United States are affected by food allergies [6]. Adverse reactions to foods are classified as either *food hypersensitivity (allergy)* or *food intolerance* [1,14].

Food allergy

Food hypersensitivity (allergy) is due to an immunologic reaction resulting from the ingestion of a food or food additive. This reaction occurs only in some patients, may occur after only a small amount of the substance is ingested, and is unrelated to any physiologic effect of the food or food additive. Food allergy occurs due to an immune response that typically involves the IgE mechanism, of which anaphylaxis is the best example. Adverse reactions to food additives are rare [11,12,15]. Several other food hypersensitivity disorders involve cell-mediated immune responses that are mixed with IgE-mediated mechanisms or may be entirely unrelated to IgE-mediated responses (Table 8.1).

Food intolerance

Food intolerance is a general term describing an abnormal physiologic response to an ingested food or food additive. This reaction has not been proven to be immunologic in nature, which distinguishes these reactions from those occurring as a result of food allergy. Food intolerance may be caused by many factors including toxic contaminants

Food Allergy: Adverse Reactions to Foods and Food Additives, 4th edition.
Edited by Dean D. Metcalfe, Hugh A. Sampson, and Ronald A. Simon.
© 2008 Blackwell Publishing, ISBN: 978-1-4501-5129-0.

Table 8.1 Food allergy disorders mediated by IgE and mixed IgE and cellular mechanisms

Immune mechanism	Disorders
IgE mediated	
Cutaneous	Urticaria
	Angioedema
	Morbiliform rashes
	Flushing/pruritus
Respiratory	Rhinoconjunctivitis
	Laryngospasm
	Wheezing/bronchospasm
Gastrointestinal	Oral allergy syndrome
	Gastrointestinal anaphylaxis
Multi-system	Generalized anaphylaxis
	Food and exercise-induced anaphylaxis
Mixed IgE and cell mediated	
Cutaneous	Atopic dermatitis
Respiratory	Asthma
Gastrointestinal	Eosinophilic esophagitis
	Eosinophilic gastroenteritis

(e.g. histamine in scromboid fish poisoning, toxins secreted by infectious agents such as Salmonella, Shigella, and Campylobacter), pharmacologic properties of the food (e.g. caffeine in coffee, tyramine in aged cheeses, sulfites in red wine), characteristics of the host such as metabolic disorders (e.g. lactase deficiency), and idiosyncratic responses.

Spectrum of food-allergic responses

The spectrum of food-allergic responses can best be understood by categorizing reactions based on the types of primary immune mechanisms responsible for these adverse reactions. The spectrum of food-induced reactions ranges from benign manifestations of disease, such as flushing or rhinorrhea, to life-threatening symptoms such as anaphylaxis or enterocolitis syndrome. In this chapter, we will examine adverse food reactions that are based on the following immune-mediated mechanisms: (1) IgE-mediated, (2) non-IgE-mediated, (3) eosinophilic disorders, and (4) allergic responses due to combinations of immune mechanisms.

IgE-mediated reactions

IgE-mediated food-allergic reactions are rapid in onset (usually within minutes to 2 hours) and are the most widely known reactions associated with foods. Symptoms are believed to be caused by preformed mediator release from tissue mast cells and circulating basophils that have been previously sensitized to a specific food antigen [14]. Specific

manifestations of IgE-mediated food hypersensitivity reactions can involve any system within the human body. These reactions frequently involve the skin, respiratory tract, gastrointestinal tract, and cardiovascular system. More severe symptoms and those involving multiple systems are defined by the term "generalized anaphylaxis" and are often life threatening. Two additional distinct presentations of IgE-mediated food-allergic reactions are the oral allergy syndrome and food-dependent, exercise-induced anaphylaxis.

Cutaneous responses

The *skin* is the most common target organ in IgE-mediated food hypersensitivity reactions, and cutaneous symptoms occur in >80% of allergic reactions to foods [16]. The ingestion of food allergens can lead either to immediate cutaneous symptoms or exacerbate chronic conditions such as AD. Acute *urticaria* and *angioedema* are the most common cutaneous manifestation of food hypersensitivity reactions, generally appearing within minutes of ingestion of the food allergen. Food allergy may account for 20% of cases of acute urticaria [17,18]. By comparison, food allergies underlying chronic urticaria and angioedema (defined as symptoms >6 weeks duration) appear to be uncommon. In adult patients with chronic urticaria evaluated by placebo-controlled food challenge, <10% of symptoms were associated with food allergy despite the perception of food involvement in as many as 50% of patients [19].

Flushing, pruritus, and morbiliform rash are other acute cutaneous manifestations that commonly occur during allergic reactions to foods. These early symptoms often precede the development of urticaria, angioedema, or more serious adverse symptoms. Food can also cause acute contact urticaria. In this condition, urticarial lesions develop only on the area of skin that is in direct contact with the food. Raw meats, seafood, raw vegetables and fruits, milk, egg, mustard, rice, and beer are among the foods that have been implicated in this form of food allergy [20–22].

Respiratory and ocular responses

Upper respiratory symptoms such as rhinorrhea, sneezing, nasal congestion, and pruritus are frequently experienced during allergic reactions to foods. Nasal symptoms typically occur in conjunction with other organ system involvement [3]. *Ocular* symptoms commonly occur concurrently with respiratory manifestations of IgE-mediated reactions to foods [14,23]. Symptoms may include periocular erythema, pruritus, conjunctival erythema, and tearing. Isolated symptoms of rhinitis and/or conjunctivitis in response to food-allergen ingestion are rare.

Lower respiratory symptoms are potentially life-threatening manifestations of IgE-mediated reactions to foods [14,24]. Symptoms can include laryngospasm, cough, and wheezing and require prompt medical intervention. In a retrospective chart review of 253 failed oral food challenges, Perry and colleagues found that 26% of participants experienced lower respiratory symptoms, and each of the tested foods carried a similar risk for eliciting lower respiratory symptoms [16]. Although lower respiratory symptoms can occur in any person experiencing anaphylaxis to foods, patients with underlying asthma are at increased risk of severe symptoms. Lower respiratory symptoms due to food allergy are temporally related to ingestion and are typically accompanied by other organ system involvement. It is rare that chronic lower respiratory symptoms or poorly controlled asthma are sole manifestations of food allergy [25,26].

These points are illustrated by a large study of 480 patients with a history of an adverse food reaction undergoing double-blind placebo-controlled oral food challenges (DBPCFCs). Positive reactions were observed in 185 patients, 39% of whom had respiratory and ocular symptoms [3]. Symptoms included combinations of periocular erythema, pruritus, and tearing; nasal congestion, pruritus, sneezing, and rhinorrhea; and coughing, voice changes, and wheezing. Isolated respiratory symptoms occurred in only 5%. One area of exception involves occupational exposure to potential food allergens. Adults working in the food processing and packing industries may develop occupational food allergies and present with rhinoconjunctivitis, with or without asthma [27–30].

Gastrointestinal responses

The signs and symptoms of food-induced IgE-mediated gastrointestinal allergy are most commonly seen as immediate gastrointestinal hypersensitivity but can also be manifested as oral allergy syndrome [23].

Immediate gastrointestinal hypersensitivity is a form of IgE-mediated food allergy, which may accompany allergic manifestations in other target organs [15,24,31,32]. The symptoms vary and may include nausea, abdominal pain or cramping, vomiting, and/or diarrhea. The onset of upper gastrointestinal symptoms (nausea, vomiting, pain) is generally minutes to 2 hours after ingestion of the offending food but lower gastrointestinal symptoms, such as diarrhea, may begin immediately or may be delayed for 2–6 hours after ingestion. Symptoms may be severe and protracted resulting in the need for fluid or electrolyte replacement.

The *oral allergy syndrome or pollen–food related syndrome* is considered to be a form of contact urticaria that is confined almost exclusively to the oropharynx and rarely involves the lower respiratory tract or other target organs [33,34]. Oral allergy syndrome is manifested by the rapid onset of pruritus and angioedema of the lips, tongue, palate, and throat. This syndrome has been reported in up to 50% of patients with pollen-induced rhinoconjunctivitis and is most commonly associated with the ingestion of fresh fruits and vegetables. For example, patients with ragweed allergy may experience symptoms following contact with melons (e.g. watermelons, cantaloupe, honeydew) and bananas.

Birch pollen-sensitive patients often have symptoms following the ingestion of raw potatoes, carrots, celery, apples, pears, cherries, and hazelnuts. Mugwort-allergic patients may react to celery or mustard. Symptoms typically resolve spontaneously within minutes after ingestion ceases. Although symptoms rarely progress to involve other organ systems, progression to systemic involvement has been noted in approximately 10% of patients with anaphylaxis reported in not more than 1–2% [33,35,36]. Tree nuts and peanuts causing oral symptoms are best avoided because of the frequency with which these foods cause more severe reactions. Peanut and tree nut associated oral symptoms are not usually defined as part of the oral allergy symptom, rather serve as a precursor "warning sign" for more advanced symptoms to follow [37].

Generalized anaphylaxis

Anaphylaxis is defined as a "severe, potentially fatal, systemic-allergic reaction that occurs suddenly after contact with an allergy-causing substance [38]." Food-induced generalized anaphylaxis involves multiple organ systems and has been estimated to account for 30–50% of all anaphylaxis treated in emergency department settings [24,39,40]. Peanuts, tree nuts, fish, and shellfish account for more anaphylactic reactions than any other foods. In generalized anaphylaxis, the onset of symptoms is abrupt, often occurring within minutes of ingestion. Symptoms are due to the effects of potent intracellular mediators such as histamine, tryptase, and leukotrienes that are released from mast cells and basophils during an allergic reaction and can involve any organ system. Severe or life-threatening anaphylactic reactions involving the respiratory and cardiovascular systems can culminate in respiratory failure, hypotension, cardiac dysrhythmias, shock, and death if left untreated. In 25–30% of cases of food-induced anaphylaxis, a biphasic course is noted with a recurrence of symptoms hours after the initial onset. This second phase may follow a quiescent, asymptomatic interval [24,37].

Fatal and near-fatal reactions to foods have been described [37,41,42]. Peanuts and tree nuts are the most common allergens reported in such cases. Risk factors associated with fatal food-induced anaphylaxis include adolescent or young adult age group, co-existent asthma, history of previous serious reaction, delayed administration of epinephrine, and absence of skin symptoms. In a series of 13 children with fatal or near-fatal anaphylactic reactions to food, all were known to have food allergies and had accidentally ingested peanuts (four patients), nuts (six patients), eggs (one patient), or milk (two patients) [37]. Twelve of the 13 had asthma that was well controlled. Six patients died, with only two of those receiving epinephrine within the first hour. By comparison, six of the seven survivors received epinephrine within 30 minutes. The correlation between absence of skin findings and fatal anaphylaxis has not been systematically studied, although it is postulated to result from the rapid development of hypotension, resulting in poor skin perfusion and minimal skin symptoms. An alternative explanation may be that patients lacking skin symptoms are not recognized as having anaphylaxis as quickly, leading to a delay in treatment and consequently poor outcome.

Food-associated, exercise-induced anaphylaxis

There have been increasingly more reports of patients with anaphylaxis that occur only when the ingestion of food is coupled with exercise within a 2–4 hour time interval. This syndrome is known as food-associated, exercise-induced anaphylaxis [43–47]. It appears to be most prevalent in adolescents and young adults, although there have been reports in middle aged patients as well. Most patients react to one or two specific foods. Common causative foods include wheat, celery, and seafood [44–47]. Classically, the food can be ingested in the absence of exercise without development of symptoms. Alternatively, patients may exercise without eating the specific food without induction of symptoms. The coupling of specific food ingestion and exercise, however, produces a potential life-threatening anaphylaxis.

Non-IgE-mediated reactions

Non-IgE-mediated food allergies typically present with more subacute or chronic symptoms isolated to the gastrointestinal tract that present within hours or days of food ingestion. Affected patients commonly present with a classic constellation of features that are consistent with well-described clinical disorders. These disorders include food protein-induced enterocolitis, food protein-induced proctocolitis, food protein-induced gastroenteropathy, food-induced contact dermatitis, celiac disease with or without dermatitis herpetiformis (DH), and food-induced pulmonary hemosiderosis. Although the precise immune mechanisms have not been described, evidence suggests a cell-mediated hypersensitivity response associated with all of these disorders (Table 8.2).

Cutaneous responses

Food-induced contact dermatitis has been reported in individuals without IgE antibodies to the causal food [48]. This

Table 8.2 Food allergies mediated by cellular (non-IgE) mechanisms

Cutaneous	Contact dermatitis
	Dermatitis herpetiformis
Respiratory	Food-induced pulmonary hemosiderosis (Heiner's syndrome)
Gastrointestinal	Celiac disease
	Food protein enterocolitis
	Food protein-induced enteropathy
	Food protein-induced proctocolitis

reaction typically occurs in food handlers and can be confirmed by patch testing, thus indicating a cell-mediated immune response. Implicated foods frequently include fish, shellfish, meats, and eggs [20–22,24].

DH is a skin manifestation of celiac disease (gluten-sensitive enteropathy). DH is a chronic blistering skin rash characterized by chronic, pruritic papulovesicular lesions that are symmetrically distributed over the extensor surfaces of the extremities and on the buttocks [49–51]. Gastrointestinal symptoms and histopathologic findings within the gut mucosa are generally milder than those seen in patients presenting with primary gastrointestinal disease. Elimination of gluten from the diet typically results in resolution of skin and gastrointestinal lesions.

Gastrointestinal responses

Food protein-induced enterocolitis syndrome (FPIES) is a disorder which presents most commonly in early infancy [52]. Acute symptoms are typically isolated to the gastrointestinal tract and consist of profuse, repetitive vomiting, and not infrequently diarrhea. Symptoms are often severe and may cause dehydration and shock, often leading to an erroneous diagnosis of sepsis. Cow's milk and/or soy protein in infant formulas or maternal breast milk are most often responsible for induction of symptoms, although FPIES due to solid food (e.g. rice) is being reported more frequently [52,53]. Objective findings on stool examination consist of gross or occult blood, polymorphonuclear neutrophils, eosinophils, Charcot–Leyden crystals, and positive reducing substances. IgE testing for food proteins is characteristically negative. Jejunal biopsies often reveal flattened villi, edema, and increased numbers of lymphocytes, eosinophils, and mast cells. A food challenge with the responsible protein generally results in vomiting and occasionally diarrhea within minutes to several hours, and occasionally leads to shock [15,23,54].

Infants and children with FPIES are often allergic to both cow's milk and soy protein. Approximately 50% of children with cow's milk allergy will have concomitant soy allergy, therefore it is recommended that infants with FPIES due to cow's milk also avoid soy products during the first year of life [23,52,55]. Elimination of the offending allergen generally results in resolution of the symptoms within 72 hours although secondary disaccharidase deficiency may persist longer. This disorder tends to subside by 18–24 months of age.

Food protein-induced enteropathy is characterized by diarrhea, vomiting, malabsorption, and poor weight gain [56]. It is clinically distinguishable from FPIES due to the presence of non-bloody stools. Vomiting is often less prominent, and re-exposure does not elicit acute symptoms after a period of avoidance. Onset of symptoms is typically delayed for days to weeks and may require continual feeding of the culprit food protein. Other clinical features include abdominal pain and distension, hypoproteinemia, and edema. Patients typically present in the first year of life. The most common causal food is cow's milk although other foods such as soy, egg, and grains have been associated with food protein-induced enteropathy. Histologic examination reveals patchy villous atrophy, mononuclear cell infiltrates, and few eosinophils. Symptoms typically resolve within 72 hours after dietary elimination and is usually outgrown within 12–24 months of dietary-allergen avoidance.

Food protein-induced proctocolitis generally presents in the first few months of life and, like FPIES, is often secondary to cow's milk and/or soy protein hypersensitivity [23,31]. Infants with this disorder often do not appear ill and generally present with bloody stools. Other distinguishing features include normal growth and absence of vomiting. Gastrointestinal lesions are usually confined to the rectum but can involve the entire large bowel and consist of eosinophilic infiltrates (5–20 eosinophils per HPF), or eosinophilic abscesses in the epithelium and lamina propria. If lesions are severe with crypt destruction, polymorphonuclear leukocytes (PMNs) are also prominent in this disorder [57]. Food protein-induced proctocolitis typically resolves after 6–12 months of dietary-allergen avoidance. Elimination of the offending food allergen leads to resolution of hematochezia within 72 hours, but the mucosal lesions may take up to 1 month to disappear and range from patchy mucosal injection to severe friability with small aphthoid ulcerations and bleeding.

Celiac disease (or gluten-sensitive enteropathy) is an extensive enteropathy leading to malabsorption [58]. Total villous atrophy and an extensive cellular infiltrate are associated with sensitivity to gliadin, the alcohol-soluble portion of gluten found in wheat, rye, and barley. Celiac disease is almost exclusively limited to genetically predisposed individuals who express the HLA-DQ2 and/or HLA-DQ8 heterodimers [59,60]. Patients often have presenting symptoms of diarrhea or frank steatorrhea, abdominal distention and flatulence, failure to thrive, and occasionally nausea and vomiting. Oral ulcers and other extra-intestinal symptoms secondary to malabsorption are sometimes associated. Serologic testing aids in the diagnosis and includes measurement of anti-IgA antibodies to human tissue transglutaminase (TTG) and anti-endomysial (EMA) [58]. Serologic testing to rule out low total serum IgA (IgA deficiency) is essential for the diagnosis of celiac disease. Confirmation with endoscopic biopsies is necessary for diagnosis and reveals total villous atrophy and inflammatory infiltrates. Clinical symptoms and endoscopic findings resolve with strict dietary elimination of gluten that must be maintained for life.

Respiratory responses

Food-induced pulmonary hemosiderosis (Heiner's syndrome) is a rare syndrome in infants characterized by recurrent pneumonia with pulmonary infiltrates, hemosiderosis, gastrointestinal blood loss, iron-deficiency anemia, and failure to thrive [61,62]. Symptoms are associated with non-IgE-mediated hypersensitivity to cow's milk with evidence of peripheral eosinophilia and the presence of cow's milk precipitins on diagnostic testing. Deposits of immunoglobulins and C3 may also be found on lung biopsy. Strict dietary elimination of milk results in reversal of symptoms.

Adverse food reactions associated with eosinophilic disease

Allergic eosinophilic gastroenteropathies are a group of disorders characterized by symptoms of post-prandial gastrointestinal dysfunction associated with eosinophilic infiltration of at least one layer of the gastrointestinal tract, absence of vasculitis, and peripheral eosinophilia in about 50% of cases [2,23,55]. These disorders are defined by the site(s) of involvement and include eosinophilic esophagitis (EE) and eosinophilic gastroenteritis. Symptoms for each of these syndromes are related to the specific anatomical site of involvement. The pathogenesis of these disorders likely involves both IgE-mediated and cellular immune mechanisms.

Eosinophilic esophagitis

EE is characterized by severe or refractory gastrointestinal symptoms that are suggestive of gastroesophageal reflux disease (GERD) and include dysphagia, epigastric pain, and post-prandial nausea and vomiting [63]. This disorder should be considered in patients of any age presenting with esophageal symptoms, especially when recalcitrant to symptomatic treatment, such as antacids or anti-reflux medications. Very young children may present with feeding disorders; whereas, older children and adults present with dysphagia, vomiting, and abdominal pain. A history of food impaction is common.

Many patients with EE have other atopic diseases. In a series of 103 children with EE, rhinoconjunctivitis was present in 57% and wheezing was noted in 37%, while possible food allergy was cited in 46% [64]. In a retrospective review of 381 children with EE, the most commonly implicated foods were cow's milk, egg, soy, corn, wheat, and beef. Most patients with evidence of food sensitivity tested positive for multiple foods [63]. Elimination of these foods or the use of elemental diets typically results in clinical and histologic improvement. However, the pathophysiologic relationship between EE and allergens, such as foods or aeroallergens, remains unclear.

Eosinophils are not normally found in the esophageal mucosa and symptoms are likely due to the release of eosinophilic mediators. EE is clinically distinguishable from GERD due to its feature of being refractory to aggressive management with antacids, protein pump inhibitors (PPI), and pro-motility medications that are typically effective in the treatment of GERD. Other distinguishing characteristics include normal pH probe results, the presence of patient or family history of atopy, and peripheral eosinophilia. On endoscopy, EE patients may have visually normal-appearing esophageal mucosa although esophageal furrowing and rings have been reported [65]. On histologic examination, esophageal biopsies in patients with EE typically contain >20 eosinophils per HPF as compared with <5 eosinophils per HPF in patients with GERD. Proximal and mid-esophageal lesions are common in EE whereas reactive eosinophilic infiltrates due to GERD are mainly limited to the distal esophagus [66].

Eosinophilic gastroenteritis

Eosinophilic gastroenteritis can present at any age with abdominal pain, nausea, diarrhea, malabsorption, and weight loss. In infants, it may present as outlet obstruction with postprandial projectile vomiting. In adolescents and adults, it can mimic irritable bowel syndrome [67]. Approximately one-half of patients have allergic disease, such as defined food allergies, asthma, eczema, or rhinitis [68]. However, in contrast to EE, avoidance of implicated foods may have limited value [69,70]. Eosinophilic gastroenteritis is characterized by eosinophilic infiltration of the stomach, small intestine, or both with variable involvement of the large intestine [71]. Symptoms may include vomiting, abdominal pain, diarrhea, malabsorption, and failure to thrive. Severe symptoms can mimic pyloric stenosis or other forms of gastric outlet obstruction when duodenal involvement is present. Since eosinophils may normally be found in the stomach and intestine, endoscopic findings are more difficult to interpret as compared to EE. In addition, multiple sites may need to be biopsied to effectively exclude eosinophilic gastroenteritis due to the patchy nature of eosinophilic infiltration. Biopsies in eosinophilic gastroenteritis will typically show 20–40 eosinophils per HPF. Treatment may involve elimination of the potential offending food(s) or institution of an elemental diet with slow addition of foods. Similar to EE, eosinophilic gastroenteritis usually follows a prolonged course requiring protracted therapy and dietary intervention for months to years. After dietary restriction, foods can be re-introduced slowly after avoidance and based on endoscopic and clinical evidence of disease resolution.

Conditions associated with multiple immune mechanisms

Asthma

Asthma alone is an infrequent manifestation of food allergy. Although ingestion of food allergens is rarely the main aggravating factor in chronic asthma, there is some evidence to suggest that food antigens can provoke bronchial hyperreactivity [25,26]. An exception is occupational asthma (often with accompanying rhinitis) in food-industry workers. "Baker's asthma," caused by IgE-mediated allergy to inhaled wheat proteins, is an example [72]. Patients with these conditions may not react to the food upon ingestion, rather only with inhalation exposure. More typically, asthma is seen as a component of more generalized, IgE-mediated reactions. Asthmatic reactions secondary to airborne food allergens have been reported in cases where susceptible individuals are exposed to vapors or steam emitted from cooking food (e.g. fish, mollusks, crustacea, eggs, and garbanzo beans) [27–30].

Another relationship between food allergy and asthma is that co-existing asthma is a significant risk factor for death from food-induced anaphylaxis. Conversely, substantially higher rates of food allergy are noted among children requiring intubation for asthma compared to a control group of asthmatic children [73].

Atopic dermatitis

Atopic dermatitis (AD) is a chronic skin disorder that generally begins in early infancy and is characterized by typical distribution, extreme pruritus, chronically relapsing course, and association with asthma and allergic rhinitis [9]. Food allergy has been correlated with the development and persistence of AD, especially during infancy and early childhood. In children <5 years old, 35–40% will be allergic to at least one food [9,74–76]. These patients typically fail to respond to conventional medical therapy or may have frequent exacerbations of underlying skin disease if causal foods are not strictly avoided. The most common foods associated with AD include cow's milk, egg, peanut, soy, wheat, fish, and tree nuts. Due to the chronicity of symptoms, a trial of dietary elimination of the suspected food allergen and the use of diagnostic food challenges may be warranted to aid in the accurate diagnosis of food allergy in these children. Dietary elimination of relevant food allergens may result in clearing of the skin. However, some patients continue to have ongoing skin disease due to concomitant sensitization to aeroallergens or due to non-allergic triggers.

In one well-designed report, 113 patients with marked AD underwent DBPCFC [76]. Among the 101 positive food challenges observed in 63 children skin, gastrointestinal, and respiratory symptoms were observed in 84%, 52%, and 32% oral food challenges, respectively. Some patients were subsequently placed on elimination diets based on these findings, with most exhibiting significant clinical improvement in skin symptoms. Although egg, peanut, and milk were responsible for most reactions, it was difficult to predict the patients with food allergy based on history and laboratory information alone.

In a single center's experience evaluating over 2000 food challenges in 600 children with AD, approximately 40% of the DBPCFCs were positive [74]. Nearly 75% of the positive tests included cutaneous manifestations, principally consisting of macular, morbilliform, and/or pruritic rashes located in areas commonly affected by AD. Approximately 30% of positive tests consisted of skin rashes alone.

Summary

The ingestion of food represents the greatest foreign antigenic load confronting the human immune system. In the vast majority of individuals, tolerance develops to food antigens, which are constantly gaining access to the body proper. However, when tolerance fails to develop, the immune system responds with a hypersensitivity reaction. Inadvertent ingestion of food allergens may provoke various cutaneous, respiratory, gastrointestinal symptoms, and/or systemic anaphylaxis with shock. Investigations in the past have characterized the food hypersensitivity disorders, but our understanding of the basic immunopathologic mechanisms is incomplete and requires further investigation in order to provide target sites for therapeutic interventions.

References

1 Anderson J, Sogn D. Adverse reactions to foods. American Academy of Allergy and Immunology Committee on Adverse Reactions to Foods and the National Institute of Allergy and Infectious Disease. National Institutes of Health Publication No. 84-2442, 1984.

2 Bock SA. Prospective appraisal of complaints of adverse reactions to foods in children during the first 3 years of life. *Pediatrics* 1987;79:683–8.

3 Bock SA, Atkins FM. Patterns of food hypersensitivity during sixteen years of double-blind, placebo-controlled food challenges. *J Pediatr* 1990;117:561–7.

4 Young E, Stoneham MD, Petruckevitch A, *et al.* A population study of food intolerance. *Lancet* 1994;343:1127–30.

5 Jansen JJ, Kardinaal AF, Huijbers G, *et al.* Prevalence of food allergy and intolerance in the adult Dutch population. *J Allergy Clin Immunol* 1994;93:446–56.

6 Sampson HA. Food allergy. Part 1. Immunopathogenesis and clinical disorders. *J Allergy Clin Immunol* 1999;103:717–28.

7 Sicherer SH, Munoz-Furlong A, Sampson HA. Prevalence of peanut and tree nut allergy in the United States determined by means of a random digit dial telephone survey: a 5-year follow-up study. *J Allergy Clin Immunol* 2003;112:1203–7.

8 Grundy J, Matthews S, Bateman B, *et al.* Rising prevalence of allergy to peanut in children: data from 2 sequential cohorts. *J Allergy Clin Immunol* 2002;110:784–9.

9 Eigenmann PA, Sicherer SH, Borkowski TA, *et al.* Prevalence of IgE-mediated food allergy among children with atopic dermatitis. *Pediatrics* 1998;101:E8.

10 Novembre E, de Martino M, Vierucci A. Foods and respiratory allergy. *J Allergy Clin Immunol* 1988;81:1059–65.

11 Young E, Patel S, Stoneham M, *et al.* The prevalence of reaction to food additives in a survey population. *J Roy Coll Phys Lond* 1987;21:241–7.

12 Simon RA. Adverse reactions to food additives. *Curr Allergy Asthma Rep* 2003;3:62–6.

13 Fuglsang G, Madsen G, Halken S, *et al.* Adverse reactions to food additives in children with atopic symptoms. *Allergy* 1994;49:31–7.

14 Sampson HA, Burks AW. Mechanisms of food allergy. *Annu Rev Nutr* 1996;16:161–77.

15 Nettis E, Colanardi MC, Ferrannini A, Tursi A. Suspected tartrazine-induced acute urticaria/angioedema is only rarely reproducible by oral rechallenge. *Clin Exp Allergy* 2003;33: 1725–9.

16 Perry TT, Matsui EC, Conover-Walker MK, Wood RA. Risk of oral food challenges. *J Allergy Clin Immunol* 2004;114:1164–8.

17 Champion RH, Roberts SO, Carpenter RG, Roger JH. Urticaria and angio-oedema. A review of 554 patients. *Br J Dermatol* 1969;81:588–97.

18 Sehgal VN, Rege VL. An interrogative study of 158 urticaria patients. *Ann Allergy* 1973;31:279–83.

19 Kobza BA, Greaves MW, Champion RH, Pye RJ. The urticarias 1990. *Br J Dermatol* 1991;124:100–8.

20 Jovanovic M, Oliwiecki S, Beck MH. Occupational contact urticaria from beef associated with hand eczema. *Contact Dermatitis* 1992;27:188–9.

21 Delgado J, Castillo R, Quiralte J, *et al.* Contact urticaria in a child from raw potato. *Contact Dermatitis* 1996;35:179–80.

22 Fisher AA. Contact urticaria from handling meats and fowl. *Cutis* 1982;30:726–9.

23 Sampson HA, Anderson JA. Summary and recommendations: classification of gastrointestinal manifestations due to immunologic reactions to foods in infants and young children. *J Pediatr Gastroenterol Nutr* 2000;30:S87–94.

24 Sampson HA. Adverse reactions to foods. In: Adkinson N, Bochner BS, Yunginger JW, *et al.* (eds.) *Middleton's Allergy Principles and Practice.* St. Louis, MO: Mosby, 2003:1619–43.

25 James JM. Respiratory manifestations of food allergy. *Pediatrics* 2003;111:1625–30.

26 James JM. Food allergy, respiratory disease, and anaphylaxis. In: Leung DY, Sampson HA, Geha RS, Szefler SJ (eds.) *Pediatric allergy: principles and practice.* St. Louis, MO: Mosby, 2003:529–37.

27 Toskala E, Piipari R, Aalto-Korte K, *et al.* Occupational asthma and rhinitis caused by milk proteins. *J Occup Environ Med* 2004;46:1100–101.

28 Sherson D, Hansen I, Sigsgaard T. Occupationally related respiratory symptoms in trout-processing workers. *Allergy* 1989;44:336–41.

29 Hudson P, Cartier A, Pineau L, *et al.* Follow-up of occupational asthma caused by crab and various agents. *J Allergy Clin Immunol* 1985;76:682–8.

30 Storaas T, Steinsvag SK, Florvaag E, *et al.* Occupational rhinitis: diagnostic criteria, relation to lower airway symptoms and IgE sensitization in bakery workers. *Acta Otolaryngol* 2005;125:1211–17.

31 Crowe SE, Perdue MH. Gastrointestinal food hypersensitivity: basic mechanisms of pathophysiology. *Gastroenterology* 1992; 103:1075–95.

32 Bush RK, Taylor S, Hefle S. Adverse reactions to food and drug additives. In: Adkinson N, Yunginger JW, Busse W, *et al.* (eds.) *Middleton's Allergy: Principles and Practice.* St. Louis, MO: Mosby, 2003:1619–63.

33 Egger M, Mutschlechner S, Wopfner N, *et al.* Pollen–food syndromes associated with weed pollinosis: an update from the molecular point of view. *Allergy* 2006;61:461–76.

34 Garcia-Careaga Jr M, Kerner Jr JA. Gastrointestinal manifestations of food allergies in pediatric patients. *Nutr Clin Pract* 2005;20:526–35.

35 Bruijnzeel-Koomen C, Ortolani C, Aas K, *et al.* Adverse reactions to food. European Academy of Allergology and Clinical Immunology Subcommittee. *Allergy* 1995;50:623–35.

36 Caballero T, San Martin MS, Padial MA, *et al.* Clinical characteristics of patients with mustard hypersensitivity. *Ann Allergy Asthma Immunol* 2002;89:166–71.

37 Sampson HA, Mendelson L, Rosen JP. Fatal and near-fatal anaphylactic reactions to food in children and adolescents. *N Engl J Med* 1992;327:380–4.

38 Sampson HA, Munoz-Furlong A, Campbell RL, *et al.* Second symposium on the definition and management of anaphylaxis: summary report – *Second National Institute of Allergy and Infectious Disease/Food Allergy and Anaphylaxis Network Symposium. J Allergy Clin Immunol* 2006;117:391–7.

39 Yocum MW, Butterfield JH, Klein JS, *et al.* Epidemiology of anaphylaxis in Olmsted County: a population-based study. *J Allergy Clin Immunol* 1999;104:452–6.

40 Clark S, Bock SA, Gaeta TJ, *et al.* Multicenter study of emergency department visits for food allergies. *J Allergy Clin Immunol* 2004;113:347–52.

41 Bock SA, Munoz-Furlong A, Sampson HA. Fatalities due to anaphylactic reactions to foods. *J Allergy Clin Immunol* 2001;107:191–3.

42 Yunginger JW, Nelson DR, Squillace DL, *et al.* Laboratory investigation of deaths due to anaphylaxis. *J Forensic Sci* 1991;36:857–65.

43 Sampson HA. Anaphylaxis and emergency treatment. *Pediatrics* 2003;111:1601–8.

44 Dohi M, Suko M, Sugiyama H, *et al.* Food-dependent, exercise-induced anaphylaxis: a study on 11 Japanese cases. *J Allergy Clin Immunol* 1991;87:34–40.

45 Romano A, Di Fonso M, Giuffreda F, *et al.* Diagnostic work-up for food-dependent, exercise-induced anaphylaxis. *Allergy* 1995;50:817–24.

46 Kushimoto H, Aoki T. Masked type I wheat allergy. Relation to exercise-induced anaphylaxis. *Arch Dermatol* 1985;121:355–60.

47 Horan R, Sheffer A. Food-dependent exercise-induced anaphylaxis. *Immunol Allergy Clin North Am* 1991:757–66.

48 Hjorth N, Roed-Petersen J. Occupational protein contact dermatitis in food handlers. *Contact Dermatitis* 1976;2:28–42.

49 Oxentenko AS, Murray JA. Celiac disease and dermatitis herpetiformis: the spectrum of gluten-sensitive enteropathy. *Int J Dermatol* 2003;42:585–7.

50 Zone JJ. Skin manifestations of celiac disease. *Gastroenterology* 2005;128:S87–91.

51 Fasano MB. Dermatologic food allergy. *Pediatr Ann* 2006; 35:727–31.

52 Sicherer SH. Food protein-induced enterocolitis syndrome: case presentations and management lessons. *J Allergy Clin Immunol* 2005;115:149–56.

53 Nowak-Wegrzyn A, Sampson HA, Wood RA, Sicherer SH. Food protein-induced enterocolitis syndrome caused by solid food proteins. *Pediatrics* 2003;111:829–35.

54 Goldman AS, Anderson Jr DW, Sellers WA, *et al.* Milk allergy. I. Oral challenge with milk and isolated milk proteins in allergic children. *Pediatrics* 1963;32:425–43.

55 Chehade M, Magid MS, Mofidi S, *et al.* Allergic eosinophilic gastroenteritis with protein-losing enteropathy: intestinal pathology, clinical course, and long-term follow-up. *J Pediatr Gastroenterol Nutr* 2006;42:516–21.

56 Lake A. Food protein-induced gastroenteropathy in infants and children. In: Metcalfe DD, Sampson HA, Simon R (eds.) *Food allergy adverse reactions to foods and food additives.* St. Louis, MO: Mosby, 1991:173–85.

57 Jenkins HR, Pincott JR, Soothill JF, *et al.* Food allergy: the major cause of infantile colitis. *Arch Dis Child* 1984;59:326–9.

58 Hill ID, Dirks MH, Liptak GS, *et al.* Guideline for the diagnosis and treatment of celiac disease in children: recommendations of the North American Society for Pediatric Gastroenterology, Hepatology and Nutrition. *J Pediatr Gastroenterol Nutr* 2005; 40:1–19.

59 Papadopoulos GK, Wijmenga C, Koning F. Interplay between genetics and the environment in the development of celiac disease: perspectives for a healthy life. *J Clin Invest* 2001; 108:1261–6.

60 Sollid LM, Thorsby E. HLA susceptibility genes in celiac disease: genetic mapping and role in pathogenesis. *Gastroenterology* 1993;105:910–22.

61 Heiner DC, Sears JW, Kniker WT. Multiple precipitins to cow's milk in chronic respiratory disease. A syndrome including poor growth, gastrointestinal symptoms, evidence of allergy, iron deficiency anemia, and pulmonary hemosiderosis. *Am J Dis Child* 1962;103:634–54.

62 Lee SK, Kniker WT, Cook CD, Heiner DC. Cow's milk-induced pulmonary disease in children. *Adv Pediatr* 1978;25:39–57.

63 Liacouras CA, Spergel JM, Ruchelli E, *et al.* Eosinophilic esophagitis: a 10-year experience in 381 children. *Clin Gastroenterol Hepatol* 2005;3:1198–206.

64 Noel RJ, Putnam PE, Rothenberg ME. Eosinophilic esophagitis. *N Engl J Med* 2004;351:940–1.

65 Liacouras CA, Ruchelli E. Eosinophilic esophagitis. *Curr Opin Pediatr* 2004;16:560–6.

66 Fox VL, Nurko S, Furuta GT. Eosinophilic esophagitis: it's not just kid's stuff. *Gastrointest Endosc* 2002;56:260–70.

67 Talley NJ, Shorter RG, Phillips SF, Zinsmeister AR. Eosinophilic gastroenteritis: a clinicopathological study of patients with disease of the mucosa, muscle layer, and subserosal tissues. *Gut* 1990;31:54–8.

68 Ureles AL, Alschibaja T, Lodico D, Stabins SJ. Idiopathic eosinophilic infiltration of the gastrointestinal tract, diffuse and

circumscribed; a proposed classification and review of the literature, with two additional cases. *Am J Med* 1961;30:899–909.

69 Klein NC, Hargrove RL, Sleisenger MH, Jeffries GH. Eosinophilic gastroenteritis. *Medicine (Baltimore)* 1970;49:299–319.

70 Leinbach GE, Rubin CE. Eosinophilic gastroenteritis: a simple reaction to food allergens? *Gastroenterology* 1970;59:874–89.

71 Rothenberg ME. Eosinophilic gastrointestinal disorders (EGID). *J Allergy Clin Immunol* 2004;113:11–28.

72 Roberts G, Lack G. Relevance of inhalational exposure to food allergens. *Curr Opin Allergy Clin Immunol* 2003;3:211–15.

73 Roberts G, Patel N, Levi-Schaffer F, *et al.* Food allergy as a risk factor for life-threatening asthma in childhood: a case-controlled study. *J Allergy Clin Immunol* 2003;112:168–74.

74 Sicherer SH, Sampson HA. Food hypersensitivity and atopic dermatitis: pathophysiology, epidemiology, diagnosis, and management. *J Allergy Clin Immunol* 1999;104:S114–22.

75 Burks AW, James JM, Hiegel A, *et al.* Atopic dermatitis and food hypersensitivity reactions. *J Pediatr* 1998;132:132–6.

76 Sampson HA, McCaskill CC. Food hypersensitivity and atopic dermatitis: evaluation of 113 patients. *J Pediatr* 1985;107:669–75.

9

CHAPTER 9

Eczema and Food Hypersensitivity

David M. Fleischer and Donald Y.M. Leung

KEY CONCEPTS

- Food allergy plays a role in the pathogenesis of atopic dermatitis (AD) in a subset of patients.

- Approximately one-third of children with moderate to severe AD are affected by food allergy. Studies in adults with AD have not clearly shown a significant role for food allergy.

- Eighty percent of food allergy diagnosed by food challenge in children with AD is caused by milk, egg, and peanut. The most common food allergens in adults are peanut, tree nuts, fish, and shellfish.

- By correctly diagnosing food allergy and eliminating the offending food allergen(s), eczematous lesions can significantly improve and even clear in children with AD and food allergy.

- Infants and children with AD and food allergy are at high risk for the development of allergic rhinitis and asthma.

Introduction

Atopic dermatitis (AD) is one type of eczema that usually begins in early infancy and is typified by extreme pruritus, a chronic relapsing course, and a distinctive pattern of skin distribution. AD is a global problem that affects a large number of children and adults around the world [1]. Prevalence of AD ranges from 1% to 20% based on data from the Global International Study of Asthma and Allergies in Childhood trial, with the highest prevalence in Northern Europe [2]. The most recent data from school-aged children in the United States indicate that the prevalence in this population approaches 17% [3]. The onset of AD occurs during the first 6 months of life in 45% of children, during the first year of life in 60%, and before the age of 5 years in 85% of affected individuals [4]; only approximately 17% of adults with AD have onset after adolescence [5,6]. AD is often the first step in the atopic march, with more than 50% of affected children developing asthma and allergic rhinitis [7,8].

Numerous triggers for AD have been identified over the past few decades, including food allergens, inhalant respiratory allergens, irritant substances, and infectious organisms such as *Staphylococcus aureus* [9] and *Malassezia furfur* [10] (Table 9.1). Food allergy has been strongly correlated with the development and persistence of AD, especially in infants and young children. In this chapter, we will focus on how

Table 9.1 Allergic triggers of AD (Reproduced from Leung D. *Pediatric Allergy*: principles and practice. St. Louis: Mosby, 2003, with permission from Elsevier.)

Food allergens (most common)	Microorganisms
Cow's milk	Bacteria
Egg	*Staphylococcus aureus*
Soy	*Streptococcus* species
Wheat	
Peanut	Fungi/yeasts
Tree nuts	*Trichophyton* species
Fish	*Malassezia* (formerly known
Shellfish	as *pityrosporum orbiculare/ ovale*) species
Aeroallergens	*Candida* species
Pollen	
Mold	
Dust mite	
Animal dander	
Cockroach	

the ingestion of certain foods can trigger AD. Laboratory and clinical investigations that demonstrate how food hypersensitivity plays a pathophysiologic role in AD will be reviewed. The epidemiology, diagnosis, management, natural history, and prevention of food hypersensitivity with respect to AD will also be discussed.

Immunopathophysiology of atopic dermatitis

The pathophysiology of AD involves an intricate interaction between various susceptibility genes, host environments,

Food Allergy: Adverse Reactions to Foods and Food Additives, 4th edition.
Edited by Dean D. Metcalfe, Hugh A. Sampson, and Ronald A. Simon.
© 2008 Blackwell Publishing, ISBN: 978-1-4501-5129-0.

infectious agents, defects in skin barrier function, and immunologic responses. It also involves multiple cell types including T-lymphocytes, dendritic cells (DCs), macrophages, keratinocytes, mast cells, and eosinophils. While a full understanding is not yet complete, some important insights into the allergic mechanisms involved in the initiation and maintenance of skin inflammation in AD have been elucidated [11–13].

Acute AD skin lesions are associated with an increased number of T_H2 cytokines, notably IL-4 and IL-13. IL-4 and IL-13 mediate antibody isotype switching to IgE synthesis and upregulation of adhesion molecules on endothelial cells. T-lymphocytes in chronic AD lesions express increased IL-5, which is involved in eosinophil development [14], as well as IFN-γ, which potentiates effector function of pro-inflammatory cells. The maintenance of chronic AD also involves increased production of GM-CSF [15], IL-12 [16], and IL-18, as well as several remodeling-associated cytokines IL-11, IL-17, and TGF-β1 [17]. The T_H2 cytokines help promote recruitment and subsequently allergic inflammation by upregulating adhesion molecules on vascular endothelial cells, such as vascular adhesion molecule-1 (VCAM-1), E-selectin, and intercellular adhesion molecule-1 (ICAM-1) [18,19]. Studies have shown that adhesion molecules are not expressed in the skin of non-atopic individuals; however, they are expressed in normal-appearing skin of patients with AD and are markedly upregulated in lesional skin or upon epicutaneous application of allergen in sensitized AD patients [20].

Increased expression of chemokines such as CCL5 (RANTES), CCL13 (monocyte chemoattractant 4), and CCL11 (eotaxin) contribute to the infiltration of T-cells, macrophages, and eosinophils into AD skin [21]. IL-16, produced by epidermal Langerhans' cells (LCs), is a cytokine that induces chemotactic responses in CD4$^+$ T-cells, monocytes, and eosinophils [22,23].

Serum IgE levels are elevated in approximately 85% of patients with AD, and often contain food-allergen-specific and aeroallergen-specific IgE antibodies [24]. Some patients have IgE sensitization to microbial antigens, such as *Staphylococcus aureus* [9] enterotoxins and *Candida albicans* or *Malassezia sympodialis* [10]. The role of allergen-specific IgE in the pathogenesis of AD involves a number of cell types. LCs in AD lesions have allergen-specific IgE antibodies on their surface [25], and this makes them 100- to 1000-fold more efficient at presenting allergen to T-cells than LCs which do not express the high-affinity IgE receptor (FcεRI) [26,27]. T_H2 cytokines upregulate FcεRI on LCs and other antigen-presenting cells (APCs), and promote local IgE synthesis [28]. IgE-bearing FcεRI$^+$ inflammatory dendritic epidermal cells (IDECs) are prominent in chronic AD skin lesions. It is believed that IDECs are not only involved in cell recruitment and IgE-mediated antigen presentation to T-cells, but that they also release IL-12 and IL-18 and promote T_H1 cytokine production by priming naive T-cells

into IFN-γ-producing T-cells, which together may lead to the switch from an initial T_H2-type immune response to a T_H1-type immune response [29].

AD is associated with abnormalities in keratinocyte differentiation. This results in skin barrier dysfunction and frequent skin infections. Microarray analysis demonstrated that decreased expression of a group of antimicrobial genes, including human β-defensin, IL-8, and inducible nitric oxide synthetase, occurs as the result of local upregulation of T_H2 cytokines and the lack of elevated amounts of TNF-α and IFN-γ under inflammatory conditions in AD skin. This could explain the increased susceptibility of AD skin to microorganisms [30]. Reduced expression of skin barrier genes, such as filaggrin and lipids, may account for the characteristic skin dryness found in AD [12].

Eosinophils are thought to play a significant role in AD [13]. Inhibition of eosinophil apoptosis in AD, probably mediated by an autocrine release of IL-5 and GM-CSF, appears to be a mechanism for the eosinophil accumulation in AD [31]. Several studies indicate that eosinophils are recruited to and activated at tissue sites by T_H2 cytokines, such as IL-5 and IL-13 [32]. Once activated, eosinophils are capable of releasing an arsenal of potent cytotoxic granule proteins and chemical mediators, which contribute to tissue inflammation, as shown by the deposition of eosinophil products in the inflamed skin [32,33]. One of these products is eosinophil major basic protein (MBP), which is known to damage skin epithelial cells [34] and promote mast cell degranulation [29,35].

Role of food allergy in atopic dermatitis

The causal link between food allergy and AD has been the subject of debate for many years and still remains controversial [36]. There is, however, a large and growing body of evidence that supports the pathogenic role of food allergy in AD in at least a subset of patients, particularly in children (Table 9.2). Three patterns of cutaneous reactions to food may occur in patients with AD: (1) immediate-type allergic reactions, such as urticaria and angioedema, which occur within 2 hours after food ingestion, and suggests an IgE-mediated mechanism; (2) pruritus within 2 hours soon after food ingestion, which also suggests an IgE-mediated mechanism, with subsequent scratching leading to an AD exacerbation; and (3) delayed reactions with AD exacerbations that occur after 6–48 hours, either with or without a previous immediate-type response, suggestive of a non-IgE-mediated reaction or a cutaneous late-phase reaction of IgE-mediated hypersensitivity [37]. The following sections will review the evidence and methods used to evaluate the role of food allergy in AD.

Clinical evidence

Recent clinical evidence supporting the pathogenic role of food allergy in AD is based on three areas of clinical

Table 9.2 Association between AD and food allergy (Modified from Sicherer SH and Sampson HA [46], with permission from the American Academy of Allergy, Asthma and Immunology.)

Clinical studies
- Appropriate dietary elimination leads to improvement in AD
- Double-blind, placebo-controlled food challenges reproduce skin symptoms
- Breast-feeding for at least 3–4 months decreases the risk of the development of AD in high-risk infants
- The use of a hydrolyzed formula compared to a cow's milk formula in high-risk infants who are not able to be completely breastfed reduces infant and childhood allergy and infant cow's milk allergy

Laboratory studies
- Presence of elevated total IgE and food-specific IgE antibodies
- LCs bear high-affinity IgE receptors and can present allergen to T-cells
- Food allergens can activate skin mast cells after ingestion
- Plasma histamine elevation during positive OFCs
- Elevated histamine releasing factors in children when consuming diet with allergenic food
- Increased spontaneous basophil histamine release while ingesting causal food
- AD lesions contain eosinophil products: MBP and eosinophil cationic protein
- Eosinophils are activated during positive food challenge
- T-cells, cloned from active lesions of AD, can react to food allergen
- Children allergic to milk with AD have CLA+, milk-reactive T-cells.

investigation: elimination diet studies, oral food challenge (OFC) studies, and preventive studies of AD. Multiple clinical studies have shown that elimination of pertinent food allergens can lead to improvement in AD symptoms, that repeat oral challenge with the offending food(s) can lead to redevelopment of skin symptoms, and that AD and food hypersensitivity can be partially prevented by prophylactic elimination of highly allergic foods from infant diets and possibly from diets of breast-feeding mothers.

Elimination diet studies

Numerous studies have addressed the therapeutic effect of dietary elimination on the treatment of AD. Atherton *et al.* [38] showed that 14 of 20 subjects (70%) with AD between the ages of 2 and 8 years showed significant improvement after completing a 12-week, double-blind, controlled, cross-over trial of an egg and cow's milk (CM) exclusion diet. However, there were notable problems in this study, including 16 of the 36 subjects who did not complete the study (44% dropout) and poor control of confounding variables such as environmental factors and other triggers of AD. Neild *et al.* [39] studied 53 subjects with AD in another trial using a similar design as Atherton and colleagues. Forty of the 53 subjects (75%) complied adequately with the trial regimen, but only 10 of the 40 subjects benefited from the egg and CM exclusion diet, yielding a response rate to the

diet that was not statistically significant. Juto *et al.* [40] studied 21 infants with AD, of which only 20 were treated with a strict elimination diet for up to 6 weeks. Seven infants had complete resolution of their rash, 12 had some skin improvement while on the diet, and the remaining infant had no change in skin condition. While the cumulative results of the above studies provide support for the role of food allergy in AD, most of the trials failed to control confounding factors such as other potential AD triggers, placebo effect, or observer bias.

In one of the original prospective follow-up studies of the natural history of food hypersensitivity in children with AD, Sampson and Scanlon [41] studied 34 subjects with AD, of whom 17 had food allergy diagnosed by double-blind, placebo-controlled food challenges (DBPCFCs). These 17 subjects were placed on appropriate elimination diets and experienced significant improvement in their clinical symptoms. Comparisons made at 1–2-year and 3–4-year follow-ups with 12 control subjects who did not have food allergy and 5 subjects with food allergy who were noncompliant with their diet showed that the 17 food-allergic subjects with appropriate dietary restriction demonstrated highly significant improvement in their AD compared with the control groups. The amount of time for resolution of their food hypersensitivity was also reduced.

Lever *et al.* [42] performed a randomized, controlled trial of an egg exclusion diet in 55 children who presented to a dermatology clinic with AD and possible egg sensitivity identified by radioallergosorbent (RAST) testing before randomization. True egg sensitivity was confirmed by DBPCFC after the trial. The 55 children were randomized either to a 4-week regimen in which mothers received general advice on the care of AD and additional specific advice from a dietician about an egg elimination diet (diet group), or to a control group in which only general advice was provided. There was a significantly greater mean reduction in surface area affected by AD in the diet group (from 19.6% to 10.9% area affected; $p = 0.02$) than in the control group (from 21.9% to 18.9%). There was also significant improvement in symptom severity scores from 33.9 to 24.0 ($p = 0.04$) for the diet group, compared with a decrease from 36.7 to 33.5 in the control group.

Oral food challenge studies

For almost 30 years, researchers have used OFCs to demonstrate that food allergens can cause symptoms of rash and pruritus in children with food-allergy-associated AD. Bock *et al.* [43], in their studies of children with suspected food and respiratory allergies, reported that 4 of 7 children with a history of developing eczematous reactions to food developed skin rashes within 2 hours of a DBPCFC. In two studies, Burks *et al.* [44,45] also used the DBPCFC to study 165 children with mild to severe AD who presented to university allergy and dermatology clinics. Sixty percent of the subjects with AD had a positive skin prick test (SPT) to at least one of the following foods: milk, egg, soy, wheat, peanut, cashew, and codfish. They performed 266 DBPCFCs, and 64 subjects, 38.7% of the total group with AD, were found to have food allergy. Using a similar challenge protocol, Sampson and colleagues have studied over 600 subjects who were referred for evaluation of severe AD, and have performed more than 2000 OFCs [46].

Sampson and Scanlon [41], Sampson and McCaskill [47], Sampson and Metcalfe [48] and Eigenmann *et al.* [49] published a number of articles spanning over 17 years using DBPCFCs to identify foods that are trigger factors of AD. In the initial evaluation of 470 subjects with a median age of 4.1 years (range 3 months to 24 years), serum total IgE concentration was elevated in 376 subjects (80%), with a median of 3410 IU/ml and range of 1.5–45,000 IU/ml. Foods used in the DBPCFCs were selected based on skin and RAST testing results and/or a clinical history suggestive of food allergy, and these foods were eliminated from the subject's diet for at least 7–10 days prior to admission. A total of 1776 DBPCFCs were performed during the studies and 714 (40%) were positive and 1062 were negative. Cutaneous reactions during challenges developed in the vast majority of subjects (529 [74%] of the 714 DBPCFC-positive cases). The cutaneous reactions comprised a pruritic, erythematous, macular, or morbilliform rash that occurred primarily in previously affected AD sites. The development of skin symptoms only occurred in 214 (30%) of the positive reactions, and typical urticaria were rarely seen, and if present, consisted of only a few lesions. However, intense pruritus and scratching often led to superficial excoriations and occasionally bleeding.

Almost all symptoms during the DBPCFCs began between 5 minutes and 2 hours after starting the challenge. Immediate-type response symptoms generally occurred abruptly and lasted 1–2 hours. A few patients had a delayed second episode of pruritus, scratching, and transient morbilliform rash 6–10 hours after the initial challenge. This morbilliform rash may represent the acute phase of AD, and it is induced in the OFCs by acute consumption of a food that previously caused symptoms on a chronic basis [50]. Clinical reactions to milk, egg, soy, and wheat accounted for nearly 75% of the reactions in the studies. Some subjects had repeated reactions during a series of daily OFCs and subsequently had an increasingly severe AD exacerbation. This data provide further evidence that ingestion of a causal food can trigger itching, scratching, and the reappearance of typical AD lesions.

Prevention of food hypersensitivity and atopic dermatitis through diet

In addition to the above-mentioned studies that have shown that AD can improve through elimination diets of offending foods and that reintroduction of these foods during DBPCFCs can elicit symptoms, many studies have been performed in an attempt to prevent food allergy and AD through dietary means during pregnancy, lactation, and early infant feeding. Although it can be argued that all families should practice primary allergy prevention, this method can be so difficult that it is typically recommended only for those at "high risk" for developing allergy, defined as infants with at least one first-degree relative (parent or sibling) with documented allergic disease.

Maternal and/or infant elimination diets

Studies attempting to prevent CM and egg allergies by maternal CM and egg avoidance during late pregnancy have failed to show a reduction in food allergy, any other atopic disorder, or sensitization from birth through age 5 years. Additionally, maternal weight gain during pregnancy was negatively affected by these dietary restrictions. A recent Cochrane meta-analysis [51] confirmed the above findings, and the authors concluded that the prescription of an antigen avoidance diet to a high-risk woman during pregnancy is unlikely to substantially reduce the child's risk of atopic diseases, and such a diet may adversely affect maternal or fetal nutrition, or both. Another recent review of this issue by Muraro *et al.* [52] stated that there is no conclusive evidence for a protective effect of a maternal exclusion diet during pregnancy. Therefore, both the American and European guidelines do not recommend maternal avoidance diets that exclude essential foods during pregnancy.

Breast-feeding

For quite some time, it has been suggested that the presence of food antigens in breast milk might sensitize an infant if the mother does not avoid these foods in her diet during lactation. However, results of studies during the 1980s and 1990s examining this hypothesis have been contradictory. These contradictory studies, along with consideration of many others, led both a Cochrane analysis [51] and a recent meta-analysis [52] to conclude that while the prescription of an antigen avoidance diet to high-risk women during lactation may reduce the child's risk of developing AD, there is insufficient conclusive evidence to show a preventative effect of maternal diet during lactation on atopic disease in childhood. Furthermore, one cannot state for certain whether food antigens in breast milk will induce allergy or be immunoprotective in any given recipient [53].

Great debate exists today regarding the degree to which breast-feeding prevents, reduces, delays, or increases the development of allergic disease. Some trends can be observed and conclusions drawn from a review of the literature on the effects of human milk and breast-feeding on AD and food allergy. Of the many studies regarding the association between breast-feeding and AD, some have shown a protective effect [54,55], whereas others have shown a lack of association [56], and some have even shown a positive association [57]. To assist in sorting out the discrepancies in the above studies, Gdalevich *et al.* [58] performed a systematic review and meta-analysis of prospective studies in developed countries that compared breast-feeding with CM formula feeding on the development of AD. Statistical analysis revealed a significant overall protective effect of breast-feeding for 3 months on AD, with an OR of 0.68 (95% CI, 0.52–0.88) in the cohort as a whole. The effect was even stronger in children with a family history of atopy (OR, 0.58; 95% CI, 0.41–0.92). No protective effect was demonstrated in children without at least a first-degree relative with atopy (OR, 1.43; 95% CI, 0.72–2.86). In summary, despite contradictory study results, the preponderance of evidence suggests that exclusive breast-feeding for at least 3–4 months decreases the risk of the development of AD in high-risk infants. Based on the current data, there is lack of evidence that this statement holds true for infants not at risk for atopy.

The effect of breast-feeding on the development of food allergy is difficult to determine, as both AD and asthma are closely associated with the development of food allergy. There are a limited number of studies that have examined breast-feeding's role on the outcomes of specific food allergies, and the results may be affected by other dietary variables such as the length and extent of exclusivity of breast-feeding. After reviewing the existing studies, Muraro *et al.* [52] determined that exclusive breast-feeding for at least 4 months is related to a lower cumulative incidence of CM allergy until 18 months of age. However, no firm conclusions about the role of breast-feeding in either the primary prevention of or delay in onset of other specific food allergies can be made at this time.

Infant formula selection

Many studies have been performed exploring the use of various infant formulas, including conventional CM formula, partial whey hydrolysate formula (pHF), extensive casein hydrolysate formulas (eHF), and soy-protein-based formulas in the prevention of allergy. A recent Cochrane review [59] determined that there is no evidence to support prolonged feeding with a hydrolyzed formula to prevent allergy in preference to exclusive breast-feeding. In high-risk infants who are not able to be completely breastfed, there is evidence that the use of a hydrolyzed formula compared to a CM formula reduces infant and childhood allergy and infant CM allergy. Although some studies show a slight benefit of eHFs compared with pHFs, there is inconclusive evidence at this time to determine whether feeding with an eHF has any advantage over a pHF [60]. There is convincing evidence that feeding with a soy formula is not recommended in high-risk infants for the prevention of allergy [61]. Amino-acid-based formulas have not been studied in the primary prevention of allergy.

Introduction of solids

Early studies regarding the timing of solid food introduction demonstrated some benefit in delaying early solid food introduction [62,63], but more recent studies have shown a lack of protective effect [64]. The conflicting data from the studies taken as a whole does not currently allow an authoritative statement regarding the relation between the introduction of solids and the development of allergy to be made. Therefore, the advantage of delaying highly allergic solid food introduction beyond 4–6 months is unconfirmed. Delaying solid food introduction may even increase the risk of allergy (e.g. wheat allergy [65]).

Laboratory evidence

There are several other lines of laboratory evidence in addition to those presented previously in the immunopathophysiologic role of allergy in AD section that provide support for the role of food-specific IgE in the pathogenesis of AD. To show that food antigen ingestion led to IgE-mediated reactions, Sampson and Jolie [66] sought markers of mast cell activation in 33 subjects with AD who underwent DBPCFCs to evaluate the role of histamine in food hypersensitivity by monitoring changes in circulating plasma histamine. Only the group of subjects with positive DBPCFCs demonstrated a significant rise in plasma histamine, from 296 + 80pg/ml before challenge to 1055 + 356pg/ml ($p < 0.001$); subjects who consumed placebo or had negative DBPCFCs showed no demonstrable rise in plasma histamine. The rise in plasma histamine that was observed implicated the role of mast cell or basophil mediators in the pathogenesis of food allergy in AD.

Mechanisms that involve IgE antibody, other than direct IgE-mediated activation of cutaneous mast cells, may also play a role in the inflammatory process in AD. Sampson *et al.* [67] studied 63 subjects with AD and food hypersensitivity documented by DBPCFCs, 20 subjects with AD but no food allergy based on negative DBPCFCs, and 18 normal controls. Subjects with AD and food allergy had higher rates of mean spontaneous histamine release than the other two subject groups: 35.1% + 3.9% versus 1.8% + 0.2% (AD, no food allergy) and 2.3% + 0.2% (controls); $p < 0.001$. The high rate of histamine release appeared to depend on continued ingestion of the offending food, because once a subject was placed on the appropriate elimination diet for 9–12 months, the spontaneous histamine release returned to normal levels. Another important finding was the identification of spontaneously produced cytokines called histamine releasing factors (HRFs) from peripheral blood mononuclear cells (PBMCs) of food-allergic subjects with high spontaneous histamine release. HRF *in vitro* could activate basophils from other food-allergic subjects, but not from non-food-allergic subjects. Normal controls did not produce HRFs, and subjects with food allergy who adhered to an elimination diet had a decrease in the rate of spontaneous HRF production. The HRF was found to activate basophils through surface-bound IgE. Several different forms of IgE have been identified [68], and it has been proposed that HRFs may interact with certain of these IgE isoforms.

Basophil histamine release (BHR) had been proposed as an *in vitro* correlate to *in vivo* allergic responses [69]. BHR as a method of diagnosing food allergy was reported by Nolte [70] to correlate well with SPTs, RASTs, and open OFCs, but not with histamine release from intestinal mast cells obtained by duodenal biopsy in children. Another study by Sampson and Ho comparing BHR, SPTs, and DBPCFCs, however, showed that the BHR assay was no more effective in predicting clinical sensitivity than SPTs [71]. The clinical application of BHR is further complicated by several factors: it is not a widely available test, blood needs to be processed within a certain amount of time for cells to be viable, and there are no standardized methods for performing BHR. BHR assays are now primarily used in research settings.

A relatively new technique used to study the mediator effects of basophils, the basophil activation test (BAT), has the potential to overcome the pitfalls of BHR. The emerging ability to measure basophil activation as an assay for immediate hypersensitivity has the potential to provide diagnostic or prognostic utility in food allergy [72]. Allergen desensitization in studies has been shown to induce basophil hyporesponsiveness to allergen-induced degranulation [73,74], and *in vivo* constitutive activation of basophils correlates with CD203c expression measured directly *ex vivo* by flow cytometry [72]. Some have found that CD203c is expressed at very high levels in patients with AD and food allergy [72]. The assessment of BAT as a clinical diagnostic tool for food allergy in AD is still in its early stages, however. Monitoring the BAT for patients with food allergy on various elimination diets or following OFCs with subjective or late-phase reactions may also prove to be an important clinical tool, but further studies are needed.

Other data support a key role of eosinophils in the pathogenesis of food-sensitive AD, particularly in the late-phase IgE response. Studies of the late-phase reactions after the initial mast cell activation have shown that the terminal stages of IgE-mediated allergic reactions are characterized by infiltration of inflammatory cells, including eosinophils [75,76]. Although blood eosinophilia is common in AD patients, increased numbers of activated eosinophils have not always been found in biopsies of AD lesions. However, eosinophil degranulation and release of potent mediators clearly occurs. Leiferman *et al.* [77] found extensive dermal deposition of eosinophil-derived MBP in lesional biopsies of 18 subjects with AD but not in normal-appearing skin in affected subjects, suggesting that the assessment of eosinophil involvement cannot be based simply on the eosinophil numbers in tissue. Suomalainen *et al.* [78] studied 28 challenge-proven CM-allergic subjects and showed increased levels of eosinophil cationic protein (ECP) in the subjects with cutaneous symptoms only, which indicated that ingestion of an offending food in an allergic patient can lead to activation of circulating eosinophils that may then infiltrate the skin of AD patients. Another study confirmed the finding of significantly elevated plasma ECP levels in subjects with AD [79].

Several important studies have helped clarify the role of food-allergen-specific T-cells in the underlying inflammatory process in AD, showing that cell-mediated immunity also occurs in patients with food-sensitive AD in addition to IgE-mediated hypersensitivity. Food-antigen-specific T-cells have been isolated and cloned from active AD lesions [80–82]. Researchers have also been able to routinely identify food-antigen-specific T-cells from peripheral blood in subjects with food-allergy-associated AD [81–83]. There has been disagreement in the literature, though, about the validity of *in vitro* T-lymphocyte proliferation responses to specific foods in AD. Kondo, Agata, and colleagues [84,85] demonstrated that proliferative responses of PBMCs to the offending food antigen in subjects with non-immediate types of food allergy (rash developing at least 2 hours after OFC) were significantly higher than those of healthy controls and subjects with immediate types of food allergy, respectively, indicating that the proliferative response of PBMCs to food antigens is specific to each offending food antigen in non-immediate types of food-allergy-related AD. On the other hand, others have found increased lymphocyte proliferative responses to relevant foods also in subjects with immediate reactions [82]. Overall, the clinical utility of lymphocyte proliferation assays in food-allergic patients is considered marginal due to considerable overlap in individual responses to the test, as Hoffman *et al.* [86] found them to be neither diagnostic nor predictive of clinical reactivity in individual subjects with milk allergy because lymphocytes of many control patients were highly responsive to milk antigens, and lymphocytes of many subjects with milk allergy were not.

Further evidence of T-lymphocyte involvement in the development of AD in food-allergic patients relates to the homing of allergen-specific T-cells to the skin [81]. The extravasation of T-cells at sites of inflammation is critically dependent on the activity of homing receptors that are involved in endothelial cell recognition and binding. Two such homing receptors, cutaneous lymphocyte-associated antigen (CLA) and L-selectin, have been shown to be selectively involved in T-cell migration to the skin and peripheral lymph nodes, respectively. Significantly higher expression of CLA occurred in casein-reactive T-cells from children with milk-induced AD than *Candida albicans*-reactive T-cells from the same subjects, and from either casein- or *Candida albicans*-reactive T-cells from the control groups. In contrast, the percentage of L-selectin-expressing T-cells did not significantly differ among the three groups.

The role of non-IgE-mediated food-induced hypersensitivity in AD remains unclear [28], likely in part due to the raging debate for several decades whether food can act as a provocation factor for late eczematous reactions. Atopy patch tests (APTs) have been proposed as a mode of diagnosis of non-IgE-mediated food allergy and in identifying allergens in delayed-onset clinical reactions. The patch test reaction seems to be specific for sensitized patients with AD, as it does not occur in healthy volunteers or in patients suffering from asthma or rhinitis (87). The outcome of APTs in different studies shows large variations due to differences in patient selection and, more importantly, differences in methodology. These facts make interpretation of studies somewhat difficult due to reliability issues, but a number of investigators, as discussed in the diagnostic section below, have examined the use of the APTs in addition to SPTs for the diagnosis of non-IgE-mediated food allergy, primarily in patients with AD.

Epidemiology of food allergy in atopic dermatitis

The prevalence of food allergy in patients with AD differs depending on the age of the patient and the severity of AD. Burks et al. [44], using DBPCFCs, diagnosed food allergy in 15 of 46 children (33%) with AD ranging from mild to severe that were referred to allergy or dermatology clinics. In a larger study published 10 years later of 165 children with AD referred to the allergy clinic, Burks and colleagues [45] diagnosed food allergy in 64 children (38.7%) utilizing DBPCFCs. Ascertainment bias could have affected the results of these two studies since many of the patients were referred to an allergist, so Eigenmann et al. [49] addressed this potential bias by evaluating 63 unselected children referred to a university-based dermatologist for assessment of moderate to severe AD. Again OFCs were used as part of the evaluation, and ultimately 23 of 63 (37%; 95% CI, 25–50%) were found to have clinically significant IgE-mediated food hypersensitivity. In an epidemiologic study of IgE-mediated food allergy in 74 Swiss children with AD referred to an allergist or dermatologist, Eigenmann and Calza [88] found that 25 of the 74 children (33.8%) were food allergic using OFCs and other tests. While the above studies did not stratify children by the severity of AD [44,49,87] or demonstrate a direct relationship between severity of AD and presence of food allergy [45], Guillet and Guillet [89] attempted this in a study of 250 children with AD. They found that increased severity of AD and younger age of children directly correlated with the presence of food allergy. Finally, two more studies, neither of which performed OFCs, looked at the prevalence of food allergy in two prospective birth cohorts in Australia. In the first, Hill et al. [90] found a cumulative prevalence of AD of 24%. The contribution of IgE food sensitization to the burden of AD was calculated as an attributable risk percent; this calculation estimated that IgE food sensitization was responsible for 65% and 64% of

AD in the at-risk cohort at 6 and 12 months, respectively. In the second study, Hill and Hosking [91] discovered a cumulative prevalence of AD of 28.9%. The association between IgE-mediated food allergy and AD was assessed using only SPT cut-offs and was stratified by groups of AD severity. As the severity of AD increased, so did the frequency of IgE-mediated food allergy and reported adverse food reactions, from 12% in the least severe AD group, up to 69% in the most severe AD group.

Epidemiologic studies of food allergy in adults with severe AD are comparatively limited, which may in part be due to the fact that most food allergy is outgrown in children, with the notable exceptions of peanut, tree nuts, fish, and shellfish. In a double-blind, controlled study using an antigen-free formula (Vivasorb) compared with placebo diet in 33 severe AD adults, Munkvad et al. [92] found that food allergy played little role in the etiology of AD in adults because the antigen-free diet did not significantly reduce symptoms. de Maat-Bleeke be De and Bruijnzeel-Koomen [93] also failed to discover a significant role of food allergy in adult AD. However, one study from Japan found that 44% of the 195 adults with AD had positive challenges to foods, although the causative foods listed were uncommon allergens, including chocolate, coffee, and rice [94]. Finally, a recent German study by Worm et al. [95] found that certain adult subjects were sensitized to pollen allergens, and according to those pollen allergens, also sensitized to pollen-associated food allergens; this trend was not frequently found though.

Diagnosis of food hypersensitivity in patients with atopic dermatitis

General approach
The diagnosis of food allergy (Fig. 9.1) must first begin with a careful medical history since the information gathered will be used to guide the best mode of diagnosis, or it could lead to dismissal of the problem by history alone. In fact, it is well documented in several studies where DBPCFCs were used to diagnose food allergy that only about 40% of patient histories of suspected food-induced allergic reactions could be verified [96]. The history should focus on the food(s) and quantity of food suspected of provoking the reaction, the type of symptoms attributed to food ingestion (acute versus chronic), the timing between ingestion and onset of symptoms, patterns of reactivity, the most recent reaction, and whether other associated activities play a role in inducing symptoms (e.g. exercise, alcohol ingestion). When gathering the history, one must also be aware of other foods eaten at the same time, potentially contaminated foods that may have been packaged on non-dedicated lines, and hidden sources of ingredients.

Once a symptom history is established, the search for a food-related etiology needs to be put in context with the

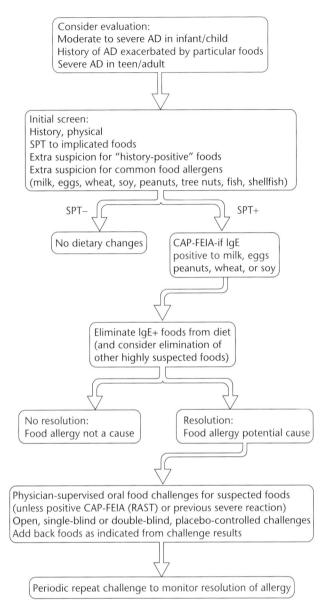

Figure 9.1 General approach to the evaluation of food allergy in AD. (Reproduced from Leung D. *Pediatric Allergy: Principles and Practice*. St. Louis: Mosby, 2003, with permission from Elsevier.)

prevalence that food allergy is implicated as the causative factor. The prevalence of food hypersensitivities is greatest in the first few years of life, affecting about 6% of children less than 3 years of age, then decreasing to a steady prevalence of 3.7% by late childhood through adulthood [97]. Furthermore, although any food could theoretically cause an allergic reaction, a small number of foods account for about 90% of verified food reactions: milk, egg, soy, wheat, peanut, tree nuts, and fish in children; and peanuts, tree nuts, fish, and shellfish in adults.

Once a thorough history has been obtained, the physical examination should focus on detecting other atopic features,

which are more commonly found in patients with IgE-mediated allergic reactions. After completing the history and physical, the physician should determine whether the patient's findings implicate a food-induced disorder and whether an IgE-mediated or non-IgE-mediated mechanism is most likely responsible. When food allergy has been identified as the likely cause of symptoms, confirmation of the diagnosis and identification of the implicated food(s) can begin. A number of tools exist that aid in the diagnosis of food allergy. In general, laboratory tests are more useful in delineating the specific foods responsible for IgE-mediated reactions, whereas they are of limited or no value in non-IgE-mediated disorders. Available studies include *in vivo* tests such as SPT, OFCs, elimination diets, and APTs, and *in vitro* tests such as quantification of food-specific IgE and the BAT (discussed previously). The utility of these test modalities will be briefly discussed.

In vivo and *in vitro* laboratory testing

SPTs are commonly used to screen patients with suspected IgE-mediated food reactions. When an SPT is positive, it indicates the possible association between the food tested and the patient's reactivity to that food because the positive predictive accuracies of SPTs are less than 50% compared to DBPCFCs. However, a positive SPT may be considered diagnostic in patients who have experienced a systemic anaphylactic reaction to an isolated food. On the other hand, negative responses virtually exclude the possibility of an IgE-mediated reaction because their negative predictive value (NPV) exceeds 95% [98]. The accuracy of SPTs varies depending on which food antigen is being studied, the quality of the food extract, and the technical skills of the tester. As a result of a study by Bock *et al.* [99], intradermal skin tests (ISTs) to food extracts were found to have no positive advantage over SPTs, and it was concluded that the increased sensitivity of ISTs would lead to even more false-positive tests than seen with the prick technique [100]. Fresh food skin prick tests (FFSPTs) may be performed because some commercially prepared extracts frequently lack the labile proteins that are responsible for IgE-mediated sensitivity to many fruits and vegetables because they are degraded or lose allergenicity during extract preparation [101]. Negative SPTs with commercially available extracts that contradict a convincing history of a food-induced allergic reaction should be repeated with the fresh food before concluding that food-specific IgE is absent [102].

Another way to identify food-specific IgE that is more widely available to the general practitioner is the CAP-System fluorescent-enzyme immunoassay (FEIA), although the sensitivity is slightly less than SPTs. The development of the CAP-System FEIA allowed better quantitation of food-specific IgE antibodies, which have been shown in key studies to be more predictive of symptomatic IgE-mediated food hypersensitivity. In a retrospective study on 196 children

Conclusions

The triggers associated with disease pathogenesis and clinical symptoms in patients with AD are numerous. Early in life, the role of allergens, especially food allergens, is clearly important. A careful history with appropriate diagnostic testing coupled with a comprehensive treatment program can alter the disease and life for patients with AD and food hypersensitivity.

References

1 Williams H, Robertson C, Stewart A, *et al.* Worldwide variations in the prevalence of symptoms of atopic eczema in the International Study of Asthma and Allergies in Childhood. *J Allergy Clin Immunol* 1999;103:125–38.

2 The International Study of Asthma and Allergies in Childhood (ISAAC) Steering Committee. Worldwide variation in prevalence of symptoms of asthma, allergic rhinoconjunctivitis, and atopic eczema: ISAAC. *Lancet* 1998;351:1225–32.

3 Laughter D, Istvan JA, Tofte SJ, *et al.* The prevalence of atopic dermatitis in Oregon schoolchildren. *J Am Acad Dermatol* 2000; 43:649–55.

4 Kay J, Gawkrodger DJ, Mortimer MJ, *et al.* The prevalence of childhood atopic eczema in a general population. *J Am Acad Dermatol* 1994;30:35–9.

5 Williams HC, Strachan DP. The natural history of childhood eczema: observations from the British 1958 birth cohort study. *Br J Dermatol* 1998;139:834–9.

6 Ozkaya E. Adult-onset atopic dermatitis. *J Am Acad Dermatol* 2005;52:579–82.

7 Lau S, Nickel R, Niggeman B, *et al.* The development of childhood asthma: lessons from the German Multicentre Allergy Study (MAS). *Paediatr Respir Rev* 2002;3:265–72.

8 Spergel JM, Paller JS. Atopic dermatitis and the atopic march. *J Allergy Clin Immunol* 2003;112:S118–27.

9 Novak N, Allam JP, Bieber T. Allergic hyperreactivity to microbial components: a trigger factor of "intrinsic" atopic dermatitis? *J Allergy Clin Immunol* 2003;112:215–16.

10 Scheynius A, Johansson C, Buentke E, *et al.* Atopic eczema/dermatitis syndrome and *Malassezia*. *Int Arch Allergy Immunol* 2002;127:161–9.

11 Morar N, Willis-Owen SA, Moffatt MF, *et al.* The genetics of atopic dermatitis. *J Allergy Clin Immunol* 2006;118:24–34.

12 Cork MJ, Robinson DA, Vasilopoulos Y, *et al.* New perspectives on epidermal barrier dysfunction in atopic dermatitis: gene – environment interactions. *J Allergy Clin Immunol* 2006;118:3–21.

13 Akdis CA, Akdis M, Bieber T, *et al.* Diagnosis and treatment of atopic dermatitis in children and adults: European Academy of Allergology and Clinical Immunology/American Academy of Allergy, Asthma and Immunology/PRACTALL Consensus Report. *J Allergy Clin Immunol* 2006;118:152–69.

14 Hamid Q, Boguniewicz M, Leung DY. Differential *in situ* cytokine gene expression in acute versus chronic atopic dermatitis. *J Clin Invest* 1994;94:870–6.

15 Bratton DL, Hamid Q, Boguniewicz M, *et al.* Granulocyte macrophage colony-stimulating factor contributes to enhanced monocyte survival in chronic atopic dermatitis. *J Clin Invest* 1995;95;211–18.

16 Hamid Q, Naseer T, Minshall EM, *et al. In vivo* expression of IL-12 and IL-13 in atopic dermatitis. *J Allergy Clin Immunol* 1996;98:225–31.

17 Toda M, Leung DY, Molet S, *et al.* Polarized *in vivo* expression of IL-11 and IL-17 between acute and chronic skin lesions. *J Allergy Clin Immunol* 2003;111:875–881.

18 Wakita H, Sakamoto T, Tokura Y, *et al.* E-selectin and vascular cell adhesion molecule-1 as critical adhesion molecules for infiltration of T lymphocytes and eosinophils in atopic dermatitis. *J Cutan Pathol* 1994;1:33–9.

19 Schon MP, Zollner TM, Henning-Boehncke. The molecular basis of lymphocyte recruitment to the skin: clues for pathogenesis and selective therapies of inflammatory disorders. *J Invest Dermatol* 2003;121:951–62.

20 Kallos P, Kallos L. Experimental asthma in guinea pigs revisited. *Int Arch Allergy Appl Immunol* 1984;73:77–85.

21 Taha RA, Minshall EM, Leung DYM, *et al.* Evidence for increased expression of eotaxin and monocyte chemotactic protein-4 in atopic dermatitis. *J Allergy Clin Immunol* 2000; 105:1002–7.

22 Laberge S, Ghaffar O, Boguniewicz M, *et al.* Association of increased CD4+ T-cell infiltration with increased IL-16 gene expression in atopic dermatitis. *J Allergy Clin Immunol* 1998; 102:645–50.

23 Reich K, Hugo S, Middel P, *et al.* Evidence for a role of Langerhans cell-derived IL-16 in atopic dermatitis. *J Allergy Clin Immunol* 2002;109:681–7.

24 Sampson HA. Food sensitivity and the pathogenesis of atopic dermatitis. *J Roy Soc Med* 1997;90:S3–9.

25 Bruynzeel-Koomen C, Van Wicker DF, Toonstra J, *et al.* The presence of IgE molecules on epidermal Langerhans cells in patients with atopic dermatitis. *Arch Dermatol Res* 1986;297:205.

26 Mudde G, Bheekha R, Bruijnzeel-Koomen C. Consequences of IgE/CD-23-mediated antigen presentation in allergy. *Immunol Today* 1995;16:380–3.

27 Mudde G, van Reijsen F, Boland G, *et al.* Allergen presentation by epidermal Langerhan's cells from patients with atopic dermatitis is mediated by IgE. *Immunology* 1990;69:335–41.

28 Sampson HA. Eczema and food hypersensitivity. In: Metcalfe DD, Sampson HA, Simon RA (eds.) *Food Allergy: Adverse Reactions to Foods and Food Additives*, 3rd edn. Malden: Blackwell Publishing, Inc., 2003:144–59.

29 Novak N, Valenta R, Bohle B, *et al.* FcεRI engagement of Langerhans cell-like dendritic cells and inflammatory dendritic epidermal cell-like dendritic cells induces chemotactic signals and different T-cell phenotypes *in vitro*. *J Allergy Clin Immunol* 2004;113:949–57.

30 Nomura I, Goleva E, Howell MD, *et al.* Cytokine milieu of atopic dermatitis, as compared to psoriasis, skin prevents induction of innate immune response genes. *J Immunol* 2003; 171:3262–9.

31 Wedi B, Raap U, Lewrick H, *et al.* Delayed eosinophil programmed cell death *in vitro*: a common feature of inhalant allergy and extrinsic and intrinsic atopic dermatitis. *J Allergy Clin Immunol* 1997;100:536–43.

32 Simon D, Braathen LR, Simon HU. Eosinophils and atopic dermatitis. *Allergy* 2004;59:561–70.

33 Kapp A. The role of eosinophils in the pathogenesis of atopic dermatitis – eosinophil granule proteins as markers of disease activity. *Allergy* 1993;48:1–5.

34 Gleich G, Frigas E, Loegering DA, *et al.* Cytotoxic properties of eosinophilic major basic protein. *J Immunol* 1979;123: 2925–7.

35 O'Donnell MC, Ackerman S, Gleich G, *et al.* Activation of basophil and mast cell histamine release by eosinophil granule major basic protein. *J Exp Med* 1983;157:1981–91.

36 Rowlands D, Tofte SJ, Hanifin JM. Does food allergy cause atopic dermatitis? Food challenge testing to dissociate eczematous from immediate reactions. *Dermatol Ther* 2006;19:97–103.

37 Wuthrich B. Food-induced cutaneous adverse reactions. *Allergy* 1998;53:S56–60.

38 Atherton DJ, Sewell M, Soothill JF, *et al.* A double-blind controlled crossover trial of an antigen-avoidance diet in atopic eczema. *Lancet* 1978;1:401–3.

39 Neild VS, Marsden RA, Bailes JA, *et al.* Egg and milk exclusion diets in atopic eczema. *Br J Dermatol* 1986;114:117–23.

40 Juto P, Engberg S, Winberg J. Treatment of infantile atopic dermatitis with a strict elimination diet. *Clin Allergy* 1978;8: 493–500.

41 Sampson HA, Scanlon SM. Natural history of food hypersensitivity in children with atopic dermatitis. *J Pediatr* 1989;115:23–7.

42 Lever R, MacDonald C, Waugh P, *et al.* Randomised controlled trial of advice on an egg exclusion diet in young children with atopic eczema and sensitivity to eggs. *Pediatr Allergy Immunol* 1998;9:13–9.

43 Bock S, Lee W, Remigio L, *et al.* Studies of hypersensitivity reactions to food in infants and children. *J Allergy Clin Immunol* 1978;62:3327–34.

44 Burks AW, Mallory SB, Williams LW, *et al.* Atopic dermatitis: clinical relevance of food hypersensitivity reactions. *J Pediatr* 1988;113:447–51.

45 Burks AW, James JM, Hiegel A, *et al.* Atopic dermatitis and food hypersensitivity reactions. *J Pediatr* 1998;132:132–6.

46 Sicherer SH, Sampson HA. Food hypersensitivity and atopic dermatitis: pathophysiology, epidemiology, diagnosis, and management. *J Allergy Clin Immunol* 1999;104:S114–22.

47 Sampson HA, McCaskill CC. Food hypersensitivity and atopic dermatitis: Evaluation of 113 patients. *J Pediatr* 1985;107: 669–75.

48 Sampson HA, Metcalfe DD. Food allergies [Review]. *JAMA* 1992;268:2840–4.

49 Eigenmann PA, Sicherer SH, Borkowski TA, *et al.* Prevalence of IgE-mediated food allergy among children with atopic dermatitis. *Pediatrics* 1998;101:e8.

50 Sicherer SH, Sampson HA. Role of food allergens. In: Leung DY, Greaves MW (eds.) *Allergic Skin Disease: A Multidisciplinary Approach,* 1st edn. Philadelphia, PA: Marcel Dekker, Inc, 2000: 403–422.

51 Kramer MS, Kakuma R. Maternal dietary antigen avoidance during pregnancy or lactation, or both, for preventing or treating atopic disease in the child. *Cochrane Database Syst Rev* 2003;4: CD0001333.

52 Muraro A, Dreborg S, Halken S, *et al.* Dietary prevention of allergic diseases in infants and small children. Part III. Critical review of published peer-reviewed observational and interventional studies and final recommendations. *Pediatr Allergy Immunol* 2004;15:291–307.

53 Friedman NJ, Zeiger RS. The role of breast-feeding in the development of allergies and asthma. *J Allergy Clin Immuol* 2005; 115:1238–48.

54 Kull I, Bohme M, Wahlgren C-F, *et al.* Breast-feeding decreases the risk for childhood eczema. *J Allergy Clin Immunol* 2005;116: 657–61.

55 Laubereau B, Brockow I, Zirngibl A, *et al.* Effect of breast-feeding on the development of atopic dermatitis during the first 3 years of life – results from the GINI-birth cohort study. *J Pediatr* 2004;144:602–7.

56 Ludvigsson JF, Mostrom M, Ludvigsson J, *et al.* Exclusive breast-feeding and the risk of atopic dermatitis in some 8300 infants. *Pediatr Allergy Immunol* 2005;16:201–8.

57 Pesonen M, Kallio MJ, Ranki A, *et al.* Prolonged exclusive breastfeeding is associated with increased atopic dermatitis: a prospective follow-up study of unselected healthy newborns from birth to age 20 years. *Clin Exp Allergy* 2006;36: 1011–8.

58 Gdalevich M, Mimouni D, David M, *et al.* Breast-feeding and the onset of atopic dermatitis in childhood: a systematic review and meta-analysis of prospective studies. *J Am Acad Dermatol* 2001;45:520–7.

59 Osborn DA, Sinn J. Formulas containing hydrolyzed protein for prevention of allergy and food intolerance in infants. *Cochrane Database Syst Rev* 2006;4:CD003664.

60 von Berg A, Koletzko S, Filipiak-Pittroff B, *et al.* Certain hydrolyzed formulas reduce the incidence of atopic dermatitis but not that of asthma: three-year results of the German Infant Nutritional Intervention Study. *J Allergy Clin Immunol* 2007;119:718–25.

61 Osborn DA, Sinn J. Soy formula for the prevention of allergy and food intolerance in infants. *Cochrane Database Syst Rev* 2006;3:CD003741.

62 Fergusson DM, Horwood LJ, Shannon FT. Early solid feeding and recurrent childhood eczema: a 10-year longitudinal study. *Pediatrics* 1990;86:541–6.

63 Kajosaari M. Atopy prophylaxis in high-risk infants: prospective 5-year follow-up study of children with six months exclusive breastfeeding and solid food elimination. *Adv Exp Med Biol* 1991;310:453–8.

64 Zutavern A, Brockow I, Schaaf B, *et al.* Timing of solid food introduction in relation to atopic dermatitis and atopic sensitization: results from a prospective birth cohort study. *Pediatrics* 2006;117:401–11.

65 Poole JA, Barriga K, Leung DY, *et al.* Timing of initial exposure to cereal grains and the risk of wheat allergy. *Pediatrics* 2006;117:2175–82.

66 Sampson HA, Jolie PL. Increased plasma histamine concentrations after food challenges in children with atopic dermatitis. *N Engl J Med* 1984;311:372–6.

67 Sampson HA, Broadbent KR, Bernhisel-Broadbent J. Spontaneous release of histamine from basophils and histamine-releasing factor in patients with atopic dermatitis and food hypersensitivity. *N Engl J Med* 1989;321:228–32.

68 Lyczak JB, Zhang K, Saxon A, *et al.* Expression of novel secreted isoforms of human immunoglobulin E proteins. *J Biol Chem* 1996;271:3428–36.

69 Du Buske LM. Introduction: basophil histamine release and the diagnosis of food allergy. *Allergy Proc* 1993;14:243–9.

70 Nolte H. The clinical utility of basophil histamine release. *Allergy Proc* 1993;14:251–4.

71 Sampson HA, Ho DG. Relationship between food-specific IgE concentrations and the risk of positive food challenges in children and adolescents. *J Allergy Clin Immunol* 1997; 100:444–51.

72 Shreffler WG. Evaluation of basophil activation in food allergy: present and future applications. *Curr Opin Allergy Clin Immunol* 2006;6:226–33.

73 Sobotka AK, Dembo M, Goldstein B, *et al.* Antigen-specific desensitization of human basophils. *J Immunol* 1979; 122:511–17.

74 Satti MZ, Cahen P, Skov PS, *et al.* Changes in IgE- and antigen-dependent histamine-release in peripheral blood of Schistosoma mansoni-infected Ugandan fishermen after treatment with praziquantel. *BMC Immunol* 2004;5:6.

75 Demoly P, Piette V, Bousquet J. *In vivo* methods for study of allergy. In: Adkinson NF, Yunginger JW, Busse WW, *et al.* (eds.) *Middleton's Allergy: Principles and Practice*, 6th edn. Philadelphia, PA: Mosby, Inc., 2003:631–2.

76 Abramovits W. Atopic dermatitis. *J Am Acad Dermatol* 2005;53: S86–93.

77 Leiferman KM, Ackerman SJ, Sampson HA, *et al.* Dermal deposition of eosinophil-granule major basic protein in atopic dermatitis. Comparison with onchocerciasis. *N Engl J Med* 1985; 313:282–5.

78 Suomalainen H, Soppi E, Isolauri E. Evidence for eosinophil activation in cow's milk allergy. *Pediatr Allergy Immunol* 1994; 5:27–31.

79 Magnarin M, Knowles A, Ventura A, *et al.* A role for eosinophils in the pathogenesis of skin lesions in patients with food-sensitive atopic dermatitis. *J Allergy Clin Immunol* 1995; 96:200–8.

80 van Reijsen FC, Felius A, Wauters EA. T-cell reactivity for a peanut-derived epitope in the skin of a young infant with atopic dermatitis. *J Allergy Clin Immunol* 1998;101:207–9.

81 Abernathy-Carver KJ, Sampson HA, Parker LJ, *et al.* Milk-induced eczema is associated with the expansion of T cells expressing cutaneous lymphocyte antigen. *J Clin Invest* 1995; 95:913–18.

82 Reekers R, Beyer K, Niggemann B, *et al.* The role of circulating food antigen-specific lymphocytes in food allergic children with atopic dermatitis. *Br J Dermatol* 1996;135:935–41.

83 Werfel T, Ahlers G, Schmidt P, *et al.* Detection of kappa-casein-specific lymphocyte response in milk-responsive atopic dermatitis. *Clin Exp Allergy* 1996;26:1380–6.

84 Kondo N, Fukutomi O, Agata H, *et al.* Proliferative responses of lymphocytes to food antigens are useful for detection of allergens in nonimmediate types of food allergy. *J Investig Allergol Clin Immunol* 1997;7:122–6.

85 Agata H, Kondo N, Fukutomi O, *et al.* Effect of elimination diets in food-specific IgE antibodies and lymphocyte proliferative responses to food antigens in atopic dermatitis patients exhibiting sensitivity to food allergens. *J Allergy Clin Immunol* 1993;91:668–79.

86 Hoffman KM, Ho DG, Sampson HA. Evaluation of the usefulness of lymphocyte proliferation assays in the diagnosis of allergy to cow's milk. *J Allergy Clin Immunol* 1997;99:360–6.

87 De Bruin-Weller MS, Knol EF, Bruijnzeel-Koomen C. Atopy patch testing – a diagnostic tool? *Allergy* 1999;54:784–91.

88 Eigenmann PA, Calza A-M. Diagnosis of IgE-mediated food allergy among Swiss children with atopic dermatitis. *Pediatr Allergy Immunol* 2000;11:95–100.

89 Guillet G, Guillet M-H. Natural history of sensitizations in atopic dermatitis. A 3-year follow-up in 250 children: food allergy and high risk of respiratory symptoms. *Arch Dermatol* 1992;128:187–92.

90 Hill DJ, Sporik R, Thorburn J, *et al.* The association of atopic dermatitis in infancy with immunoglobulin E food sensitization. *J Pediatr* 2000;137:475–9.

91 Hill DJ, Hosking CS. Food allergy and atopic dermatitis in infancy: an epidemiologic study. *Pediatr Allerg Immunol* 2004; 15:421–7.

92 Munkvad M, Danielsen L, Hoj L, *et al.* Antigen-free diet in adult patients with atopic dermatitis. A double-blind controlled study. *Acta Derm Venereol* 1984;64:524–8.

93 de Maat-Bleeker F, Bruijnzeel-Koomen C. Food allergy in adults with atopic dermatitis. *Monogr Allergy Basel Karger* 1996; 32:157–63.

94 Uenishi T, Sugiura H, Uehara M. Role of foods in irregular aggravation of atopic dermatitis. *J Dermatol* 2003;30:91–7.

95 Worm M, Forschner K, Lee HH, *et al.* Frequency of atopic dermatitis and relevance of food allergy in adults in Germany. *Acta Derm Venereol* 2006;86:119–22.

96 Bock SA, Atkins FM. Patterns of food hypersensitivity during sixteen years of double-blind, placebo-controlled food challenges. *J Pediatr* 1990;117:561–7.

97 Sicherer SH, Sampson HA. Food allergy. *J Allergy Clin Immunol* 2006;117:S470–5.

98 Sampson HA. Food allergy. Part 2. Diagnosis and management. *J Allergy Clin Immunol* 1999;103:981–9.

99 Bock SA, Lee WY, Remigio L, *et al.* Appraisal of skin tests with food extracts for diagnosis of food hypersensitivity. *Clin Allergy* 1978;8:559–64.

100 Sampson HA. Utility of food-specific IgE concentrations in predicting symptomatic food allergy. *J Allergy Clin Immunol* 2001; 107:891–6.

101 Ortolani C, Ispano M, Pastorello EA, *et al.* Comparison of results of skin prick tests (with fresh foods and commercial food extracts) and RAST in 100 patients with oral allergy syndrome. *J Allergy Clin Immunol* 1989;83:683–90.

102 Eigenmann PA, Sampson HA. Interpreting skin prick tests in the evaluation of food allergy in children. *Pediatr Allergy Immunol* 1998;9:186–91.

103 Roehr CC, Reibel S, Ziegert M, *et al.* Atopy patch tests, together with determination of specific IgE levels, reduce the need for oral food challenges in children with atopic dermatitis. *J Allergy Clin Immunol* 2001;107:548–53.

104 Breuer K, Heratizadeh A, Wulf A, *et al.* Late eczematous reactions to food in children with atopic dermatitis. *Clin Exp Allergy* 2004;34:817–24.

105 Mehl A, Rolinck-Werninhaus C, Staden U, *et al.* The atopy patch test in the diagnostic workup of suspected food-related symptoms in children. *J Allergy Clin Immunol* 2006;118:923–9.

106 Turjanmaa K. The role of atopy patch tests in the diagnosis of allergy in atopic dermatitis. *Curr Opin Allergy Clin Immunol* 2005;5:425–8.

107 Sicherer SH, Bock SA. An expanding evidence base provides food for thought to avoid indigestion in managing difficult dilemmas in food allergy. *J Allergy Clin Immunol* 2006; 117:1419–22.

108 Bock SA, Sampson HA, Atkins FA, *et al.* 1988. Double-blind, placebo-controlled food challenge (DBPCFC) as an office procedure: a manual. *J Allergy Clin Immunol* 1988;82:986–97.

109 Sicherer SH. Food allergy: when and how to perform oral food challenges. *Pediatr Allergy Immunol* 1999;10:226–34.

110 Sicherer SH. Food allergy. *Lancet* 2002;360:701–10.

111 Sampson HA. Use of food-challenge tests in children. *Lancet* 2001;358:1832–3.

112 Sampson HA, Mendelson LM, Rosen JP. Fatal and near-fatal anaphylactic reactions to foods in children and adolescents. *N Eng J Med* 1992;327:380–4.

113 Bock SA. The natural history of food sensitivity. *J Allergy Clin Immunol* 1982;69:173–7.

114 Skolnick HS, Conover-Walker MK, Sampson HA, *et al.* The natural history of peanut allergy. *J Allergy Clin Immunol* 2002; 107:367–74.

115 Fleischer DM, Conover-Walker MK, Christie L, *et al.* The natural progression of peanut allergy: resolution and the possibility of recurrence. *J Allergy Clin Immunol* 2003;112:183–9.

116 Fleischer DM, Conover-Walker MK, Matsui EC, *et al.* The natural history of tree nut allergy. *J Allergy Clin Immunol* 2005; 116:1087–93.

117 Fleischer DM, Conover-Walker MK, Christie L, *et al.* Peanut allergy: recurrence and its management. *J Allergy Clin Immunol* 2004;114:1195–1201.

118 Nickel R, Kulig M, Forster G, *et al.* Sensitization to hen's egg at the age of 12 months is predictive for allergen sensitization to common indoor and outdoor allergens at the age of 3 years. *J Allergy Clin Immunol* 1997;99:613–7.

10 CHAPTER 10

Other IgE- and Non-IgE-Mediated Reactions of the Skin

Carsten Bindslev-Jensen and Morten Osterballe

KEY CONCEPTS

- Acute urticaria is one of the most common findings in food allergy.
- Acute urticaria may vary from local contact urticaria to generalized urticaria.
- Presence of generalized urticaria is a danger signal in food-allergic patients.
- Chronic urticaria is only rarely of allergic origin.

IgE- and non-IgE-mediated reactions of the skin exclusive of eczema usually present as urticaria and/or angioedema. This heterogeneous group of disorders is often classified by duration and trigger factors. A classification based on clinical grounds and by trigger factors is convenient, but with inherent inconsistencies (Fig. 10.1). The distinction between acute and chronic urticaria is arbitrarily chosen and the duration of acute urticaria is normally limited to 6 weeks [1]. Classification of the many instances of recurrent acute attacks is difficult in cases of food-associated urticaria. Elicitation of wheals by direct contact between immunological or non-immunological stimuli, known as contact urticaria, is an important disease entity and is characterized by wheals confined to the area of contact. In contrast, wheals may erupt anywhere on the skin in the other types of acute urticaria [1,2].

Chronic urticaria can be further subdivided into primary urticaria and urticaria associated with disease (thyroid diseases, infection, or syndromes such as Schnitzler's or Muckle–Wells) [1,3,4]. Primary chronic urticarias are further classified into physical urticarias, which are elicited by factors such as cold, pressure, heat, ultraviolet light; autoimmune urticaria, in which antibodies against IgE or against the FcεR1 receptor on the mast cell (MC) are present [5]; and chronic idiopathic urticaria (CIU) (Fig. 10.1). The term "idiopathic" has, however, been left out in the new classifications [1]. This classification is suitable from a clinical point of view,

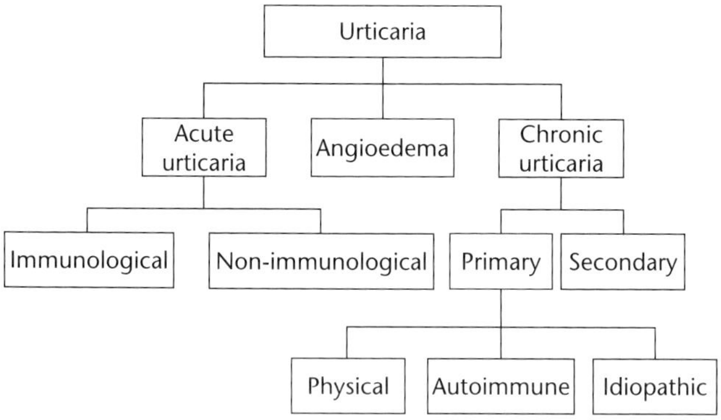

Figure 10.1 Classification of the urticarias and angioedema.

because the physical urticarias are rarely associated with any other disease (including food allergy), thus extensive investigations are rarely needed [1,6]. It is, however, important to emphasize that physical urticaria and CIU often occur in the same patient [7–9].

An urticarial wheal is present on the skin for less than 24 hours. If it persists longer, urticarial vasculitis, which rarely has an allergic etiology, must be suspected [8]. Diseases such as urticaria pigmentosa, a cutaneous form of mastocytosis, are usually not associated with an IgE-dependent mechanism.

Angioedema is a variant of urticaria in which mainly the subcutaneous tissues, rather than the dermis, are involved. The same situation with multiple etiologies and lack of a precise diagnosis that applies to chronic urticarias also applies to angioedema [10], with the exception of a hereditary form that accounts for about 1% of all angioedema

Food Allergy: Adverse Reactions to Foods and Food Additives, 4th edition.
Edited by Dean D. Metcalfe, Hugh A. Sampson, and Ronald A. Simon.
© 2008 Blackwell Publishing, ISBN: 978-1-4501-5129-0.

cases without concomitant urticaria. In this form, the pathological basis is a deficiency of the complement C1 esterase inhibitor. This disease is not associated with allergy [11].

Pathophysiology

Skin biopsies of urticarial wheals reveal only sparse pathological findings. The number of MCs is within the normal range and by light microscopy usually only vascular and lymphatic dilation are found. There is a variable perivascular cellular infiltrate consisting of lymphocytes, monocytes, neutrophils, and eosinophils.

The cutaneous MC is central to the pathophysiology of urticaria and angioedema. These cells may be activated by both immunological and non-immunological stimuli. Interestingly, using a microdialysis technique, histamine release has been found to be confined to the wheal area; no histamine was found in the surrounding flare area [12].

Acute urticaria

The most common cause of acute urticaria is infection, especially in infants and children [13]. In food allergy, acute urticaria is normally present together with symptoms and signs from other sites, such as the respiratory or gastrointestinal (GI) tract [14]. As can be seen in Table 10.1, urticaria is elicited by challenge in about 14% of the challenges that have been reported. Although data on the exact incidence of type I food allergy in the population are not available, a reported prevalence of 7–10% in children [14] suggests that the incidence of acute food-dependent urticaria is about 1–2% in children.

Food additives can elicit acute urticaria in children, as was demonstrated by double-blind challenge with colorants and other additives. In two trials, the incidence of acute urticaria in children attending a pediatric allergy clinic was found to be 1–2% [15,16].

Acute urticaria as the only sign of a food allergy is unusual. In rare cases, monosymptomatic acute urticaria can be elicited by skin prick test (SPT) in highly sensitive patients, especially with non-standardized extracts (Fig. 10.2(a, b)). A 31-year-old female with known allergy to Brazil nut and no history of urticaria experienced generalized urticaria requiring treatment with antihistamines and glucocorticoid during skin testing with Brazil nut and other nuts. From a stochiometric point of view, the total dose in this case of absorbed allergens would be <1 ng.

The mechanisms underlying elicitation of non-localized urticarial wheals on the skin immediately after oral challenge with non-tolerated foods remain obscure. Wheals often develop within less than 1–2 minutes after ingestion of the food. Thus, direct contact between absorbed proteins (via the bloodstream) from the food and IgE on the MC in the skin is very rapid or there are ancillary mechanisms.

Urticaria may develop anywhere on the skin, but special attention should be paid to itching of the palms and soles, where wheals are often difficult to see because of the tightly bound epidermis. This sign may be a special warning signal for subsequent development of systemic anaphylaxis [17].

Contact urticaria

In contact urticaria, an immediate wheal and flare response develops upon topical application of a substance to the skin. The substances involved are numerous and may be chemically defined molecules such as cinnamic acid, benzoic acid, or parabens; or chemically undefined, as are found in arthropods, plants, spices, fruits, or fish [18].

Contact urticaria can be subdivided into immunological and non-immunological contact urticaria [2,18]. In immunological contact urticaria, wheals are elicited by direct contact with proteins to which the patient is sensitized; for example, on the hands of a latex-sensitive patient wearing latex gloves, or periorally in a food-allergic infant. This condition should not be confused with non-immonological perioral contact urticaria elicited by sorbic and ascorbic acids in tomatoes and citrus fruits [2]. This generally harmless phenomenon, which reportedly rarely is followed by a systemic reaction, is often misinterpreted by parents and physicians as an allergic reaction. Unnecessary avoidance of the offending food can result. True allergic contact urticaria can proceed to a systemic reaction. Therefore, a thorough diagnostic work-up to rule out or demonstrate involvement of the immune system is important so that the patient (or most often the parents) is properly informed.

Contact urticaria to foods is also common in cooks and food handlers [19]. A characteristic feature in these patients is that, although skin contact with the foods such as fish or meat may cause wheals, oral intake of the same food is often tolerated [20].

In the vast majority of patients, contact dermatitis (an immunological type IV reaction in the skin) is due to sensitization to small molecules such as nickel. Additionally, protein contact dermatitis may be seen, especially in food handlers, where allergic hand eczema may develop over 2–3 days of contact between the skin and the food in question [19].

Treatment of immunological contact urticaria is avoidance, because a systemic reaction may follow the localized reaction. Non-immunological contact urticaria normally is harmless and may be thus prevented, for example, by application of an ointment around the mouth of an infant prior to feeding.

Chronic urticaria

Although there is little doubt that acute urticaria in food-allergic patients belongs to the Th_2-related diseases, new data point toward chronic urticarias belonging to the TH_0 diseases [6].

Table 10.1 Incidence of acute urticaria in food allergy; urticaria reactions to food and additives

Food	Number of studies (OFC/SBFC/DBPCFC)	Number of patients reacting with urticaria	References
Cow's milk	18/1/52	339 of 2061	[21–83]
Egg	2/1/41	229 of 1491	[24,25,33,35,39–51,53,55,57,58,60–67,69–72,76,77,80,81,83–95]
Peanut	15/1/19	150 of 639	[25,33,49–51,55,60,62–64,69–71,76,83,87,90,93,96–106]
Additives	4/2/2	47 of 226	[15,107–118]
Mustard	0/2/1	36 of 102	[55,111,120]
Cod fish	0/1/7	21 of 188	[43–45,47,49–51,55,60,61,63,64,69,72,76,77,81,87,121–124]
Wheat	6/1/33	19 of 283	[24,35,40–42,44–51,55,60,61,63–67,70,72,76,77,80,93,104,105,125–131]
Goat's milk	0/1/1	15 of 27	[29,55]
Kiwi	2/1/3	9 of 112	[55,105,132–135]
Sesame seeds	2/1/1	6 of 51	[46,136–138]
Soy	6/1/23	5 of 281	[23,25,35,43–51,55,60,62,64–67,69,70,76,77,80,87,92,139–141]
Hazelnut	3/1/5	5 of 179	[24,55,61,69,87,99,142–145]
Cashew	1/0/2	5 of 14	[25,44,146]
Apple	8/1/3	3 of 185	[55,70,98,104,148–152]
Orange	4/0/3	3 of 49	[61,65,70,80,99,104,133]
Celery	5/0/6	3 of 44	[87,93,99,105,153,154]
Shrimp	1/1/6	2 of 33	[38,44,55,69,83,90,93,155]
Potato	4/0/3	2 of 16	[24,64,65,77,99,156]
Garlic	3/0/1	2 of 4	[24,87,105,157]
Pea	2/1/3	1 of 46	[55,63,69,92,156]
Corn	3/0/4	1 of 35	[70,72,129,131,156,158]
Walnut	3/0/0	1 of 6	[99,105,159]
Pineapple	1/0/0	1 of 1	[83]
Almond	2/1/1	0 of 36	[55,104,105,151]
Apricot	2/0/1	0 of 12	[105,151,160]
Avocado	1/0/0	0 of 1	[156]
Banana	2/1/1	0 of 6	[40,55,69,156]
Barley	1/0/2	0 of 9	[45,80,129]
Bean	2/0/0	0 of 2	[105,156]
Beef	2/1/4	0 of 30	[44,51,63,77,80,161]
Beer	0/0/1	0 of 1	[90]
Carrot	3/0/2	0 of 14	[90,99,104,105,156]
Citrus	1/0/0	0 of 10	[124]
Coconut	0/0/1	0 of 1	[38]
Fennel	2/0/0	0 of 5	[99,105]
Fenugreek	2/0/0	0 of 5	[162]
Lamb	2/0/0	0 of 7	[156]
Lentil	0/1/1	0 of 7	[55]
Lettuce	1/0/0	0 of 1	[154]
Lupinflour	0/1/0	0 of 7	[55]
Melon	1/0/1	0 of 18	[99,163]
Oat	0/0/3	0 of 8	[38,45,129]
Onion	1/0/0	0 of 1	[105]
Peach	3/0/2	0 of 101	[99,151]
Plum	1/0/1	0 of 12	[151,160]
Pork	3/1/1	0 of 25	[38,55,77]
Rabbit	1/0/1	0 of 1	[156]
Rice	2/1/2	0 of 11	[24,80,129,156,164]
Rye	1/0/5	0 of 9	[41,63,69,87,129]
Strawberry	1/0/1	0 of 23	[105,151]
Sunflower	1/0/0	0 of 25	[104]
Tomato	5/0/3	0 of 25	[24,38,65,80,99,104,105,165]
Turkey	0/0/0	0 of 1	[69]
Vanilla	0/1/0	0 of 4	[55]
Yeast	0/0/1	0 of 1	[59]
Zucchini	0/0/2	0 of 5	[69,166]
Total	136/25/256	905 of 6497	

The average number of patients demonstrating urticaria upon challenge is 13.9%.

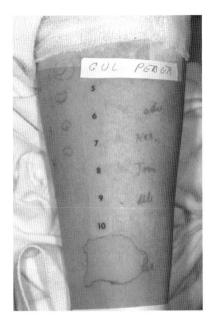

(a)

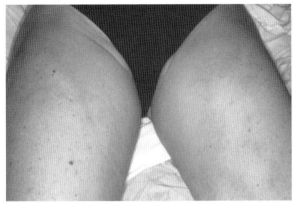

(b)

Figure 10.2 (a) SPT with fresh foods. Wheal elicited by Brazil nut is presented below number 10; it measures 32 × 49 mm. (b) Generalized acute urticaria elicited by SPT in the same patient depicted in (a), 20 minutes after administration of SPT. Note the typical wheal and flare on right thigh and confluent wheals proximally.

According to Greaves [5], food additives are causative in less than 5% of the cases of chronic urticaria seen in his clinic. Therefore, most of the chronic urticarias (and all of the purely physical urticarias) seem not to be associated with hypersensitivity to foods or additives. In a study in children, foods were incriminated in 4% of the cases, whereas additives were thought to be involved in only 2.6% of the cases [167]. In contrast, Henz and Zuberbier [168] believe most chronic urticaria to be food dependent and not idiopathic. On a diet eliminating preservatives, dyes, and natural "pseudo-allergens," 73% of their adult patients experienced remission over a period of 6 months, compared to a 24% spontaneous remission rate. Subsequent double-blind challenges revealed that 18% of the patients reacted to dyes and preservatives, whereas 71% reacted to pureed tomatoes. In a subsequent

study, Zuberbier [169] concluded that low molecular weight substances (salicylate, histamine, aldehydes, and ketones) were responsible for the reactions. Abnormal histamine metabolism has been described in chronic urticaria, but the nature of the abnormality remains to be clearly elucidated [170]. Ehlers [171] reported about the same percentage (75%) of reactors to additives in children.

The discrepancies between the reported incidences are too large to be attributed to differences in patient populations, although at present no epidemiological studies on the actual incidence of urticarias in different populations exist. Differences in patient selection criteria may play a central role.

More well-controlled epidemiological trials focusing on food additives and chronic urticaria are needed to establish their role in the disease. Currently the question is unresolved. Therefore, a diet omitting additives may be worth trying in severe cases of chronic urticaria unresponsive to conventional antihistamine therapy. No data exists on a possible relationship between additive-dependent and autoimmune urticaria.

Although aspirin is degraded to salicylates in plasma and aspirin may augment some food-allergic reactions [172], no conclusive data demonstrating a role for salicylates in adverse reactions to foods exists. Aspirin-intolerant asthmatics tolerate salicylate in high amounts, so at least in these patients, it is not likely that the salicylate component is involved [173].

Treatment

Once the diagnosis of a food-dependent urticaria is established, the only available preventative treatment is avoidance of the food or additive in question. Food-dependent acute urticaria can often be effectively treated with antihistamines, but these drugs should be used with caution in food-allergic patients because they also block the warning signs preceding a systemic reaction. The oral allergy syndrome (OAS), which most often is the initial warning sign, is prevented by prior intake of antihistamines [174] and careful instruction of the patient is necessary.

Conclusions

Acute urticaria is a frequent part of the symptoms and signs elicited in food-allergic patients. Contact urticaria can also be attributed to direct contact with foods, but the distinction between an immunological and a non-immunological contact urticaria is important.

The role of food hypersensitivity in chronic urticarias remains unsettled. In severe cases, a trial diet avoiding additives may be considered; but it is our view that, although we frequently use such a diet in the diagnostic workup in our patients, we rarely see a clear-cut response to an additive-free diet.

References

1 Zuberbier T, Bindslev-Jensen C, Canonica W, *et al.* EAACI/ GA2LEN/EDF guideline: definition, classification and diagnosis of urticaria. *Allergy* 2006;61:316–20.

2 Lahti A. Non-immunologic contact urticaria. *Acta Derm Venereol Suppl (Stockh)* 1980;91:1–49.

3 Muckle TJ, Wells MV. Urticaria, deafness and amyloidosis: a new heredofamilial syndrome. *Q J Med* 1961;50:235–48.

4 Schnitzler I, Schbert B, Boasson I. Urticaire chronique, lesions osseuses, macroglobulinemie IgM: maladie de waldestrom. *Fr Dermatol Syphilol* 1974;81:363.

5 Greaves M. Chronic urticaria. *J Allergy Clin Immunol* 2000;105:664–72.

6 Ying S, Kikuchi Y, Meng Q, *et al.* TH1/TH2 cytokines and inflammatory cells in skin biopsy specimens from patients with chronic idiopathic urticaria: comparison with the allergen-induced late-phase cutaneous reaction. *J Allergy Clin Immunol* 2002;109:694–700.

7 Humphreys F, Hunter JA. The characteristics of urticaria in 390 patients. *Br J Dermatol* 1998;138:635–8.

8 Black AK. Urticarial vasculitis. *Clin Dermatol* 1999;17:565–9.

9 Brockow K, Metcalfe DD. Mastocytosis. *Curr Opin Allergy Clin Immunol* 2001;1:449–54.

10 Champion RH, Roberts SO, Carpenter RG, *et al.* Urticaria and angio-oedema. A review of 554 patients. *Br J Dermatol* 1969;81:588–97.

11 Donaldson VH, Rosen FS. Hereditary angioneurotic edema: a clinical survey. *Pediatrics* 1966;37:1017–27.

12 Petersen LJ. Measurement of histamine release in intact human skin by microdialysis technique. Clinical and experimental findings. *Dan Med Bull* 1998;45:383–401.

13 Mortureux P, Leaute-Labreze C, Legrain-Lifermann V, *et al.* Acute urticaria in infancy and early childhood: a prospective study. *Arch Dermatol* 1998;134:319–23.

14 Bruijnzeel-Koomen C, Ortolani C, Aas K, *et al.* Adverse reactions to food. European Academy of Allergology and Clinical Immunology Subcommittee. *Allergy* 1995;50:623–35.

15 Fuglsang G, Madsen C, Saval P, *et al.* Prevalence of intolerance to food additives among Danish school children. *Pediatr Allergy Immunol* 1993;4:123–9.

16 Fuglsang G, Madsen G, Halken S, *et al.* Adverse reactions to food additives in children with atopic symptoms. *Allergy* 1994;49:31–7.

17 Moneret-Vautrin DA, Kanny G, Morisset M, *et al.* Food anaphylaxis in schools: evaluation of the management plan and the efficiency of the emergency kit. *Allergy* 2001;56:1071–6.

18 von Krogh G, Maibach HI. The contact urticaria syndrome – an updated review. *J Am Acad Dermatol* 1981;5:328–42.

19 Wuthrich B. Food-induced cutaneous adverse reactions. *Allergy* 1998;53:131–5.

20 Halkier-Sorensen L, Heickendorff L, Dalsgaard I, *et al.* Skin symptoms among workers in the fish processing industry are caused by high molecular weight compounds. *Contact Dermatitis* 1991;24:94–100.

21 Baehler P, Chad Z, Gurbindo C, *et al.* Distinct patterns of cow's milk allergy in infancy defined by prolonged, two-stage double-blind, placebo-controlled food challenges. *Clin Exp Allergy* 1996;26:254–61.

22 Hill DJ, Duke AM, Hosking CS, *et al.* Clinical manifestations of cows' milk allergy in childhood. II. The diagnostic value of skin tests and RAST. *Clin Allergy* 1988;18:481–90.

23 Powell GK. Milk- and soy-induced enterocolitis of infancy. Clinical features and standardization of challenge. *J Pediatr* 1978;93:553–60.

24 Pastorello EA, Stocchi L, Pravettoni V, *et al.* Role of the elimination diet in adults with food allergy. *J Allergy Clin Immunol* 1989;84:475–83.

25 Bock SA, Lee WY, Remigio LK, *et al.* Studies of hypersensitivity reactions to foods in infants and children. *J Allergy Clin Immunol* 1978;62:327–34.

26 Host A, Halken S. A prospective study of cow milk allergy in Danish infants during the first 3 years of life. Clinical course in relation to clinical and immunological type of hypersensitivity reaction. *Allergy* 1990;45:587–96.

27 Suomalainen H, Isolauri E, Kaila M, *et al.* Cow's milk provocation induces an immune response to unrelated dietary antigens. *Gut* 1992;33:1179–83.

28 Vanto T, Juntunen-Backman K, Kalimo K, *et al.* The patch test, skin prick test, and serum milk-specific IgE as diagnostic tools in cow's milk allergy in infants. *Allergy* 1999;54:837–42.

29 Bellioni-Businco B, Paganelli R, Lucenti P, *et al.* Allergenicity of goat's milk in children with cow's milk allergy. *J Allergy Clin Immunol* 1999;103:1191–4.

30 Eggesbo M, Botten G, Halvorsen R, *et al.* The prevalence of CMA/CMPI in young children: the validity of parentally perceived reactions in a population-based study. *Allergy* 2001;56:393–402.

31 Sutas Y, Kekki OM, Isolauri E. Late onset reactions to oral food challenge are linked to low serum interleukin-10 concentrations in patients with atopic dermatitis and food allergy. *Clin Exp Allergy* 2000;30:1121–8.

32 Isolauri E, Turjanmaa K. Combined skin prick and patch testing enhances identification of food allergy in infants with atopic dermatitis. *J Allergy Clin Immunol* 1996;97:9–15.

33 May CD. Objective clinical and laboratory studies of immediate hypersensitivity reactions to foods in asthmatic children. *J Allergy Clin Immunol* 1976;58:500–15.

34 Norgaard A, Skov PS, Bindslev-Jensen C. Egg and milk allergy in adults: comparison between fresh foods and commercial allergen extracts in skin prick test and histamine release from basophils. *Clin Exp Allergy* 1992;22:940–7.

35 Van Bever HP, Docx M, Stevens WJ. Food and food additives in severe atopic dermatitis. *Allergy* 1989;44:588–94.

36 Carroccio A, Montalto G, Custro N, *et al.* Evidence of very delayed clinical reactions to cow's milk in cow's milk-intolerant patients. *Allergy* 2000;55:574–9.

37 Iacono G, Cavataio F, Montalto G, *et al.* Intolerance of cow's milk and chronic constipation in children. *N Engl J Med* 1998;339:1100–4.

38 Bernstein M, Day JH, Welsh A. Double-blind food challenge in the diagnosis of food sensitivity in the adult. *J Allergy Clin Immunol* 1982;70:205–10.

39 Roesler TA, Barry PC, Bock SA. Factitious food allergy and failure to thrive. *Arch Pediatr Adolesc Med* 1994;148:1150–5.

40 Gerrard JW. Food intolerance. *Lancet* 1984;2:413.

41 Bengtsson U, Nilsson-Balknas U, Hanson LA, *et al.* Double blind, placebo controlled food reactions do not correlate to IgE allergy in the diagnosis of staple food related gastrointestinal symptoms. *Gut* 1996;39:130–5.

42 Caffarelli C, Romanini E, Caruana P, *et al.* Clinical food hypersensitivity: the relevance of duodenal immunoglobulin E-positive cells. *Pediatr Res* 1998;44:485–90.

43 Chandra RK. Five-year follow-up of high-risk infants with family history of allergy who were exclusively breast-fed or fed partial whey hydrolysate, soy, and conventional cow's milk formulas. *J Pediatr Gastroenterol Nutr* 1997;24:380–8.

44 Burks AW, James JM, Hiegel A, *et al.* Atopic dermatitis and food hypersensitivity reactions. *J Pediatr* 1998;132:132–6.

45 Eigenmann PA, Calza AM. Diagnosis of IgE-mediated food allergy among Swiss children with atopic dermatitis. *Pediatr Allergy Immunol* 2000;11:95–100.

46 Niggemann B, Sielaff B, Beyer K, *et al.* Outcome of double-blind, placebo-controlled food challenge tests in 107 children with atopic dermatitis. *Clin Exp Allergy* 1999;29:91–6.

47 James JM, Eigenmann PA, Eggleston PA, Sampson HA. Airway reactivity changes in asthmatic patients undergoing blinded food challenges. *Am J Respir Crit Care Med* 1996;153:597–603.

48 Sampson HA, Albergo R. Comparison of results of skin tests, RAST, and double-blind, placebo-controlled food challenges in children with atopic dermatitis. *J Allergy Clin Immunol* 1984;74:26–33.

49 James JM, Bernhisel-Broadbent J, Sampson HA. Respiratory reactions provoked by double-blind food challenges in children. *Am J Respir Crit Care Med* 1994;149:59–64.

50 Sampson HA, Ho DG. Relationship between food-specific IgE concentrations and the risk of positive food challenges in children and adolescents. *J Allergy Clin Immunol* 1997;100:444–51.

51 Sampson HA, McCaskill CC. Food hypersensitivity and atopic dermatitis: evaluation of 113 patients. *J Pediatr* 1985;107:669–75.

52 James JM, Sampson HA. Immunologic changes associated with the development of tolerance in children with cow milk allergy. *J Pediatr* 1992;121:371–7.

53 Yazicioglu M, Baspinar I, Ones U, *et al.* Egg and milk allergy in asthmatic children: assessment by immulite allergy food panel, skin prick tests and double-blind placebo-controlled food challenges. *Allergol Immunopathol (Madr)* 1999;27:287–93.

54 Jakobsson I, Lindberg T. A prospective study of cow's milk protein intolerance in Swedish infants. *Acta Paediatr Scand* 1979;68:853–9.

55 Rance F, Kanny G, Dutau G, Moneret-Vautrin DA. Food hypersensitivity in children: clinical aspects and distribution of allergens. *Pediatr Allergy Immunol* 1999;10:33–8.

56 Ragno V, Giampietro PG, Bruno G, Businco L. Allergenicity of milk protein hydrolysate formulae in children with cow's milk allergy. *Eur J Pediatr* 1993;152:760–2.

57 Niggemann B, Beyer K, Wahn U. The role of eosinophils and eosinophil cationic protein in monitoring oral challenge tests in children with food-sensitive atopic dermatitis. *J Allergy Clin Immunol* 1994;94:963–71.

58 Beyer K, Renz H, Wahn U, Niggemann B. Changes in blood leukocyte distribution during double-blind, placebo-controlled food challenges in children with atopic dermatitis and suspected food allergy. *Int Arch Allergy Immunol* 1998;116:110–15.

59 Bentley SJ, Pearson DJ, Rix KJ. Food hypersensitivity in irritable bowel syndrome. *Lancet* 1983;2:295–7.

60 Baker JC, Duncanson RC, Tunnicliffe WS, Ayres JG. Development of a standardized methodology for double-blind, placebo-controlled food challenge in patients with brittle asthma and perceived food intolerance. *J Am Diet Assoc* 2000;100:1361–7.

61 Vatn MH, Grimstad IA, Thorsen L, *et al.* Adverse reaction to food: assessment by double-blind placebo-controlled food challenge and clinical, psychosomatic and immunologic analysis. *Digestion* 1995;56:421–8.

62 Bock SA. Prospective appraisal of complaints of adverse reactions to foods in children during the first 3 years of life. *Pediatrics* 1987;79:683–8.

63 Sampson HA, Jolie PL. Increased plasma histamine concentrations after food challenges in children with atopic dermatitis. *N Engl J Med* 1984;311(6):372–6.

64 Sampson HA. Role of immediate food hypersensitivity in the pathogenesis of atopic dermatitis. *J Allergy Clin Immunol* 1983;71(5):473–80.

65 Sloper KS, Wadsworth J, Brostoff J. Children with atopic eczema. I: clinical response to food elimination and subsequent double-blind food challenge. *Q J Med* 1991;80(292):677–93.

66 Roehr CC, Reibel S, Ziegert M, *et al.* Atopy patch tests, together with determination of specific IgE levels, reduce the need for oral food challenges in children with atopic dermatitis. *J Allergy Clin Immunol* 2001;107:548–53.

67 Niggemann B, Reibel S, Wahn U. The atopy patch test (APT) – a useful tool for the diagnosis of food allergy in children with atopic dermatitis. *Allergy* 2000;55:281–5.

68 Schrander JJ, van den Bogart JP, Forget PP, *et al.* Cow's milk protein intolerance in infants under 1 year of age: a prospective epidemiological study. *Eur J Pediatr* 1993;152:640–4.

69 Bock SA, Atkins FM. Patterns of food hypersensitivity during sixteen years of double-blind, placebo-controlled food challenges. *J Pediatr* 1990;117:561–7.

70 Nsouli TM, Nsouli SM, Linde RE, *et al.* Role of food allergy in serous otitis media. *Ann Allergy* 1994;73:215–19.

71 Sporik R, Hill DJ, Hosking CS. Specificity of allergen skin testing in predicting positive open food challenges to milk, egg and peanut in children. *Clin Exp Allergy* 2000;30:1540–6.

72 Onorato J, Merland N, Terral C, *et al*. Placebo-controlled double-blind food challenge in asthma. *J Allergy Clin Immunol* 1986;78:1139–46.

73 Burks AW, Williams LW, Casteel HB, *et al*. Antibody response to milk proteins in patients with milk-protein intolerance documented by challenge. *J Allergy Clin Immunol* 1990;85:921–7.

74 Cavataio F, Iacono G, Montalto G, *et al*. Gastroesophageal reflux associated with cow's milk allergy in infants: Which diagnostic examinations are useful? *Am J Gastroenterol* 1996;91:1215–20.

75 Pelto L, Salminen S, Lilius EM, *et al*. Milk hypersensitivity – key to poorly defined gastrointestinal symptoms in adults. *Allergy* 1998;53:307–10.

76 Burks AW, Mallory SB, Williams LW, Shirrell MA. Atopic dermatitis: clinical relevance of food hypersensitivity reactions. *J Pediatr* 1988;113:447–51.

77 Lee SS, Noh GW, Lee KY. Clinical application of histamine prick test for food challenge in atopic dermatitis. *J Korean Med Sci* 2001;16:276–82.

78 Burks AW, Casteel HB, Fiedorek SC, *et al*. Prospective oral food challenge study of two soybean protein isolates in patients with possible milk or soy protein enterocolitis. *Pediatr Allergy Immunol* 1994;5:40–5.

79 Juto P, Engberg S, Winberg J. Treatment of infantile atopic dermatitis with a strict elimination diet. *Clin Allergy* 1978;8:493–500.

80 Gerrard JW, MacKenzie JW, Goluboff N, *et al*. Cow's milk allergy: prevalence and manifestations in an unselected series of newborns. *Acta Paediatr Scand Suppl* 1973;234:1–21.

81 Patriarca G, Nucera E, Pollastrini E, *et al*. Oral specific desensitization in food-allergic children. *Dig Dis Sci* 2007;52:1662–1672.

82 Martorell A, Plaza AM, Bone J, *et al*. Cow's milk protein allergy. A multi-centre study: clinical and epidemiological aspects. *Allergol Immunopathol (Madr)* 2006;34:46–53.

83 Osterballe M, Hansen TK, Mortz CG, *et al*. The prevalence of food hypersensitivity in an unselected population of children and adults. *Pediatr Allergy Immunol* 2005;16:567–73.

84 Norgaard A, Bindslev-Jensen C. Egg and milk allergy in adults. Diagnosis and characterization. *Allergy* 1992;47:503–9.

85 Eggesbo M, Botten G, Halvorsen R, Magnus P. The prevalence of allergy to egg: a population-based study in young children. *Allergy* 2001;56:403–11.

86 Caffarelli C, Cavagni G, Giordano S, *et al*. Relationship between oral challenges with previously uningested egg and egg-specific IgE antibodies and skin prick tests in infants with food allergy. *J Allergy Clin Immunol* 1995;95:1215–20.

87 Moneret-Vautrin DA, Halpern GM, Brignon JJ, *et al*. Food specific IgE antibodies: a comparative study of AlaSTAT and Pharmacia RAST Phadebas CAP systems in 49 patients with food allergies. *Ann Allergy* 1993;71:107–14.

88 Urisu A, Ando H, Morita Y, *et al*. Allergenic activity of heated and ovomucoid-depleted egg white. *J Allergy Clin Immunol* 1997;100:171–6.

89 Fukutomi O, Kondo N, Agata H, *et al*. Timing of onset of allergic symptoms as a response to a double-blind, placebo-controlled food challenge in patients with food allergy combined with a radioallergosorbent test and the evaluation of proliferative lymphocyte responses. *Int Arch Allergy Immunol* 1994;104:352–7.

90 Atkins FM, Steinberg SS, Metcalfe DD. Evaluation of immediate adverse reactions to foods in adult patients. I. Correlation of demographic, laboratory, and prick skin test data with response to controlled oral food challenge. *J Allergy Clin Immunol* 1985;75:348–55.

91 Lever R, MacDonald C, Waugh P, Aitchison T. Randomised controlled trial of advice on an egg exclusion diet in young children with atopic eczema and sensitivity to eggs. *Pediatr Allergy Immunol* 1998;9:13–19.

92 Bernhisel-Broadbent J, Sampson HA. Cross-allergenicity in the legume botanical family in children with food hypersensitivity. *J Allergy Clin Immunol* 1989;83:435–40.

93 Martin ME, Guthrie LA, Bock SA. Serum complement changes during double-blind food challenges in children with a history of food sensitivity. *Pediatrics* 1984;73:532–7.

94 Buchanan AD, Green TD, Jones SM, *et al*. Egg oral immunotherapy in nonanaphylactic children with egg allergy. *J Allergy Clin Immunol* 2007;119:199–205.

95 Osterballe M, Bindslev-Jensen C. Threshold levels in food challenge and specific IgE in patients with egg allergy: Is there a relationship? *J Allergy Clin Immunol* 2003;112:196–201.

96 Hourihane JO, Kilburn SA, Nordlee JA, *et al*. An evaluation of the sensitivity of subjects with peanut allergy to very low doses of peanut protein: a randomized, double-blind, placebo-controlled food challenge study. *J Allergy Clin Immunol* 1997;100:596–600.

97 Moneret-Vautrin DA, Rance F, Kanny G, *et al*. Food allergy to peanuts in France – evaluation of 142 observations. *Clin Exp Allergy* 1998;28:1113–9.

98 Moneret-Vautrin DA, Hatahet R, Kanny G, Ait-Djafer Z. Allergenic peanut oil in milk formulas. *Lancet* 1991;338:1149.

99 Ortolani C, Ispano M, Pastorello EA, *et al*. Comparison of results of skin prick tests (with fresh foods and commercial food extracts) and RAST in 100 patients with oral allergy syndrome. *J Allergy Clin Immunol* 1989;83:683–90.

100 Hourihane JO, Bedwani SJ, Dean TP, Warner JO. Randomised, double blind, crossover challenge study of allergenicity of peanut oils in subjects allergic to peanuts. *BMJ* 1997;314:1084–8.

101 Pucar F, Kagan R, Lim H, Clarke AE. Peanut challenge: a retrospective study of 140 patients. *Clin Exp Allergy* 2001;31:40–6.

102 Baker H, Luyt D, Stern M. Open challenge to nuts in children. *Allergy* 1999;54:79–80.

103 Armstrong D, Rylance G. Definitive diagnosis of nut allergy. *Arch Dis Child* 1999;80:175–7.

104 Kivity S, Dunner K, Marian Y. The pattern of food hypersensitivity in patients with onset after 10 years of age. *Clin Exp Allergy* 1994;24:19–22.

105 Boccafogli A, Vicentini L, Camerani A, *et al*. Adverse food reactions in patients with grass pollen allergic respiratory disease. *Ann Allergy* 1994;73:301–8.

106 Flinterman AE, Pasmans SG, Hoekstra MO, *et al*. Determination of no-observed-adverse-effect levels and eliciting doses in a

representative group of peanut-sensitized children. *J Allergy Clin Immunol* 2006;117:448–54.

107 Veien NK, Hattel T, Justesen O, Norholm A. Oral challenge with food additives. *Contact Dermatitis* 1987;17:100–3.

108 Hannuksela M, Haahtela T. Hypersensitivity reactions to food additives. *Allergy* 1987;42:561–75.

109 Malanin G, Kalimo K. The results of skin testing with food additives and the effect of an elimination diet in chronic and recurrent urticaria and recurrent angioedema. *Clin Exp Allergy* 1989;19:539–43.

110 Moneret-Vautrin DA. Food antigens and additives. *J Allergy Clin Immunol* 1986;78:1039–46.

111 Allen DH, Delohery J, Baker G. Monosodium L-glutamate-induced asthma. *J Allergy Clin Immunol* 1987;80:530–7.

112 Berglund F. Food additives. *Arch Toxicol Suppl* 1978:33–46.

113 Taylor SL, Bush RK, Selner JC, *et al*. Sensitivity to sulfited foods among sulfite-sensitive subjects with asthma. *J Allergy Clin Immunol* 1988;81:1159–67.

114 Ortolani C, Pastorello E, Luraghi MT, *et al*. Diagnosis of intolerance to food additives. *Ann Allergy* 1984;53:587–91.

115 Kanny G, Hatahet R, Moneret-Vautrin DA, *et al*. Allergy and intolerance to flavouring agents in atopic dermatitis in young children. *Allerg Immunol (Paris)* 1994;26:204–10.

116 Wuthrich B, Kagi MK, Hafner J. Disulfite-induced acute intermittent urticaria with vasculitis. *Dermatology* 1993;187:290–2.

117 Wuthrich B. Adverse reactions to food additives. *Ann Allergy* 1993;71:379–84.

118 Nettis E, Colanardi MC, Ferrannini A, Tursi A. Sodium benzoate-induced repeated episodes of acute urticaria/angio-oedema: randomized controlled trial. *Br J Dermatol* 2004;151:898–902.

119 Rance F, Dutau G, Abbal M. Mustard allergy in children. *Allergy* 2000;55:496–500.

120 Figueroa J, Blanco C, Dumpierrez AG, *et al*. Mustard allergy confirmed by double-blind placebo-controlled food challenges: clinical features and cross-reactivity with mugwort pollen and plant-derived foods. *Allergy* 2005;60:48–55.

121 Hansen TK, Bindslev-Jensen C. Codfish allergy in adults. Identification and diagnosis. *Allergy* 1992;47:610–7.

122 Bernhisel-Broadbent J, Scanlon SM, Sampson HA. Fish hypersensitivity. I. *In vitro* and oral challenge results in fish-allergic patients. *J Allergy Clin Immunol* 1992;89:730–7.

123 Helbling A, Haydel RJ, McCants ML, *et al*. Fish allergy: Is cross-reactivity among fish species relevant? Double-blind placebo-controlled food challenge studies of fish allergic adults. *Ann Allergy Asthma Immunol* 1999;83:517–23.

124 Saarinen UM, Kajosaari M. Does dietary elimination in infancy prevent or only postpone a food allergy? A study of fish and citrus allergy in 375 children. *Lancet* 1980;1:166–7.

125 Majamaa H, Moisio P, Holm K, Turjanmaa K. Wheat allergy: diagnostic accuracy of skin prick and patch tests and specific IgE. *Allergy* 1999;54:851–6.

126 Kanny G, Chenuel B, Moneret-Vautrin DA. Chronic urticaria to wheat. *Allergy* 2001;56:356–7.

127 Hanakawa Y, Tohyama M, Shirakata Y, *et al*. Food-dependent exercise-induced anaphylaxis: a case related to the amount of food allergen ingested. *Br J Dermatol* 1998;138:898–900.

128 Gall H, Steinert M, Peter RU. Exercise-induced anaphylaxis to wheat flour. *Allergy* 2000;55:1096–7.

129 Jones SM, Magnolfi CF, Cooke SK, Sampson HA. Immunologic cross-reactivity among cereal grains and grasses in children with food hypersensitivity. *J Allergy Clin Immunol* 1995;96:341–51.

130 Scibilia J, Pastorello EA, Zisa G, *et al*. Wheat allergy: a double-blind, placebo-controlled study in adults. *J Allergy Clin Immunol* 2006;117:433–9.

131 Weichel M, Vergoossen NJ, Bonomi S, *et al*. Screening the allergenic repertoires of wheat and maize with sera from double-blind, placebo-controlled food challenge positive patients. *Allergy* 2006;61:128–35.

132 Jansen JJ, Kardinaal AF, Huijbers G, *et al*. Prevalence of food allergy and intolerance in the adult Dutch population. *J Allergy Clin Immunol* 1994;93:446–56.

133 Osterballe M, Hansen TK, Mortz CG, Bindslev-Jensen C. The clinical relevance of sensitization to pollen-related fruits and vegetables in unselected pollen-sensitized adults. *Allergy* 2005;60:218–25.

134 Lucas JS, Grimshaw KE, Collins K, *et al*. Kiwi fruit is a significant allergen and is associated with differing patterns of reactivity in children and adults. *Clin Exp Allergy* 2004;34:1115–21.

135 Aleman A, Sastre J, Quirce S, *et al*. Allergy to kiwi: a double-blind, placebo-controlled food challenge study in patients from a birch-free area. *J Allergy Clin Immunol* 2004;113:543–50.

136 Pajno GB, Passalacqua G, Magazzu G, *et al*. Anaphylaxis to sesame. *Allergy* 2000;55:199–201.

137 Venter C, Pereira B, Grundy J, *et al*. Prevalence of sensitization reported and objectively assessed food hypersensitivity amongst six-year-old children: a population-based study. *Pediatr Allergy Immunol* 2006;17:356–63.

138 Agne PS, Bidat E, Agne PS, *et al*. Sesame seed allergy in children. *Allerg Immunol (Paris)* 2004;36:300–5.

139 Zeiger RS, Sampson HA, Bock SA, *et al*. Soy allergy in infants and children with IgE-associated cow's milk allergy. *J Pediatr* 1999;134:614–22.

140 Magnolfi CF, Zani G, Lacava L, *et al*. Soy allergy in atopic children. *Ann Allergy Asthma Immunol* 1996;77:197–201.

141 Bardare M, Magnolfi C, Zani G. Soy sensitivity: personal observation on 71 children with food intolerance. *Allerg Immunol (Paris)* 1988;20:63–6.

142 Ortolani C, Ballmer-Weber BK, Hansen KS, *et al*. Hazelnut allergy: a double-blind, placebo-controlled food challenge multicenter study. *J Allergy Clin Immunol* 2000;105:577–81.

143 Martin MF, Lopez CJ, Villas F, *et al*. Exercise-induced anaphylactic reaction to hazelnut. *Allergy* 1994;49:314–6.

144 Wensing M, Penninks A, Hefle SL, *et al*. The range of minimun provoking doses in hazelnut-allergic patients as determined by double-blind placebo-controlled food challenges (DBPCFCs). *Clin Exp Allergy* 2002:1757–62

145 Flinterman AE, Hoekstra MO, Meijer Y, *et al.* Clinical reactivity to hazelnut in children: association with sensitization to birch pollen or nuts? *J Allergy Clin Immunol* 2006;118:1186–9.

146 Rance F, Bidat E, Bourrier T, Sabouraud D. Cashew allergy: observations of 42 children without associated peanut allergy. *Allergy* 2003;58:1311–14.

147 Pastorello EA, Pravettoni V, Farioli L, *et al.* Clinical role of a lipid transfer protein that acts as a new apple-specific allergen. *J Allergy Clin Immunol* 1999;104:1099–106.

148 Asero R. Effects of birch pollen-specific immunotherapy on apple allergy in birch pollen-hypersensitive patients. *Clin Exp Allergy* 1998;28:1368–73.

149 Anibarro B, Dominguez C, Diaz JM, *et al.* Apple-dependent exercise-induced anaphylaxis. *Allergy* 1994;49:481–2.

150 Vieths S, Jankiewicz A, Schoning B, Aulepp H. Apple allergy: the IgE-binding potency of apple strains is related to the occurrence of the 18-kDa allergen. *Allergy* 1994;49:262–71.

151 Rodriguez J, Crespo JF, Lopez-Rubio A, *et al.* Clinical cross-reactivity among foods of the Rosaceae family. *J Allergy Clin Immunol* 2000;106:183–9.

152 Skamstrup HK, Vestergaard H, Stahl SP, *et al.* Double-blind, placebo-controlled food challenge with apple. *Allergy* 2001;56:109–17.

153 Ballmer-Weber BK, Vieths S, Luttkopf D, *et al.* Celery allergy confirmed by double-blind, placebo-controlled food challenge: a clinical study in 32 subjects with a history of adverse reactions to celery root. *J Allergy Clin Immunol* 2000;106:373–8.

154 Franck P, Kanny G, Dousset B, *et al.* Lettuce allergy. *Allergy* 2000;55:201–2.

155 Daul CB, Morgan JE, Hughes J, Lehrer SB. Provocation-challenge studies in shrimp-sensitive individuals. *J Allergy Clin Immunol* 1988;81:1180–6.

156 Devlin J, David TJ, Stanton RH. Elemental diet for refractory atopic eczema. *Arch Dis Child* 1991;66:93–9.

157 Pires G, Pargana E, Loureiro V, *et al.* Allergy to garlic. *Allergy* 2002;57:957–8.

158 Tanaka LG, El-Dahr JM, Lehrer SB. Double-blind, placebo-controlled corn challenge resulting in anaphylaxis. *J Allergy Clin Immunol* 2001;107:744.

159 Green TD, Palmer KP, Burks AW. Delayed anaphylaxis to walnut following epinephrine administration. *J Pediatr* 2006;149:733–4.

160 Pastorello EA, Ortolani C, Farioli L, *et al.* Allergenic cross-reactivity among peach, apricot, plum, and cherry in patients with oral allergy syndrome: an *in vivo* and *in vitro* study. *J Allergy Clin Immunol* 1994;94:699–707.

161 Werfel SJ, Cooke SK, Sampson HA. Clinical reactivity to beef in children allergic to cow's milk. *J Allergy Clin Immunol* 1997;99:293–300.

162 Patil SP, Niphadkar PV, Bapat MM. Allergy to fenugreek (*Trigonella foenum-graecum*). *Ann Allergy Asthma Immunol* 1997;78:297–300.

163 Rodriguez J, Crespo JF, Burks W, *et al.* Randomized, double-blind, crossover challenge study in 53 subjects reporting adverse reactions to melon (*Cucumis melo*). *J Allergy Clin Immunol* 2000;106:968–72.

164 Borchers SD, Li BU, Friedman RA, McClung HJ. Rice-induced anaphylactoid reaction. *J Pediatr Gastroenterol Nutr* 1992;15:321–4.

165 Acciai MC, Brusi C, Francalanci S, *et al.* Skin tests with fresh foods. *Contact Dermatitis* 1991;24:67–8.

166 Reindl J, Anliker MD, Karamloo F, *et al.* Allergy caused by ingestion of zucchini (*Cucurbita pepo*): characterization of allergens and cross-reactivity to pollen and other foods. *J Allergy Clin Immunol* 2000;106:379–85.

167 Volonakis M, Katsarou-Katsari A, Stratigos J. Etiologic factors in childhood chronic urticaria. *Ann Allergy* 1992;69:61–5.

168 Henz BM, Zuberbier T. Most chronic urticaria is food-dependent, and not idiopathic. *Exp Dermatol* 1998;7:139–42.

169 Zuberbier T, Pfrommer C, Specht K, *et al.* Aromatic components of food as novel eliciting factors of pseudoallergic reactions in chronic urticaria. *J Allergy Clin Immunol* 2002;109:343–8.

170 Kanny G, Moneret-Vautrin DA, Schohn H, *et al.* Abnormalities in histamine pharmacodynamics in chronic urticaria. *Clin Exp Allergy* 1993;23:1015–20.

171 Ehlers I, Niggemann B, Binder C, *et al.* Role of nonallergic hypersensitivity reactions in children with chronic urticaria. *Allergy* 1998;53:1074–7.

172 Paul E, Gall HM, Muller I, *et al.* Dramatic augmentation of a food allergy by acetylsalicylic acid. *J Allergy Clin Immunol* 2000;105:844.

173 Dahlen B, Boreus LO, Anderson P, *et al.* Plasma acetylsalicylic acid and salicylic acid levels during aspirin provocation in aspirin-sensitive subjects. *Allergy* 1994;49:43–9.

174 Bindslev-Jensen C, Vibits A, Stahl SP, *et al.* Oral allergy syndrome: the effect of astemizole. *Allergy* 1991;46:610–3.

11

CHAPTER 11
Oral Allergy Syndrome

Julie Wang

KEY CONCEPTS

- Oral allergy syndrome is a subset of plant cross-reactivity syndromes.

- Pollen–fruit syndrome explains the relationship between allergic rhinitis and certain fruit allergies through homologous proteins in the plant kingdom.

- Wide regional variability exists in plant cross-reactivity syndromes.

- The diagnosis of plant cross-reactivity syndrome is currently suboptimal, as *in vivo* and *in vitro* tests are poor predictors of clinical reactivity.

- The management of plant cross-reactivity syndromes currently relies on food avoidance, but may evolve to include immunotherapy in the future.

The first report of hypersensitivity to fruits and vegetables in patients with pollinosis occurred in 1942 when Tuft *et al.* described four individuals with hay fever who experienced localized symptoms with fresh fruits and vegetables [1]. In 1970, the observation that ragweed allergy was commonly associated with allergy to melon and banana was described [2]. Ragweed-allergic patients experienced immediate oral symptoms after eating melons or bananas. There were no reports of anaphylaxis and none of the non-pollinosis patients reported symptoms with these fruits. Soon after, similar associations were reported for birch pollen and apple allergy [3] as well as for celery and mugwort allergy [4]. These pollen–fruit–vegetable associations have similar characteristics of localized oropharyngeal symptoms following the ingestion of fresh plant-derived products.

The term oral allergy syndrome (OAS) has been used to describe such symptoms with ingestion of fresh fruits and vegetables in pollinosis patients. This is an IgE-mediated allergy that is generally due to cross-reacting, homologous proteins found in the food proteins and pollens [5]. Since conserved proteins are widely expressed throughout the plant kingdom, it is not surprising that homologous proteins are being identified in a growing number of plant-derived foods. In fact, cross-reactivities between fruits and vegetables and pollens have been increasingly reported in recent

years, coincident with the increased prevalence of allergic rhinitis. There has been tremendous progress in the characterization of these proteins in the last two decades leading to a better understanding of these cross-reacting allergens.

Epidemiology

OAS is the most common form of food allergy in adults, with more than half of food-allergic individuals reporting oropharyngeal symptoms to fresh fruits and vegetables [6,7]. Recently, a study of an unselected adult population in Denmark revealed that 10% of adults have both allergic rhinitis and OAS [8]. Among individuals with allergic rhinitis, the prevalence of OAS ranges from 30% to 70% depending on location, likely due to differences in pollens and dietary habits [8–10]. Osterballe *et al.* [8] found that a higher probability of clinical allergy to plant-derived foods occurs in individuals who have sensitization to multiple pollens (birch, grass, and/or mugwort). Fewer studies have reported the prevalence of OAS in children. However, it appears relatively common in the pediatric population, with 29% of Italian children with allergic rhinitis to grass reporting food allergy symptoms [11].

In addition to regional variations in prevalence, different foods are responsible for OAS in different locations. In a study of 274 adults in England who were allergic to at least one pollen (birch, grass, and/or mugwort), 34% were sensitive to apple, 25% to potato, 23% to carrot, 23% to celery, 22% to peach, and 16% to melon [9]. In contrast, OAS was most commonly due to hazelnut, kiwi, apple (Golden

Food Allergy: Adverse Reactions to Foods and Food Additives, 4th edition.
Edited by Dean D. Metcalfe, Hugh A. Sampson, and Ronald A. Simon.
© 2008 Blackwell Publishing, ISBN: 978-1-4501-5129-0.

Delicious), and celery root in Italy [8]. Pollen-allergic adults in Sweden most often reported symptoms with hazelnut, apple, tomato, carrot, and peanut [12]. In Spain, peach is the most common fruit which causes allergy [13].

Regional differences also exist in the patterns of associations. Patients with allergy to apple, but not birch, have not been reported in northern and middle Europe, but are usually seen in Spain [14]. In Spain, Rosaceae fruit allergy is instead associated with grass allergy [15]. Different patterns of kiwi allergen recognition are evident in different parts of Europe as well [16]. Kiwi is associated with grass pollen allergy in Italy, but with birch pollen allergy in Spain [11]. New sensitizations have also been reported when people are exposed to new environments. Two patients who tolerated jackfruit in the Philippines, a birch-free environment, reportedly reacted to jackfruit when they were sensitized to birch in Switzerland [17]. This highlights the role of regional exposures on the development of cross-sensitization.

Clinical features

OAS is an IgE-mediated allergy that is generally mild. It is a contact allergy resulting in local symptoms such as lip/mouth pruritus, swelling, hoarseness, papulae, and in rare cases, blisters [14]. The onset of symptoms is rapid, with most symptoms appearing within 5 minutes of exposure to the food [18]. However, symptoms may be delayed, appearing after 30 minutes in 7% of cases [18]. The degree of clinical reactivity has seasonal variations; birch pollen-allergic individuals were shown to have higher symptom scores to apple during the birch pollen season [19]. This may be due to upregulation of birch pollen allergens (Bet v 1 and 2) in pollen during maturation [20].

Symptoms can occur outside the oropharynx as well (Table 11.1). In a study of 706 patients with plant food allergy, 13.6% had extra-oral gastrointestinal symptoms, 13.9% reported laryngeal edema, and 2.1% of individuals experienced

Table 11.1 Symptoms of pollen–food syndrome

Oropharyngeal
Lip/mouth swelling
Lip/mouth pruritus
Hoarseness
Papulae
Laryngeal edema

Systemic
Cutaneous – urticaria/angioedema, atopic dermatitis flare
Rhinitis
Conjunctivitis
Wheezing
Gastrointestinal symptoms – abdominal pain/cramps, nausea, vomiting, diarrhea
Anaphylaxis

anaphylaxis [21]. However, only 71% of these patients had evidence of allergic rhinitis, as this study selected for patients with plant food allergy, not OAS. Since symptoms can extend beyond the oropharyngeal area and symptoms are elicited from cross-reactive proteins between pollens and foods, the more inclusive term pollen–food syndrome (PFS) may be more appropriate.

Molecular basis/pathogenesis

IgE-mediated food allergies can be classified according to the route of sensitization [22]. Class I allergy is due to sensitization via the gastrointestinal tract, whereas class II allergy indicates that the primary allergic sensitization is to inhalant allergens. Class I allergy often presents in childhood, while class II allergy is more commonly observed in adults. Complete food allergens, which have the ability to both sensitize and elicit symptoms, induce class I allergy. In contrast, class II allergy is a result of incomplete food allergens, which cannot cause sensitization, but can elicit symptoms because of cross-reactivity to the homologous sensitizer [23]. PFS is classified as class II allergy, since the pollen allergens are the sensitizers and homologous proteins in plant-derived foods elicit symptoms. These food allergens are generally heat labile and susceptible to gastric digestion, thus inducing symptoms limited to the oropharynx.

There are several hypotheses explaining the localized symptoms present in PFS. Amlot *et al.* proposed that the local oral symptoms occur because there is a high concentration of mast cells in oropharyngeal mucosa [5]. Local symptoms may also be due to a high concentration of allergens in the oral mucosa that are rapidly released when in contact with saliva [14]. Alternatively, high concentrations of T-cells in the oropharyngeal lymphoid tissue can have food-specific T-cell responses since cross-reactivity has been found at the T-cell level [24,25].

Allergens

A variety of plant proteins have been identified to play a role in food allergy. These include pathogenesis-related (PR) proteins, proteinase and α-amylase inhibitors, peroxidases, profilins, seed storage proteins, thiol proteases, and lectins [26]. Many of these are distributed throughout the plant kingdom, accounting for the extensive IgE cross-reactivity between taxonomically unrelated plant foods.

Several plant allergens belong to the PR protein family. These are plant defense proteins that are expressed in response to stress from the environment, chemicals, or infection [27]. IgE to the major birch pollen, Bet v 1, cross-reacts with homologous plant food allergens belonging to the PR-10 protein family. Symptoms are often mild, due to the heat liability of these Bet v 1-related proteins [28,29]. The most common fruits causing symptoms in Bet v 1-allergic individuals include members of the order Rosaceae, such as apple, pear, cherry, and apricot (Table 11.2). Homologous proteins are also found in celery, carrot, hazelnut, soy, and peanut.

Profilin is another family of allergens involved in many cross-reactivities between pollens and plant foods (Table 11.2) [22]. They are small (12–15 kDa) proteins that bind actin and have an important role regulating the cytoskeleton. Profilins also are sensitive to heat and gastric digestion [30]. The first profilin identified was a minor birch pollen protein, Bet v 2 [31]. Patients with pollinosis and plant food allergy have a high frequency of IgE reactivity to Bet v 2. Patients sensitized to Bet v 2 also had reactivity to latex, grass, olive tree, and mugwort pollens, suggesting that reactivity to Bet v 2 may be a marker for broad aeroallergen sensitization [32]. Wensing *et al.* [33] similarly reported that profilin is responsible for a broader spectrum of cross-reactivity than Bet v 1. The authors found that those sensitized to both Bet v 1 and profilin had significantly more

Table 11.2 List of allergens mentioned in this chapter (scientific names in parenthesis)

Bet v 1 homologs
Apple (Mal d 1)
Apricot (Pru ar 1)
Carrot (Dau c 1)
Celery (Api g 1)
Cherry (Pru av 1)
Hazelnut (Cor a 1.04)
Jackfruit (Art i)
Peanut (Ara h 8)
Pear (Pyr c 1)
Soy (Gly m 4) (starvation-associated message 22)
Strawberry (Fra a 1)

Profilin
Almond (Pru du 4)
Apple (Mal d 4)
Banana (Mus xp 1)
Bell pepper (Cap a 2)
Birch (Bet v 2)
Carrot (Dau c 4)
Celery (Api g 4)
Hazelnut (Cor a 2)
Latex (Hev b 8)
Melon (Cuc m 2)
Mugwort (Art v 4)
Peach (Pru p 4)
Ragweed (Amb a 8)
Soy (Gly m 3)
Strawberry (Fra a 4)
Timothy grass (Phl p 12)
Tomato (Lyc e 1)

Adapted from the International Union of Immunological Societies (IUIS) List of Allergens. A complete list can be found at www.allergen.org.

specific IgE to foods than those sensitized only to Bet v 1. However, this broad sensitization was not always correlated with clinical reactivity. Therefore, the clinical role for profilin remains unclear, since sensitization to profilin is rarely associated with clinical symptoms [34].

A group of high molecular weight allergens (45–60 kDa) has recently been identified in various pollen and foods [35]. These are highly cross-reactive IgE-binding structures, and have been named cross-reactive carbohydrate determinants (CCDs) [35]. They are ubiquitous in pollen and plant-derived foods and have also been identified in hymenoptera venom [35]. Thirty to forty percent of pollen-allergic individuals have evidence of IgE against CCDs. CCDs exhibit broad *in vitro* cross-reactivity [36] and are heat stable [37]. Their immunological activity was demonstrated by Foetisch *et al.* [38] who showed that the tomato glycoprotein, β-fructofuranosidase, could induce histamine release when basophils were sensitized by serum from tomato-allergic patients. However, the role of CCDs in PFS remains uncertain as the *in vivo* relevance has not been demonstrated.

Pollen–food syndromes

Birch–fruit–vegetable syndrome

Foods belonging to the order Rosaceae, which include apple, pear, peach, and almond, most commonly cause symptoms in birch-allergic patients. Bet v 1, the major birch tree allergen, accounts for most of this cross-reactivity [39]. The prevalence birch–fruit syndrome is variable depending on geographic location. A US study reported that 75.9% of birch pollen-allergic patients had clinical symptoms with apple [40]. Lower rates have been reported in Europe, with 34% of birch pollen patients in Denmark reporting symptoms to apple [3], and 9% of birch pollen patients in Italy having symptoms following ingestion of apple [8].

The primary sensitization in birch–fruit syndrome is to birch pollen, and the symptoms elicited by foods is a secondary phenomenon [20]. A Bet v 1 homolog was identified in apple in 1991 (Mal d 1) [40]. Other Bet v 1 homologs have subsequently been identified in various fruits and vegetables, including celery, pear, carrot, apricot, cherry, and hazelnut (Table 11.2) [26]. There is a high degree of homology between Bet v 1 and the plant food allergens. Bet v 1 and Mal d 1 share 64.5% sequence homology [14], and Cor a 1 (hazelnut) is 72% homologous with Bet v 1 [28]. Bet v 1-related proteins have also been identified in peanut [29] and soy [41].

Celery–birch–mugwort–spice syndrome

Celery has been found to have cross-reactivity with both birch and mugwort pollens. In areas where birch trees are prevalent, celery allergy is due to Bet v 1 homologs. However, celery allergy does exist in birch-free areas; in these cases, mugwort pollen allergens may be the primary sensitizer [22]. Wuthrich *et al.* [42] reported that patients with celery–birch allergy had negative or low specific IgE to cooked and uncooked celery. In contrast, patients with celery–mugwort association had positive IgE to cooked and uncooked celery, suggesting that different allergens are involved in these two associations. Similarly, Hoffmann-Sommergruber *et al.* [43] examined two groups of celery-allergic individuals from two different geographic locations, one from Switzerland (birch trees present) and one from southern France (birch free). The authors found that in Switzerland, all the patients had positive skin testing to birch and commercial celery extract. In contrast, only 25% of patients in southern France had positive skin testing to birch pollen and commercial celery extract, but all had sensitization to mugwort pollen. Immunoblots from these patients revealed IgE against high molecular weight proteins in the range of 28–69 kDa and two had IgE reactivity to a 12–13 kDa protein, suggesting that CCDs and profilin may be playing a role, rather than Bet v 1 homologs.

Bet v 1 and profilins have also been identified in various spices, including anise (Pim a 1 and 2), coriander (Cor s 1 and 2), cumin (Cum c 1 and 2), fennel (Foe v 1 and 2), and parsley (Pet c 1 and 2) [44]. Cross-reactivity between mugwort and mustard has been demonstrated recently [45]. Thus, the term celery–birch–mugwort–spice syndrome has been used to describe these cross-reactivities.

Ragweed–melon–banana association

Up to 50% of ragweed-allergic patients have specific IgE to at least one member of the gourd family (Cucurbitaceae, e.g. watermelon, cantaloupe, honeydew, zucchini, cucumber) [46]. In fact, this association was the first report linking pollen and fruit allergy [2]. Melon allergy occurs mainly in association with pollinosis, even in ragweed-free locations [47].

Profilin has been identified in both melon [22] and banana [48]. Melon profilin is highly susceptible to pepsin digestion [49], and therefore melon allergy usually causes oropharyngeal symptoms. However, one study reported that almost 20% of melon-allergic individuals experienced symptoms outside the mouth [50], and in another study, 11% had anaphylaxis [51], suggesting that other more stable allergens such as lipid-transfer proteins (LTPs) may be involved as well. It has also been reported that pollen-allergic patients with melon allergy have higher rates of asthma than pollen-allergic individuals without melon allergy [50].

Other associations

PFS are becoming more complex as new associations are being described. Additional associations include mugwort–peach association, plantain–melon association, pellitory–pistachio association, goosefoot–fruit association, and Russian thistle–saffron association. With this continually expanding knowledge, allergen-based classification has been proposed as a more appropriate categorization [22].

Other cross-reactivity associations

Latex–fruit syndrome

The first report of an allergic reaction to banana in a latex-allergic patient was published in 1991 [52]. Soon thereafter, cross-reactivity between latex and various fruits was demonstrated, and this was termed latex–fruit syndrome [53]. Significant cross-reactivity between the latex and fruit allergens was demonstrated by Blanco *et al.* [53] who reported that 13 of 25 patients (52%) with latex allergy had specific IgE (prick skin test or *in vitro* test) to fruits. Similar studies have reported up to 88% of latex-allergic adults have evidence of specific IgE to plant-derived foods [54,55]. Although there is a high degree of immunological cross-reactivity between the latex and fruit allergens, the clinical significance appears to be much lower. A study from Germany of 136 latex-allergic patients showed that although 69% had specific IgE to fruits, only 32% had clinical symptoms [56]. Similarly, among melon-allergic patients, 68% had detectable latex-specific IgE, but only 26% were clinically reactive [51].

The primary sensitization is believed to be due to latex, generally via inhalation. In a study of children with atopic dermatitis, all of the children who had latex-specific IgE also had IgE to various foods, mostly potato, tomato, sweet pepper, and avocado [57]. However, none of the children with elevated IgE to avocado, chestnut, and kiwi ever had exposure to these foods.

Several latex allergens have been implicated in the latex–fruit syndrome (Table 11.3). Class I chitinases (Hev b 11) belonging to the PR-3 protein family have been identified in chestnut, avocado, and banana [58]. The *N*-terminal region of Hev b 11 is related to hevein (Hev b 6.02), which is an important latex allergen that has several cross-reactive epitopes.

Table 11.3 Latex allergens involved in latex–fruit syndrome and the plant foods that have homologous proteins

Hev b 2 (β-1,3-glucanase)
Bell pepper

Hev b 11 (class I chitinase)
Avocado (Prs a 1)
Banana
Cherimoya
Chestnut (Cas s 1)
Kiwi
Mango
Papaya
Passion fruit
Tomato

Hev b 8 (profilin)
Banana
Bell pepper
Celery
Pineapple

Low-level inhibition of IgE binding to hevein, a major latex allergen, can be demonstrated with class I chitinases from several fruits [59], suggesting that these two allergens share some IgE-binding epitopes. In fact, Hev b 11 and hevein share 58% sequence identity at the chitin-binding domain [59]. Another major latex allergen, Hev b 2 (β-1,3-glucanase, PR-2 protein family), is also involved in the latex–fruit syndrome and has been identified in bell peppers [60]. Furthermore, Hev b 8 (profilin), a minor latex allergen, has been demonstrated to have cross-reactivity with some fruits [61]. Thus, many latex allergens may contribute to food allergies in latex-sensitive individuals.

Individuals with latex–fruit syndrome can experience more generalized symptoms in addition to oral symptoms, distinguishing this from OAS [62]. These more severe symptoms may be due to the stability of some latex allergens. Hevein has been demonstrated to be stable in simulated gastric fluid [23]. In addition, although class I chitinase in avocado is extensively degraded in simulated gastric fluid, the peptides have been shown to retain their IgE-binding epitopes, and can induce positive skin test results [63].

Differences have been observed between patients allergic to latex (without fruit allergy) and those with allergy to both latex and fruit. Blanco *et al.* [58] showed that chestnut and avocado class I chitinases were able to induce positive prick skin test responses in more than 60% of patients with latex–fruit allergy, but did not result in positive tests in control subjects who were latex, but not fruit allergic. Pooled serum from latex-allergic and not fruit-allergic individuals also do not detect class I chitinases in several fruit extracts [58]. In addition, different human leukocyte antigen (HLA) associations have been identified for those with latex–fruit syndrome as compared to those with only latex allergy, suggesting a genetic basis for the latex–fruit syndrome [64].

Lipid-transfer protein syndrome

Approximately 15–20% of patients with allergies to fruits and/or vegetables have no reported symptoms of allergic rhinitis and negative skin tests to pollens [18,65]. In fact, up to 20% of peach allergy is not associated with pollinosis [13]. Since sensitization is found in patients who do not have pollinosis, this suggests that the primary sensitization in this group may occur via the gastrointestinal tract (class I allergy) [17,66].

Individuals with allergies to plant-derived foods without associated pollinosis were found to have several features distinguishing them from those with OAS-associated pollinosis [15]. In a study comparing the two groups, individuals without pollinosis had significantly more systemic symptoms (82% versus 45%), including anaphylaxis (73% versus 18%) and had fewer oral symptoms (64% versus 91%) when compared to those with pollinosis. Individuals without pollinosis were older at the onset of symptoms to fruits and vegetables (19 years of age versus ~12 years). In addition, those without pollinosis mainly reacted to fruits in the order Rosaceae whereas those with pollinosis had more diverse sensitizations to different families of fruits and had reactions to a greater number of foods in general. Although the non-pollen-allergic group is more likely to have systemic reactions, those with pollinosis appear to have a higher risk of asthma [22].

LTPs, belonging to the PR-14 family [66], have been identified as major allergens involved in non-pollinosis plant food allergies; the term LTP syndrome has since been used to describe these patients. LTPs comprise a family of polypeptides that have the ability to transfer phospholipids from liposomes to mitochondria and are found throughout the plant kingdom [22]. They are defense proteins upregulated by some plants in response to fungal infection [67].

They were first identified as the major allergen in peach as well as an allergen for apple in 1999 [68,69], and have since been discovered in other related foods, including apricot [70], plum [71], and cherry (Table 11.4) [72]. LTPs have also been identified in various unrelated plant products such as corn, asparagus, grape, lettuce, sunflower seeds, latex, and mugwort [17,73].

A recent study reported that apple allergy in Spain (birch-free area) is more severe (>35% systemic reactions) than apple allergy in other locations, and the major allergen in these cases has been identified as Mal d 3, a LTP [74]. The authors proposed that apple allergy in Spain is a result of cross-reactivity with peach proteins rather than with birch pollen proteins because peach is introduced in early childhood in that country and consumed in large quantities. Peach allergy develops at a younger age than apple allergy; therefore, the primary sensitization is likely to peach LTP, Pru p 3. This is consistent with the hypothesis that LTP syndrome is a class I allergy.

The reactions that occur with LTP syndrome are more systemic, and are likely due to the stability of LTPs in acidic and proteolytic conditions of the gastrointestinal tract [75] as well

Table 11.4 LTPs found in plant foods and pollens

Asparagus (Asp a o 1)
Apple (Mal d 3)
Apricot (Pru ar 3)
Cherry (Pru av 3)
Grape (Vit v 1)
Hazelnut (Cor a 8)
Lettuce (Lac s 1)
Maize, corn (Zea m 14)
Mugwort (Art v 3)
Parietaria (Par j 1 and 2)
Peach (Pru p 3)
Strawberry (Fra a 3)
Tomato (Lyc e 3)
Walnut (Jug r 3)

as their resistance to heating [28,37]. For example, celery-allergic patients have been shown to have positive food challenges to cooked celery under double-blind, placebo-controlled conditions [37]. The heat resistance of LTP has also been demonstrated for hazelnut, maize, and cherry [28,66,76]. Thus, commercial foods that have been thermally processed may still cause symptoms in some sensitized individuals.

Recent reports have indicated that LTPs may sensitize via the inhalation route as well, thus suggesting that LTP syndrome may be a class II allergy in some cases. Lombardero *et al.* [77] demonstrated that in some mugwort-allergic individuals, mugwort LTP (Art v 3) is the primary sensitizing agent since these patients were sensitized to Art v 3, but demonstrated no sensitization to Pru p 3 (peach LTP). In a subset of these patients, Art v 3 was able to partially inhibit IgE binding to Pru p 3; however, Pru p 3 was not able to inhibit IgE binding to Art v 3, suggesting that Art v 3 was the primary allergen.

Diagnosis

The primary diagnostic tools for food allergy are prick skin tests and serum-specific IgE levels. However, these tests are not very reliable for the diagnosis of PFS. The results may be variable depending on which food is being tested since there can be a great deal of cross-reactivity between allergens that have common epitopes in different foods.

Skin tests and *in vitro* tests are poor predictors of clinical reactivity. Skin tests rely on extracts that may not contain all of the relevant allergens. Some plant food allergens are heat labile [28,29] and lose potency, and thus sensitivity, during processing of the extracts. Proteases from the fruits themselves can play a role in allergen degradation, as has been demonstrated for pineapple. The pineapple protease bromelain destroys pineapple profilin in extracts prepared without protease inhibitor [61]. In addition, low yield of protein for extracts has been a problem for some exotic fruits [61].

Skin testing with fresh fruits and vegetables is generally a better predictor of clinical reactivity when compared to commercial extracts, but this type of testing is not standardized [78,79]. A study by Anhoej *et al.* [80] showed that the negative predictive value for skin testing with fresh hazelnut, apple, and melon was greater than 90%. The positive predictive value was more variable, ranging from 50% to 85%. Sensitivity was high for all three (89–97%) and the specificities were greater than 70%. Of note, ripeness of the plant food can affect the sensitivity of *in vivo* tests, since allergenicity has been demonstrated to increase with ripening in banana [81] and peach [82]. Additionally, differences in storage and different cultivars (e.g. Golden Delicious apples, Granny Smith apples) can lead to variations in allergenicity [83,84]. Apples in prolonged cold storage under controlled atmosphere conditions are less allergenic than apples stored at 2°C in normal air, and Golden Delicious apples are generally more allergenic than Santana apples [83].

Skin and *in vitro* testing can indicate allergic sensitization, but positive results do not always correlate with clinical reactivity. Therefore, double-blind, placebo-controlled food challenge remains the gold standard for the diagnosis of food allergy. However, there are no standardized protocols for oral food challenges for PFS, and issues such as adequate blinding of fresh foods are a concern.

Management

There are currently no consensus guidelines for the management of PFS. A survey of allergists revealed that there is tremendous variation in management strategies used [85]. These authors suggest that this may be due, in part, to the imprecise definition of PFS and lack of accurate and standardized diagnostic tests.

Recommendations range from avoidance of only the offending fruits or vegetables to eliminating the entire botanical family. Allergy to one food, however, does not necessarily indicate allergy to all members of the botanical family. For example, 63% of peach-allergic individuals react to more than one Prunoideae fruit [86], and 46% have clinical cross-reactivity with other Rosaceae fruits [87]. A study of 65 adults in Madrid with PFS revealed that only 8% of the positive *in vivo* and *in vitro* tests for cross-reacting foods resulted in positive food challenges [88]. This supports the recommendation not to eliminate entire families of cross-reactive foods, which would be unnecessarily restrictive. However, the authors noted that in this series, patients reacted to an additional 18 allergens, which were previously unknown to the patients and were detected only because of further testing and food challenges. Therefore, they suggest that oral challenges be performed to related foods that the patients have not eaten since the most recent allergic reaction in order to rule out other sensitivities to related foods.

Allergenicity can vary between different cultivars of fruits (Table 11.5). For example, Golden Delicious and Gala apples are highly allergenic, whereas Santana apples have been found to have low allergenicity [83]. Therefore, it may be possible that some individuals can tolerate lower allergenic cultivars. In addition, this information may be useful in breeding novel, lower allergenic cultivars. Allergen distribution within the fruit has also been investigated. Mal d 1 (Bet v 1 homolog) is present in both the peel and pulp of

Table 11.5 Allergenicity of different apple cultivars

Golden Delicious, Jonagold, Gala – high allergenic
Elstar, Fuji, Granny Smith – moderate allergenic
Santana, Elize, Braeburn – low allergenic

Ranking from nine Dutch patients (northern Europe) – based on prick–prick testing and double-blind, placebo-controlled food challenges. (Adapted from Bolhaar ST *et al.* [83].)

apples, however, Mal d 3 (LTP) is most abundant in peel. This suggests that some patients may be able to tolerate certain parts of each fruit.

For individuals with PFS due to heat-labile proteins, such as Bet v 1 homologs, cooked versions of the fruits and vegetables can denature the relevant proteins, thus allowing symptom-free consumption. Anecdotal evidence has suggested that briefly heating apples (e.g. by microwaving) may be sufficient to denature Mal d 1 allergens, without compromising the integrity of the fruit, however, this has not been investigated by controlled studies.

Risk factors for systemic reactions to plant-derived foods include a history of systemic reactions to the food, reactions to cooked forms of the food [37,66], positive skin test results to the food extract [89], lack of pollen sensitization [15], and peach allergy/LTP syndrome (Table 11.6) [68]. Therefore, self-injectable epinephrine should be prescribed for such individuals, and patients should be educated on the management of severe reactions.

In addition, physicians should be aware of whether their patients use antihistamines. This may mask mild symptoms, prompting increased consumption of the triggering foods, which may lead to more severe systemic symptoms. This may be a concern for patients who are already taking allergy medications for their allergic rhinitis symptoms [90].

Future directions

More research is needed to characterize the various allergens and clinical cross-reactivity syndromes. An alternative classification of associations based on the major allergens, rather than botanical relationships has been suggested, and this may facilitate the identification of individuals for different forms of therapy [91]. This classification would also encompass the other cross-reactivity syndromes, including latex–fruit allergy and LTP syndrome.

It would also be helpful to understand why individuals are increasingly experiencing these cross-reactivity syndromes. Since many of the allergens are PR proteins and are induced when plants undergo stress, it is possible that pollution and chemicals may be inducing novel proteins (PR family) or upregulating allergenic proteins [62]. Breeding and genetic modification of plants may also lead to the development of novel allergens, potentially contributing to the recent increase in prevalence of affected individuals.

Table 11.6 Risk factors for severe symptoms of cross-reactivity syndromes

- History of systemic reaction to the food.
- Reaction to cooked forms of the food [37,66].
- Positive skin test result to the food extract [89].
- Lack of pollen sensitization [15].
- Peach allergy/LTP syndrome [68].

Immunotherapy

Immunotherapy is an effective treatment for allergic rhinitis. Since pollen–fruit syndrome is, in many cases, due to cross-reactivity with pollens, immunotherapy would seem to be a logical treatment for PFS. A study of birch immunotherapy for apple allergy in adults found a reduction of oral symptoms in 11/14 and decreased skin test sizes in 12/14, but an increase in apple-specific IgE was observed in 6/14 [92]. This study was limited by the self-reported symptoms and lack of placebo controls. Another study of birch subcutaneous immunotherapy (SCIT) found decreased symptoms (based on double-blind, placebo-controlled food challenges) and skin test sizes in the treated group, but there was no placebo SCIT group for comparison [93]. Instead, the comparison was made with a group of patients who used medication for symptomatic treatment. A case report of a patient with improved oral symptoms to fennel, cucumber, and melon after 3.5 years of SCIT with grass, mugwort, and ragweed has also been reported [94].

In contrast, several studies have not shown similar efficacy of immunotherapy for PFS. Bucher et al. [95] placed 15 adults on SCIT for birch to treat PFS to apple and hazelnut. Open challenges were performed before and after SCIT. The authors found limited benefit of immunotherapy with birch for PFS. Similarly, another study found no benefit of subcutaneous and sublingual immunotherapy to birch for PFS to apple [96]. A pediatric study from Sweden indicated no beneficial effect of birch SCIT or oral immunotherapy for food-allergic symptoms [97]. In addition to difficulties in objective evaluations for improvement in symptoms, there is no consensus for target doses and thus immunotherapy remains an unproven therapeutic approach for PFS.

Purified or recombinant allergens

Improved diagnostic tools may facilitate diagnosis and management of PFS. Purified or recombinant allergens are being developed for several foods and have shown potential. Pauli et al. [34] found that individuals with PFS to cherry, apple, or hazelnut reacted to recombinant Bet v 1 (rBet v 1), thus concluding that rBet v 1 is specific for birch and Rosaceae allergy. Mittag et al. [41] showed that 45% of 22 patients with pollen–soy allergy had IgE to soy extract, but 96% were positive to the recombinant allergen, rGly m 4, a Bet v 1-related protein. In a study of peanut and birch-allergic patients, 17 of 20 had specific IgE to recombinant Ara h 8 (Bet v 1 homolog) [29]. Interestingly, six of these did not have detectable IgE to the major peanut allergens, Ara h 1–3. The development of new recombinant allergens may thus help standardize the diagnosis of PFS.

T-cell cross-reactivity

PR-10 proteins have been shown to have cross-reactivity at the T-cell level [24,25]. Reekers et al. [98] reported that some patients with hypersensitivity to birch pollen and atopic dermatitis developed worsening of their eczema after oral challenge with birch pollen-related foods. The authors also found birch pollen-specific T-cell responses in the eczematous skin of these patients. The C-terminal end of Bet v 1 (142–156) has been identified as an immunodominant T-cell epitope in many patients with birch–fruit–vegetable syndrome [99]. Bet v 1 (142–156)-specific T-cell clones cross-reacted with Rosaceae fruit allergens in apple and cherry, but less cross-reactivity occurred with vegetables of the Apiaceae family, celery and carrot. Interestingly, celery and carrot allergens were more potent activators of the T-cell clones than apple and peach allergens.

A recent study showed that in patients who have birch allergy and atopic dermatitis, worsening of skin lesions without oral symptoms can be observed when eating cooked fruits and vegetables (i.e. apple, carrot, and celery) [100]. These authors suggest that eating birch related fruits and vegetables outside the birch season can lead to pollen-specific T-cell activation (high IL-4 and thus elevated IgE) and maintenance of the allergic immune response perennially. This raises the question of whether patients should continue to consume the related plant food products outside of the pollen season despite lack of immediate symptoms.

Conclusions

The term oral allergy syndrome was first coined in 1987 [5], but has since evolved to encompass a larger family of cross-reactivity syndromes, including pollen–fruit syndromes, latex–fruit syndrome, and LTP syndrome. The literature on this topic has suffered from an evolving definition and a lack of reliable diagnostic tools. The common unifier to these cross-reactivity syndromes is the presence of a plant-derived food allergy, which can often be attributed to homologous plant proteins. Cross-reactivity syndromes will pose an ongoing challenge as allergens are continually being identified in plant foods and demonstrate regional variability. Finally, effective treatments have yet to be identified as immunotherapy remain unproven.

References

1 Tuft L, Blumstein GI. Studies in food allergy. II. Sensitization in fresh fruits: clinical and experimental observations. *J Allergy* 1942;13:574–81.

2 Anderson Jr LB, Dreyfuss EM, Logan J, *et al*. Melon and banana sensitivity coincident with ragweed pollinosis. *J Allergy* 1970;45:310–19.

3 Hannuksela M, Lahti A. Immediate reactions to fruits and vegetables. *Contact Dermatitis* 1977;3:79–84.

4 Wuthrich B, Hofer T. Food allergy: the celery–mugwort–spice syndrome. Association with mango allergy? *Dtsch Med Wochenschr* 1984;109:981–6.

5 Amlot PL, Kemeny DM, Zachary C, *et al*. Oral allergy syndrome (OAS): symptoms of IgE-mediated hypersensitivity to foods. *Clin Allergy* 1987;17:33–42.

6 Castillo R, Delgado J, Quiralte J, *et al*. Food hypersensitivity among adult patients: epidemiological and clinical aspects. *Allergol Immunopathol (Madr)* 1996;24:93–7.

7 Mattila L, Kilpelainen M, Terho EO, *et al*. Food hypersensitivity among finnish university students: association with atopic diseases. *Clin Exp Allergy* 2003;33:600–6.

8 Osterballe M, Hansen TK, Mortz CG, Bindslev-Jensen C. The clinical relevance of sensitization to pollen-related fruits and vegetables in unselected pollen-sensitized adults. *Allergy* 2005;60:218–25.

9 Bircher AJ, Van Melle G, Haller E, *et al*. IgE to food allergens are highly prevalent in patients allergic to pollens, with and without symptoms of food allergy. *Clin Exp Allergy* 1994;24: 367–74.

10 Eriksson NE, Formgren H, Svenonius E. Food hypersensitivity in patients with pollen allergy. *Allergy* 1982;37:437–43.

11 Ricci G, Righetti F, Menna G, *et al*. Relationship between bet v 1 and bet v 2 specific IgE and food allergy in children with grass pollen respiratory allergy. *Mol Immunol* 2005;42:1251–7.

12 Ghunaim N, Gronlund H, Kronqvist M, *et al*. Antibody profiles and self-reported symptoms to pollen-related food allergens in grass pollen-allergic patients from northern Europe. *Allergy* 2005;60:185–91.

13 Cuesta-Herranz J, Lazaro M, Martinez A, *et al*. Pollen allergy in peach-allergic patients: sensitization and cross-reactivity to taxonomically unrelated pollens. *J Allergy Clin Immunol* 1999;104:688–94.

14 Pastorello EA, Ortolani C. Oral allergy syndrome. In: Metcalfe DD, Sampson HA, Simon RA (eds.), Food Allergy: Adverse Reactions to Foods and Food Additives 3rd edn. MA: Blackwell Publishing, 2003:169–82.

15 Fernandez-Rivas M, van Ree R, Cuevas M. Allergy to rosaceae fruits without related pollinosis. *J Allergy Clin Immunol* 1997;100:728–33.

16 Bublin M, Mari A, Ebner C, *et al*. IgE sensitization profiles toward green and gold kiwifruits differ among patients allergic to kiwifruit from 3 European countries. *J Allergy Clin Immunol* 2004;114:1169–75.

17 van Ree R. Clinical importance of cross-reactivity in food allergy. *Curr Opin Allergy Clin Immunol* 2004;4:235–40.

18 Ortolani C, Ispano M, Pastorello E, *et al*. The oral allergy syndrome. *Ann Allergy* 1988;61:47–52.

19 Skamstrup Hansen K, Vieths S, Vestergaard H, *et al*. Seasonal variation in food allergy to apple. *J Chromatogr B Biomed Sci Appl* 2001;756:19–32.

20 Valenta R, Kraft D. Type 1 allergic reactions to plant-derived food: a consequence of primary sensitization to pollen allergens. *J Allergy Clin Immunol* 1996;97:893–5.

21 Ortolani C, Pastorello EA, Farioli L, *et al*. IgE-mediated allergy from vegetable allergens. *Ann Allergy* 1993;71:470–6.

22 Egger M, Mutschlechner S, Wopfner N, *et al*. Pollen–food syndromes associated with weed pollinosis: an update from the molecular point of view. *Allergy* 2006;61:461–76.

23 Yagami T, Haishima Y, Nakamura A, *et al*. Digestibility of allergens extracted from natural rubber latex and vegetable foods. *J Allergy Clin Immunol* 2000;106:752–62.

24 Bohle B, Radakovics A, Jahn-Schmid B, *et al*. Bet v 1, the major birch pollen allergen, initiates sensitization to api g 1, the major allergen in celery: evidence at the T cell level. *Eur J Immunol* 2003;33:3303–10.

25 Fritsch R, Bohle B, Vollmann U, *et al*. Bet v 1, the major birch pollen allergen, and mal d 1, the major apple allergen, cross-react at the level of allergen-specific T helper cells. *J Allergy Clin Immunol* 1998;102:679–86.

26 Breiteneder H, Ebner C. Molecular and biochemical classification of plant-derived food allergens. *J Allergy Clin Immunol* 2000;106:27–36.

27 Hoffmann-Sommergruber K. Plant allergens and pathogenesis-related proteins. What do they have in common? *Int Arch Allergy Immunol* 2000;122:155–66.

28 Pastorello EA, Vieths S, Pravettoni V, *et al*. Identification of hazelnut major allergens in sensitive patients with positive double-blind, placebo-controlled food challenge results. *J Allergy Clin Immunol* 2002;109:563–70.

29 Mittag D, Akkerdaas J, Ballmer-Weber BK, *et al*. Ara h 8, a bet v 1-homologous allergen from peanut, is a major allergen in patients with combined birch pollen and peanut allergy. *J Allergy Clin Immunol* 2004;114:1410–17.

30 Breiteneder H, Radauer C. A classification of plant food allergens. *J Allergy Clin Immunol* 2004;113:821–30; quiz 831.

31 Valenta R, Duchene M, Pettenburger K, *et al*. Identification of profilin as a novel pollen allergen; IgE autoreactivity in sensitized individuals. *Science* 1991;253:557–60.

32 Diez-Gomez ML, Quirce S, Cuevas M, *et al*. Fruit–pollen–latex cross-reactivity: implication of profilin (bet v 2). *Allergy* 1999;54:951–61.

33 Wensing M, Akkerdaas JH, van Leeuwen WA, *et al*. IgE to bet v 1 and profilin: cross-reactivity patterns and clinical relevance. *J Allergy Clin Immunol* 2002;110:435–42.

34 Pauli G, Oster JP, Deviller P, *et al*. Skin testing with recombinant allergens rBet v 1 and birch profilin, rBet v 2: diagnostic value for birch pollen and associated allergies. *J Allergy Clin Immunol* 1996;97:1100–9.

35 Ebo DG, Hagendorens MM, Bridts CH, *et al*. Sensitization to cross-reactive carbohydrate determinants and the ubiquitous protein profilin: mimickers of allergy. *Clin Exp Allergy* 2004;34:137–44.

36 Mari A. Multiple pollen sensitization: a molecular approach to the diagnosis. *Int Arch Allergy Immunol* 2001;125:57–65.

37 Ballmer-Weber BK, Hoffmann A, Wuthrich B, *et al*. Influence of food processing on the allergenicity of celery: DBPCFC with celery spice and cooked celery in patients with celery allergy. *Allergy* 2002;57:228–35.

38 Foetisch K, Westphal S, Lauer I, *et al*. Biological activity of IgE specific for cross-reactive carbohydrate determinants. *J Allergy Clin Immunol* 2003;111:889–96.

39 Breiteneder H, Pettenburger K, Bito A, *et al*. The gene coding for the major birch pollen allergen Betv1, is highly homologous to a pea disease resistance response gene. *EMBO J* 1989;8:1935–8.

40 Ebner C, Birkner T, Valenta R, *et al*. Common epitopes of birch pollen and apples – studies by western and northern blot. *J Allergy Clin Immunol* 1991;88:588–94.

41 Mittag D, Vieths S, Vogel L, *et al*. Soybean allergy in patients allergic to birch pollen: clinical investigation and molecular characterization of allergens. *J Allergy Clin Immunol* 2004;113:148–54.

42 Wuthrich B, Stager J, Johansson SG. Celery allergy associated with birch and mugwort pollinosis. *Allergy* 1990;45:566–71.

43 Hoffmann-Sommergruber K, Demoly P, Crameri R, *et al*. IgE reactivity to api g 1, a major celery allergen, in a central european population is based on primary sensitization by bet v 1. *J Allergy Clin Immunol* 1999;104:478–84.

44 Scholl I, Jensen-Jarolim E. Allergenic potency of spices: hot, medium hot, or very hot. *Int Arch Allergy Immunol* 2004;135:247–61.

45 Figueroa J, Blanco C, Dumpierrez AG, *et al*. Mustard allergy confirmed by double-blind placebo-controlled food challenges: clinical features and cross-reactivity with mugwort pollen and plant-derived foods. *Allergy* 2005;60:48–55.

46 Enberg RN, Leickly FE, McCullough J, *et al*. Watermelon and ragweed share allergens. *J Allergy Clin Immunol* 1987;79:867–75.

47 Cuesta-Herranz J, Lazaro M, Figueredo E, *et al*. Allergy to plant-derived fresh foods in a birch- and ragweed-free area. *Clin Exp Allergy* 2000;30:1411–6.

48 Grob M, Reindl J, Vieths S, *et al*. Heterogeneity of banana allergy: characterization of allergens in banana-allergic patients. *Ann Allergy Asthma Immunol* 2002;89:513–6.

49 Rodriguez-Perez R, Crespo JF, Rodriguez J, Salcedo G. Profilin is a relevant melon allergen susceptible to pepsin digestion in patients with oral allergy syndrome. *J Allergy Clin Immunol* 2003;111:634–9.

50 Figueredo E, Cuesta-Herranz J, De-Miguel J, *et al*. Clinical characteristics of melon (cucumis melo) allergy. *Ann Allergy Asthma Immunol* 2003;91:303–8.

51 Rodriguez J, Crespo JF, Burks W, *et al*. Randomized, double-blind, crossover challenge study in 53 subjects reporting adverse reactions to melon (cucumis melo). *J Allergy Clin Immunol* 2000;106:968–72.

52 M'Raihi L, Charpin D, Pons A, *et al*. Cross-reactivity between latex and banana. *J Allergy Clin Immunol* 1991;87:129–30.

53 Blanco C, Carrillo T, Castillo R, *et al*. Latex allergy: clinical features and cross-reactivity with fruits. *Ann Allergy* 1994;73:309–14.

54 Beezhold DH, Sussman GL, Liss GM, Chang NS. Latex allergy can induce clinical reactions to specific foods. *Clin Exp Allergy* 1996;26:416–22.

55 Ebo DG, Bridts CH, Hagendorens MM, *et al*. The prevalence and diagnostic value of specific IgE antibodies to inhalant, animal and plant food, and ficus allergens in patients with natural rubber latex allergy. *Acta Clin Belg* 2003;58:183–9.

56 Brehler R, Theissen U, Mohr C, Luger T. "Latex–fruit syndrome": frequency of cross-reacting IgE antibodies. *Allergy* 1997;52:404–10.

57 Tucke J, Posch A, Baur X, *et al*. Latex type I sensitization and allergy in children with atopic dermatitis. Evaluation of cross-reactivity to some foods. *Pediatr Allergy Immunol* 1999;10:160–7.

58 Blanco C, Diaz-Perales A, Collada C, *et al*. Class I chitinases as potential panallergens involved in the latex–fruit syndrome. *J Allergy Clin Immunol* 1999;103:507–13.

59 Wagner S, Breiteneder H. The latex–fruit syndrome. *Biochem Soc Trans* 2002;30:935–40.

60 Wagner S, Radauer C, Hafner C, *et al*. Characterization of cross-reactive bell pepper allergens involved in the latex–fruit syndrome. *Clin Exp Allergy* 2004;34:1739–46.

61 Reindl J, Rihs HP, Scheurer S, *et al*. IgE reactivity to profilin in pollen-sensitized subjects with adverse reactions to banana and pineapple. *Int Arch Allergy Immunol* 2002;128:105–14.

62 Yagami T. Allergies to cross-reactive plant proteins. Latex–fruit syndrome is comparable with pollen–food allergy syndrome. *Int Arch Allergy Immunol* 2002;128:271–9.

63 Diaz-Perales A, Blanco C, Sanchez-Monge R, *et al*. Analysis of avocado allergen (prs a 1) IgE-binding peptides generated by simulated gastric fluid digestion. *J Allergy Clin Immunol* 2003;112:1002–7.

64 Blanco C, Sanchez-Garcia F, Torres-Galvan MJ, *et al*. Genetic basis of the latex–fruit syndrome: association with HLA class II alleles in a spanish population. *J Allergy Clin Immunol* 2004;114:1070–6.

65 Hernandez J, Garcia Selles FJ, Pagan JA, Negro JM. Immediate hypersensitivity to fruits and vegetables and pollenosis. *Allergol Immunopathol (Madr)* 1985;13:197–211.

66 Pastorello EA, Pompei C, Pravettoni V, *et al*. Lipid-transfer protein is the major maize allergen maintaining IgE-binding activity after cooking at 100 degrees C, as demonstrated in ana-phylactic patients and patients with positive double-blind, pla-cebo-controlled food challenge results. *J Allergy Clin Immunol* 2003;112:775–83.

67 Molina A, Segura A, Garcia-Olmedo F. Lipid transfer pro-teins (nsLTPs) from barley and maize leaves are potent inhibi-tors of bacterial and fungal plant pathogens. *FEBS Lett* 1993 Jan 25;316:119–22.

68 Pastorello EA, Farioli L, Pravettoni V, *et al*. The major allergen of peach (prunus persica) is a lipid transfer protein. *J Allergy Clin Immunol* 1999;103:520–6.

69 Sanchez-Monge R, Lombardero M, Garcia-Selles FJ, *et al*. Lipid-transfer proteins are relevant allergens in fruit allergy. *J Allergy Clin Immunol* 1999;103:514–9.

70 Pastorello EA, D'Ambrosio FP, Pravettoni V, *et al*. Evidence for a lipid transfer protein as the major allergen of apricot. *J Allergy Clin Immunol* 2000;105:371–7.

71 Pastorello EA, Farioli L, Pravettoni V, *et al*. Characterization of the major allergen of plum as a lipid transfer protein. *J Chromatogr B Biomed Sci Appl* 2001;756:95–103.

72 Scheurer S, Pastorello EA, Wangorsch A, *et al*. Recombinant allergens pru av 1 and pru av 4 and a newly identified lipid transfer protein in the *in vitro* diagnosis of cherry allergy. *J Allergy Clin Immunol* 2001;107:724–31.

73 Pastorello EA, Farioli L, Pravettoni V, *et al*. The maize major aller-gen, which is responsible for food-induced allergic reactions, is a lipid transfer protein. *J Allergy Clin Immunol* 2000;106:744–51.

74 Fernandez-Rivas M, Bolhaar S, Gonzalez-Mancebo E, *et al*. Apple allergy across europe: how allergen sensitization profiles determine the clinical expression of allergies to plant foods. *J Allergy Clin Immunol* 2006;118:481–8.

75 Asero R, Mistrello G, Roncarolo D, *et al*. Lipid transfer protein: a pan-allergen in plant-derived foods that is highly resistant to pepsin digestion. *Int Arch Allergy Immunol* 2000;122:20–32.

76 Scheurer S, Lauer I, Foetisch K, *et al*. Strong allergenicity of pru av 3, the lipid transfer protein from cherry, is related to high stability against thermal processing and digestion. *J Allergy Clin Immunol* 2004;114:900–7.

77 Lombardero M, Garcia-Selles FJ, Polo F, *et al*. Prevalence of sen-sitization to artemisia allergens art v 1, art v 3 and art v 60kDa. Cross-reactivity among art v 3 and other relevant lipid-transfer protein allergens. *Clin Exp Allergy* 2004;34:1415–21.

78 Ortolani C, Ispano M, Pastorello EA, *et al*. Comparison of results of skin prick tests (with fresh foods and commercial food extracts) and RAST in 100 patients with oral allergy syndrome. *J Allergy Clin Immunol* 1989;83:683–90.

79 Osterballe M, Scheller R, Stahl Skov P, *et al*. Diagnostic value of scratch-chamber test, skin prick test, histamine release and spe-cific IgE in birch-allergic patients with oral allergy syndrome to apple. *Allergy* 2003;58:950–3.

80 Anhoej C, Backer V, Nolte H. Diagnostic evaluation of grass- and birch-allergic patients with oral allergy syndrome. *Allergy* 2001;56:548–52.

81 Clendennen SK, May GD. Differential gene expression in ripen-ing banana fruit. *Plant Physiol* 1997;115:463–9.

82 Brenna OV, Pastorello EA, Farioli L, *et al*. Presence of aller-genic proteins in different peach (prunus persica) cultivars and dependence of their content on fruit ripening. *J Agric Food Chem* 2004 Dec 29;52:7997–8000.

83 Bolhaar ST, van de Weg WE, van Ree R, *et al*. *In vivo* assessment with prick-to-prick testing and double-blind, placebo-controlled food challenge of allergenicity of apple cultivars. *J Allergy Clin Immunol* 2005;116:1080–6.

84 Carnes J, Ferrer A, Fernandez-Caldas E. Allergenicity of 10 differ-ent apple varieties. *Ann Allergy Asthma Immunol* 2006;96:564–70.

85 Ma S, Sicherer SH, Nowak-Wegrzyn A. A survey on the man-agement of pollen–food allergy syndrome in allergy practices. *J Allergy Clin Immunol* 2003;112:784–8.

86 Pastorello EA, Ortolani C, Farioli L, *et al*. Allergenic cross-reactivity among peach, apricot, plum, and cherry in patients with oral allergy syndrome: an *in vivo* and *in vitro* study. *J Allergy Clin Immunol* 1994;94:699–707.

87 Rodriguez J, Crespo JF, Lopez-Rubio A, *et al*. Clinical cross-reactivity among foods of the rosaceae family. *J Allergy Clin Immunol* 2000;106:183–9.

88 Crespo JF, Rodriguez J, James JM, *et al*. Reactivity to potential cross-reactive foods in fruit-allergic patients: implications for prescribing food avoidance. *Allergy* 2002;57:946–9.

89 Asero R. Detection and clinical characterization of patients with oral allergy syndrome caused by stable allergens in rosaceae and nuts. *Ann Allergy Asthma Immunol* 1999;83:377–83.

90 Mari A, Ballmer-Weber BK, Vieths S. The oral allergy syn-drome: improved diagnostic and treatment methods. *Curr Opin Allergy Clin Immunol* 2005;5:267–73.

91 Mothes N, Horak F, Valenta R. Transition from a botanical to a molecular classification in tree pollen allergy: implications for diagnosis and therapy. *Int Arch Allergy Immunol* 2004; 135:357–73.

92 Asero R. Effects of birch pollen-specific immunotherapy on apple allergy in birch pollen-hypersensitive patients. *Clin Exp Allergy* 1998;28:1368–73.

93 Bolhaar ST, Tiemessen MM, Zuidmeer L, *et al*. Efficacy of birch–pollen immunotherapy on cross-reactive food allergy confirmed by skin tests and double-blind food challenges. *Clin Exp Allergy* 2004;34:761–9.

94 Asero R. Fennel, cucumber, and melon allergy successfully treated with pollen-specific injection immunotherapy. *Ann Allergy Asthma Immunol* 2000;84:460–2.

95 Bucher X, Pichler WJ, Dahinden CA, Helbling A. Effect of tree pollen specific, subcutaneous immunotherapy on the oral allergy syndrome to apple and hazelnut. *Allergy* 2004;59:1272–6.

96 Skamstrup Hansen K, Sondergaard KM, Stahl SP, *et al*. Food allergy to apple and specific immunotherapy with birch pollen. *Mol Nutr Food Res* 2004;48:441–8.

97 Moller C. Effect of pollen immunotherapy on food hypersensitivity in children with birch pollinosis. *Ann Allergy* 1989;62:343–5.

98 Reekers R, Busche M, Wittmann M, *et al*. Birch pollen-related foods trigger atopic dermatitis in patients with specific cutaneous T-cell responses to birch pollen antigens. *J Allergy Clin Immunol* 1999;104:466–72.

99 Jahn-Schmid B, Radakovics A, Luttkopf D, *et al*. Bet v 1 142-156 is the dominant T-cell epitope of the major birch pollen allergen and important for cross-reactivity with bet v 1-related food allergens. *J Allergy Clin Immunol* 2005;116:213–9.

100 Bohle B, Zwolfer B, Heratizadeh A, *et al*. Cooking birch pollen-related food: divergent consequences for IgE- and T cell-mediated reactivity *in vitro* and *in vivo*. *J Allergy Clin Immunol* 2006;118:242–9.

12

CHAPTER 12

The Respiratory Tract and Food Hypersensitivity

Philippe A. Eigenmann and John M. James

KEY CONCEPTS

- The medical history supplemented with appropriate laboratory testing and well-designed food challenges can provide useful information in the workup of patients with respiratory symptoms that may be induced by food allergy. A diagnosis based solely on history, skin testing, or *in vitro* measurements of specific IgE to a given food allergen(s) is not acceptable.

- There continues to be an elevated public perception of food allergy, including an elevated public perception of food allergy-induced asthma and other respiratory disorders. The true prevalence established by standardized challenges is much lower.

- Skin sensitivity to certain food allergens (e.g. hen's egg, cow's milk, or both) in the first several years of life may be predictive of later respiratory allergic disease, including allergic rhinitis and asthma.

- Several recent investigations have highlighted cases of respiratory allergic disease that have been precipitated by the inhalation exposure to airborne food allergens, as opposed to the ingestion of the implicated food allergen.

- If no specific foods are implicated in the history and if skin tests to foods are negative, further workup for IgE-mediated allergy is not generally indicated. If respiratory symptoms persist after food elimination diets are implemented, food is not likely to be the problem, except in some cases of atopic dermatitis or chronic asthma. Respiratory symptoms recurring after a regular diet is resumed should be evaluated with a properly designed food challenge.

- The vital prognosis of food-induced anaphylaxis is determined by respiratory symptoms. Epinephrine can be life-saving and should be made available to patients with asthma and food allergy, and to patients at risk for food-induced respiratory reactions.

Introduction

The skin, with urticaria and atopic dermatitis, is the organ which classically harbors IgE-mediated manifestations of food allergy. However, more recently, food-induced anaphylaxis has received major public and scientific attention. It also has been well established that respiratory manifestations of food-induced anaphylaxis often determine the outcome of the reaction, since the severity of the reaction is mainly determined by upper or lower airway obstruction. Recognizing the severity of a food-induced allergic reaction by assessing the importance of airway involvement has become a major task not only to allergists, but also to primary care physicians. In addition, food-induced allergic reactions are frequently suspected in patients with recurrent

episodic or chronic asthma, or in patients with recurrent upper airway infections. Although few patients with these conditions benefit from a food-exclusion diet, it is a major challenge to properly identify and diagnose the few patients who might suffer from chronic respiratory manifestations. This chapter will review various aspects of respiratory manifestations of food allergy, including the less commonly suspected reactions by inhalation of the offended food.

Epidemiology/etiology

Overview of adverse food reactions

Understanding the terminology and basic classification of adverse food reactions will aid in the interpretation of the scientific studies implicating food hypersensitivity and respiratory tract symptoms [1]. The two broad groups of immune reactions are IgE mediated and non-IgE mediated. The IgE-mediated reactions are usually divided into immediate-onset reactions and immediate plus late-phase reactions (i.e. in

Food Allergy: Adverse Reactions to Foods and Food Additives, 4th edition.
Edited by Dean D. Metcalfe, Hugh A. Sampson, and Ronald A. Simon.
© 2008 Blackwell Publishing, ISBN: 978-1-4501-5129-0.

which the immediate-onset symptoms are followed by pro-longed, in time, or ongoing symptoms). The former have been well characterized in many studies, whereas the latter are under more intense scrutiny to determine their mechanisms and to unravel the role of the immune system. Non-IgE-mediated reactions are typically delayed in onset (i.e. 4–48 hours) and most frequently involve the gastrointestinal tract (Fig 12.1).

Prevalence

While there has been an increase in the prevalence of food allergy and its clinical expression in westernized societies over the past two decades [2], there continues to be an elevated public perception of food allergy, including an elevated public perception of food allergy-induced asthma [3]. These public perceptions, however, have not always been substantiated when careful objective investigations, including food challenges, have been undertaken to confirm patient histories [4,5]. It is generally assumed that questionnaire-based studies vastly overestimate the prevalence of food hypersensitivity. For example, the reported, perceived prevalence of food hypersensitivity varied from 3.24% to 34.9%, which may be explained partly by the difference in reporting lifetime prevalence compared with point prevalence. The high prevalence of pollen-related food allergy in younger adults in the population suggests that the increase in pollen allergy is also being accompanied by an increase in pollen-related food allergy [6]. Adult food allergy has been estimated at approximately 3.2% worldwide. Factors favoring the acquisition of allergy could be sensitization to pollens and occupational sensitization by inhalation [7].

A group of investigators in Denmark evaluated a cohort of 898 patients by questionnaire, skin prick test, histamine release test, and specific IgE followed by oral challenge to the most common allergenic foods. The prevalence of food hypersensitivity confirmed by oral challenge was 2.3% in children 3 years of age, 1% in children older than 3 years of age, and 3.2% in adults. The prevalence of clinical reactions to pollen-related foods in pollen-sensitized adults was estimated to be 32% [8]. Likewise, an investigation in the United Kingdom measured the prevalence of allergic sensitization in a large birth cohort (n = 13,638) and examined the associations between sensitization to different allergens. Seven-year-old children were primarily sensitized to aeroallergens (e.g. grass pollen, dust mites, animal dander), but also to peanut and tree nuts. A relationship was observed between aeroallergen and food-allergen sensitization in these children [9]. Finally, a total of 94 (11.8%) 6-year olds in the Isle of Wight, UK, reported a problem with a food or food ingredient. The rate of sensitization to the predefined panel of food allergens was 25/700 (3.6%). Based on open food challenge and/or suggestive histories and skin tests, the prevalence of food allergy was 2.5% (95% CI: 1.5–3.8). Based on double-blind challenges, a clinical diagnosis or

suggestive history and positive skin tests, the prevalence was 1.6% (95% CI: 0.9–2.7). Milk, egg, and peanut were the key food allergens among those with positive challenges [10].

A few population-based studies have investigated the incidence of food hypersensitivity in the first year of life. One birth cohort (n = 969) was recruited and the investigators examined feeding practices and reported symptoms of allergy at 3, 6, 9, and 12 months. At 1 year, infants underwent a medical examination and skin prick testing to a battery of allergens. Symptomatic infants underwent food challenges. Of these infants, 1% was sensitized to aeroallergens and 2.2% to food allergens. The cumulative incidence of food hypersensitivity by 12 months was 4% on the basis of open food challenges and 3.2% on the basis of double-blind, placebo-controlled food challenges (DBPCFCs). Using this data, the investigators were able to conclude that the rate of parental perception of food hypersensitivity was higher than the prevalence of atopic sensitization to major food allergens or objectively assessed food allergy [11]. In another investigation by the same group, it was determined that 2.3% of both 11- and 15-year-old children had food hypersensitivity as determined by objective assessment including food challenges [12].

When the specific focus has been on the role of food allergy and respiratory tract manifestations, the incidence has been estimated to be between 2% and 8% in children and adults with asthma [13,14]. Children with a family history of atopy and sensitization to food proteins in early infancy are at high risk of subsequent respiratory allergic disease and they may require specific prevention measures [15].

A French population study of food allergy determined the prevalence, clinical features, specific allergens, and risk factors of food allergy [16]. The overall prevalence of food allergy was estimated to be 3.24%. Of the respiratory reactions reported, rhinitis and asthma were documented in 6.5% and 5.7% of cases, respectively. In addition, the clinical expression of food allergy was dependent on the existence of sensitization to pollens and was typically expressed in the form of rhinitis, asthma, and angioedema. A different survey found that 17% of 669 adult respondents in Australia reported food-induced respiratory symptoms [17].

Investigators from the Isle of Wight have reported that egg allergy in infancy predicts respiratory allergic disease by 4 years of age [18]. A cohort of 1218 consecutive births was recruited and followed until 4 years of age. Of these, 29 (2.4%) developed egg allergy by 4 years of age. Increased respiratory allergy (e.g. rhinitis, asthma) was associated with egg allergy (OR: 5.0; 95% CI: 1.1–22.3; p < 0.05) with a positive predictive value of 55%. Furthermore, the addition of the diagnosis of eczema to egg allergy increased the positive predictive value to 80%. The investigators concluded that egg allergy in infancy, especially when associated with eczema, increases respiratory allergic symptoms in

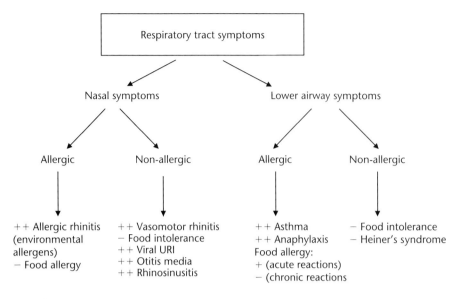

Common : ++
Uncommon : +
Rare : −

Figure 12.1 Respiratory tract symptoms
and food allergy: differential diagnosis.

early childhood. In addition, Rhodes *et al.* conducted a prospective cohort study of subjects at risk of asthma and atopy in England [19]. Of the 100 babies of atopic parents who were recruited at birth, 73 were followed up at 5 years, 67 at 11 years, and 63 at 22 years. Skin sensitivity to hen's egg, cow's milk, or both in the first 5 years of life was predictive of asthma (OR: 10.7; 95% CI: 2.1–55.1; $p = 0.001$; sensitivity 57%; specificity 89%).

Recently, investigators examined the degree of food-allergen sensitization in inner-city patients with asthma included in the National Cooperative Inner City Asthma Study in the United States [20]. The children ranged in age from 4 to 9 years (median age 6 years) and 504 random serum samples were evaluated for specific IgE to six common food allergens (e.g. egg, milk, soy, peanut, wheat, and fish). There was a significant correlation between sensitization to foods and sensitization to aeroallergens, with sensitization to the highest number of aeroallergens correlating with sensitization to soy, wheat, and peanut. Children sensitized to foods had higher rates of asthma hospitalization ($p < 0.01$) and required more steroid medications ($p = 0.25$). In addition, sensitization to foods was correlated with sensitization to more indoor and outdoor aeroallergens ($p < 0.001$). The association of increased asthma morbidity with at least one food sensitization, and findings that patients with sensitization to multiple foods had significantly more asthma morbidity than those with single-food sensitization, suggests that food-allergen sensitivity may be a marker for increased asthma severity.

An investigation by Sicherer and colleagues summarized data from a voluntary registry of 5149 individuals (median age: 5 years) with peanut and/or tree nut allergy [21].

Respiratory reactions, including wheezing, throat tightness, and nasal congestion, were reported in 42% and 56% of respondents as part of their initial reactions to peanuts and tree nuts, respectively. One-half of the reactions involved more than one system and more than 75% of those surveyed required some form of medical treatment. Interestingly, registrants with asthma were significantly more likely than those without asthma to have severe reactions (33% versus 21%; $p < 0.0001$). A more recent, yet related investigation by the same group of investigators estimated the prevalence of seafood allergy in the United States using a nationwide, cross-sectional, random telephone survey and standardized questionnaire. A total of 5529 households completed the survey, representing a census of 14,948 individuals. Fish or shellfish allergy defined by established criteria was reported in 5.9% of households. Recurrent reactions were common. Shortness of breath and throat tightness were reported by more than 50% of those surveyed and 16% were treated with epinephrine. The investigators concluded that physician-diagnosed and/or convincing seafood allergy is reported by 2.3% of the general population, or approximately 6.6 million Americans [22].

Pathogenesis

It has become evident in recent years that the gut, which is the classic site of sensitization to foods, is only responsible for primary sensitization in a subset of the patients. These patients are mainly young children who exhibit the first symptoms shortly after initial feedings with the food. The newly recognized route of sensitization in food allergy is by initial exposure to allergens through inhalation, mostly pollens, with secondary clinical reaction upon ingestion of specific cross-reactive foods. In these patients, many years may elapse before the first respiratory symptoms appear. Pathogenic mechanisms in relation to food allergy due to cross-reacting respiratory allergens will be developed in the corresponding sections.

In food allergy with initial sensitization to foods in the gut, the site of antigen-specific activation for the immune system is believed to be mostly the Peyer's patches [23,24]. The risk that a specific antigen may act as the sensitizing protein is very low. Physical "barriers" such as acidic and proteolytic digestion, the gastrointestinal peristalsis, mucous coating of the epithelium, secretory IgA antibodies, and the epithelial barrier prevent most potentially pathogenic proteins from entering the sub-mucosa of the gut [25,26]. Potential allergens will be taken over by antigen-presenting cells such as dendritic cells of the sub-mucosa, and presented to naive T-cells via their T-cell receptors generating the initial priming of the immune system. In IgE-mediated food allergy, the immune mechanism mostly involved in respiratory reactions to foods, primed allergen-specific CD4+ cells, will facilitate antigen-specific IgE antibodies by plasmocytes. Circulating antigen-specific IgE antibodies will be distributed in the various organs and attached to organ-resident mast cells. Further ingestion of the offending allergen will then directly, by bridging IgE on the Fcε receptor on mast cells, trigger mast cell degranulation and liberation of vasoactive substances such as histamine or tryptase [27].

Unlike in respiratory allergy, most patients with food allergy will experience mostly symptoms in organs distal to the site of primary sensitization, suggesting that a specific tropism of inflammatory cells might favor organ-specific reactions. It has been shown that patients with atopic dermatitis as a symptom of food allergy exhibit a much larger number of circulating antigen-specific cutaneous lymphocyte antigen (CLA)-expressing T-cells than patients with gastrointestinal symptoms [28]. Likewise, patients with immediate-type IgE-mediated food allergy have a high number of the mucosal homing integrin, α4β7 expressing lymphocytes [29]. These observations suggest that memory T-cells could play a role in the preferential localization of allergic reactions. However, it is not clear if homing receptor expressing T-cells favor local IgE production and secondarily mast cells degranulation, or if they may help to prime the allergic reaction. A specific feature of the food-induced respiratory reaction, similarly to atopic dermatitis, is the possibility of the occurrence of a late-phase reaction mostly related to the inflammatory response [30].

Allergens

A short list of specific foods has been implicated in allergic reactions, including cutaneous, gastrointestinal, and respiratory symptoms that have been subsequently confirmed in well-controlled, blinded food challenges [4,31–33]. Anaphylactic reactions to foods including significant respiratory symptoms, and in some cases, fatal and near-fatal anaphylactic reactions have been reported [34–36]. Some food allergens seem to be more prone to present with respiratory tract symptoms. Respiratory reactions, including wheezing, throat tightness, and nasal congestion, were reported in 42% and 56% of respondents as part of their initial reactions to peanuts and tree nuts, respectively [21]. The presence of asthma was a risk factor for these patients to have more severe reactions (33% versus 21%; $p < 0.0001$). Fish or shellfish allergy defined by established criteria was reported in 5.9% of households using a nationwide, cross-sectional, random telephone survey and standardized questionnaire [22]. Respiratory symptoms included shortness of breath and throat tightness and they were reported by more than 50% of those surveyed. Moreover, sesame allergy is a significant, serious, and growing problem. Immediate hypersensitivity, including respiratory symptoms and systemic anaphylaxis, has been observed [37].

Other food allergens have been implicated by the inhalation route as opposed to the ingestion route as a cause for respiratory tract symptoms secondary to food hypersensitivity. Investigations confirming this have included foods including poppy seed [38], carrot [39], sunflower seeds [40], lupine [41,42], asparagus [43], and soybean [44]. For example, asthma attacks and mortality due to inhalation of soybean antigens in Barcelona, Spain, have been well documented. Strict protective measures in the unloading process were established in 1998 to avoid the release of soybean dust into the atmosphere. These measures have reduced the concentration of soybean dust in the atmosphere and have demonstrated the effectiveness of these measures [44].

A high percentage of patients with asthma perceive that food additives contribute to a worsening of their respiratory symptoms [45]. Several different food additives, including monosodium glutamate (MSG), sulfites, and aspartame, have been implicated in adverse respiratory reactions [46]. Well-controlled investigations in this area, however, have reported a prevalence rate of less than 5% [14,31].

There is conflicting evidence that some people with asthma are more likely to have adverse effects from MSG compared to the general population. Woods and co-workers [47] designed a randomized, double-blind, placebo-controlled, MSG challenge protocol for identifying early and late asthmatic reactions. They were unable to demonstrate MSG-induced immediate or late asthmatic reactions in a group of 12 adult asthmatic subjects who perceived that MSG adversely affected their overall asthma control. In addition, these investigators observed no significant changes in bronchial hyperresponsiveness or soluble inflammatory markers (e.g. eosinophil cationic protein, tryptase) during this investigation. In addition, another recent investigation performed double-blind, placebo-controlled oral challenges with MSG in subjects who had histories of adverse reactions [48]. While the participants experienced no specific upper or lower respiratory complaints, 22 (36.1%) of the 61 enrolled subjects had confirmed adverse reactions to MSG including headache, muscle tightness, numbness, general weakness, and flushing.

Routes of exposure and subsequent respiratory symptoms

Oral ingestion of food allergens

Oral ingestion is the primary route of exposure to food that can cause or exacerbate respiratory symptoms (e.g. asthma). The vast majority of published reports, which are highlighted in this chapter, focus on respiratory tract symptoms following the ingestion of food allergens. These reactions will be discussed in more detail throughout this chapter and in other chapters.

Common food allergens implicated in respiratory reactions	
All respiratory reactions	*Near-fatal and fatal anaphylaxis*
Hen's egg	Peanuts
Cow's milk	Tree nuts
Peanut	Shellfish
Fish	
Shellfish	
Tree nuts	

Inhalation of food allergens

As opposed to the oral ingestion of food allergens, several investigations have highlighted cases of respiratory allergic disease that have been precipitated by the inhalation exposure to airborne food allergens. Highly allergic persons may react when exposed to clinically relevant levels of allergenic food in a seafood restaurant, or when fish, shellfish, or eggs are cooked in a confined area [49]. Seafood allergens aerosolized during food preparation are a source of potential respiratory and contact allergens. Shrimp and scallops demonstrate significant cross-reactivity. The primary cross-reactive allergen of these two foods is the 35–39kDa heat-stable allergen, previously demonstrated to be muscle tropomyosin [50]. Another report highlighted allergic reactions associated with airborne fish particles in patients with fish allergy [51]. These investigators evaluated children who reported allergic reactions upon incidental inhalation of fish odors or fumes. By using air sampling and an immunochemical analytic technique, fish allergen was detectable in the air of an open-air fish market. Avoidance of a food allergen, such as fish, should include the prevention of the exposure to aerosolized particles through inhalation in relevant environments [52]. An Internet-based survey of

51 anaphylactic reactions to foods revealed that most reactions (40 (78%)) occurred after ingestion, while eight (16%) reactions occurred after exclusive skin contact and three (6%) after inhalation [53]. Of interest, anaphylaxis after inhalation was graded as severe in three of eight subjects (38%).

Roberts *et al.* recently reported that a group of children with food allergies also developed asthma when exposed to the aerosolized form of the food [54]. Children with IgE-mediated food allergy developed asthma on inhalational exposure to the relevant food allergen while it was being cooked. Subjects were exposed for 20 minutes to the aerosolized form of the allergen and adverse clinical symptoms and lung functions were monitored. Twelve children with food allergy developed asthma on inhalational exposure to relevant food allergens. The implicated foods were fish, chickpea, milk, egg, or buckwheat. Nine of the 12 children consented to undergo a bronchial food challenge. Five challenges were positive with objective clinical features of asthma. In addition, two children developed late-phase symptoms with a decrease in lung function. Positive reactions were seen with fish, chickpea, and buckwheat. There were no reactions to the seven placebo challenges. These data demonstrate that, as in the case of other aeroallergens, inhaled food allergens can produce both early- and late-phase asthmatic responses. The investigators highlighted the importance of considering foods as aeroallergens in children with co-existent food allergy and allergic asthma. For these children, dietary avoidance alone may not be sufficient and further environmental measures may be required to limit exposure to aerosolized food.

Occupational as well as non-occupational exposures to food allergens by the inhalation route have been investigated. For example, a recent investigation from Greece examined the prevalence, work-related symptoms and possible risk factors for IgE-mediated sensitization in seafood-processing workers [55]. Sixty-four fish and seafood-processing workers were compared with 60 controls regarding sensitization to seafood allergens. Twenty-three of 64 workers (35.9%) were sensitive to at least one of the seafood allergens tested, as opposed to 10% of the controls. Presence of atopy ($p = 0.02$) and the intensity ($p = 0.03$) and duration of exposure ($p = 0.03$) were found to be the potential risk factors for sensitization. Four of 64 (6.25%) workers reported work-related symptoms. Therefore, occupational exposure to fish and seafood may increase the likelihood of sensitization to these important allergens, and atopy and the duration and intensity of exposure are the associated risk factors. Moreover, another report focused on three patients who developed asthma and rhinitis caused by exposure to raw, but not cooked, green beans and chards in a non-occupational environment [56]. Minor differences were observed in IgE reactivity between nitrocellulose-blotted raw and boiled green bean extracts. Rhinitis symptoms among bell pepper greenhouse employees can be caused by an allergy to occupational allergens, such as green pepper pollen. Sensitization to bell pepper pollen had a significant negative effect on all the domain and mean quality of life scores tested. Bell pepper greenhouse employees have impaired overall quality of life assessments because of their sensitization to bell pepper pollen [57]. One case report highlighted a 40-year-old female cook who experienced sneezing, rhinorrhea, contact urticaria, and wheezing within a few minutes of handling or cutting raw carrots. IgE sensitization to carrot and an inhalation provocation test while handling carrots were both positive [58]. Finally, another case report implicated lupine inhalation as a provocative trigger for asthma in a child [42].

Allergic sensitizations to other foods have been reported through the inhalation route. A case of oral syndrome after eating sunflower seeds has been reported. Allergic sensitization most likely occurred through inhalant route when these seeds were used to feed birds [40]. In addition, airborne carrot allergens have been implicated in patients with carrot-induced asthma. Airborne carrot allergens were able to sensitize these patients without the implication of a previous birch pollen allergy [39]. Finally, Sicherer and colleagues have reported that patients with peanut allergy might experience adverse respiratory reactions when they are exposed to peanut dust on airline flights serving peanut snacks [59].

Occupational exposures to airborne food allergens can also result in chronic asthma. For example, Baker's asthma is caused by occupational exposure to airborne cereal grain dust [60]. Published data suggest that a significant percentage of bakers develop occupational asthma and chronic obstructive bronchitis. Interestingly, the frequency of a positive methacholine test was 33% in bakers with atopic status, compared to 6.1% ($p < 0.01$) in those without atopic status. In another investigation involving bakers who displayed a positive skin test to wheat flour, a specific bronchial challenge test with flour was positive in two (13.3%) bakers versus none in the bakers with a negative skin test to wheat [61]. Inhalation of dust from different enzymes can be the cause of occupational asthma in exposed workers. One study characterized exposure to inhalation dust, wheat flour, and α-amylase allergens in industrial and traditional bakeries [62]. Furthermore, occupational allergens including wheat and fungal α-amylase can be found in house dust from the homes of bakers and levels are associated with hygienic behavior and distance to the bakery [63].

Bakery workers have been reported to develop IgE-mediated occupational asthma to soybean flour. The allergens involved are predominantly high-molecular-weight proteins that are present in both soybean hull and flour, and they are different from the allergens causing asthma outbreaks, which are mainly low-molecular-weight proteins concentrated in the hull [64]. Sensitization to soybean hull allergens has been reported in subjects from Argentina, a soybean producing country. Specific IgE and IgG4 to an identified soybean hull allergen are common in serum samples from allergic individuals living in rural areas in this country. Sensitization to this allergen is common in subjects who are repeatedly exposed to soybean dust inhalation [64,65]. Furthermore, bakery workers may develop IgE-mediated allergy to liquid and aerosolized hen's egg proteins that are commonly used in the baking and confectionery industries. Four bakery workers were studied who had work-related allergic respiratory symptoms upon exposure to egg aerosols. Specific IgE determinations to egg white were positive in all patients, to lysozyme in two, to ovalbumin in three, to ovomucoid in two, and to egg yolk in two of them. Methacholine inhalation challenges revealed bronchial hyperresponsiveness in all workers. Specific inhalation challenges elicited early asthmatic reactions in all subjects, and DBPCFCs with raw egg white were positive in three subjects. Therefore, these bakery workers had developed IgE-mediated occupational asthma to hen's egg white proteins [66].

Another report highlighted an observation that inhalation of lupine flour may be an important cause of allergic sensitization in exposed workers and may actually give rise to occupational asthma and food allergy [41]. Therefore, lupine seed flour may be a potential sensitizing agent by inhalation in exposed workers and may give rise to occupational asthma and food allergy. Finally, asparagus is a relevant source of occupational allergy. Severe disease (e.g. anaphylaxis or asthma) has been reported [43].

Differential diagnosis of food-induced respiratory syndromes

Many open questions remain when evaluating respiratory manifestations possibly related to foods. Unlike common skin symptoms such as urticaria, respiratory manifestations are typically chronic or may be delayed mostly due to the pattern of inflammatory manifestations of the respiratory tract. This section will review potential manifestations of food allergy in the respiratory tract according to questions most frequently raised by the clinician.

Which respiratory symptoms could be due to food allergy?
Recurrent or chronic rhinitis induced by food allergy

Acute symptoms of rhinitis accounted for 70% of the overall respiratory symptoms observed in a large group of children undergoing DBPCFCs [67]. These symptoms typically occur in association with other clinical manifestations (i.e. cutaneous and/or gastrointestinal symptoms) during allergic reactions to foods, and rarely occur in isolation [31,67]. Chronic or recurrent rhinitis, mostly in pre-school children, is sometimes associated to allergic reactions mostly to milk. While some patients claim of a significant decrease of the symptoms on an avoidance diet, a clear relation has not been reproduced by validated studies. Some patients also link consumption of milk-protein-containing products to increased amounts of secretion of the nose and the upper respiratory tract. Again there is no evidence of an allergy-related mechanism.

Recurrent or chronic otitis media induced by food allergy

Serous otitis media has multiple etiologies, of which the most common is viral upper respiratory tract infections. Allergic inflammation in the nasal mucosa may cause Eustachian tube dysfunction and subsequent otitis media with effusion. The few studies that have investigated an allergic mechanism for the role of food allergy in recurrent serous otitis media are controversial both by the study design and by interpretation of the results [68,69].

Dyspnea associated to anemia in infants

In 1960, Heiner reported a syndrome in infants consisting of recurrent episodes of pneumonia associated with pulmonary infiltrates, hemosiderosis, gastrointestinal blood loss, iron-deficiency anemia, and failure to thrive [70]. This syndrome is most often associated with a non-IgE-mediated hypersensitivity to cow's milk proteins. While increased peripheral blood eosinophils and multiple serum precipitins to cow's milk are commonly observed, the specific immunologic mechanisms responsible for this disorder are not known [71]. The diagnosis is suggested by infiltrates on the chest X-ray, anemia, hemosiderosis evidenced by bronchioalveolar lavages and elimination of the precipitating allergen leading to subsequent resolution of symptoms. The presence of characteristic laboratory data including precipitating antibodies to cow's milk is also considered necessary to make the diagnosis. This food-induced syndrome with respiratory manifestations has not led to any recent publications and is only very rarely observed even in referral clinics for childhood food allergy.

Acute asthma induced by food allergy

The wide use of standardized food challenges has provided a better view of the type and the frequency of respiratory reactions in food allergy. Hill and colleagues challenged 100 milk-allergic patients with a mean age of 16.2 months and elicited cough and/or wheeze in 20 patients, rhinitis in 12 patients, and stridor in 2 patients. Cough and wheezing were more frequent in the groups of patients who initially presented with chronic eczema and recurrent bronchitis, and with urticaria and eczema. Lower respiratory symptoms were only observed in 2 of the 53 patients (4%) with mostly gastrointestinal symptoms [72]. Respiratory reactions induced by food challenges in children with pulmonary disease at National Jewish Center for Immunology and Respiratory Medicine have been reported by Bock [73]. Of

the 410 children with a history of asthma, 279 (68%) had a history of food-induced asthma. There were positive food challenges in 168 (60%) of the 279 patients. This investigation documented that 67 (24%) of the 279 children with a history of food-induced asthma had a positive blinded food challenge that included wheezing. The most common foods that were responsible for these reactions included: peanut 19, cow's milk 18, egg 13, and tree nuts 10. Interestingly, only 5 (2%) of these patients had wheezing as their only objective adverse symptom. In addition, 10 of the group of 188 children without a history of asthma had wheezing elicited by the food challenge, showing a tendency for a bronchial response in the absence of a concomitant asthma.

A total of 320 children predominantly presenting with atopic dermatitis undergoing blinded food challenges at Johns Hopkins Hospital were monitored for respiratory reactions [67]. The patients, aged 6 months to 30 years, were highly atopic, had multiple allergic sensitivities to foods, and over one-half had a prior diagnosis of asthma. In the 205 (64%) patients with food allergy confirmed by blinded challenges, almost two-thirds experienced respiratory reactions during their positive food challenges (e.g. nasal 70%, laryngeal 48%, pulmonary 27%). Overall, 34 (17%) of 205 children with positive food challenges developed wheezing as part of their reaction. Furthermore, 88 of these patients were monitored with pulmonary function testing during positive and negative food challenges. Thirteen (15%) developed lower respiratory symptoms including wheezing in 10 patients, however, only six patients had a >20% decrease in forced expiratory volume in 1 second (FEV1). As documented in the investigations cited earlier, wheezing as the only manifestation of the respiratory reaction was a rare observation.

In 2002, Rancé and Duteau reported a series of 163 children in which 385 DBPCFCs were performed [74]. Overall, 250 (65%) tests were positive to mostly peanuts (31%), hen's egg (23%), and cow's milk (9%). Cutaneous symptoms were observed in most positive challenges (59%), but respiratory reactions were also frequent (24%). Among the respiratory reactions, oral symptoms (5%), rhinitis and conjunctivitis (6%), and asthma (10%) were observed. Again, isolated asthma was rare, as it was documented as the sole manifestation in only 2.8% of the challenges.

If lower respiratory reactions are present in patients without asthma, does food allergy predispose to bronchial hyperreactivity?

It has been observed in patients with atopic dermatitis and food allergy that the food avoidance diet significantly improved their asthma, despite absence of respiratory symptoms during food challenges. This prompted a series of investigation on bronchial hyperreactivity (BHR) in food-allergic patients without overt respiratory symptoms. In one investigation, 26 adolescents and young adults with asthma and food allergy were evaluated using methacholine inhalation challenges for changes in their BHR before and after blinded food challenges [75]. Of the 22 positive blinded food challenges, 12 (55%) involved chest symptoms (cough, laryngeal reactions, and/or wheezing). Another 10 (45%) positive food challenges included laryngeal, gastrointestinal, and/or skin symptoms without any chest symptoms. Significant increases in BHR were documented several hours after positive food challenges in 7 of the 12 (58%) patients who experienced chest symptoms during these challenges. During the actual food challenges decreases in FEV1 were not observed in these seven patients suggesting that significant changes in BHR can occur without demonstrable pulmonary function changes in a preceding food challenge. These data confirmed that food-induced allergic reactions may increase airway reactivity in a subset of patients with moderate to severe asthma, and may do so without inducing acute asthma symptoms.

In contrast, another investigation concluded that food allergy is an unlikely cause of increased airway reactivity [76]. Eleven adults with asthma, a history of food-induced wheezing, and positive prick skin tests to the suspected foods were evaluated. An equal number of patients had increased BHR, as determined by methacholine inhalation challenges, 24 hours after blinded food challenges to either food allergen or placebo. Unfortunately, the small number of patients investigated and the lack of environmental controls prior to the repeat methacholine challenges limit their conclusions. Overall these studies suggest induction of BHR for a limited time (<24 hours) after a single exposure to a food.

Two more recent studies indicate that patients with food allergy in the absence of asthma might have increased BHR. Thaminy *et al.* studied 35 non-asthmatic patients with food allergy, and found BHR by methacholine inhalation challenges in 10 of 19 patients (53%) [77]. Similarly, Kivity *et al.* investigated patients with food allergy with or without asthma and/or allergic rhinitis by spirometry, methacholine challenges, and sputum-induced cell analysis [78]. BHR by methacholine challenge was observed in all patients with asthma, and in 40% of patients with food allergy alone. They also found mainly eosinophils in the sputum of patients with asthma, and neutrophils in the patients with food allergy but no asthma. This observation has been confirmed by other investigators, who in addition to an increased proportion of neutrophils in non-asthmatic food-allergic patients found also increased levels of IL-8 [79].

An animal study came to a similar conclusion, as mice sensitized by intraperitoneal injection of ovalbumin in the presence of alum and then exposed to intratracheal ovalbumin had a significant airway inflammation for up to 12 days after a single intranasal challenge to ovalbumin [80]. Interestingly, an unrelated antigen, house dust mite, induced a similar inflammatory response. Taken together, these observations suggest that food sensitization with non-respiratory manifestations of food allergy might also enhance inflammation

in other mucosal tissues. Hence, non-asthmatic patients diagnosed with food allergy should be carefully evaluated for bronchial inflammation in order not to delay appropriate anti-inflammatory treatment if necessary.

Do respiratory symptoms contribute to the severity of acute allergic reactions to foods?

Until two decades ago, fatal food-induced anaphylaxis had mainly consisted of anecdotal reports of isolated cases. In 1988, Yuninger *et al.* reported a series of seven cases identified over a 16-month period [35]. Five patients reacted to a nut or to peanuts. The authors highlighted the fact that "the majority were highly atopic individuals with histories of asthma, eczema, and/or rhinitis." Only 4 years later, Sampson *et al.* reported on the circumstances of 13 fatal and near-fatal anaphylactic reactions in children and adolescents [34]. Again, most patients reacted to a nut or to peanuts, and all patients had a history of asthma. This report provided additional information on current asthma medication in these patients. Inhaled β-adrenergic drugs were taken by all but one, and most were either on inhaled beclomethasone or cromolyn and/or theophylline. Taken together these reports revealed that chronic bronchial inflammation may have contributed to the acute reaction to the food. Moreover, respiratory symptoms were prominent in all patients, and most probably determined the outcome of the reaction. More recently Bock *et al.* analyzed the circumstances of 32 fatal cases after food-induced anaphylaxis reported to a national registry [81]. Similar results to the two publications described above were reported, as allergies to peanuts and tree nuts elicited most fatalities. In addition, all patients with adequate information but one were known to have asthma. These reports highlight an increased risk for severe food-induced anaphylaxis in patients with asthma, in particular those needing chronic medications. Follow-up visits in these patients should emphasize the importance of a good asthma control plan, and should assure availability and proper instruction of the use of self-injectable epinephrine.

Should patients with recurrent or chronic asthma be routinely tested for food allergy?

Food allergy is often suspected in the quest for allergic triggers of recurrent or chronic asthma. However, a clear link between ingestion of a specific food and worsening of asthma is only exceptionally reported. In one investigation, 300 consecutive patients with asthma (age range: 7 months to 80 years) were evaluated in a pulmonary clinic [14]. Twenty-five (12%) patients had a history of food allergy suggested by clinical symptoms, and/or positive tests of food-specific IgE antibodies. Food-induced wheezing was documented in 6 (2%) of the cases; all were children aged 4–17 years. In another investigation, 140 children, aged

2–9 years, with asthma were screened by clinical history, and testing for food-specific IgE antibodies [82]. Of these children, 32 patients were able to undergo blinded food challenges: 13 (9.2%) had food-induced respiratory symptoms and 8 (5.7%) had specific asthmatic reactions documented during food challenges. Only one patient had asthma as the sole symptom during a positive food challenge. Interestingly, the patients with food allergy and asthma were generally younger and had a past medical history of atopic dermatitis.

Estimated prevalence of food allergy-induced asthmatic reactions	
Clinical population	*Estimated prevalence (%)*
Infants with cow's milk allergy	29
Food-induced wheezing	2–24
Food additive-induced wheezing	<5
Patients with atopic dermatitis	17–27

In a similar investigation, Oehling and co-workers reported that food-induced bronchospasm was present in 8.5% of 284 asthmatic children evaluated [83]. The majority of the allergic sensitization occurred in the first year of life and was caused by a single food, especially egg. In addition, Businco and colleagues evaluated 42 children (age range: 10–76 months) with atopic dermatitis and milk allergy [84]. Eleven (27%) of these patients developed asthmatic symptoms during a positive food challenge. Finally, an investigation from Turkey confirmed that food allergy can elicit asthma in children less than 6 years; the incidence was 4%. The most common food allergens implicated were egg and cow's milk [85].

In order to evaluate food allergy as a risk factor for severe asthma, Roberts and colleagues investigated 19 children with exacerbations of asthma requiring ICU ventilation [86]. When compared to controls, these patients had an increased risk of food allergy (OR: 8.58; 95% CI: 1.85–39.71), multiple allergic diagnoses (OR: 4.42; 95% CI: 1.17–16.71), and frequent asthma admissions (OR: 14.2; 95% CI: 1.77–113.59). The authors concluded that food allergy and frequent asthma admissions appear to be significant, independent risk factors for life-threatening asthmatic events.

A different population, mostly young women with brittle asthma, was investigated for food allergy triggers by Baker *et al.* [87]. They randomized patients into groups with open or blinded food challenges. Challenges were performed with specific foods or a mix of potentially allergenic foods (egg, milk, wheat, fish, orange, peanut, soy) over a 5–9 day period. Peak expiratory flow and FEV1 measures were performed at regular intervals during and after the challenges. More than half of the patients (52–62% according to the groups) had positive tests with significant respiratory reactions. All foods tested elicited reactions: most frequently oranges (20–58%), wheat (33–62%), egg (17–77%), and milk (42–62%).

In summary, these results suggest that respiratory symptoms may be provoked in a subset of patients with asthma. However, the patient group most frequently tested for food allergy, namely pre-school children with BHR, and mostly virus-triggered asthma, is the one least likely to have food allergy as a trigger of asthma.

Evaluation/management

Medical history

A comprehensive medical history should be obtained in patients suspected of having food allergy-induced respiratory tract symptoms or anaphylaxis [49]. The history should include questions about the timing of the reaction in relation to food ingestion, the minimum quantity of food required to cause symptoms, specific upper and lower respiratory signs and symptoms, the reproducibility of the symptoms, and a current or past clinical history of allergy to specific food allergens (e.g. egg). A family history positive for allergy and/or asthma can be a useful historical point. When there is a history of an unexplained sudden asthma exacerbation, details about preceding food ingestion should be elicited. A history of a severe or anaphylactic reaction following the ingestion of a food may be sufficient to indicate a causal relationship. Finally, documentation of the specific treatment received and its response should be compiled.

Physical examination

In evaluating patients with respiratory system complaints that may be induced by food allergy, the physical examination can be useful. Findings here are helpful in assessing overall nutritional status, growth parameters, and any signs of allergic disease, especially atopic dermatitis. Moreover, this examination will help rule out other conditions that may mimic food allergy.

Skin testing for food allergy

When used in conjunction with standard criterion of interpretation, skin testing (e.g. percutaneous) can give reliable clinical information in a short period of time (i.e. 15–20 minutes), and should provide reliable clinical information in the overall workup of a patient with suspected food allergy-induced respiratory tract reactions. The routine use of skin testing to foods in patients presenting with asthma, however, is not practical. Of children evaluated in a tertiary care hospital emergency room, 97 patients with asthma or bronchiolitis were skin tested to common foods and aeroallergens and compared to similar testing in 60 control patients without any respiratory disease [88]. Most specific IgE antibody responses among wheezing children were to aeroallergens; the prevalence of specific IgE antibodies to food allergens was low.

Other testing

Laboratory assessment of food allergy may include the measurement of food-specific IgE in the serum (e.g. IgE RAST, radioallergosorbent testing or quantitative IgE (UniCap; Phadia, Uppsala, Sweden)). When highly sensitive assays are used, the sensitivity is similar to that of skin tests [89–92]. In contrast, basophil histamine release assays, which are mainly limited to research settings, have not been shown conclusively to be a reproducible, diagnostic test for food allergy [93]. The diagnostic values of the following tests are not currently supported by objective scientific evidence: food-specific IgG or IgG subclass antibody concentrations, food antigen–antibody complexes, cytotoxic food tests, and subcutaneous provocation and neutralization [94,95].

Food challenges

When there is a clinical suspicion of a food-induced respiratory tract reaction and the test for specific IgE antibody to the food is positive, an elimination diet may be implemented to see if there is a resolution of clinical symptoms. Confirming this association, however, can be very difficult. Food challenges can be very useful and reliable in the diagnostic evaluation of a patient with food-induced respiratory symptoms. An excellent publication has reviewed the combined clinical experience of six centers conducting food challenges [96]. Of these procedures, the DBPCFC is the best method to diagnose and confirm food allergy and other adverse food reactions. These challenges should be conducted in a clinic or hospital setting with available personnel and equipment for treating systemic anaphylaxis. If the clinical history does not suggest a high risk of a severe reaction, an oral food challenge can be performed in the office setting.

Treatment

Once a food allergy has been confirmed as a cause for respiratory tract symptoms, strict avoidance of the offending food is necessary [31,90,93]. A properly managed elimination diet can lead to resolution of clinical symptoms, such as chronic asthma. Appropriate nutritional counseling is important to ensure that an elimination diet is well balanced, to provide appropriate substitutes for foods that are eliminated from the diet, and to avoid any anticipated nutritional deficiencies, such as calcium deficiency [97–99]. Growth parameters should be closely monitored, especially in infants and children on elimination diets. Woods and co-workers were unable to prove that the ingestion of dairy products induced bronchoconstriction in a group of adults with asthma. They recommended that patients with asthma should not be unnecessarily restricting their dairy product intake, which could lead to the development of nutritional deficiencies [47]. Therefore, restriction diets should exclude only those foods proven to provoke food allergy [31,90].

An emergency plan should be written to help patients manage their clinical symptoms caused by accidental ingestion of a relevant food allergen [34,90,100]. For children, the written plan should be given to the appropriate school personnel. Self-injectable epinephrine and antihistamines must be immediately available to treat allergic reactions after accidental ingestions. Epinephrine is the drug of choice to treat acute, severe reactions and to allow time to seek immediate medical attention.

Summary and conclusions

Previous investigations have clearly established the pathogenic role of food allergy in respiratory tract symptoms in a subset of patients. These symptoms are typically accompanied by skin and gastrointestinal manifestations and rarely occur in isolation. Specific foods have been implicated in these reactions. Allergic sensitization to foods in infancy predicts the later development of respiratory allergies and asthma. The role of food allergy in otitis media is controversial and probably is very rare. Likewise, asthmatic reactions to food additives can occur but are very uncommon. Food-induced asthma is more common in young pediatric patients, especially those with atopic dermatitis, than in adolescents and adults and can be triggered by inhalation of a relevant food allergen. Respiratory symptoms, especially asthma, induced by food allergens are considered risk factors for fatal and near-fatal anaphylactic reactions.

Studies have demonstrated that foods can elicit airway hyperreactivity and asthmatic responses; therefore, evaluation for food allergy should be considered among patients with recalcitrant or otherwise unexplained acute severe asthma exacerbations, asthma triggered following ingestion or inhalation of particular foods, and in patients with asthma and other manifestations of food allergy (e.g. anaphylaxis, moderate to severe atopic dermatitis). Practice parameters for the diagnosis and treatment of asthma have recently highlighted the potential role of food allergy in asthma in some patients [101].

References

1 Bock SA, Sampson HA. Evaluation of food allergy. In: Leung DYM, Sampson HA, Geha RS, Szefler SJ (eds.) *Pediatric Allergy: Principles and Practice*. St. Louis, MO: Mosby, 2003:478–87.

2 Nowak-Wegrzyn A, Sampson HA. Adverse reactions to foods. *Med Clin N Am* 2006;90:97–127.

3 Woods RK, Weiner J, Abramson M, *et al*. Patients' perceptions of food-induced asthma. *Aust N Z J Med* 1996;26:504–12.

4 Bock SA. Prospective appraisal of complaints of adverse reactions to foods in children during the first 3 years of life. *Pediatrics* 1987;79:683–8.

5 Niestijl Jansen JJ, Kardinaal AFM, Huijbers GH, *et al.* Prevalence of food allergy and intolerance in the adult Dutch population. *J Allergy Clin Immunol* 1994;93:446–56.

6 Madsen C. Prevalence of food allergy: an overview. *Proc Nutr Soc* 2005;64:413–17.

7 Moneret-Vautrin DA, Morisset M. Adult food allergy. *Curr Allergy Asthma Rep* 2005;5:80–5.

8 Osterballe M, Hansen TK, Mortz CG, *et al.* The prevalence of food hypersensitivity in an unselected population of children and adults. *Pediatr Allergy Immunol* 2005;16:567–73.

9 Roberts G, Peckitt C, Northstone K, *et al.* Relationship between aeroallergen and food allergen sensitization in childhood. *Clin Exp Allergy* 2005;35:933–40.

10 Venter C, Pereira B, Grundy J, *et al.* Prevalence of sensitization reported and objectively assessed food hypersensitivity amongst six-year-old children: a population-based study. *Pediatr Allergy Immunol* 2006;17:356–63.

11 Venter C, Pereira B, Grundy J, *et al.* Incidence of parentally reported and clinically diagnosed food hypersensitivity in the first year of life. *J Allergy Clin Immunol* 2006;117:1118–24.

12 Pereira B, Venter C, Grundy J, *et al.* Prevalence of sensitization to food allergens, reported adverse reaction to foods, food avoidance, and food hypersensitivity among teenagers. *J Allergy Clin Immunol* 2005;116:884–92.

13 Nekam KL. Nutritional triggers in asthma. *Acta Microbiol Immunol Hung* 1998;45:113–17.

14 Onorato J, Merland N, Terral C, *et al.* Placebo-controlled double-blind food challenge in asthma. *J Allergy Clin Immunol* 1986;78:1139–46.

15 Peroni DG, Chatzimichail A, Boner AL. Food allergy: What can be done to prevent progression to asthma? *Ann Allergy Asthma Immunol* 2002;89:44–51.

16 Kanny G, Moneret-Vautrin DA, Flabbee J, *et al.* Population study of food allergy in France. *J Allergy Clin Immunol* 2001; 108:133–40.

17 Woods RK, Abramson M, Raven JM, *et al.* Reported food intolerance and respiratory symptoms in young adults. *Eur Respir J* 1998;11:151–5.

18 Tariq SM, Matthews SM, Hakim EA, Arshad SH. Egg allergy in infancy predicts respiratory allergic disease by 4 years of age. *Pediatr Allergy Immunol* 2000;11:162–7.

19 Rhodes HL, Sporik R, Thomas P, *et al.* Early life risk factors for adult asthma: a birth cohort study of subjects at risk. *J Allergy Clin Immunol* 2001;108:720–5.

20 Wang J, Visness CM, Sampson HA. Food allergen sensitization in inner-city children with asthma. *J Allergy Clin Immunol* 2005;115:1076–80.

21 Sicherer SH, Furlong TJ, Munoz-Furlong A, *et al.* A voluntary registry for peanut and tree nut allergy: characteristics of the first 5149 registrants. *J Allergy Clin Immunol* 2001;108: 128–32.

22 Sicherer SH, Munoz-Furlong A, Sampson HA. Prevalence of seafood allergy in the United States determined by a random telephone survey. *J Allergy Clin Immunol* 2004;114:159–65.

23 Frossard CP, Tropia L, Hauser C, Eigenmann PA. Lymphocytes in Peyer's patches regulate clinical tolerance in a murine model of food allergy. *J Allergy Clin Immunol* 2004;113:958–64.

24 Chehade M, Mayer L. Oral tolerance and its relation to food hypersensitivities. *J Allergy Clin Immunol* 2005;115:3–12.

25 Poley JR. Loss of the glycocalyx of enterocytes in small intestine: a feature detected by scanning electron microscopy in children with gastrointestinal intolerance to dietary protein. *J Pediatr Gastroenterol Nutr* 1988;7:386–94.

26 Shub MD, Pang KY, Swann DA, Walker WA. Age-related changes in chemical composition and physical properties of mucus glycoproteins from rat small intestine. *Biochem J* 1983;215:405–11.

27 Sampson HA. Food allergy. Part 1. Immunopathogenesis and clinical disorders. *J Allergy Clin Immunol* 1999;103:717–28.

28 Abernathy-Carver KJ, Sampson HA, Picker LJ, Leung DYM. Milk-induced eczema is associated with the expansion of T cells expressing cutaneous lymphocyte antigen. *J Clin Invest* 1995;95:913–18.

29 Eigenmann PA, Tropia L, Hauser C. The mucosal adhesion receptor alpha4beta7 integrin is selectively increased in lymphocytes stimulated with beta-lactoglobulin in children allergic to cow's milk. *J Allergy Clin Immunol* 1999;103:931–6.

30 Adel-Patient K, Nahori MA, Proust B, *et al.* Elicitation of the allergic reaction in beta-lactoglobulin-sensitized Balb/c mice: biochemical and clinical manifestations differ according to the structure of the allergen used for challenge. *Clin Exp Allergy* 2003;33:376–85.

31 Bock SA, Atkins FM. Patterns of food hypersensitivity during sixteen years of double-blind, placebo-controlled food challenges. *J Pediatr* 1990;117:561–7.

32 Burks AW, James JM, Hiegel A, *et al.* Atopic dermatitis and food hypersensitivity reactions. *J Pediatr* 1998;132:132–6.

33 Sampson HA. Food hypersensitivity and atopic dermatitis. *Allergy Proc* 1991;12:327–31.

34 Sampson HA, Mendelson LM, Rosen JP. Fatal and near-fatal anaphylactic reactions to food in children and adolescents. *N Engl J Med* 1992;327:380–4.

35 Yunginger JW, Sweeney KG, Sturner WQ, *et al.* Fatal food-induced anaphylaxis. *JAMA* 1988;260:1450–2.

36 James JM. Anaphylactic reactions to foods. *Immunol Allergy Clin North Am* 2001;21:653–67.

37 Gangur V, Kelly C, Navuluri L. Sesame allergy: A growing food allergy of global proportions? *Ann Allergy Asthma Immunol* 2005;95:4–11.

38 Keskin O, Sekerel BE. Poppy seed allergy: a case report and review of the literature. *Allergy Asthma Proc* 2006;27:396–8.

39 Moreno-Ancillo A, Gil-Adrados AC, Cosmes PM, *et al.* Role of Dau c 1 in three different patterns of carrot-induced asthma. *Allergol Immunopathol (Madr)* 2006;34:116–20.

40 Palma-Carlos AG, Palma-Carlos ML, Tengarrinha F. Allergy to sunflower seeds. *Allerg Immunol (Paris)* 2005;37:183–6.

41 Crespo JF, Rodriguez J, Vives R, *et al.* Occupational IgE-mediated allergy after exposure to lupine seed flour. *J Allergy Clin Immunol* 2001;108:295–7.

42 Moreno-Ancillo A, Gil-Adrados AC, Dominguez-Noche C, Cosmes PM. Lupine inhalation induced asthma in a child. *Pediatr Allergy Immunol* 2005;16:542–4.

43 Tabar AI, Alvarez-Puebla MJ, Gomez B, *et al*. Diversity of asparagus allergy: clinical and immunological features. *Clin Exp Allergy* 2004;34:131–6.

44 Rodrigo MJ, Cruz MJ, Garcia MD, *et al*. Epidemic asthma in Barcelona: an evaluation of new strategies for the control of soybean dust emission. *Int Arch Allergy Immunol* 2004;134:158–64.

45 Abramson MJ, Kutin JJ, Rosier MJ, Bowes G. Morbidity, medication and trigger factors in a community sample of adults with asthma. *Med J Aust* 1995;162:78–81.

46 Weber RW. Food additives and allergy. *Ann Allergy* 1993; 70:183–90.

47 Woods RK, Weiner JM, Abramson M, *et al*. Do dairy products induce bronchoconstriction in adults with asthma? *J Allergy Clin Immunol* 1998;101:45–50.

48 Yang WH, Drouin MA, Herbert M, Mao Y, Karsh J. The monosodium glutamate symptom complex: assessment in a double-blind, placebo-controlled, randomized study. *J Allergy Clin Immunol* 1997;99:757–62.

49 Sicherer SH. Is food allergy causing your patient's asthma symptoms? *J Resp Dis* 2000;21:127–36.

50 Goetz DW, Whisman BA. Occupational asthma in a seafood restaurant worker: cross-reactivity of shrimp and scallops. *Ann Allergy Asthma Immunol* 2000;85:461–6.

51 Crespo JF, Pascual C, Dominguez C, *et al*. Allergic reactions associated with airborne fish particles in IgE-mediated fish hypersensitive patients. *Allergy* 1995;50:257–61.

52 Taylor AV, Swanson MC, Jones RT, *et al*. Detection and quantitation of raw fish aeroallergens from an open-air fish market. *J Allergy Clin Immunol* 2000;105:166–9.

53 Eigenmann PA, Zamora SA. An internet-based survey on the circumstances of food-induced reactions following the diagnosis of IgE-mediated food allergy. *Allergy* 2002;57:449–53.

54 Roberts G, Golder N, Lack G. Bronchial challenges with aerosolized food in asthmatic, food-allergic patients. *Allergy* 2002;57: 713–7.

55 Kalogeromitros D, Makris M, Gregoriou S, *et al*. IgE-mediated sensitization in seafood processing workers. *Allergy Asthma Proc* 2006;27:399–403.

56 Daroca P, Crespo JF, Reano M, *et al*. Asthma and rhinitis induced by exposure to raw green beans and chards. *Ann Allergy Asthma Immunol* 2000;85:215–18.

57 Groenewoud GC, de Groot H, van Wijk RG. Impact of occupational and inhalant allergy on rhinitis-specific quality of life in employees of bell pepper greenhouses in the Netherlands. *Ann Allergy Asthma Immunol* 2006;96:92–7.

58 Moreno-Ancillo A, Gil-Adrados AC, Dominguez-Noche C, *et al*. Occupational asthma due to carrot in a cook. *Allergol Immunopathol (Madr)* 2005;33:288–290.

59 Sicherer SH, Furlong TJ, DeSimone J, Sampson HA. Self-reported allergic reactions to peanut on commercial airliners. *J Allergy Clin Immunol* 1999;104:186–9.

60 Baur X, Posch A. Characterized allergens causing bakers' asthma. *Allergy* 1998;53:562–6.

61 Pavlovic M, Spasojevic M, Tasic Z, Tacevic S. Bronchial hyperactivity in bakers and its relation to atopy and skin reactivity. *Sci Total Environ* 2001;270:71–5.

62 Bulat P, Myny K, Braeckman L, *et al*. Exposure to inhalable dust, wheat flour and alpha-amylase allergens in industrial and traditional bakeries. *Ann Occup Hyg* 2004;48:57–63.

63 Vissers M, Doekes G, Heederik D. Exposure to wheat allergen and fungal alpha-amylase in the homes of bakers. *Clin Exp Allergy* 2001;31:1577–82.

64 Quirce S, Polo F, Figueredo E, *et al*. Occupational asthma caused by soybean flour in bakers – differences with soybean-induced epidemic asthma. *Clin Exp Allergy* 2000;30:839–46.

65 Codina R, Ardusso L, Lockey RF, *et al*. Identification of the soybean hull allergens involved in sensitization to soybean dust in a rural population from Argentina and *N*-terminal sequence of a major 50 KD allergen. *Clin Exp Allergy* 2002; 32:1059–63.

66 Escudero C, Quirce S, Fernandez-Nieto M, *et al*. Egg white proteins as inhalant allergens associated with baker's asthma. *Allergy* 2003;58:616–20.

67 James JM, Bernhisel-Broadbent J, Sampson HA. Respiratory reactions provoked by double-blind food challenges in children. *Am J Respir Crit Care Med* 1994;149:59–64.

68 Bernstein JM. The role of IgE-mediated hypersensitivity in the development of otitis media with effusion: a review. *Otolaryngol Head Neck Surg* 1993;109:611–20.

69 Nsouli TM, Nsouli SM, Linde RE, *et al*. Role of food allergy in serous otitis media. *Ann Allergy* 1994;73:215–19.

70 Heiner DC, Sears JW. Chronic respiratory disease associated with multiple circulation precipitins to cow's milk. *Am J Dis Child* 1960;100:500–2.

71 Heiner DC, Sears JW, Knicker WT. Multiple precipitins to cow's milk in chronic respiratory disease. *Am J Dis Child* 1962; 103:634–54.

72 Hill DJ, Firer MA, Shelton MJ, Hosking CS. Manifestations of milk allergy in infancy: clinical and immunological findings. *J Pediatr* 1986;109:270–6.

73 Bock SA. Respiratory reactions induced by food challenges in children with pulmonary disease. *Pediatr Allergy Immunol* 1992; 3:188–94.

74 Rance F, Dutau G. Asthma and food allergy: report of 163 pediatric cases. *Arch Pediatr* 2002;9:402s–7s.

75 James JM, Eigenmann PA, Eggleston PA, Sampson HA. Airway reactivity changes in food-allergic, asthmatic children undergoing double-blind placebo-controlled food challenges. *Am J Respir Crit Care Med* 1996;153:597–603.

76 Zwetchkenbaum JF, Skufca R, Nelson HS. An examination of food hypersensitivity as a cause of increased bronchial responsiveness to inhaled methacholine. *J Allergy Clin Immunol* 1991; 88:360–4.

77 Thaminy A, Lamblin C, Perez T, *et al*. Increased frequency of asymptomatic bronchial hyperresponsiveness in nonasthmatic patients with food allergy. *Eur Respir J* 2000;16:1091–4.

78 Kivity S, Fireman E, Sade K. Bronchial hyperactivity, sputum analysis and skin prick test to inhalant allergens in patients with symptomatic food hypersensitivity. *Isr Med Assoc J* 2005; 7:781–4.

79 Wallaert B, Gosset P, Lamblin C, *et al.* Airway neutrophil inflammation in nonasthmatic patients with food allergy. *Allergy* 2002;57:405–10.

80 Brandt EB, Scribner TA, Akei HS, Rothenberg ME. Experimental gastrointestinal allergy enhances pulmonary responses to specific and unrelated allergens. *J Allergy Clin Immunol* 2006;118:420–7.

81 Bock SA, Munoz-Furlong A, Sampson HA. Fatalities due to anaphylactic reactions to foods. *J Allergy Clin Immunol* 2001; 107:191–3.

82 Novembre E, de Martino M, Vierucci A. Foods and respiratory allergy. *J Allergy Clin Immunol* 1988;81:1059–65.

83 Oehling A, Cagnani CEB. Food allergy and child asthma. *Allergol Immunopathol* 1980;8:7–14.

84 Businco L, Falconieri P, Giampietro P, Bellioni B. Food allergy and asthma. *Pediatr Pulmonol Suppl* 1995;11:59–60.

85 Yazicioglu M, Baspinar I, Ones U, *et al.* Egg and milk allergy in asthmatic children: assessment by immulite allergy food panel, skin prick tests and double-blind placebo-controlled food challenges. *Allergol Immunopathol (Madr)* 1999;27:287–93.

86 Roberts G, Patel N, Levi-Schaffer F, *et al.* Food allergy as a risk factor for life-threatening asthma in childhood: a case-controlled study. *J Allergy Clin Immunol* 2003;112:168–74.

87 Baker JC, Duncanson RC, Tunnicliffe WS, Ayres JG. Development of a standardized methodology for double-blind, placebo-controlled food challenge in patients with brittle asthma and perceived food intolerance. *J Am Diet Assoc* 2000;100:1361–7.

88 Price GW, Hogan AD, Farris AH, *et al.* Sensitization (IgE antibody) to food allergens in wheezing infants and children. *J Allergy Clin Immunol* 1995;96:266–70.

89 Sampson HA, Ho DG. Relationship between food-specific IgE concentrations and the risk of positive food challenges in children and adolescents. *J Allergy Clin Immunol* 1997;100:444–51.

90 Sampson HA. Food allergy. Part 2. Diagnosis and management. *J Allergy Clin Immunol* 1999;103:981–9.

91 Sampson HA. Utility of food-specific IgE concentrations in predicting symptomatic food allergy. *J Allergy Clin Immunol* 2001; 107:891–6.

92 Wraith DG, Merrett J, Roth A, *et al.* Recognition of food-allergic patients and their allergens by the RAST technique and clinical investigation. *Clin Allergy* 1979;9:25–36.

93 James JM, Sampson HA. An overview of food hypersensitivity. *Pediatr Allergy Immunol* 1992;3:707–870.

94 Condemini JJ. Unproved diagnostic and therapeutic techniques. In: Metcalfe DD, Sampson HA, Simon RA (eds.) *Food Allergy: Adverse Reactions to Foods and Food Additives.* Cambridge, MA, USA: Blackwell Scientific Publications, 1997:541–50.

95 James JM. Unproven diagnostic and therapeutic techniques. *Curr Allergy Asthma Rep* 2002;2:87–91.

96 Bock SA, Sampson HA, Atkins FM, *et al.* Double-blind, placebo-controlled food challenge (DBPCFC) as an office procedure: a manual. *J Allergy Clin Immunol* 1988;82:986–97.

97 David TJ, Waddington E, Stanton RH. Nutritional hazards of elimination diets in children with atopic eczema. *Arch Dis Child* 1984;59:323–5.

98 Davidovits M, Levy Y, Avramovitz T, Eisenstein B. Calcium-deficiency rickets in a four-year-old boy with milk allergy. *J Pediatr* 1993;122:249–51.

99 McGowan M, Gibney MJ. Calcium intakes in individuals on diets for the management of cows' milk allergy: a case control study. *Eur J Clin Nutr* 1993;47:609–16.

100 Hallett R, Teuber SS. Food allergies and sensitivities. *Nutr Clin Care* 2004;7:122–9.

101 Spector SL, Nicklas RA. Practice parameters for the diagnosis and treatment of asthma. *J Allergy Clin Immunol* 1995;96:707–870.

13 CHAPTER 13

Anaphylaxis and Food Allergy

Hugh A. Sampson

KEY POINTS

- Food allergy is the leading single cause of anaphylaxis treated in emergency departments in the United States.

- Any food may cause an anaphylactic reaction, but peanut, tree nuts, fish, and shellfish are most often implicated in severe and fatal reactions.

- A careful clinical history is critical for the accurate diagnosis of food-induced anaphylaxis; an algorithm of clinical symptoms has been proposed, which provides a universal standard for accurately diagnosing anaphylaxis.

- Laboratory studies are not diagnostic of anaphylaxis, simply supportive.

- All patients at risk for a food-induced anaphylactic reaction should be provided with an emergency plan and appropriate medications, for example epinephrine autoinjector, to initiate therapy in case of an accidental allergen ingestion.

Introduction

Although fatal allergic reactions have been recognized for over 4500 years [1], it was not until the 20th century that the syndrome of anaphylaxis was fully characterized. In their classic studies, Portier and Richet described the rapid death of several dogs that they were attempting to immunize against the toxic sting of the sea anemone [2]. Since this reaction represented the opposite of their intended "prophylaxis," they coined the term "anaphylaxis," or "without or against protection." From these studies, they concluded that anaphylaxis required a latent period for sensitization and re-exposure to the sensitizing material. Shortly thereafter Schlossman reported a patient who developed acute shock after the ingestion of cow's milk [3]. The first modern-day series of food anaphylaxis in man was published in 1969 by Golbert and colleagues [4]. They described 10 cases of anaphylaxis following the ingestion of various foods, including different legumes, fish, and milk. The reports by Yunginger [5] and then by Sampson [6] and Bock [7,8] further characterized the natural course of near-fatal and fatal food-induced anaphylactic reactions.

Definitions

The term "food-induced anaphylaxis" refers to a serious allergic reaction following the ingestion of a food, typically IgE mediated, which is generally rapid in onset and may progress to death [9]. Typically the term *anaphylaxis* connotes an immunologically mediated event that occurs after exposure to certain foreign substances, whereas the term *anaphylactoid* indicates a clinically indistinguishable reaction that is not believed to be IgE mediated but probably involves many of the same mediators, for example, histamine. The syndrome results from the generation and release of a variety of potent biologically active mediators and their concerted effects on various target organs. "Biphasic anaphylaxis" is defined as a recurrence of symptoms that develop following the apparent resolution of the initial anaphylactic event. Biphasic reactions have been reported to develop in 1–20% of anaphylactic reactions and typically occur within 1–4 hours following the resolution of the initial symptoms, although some cases have been reported up to 72 hours later [10]. "Protracted anaphylaxis" is defined as an anaphylactic reaction that lasts for hours or in extreme cases, days [6]. "Food-associated, exercise-induced anaphylaxis" refers to a food-induced anaphylactic reaction that occurs only when the patient exercises within several hours of ingesting a food; when the food is consumed without subsequent exercise or when exercise occurs without the ingestion of the food allergen, the patient will not experience allergic symptoms [11,12].

Anaphylaxis is recognized by a constellation of cutaneous, respiratory, cardiovascular, and gastrointestinal signs and symptoms occurring singly or in combination. To facilitate and standardize the diagnosis of anaphylaxis, the National Institute of Allergy and Infectious Diseases (NIAID) and Food Allergy & Anaphylaxis Network (FAAN) convened

Food Allergy: Adverse Reactions to Foods and Food Additives, 4th edition.
Edited by Dean D. Metcalfe, Hugh A. Sampson, and Ronald A. Simon.
© 2008 Blackwell Publishing, ISBN: 978-1-4501-5129-0.

Table 13.1 Diagnostic criteria for anaphylaxis (Reproduced from Sampson *et al.* [13], with permission from Elsevier.)

Anaphylaxis is highly likely when any *one* of the following three criteria is fulfilled:

(1) Acute onset of an illness (minutes to several hours) with involvement of the skin, mucosal tissue, or both (e.g. generalized hives, pruritus, or flushing, swollen lips–tongue–uvula)
  And at least one of the following:
  (a) Respiratory compromise (e.g. dyspnea, wheeze-bronchospasm, stridor, reduced peak expiratory flow, hypoxemia)
  (b) Reduced blood pressure or associated symptoms of end-organ dysfunction (e.g. hypotonia (collapse), syncope, incontinence)

(2) Two or more of the following that occur rapidly after exposure *to a likely allergen for that patient* (minutes to several hours):
  (a) Involvement of the skin-mucosal tissue (e.g. generalized hives, itch-flush, swollen lips–tongue–uvula)
  (b) Respiratory compromise (e.g. dyspnea, wheeze-bronchospasm, stridor, reduced peak expiratory flow, hypoxemia)
  (c) Reduced blood pressure or associated symptoms of end-organ dysfunction (e.g. hypotonia (collapse), syncope, incontinence)
  (d) Persistent gastrointestinal symptoms (e.g. crampy abdominal pain, vomiting)

(3) Reduced BP after exposure *to known allergen for that patient* (minutes to several hours):
  (a) Infants and children: low systolic blood pressure (age-specific) or greater than 30% decrease in systolic blood pressure*
  (b) Adults: systolic blood pressure <90 mmHg or >30% decrease from that patient's baseline

BP: blood pressure; PEF: Peak expiratory flow.
*Low systolic BP for children: 1 month–1 year < 70 mmHg; 1–10 years < (70 mmHg + (2 × age)); 11–17 years < 90 mmHg.

Table 13.2 Grading severity of anaphylaxis

Grade	Defined by
(1) *Mild* (skin and subcutaneous tissues, GI, and/or mild respiratory)	Flushing, urticaria, periorbital erythema, or angioedema; mild dyspnea, wheezing, and upper respiratory symptoms; mild abdominal pain and/or emesis
(2) *Moderate* (mild symptoms + features suggesting moderate respiratory, cardiovascular, or GI symptoms)	Marked dysphagia, hoarseness, and/or stridor; SOB, wheezing, and retractions; crampy abdominal pain, recurrent vomiting, and/or diarrhea; and/or mild dizziness
(3) *Severe* (hypoxia, hypotension, or neurological compromise)	Cyanosis or SpO_2 ≤92% at any stage, hypotension, confusion, collapse, loss of consciousness; or incontinence

an international panel of experts from various medical specialties that deal with anaphylactic cases. An algorithm was proposed, as depicted in Table 13.1 [13]. Since anaphylactic reactions may present with varied degrees of severity, which may influence the form of treatment rendered, Table 13.2 presents a simplified scoring system based on the diagnostic algorithm of anaphylaxis proposed by the NIAID–FAAN working group. This chapter focuses on allergic reactions to foods that manifest as signs and symptoms fulfilling the proposed definition of anaphylaxis.

Prevalence

The prevalence of anaphylaxis is unknown since unlike many disorders, there is no requirement to report such reactions to a national registry. In addition, it is likely that many cases are misdiagnosed [14,15]. Also contributing to this lack of scientific data is the fact that many patients who experience a mild anaphylactic reaction recognize the causative relationship to a specific food, self-medicate, and simply attempt to avoid that food rather than consult a physician.

Only in the past few years has an *International Classification of Diseases* (*ICD*) code for food-induced anaphylaxis become available, prior to which it has been extremely difficult to obtain any reliable information regarding the prevalence, incidence, or mortality rates for these reactions. In a retrospective survey, Yocum and Khan [16] reviewed all cases of anaphylaxis treated in the Mayo Clinic Emergency Department (United States) over a 3.5-year period. Records were reviewed on all patients experiencing respiratory obstructive symptoms and/or cardiovascular symptoms plus evidence of allergic mediator release, for example, urticaria. Overall, 179 patients were identified; 66% were female, 49% were atopic, and 37% had experienced an immediate reaction to the responsible allergen in the past. A probable cause was identified in 142 cases (Table 13.3). Allergic reactions to food were found to be the most common single cause of anaphylactic reactions outside of the hospital, more frequent than reactions to bee sting and drugs combined. Bock surveyed 73 emergency departments in Colorado over a 2-year period and identified 25 cases of severe anaphylactic reactions to food with one death [17]. From this it was concluded that at least 950 cases of severe food-induced anaphylaxis occur in the United States every year. However, Bock cautioned that his survey was an underestimate of the problem since patients had been referred to him who were not included in the survey, and the proportion of reactions was higher in rural emergency departments serving smaller populations than in the busier metropolitan departments. In a more recent US survey, Yocum reported an annual incidence of food-induced anaphylaxis of 7.6 cases per 100,000 person-years and a food-induced anaphylaxis occurrence rate of 10.8 per 100,000 person-years [18]. The figures were based on a review of the medical records of Olmsted County inhabitants followed in the Rochester Epidemiology Study from 1983 to 1987.

Table 13.3 Three-year retrospective survey of anaphylaxis occurring outside of the hospital treated by the Mayo Clinic Emergency Department (From Yocum and Khan [16], with permission from Elsevier.)

Presumed etiology of anaphylaxis	Number	%
Food	59	33
Idiopathic	34	19
Hymenoptera	25	14
Medications	23	13
Exercise	12	7
Other	8	4
False diagnosis	18	10
Foods implicated in 18 patients who were skin tested:		
Peanut	4	
Cereals	6	
Egg	2	
Nuts	9	
Milk	2	

Assuming that the US population is now 280 million and that the prevalence of food allergy did not increase since the late 1980s (although peanut allergy has been shown to have increased [19,20]) one could estimate that about 30,000 food-induced anaphylactic episodes occur in the United States every year resulting in approximately 2000 hospitalizations and 150 deaths [11]. Food-induced anaphylactic reactions account for over one-third of the anaphylactic reactions treated in emergency departments and are most often due to peanut, tree nuts, fish, or shellfish. Pumphrey [21] and Moneret-Vautrin [22] reported similar findings in the United Kingdom and France, respectively. In Italy, Novembre reported that food allergy was responsible for about one-half of severe anaphylactic episodes in children treated in emergency departments [23]. Similarly, a survey of South Australian pre-school and school-age children revealed a parent-reported food-induced anaphylaxis rate of 0.43 per 100 school children, which accounted for over one-half of all cases of anaphylaxis in this age group [24]. Similarly, the Canadian Pediatric Surveillance Program reported that 81% of anaphylaxis cases in children were due to food [25]. A 5-year survey of anaphylactic reactions treated at the Children's Hospital of Philadelphia also showed that food allergy was the most common cause of anaphylaxis outside of the hospital [26]. In a more recent survey from Australia, 526 children with generalized allergic reactions were seen in a local emergency department and 57 were diagnosed with anaphylaxis. This represented an incidence of 9.3 in 1000 emergency department visits for generalized allergic reactions and an anaphylaxis incidence of 1 in 1000 [27]. In a similar series of 304 adults attending an emergency department in the same city over a 1-year period, 162 were diagnosed with acute allergic reactions and 142 with anaphylaxis, including 60 whose anaphylaxis was severe and one of whom died, for an anaphylaxis presentation incidence of 1 in 439 [28].

The first of several reports on fatal food-induced anaphylaxis was in 1988 by Yunginger and colleagues who reported seven cases of fatal anaphylaxis evaluated during a 16-month period [5]. In all but possibly one case, the victims unknowingly ingested a food which had provoked a previous allergic reaction. Similarly six fatal and seven near-fatal food-induced anaphylactic reactions in children (aged 2–17 years) were accumulated from three metropolitan areas over a 14-month period [6]. Common risk factors were noted in these cases: all patients had asthma (although generally well controlled); all patients were unaware that they were ingesting the food allergen; all patients had experienced previous allergic reactions to the incriminated food, although in most cases symptoms had been much milder; and all patients had immediate symptoms with about half experiencing a quiescent period prior to a major respiratory collapse. In both these early series, no patient who died received adrenaline immediately; however, three patients with near-fatal reactions did receive adrenaline within 15 minutes of developing symptoms but still went on to develop respiratory collapse and hypotension requiring mechanical ventilation and vasopressor support for 12 hours to 3 weeks. None of these patients investigated had a significant increase in serum tryptase.

In two reports by Bock and co-workers [7,8], 63 cases of fatal food-induced anaphylaxis were evaluated. As in earlier series, peanuts and tree nuts accounted for more than 90% of the fatalities, but in the second report, milk accounted for 4 of 31 deaths. In these series, all but 2 of the patients were known to have asthma and most of the individuals did not have epinephrine available at the time of their fatal reaction. Of the cumulative 63 fatal food anaphylaxis cases reported, however, 6 individuals (~10%) had received epinephrine in a timely manner but failed to respond. In an earlier series of 48 fatal cases reviewed by Pumphrey, 3 patients (~6%) died despite receiving epinephrine from a self-administration kit appropriately at the onset of their reaction [21].

The incidence of food-dependent exercise-induced anaphylaxis appears to be increasing, possibly due to the increased popularity of exercising over the past decade. Two forms of food-dependent exercise-induced anaphylaxis have been described: reactions following the ingestion of specific foods (e.g. egg, celery, shellfish, wheat) [29–35] and rarely reactions following the ingestion of any food [30]. Anaphylaxis will occur when a patient exercises within 2–4 hours of ingesting a food, but otherwise the patient can ingest the food without any apparent reaction and can exercise without any apparent reaction as long as the specific food (or any food in the case of non-specific reactors) has not been ingested within the past several hours. This disorder is twice as common in females and greater than 60% of cases occur in individuals less than 30 years of age.

In a survey of 199 individuals experiencing exercise-induced anaphylaxis, ingestion of food within 2 hours of exercise was felt to be a factor in the development of attacks in 54% of the cases [32]. More recently, several cases of food- and aspirin-dependent exercise-induced anaphylaxis have been reported [36–38]. Symptoms generally start with a sensation of generalized pruritus that progresses to urticaria and erythema, respiratory obstruction, and cardiovascular collapse. Patients with specific food-dependent exercise-induced anaphylaxis generally have positive prick skin tests to the food and occasionally these patients will have a history of "outgrowing" an allergy to the causative food when they were younger. As discussed below, specific management of this disorder involves identifying the food(s) which cause the reaction (i.e. DBPCFC with exercise).

Several factors appear to predispose an individual to food-induced anaphylaxis including a personal history of atopy, family history of atopy, age, and dietary exposure. Atopic patients with asthma are at increased risk of developing more severe food-allergic reactions [6,9,39]. In the reports of Yunginger et al. [5], Sampson et al. [6], and Bock et al. [7,8] the majority of individuals were highly atopic, and all had histories of asthma. Although atopy reportedly does not predispose individuals to an increased risk of anaphylaxis [40], it does tend to predispose to more severe reactions. In general, it has been thought that individuals inherit the ability to produce antigen-specific IgE to food proteins and that hypersensitivity to a specific food is not inherited. However, in a report evaluating twins with peanut allergy, there was a significant concordance rate of peanut allergy among monozygotic twins compared to dizygotic twins suggesting strongly that there is a major genetic influence on the inheritance of peanut allergy [41].

Age may play a factor in predisposing an individual to food-induced anaphylaxis. The prevalence of food allergy appears greatest in the first 2 years of life and decreases with age [12]. Consequently foods introduced during the first year (e.g. cow's milk, egg, soy, wheat, and peanut (as peanut butter in the United States)) are more apt to induce hypersensitization. Allergic reactions to milk, egg, soybean, and wheat are generally "outgrown" with age [12]. The age of onset of milk allergy is usually in the first year of life, with about 85% of infants "outgrowing" their sensitivity by 7–8 years of age [42,43]. While most food hypersensitivities are outgrown during childhood, food sensitivity to peanuts, tree nuts, fish, and shellfish often persist into adulthood [44,45]. It had been thought to be quite rare to find a patient who develops clinical tolerance to peanuts and tree nuts, although studies now suggest that 20% of children diagnosed with peanut allergy early in life do outgrow their peanut allergy [46,47] and about 10% outgrow their tree nut allergy [48].

Dietary exposure can influence the occurrence of food-induced anaphylaxis in several ways. Different populations and nationalities may consume more of certain foods, and the increased exposure may result in an increased prevalence of that specific food allergy. In the United States peanut is one of the most common food allergies [49], Americans ingest several tons of peanuts daily (FDA, 1986). By contrast, in Scandinavia, where fish consumption is high, the incidence of allergic reactions to codfish is increased (FDA,1986). Rice and buckwheat allergy are quite rare in the United States but not uncommon in Japan where these foods are frequently ingested [50].

Etiology

Foods

A large variety of foods have been reported to have precipitated an anaphylactic reaction. The list of foods that may induce an anaphylactic reaction is unlimited, and in theory, any food protein is capable of causing an anaphylactic reaction. As indicated in Table 13.4, certain foods tend to be cited most frequently as the cause of anaphylaxis, although any food may be the cause. Foods most often responsible for anaphylactic reactions include peanuts (and to a much lesser extent other legumes: soybeans, lupine, lentils, peas, garbanzo beans), fish (e.g. cod, whitefish, salmon), shellfish (shrimp, lobster, crab, scallops, oyster), tree nuts (hazelnuts, cashews, pistachio, walnuts, pecans, Brazil nuts, almonds), cow's milk, egg, fruits (banana, kiwi), seeds (sesame seed, mustard), and cereals or grains (wheat, rice, rye, millet, buckwheat) [12]. The potency of particular foods to induce an anaphylactic reaction appears to vary and is also dependent on the sensitivity of the individual. In general, it appears that for some foods such as peanuts, microgram quantities may be sufficient to induce a reaction.

In oral food-challenge studies where food-allergic patients are challenged on a regular basis (e.g. annually) over a period of years, patients who eventually become tolerant to a food often appear to tolerate more of the antigen in successive years. For example, the initial challenge may

Table 13.4 Foods most frequently implicated in food-induced anaphylaxis

Peanut	
Tree nuts	(hazel nuts (filberts), walnuts, cashews, pistachios, Brazil nuts)
Fish	(less often tuna)
Shellfish	(shrimp, crab, lobster, oyster, scallop)
Cow's milk	(goat's milk)
Hen's egg	
Seeds	(cotton seed, sesame seed, pine nuts, sunflower seed)
Beans	(soybeans, green peas, pinto beans, garbanzo beans, green beans)
Fruit	(banana, kiwi)
Cereal grains	(wheat, barley, oat, buckwheat)
Potato	

be positive after 500 mg of the food and then in the subsequent challenge 1 year later the patient may tolerate 5 g of the food. The next challenge the following year may reveal that the patient is no longer sensitive to that food.

Prior exposure and sensitization to food allergens theoretically must precede the initial anaphylactic reaction. However, there have been numerous reports of an anaphylactic reaction occurring after the first known exposure to a food substance. In one series of children allergic to peanuts and tree nuts, a significant number of these patients reacted on their first known exposure to the food [51,52]. Several possibilities may account for this apparent paradox: most often infants are sensitized to foods passed in maternal breast milk during lactation; sensitization following allergen contact on the skin in infants with atopic dermatitis [53], sensitization may occur following an unknown exposure to a food antigen (e.g. milk formula given during the night in the newborn nursery, food given by another caregiver (e.g. babysitter or grandparent), or food contained in another product which was not suspected of containing the antigen in question); and sensitization may occur because of cross-sensitization to a similar allergen (e.g. kiwi or banana allergy in a latex-sensitive individual) [54]. Some data suggest that sensitization may occur *in utero* [55].

Food additives

Although food additives are often suspected of provoking anaphylactic reactions, the only food additives for which there is significant evidence of precipitating an anaphylactic reaction are sulfites and papain, both of which are quite rare. One of the initial reports detailed an atopic, non-asthmatic patient who experienced an anaphylactic reaction after consuming a restaurant meal which contained significant sodium bisulfite [56]. Specific IgE to sodium bisulfite was demonstrated by skin testing and transfer of passive cutaneous anaphylaxis, and an oral food challenge produced itching of the ears and eyes, nausea, warmness, cough, tightness in the throat, and erythema of the shoulders. These symptoms resolved following treatment with epinephrine. There have been other scattered case reports in the literature confirming sulfite-induced anaphylaxis [57,58].

One patient has been reported with papain-induced anaphylaxis following the ingestion of a beefsteak that had been treated with papain as a meat tenderizer [59]. The patient was found to have specific IgE to papain by prick skin testing and experienced a positive oral challenge to papain with palatal itching and throat tightness. One study suggested that MSG could provoke asthma and anaphylaxis in some patients, but this remains controversial [60].

Clinical features

The hallmark of a food-induced anaphylactic reaction is the onset of symptoms within seconds to minutes following the ingestion of the food allergen. The time course of the appearance and perception of symptoms and signs will differ among individuals. Almost invariably, at least some symptoms will begin within the first hour after the exposure. Generally the later the onset of anaphylactic signs and symptoms, the less severe the reaction. About 25–30% of patients will experience a biphasic reaction [6,61,62], where patients typically develop classical symptoms initially, appear to be recovering (and may become asymptomatic), and then experience the recurrence of significant, often catastrophic symptoms, which may be more refractory to standard therapy. The intervening quiescent period may last up to 1–3 hours. In the report by Sampson and colleagues, three of seven patients with near-fatal anaphylaxis experienced protracted anaphylaxis, with symptoms lasting from 1 day to 21 days [6]. Most reports suggest that the earlier epinephrine is administered in the course of anaphylaxis the better the chance of a favorable prognosis, but there is no data to indicate that the timing of epinephrine affects the prevalence of biphasic or protracted symptoms [61]. In addition, it should be noted that in about 5–10% of cases in which patients have received an initial injection of epinephrine in a timely manner, they still progressed to fatal anaphylaxis [7,8]. Even with appropriate treatment in a medical facility, it rarely may be impossible to reverse an anaphylactic reaction once it has begun.

The symptoms of anaphylaxis are generally related to the gastrointestinal, respiratory, cutaneous, and cardiovascular systems [9]. Other organ systems may be affected but much less commonly. The sequence of symptom presentation and severity will vary from one individual to the other. Additionally, one patient who experiences anaphylaxis to more than one type of food may experience a different sequence of symptoms with each food. While many patients will develop similar allergic symptoms on subsequent occasions following the ingestion of a food allergen, patients with asthma and peanut and/or nut allergy seem to be less predictable. There are many cases of peanut-allergic children who reacted with minimal cutaneous and gastrointestinal symptoms as a young child who later developed asthma and then experienced a catastrophic anaphylactic event after ingesting peanut in their teenage years.

The first symptoms experienced often involve the oropharynx. Symptoms may include edema and pruritus of the lips, oral mucosa, palate, and pharynx [9,63]. Young children may be seen scratching at their tongue, palate, anterior neck, or external auditory canals (presumably from referred pruritus of the posterior pharynx). Evidence of laryngeal edema includes a "dry staccato" or croupy cough and/or dysphonia and dysphagia. Gastrointestinal symptoms include nausea, vomiting, crampy abdominal pain, and diarrhea. Emesis generally contains large amounts of "stringy" mucus. Respiratory symptoms may consist of a deep repetitive cough, stridor, dyspnea, and/or wheezing. Cutaneous symptoms of anaphylaxis may include flushing, urticaria, angioedema, and/or an erythematous macular rash. The development of cardiovascular symptoms, along with airway obstruction, is of greatest concern in anaphylactic reactions. Although cardiovascular symptoms occur less frequently in food-induced anaphylactic reactions compared to insect-sting or medication-induced anaphylaxis, it is important to recognize the symptoms early and the potential complications. Symptoms associated with hypotension can include nausea, vomiting, diaphoresis, dyspnea, hypoxia, dizziness, seizures and collapse [64]. Extravasation of fluid and vasodilation can lead to a decrease in circulating blood volume of up to 35% within 10 minutes [65]. In addition, cardiac dysfunction associated with nonspecific electrocardiographic changes and normal coronary arteries has been reported [66]. Therefore, aggressive fluid resuscitation, as well as placing the patient in a supine position and elevating the legs to prevent pooling of blood in the lower extremities, is recommended. In fact, upright posture has been found to lead to fatalities in cases of food-induced anaphylactic shock [67].

Other signs and symptoms reported frequently in anaphylaxis include periocular and nasal pruritus, sneezing, diaphoresis, disorientation, fecal or urinary urgency or incontinence, and uterine cramping (manifested as lower back pain similar to "labor" pains). Patients often report an impending "sense of doom." In some instances the initial manifestation of anaphylaxis may be the loss of consciousness. Death may ensue in minutes but has been reported to occur days to weeks after anaphylaxis [7,8,21], with late deaths generally resulting from organ damage experienced early in the course of anaphylaxis.

Several factors appear to increase the risk of more severe anaphylactic reactions. Patients taking β-adrenergic antagonists or calcium channel blockers may be resistant to standard therapeutic regimens and therefore at increased risk for severe anaphylaxis [9]. Patients with asthma appear to be at increased risk for severe symptoms as noted in a number of recent reports concerning fatal and near-fatal food anaphylactic reactions [7]. Similar findings have been reported in patients with insect-sting allergy [68] and from patients experiencing anaphylaxis as a result of immunotherapy [69,70]. In these patients significant, acute bronchospasm developed along with other symptoms of anaphylaxis.

The skin is the most commonly affected organ in anaphylaxis, appearing in more than 80% of cases [9,62]. However, up to 20% of cases do not present with skin findings, particularly in children reacting to foods [6,27]. In these cases, a history of allergy and possible exposure, along with symptoms consistent with criteria no. 2 listed in Table 13.1 would establish the diagnosis. In rare cases, hypotension has been reported to be the primary symptom of anaphylaxis. These situations would satisfy the third criteria if the patient had exposure to a known allergen. The annual incidence of anaphylaxis with cardiovascular compromise is 8–10 per 100,000 inhabitants [18,71]. In six cases of fatal food-induced

anaphylaxis [6], initial symptoms developed within 3–30 minutes and severe respiratory symptoms within 20–150 minutes. Symptoms involved the lower respiratory tract in 6 of 6 children, the gastrointestinal tract in 5 of 6 patients, and the skin in only 1 of 6 children. *Anaphylaxis should never be considered ruled-out on the basis of absent skin symptoms.*

Diagnosis

Using the algorithm presented in Table 13.1, the diagnosis of anaphylaxis should be readily apparent [13]. Young children presenting with anaphylaxis most often present with cutaneous and gastrointestinal symptoms [27], whereas adults will often have respiratory and cardiovascular symptoms [66]. In many cases where a food is implicated, the inciting food is obvious from the temporal relationship between the ingestion and the onset of symptoms. The initial step in determining the cause of an episode of anaphylaxis is a very careful history, especially when the cause of the episode is not straightforward [39]. Specific questions to address include the type and quantity of food eaten, the last time the food was ingested, the time frame between ingestion and the development of symptoms, the nature of the food (cooked or uncooked), other times when similar symptoms occurred (and if the food in question was eaten on those occasions), and whether any other precipitating factors appear to be involved, for example, exercise, alcohol, NSAIDs.

Basically, any food may precipitate an anaphylactic reaction, but there are a few specific foods which appear to be most often implicated in the etiology of food-induced anaphylactic reactions: peanuts, tree nuts, fish, and shellfish. In cases where the etiology of the anaphylactic reaction is not apparent, a dietary history should review all ingredients of the suspected meal including any possible concealed ingredients or food additives. The food provoking the reaction may be merely a contaminant (knowingly or unknowingly) in the meal. For example, peanuts or peanut butter are frequently added to cookies, candies, pastries, or sauces such as chili, spaghetti, and barbecue sauces. Chinese restaurants frequently use peanut butter to "glue" the overlapping ends of an egg roll, pressed or "extruded" peanut oil in their cooking, and the same wok to cook a variety of different meals resulting in residual contaminant carry-over. Another infrequent (but not rare) cause of food contamination occurs during the manufacturing process. This contamination may happen with scraps of candy or dough that are "reworked" into the next batch of candy or cookies, or in processing plants where there is a production change from one product to the next. As an example, a reaction to almond butter by a peanut-allergic patient started an investigation which determined that 10% of the almond butter produced in that plant was contaminated with peanut butter (FDA, 1986). This occurred after a production change in the manufacturing process from peanut butter to almond butter. Other examples include popsicles run on the same line as creamsicles (milk), fruit juices packaged in individual cartons where milk products have been packaged, milk-free desserts packaged in dairy plants [72], etc. Food items with "natural flavoring" designated on the label may contain an unsuspected allergen, for example casein in canned tuna fish, hot-dogs, or bologna, soy in a variety of baked goods, etc. However, the *Food Allergen Labeling and Consumer Protection Act* (*FALCPA*) became law on January 1, 2006 in the United States and mandated that foods containing any amount of milk, egg, peanut, tree nuts, fish, shellfish, soy, or wheat must declare the food in plain language on the ingredient label, that is "milk" and not "sodium caseinate." FALCPA has made label reading to ascertain ingredients much easier for millions of Americans. In the European Common Market countries, similar legislation has been enacted.

Food allergy can develop at any age, although it appears more commonly in the first 3 years of life. Not uncommonly a patient will present who has tolerated a food (i.e. shrimp) for his/her entire life and then at some point in mid-adulthood experiences a major allergic reaction after ingestion of the food. These patients may experience no forewarning of their impending episode, but on detailed questioning will not infrequently describe some minor symptoms previously, such as oral pruritus or nausea and cramping. It is also possible that cooking or processing of some foods may remove, diminish, or even enhance their allergenicity.

Some conditions may be confused with food anaphylaxis. Among these clinical problems are scromboid poisoning, factitious allergic emergency, and vasovagal collapse. In the absence of urticaria and angioedema one must consider arrhythmia, myocardial infarction, hereditary angioedema, aspiration of a bolus of food, pulmonary embolism, and seizure disorders. Following the algorithm in Table 13.1 should enable physicians to accurately identify individuals with anaphylaxis.

With the presence of laryngeal edema, especially when accompanied by abdominal pain, the diagnosis of hereditary angioedema must be considered. In general, this disorder is slower in onset, does not include urticaria, and often there is a family history of similar reactions [73,74]. Systemic mastocytosis results in flushing, tachycardia, pruritus, headache, abdominal pain, diarrhea, and syncope. A factitious allergic emergency may occur when patients knowingly and secretively ingest a food substance to which they are known to be allergic.

In vasovagal syncope, the patient may collapse after an injection or a painful or disturbing situation. The patient typically looks pale and complains of nausea prior to the syncopal episode, but does not complain of pruritus or become cyanotic. Respiratory difficulty does not occur and symptoms are almost immediately relieved by recumbency. Profuse diaphoresis, slow pulse, and maintenance of blood pressure generally complete the syndrome [75], but asystole

and bradycardia have been reported to be associated with blood drawing [76]. Hyperventilation may cause breathlessness and collapse. It is usually not associated with other signs and symptoms of anaphylaxis, except peripheral and perioral tingling sensations.

Laboratory evaluation

The laboratory evaluation of patients with an anaphylactic reaction should be directed at identifying specific IgE antibodies to the food in question. IgE antibody can be recognized *in vivo* by prick or puncture skin testing. Although not absolute, a negative prick/puncture skin test is an excellent predictor for a negative IgE-mediated food reaction to the suspected food. In contrast, a positive prick skin test does not necessarily mean that the food is the inciting agent, but in a patient with a classic history of anaphylaxis to ingestion of an isolated food and a positive prick/puncture skin test to that food, this laboratory test appears to be a good positive predictor of allergic reactivity. In cases of food-associated or aspirin-associated exercise-induced anaphylaxis, prick skin tests performed following exercise/ingestion of aspirin are enhanced compared to tests done prior to exercise/aspirin ingestion in many patients [37].

There are some limitations to skin testing which need to be recognized. There is speculation that skin testing shortly following the anaphylactic event may fail to yield a positive response owing to temporary anergy. Although not demonstrated in food allergy, this phenomenon has been demonstrated in Hymenoptera sensitivity following an insect sting [77]. Possible causes of false-negative prick skin tests include improper skin test technique, concomitant use of antihistamines, or the use of food extracts with reduced or inadequate allergenic potential. With some foods, the processing of the food for commercial extracts may diminish antigenicity [78]. This is especially true for some fruits and vegetables, and occasionally shellfish. However, if there is a high index of suspicion that a food may have precipitated an anaphylactic reaction even though the prick skin test is negative, the patient should be tested with the natural food utilizing the "prick-plus-prick" method to ensure an absence of detectable IgE antibody [79]. Some caution should be exercised in doing this procedure since the amount of antigen on the prick device will not be controlled, and appropriate negative controls should also be performed.

Appropriate skin testing is indicated in each patient, although *in vitro* measurement of food-specific IgE may be evaluated initially. In many patients with anaphylaxis, limited prick skin testing is necessary to confirm the etiology of the anaphylactic reaction. In cases of idiopathic anaphylaxis, more extensive prick testing may occasionally prove helpful in making the diagnosis [80]. The clinician must decide how many skin tests are practical and justified, taking into account the anticipated low yield of positive results in idiopathic anaphylaxis and the value of discovering an etiology in this serious disorder.

Intradermal skin tests are sometimes performed following negative prick/puncture skin tests in other allergic diseases, but the diagnostic significance of a positive intradermal test to food following a negative prick/puncture test is dubious and of no clinical benefit [81]. Fatal anaphylactic reactions have been documented following intradermal skin tests to foods [69,82], so extra caution should be exercised if intradermal tests are performed (if done at all). *Under no circumstances should an intradermal skin test be performed prior to performing a prick/puncture test.* In cases where extreme hypersensitivity is suspected, alternative approaches may be warranted including the further dilution of the food extract prior to prick skin testing or the use of a food-specific IgE *in vitro* tests, for example, UniCAP®; Phadia, Uppsala, Sweden. The UniCAP System appears to be slightly more sensitive than the older standard RAST. In a number of studies, predictive curves and diagnostic decision points have been established using the UniCAP System for predicting a positive food challenge for at least milk, egg, and peanuts [83,84]. At the present time there is no laboratory test that will predict the potential severity of an allergic reaction. A study investigating peanut-allergic patients' IgE binding to allergenic peanut epitopes demonstrated that individuals with binding to large numbers of epitopes (epitope diversity) tended to have more severe reactions than those binding fewer epitopes [85].

Massive activation of mast cells during anaphylaxis results in a dramatic rise in plasma histamine and somewhat later a rise in plasma serum tryptase [86,87]. Plasma histamine rises over the first several minutes of a reaction, generally remains elevated for only several minutes, requires special collection techniques, and will breakdown unless the plasma sample is frozen immediately. Consequently, measurement of plasma histamine to document anaphylaxis is often impractical except in research situations. Whether measurement of urinary methyl histamine will be useful in the documentation of anaphylaxis remains to be demonstrated. Serum tryptase rises over the first hour and may remain elevated for many hours. It is fairly stable at room temperature and can be obtained from post-mortem specimens [87]. Total tryptase has been shown to be markedly elevated in some cases of bee-sting or drug-induced anaphylaxis [87], but several recent studies have found it less often elevated than plasma histamine [39,88,89]. Unfortunately, total tryptase is rarely elevated in food-induced anaphylaxis [6]. Mature β-tryptase is a better indicator of mast cell activation, and if the assay for β-tryptase becomes more available, it may prove to be a better indicator of anaphylaxis than total tryptase [39]. Other mediators being evaluated for potential use as a laboratory marker of anaphylaxis include carboxypeptidase and platelet-activating factor [39].

Double-blind placebo-controlled food challenges are the "gold standard" for diagnosing food allergy, but are contraindicated in patients with an unequivocal history of anaphylaxis following the isolated ingestion of a food to which they have evidence of significant IgE antibodies. However, if several foods were ingested and the patient has positive skin tests to several foods, it is essential that the responsible food be identified. Patients have been reported who experienced repeated anaphylactic reactions because physicians incorrectly assumed that they had identified the responsible food [6]. Young children who experience anaphylactic reactions to foods other than peanuts, tree nuts, fish, and shellfish may eventually outgrow their clinical reactivity, so an oral food challenge may be warranted following an extended period of food elimination with no history of reactions to accidental ingestions.

Treatment

Treatment of food-induced anaphylaxis may be subdivided into acute and long-term management. While management of an acute attack is something physicians spend hours preparing for, it is the long-term measures that provide the best quality of life for the food-allergic patient.

Acute management (Table 13.5)

Fatalities may occur if treatment of a food-induced anaphylactic reaction is not immediate [5–8]. Data from the review of fatal bee-sting-induced anaphylactic reactions indicate that the longer the initial therapy is delayed, the greater the incidence of complications and fatalities [90]. Although epinephrine is clearly the medicine of first choice for the treatment of anaphylaxis, a multi-center study of US emergency room visits for food allergies revealed that only 16% of 678 patients presenting to the emergency room with acute allergic reactions to foods received epinephrine. Even in the group determined to have anaphylaxis (51%), only 22% received epinephrine [91]. Initial treatment must be preceded by a rapid assessment to determine the extent and severity of the reaction, the adequacy of oxygenation, cardiac output and tissue perfusion, any potential confounding medications (e.g. β-blockers), and the suspected cause of the reaction [9]. The patient should be placed in the supine position with the legs elevated, if tolerated, to help maintain adequate perfusion and blood pressure [67]. Initial therapy should be directed at the maintenance of an effective airway and circulatory system. The first step in the acute management of anaphylaxis is the intramuscular injection of 0.01 ml/kg of aqueous epinephrine 1:1000 (maximal dose 0.3–0.5 ml, or 0.3–0.5 mg). Intravenous administration of epinephrine may cause fatal arrhythmias or myocardial infarction, particularly in adults, and should be reserved for refractory hypotension requiring cardiopulmonary resuscitation [92]. In patients with pulmonary symptoms, supplemental oxygen should be administered.

In order to ensure that patients receive epinephrine as early as possible, it is important that they, their family members,

Table 13.5 Acute management of anaphylaxis

Rapid assessment of	Extent and severity of symptoms
	Adequacy of oxygenation, cardiac output, and tissue perfusion potential confounding medications
	Suspected cause of the reaction
Initial therapy	*Epinephrine* – 0.01 mg/kg/dose up to 0.3–0.5 mg i.m. up to 3 times every 15–20 minutes (EpiPen®, Twinject®, epinephrine ampule – 1:1000)
	Oxygen – 40–100% by mask
	Lie patient in supine position with legs elevated, if tolerated
	Intravenous fluids – 30 ml/kg of crystalloid up to 2 l (or more depending on blood pressure and response to medications)
Secondary medications	Nebulized albuterol – may be continuous
	Antihistamines: H1 antagonist (diphenhydramine – 1 mg/kg up to 75 mg; cetirizine – 0.25 mg/kg up to 10 mg)
	H$_2$ antagonist (cimetidine – 4 mg/kg up to 300 mg; ranitidine – 1–2 mg/kg up to 150 mg)
	Corticosteroids: solumedrol – 1–2 mg/kg/dose
	Dopamine – for hypotension refractory to epinephrine (2–20 μg/kg/min)
	Norepinephrine – for hypotension refractory to epinephrine
	Glucagon – (5–15 μg/min) for hypotension refractory to epinephrine and
	Norepinephrine; especially patients on β-blockers
Discharge	Emergency plan and medications
	Appointment for evaluation of cause if not known

and other care providers are instructed in the self-administration of epinephrine. Preloaded syringes with epinephrine are available and should be given to any patient at risk for food-induced anaphylaxis, that is patients with a history of a previous anaphylactic reaction and patients with asthma and food allergy, especially if they are allergic to peanuts, nuts, fish, or shellfish. In the United States, premeasured doses of epinephrine can be obtained from two sources in two doses: Epi-Pen® (0.3 mg) and Epi-Pen, Jr® (0.15 mg) distributed by Dey Laboratories (Napa, CA) and Twinject® (0.3 mg) and Twinject Jr® (0.15 mg) distributed by Verus Pharmaceuticals (San Diego, CA). Both devices are a disposable drug delivery system with a spring-activated concealed needle. The Epi-Pen is intended for a single intramuscular injection while the Twinject disassembles to provide a second dose administered with a small syringe. Both are obtained in two doses: 0.3 mg for those weighing over 28 kg and 0.15 mg for those weighing less than 28 kg. Children are generally advanced to the 0.3-mg dose when they reach 23–28 kg [93], depending on the severity of previous reactions. Since parent or caregivers attempting to measure and administer epinephrine from a vial is so inaccurate [94], the 0.15-mg epinephrine dose is often used in small children weighing 8 kg or more. Those individuals who experienced previous severe symptoms should be advanced to the 0.3-mg dose earlier than those with a history of milder reactions. Since the Epi-Pen® can deliver only a single dose, two Epi-Pens may be prescribed for patients who have experienced a previous anaphylactic reaction or who are at high risk and do not have ready access to a medical center. It is imperative that the patient and/or family members practice with appropriate training devices to ensure their ability to use the device proficiently in case of an emergency. Also, it should be made clear to the patients that

these preloaded devices carry a 1-year shelf life and therefore should be renewed every year.

Sustained-release preparations of epinephrine are not appropriate treatment for acute anaphylaxis. While inhaled epinephrine (either nebulized or via metered-dose inhaler; Primatine Mist® in the United States) has been recommended in the past [95], a minimum of 20 puffs inhaled correctly by adults or 10–15 puffs by children are necessary to produce blood levels similar to an injection of 0.3 mg or 0.15 mg, respectively [96]. However, a study by Simon and co-workers demonstrated that most children are unable to inhale sufficient epinephrine to produce adequate systemic levels [97]. Lesser doses may be beneficial to reverse laryngeal edema or persistent bronchospasm.

Once epinephrine has been administered, other therapeutic modalities may be of benefit. Studies have suggested that the combination of an H1 antihistamines (i.e. diphenhydramine – 1 mg/kg up to 75 mg) either intramuscularly or intravenously and an H2 antihistamine (i.e. 4 mg/kg up to 300 mg of cimetidine) administered intravenously may be more effective than either administered alone [98]. Both histamine antagonists should be infused slowly if given intravenously since rapid infusion of diphenhydramine is associated with arrhythmias and cimetidine with fall in blood pressure. The role of corticosteroids in the treatment of anaphylaxis remains unclear. However, most authorities recommend giving prednisone (1 mg/kg orally) for mild to moderate episodes of anaphylaxis and solumedrol (1–2 mg/kg intravenously) for severe anaphylaxis in an attempt to modulate the late-phase response [9]. Patients who have been receiving glucocorticosteroid therapy for other reasons should be assumed to have hypothalamic–pituitary–adrenal axis suppression and should be administered stress doses of hydrocortisone intravenously during resuscitation. If wheezing is prominent, an aerosolized $\tilde{\beta}$-adrenergic agent (e.g. albuterol) is recommended intermittently or continuously depending on the patient's symptoms and the availability of cardiac monitoring. Intravenous aminopylline may also be useful for recalcitrant respiratory symptoms. Aerosolized epinephrine may be useful for preventing life-threatening upper airway edema, however in about 10%, a tracheotomy may be required to prevent fatal laryngeal obstruction [99]. Hypotension, due to a shift in fluid from the intravascular to extravascular space, may be severe and refractory to epinephrine and antihistamines. Depending on the blood pressure, large volumes of crystalloid (e.g. lactated Ringer's solution or normal saline) infused rapidly are frequently required to reverse the hypotensive state [100]. An alternative to crystalloid solution is the colloid, hydroxyethal starch. Children may need up to 30 ml/kg of crystalloid over the first hour [101] and adults up to 2 l [66] over the first hour to control hypotension. Patients taking $\tilde{\beta}$-blockers may require much larger volumes (e.g. 5–7 l) of fluid before pressure is stabilized [102].

Although epinephrine and fluids are the mainstay of treatment for hypotension, the use of other vasopressor drugs may be necessary [11,103]. Dopamine administered at a rate of 2–20 μg/kg/minute while carefully monitoring the blood pressure may be lifesaving. In addition, 1–5 mg of glucagon given as a bolus followed by an infusion of 5–15 μg/minute titrated against clinical response may be helpful in refractory cases or in patients taking $\tilde{\beta}$-blockers. The best approach to treating patients experiencing anaphylaxis while taking β-adrenergic blocking drugs remains uncertain. If combined β_1 and β_2 receptor blockers (e.g. propranolol) are used, it may be possible to administer epinephrine for its α-adrenergic activity and isoproterenol to attempt to overcome the β-blockade. Since patients may experience a biphasic response, all patients should be monitored for a minimum of 4 hours, longer in cases of more severe anaphylaxis [9].

Although controversial, some authorities have suggested the use of activated charcoal in an attempt to prevent further absorption of food allergens from the gut [104]. However, the volume required and the disagreeable taste often precludes patients from taking adequate quantities and the consequences of aspiration are grave. Others have suggested that some attempt should be made to evacuate the stomach, if vomiting has not already occurred, such as gastric lavage when large amounts of the allergen have been ingested. Whether or not these measures are beneficial in ameliorating food-induced anaphylaxis remains to be demonstrated.

Patients who are at risk for food-induced anaphylaxis should have medical information concerning their condition available to them at all times, for example, Medic Alert™ bracelet or necklace. This information may be lifesaving since it will expedite the diagnosis and appropriate treatment for a patient experiencing an anaphylactic reaction.

Long-term management (Table 13.6)

The life-threatening nature of anaphylaxis makes prevention the cornerstone of therapy. If the causative food allergen is not clearly delineated, an evaluation to determine the etiology should be promptly initiated so that a lethal reoccurrence can be prevented, as discussed above. The central focus of prevention of food-induced anaphylaxis requires the appropriate identification and complete dietary avoidance of the specific food allergen [9], especially those at higher risk for anaphylaxis, as discussed previously. An educational process is imperative to ensure the patient and family understands how to avoid all forms of the food allergen and the potential severity of a reaction if the food is inadvertently ingested. The *Food Allergy and Anaphylaxis Network* is a non-profit organization in Fairfax, Virginia, USA (Phone: 703-691-3179 or 800-929-4040; Fax: 703-691-2713; http://www.foodallergy.org) which can assist in providing patients information about food allergen avoidance and which has several programs for schools and parents of children with food allergies and anaphylaxis. Self-injectable epinephrine should be prescribed and patients/parents should be thoroughly educated in the use of the device.

It is not uncommon for patients experiencing a previous food-allergic reaction to subsequently demonstrate some instinctive avoidance measure. This may be typified by extreme dislike for the taste or even smell of the offending food. A very proactive role is required for the sensitized person to completely avoid a food that has caused a previous anaphylactic reaction. For many this may even require total removal of the food from the household. Educational measures must be directed at the patient, his/her family, and school personnel and other caretakers or fellow workers so that they understand the potential severity and scope of the problem. If a patient ingests a food prepared outside the home, they must always be very cautious and not hesitate to ask very specific and detailed questions concerning ingredients of foods they are planning to eat. Unfortunately, it is not uncommon for patients dining in restaurants to ingest a food that they were assured did not exist in the meal they were eating.

Table 13.6 Long-term management of food-induced anaphylaxis

- Identify positive food which provoked anaphylactic reaction
- Educate patient, family, and/or care providers how to avoid all exposure to food allergen
- Provide patient at risk with self-injectable epinephrine and thoroughly teach them when and how to use this medication (i.e. practice with Epi-Pen[R] trainer)
- Provide patient with liquid antihistamine (diphenhydramine or hydroxyzine) and teach them when and how to use this medication
- Establish a formal *Emergency Plan* in case of a reaction: proper use of "emergency medications" transportation to nearest emergency facility (capable of resuscitation and endotracheal tube placement)

Although changes in food labeling laws in the United States have simplified somewhat the reading of labels for food-allergic individuals, several problems still remain. These problems fall into one of the four categories: (1) misleading labels, for example "non-dairy" creamers usually contain some milk proteins; (2) ingredient switches, for example a name brand food may alter the ingredients with no significant change on the label; (3) "natural flavoring" designation often allows a product to contain a small amount of other food proteins for purposes of flavoring without having to identify that protein, for example casein in canned tuna fish; and (4) inadvertent contamination which may occur when more than one product is run on a line and residual protein from the previous run adulterates the subsequent run, for example non-dairy ice cream desserts. It is still imperative that patients and their families scrupiously read all labels of products because certain food allergens may unexpectedly occur.

Prognosis

For many young children diagnosed with anaphylaxis to foods such as milk, egg, wheat, and soybeans, there is a good possibility that the clinical sensitivity may be outgrown after several years. Children who develop their food sensitivity after 3 years of age are less likely to lose their food reactions over a several year period. Approximately 20% of children who develop peanut allergy early in life [46,47] will outgrow this sensitivity. There are rare reports of children who appear to outgrow their peanut allergy only to have allergic reactivity recur at a later date [105,106]. Allergies to foods such as tree nuts, fish, and seafood are generally not outgrown and these individuals appear likely to retain their allergic sensitivity for a lifetime. With better characterization of allergens and understanding of the immunological mechanism involved in this reaction, investigators have developed several therapeutic modalities potentially applicable to the treatment and eventual prevention of food allergy. Among the therapeutic options currently under investigation, there is peptide immunotherapy, mutated allergen protein immunotherapy, DNA immunization, immunization with immunostimulatory sequences, a Chinese herbal formulation, and anti-IgE therapy [107–109]. These novel forms of treatment for allergic disease hold promise for the safe and effective treatment of food-allergic individuals and the prevention of food allergy in the future.

References

1 Sheffer A. Anaphylaxis. *J Allergy Clin Immunol* 1985;75:227–33.

2 Portier P, Richet C. De l'action anaphylactique de certains venins. *C R Soc Biol (Paris)* 1902;54:170–2.

3 Anderson J, Sogn D. *Adverse Reactions to Foods.* In: Anderson J, Sogn D (eds.) NIH Publication No. 84-2442, 2. Bethesda, MD: National Institute of Allergy and Infectious Disease, 1984.

4 Golbert TM, Patterson R, Pruzansky JJ. Systemic allergic reactions to ingested antigens. *J Allergy* 1969;44:96–107.

5 Yunginger JW, Sweeney KG, Sturner WQ, *et al.* Fatal food-induced anaphylaxis. *JAMA* 1988;260:1450–2.

6 Sampson HA, Mendelson LM, Rosen JP. Fatal and near-fatal anaphylactic reactions to food in children and adolescents. *N Engl J Med* 1992;327:380–4.

7 Bock SA, Munoz-Furlong A, Sampson HA. Fatalities due to anaphylactic reactions to foods. *J Allergy Clin Immunol* 2001;107:191–3.

8 Bock SA, Munoz-Furlong A, Sampson HA. Further fatalities caused by anaphylactic reactions to food, 2001–2006. *J Allergy Clin Immunol* 2007;119:1016–18.

9 Sampson HA, Munoz-Furlong A, Bock A, *et al.* Symposium on the definition and management of anaphylaxis: summary report. *J Allergy Clin Immunol* 2005;115:584–91.

10 Lieberman P. Biphasic anaphylactic reactions. *Ann Allergy Asthma Immunol* 2005;95:217–26.

11 Sampson HA. Anaphylaxis and emergency treatment. *Pediatrics* 2003;111:1601–8.

12 Sicherer SH, Sampson HA. Food allergy. *J Allergy Clin Immunol* 2006;117:S470–5.

13 Sampson HA, Munoz-Furlong A, Campbell RL, *et al.* Second symposium on the definition and management of anaphylaxis: summary report – second National Institute of Allergy and Infectious Disease/Food Allergy and Anaphylaxis Network Symposium. *Ann Emerg Med* 2006;47:373–80.

14 Klein JS, Yocum MW. Underreporting of anaphylaxis in a community emergency room. *J Allergy Clin Immunol* 1995;95:637–8.

15 Sorensen H, Nielsen B, Nielsen J. Anaphylactic shock occurring outside hospitals. *Allergy* 1989;44:288–90.

16 Yocum MW, Khan DA. Assessment of patients who have experienced anaphylaxis: a 3-year survey. *Mayo Clin Proc* 1994;69:16–23.

17 Bock S. The incidence of severe adverse reactions to food in Colorado. *J Allergy Clin Immunol* 1992;90:683–5.

18 Yocum MW, Butterfield JH, Klein JS, *et al.* Epidemiology of anaphylaxis in Olmsted County: a population-based study. *J Allergy Clin Immunol* 1999;104:452–6.

19 Grundy J, Matthews S, Bateman B, *et al.* Rising prevalence of allergy to peanut in children: data from 2 sequential cohorts. *J Allergy Clin Immunol* 2002;110:784–9.

20 Sicherer SH, Munoz-Furlong A, Sampson HA. Prevalence of peanut and tree nut allergy in the United States determined by means of a random digit dial telephone survey: a 5-year follow-up study. *J Allergy Clin Immunol* 2003;112:1203–7.

21 Pumphrey RSH, Stanworth SJ. The clinical spectrum of anaphylaxis in north-west England. *Clin Exper Allergy* 1996;26:1364–70.

22 Moneret-Vautrin DA, Kanny G. Food-induced anaphylaxis. A new French multicenter survey. *Ann Gastroenterol Hepatol (Paris)* 1995;31:256–63.

23 Novembre E, Cianferoni A, Bernardini R, *et al.* Anaphylaxis in children: clinical and allergologic features. *Pediatrics* 1998;101:E8.

24 Boros CA, Kay D, Gold MS. Parent reported allergy and anaphylaxis in 4173 south Australian children. *J Paediatr Child Health* 2000;36:36–40.

25 Simons FER, Chad Z, Gold MS. Anaphylaxis in children: real-time reporting from a national network. *Allergy Clin Immunol Int J World Allergy Org* 2004;242–4.

26 Dibs SD, Baker MD. Anaphylaxis in children: a 5-year experience. *Pediatrics* 1997;99:E7.

27 Braganza SC, Acworth JP, Mckinnon DRL, *et al*. Paediatric emergency department anaphylaxis: different patterns from adults. *Arch Dis Child* 2006;91:159–63.

28 Brown AF, McKinnon D, Chu K. Emergency department anaphylaxis: a review of 142 patients in a single year. *J Allergy Clin Immunol* 2001;108:861–6.

29 Kidd J, Cohen S, Sosman A, Fink J. Food-dependent exercise-induced anaphylaxis. *J Allergy Clin Immunol* 1983;71:407–11.

30 Novey H, Fairshter R, Sainess K, *et al*. Postprandial exercise-induced anaphylaxis. *J Allergy Clin Immunol* 1983;71:498–504.

31 Dohi M, Suko M, Sugiyama H, *et al*. Food-dependent exercise-induced anaphylaxis: a study on 11 Japanese cases. *J Allergy Clin Immunol* 1991;87:34–40.

32 Horan R, Sheffer A. Food-dependent exercise-induced anaphylaxis. *Immunol Allergy Clin North Am* 1991;11:757–66.

33 Romano M, di Fonso M, Guiffreda F, *et al*. Food-dependent exercise-induced anaphylaxis: clinical and laboratory findings in 54 subjects. *Int Arch Allergy Appl Immunol* 2001;125:264–72.

34 Morita E, Kunie K, Matsuo H. Food-dependent exercise-induced anaphylaxis. *J Dermatol Sci* 2007;47:109–17.

35 Du TG. Food-dependent exercise-induced anaphylaxis in childhood. *Pediatr Allergy Immunol* 2007;18:455–63.

36 Harada S, Horikawa T, Ashida M, *et al*. Aspirin enhances the induction of type I allergic symptoms when combined with food and exercise in patients with food-dependent exercise-induced anaphylaxis. *Br J Dermatol* 2001;145:336–9.

37 Aihara M, Miyazawa M, Osuna H, *et al*. Food-dependent exercise-induced anaphylaxis: influence of concurrent aspirin administration on skin testing and provocation. *Br J Dermatol* 2002;146:466–72.

38 Matsuo H, Morimoto K, Akaki T, *et al*. Exercise and aspirin increase levels of circulating gliadin peptides in patients with wheat-dependent exercise-induced anaphylaxis. *Clin Exp Allergy* 2005;35:461–6.

39 Simons FE, Frew AJ, Ansotegui IJ, *et al*. Risk assessment in anaphylaxis: current and future approaches. *J Allergy Clin Immunol* 2007;120:S2–24.

40 Settipane G, Klein D, Boyd G. Relationship of atopy and anaphylactic sensitization: a bee sting allergy model. *Clin Allergy* 1978;8:259–64.

41 Sicherer SH, Furlong TJ, Maes HH, *et al*. Genetics of peanut allergy: a twin study. *J Allergy Clin Immunol* 2000;106:53–6.

42 Wood RA. The natural history of food allergy. *Pediatrics* 2003;111:1631–7.

43 Cantani A, Micera M. Natural history of cow's milk allergy. An eight-year follow-up study in 115 atopic children. *Eur Rev Med Pharmacol Sci* 2004;8:153–64.

44 Bock SA, Atkins FM. The natural history of peanut allergy. *J Allergy Clin Immunol* 1989;83:900–4.

45 Sampson HA. Update on food allergy. *J Allergy Clin Immunol* 2004;113:805–19.

46 Hourihane JO'B, Roberts SA, Warner JO. Resolution of peanut allergy: case-control study. *BMJ* 1998;316:1271–5.

47 Skolnick HS, Conover-Walker MK, Koerner CB, *et al*. The natural history of peanut allergy. *J Allergy Clin Immunol* 2001;107:367–74.

48 Fleischer DM, Conover-Walker MK, Matsui EC, Wood RA. The natural history of tree nut allergy. *J Allergy Clin Immunol* 2005;116:1087–93.

49 Sampson HA. Clinical practice. Peanut allergy. *N Engl J Med* 2002;346:1294–9.

50 Sampson HA. Update of food allergy. *J Allergy Clin Immunol* 2004;113:805–19.

51 Sicherer SH, Burks AW, Sampson HA. Clinical features of acute allergic reactions to peanut and tree nuts in children. *Pediatrics* 1998;102:e6.

52 Sicherer SH, Munoz-Furlong A, Burks AW, Sampson HA. Prevalence of peanut and tree nut allergy in the United States of America. *J Allergy Clin Immunol* 1999;103:559–62.

53 Lack G, Fox D, Northstone K, Golding J. Factors associated with the development of peanut allergy in childhood. *N Engl J Med* 2003;348:977–85.

54 Moneret-Vautrin D, Beaudouin E, Widmer S, *et al*. Prospective study of risk factors in natural rubber latex hypersensitivity. *J Allergy Clin Immunol* 1993;92:668–77.

55 Warner J, Miles E, Jones A, *et al*. Is deficiency of interferon gamma production by allergen triggered cord blood cells a predictor of atopic disease? *Clin Exp Allergy* 1994;24:423–30.

56 Prenner B, Stevens J. Anaphylaxis after ingestion of sodium bisulfite. *Ann Allergy* 1976;37:180–2.

57 Twarog F, Leung D. Anaphylaxis to a component of isoetharine (sodium bisulfite). *JAMA* 1982;248:2031.

58 Clayton D, Busse W. Anaphylaxis to wine. *Clin Allergy* 1980;10:341–3.

59 Mansfield L, Bowers C. Systemic reaction to papain in a nonoccupational setting. *J Allergy Clin Immunol* 1983;71:371–4.

60 Allen D, Delohery J, Baker G. Monosodium L-glutamate-induced asthma. *J Allergy Clin Immunol* 1987;80:530–7.

61 Lee JM, Greenes DS. Biphasic anaphylactic reactions in pediatrics. *Pediatrics* 2000;106:762–6.

62 Webb LM, Lieberman P. Anaphylaxis: a review of 601 cases. *Ann Allergy Asthma Immunol* 2006;97:39–43.

63 Sampson HA. Anaphylaxis and emergency treatment. *Pediatrics* 2004;111:1601–8.

64 Brown SGA. Clinical features and severity grading of anaphylaxis. *J Allergy Clin Immunol* 2004;114:371–6.

65 Fisher MM. Clinical observations on the pathophysiology and treatment of anaphylactic cardiovascular collapse. *Anaesth Intens Care* 1986;14:17–21.

66 Brown SGA. Cardiovascular aspects of anaphylaxis: implications for treatment and diagnosis. *Curr Opin Allergy Clin Immunol* 2005;5:359–64.

67 Pumphrey RSH. Fatal posture in anaphylactic shock. *J Allergy Clin Immunol* 2003;112:451–2.

68 Settipane G, Chafee R, Klein DE, *et al*. Anaphylactic reactions to Hymenoptera stings in asthmatic patients. *Clin Allergy* 1980;10:659–65.

69 Lockey R, Benedict L, Turkeltaub P, Bukantz S. Fatalities form immunotherapy and skin testing. *J Allergy Clin Immunol* 1987;79:660–7.

70 Reid MJ, Lockey RF, Turkeltaub PC, Platts-Mills TA. Survey of fatalities from skin testing and immunotherapy 1985–1989. *J Allergy Clin Immunol* 1993;92:6–15.

71 Helbling A, Hurni T, Mueller UR, Pichler WJ. Incidence of anaphylaxis with circulatory symptoms: a study over a 3-year period comprising 940,000 inhabitants of the Swiss Canton Bern. *Clin Exp Allergy* 2004;34:285–90.

72 Gern J, Yang E, Evrard H, Sampson H. Allergic reactions to milk-contaminated "non-dairy" products. *N Engl J Med* 1991;324:976–9.

73 Tricker ND, Malone KM, Ellis MM. Hereditary angioedema: a case report and literature review. *Gen Dent* 2002;50:540–3.

74 Frank MM. Hereditary angioedema: the clinical syndrome and its management in the United States. *Immunol Allergy Clin North Am* 2006;26:653–68.

75 Alboni P, Brignole M, Degli Uberti EC. Is vasovagal syncope a disease? *Europace* 2007;9:83–7.

76 Wakita R, Ohno Y, Yamazaki S, *et al*. Vasovagal syncope with asystole associated with intravenous access. *Oral Surg Oral Med Oral Pathol Oral Radiol Endod* 2006;102:e28–32.

77 Settipane G, Chafee F. Natural history of allergy of Hymenoptera. *Clin Allergy* 1979;9:385–90.

78 Ortolani C, Ispano M, Pastorello EA, *et al*. Comparison of results of skin prick tests (with fresh foods and commercial food extracts) and RAST in 100 patients with oral allergy syndrome. *J Allergy Clin Immunol* 1989;83:683–90.

79 Rosen J, Selcow J, Mendelson L, *et al*. Skin testing with natural foods in patients suspected of having food allergies: Is it necessary? *J Allergy Clin Immunol* 1994;93:1068–70.

80 Stricker W, Anorve-Lopez E, Reed C. Food skin testing in patients with idiopathic anaphylaxis. *J Allergy Clin Immunol* 1986;77:516–19.

81 Bock S, Buckley J, Holst A, May C. Proper use of skin tests with food extracts in diagnosis of food hypersensitivity. *Clin Allergy* 1978;8:559–64.

82 Lockey RF. Adverse reactions associated with skin testing and immunotherapy. *Allergy Proc* 1995;16:293–6.

83 Sampson HA. Utility of food-specific IgE concentrations in predicting symptomatic food allergy. *J Allergy Clin Immun* 2001;107:891–6.

84 Yuninger JW, Ahlstedt S, Eggleston PA, *et al*. Quantitative IgE antibody assays in allergic diseases. *J Allergy Clin Immunol* 2000;105:1077–84.

85 Shreffler WG, Beyer K, Burks AW, Sampson HA. Microarray immunoassay: association of clinical history, *in vitro* IgE function, and heterogeneity of allergenic peanut epitopes. *J Allergy Clin Immunol* 2004;113:776–82.

86 Schwartz L, Metcalfe D, Miller J, *et al*. Tryptase levels as an indicator of mast cell activation in systemic anaphylaxis and mastocytosis. *N Engl J Med* 1987;316:1622–6.

87 Schwartz L, Yuninger J, Miller J, *et al*. The time course of appearance and disappearance of human mast cell tryptase in the circulation after anaphylaxis. *J Clin Invest* 1989;83:1551–5.

88 Lin RY, Schwartz LB, Curry A, *et al*. Histamine and tryptase levels in patients with acute allergic reactions: an emergency department-based study. *J Allergy Clin Immunol* 2000;106:65–71.

89 Brown SGA, Blackmean KE, Heddle RJ. Can serum mast cell tryptase help diagnose anaphylaxis? *Emerg Med Australasia* 2004;16:120–4.

90 Barnard J. Studies of 400 Hymentoptera sting deaths in the United States. *J Allergy Clin Immunol* 1973;52:259–64.

91 Clark S, Bock SA, Gaeta TJ, *et al*. Multicenter study of emergency department visits for food allergies. *J Allergy Clin Immunol* 2004;113:347–52.

92 Brown SGA, Blackmean KE, Stenlake V, Heddle RJ. Insect sting anaphylaxis; prospective evaluation of treatment with intravenous adrenaline and volume resuscitation. *Emerg Med J* 2004;21:149–54.

93 Simons FE, Gu X, Silver NA, Simons KJ. EpiPen Jr versus EpiPen in young children weighing 15 to 30kg at risk for anaphylaxis. *J Allergy Clin Immunol* 2002;109:171–5.

94 Simons FE, Chan ES, Gu X, Simons KJ. Epinephrine for the out-of-hospital (first-aid) treatment of anaphylaxis in infants: Is the ampule/syringe/needle method practical? *J Allergy Clin Immunol* 2001;108:1040–4.

95 Muller U, Mosbech H, Aberer W, *et al*. EAACI position statement: adrenaline for emergency kits. *Allergy* 1995;50:783–7.

96 Warren J, Doble N, Dalton N, Ewan P. Systemic absorption of inhaled epinephrine. *Clin Pharmacol Ther* 1986;40:673–8.

97 Simons FE, Gu X, Johnston LM, Simons KJ. Can epinephrine inhalations be substituted for epinephrine injection in children at risk for systemic anaphylaxis? *Pediatrics* 2000;106:1040–4.

98 Kambam J, Merrill W, Smith B. Histamine-2 receptor blocker in the treatment of protamine-related anaphylactoid reactions: two case reports. *Can J Anaesth* 1989;36:463–5.

99 Delage C, Irey N. Anaphylactic deaths: a clinicopathologic study of 43 cases. *J Forensic Sci* 1972;17:525–40.

100 Brown AFT. Anaphylactic shock – mechanisms and treatment. *J Accident Emerg Med* 1995;12:89–100.

101 Saryan J, O'Loughlin J. Anaphylaxis in children. *Pediatr Ann* 1992;21:590–8.

102 Eon B, Papazian L, Gouin F. Management of anaphylaxis and anaphylactoid reactions during anesthesia. *Clin Rev Allergy* 1991;9:415–29..

103 Lieberman P, Kemp SF, Oppenheimer JJ, *et al*. The diagnosis and management of anaphylaxis: an updated practice parameter. *J Allergy Clin Immunol* 2005;115:S485–523.

104 Vadas P, Perelman B. Activated charcoal forms non-IgE binding complexes with peanut proteins. *J Allergy Clin Immunol* 2003;112:175–9.

105 Busse PJ, Nowak-Wegrzyn A, Noone SA, *et al.* Recurrent peanut allergy. *N Engl J Med* 2002;347:1535–8.

106 Fleischer DM, Connover-Walker MK, Christie DL, *et al.* Peanut allergy: recurrence and its management. *J Allergy Clin Immunol* 2004;114:1195–202.

107 Nowak-Wegrzyn A, Sampson HA. Food allergy therapy. *Immunol Allergy Clin North Am* 2004;24:705–25.

108 Pons L, Palmer K, Burks W. Towards immunotherapy for peanut allergy. *Curr Opin Allergy Clin Immunol* 2005;5: 558–62.

109 Sicherer SH, Sampson HA. Peanut allergy: emerging concepts and approaches for an apparent epidemic. *J Allergy Clin Immunol* 2007;120:491–503.

CHAPTER 14

Infantile Colic and Food Allergy

Ralf G. Heine, David J. Hill, and Clifford S. Hosking

KEY CONCEPTS

- The term "infantile colic" describes episodes of paroxysmal unexplained crying and fussing (for more than 3 hours per day) in otherwise healthy infants less than 3 months of age.

- Although the etiology of colic is multi-factorial, there is increasing evidence linking this condition to gastrointestinal food protein allergies (non-IgE-mediated).

- In breast-fed infants, hypersensitivity reactions may be caused by ingestion of intact food proteins contained in breast milk.

- In formula-fed infants, extensively hydrolyzed (casein- or whey-predominant) or amino-acid-based formulas have been shown to improve colic symptoms, whereas soy, partially hydrolyzed or lactose-free cow's milk formulas offered no therapeutic benefit.

- Maternal elimination diets have been shown to significantly reduce the crying duration in breast-fed infants with colic presenting before 6 weeks of age.

Introduction

Persistent crying is a common pediatric problem that affects up to 28% of young infants [1]. In the majority, the distressed behavior commences at 2 weeks of age, peaks at about 6 weeks, and gradually improves toward 3–4 months of age [2,3]. However, a recent Canadian study showed that 6.4% of infants still had colic at 3 months of age [4]. Although the etiology of infantile colic is multi-factorial, there is increasing evidence linking persistent crying and distress in the young infant to food allergy [5–7]. Interactive factors and behavior patterning also influence the clinical course of infantile colic [8].

Crying and fussing, especially in the evening, are normal developmental phenomena in the first months of life [2]. Unexplained paroxysms of irritability, fussing, or crying that persist for more than 3 hours per day, for more than 3 days per week, and for at least 3 weeks, are considered a separate clinical condition termed "colic" [3,9]. During such episodes the legs may be drawn up to the abdomen and the infant may become flushed. Abdominal distension and increased passage of flatus are often noted. Parents may attribute these episodes to pain. However, the infant appears generally well,

and it has been suggested that in less than 5% of infants an underlying medical etiology can be identified [8].

Epidemiology of colic

Prevalence figures for infantile colic vary greatly, depending on the definition of colic and recruitment method used in epidemiological studies [1,10]. No population-based prevalence study, using generally accepted diagnostic criteria for colic, has to date been performed. Many studies are biased toward severe colic or families presenting in crisis [1]. For example, mothers with depressive symptoms may be more likely to seek help for their crying infant [11,12]. In addition, parents perceive persistent crying as more worrisome if there are associated symptoms such as regurgitation [13] or feeding difficulties [14] which may lead to an overestimate of underlying medical conditions. Table 14.1 shows the varying prevalence of colic reported from several Western countries.

Clinical classification of crying syndromes

The etiology of infantile colic is multi-factorial. Our understanding of the mechanisms leading to distressed behavior in early infancy is incomplete. The term "colic" implies that the infants' distress is related to visceral pain or spasm, although such a mechanism has never been conclusively demonstrated. For this reason, alternative terms such as "persistent crying" or "distressed behavior" have been used.

Food Allergy: Adverse Reactions to Foods and Food Additives, 4th edition.
Edited by Dean D. Metcalfe, Hugh A. Sampson, and Ronald A. Simon.
© 2008 Blackwell Publishing, ISBN: 978-1-4501-5129-0.

In the following discussion, the term "colic" will be used interchangeably with each of these terms while not implying a particular pathological mechanism.

Barr has suggested four main crying syndromes in infancy [8]. These syndromes are difficult to define and may overlap clinically:

- Infantile colic.
- Persistent mother–infant-distress syndrome.
- The temperamentally "difficult" infant.
- The dysregulated infant.

According to this model, infantile colic is considered part of normal emotional development, in which an infant displays diminished capacity to regulate crying duration [8]. If colic is unresolved for several weeks, this may lead to disturbances in the mother–infant relationship, that is the persistent mother–infant-distress syndrome; this group often presents with associated organic manifestations. These may include feeding difficulties [14,18], gastroesophageal reflux (GER) [18–21], esophagitis [22], lactose malabsorption [23,24], or gastrointestinal motility disturbance [25–27]. Many of these manifestations have been linked to food protein allergy [28]. The temperamentally "difficult" infant may be predisposed to negative affect and have an increased tendency for persistent crying. The last category, the "dysregulated" infant, is thought to have a central dysregulation leading to poor self-calming, poor tolerance to change, and hyper-alert arousal.

Infantile and parental factors associated with infantile colic

Infantile factors

Brazelton [2] used parental recording on cry charts to document the natural history of distressed behavior in infancy. Figure 14.1 summarizes the pattern of crying and fussing in a group of 80 non-colicky infants studied in the first 12 weeks of life. Distressed behavior frequently deteriorated until infants were about 6 weeks of age, and then gradually improved. In the majority of infants, fussing behavior

occurred during the late afternoon and evening [2,9]. Barr *et al.* [28] developed 24-hour cry charts which they validated against voice-activated audiotape recordings (VAR) of crying infants. Using these validated cry charts, Hunziker and Barr [37] confirmed Brazelton's [2] findings.

Studies by our group compared the pattern and duration of distressed behavior in 30 colicky and non-colicky infants [38]. Figure 14.2 shows the higher levels of distressed behavior in the colicky infants compared to non-colicky infants. The evaluation of distressed behavior on an hour-by-hour basis found a predominance of nocturnal symptoms, but prolonged episodes of crying also occurred during other periods of the day. These prolonged and inconsolable episodes of crying appear to be features that are specific for infantile colic in the first weeks of life [39].

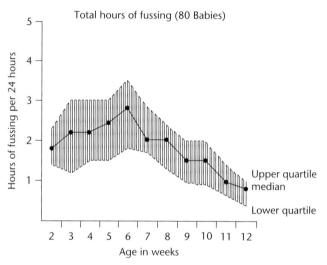

Figure 14.1 Total crying duration per 24 hours in 80 infants during the first 12 weeks of life (Reproduced from Brazelton TB [2], with permission.)

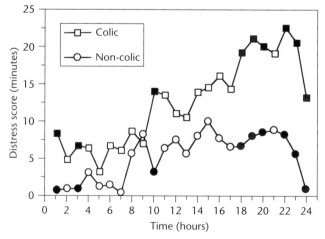

Figure 14.2 Comparison of diurnal variation in distress scores for infants with and without colic; hourly mean duration of crying and fussing time, recorded over 24 hours. Filled symbols mark periods with a significant difference in crying and fussing between groups ($p < 0.05$) [38].

Table 14.1 Prevalence of infantile colic

Author	Country	Year	Prevalence (%)
Hide and Guyer [29]	England	1982	16
Rubin and Prendergast [30]	England	1984	26
Carey [31]	USA	1984	10
Lothe [32]	Sweden	1989	17
Michelsson *et al.* [33]	Finland	1990	14
Hogdall *et al.* [34]	Denmark	1991	19
Rautava *et al.* [12]	Finland	1993	28
Lehtonen and Korvenranta [35]	Finland	1995	13
Canivet *et al.* [15]	Sweden	1996	11
Canivet *et al.* [16]	Sweden	2002	9.4
Clifford *et al.* [17]	Canada	2002	24
Wake *et al.* [36]	Australia	2006	19.1

Children with a past history of colic are at increased risk of experiencing negative emotions, negative moods, during meals and more likely to report abdominal pain in early childhood, suggesting that infant temperament may be a factor contributing to infantile colic [40]. However, the majority of colicky infants will develop normal parent–child interactions and relationships, and only a small number will progress to a more generalized "persistent mother–infant-distress syndrome" [41]. A recent Australian study of distressed infants found that persistent crying and sleep problems in the first 2 years of life are usually transient [36]. A 10-year follow-up study of 96 infants with a history of infantile colic showed a high prevalence of recurrent abdominal pain, allergic disorders, and psychological abnormalities [42]. Unremitting, severe persistent crying beyond 3 months of age may also be a marker of cognitive deficits in later childhood [43].

Maternal factors

The unpredictable, prolonged, and unexplained nature of crying in colicky infants is a source of great concern and anxiety for parents [44,45]. Maternal anxiety during late pregnancy has been shown to be a risk factor for infantile colic [46]. Studies by Rautava *et al.* in Finnish infants suggested an association between colic and maternal distress during pregnancy and childbirth or unsatisfactory sexual relationships, but not between colic and socio-demographic factors [47]. Mothers who report excessive infant crying are also more likely to perceive a lack of positive reinforcement from their infant [48].

Maternal report of a sleep problem in their infant was significantly associated with depressive symptoms [10]. This may indicate that maternal depressive symptoms during the early infant period are caused by, or compounded by, sleep deprivation. A recent study reported that persistent, rather than transient, infant distress was associated with maternal depression and parent stress [36].

Behavior interventions and parental support

Several studies have assessed the importance of behavioral and interactive factors in infantile colic. The results of these studies are summarized in Table 14.2. Taubman [49] compared parental counseling and dietary interventions in a study of 21 colicky infants. He found that increasing parental responsiveness had a similar effect on persistent crying as the introduction of a cow's milk-free diet. Interestingly, the distressed behavior of diet-responsive colicky infants decreased further with parental counseling.

Barr *et al.* [50] studied the effect of supplemental carrying on 66 colicky infants. In 6-week-old colicky infants, a significant treatment benefit of supplemental carrying could not be demonstrated. Wolke *et al.* [51] examined the effect of different supportive strategies in 92 mothers of infants with colic. After 3 months, infant distress had improved in all patients. Infants of mothers who had received advice on behavior modification improved their distress by 51%, compared with 37% in infants of mothers who were receiving empathic support, and 35% in the control group.

Colic as a manifestation of food protein allergy

Several trials have demonstrated a treatment benefit for soy and extensively hydrolyzed formulas in infants with colic, even when no other symptoms of food protein allergies were evident (Table 14.3). Irritability is a common finding in infants with allergy to cow's milk and other food proteins [5,28]. Some infants may also react to soy formula or

Table 14.2 Studies investigating disturbed family interaction as a cause of colic

Author	Study details	Outcome: change in distress (hours per 24-hour period)
Hunziker and Barr [37][a]	Carrying (n = 49) Control (n = 50)	1.2 2.2 (p < 0.001)
Barr et al. [50]	Carrying (n = 31) Control (n = 35)	3.3 3.4 (p > 0.05)
Taubman [49]	Counseling (n = 10) Diet (n = 10)	3.2 versus 1.06 (p = 0.001) 3.2 versus 2.03 (p = 0.01)
Wolke et al. [51]	Empathy (n = 27) Behavior modification (n = 21) Control (n = 44)	6.3 versus 3.7 (p < 0.001) 5.8 versus 2.8 (p < 0.001)[b] 5.7 versus 3.7 (p < 0.001)

[a]Study of non-colic infants.
[b]Behavior modification superior to empathy and control (p < 0.02).

Table 14.3 Studies supporting the role of diet as a cause of infantile colic

Author	Study details	Outcome
Jakobsson and Lindberg [52]	Breast (n = 10)	Conditional probability of 95% that intact when protein is implicated in colic
Evans et al. [53]	Breast (n = 20)	Range of maternal diet significant (p < 0.05)
Lothe and Lindberg [54]	Formula (n = 24)	Casein hydrolysate 1.0 hours versus intact whey protein 3.2 hours (p < 0.001)
Forsyth [55]	Formula (n = 17)	Cow's milk distress > casein hydrolysate distress (p < 0.01)
Lucassen et al. [56]	Formula (n = 43)	Difference in decrease of crying by 63 minutes/day for extensively hydrolyzed whey formula compared to standard formula (p < 0.05)

extensively hydrolyzed formula preparations [57,58]. In a sequential cohort of 100 patients with challenge-proven cow's milk allergy (CMA), 44% of infants displayed irritable and colicky behavior during the cow's milk challenge procedure [59].

Cow's milk allergy and colic

Cow's milk challenge in young children suspected of having CMA elicited a range of diverse manifestations [59–62]. Three clinical groups of CMA were identified based on the timing of reactions (immediate, intermediate, and late onset) [59]. Children who developed immediate reactions reacted to small volumes of cow's milk within 1 hour of commencing the challenge. Infants with intermediate reactions tolerated 60–200 ml of cow's milk, before vomiting and diarrhea developed after several hours. The third group with late-onset reactions usually tolerated greater volumes of cow's milk before gastrointestinal, cutaneous, or respiratory symptoms of CMA developed after 24–72 hours. Interestingly, the prevalence of distressed behavior after cow's milk challenge was similar in the three groups, suggesting that distressed behavior in infants with CMA may be due to several immunological mechanisms.

Food allergy in breast-fed infants

There is increasing evidence that maternal ingested food antigens are secreted into human milk and elicit clinical adverse reactions in the breast-fed infant [63–66]. Sensitization to multiple food antigens has been described in breast-fed infants [67]. Several intact dietary antigens have been demonstrated in breast milk, including β-lactoglobulin [65], ovalbumin [66], peanut [68], and gliadin [69].

Allergic IgE sensitization may occur as early as during the fetal period [70,71]. Immunological host factors appear to mediate the sensitization to food allergens in breast milk. TGF-β is considered an important immunoregulator in promoting development of oral tolerance. During early infancy, breast milk is the main source of TGF-β. Kalliomäki et al. found that TGF-β promotes specific IgA production in human colostrum [72]. IgA antibodies in human milk have a protective effect on sensitization to food allergens as they may prevent antigen entry at the intestinal surface of infants [73]. Other factors that may mediate the immune response to ingested food antigens include regulatory lymphokines, such as TNF-α and IFN-γ. TNF-α is produced by activated macrophages and T-lymphocytes in human milk and upregulates HLA class II expression. Defective TNF-α production may be a factor impeding the development of oral tolerance to ingested food antigens in breast-fed infants [74].

Differences between breast- and formula-fed infants

In contrast to breast-fed infants, formula-fed infants often develop infantile colic before 6 weeks of age [2,75]. There

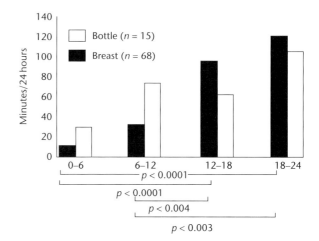

Figure 14.3 Bottle-fed infants show more distress before midday, whereas breast-fed infants have significantly more distress in the afternoon and evening [5].

are significant differences in the diurnal variation of distressed behavior between breast- and formula-fed infants. In our studies on colicky infants, we found that while the total distress levels were similar over a 24-hour period, formula-fed infants showed significantly more distress in the morning hours than breast-fed infants, whereas breast-fed infants were more distressed in the afternoon [5,38] (Fig. 14.3). Axelsson et al. [76] noted that about 4 hours after maternal cow's milk ingestion, β-lactoglobulin appeared in breast milk, and the highest concentrations of β-lactoglobulin in breast milk were found 8–12 hours after ingestion. Paganelli et al. demonstrated that cow's milk antigen appeared in serum within 1 hour of ingestion [77]. Thus, formula feeding with a large dose of ingested antigens may elicit a more rapid distress response than prolonged low-dose antigen exposure through breast milk. These observations may explain the differences in age of onset and diurnal variation of distressed behavior between breast- and formula-fed infants with colic.

Intestinal microbiota in infants with colic

There are significant differences in the composition of intestinal microbiota in infants with and without colic. Typically, bifidobacteria and lactobacilli are the predominant gut bacteria in breast-fed infants. Savino et al. [78] found that breast-fed infants with colic were less frequently colonized with lactobacilli and carried more Gram-negative gut bacteria. Also the type of lactobacilli appeared to vary between infants with and without colic. While L. lactis and L. brevis were only found in infants with colic, L. acidophilus was only found in healthy infants [69]. It remains unclear how these different bacterial microbiota are involved in the pathogenesis of infantile colic.

Development of food allergy in children with previous infantile colic

The absence of atopic manifestations in the majority of infants with colic infants suggests that non-IgE-mediated mechanisms predominate in the pathogenesis of infantile colic. However, a study from Finland suggested that infants with a history of colic are at increased risk of atopy, as compared to non-colicky infants [80]. In that study, of 116 infants with atopy at 2 years of age, 44 (38%) had presented with infantile colic. By contrast, a prospective study of 983 infants found no evidence of an increased risk for asthma and other atopic manifestations in infants with colic [81].

Infantile colic may respond to cow's milk protein elimination even in the absence of other clinical manifestations of CMA. In a study of 70 infants with severe colic, Iacono *et al.* [82] treated 70 cow's milk formula-fed infants with severe colic with soy formula. Fifty infants had improvement of colic after a change to soy formula, and their distress relapsed within 24 hours after cow's milk was reintroduced into the infants' diet [82]. Within 3 weeks, 8 of 50 infants developed soy allergy; and at the age of 9 months, 18 of 50 patients developed other symptoms of CMA at challenge. Lothe *et al.* [83] noted a similar phenomenon. Of 43 infants with colic who responded to exclusion of cow's milk, 18% showed other features of CMA by the age of 6 months, and 13% retained these features to at least 12 months of age [83]. These observations suggest that infantile colic represents an early manifestation of food allergy.

Infantile colic and gastrointestinal disorders

Gastroesophageal reflux, esophagitis, and infantile colic

Persistent distress and feeding refusal in the early infant period are frequently attributed to GER [19,20,84]. This is based on the assumption that acid reflux, even in the absence of esophagitis, may be associated with pain and feeding resistance. Crying itself does not appear to increase GER [85]. Distressed infants are often treated with anti-reflux medications on an empirical basis [18,86]. However, a causal relationship between GER and distress has never been conclusively demonstrated [19,22].

GER is considered pathological if it is associated with acid-peptic complications (esophagitis, esophageal strictures, etc.), failure to thrive, or respiratory complications (aspiration, persistent wheeze, stridor, apneic episodes). In three retrospective series of infants with severe persistent distress, abnormally frequent acid reflux was demonstrated by esophageal 24-hour pH monitoring in 15–25% of infants studied [18,22,86]. This exceeds the expected prevalence of 5–10% in young infants [87] and may in part be explained by selection bias in infants referred for gastroenterological investigation. Abnormally frequent or prolonged GER on pH monitoring usually presented with overt regurgitation and non-regurgitant "silent" GER was uncommon [18,22]. The duration of crying and fussing per day did not correlate with the severity of GER [18]. In a randomized clinical trial of infants with colic or persistent crying, treatment with ranitidine and cisapride was no better than placebo [88]. In a similar subsequent randomized trial, omeprazole, a proton pump inhibitor, was not effective in treating crying infants [89]. In that study, effective acid suppression was achieved in the infants on active medication but not on placebo. Both studies make a direct causal relationship between GER and colic unlikely [88,89].

Esophageal 24-hour pH monitoring is the definitive diagnostic test for GER. In a study of 125 distressed infants and symptoms of GER, one quarter of infants had an abnormal pH study, and one quarter had histological esophagitis. However, we found poor diagnostic agreement between abnormal pH monitoring and histological evidence of esophagitis [22]. This may indicate a non-acid-peptic etiology of the esophagitis in these infants. Esophagitis was frequently associated with gastritis or duodenitis, suggesting the presence of a more generalized upper gastrointestinal inflammatory process in infants with persistent distress [2,90].

There is evidence supporting the hypothesis that GER and esophagitis in infancy are caused by food hypersensitivity. Previous studies have provided clinical evidence of gastric dysrhythmias in infants with CMA, presenting with reflex vomiting and GER [91]. Iacono *et al.* demonstrated that in more than 42% of infants with histological esophagitis, reflux symptoms improved on hydrolyzed formula and relapsed on subsequent blinded formula challenges [92]. We have previously described a group of infants with intolerance to soy and extensively hydrolyzed formula and persistent distress attributed to reflux esophagitis, who responded to a hypoallergenic amino-acid-based formula diet (AAF) [90]. Older children with idiopathic eosinophilic esophagitis have also successfully been treated with an AAF [93]. These findings support the hypothesis of an immunologically mediated esophagitis. Recently, the infiltrate in idiopathic eosinophilic esophagitis in adult patients has been characterized as a T-helper 2-type allergic inflammatory response [94].

Colic and intestinal spasm

In a systematic review of treatments for infantile colic, dicyclomine, an anticholinergic agent, was found to be effective [6]. It is no longer used in the treatment of colic because of its potentially serious side effects in infancy [95]. The therapeutic effect in colicky infants was poorly understood but may have been due to antispasmodic properties on intestinal smooth muscle. Another anticholinergic agent, cimetropium bromide, has been shown to significantly shorten the duration of crying episodes in infants with infantile colic

[96]. This drug, a synthetic scopolamine derivative, appears to have fewer serious side effects than dicyclomine. About three quarters of infants responded to treatment with cimetropium bromide. The mean duration of crying episodes was 17.3 minutes for active medication and 47.5 minutes for placebo ($p < 0.005$). Although not conclusive, these findings may add further weight to the hypothesis that infantile colic is associated with spasmodic visceral pain that is relieved by these medications.

Animal models of food hypersensitivity have provided direct evidence of gastrointestinal spasm and motility disturbance in response to dietary antigen challenge [25]. In sensitized rats, mucosal exposure to food protein antigens resulted in gastric [97] or intestinal smooth muscle contraction [26,98]. The potential importance of disturbed gut motility in colic is further supported by the finding of increased levels of the hormone motilin, a prokinetic gastrointestinal hormone, both postnatally and at the age of onset of colicky behavior [27,99]. Maternal smoking during pregnancy and lactation has been linked to an increased risk of infantile colic and elevated serum motilin levels [100]. Serum motilin levels are higher in infants with colic, and among those infants, formula-fed infants had higher motilin levels than breast-fed infants [101]. Another gastrointestinal hormone, ghrelin, was also found to be significantly increased in infantile colic, as compared to healthy control infants [101]. These findings provide some clues to the etiology of distress in young infants and should stimulate further research into the role of abnormal gut motility in the etiology of colic in young infants.

Lactose intolerance

The role of lactose intolerance in infants with colic has remained unclear [6,7]. Lactose intolerance may occur as a result of small intestinal mucosal damage and disaccharidase depression. It is therefore possible that lactose intolerance may occur as a result of a food protein-induced enteropathy. Moore *et al.* examined the effect of lactose-containing formula on breath hydrogen production in colicky and non-colicky infants [23]. This study found that breath hydrogen concentrations, after intake of human milk or lactose-containing formula, were higher in colicky than in non-colicky infants. However, two subsequent randomized controlled trials found no significant benefit for lactase treatment of human milk or cow's milk formula [24]. A recent double-blind placebo-controlled study in 53 colicky infants has found a modest benefit of pre-incubation of feeds with lactase on colic symptoms [102]. The response to lactase treatment, however, appeared variable and the trial remained inconclusive. Low-lactose formula or pre-treatment of feeds with lactase are therefore generally not recommended as treatments for infantile colic [6,7].

Dietary treatment of colic

The self-limiting course of infantile colic makes the assessment of therapeutic interventions difficult, and no firm conclusions can be drawn unless proper double-blind placebo-controlled randomized trials are performed. However, only a few well-designed randomized trials on the treatment of colic have been conducted, and many previous studies had some shortfalls in methodology or study design. This review will focus predominantly on the role of hypoallergenic diets in the treatment of infantile colic.

Hypoallergenic formulas

Several studies have assessed the effect of dietary interventions on persistent crying, including treatment with soy- [42,103], partially hydrolyzed whey- [104], extensively hydrolyzed whey- [56], extensively hydrolyzed casein- [105], and AAFs [106,107]. Following a preliminary study, Jakobsson and Lindberg [52] noted that one-third of breast-fed infants with colic improved on maternal dietary cow's milk elimination, and relapsed on reintroduction of cow's milk into the diet. Evans *et al.* [53], however, were unable to confirm these findings. Lothe *et al.* [83] reported that 11 of 60 colic infants on cow's milk formula responded to soy formula; another 32 improved following administration of a casein hydrolysate formula. These preliminary studies have been criticized because of some methodological limitations [64,53,108].

Other more recent investigations have addressed some of these shortcomings. Lothe and Lindberg [54] implemented a 5-day cow's milk-free diet using casein hydrolysate. A marked reduction of distressed symptoms occurred in 24 of 27 colicky infants. In these infants, the total crying time decreased from 5.6 to 0.7 hours ($p < 0.001$). The 24 responding infants then entered into a randomized, double-blind, crossover trial of intact whey protein formula. Of the 24 infants challenged, 18 (two thirds of the original study population) demonstrated increased distress on whey protein challenge.

In a blinded crossover study of 17 colicky infants, casein hydrolysate alone or casein hydrolysate plus cow's milk formula were fed in sequence for four 4-day-periods [55]. Significant decreases in distressed behavior were noted after the first two formula change periods only. Over the four formula challenge periods, only 2 (11.8%) of the infants showed a reproducible effect of formula change on colic behavior. Forsyth concluded that diet was likely to be only one factor in the causation of colic [55]. He drew attention to the feelings of helplessness, frustration, and decreased confidence in parenting ability that parents of infants with colic may experience.

A recent randomized trial assessed the effect of a partially hydrolyzed whey-based formula in 199 infants with colic [104]. The formula was supplemented with prebiotic fructo- and galacto-oligosaccharides, as well as β-palmitic acid. The control group was randomized to receive either standard cow's milk formula or simethicone. Infants in the active treatment group had a significantly greater reduction in the number of crying episodes at 1 and 2 weeks than the untreated infants [104]. Further studies are required to assess the role of partially hydrolyzed formula in the prevention and treatment of colic.

The incomplete response to treatment with hypoallergenic formulas may be due to the residual allergenicity of extensively hydrolyzed whey- or casein formula [109,110]. An estimated 10–15% of infants with CMA are also intolerant of extensively hydrolyzed formula [111]. In these infants, treatment with AAF has proved effective and safe [112,113]. Recently, several groups have assessed the effect of AAF on persistent crying [58,90,106,107,114]. These preliminary studies provided evidence that AAF is effective in reducing persistent crying. However, further prospective randomized trials are required to assess the efficacy and cost-effectiveness of this approach in the community.

Maternal elimination diets

Allergen avoidance is one of the key principles in the treatment of food allergies [53]. The Melbourne Colic Study examined the role of a hypoallergenic diet on crying and fussing in a cohort of 115 colicky infants [115]. Infants were referred from community-based pediatric facilities. Mothers assigned to the active low-allergen diet excluded cow's milk and other common food allergens, such as egg, wheat, peanut, nuts, fish, and shellfish, from their diet. Formula-fed infants were randomly assigned to a casein hydrolysate preparation (low-allergen diet) or cow's milk-based formula. The response to diet was assessed on the previously validated infant-distress charts at baseline and after 1 week [28].

Clinical response to diet was defined as a reduction in distress of 25% or more. Infants on the active diet had a significantly higher response rate than those on the control diet (odds ratio 2.32; 95% confidence interval (CI) 1.07–5.0; $p = 0.03$). The treatment effect was greatest in breast-fed infants aged less than 6 weeks. These findings were confirmed in a subsequent randomized trial of a low-allergen maternal elimination diet among breast-fed infants less than 6 weeks of age with colic [116]. Again, mothers were randomly allocated to a low-allergen diet (avoiding cow's milk, soy, wheat, fish, egg, peanut, nuts, and chocolate), and a control diet. After 1 week, the clinical response rate in the low-allergen group was 74%, compared to 37% in the control group – a risk reduction of 37% in favor of the maternal elimination diet. This corresponds with a reduction in crying duration by 274 minutes/48 hours in the low-allergen group, compared to 102 minutes/48 hours in the control group; $p = 0.028$ (Fig. 14.4). This group difference demonstrates that maternally ingested food proteins

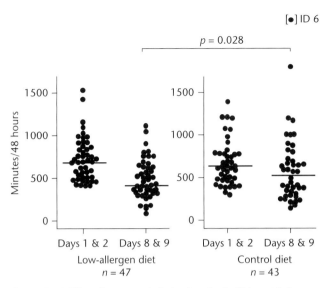

Figure 14.4 Effect of a maternal elimination diet in 90 breast-fed infants less than 6 weeks of age. There was a significantly greater reduction in cry/fuss duration for infants on the low-allergen diet, compared to infants of mothers on the unrestricted control diet [110].

are likely to be implicated in breast-fed infants with colic. However, the exact mechanisms remain to be elucidated.

Conclusion

Infantile colic is a common pediatric problem in the first months of life. No general consensus has emerged about its most likely multi-factorial etiology. Behavioral and interactional factors strongly influence the natural history of infantile colic. Infants with colic appear generally well, and in less than 5% of distressed infants a medical explanation for the distress can be found [7]. GER, esophagitis, or lactose intolerance, although sometimes present in infants with colic, are not likely to be the cause of the persistent distress, and empirical treatment with gastric acid suppressing medications or lactose-free formula is ineffective. Several trials have demonstrated a treatment benefit for hypoallergenic formulas or maternal elimination diets. Based on our community-based observations, at least 37% of young breast-fed infants with colic adversely reacted to one or several food proteins and responded to a maternal elimination diet. This may be associated with gastrointestinal inflammation and motility disturbances. The exact mechanisms by which food proteins cause persistent crying are still unclear.

In formula-fed infants with moderate to severe unremitting colic, a trial of a hypoallergenic formula should be attempted. Breast-fed infants may respond to a maternal low-allergen diet by reducing the antigen load in breast milk. The therapeutic effect of elimination diets appears to be greatest in young infants less than 6 weeks of age. After remission of symptoms, the diet can be gradually normalized and food proteins introduced into the diet, as tolerated.

Elimination diets should be closely supervised by an experienced dietician in order to prevent insufficient macro- or micronutrient intakes for both mother and infant, and growth parameters of the infant should be monitored [117]. In addition to any dietary interventions, successful management of infants with colic and their families should address the adverse effects of prolonged parental stress and maternal depression.

References

1 Lucassen PL, Assendelft WJ, van Eijk JT, et al. Systematic review of the occurrence of infantile colic in the community. *Arch Dis Child* 2001;84:398–403.

2 Brazelton TB. Crying in infancy. *Pediatrics* 1962;29:579–88.

3 Illingworth RS. Three months of colic. *Arch Dis Child* 1954; 29:165–74.

4 Clifford TJ. Sequelae of infant colic: evidence of transient infant distress and absence of lasting effects on maternal mental health. *Arch Pediatr Adolesc Med* 2002;156:1183–8.

5 Hill DJ, Hosking CS. Infantile colic and food hypersensitivity. *J Pediatr Gastroenterol Nutr* 2000,30:S67–76.

6 Lucassen PL, Assendelft WJ, Gubbels JW, et al. Effectiveness of treatments for infantile colic: systematic review. *BMJ* 1998;316:1563–9.

7 Garrison MM, Christakis DA. A systematic review of treatments for infant colic. *Pediatrics* 2000;106:184–90.

8 Barr RG. Colic and crying syndromes in infants. *Pediatrics* 1998;102:1282–6.

9 Wessel MA, Cobb JC, Jackson EB, et al. Paroxysmal fussing in infancy, sometimes called "colic". *Pediatrics* 1954;14:421–34.

10 Reijneveld SA, Brugman E, Hirasing RA. Excessive infant crying: the impact of varying definitions. *Pediatrics* 2001;108:893–7.

11 Hiscock H, Wake M. Infant sleep problems and postnatal depression: a community-based study. *Pediatrics* 2001;107:1317–22.

12 Rautava P, Helenius H, Lehtonen L. Psychosocial predisposing factors for infantile colic. *BMJ* 1993;307:600–4.

13 Nelson SP, Chen EH, Syniar GM, Christoffel KK. Prevalence of symptoms of gastroesophageal reflux during infancy. A pediatric practice-based survey. Pediatric Practice Research Group. *Arch Pediatr Adolesc Med* 1997;151:569–72.

14 Hillervik-Lindquist C. Studies on perceived breast milk insufficiency. A prospective study in a group of Swedish women. *Acta Paediatr Scand Suppl* 1991;376:1–27.

15 Canivet C, Hagander B, Jakobsson I, Lanke J. Infantile colic – less common than previously estimated? *Acta Paediatr* 1996; 85:454–8.

16 Canivet C, Jakobsson I, Hagander B. Colicky infants according to maternal reports in telephone interviews and diaries: a large Scandinavian study. *J Dev Behav Pediatr* 2002;23:1–8.

17 Clifford TJ, Campbell MK, Speechley KN, Gorodzinsky F. Infant colic: empirical evidence of the absence of an association with source of early infant nutrition. *Arch Pediatr Adolesc Med* 2002;156:1123–8.

18 Heine RG, Jordan B, Lubitz L, et al. Clinical predictors of pathological gastro-oesophageal reflux in infants with persistent distress. *J Paediatr Child Health* 2006;42:134–9.

19 Heine RG. Gastroesophageal reflux disease, colic and constipation in infants with food allergy. *Curr Opin Allergy Clin Immunol* 2006;6:220–5.

20 Putnam PE. GERD and crying: Cause and effect or unhappy coexistence? *J Pediatr* 2002;140:3–4.

21 Feranchak AP, Orenstein SR, Cohn JF. Behaviors associated with onset of gastroesophageal reflux episodes in infants. Prospective study using split-screen video and pH probe. *Clin Pediatr (Phila)* 1994;33:654–62.

22 Heine RG, Cameron DJ, Chow CW, et al. Esophagitis in distressed infants: poor correlation between esophageal pH monitoring and histological findings. *J Pediatr* 2002;140:14–19.

23 Moore DJ, Robb TA, Davidson GP. Breath hydrogen response to milk containing lactose in colicky and noncolicky infants. *J Pediatr* 1988;113:979–84.

24 Ståhlberg MR, Savilahti E. Infantile colic and feeding. *Arch Dis Child* 1986;61:1232–3.

25 Catto-Smith AG, Tan D, Gall DG, Scott RB. Rat gastric motor response to food protein-induced anaphylaxis. *Gastroenterology* 1994;106:1505–13.

26 Scott RB, Tan DT, Miampamba M, Sharkey KA. Anaphylaxis-induced alterations in intestinal motility: role of extrinsic neural pathways. *Am J Physiol* 1998;275:G812–21.

27 Lothe L, Ivarsson SA, Ekman R, Lindberg T. Motilin and infantile colic. A prospective study. *Acta Paediatr Scand* 1990;79:410–16.

28 Barr RG, Kramer MS, Boisjoly C, et al. Parental diary of infant cry and fuss behaviour. *Arch Dis Child* 1988;63:380–7.

29 Hide DW, Guyer BM. Prevalence of infant colic. *Arch Dis Child* 1982;57:559–60.

30 Rubin SP, Prendergast M. Infantile colic: incidence and treatment in a Norfolk community. *Child Care Health Dev* 1984; 10:219–26.

31 Carey WB. "Colic" – primary excessive crying as an infant-environment interaction. *Pediatr Clin North Am* 1984;31:993–1005.

32 Lothe L. *Studies on infantile colic*. Sweden: Thesis – University of Lund, 1989.

33 Michelsson K, Rinne A, Paajanen S. Crying, feeding and sleeping patterns in 1 to 12-month-old infants. *Child Care Health Dev* 1990;16:99–111.

34 Hogdall CK, Vestermark V, Birch M, et al. The significance of pregnancy, delivery and postpartum factors for the development of infantile colic. *J Perinat Med* 1991;19:251–7.

35 Lehtonen L, Korvenranta H. Infantile colic. Seasonal incidence and crying profiles. *Arch Pediatr Adolesc Med* 1995;149: 533–6.

36 Wake M, Morton-Allen E, Poulakis Z, et al. Prevalence, stability, and outcomes of cry-fuss and sleep problems in the first 2 years of life: prospective community-based study. *Pediatrics* 2006;117:836–42.

37 Hunziker UA, Barr RG. Increased carrying reduces infant crying: a randomized controlled trial. *Pediatrics* 1986;77:641–8.

38 Hill DJ, Menahem S, Hudson I, *et al.* Charting infant distress: an aid to defining colic. *J Pediatr* 1992;121:755–8.

39 Barr RG, Paterson JA, MacMartin LM, *et al.* Prolonged and unsoothable crying bouts in infants with and without colic. *J Dev Behav Pediatr* 2005;26:14–23.

40 Canivet C, Jakobsson I, Hagander B. Infantile colic. Follow-up at four years of age: still more "emotional". *Acta Paediatr* 2000;89:13–17.

41 Barr RG. Crying in the first year of life: good news in the midst of distress. *Child Care Health Dev* 1998;24:425–39.

42 Savino F, Castagno E, Bretto R, *et al.* A prospective 10-year study on children who had severe infantile colic. *Acta Paediatr Suppl* 2005;94:129.

43 Rao MR, Brenner RA, Schisterman EF, *et al.* Long term cognitive development in children with prolonged crying. *Arch Dis Child* 2004;89:989–92.

44 St James-Roberts I, Conroy S, Wilsher K. Bases for maternal perceptions of infant crying and colic behaviour. *Arch Dis Child* 1996;75:375–84.

45 Forsyth BW, Leventhal JM, McCarthy PL. Mothers' perceptions of problems of feeding and crying behaviors. A prospective study. *Am J Dis Child* 1985;139:269–72.

46 Canivet CA, Östergren PO, Rosen AS, *et al.* Infantile colic and the role of trait anxiety during pregnancy in relation to psychosocial and socioeconomic factors. *Scand J Public Health* 2005;33:26–34.

47 Rautava P, Lehtonen L, Helenius H, Sillanpaa M. Infantile colic: child and family three years later. *Pediatrics* 1995;96:43–7.

48 Beebe SA, Casey R, Pinto-Martin J. Association of reported infant crying and maternal parenting stress. *Clin Pediatr (Phila)* 1993;32:15–19.

49 Taubman B. Parental counseling compared with elimination of cow's milk or soy milk protein for the treatment of infant colic syndrome: a randomized trial. *Pediatrics* 1988;81:756–61.

50 Barr RG, McMullan SJ, Spiess H, *et al.* Carrying as colic "therapy": a randomized controlled trial. *Pediatrics* 1991;87:623–30.

51 Wolke D, Gray P, Meyer R. Excessive infant crying: a controlled study of mothers helping mothers. *Pediatrics* 1994;94:322–32.

52 Jakobsson I, Lindberg T. Cow's milk proteins cause infantile colic in breast-fed infants: a double-blind crossover study. *Pediatrics* 1983;71:268–71.

53 Evans RW, Fergusson DM, Allardyce RA, Taylor B. Maternal diet and infantile colic in breast-fed infants. *Lancet* 1981;1:1340–2.

54 Lothe L, Lindberg T. Cow's milk whey protein elicits symptoms of infantile colic in colicky formula-fed infants: a double-blind crossover study. *Pediatrics* 1989;83:262–6.

55 Forsyth BW. Colic and the effect of changing formulas: a double-blind, multiple-crossover study. *J Pediatr* 1989;115:521–6.

56 Lucassen PL, Assendelft WJ, Gubbels JW, *et al.* Infantile colic: crying time reduction with a whey hydrolysate: a double-blind, randomized, placebo-controlled trial. *Pediatrics* 2000;106:1349–54.

57 Bishop JM, Hill DJ, Hosking CS. Natural history of cow milk allergy: clinical outcome. *J Pediatr* 1990;116:862–7.

58 Hill DJ, Cameron DJ, Francis DE, *et al.* Challenge confirmation of late-onset reactions to extensively hydrolyzed formulas in infants with multiple food protein intolerance. *J Allergy Clin Immunol* 1995;96:386–94.

59 Hill DJ, Firer MA, Shelton MJ, Hosking CS. Manifestations of milk allergy in infancy: clinical and immunologic findings. *J Pediatr* 1986;109:270–6.

60 Hill DJ, Ball G, Hosking CS. Clinical manifestations of cows' milk allergy in childhood. I. Associations with *in-vitro* cellular immune responses. *Clin Allergy* 1988;18:469–79.

61 Hill DJ, Duke AM, Hosking CS, Hudson IL. Clinical manifestations of cows' milk allergy in childhood. II. The diagnostic value of skin tests and RAST. *Clin Allergy* 1988;18:481–90.

62 Hill DJ, Ball G, Hosking CS, Wood PR. Gamma-interferon production in cow milk allergy. *Allergy* 1993;48:75–80.

63 Järvinen K-M, Suomalainen H. Development of cow's milk allergy in breast-fed infants. *Clin Exp Allergy* 2001;31:978–87.

64 Järvinen K-M, Mäkinen-Kiljunen S, Suomalainen H. Cow's milk challenge through human milk evokes immune responses in infants with cow's milk allergy. *J Pediatr* 1999;135:506–12.

65 Sorva R, Mäkinen-Kiljunen S, Juntunen-Backman K. Beta-lactoglobulin secretion in human milk varies widely after cow's milk ingestion in mothers of infants with cow's milk allergy. *J Allergy Clin Immunol* 1994;93:787–92.

66 Palmer DJ, Gold MS, Makrides M. Effect of cooked and raw egg consumption on ovalbumin content of human milk: a randomized, double-blind, cross-over trial. *Clin Exp Allergy* 2005;35:173–8.

67 de Boissieu D, Matarazzo P, Rocchiccioli F, Dupont C. Multiple food allergy: a possible diagnosis in breastfed infants. *Acta Paediatr* 1997;86:1042–6.

68 Vadas P, Wai Y, Burks W, Perelman B. Detection of peanut allergens in breast milk of lactating women. *JAMA* 2001;285:1746–8.

69 Chirdo FG, Rumbo M, Anon MC, Fossati CA. Presence of high levels of non-degraded gliadin in breast milk from healthy mothers. *Scand J Gastroenterol* 1998;33:1186–92.

70 Jones CA, Holloway JA, Warner JO. Does atopic disease start in foetal life? *Allergy* 2000;55:2–10.

71 Kalayci Ö, Akpinarli A, Yigit S, Çetinkaya S. Intrauterine cow's milk sensitization. *Allergy* 2000;55:408–9.

72 Kalliomäki M, Ouwehand A, Arvilommi H, *et al.* Transforming growth factor-beta in breast milk: a potential regulator of atopic disease at an early age. *J Allergy Clin Immunol* 1999;104:1251–7.

73 Järvinen K-M, Laine ST, Järvenpää AL, Suomalainen HK. Does low IgA in human milk predispose the infant to development of cow's milk allergy? *Pediatr Res* 2000;48:457–62.

74 Järvinen K-M, Laine S, Suomalainen H. Defective tumour necrosis factor-alpha production in mother's milk is related to cow's milk allergy in suckling infants. *Clin Exp Allergy* 2000;30:637–43.

75 Lucas A, St James-Roberts I. Crying, fussing and colic behaviour in breast- and bottle-fed infants. *Early Hum Dev* 1998;53:9–18.

76 Axelsson I, Jakobsson I, Lindberg T, Benediktsson B. Bovine beta-lactoglobulin in the human milk. A longitudinal study during the whole lactation period. *Acta Paediatr Scand* 1986;75:702–7.

77 Paganelli R, Atherton DJ, Levinsky RJ. Differences between normal and milk allergic subjects in their immune responses after milk ingestion. *Arch Dis Child* 1983;58:201–6.

78 Savino F, Cresi F, Pautasso S, *et al*. Intestinal microflora in breastfed colicky and non-colicky infants. *Acta Paediatr* 2004;93:825–9.

79 Savino F, Bailo E, Oggero R, *et al*. Bacterial counts of intestinal Lactobacillus species in infants with colic. *Pediatr Allergy Immunol* 2005;16:72–5.

80 Kalliomäki M, Laippala P, Korvenranta H, *et al*. Extent of fussing and colic type crying preceding atopic disease. *Arch Dis Child* 2001;84:349–50.

81 Castro-Rodriguez JA, Stern DA, Halonen M, *et al*. Relation between infantile colic and asthma/atopy: a prospective study in an unselected population. *Pediatrics* 2001;108:878–82.

82 Iacono G, Carroccio A, Montalto G, *et al*. Severe infantile colic and food intolerance: a long-term prospective study. *J Pediatr Gastroenterol Nutr* 1991;12:332–5.

83 Lothe L, Lindberg T, Jakobsson I. Cow's milk formula as a cause of infantile colic: a double-blind study. *Pediatrics* 1982;70:7–10.

84 Hyman PE. Gastroesophageal reflux: one reason why baby won't eat. *J Pediatr* 1994;125:S103–9.

85 Orenstein SR. Crying does not exacerbate gastroesophageal reflux in infants. *J Pediatr Gastroenterol Nutr* 1992;14:34–7.

86 Heine RG, Jaquiery A, Lubitz L, *et al*. Role of gastro-oesophageal reflux in infant irritability. *Arch Dis Child* 1995;73:121–5.

87 Vandenplas Y, Goyvaerts H, Helven R, Sacré L. Gastroesophageal reflux, as measured by 24-hour pH monitoring, in 509 healthy infants screened for risk of sudden infant death syndrome. *Pediatrics* 1991;88:834–40.

88 Jordan B, Heine RG, Meehan M, *et al*. Effect of antireflux medication, placebo and infant mental health intervention on persistent crying: a randomized clinical trial. *J Paediatr Child Health* 2006;42:49–58.

89 Moore DJ, Tao BS, Lines DR, *et al*. Double-blind placebo-controlled trial of omeprazole in irritable infants with gastroesophageal reflux. *J Pediatr* 2003;143:219–23.

90 Hill DJ, Heine RG, Cameron DJ, *et al*. Role of food protein intolerance in infants with persistent distress attributed to reflux esophagitis. *J Pediatr* 2000;136:641–7.

91 Ravelli AM, Tobanelli P, Volpi S, Ugazio AG. Vomiting and gastric motility in infants with cow's milk allergy. *J Pediatr Gastroenterol Nutr* 2001;32:59–64.

92 Iacono G, Carroccio A, Cavataio F, *et al*. Gastroesophageal reflux and cow's milk allergy in infants: a prospective study. *J Allergy Clin Immunol* 1996;97:822–7.

93 Kelly KJ, Lazenby AJ, Rowe PC, *et al*. Eosinophilic esophagitis attributed to gastroesophageal reflux: improvement with an amino acid-based formula. *Gastroenterology* 1995;109:1503–12.

94 Straumann A, Bauer M, Fischer B, *et al*. Idiopathic eosinophilic esophagitis is associated with a TH2-type allergic response. *J Allergy Clin Immunol* 2001;108:954–61.

95 Williams J, Watkins-Jones R. Dicyclomine: worrying symptoms associated with its use in some small babies. *BMJ* 1984;288:901

96 Savino F, Brondello C, Cresi F, *et al*. Cimetropium bromide in the treatment of crisis in infantile colic. *J Pediatr Gastroenterol Nutr* 2002;34:417–19.

97 Catto-Smith AG, Patrick MK, Scott RB, *et al*. Gastric response to mucosal IgE-mediated reactions. *Am J Physiol* 1989;257:G704–8.

98 Oliver MR, Tan DT, Kirk DR, *et al*. Colonic and jejunal disturbances after colonic antigen challenge of sensitized rat. *Gastroenterology* 1997;112:1996–2005.

99 Lothe L, Ivarsson SA, Lindberg T. Motilin, vasoactive intestinal peptide and gastrin in infantile colic. *Acta Paediatr Scand* 1987;76:316–20.

100 Shenassa ED, Brown MJ. Maternal smoking and infantile gastrointestinal dysregulation: the case of colic. *Pediatrics* 2004;114:e497–505.

101 Savino F, Clara GE, Guidi C, *et al*. Ghrelin and motilin concentration in colicky infants. *Acta Paediatr* 2006;95:738–41.

102 Kanabar D, Randhawa M, Clayton P. Improvement of symptoms in infant colic following reduction of lactose load with lactase. *J Hum Nutr Diet* 2001;14:359–63.

103 Campbell JP. Dietary treatment of infant colic: a double-blind study. *J R Coll Gen Pract* 1989;39:11–14.

104 Savino F, Palumeri E, Castagno E, *et al*. Reduction of crying episodes owing to infantile colic: a randomized controlled study on the efficacy of a new infant formula. *Eur J Clin Nutr* 2006;60:1304–10.

105 Jakobsson I, Lothe L, Ley D, Borschel MW. Effectiveness of casein hydrolysate feedings in infants with colic. *Acta Paediatr* 2000;89:18–21.

106 Estep DC, Kulczycki Jr A. Treatment of infant colic with amino acid-based infant formula: a preliminary study. *Acta Paediatr* 2000;89:22–7.

107 Estep DC, Kulczycki Jr A. Colic in breast-milk-fed infants: treatment by temporary substitution of neocate infant formula. *Acta Paediatr* 2000;89:795–802.

108 Sampson HA. Infantile colic and food allergy: Fact or fiction? *J Pediatr* 1989;115:583–4.

109 de Boissieu D, Matarazzo P, Dupont C. Allergy to extensively hydrolyzed cow milk proteins in infants: identification and treatment with an amino acid-based formula. *J Pediatr* 1997;131:744–7.

110 Vanderhoof JA, Murray ND, Kaufman SS, *et al*. Intolerance to protein hydrolysate infant formulas: an underrecognized cause of gastrointestinal symptoms in infants. *J Pediatr* 1997;131:741–4.

111 American Academy of Pediatrics. Committee on Nutrition. Hypoallergenic infant formulas. *Pediatrics* 2000;106:346–9.

112 Isolauri E, Sütas Y, Mäkinen-Kiljunen S, *et al*. Efficacy and safety of hydrolyzed cow milk and amino acid-derived formulas in infants with cow milk allergy. *J Pediatr* 1995;127:550–7.

113 Sicherer SH, Noone SA, Barnes Koerner C, *et al*. Hypoallergenicity and efficacy of an amino acid-based formula in children with

cow's milk and multiple food hypersensitivities. *J Pediatr* 2001; 138:688–93.

114 Savino F, Cresi F, Silvestro L, Oggero R. Use of an amino-acid formula in the treatment of colicky breastfed infants. *Acta Paediatr* 2001;90:359–60.

115 Hill DJ, Hudson IL, Sheffield LJ, *et al*. A low allergen diet is a significant intervention in infantile colic: results of a community-based study. *J Allergy Clin Immunol* 1995;96:886–92.

116 Hill DJ, Roy N, Heine RG, *et al*. Effect of a low-allergen maternal diet on colic among breastfed infants: a randomized, controlled trial. *Pediatrics* 2005;116:e709–15.

117 Arvola T, Holmberg-Marttila D. Benefits and risks of elimination diets. *Ann Med* 1999;31:293–8.

15

CHAPTER 15

Eosinophilic Esophagitis, Gastroenteritis, and Colitis

James P. Franciosi, Jonathan E. Markowitz, and Chris A. Liacouras

---

KEY CONCEPTS

- Food allergens play a strong role in the pathogenesis of eosinophilic esophagitis (EoE).
- Elimination or elemental diets are highly effective treatments for EoE.
- EoE is distinct from eosinophilic gastroenteritis (EoG).
- It is essential to distinguish EoG from inflammatory bowel disease.

Primary disorders involving an accumulation of eosinophils in the gastrointestinal tract include eosinophilic esophagitis, eosinophilic gastroenteritis, and eosinophilic colitis. The goal of this chapter is to provide an overview of these conditions.

Eosinophilic esophagitis

Introduction

Our understanding of eosinophilic esophagitis (EoE) has evolved over the past 30 years from isolated case reports of patients with prominent esophageal eosinophilia (often misclassified as gastroesophageal reflux) to a well-defined clinical disorder. This disease has been given several names including EoE, allergic esophagitis, primary EoE, and idiopathic EoE.

Definition

EoE is a distinct disease defined by a clinico-pathologic diagnosis involving a localized eosinophilic inflammation of the esophagus. Since symptoms are similar to gastroesophageal reflux, esophageal endoscopic biopsies are required to establish the diagnosis. EoE is defined as the presence of 15 or more eosinophils in the most severely involved high-powered field (HPF) (400×) isolated to the esophagus and associated with characteristic clinical symptoms, which do not respond to acid blockade. Other recognized causes of esophageal eosinophilia should be excluded prior to making the diagnosis (Table 15.1).

Table 15.1 Differential diagnosis of esophageal eosinophilia

- Gastroesophageal reflux
- Inflammatory bowel disease
- Food allergy
- Eosinophilic gastroenteritis
- Celiac disease
- Parasitic infection
- Connective tissue disease
- Drug allergy
- Hypereosinophilic syndrome
- Autoimmune enteropathy
- Candida esophagitis
- Viral esophagitis (herpes or cucumber mosaic virus (CMV))
- Churg–Strauss syndrome

Incidence and prevalence

In 2003, the incidence and prevalence of EoE in children 0–19 years of age were reported to be 1 and 4.3 per 10,000 children, respectively [1]. Other studies have suggested a rising prevalence of EoE in the last 10 years [2]. In adults, the prevalence of esophageal eosinophilia has been reported to be as high as 4.8% in a random sample of the Swedish population who electively underwent esophageal endoscopy with biopsy without any clinical indication [3]. These studies lack exclusion of patients with gastroesophageal reflux, did not have uniform treatment of patients with acid blockade medications prior to establishing the diagnosis of EoE and did not follow the definition of EoE as defined above. Further studies are needed to investigate the prevalence of EoE using current definitions.

Food Allergy: Adverse Reactions to Foods and Food Additives, 4th edition. Edited by Dean D. Metcalfe, Hugh A. Sampson, and Ronald A. Simon. © 2008 Blackwell Publishing, ISBN: 978-1-4501-5129-0.

Etiology

The exact etiology of EoE is unknown; however, EoE is believed to be a mixed IgE and non-IgE mediated allergic response to food antigens, with non-IgE cell-mediated responses predominating [4]. The identified esophageal eosinophilia is thought to represent only part of a complex cellular and molecular cascade of interactions between Th2 cells, mast cells, cytokines such as IL-5 and IL-13, endogenous chemokines such as eotaxin-1 and eotaxin-3, and eosinophils [5].

While several studies have documented resolution of EoE with the strict avoidance of food antigens, in 1995, Kelly *et al.* published a sentinel paper on EoE [6]. Kelly studied 10 patients with symptoms of chronic gastroesophageal reflux who failed medical and surgical therapy (six patients had ongoing symptoms and esophageal eosinophilia despite undergoing a fundoplication). Because the suspected etiology was an abnormal immunologic response to specific unidentifiable food antigens, patients were placed on a strict diet consisting of an amino-acid-based formula for a median of 17 weeks. Symptomatic improvement was seen within an average of 3 weeks after the introduction of the elemental diet (resolution in eight patients, improvement in two). All 10 patients demonstrated a significant histologic improvement in their esophageal eosinophilia. Subsequently, all patients reverted to previous symptoms upon reintroduction of foods. Open food challenges were then conducted with a return of symptoms with challenges to milk (seven patients), soy (four patients), wheat (two patients), peanut (two patients), and egg (one patient) [6].

Several authors have suggested that aeroallergens may play a role in the development of EoE. Mishra and Rothenberg used a mouse model to show that the inhalation of Aspergillus may cause EoE [7]. They found that the allergen-challenged mice developed elevated levels of esophageal eosinophils and features of epithelial cell hyperplasia that mimic EoE. In addition, Spergel reported a case of a 21-year-old female with EoE, asthma, and allergic rhinoconjunctivitis who became symptomatic from her EoE during pollen seasons followed by resolution during winter months [8].

Clinical features

Although the current reports suggest that patients with EoE are predominantly young Caucasian males, EoE can occur at any age or race and in either sex. Those affected typically present with one or more of the following symptoms: vomiting, regurgitation, nausea, epigastric or chest pain, dysphagia, water brash, globus, or decreased appetite [9]. Less common symptoms include growth failure, hematemesis, and esophageal dysmotility. Symptoms can be frequent and severe in some patients while extremely intermittent and mild in others (Table 15.2). The majority of children experience vomiting, chronic nausea, or regurgitation while older children and adolescents develop heartburn, epigastric

Table 15.2 Clinical symptoms of eosinophilic esophagitis

– Vomiting
– Regurgitation
– Dysphagia
– Nausea
– Epigastric pain
– Chest pain
– Esophageal food impaction
– Irritability/feeding difficulties
– Night time cough

Other complications that can occur with EoE include failure to thrive, malnutrition, feeding intolerance, esophageal strictures, hiatal hernia, small caliber esophagus, and esophageal perforation. Esophageal fungal or viral superinfection may also occur. Any patient who is being considered for surgical correction of gastroesophageal reflux (fundoplication) should first be evaluated endoscopically for EoE to prevent unnecessary surgery [10].

pain, or episodes of dysphagia. Up to 50% of patients manifest additional allergy related symptoms such as asthma, eczema, or rhinitis. Furthermore, up to 50% of patients have one or more parents with history of allergy. EoE should be strongly considered in those patients who have severe or refractory symptoms of gastroesophageal reflux, especially those who are refractory to medication.

Diagnosis

Children with chronic refractory symptoms of gastroesophageal reflux disease (GERD) or dysphagia should undergo evaluation for EoE. While laboratory and radiological assessment may be appropriate in most cases, all patients should undergo an upper endoscopy with biopsy. The diagnosis of EoE is made when there is an isolated severe histologic esophagitis, unresponsive to aggressive acid blockade, associated with symptoms similar to those seen in GERD or dysphagia.

Upper endoscopy should be performed to directly visualize the esophagus and to obtain tissue samples for pathologic investigation. EoE is best defined as the presence of at least 15 eosinophils per HPF isolated strictly to the esophagus. In 1999, Ruchelli evaluated 102 patients presenting with GERD symptoms who also were found to have at least one esophageal eosinophil without any other gastrointestinal (GI) abnormalities [11]. Patients were subsequently treated with acid blockade. It was demonstrated that the treatment response could be classified into three categories. Patients who improved and had a lasting response had on average 1.1 eosinophils per HPF, patients who relapsed upon completion of therapy had 6.4 eosinophils per HPF, and patients who remained symptomatic despite therapy had on average 24.5 eosinophils per HPF.

Since EoE has been described as a patchy disease, multiple esophageal biopsies should be obtained from the mid and distal esophagus. In the past, early reports suggested that EoE patients developed proximal or mid-esophageal eosinophilia; however, recent information demonstrates that severe mucosal eosinophilia can occur in any portion (proximal, mid, distal) of the esophagus [12–14]. To make an accurate diagnosis, the remainder of the GI tract must be normal; thus, biopsies should be obtained from the gastric antrum and duodenum to rule out other diseases.

EoE has been associated with visual findings on endoscopy in 68% of patients: concentric ring formation (called "trachealization" or a "feline esophagus"), longitudinal linear furrows, and patches of small, white papules on the esophageal mucosal surface [15]. Most investigators believe that the esophageal rings and furrows are a response to full thickness esophageal tissue inflammation. The white papules appear to represent the formation of eosinophilic abscesses. However, the esophagus may be visually normal on endoscopy in over 30% of patients. Therefore, whenever the diagnosis of EoE is suspected, esophageal biopsies must be performed.

In 2000, Fox utilized high-resolution probe endosonography in patients with EoE in order to determine the extent of tissue involvement [16]. He compared eight patients with EoE to four control patients without esophagitis. He discovered that the esophageal tissue layers were thicker in EoE patients compared to controls (total wall thickness 2.8 versus 2.2 mm, $p < 0.01$; combined mucosal and submucosal thickness 1.6 versus 1.1 mm, $p < 0.01$; muscularis propria thickness 1.3 versus 1.0 mm, $p < 0.05$). These findings suggested that EoE patients had more than just surface involvement of eosinophils.

While other non-invasive tests have been used in an attempt to diagnose EoE, upper endoscopy with biopsy is the only test that can precisely determine the diagnosis of EoE. The other non-invasive GI diagnostic tests include radiographic upper GI series (UGI), pH probe, and manometry. Although radiographs demonstrate anatomic abnormalities, they do not identify tissue eosinophilia. However, in patients suspected of having esophageal strictures, an UGI can provide important information. Patients with EoE usually have normal or borderline normal pH probes. Patients may have mild GERD secondary to abnormalities in esophageal motility due to tissue eosinophilic infiltration; however, there have been no specific manometric findings of EoE to date.

Allergy testing

Once EoE is suspected, patients should be encouraged to seek an allergy consultation. Serum peripheral eosinophilia or elevated IgE levels are not present in the majority of patients. Furthermore, these tests have been found to be unreliable due to the fact that they usually respond to environmental allergens as well as ingested or inhaled allergens. Serum RAST (radioallergosorbent test) testing for food specific IgE antibodies has a very limited role in EoE due to its low sensitivity. Use of a combination of peripheral

blood absolute eosinophil count (AEC), levels of eosinophil-derived neurotoxin (EDN), and eotaxin-3 as non-invasive biomarkers are under investigation; however, these tests do not currently appear to have the sensitivity or negative predictive value needed for widespread clinical practice [17].

A combination of skin prick testing (SPT) and atopy patch testing (APT) attempts to identify IgE and non-IgE based causative food allergens, respectively. In a study population of 146 pediatric patients, elimination diet based on foods identified by a combination of SPT and APT led to resolution of esophageal eosinophilia in 67% of patients, and histologic improvement in 82% of patients [4,18]. In EoE patients, SPT most frequently identifies positive reactions to egg, milk, and soy. Given the non-IgE mediated mechanism of most of the food reactions in EoE patients, APT may play an important role in the successful identification of causative food antigens. Presently, the lack of standardization of APT methodologies in addition to variability in technique and interpretation are likely explanations for the non-uniform results of APT. Interpretation is based on a no reaction, or $1 - 3+$ scale depending on the degree of erythema, papules and/or vesicles. The most common foods identified by APT are corn, soy, and wheat [18].

Treatment
Acute management

Several treatment options are available to patients diagnosed with EoE. Currently, most investigators do not believe that esophageal acid exposure is the etiology of EoE; however, because of the severity of mucosal and submucosal disease seen in EoE, secondary acid reflux often occurs. Additionally, because there may be some histologic overlap between patients with EoE and those with GERD, it is important to exclude acid reflux as a cause of esophageal inflammation. In rare cases, acid reflux may cause significant esophageal eosinophilia. Therefore, patients suspected of having EoE should be prescribed a proton pump inhibitor so that GERD can be excluded. A case series by Ngo and colleagues have identified several patients with significant esophageal eosinophilia that resolved 1 month after taking a proton pump inhibitor medication [19]. A 4 to 6-week course of acid blockade and repeat endoscopy is important to confirm the diagnosis of EoE.

Adult gastroenterologists have reported the use of esophageal dilation for their patients who present acutely with esophageal strictures secondary to EoE. While esophageal dilation may relieve dysphagia and improve an esophageal stricture, many physicians describe esophageal tearing during endoscopy and dilation [20–23]. Higher rates of esophageal perforation after attempted esophageal endoscopic dilation have been reported in this setting [23,24]. Thus, while esophageal dilation has a role in alleviating severe esophageal strictures in patients with EoE, its results are generally temporary and the problem often recurs. Gastroenterologists should be extremely careful whenever performing endoscopy or dilation as perforation is a distinct possibility. A diagnostic endoscopy should be performed and medical or dietary therapy instituted prior to performing dilation.

Systemic corticosteroids were the first medical treatment shown to be effective in improving both symptoms and esophageal histology in patients with EoE [25]. Patients were treated with oral solumedrol (average dose 1.5 mg/kg/day; maximum dose 48 mg/day) for 1 month. Symptoms were significantly improved in 19 of 20 patients by an average of 8 days. A repeat endoscopy with biopsy (4 weeks after the initiation of therapy) demonstrated almost complete normalization of esophageal histology. However, upon discontinuation of corticosteroids, 90% had recurrence of symptoms. Oral corticosteroids should be used whenever patients have severe dysphagia (with or without strictures) or other clinical symptoms that may be contributing to possible hospitalization because of a feeding disorder, poor weight gain, or dehydration. While systemic steroids work rapidly, their disadvantages include the fact that they cannot be used chronically, that they do not cure the disease, and that they often have serious side effects with a prolonged use (bone, growth, and mood abnormalities).

Instead of prescribing systemic steroids, topical corticosteroids can be utilized [26–29]. Medications, such as fluticasone propionate, can be sprayed into the pharynx and swallowed. Within a few weeks, both clinical symptoms and esophageal histology dramatically improve. In a study by Konikoff, the authors conducted a randomized, double-blind, placebo-control trial of swallowed fluticasone in patients with active EoE [30]. Thirty-six patients were randomly assigned to receive either 880 μg of fluticasone daily or placebo. Of these, 50% of the fluticasone-treated patients achieved complete histologic remission compared to 9% of patients who received placebo. In addition, resolution of clinical symptoms occurred more frequently with fluticasone than with placebo. The authors concluded that swallowed fluticasone was effective in inducing histologic remission and clinical symptoms in EoE in a significant number of patients.

The advantage of using topical steroids is that their side effects are less than that seen with systemic steroids. The disadvantages include not treating the disease fully (the disease generally recurs when the treatment is discontinued) and the development of possible side effects such as epistaxis, dry mouth, and esophageal candidiasis. When using topical, swallowed corticosteroids, the initial dose varies from 110 to 880 μg, twice daily, depending on patient's age and size. Patients do not eat, drink, or rinse their mouth for 20–30 minutes after using this medication. Other atopic diseases should be controlled as rhinitis and environmental allergies may be linked to EoE. The patient should undergo endoscopy after 2–3 months of therapy. If improved, fluticasone can be weaned empirically. The medication can be discontinued as tolerated; however in many patients the disease

recurs. Recently, the use of a swallowed viscous budesonide solution has been reported with some effectiveness [31].

Several other medications have also been utilized. Cromolyn sodium has been used as a therapy for EoE in a small number of patients. However, cromolyn sodium did not demonstrate any histologic or clinical improvement in a series of 14 patients [32]. Leukotriene receptor antagonists have also been utilized to treat EoE [24]. Initial doses of 10–100 mg per day were prescribed with reports of symptomatic improvement; however, on repeat biopsy, there was no significant change in the patient's esophageal eosinophilia. While the advantage of using a leukotriene receptor antagonist is that it has minimal side effects and it may alleviate the patient's clinical symptoms, there have been no reports documenting improvement in the patient's histology. Additionally, the patient's clinical symptoms recur when the medication is discontinued.

Dietary therapy has been reported to be extremely effective for pediatric patients with EoE [6,7]. While there has been no definitive evidence that EoE is a food allergy, the removal of food antigens has been clearly demonstrated to successfully treat both the clinical symptoms and the underlying histopathology in well over 95% of patients with EoE. The elimination of causative foods can follow several therapeutic regimens. First, specific food elimination can be based on allergy testing and clinical history [18,33]. Second, the most likely causative foods can be removed regardless of history. Recently, a study utilized the removal of six foods (milk, eggs, wheat, soy, nuts, shellfish), without the aid of allergy testing, and demonstrated resolution of symptoms in over two-thirds of patients [8]. When comparing these studies, similar outcomes occur. In both studies, food elimination successfully improved symptoms in approximately 75% of patients. Moreover, although esophageal histology also significantly improved, in most patients it did not normalize.

While every attempt should be made to identify and eliminate potential food allergens through food elimination, a significant number of patients remain symptomatic and continue to have abnormal esophageal histology. In these cases, the administration of a strict diet utilizing an amino-acid-based formula is often necessary. As established by Kelly and Liacouras, the use of an elemental diet in children is greater than 95% successful in resolving both the clinical symptoms and histologic abnormalities of EoE [6,7]. Although the strict use of an amino acid-based formula (typically provided by nasogastric tube feeding) may be difficult for patients (and parents) to comprehend, its benefits outweigh the risks of other treatments. Once the esophagus is healed, foods are reintroduced systematically. Since the clinical symptoms are often erratic, endoscopy with biopsy should be performed in order to determine the improvement in esophageal histology.

In our experience of over 164 compliant patients, who were treated with an amino acid-based diet, 97% of patients

Table 15.3 EoE food introduction following an elemental diet

A	B	C	D
Vegetables (non-legume) Carrots, squash sweet potato, spinach, broccoli, lettuce	Other fruits Apple, banana, kiwi, pineapple, mango, watermelon, honeydew, cantaloupe, papaya, guava, avocado	Peas White potato Grains Rice, oat, barley, rye	Milk Corn Peanut Wheat Beef
Fruit Grapes, pear peaches, plum, apricot, cherries orange, grapefruit, lemon, lime, cherries, strawberries, blueberries	Legumes lima beans, chickpeas, white/ black/red beans, string beans	Meat* Lamb, chicken, turkey, pork Fish/shellfish Tree nuts Almond, walnut, hazelnut, brazil nut, pecan	Soy Egg

*Progress from well cooked to rarer.

had a clinical and histologic improvement in their EoE [32]. In those that required an elemental diet, over 84% had specific food antigens identified and were able to discontinue the elemental diet after approximately 6 months using a graded food reintroduction protocol (Table 15.3). Dietary restriction using a combination of patch and skin prick testing alone without the need for an elemental diet was successful in over 50% of 130 children. Elimination of the responsible foods usually does not lead to immediate resolution of symptoms. Rather, improvement of symptoms occurs approximately 1–3 weeks after the removal of the causative antigen. Also, in patients with EoE, symptoms do not always occur immediately after food reintroduction and may return after several days to weeks. In some cases, the responsible food antigens must be identified using a systematic approach: foods are eliminated for 6–8 weeks and repeat endoscopy is performed. New foods are typically introduced every 7 days and repeat biopsies are performed based on clinical symptoms or after 5–8 new foods are introduced. Nutritional support is also an important component in the management of EoE patients. Foods considered to be the most antigenic for EoE include milk, eggs, soy, corn, wheat, and beef.

Finally, other medications are being developed that target specific chemokines and other inflammatory mediators involved in eosinophil proliferation, recruitment, and activation. Medications such as anti-interleukin-5 (anti-IL-5), very late activating antigen, and monoclonal eotaxin antibody may benefit those patients who have severe EoE. Recently, Stein studied the use of anti-IL-5 in four patients identified with EoE [34]. These patients had long-standing dysphagia and esophageal strictures. After receiving monthly intravenous infusions of anti-IL-5 for 3 consecutive months, clinical symptoms and repeated upper endoscopy were evaluated. Anti-IL-5 therapy was associated with marked decreases of peripheral blood and esophageal eosinophilia along with improved clinical symptoms and significant resolution of dysphagia.

Long-term management

The focus of long-term management of EoE should be to provide symptom relief along with histologic healing. At this point, topical corticosteroids and dietary restriction have both been shown to be successful in the long-term treatment of EoE. Several reports have demonstrated esophageal healing and symptom resolution with dietary therapy ranging from the removal of a few foods to the use of a total elemental diet strictly using an amino acid-based formula.

Unlike infantile milk-protein allergy, the majority of patients with EoE require long-term, indefinite food antigen removal. In our series of 231 patients, only a few patients appeared to "outgrow" their food allergy; however, recent evidence suggests that an increasing number of patients may develop "tolerance" if the food antigens are removed for a prolonged period of time (years) [35].

With regard to medical therapy, because of the possibility of secondary gastroesophageal reflux due to chronic esophageal inflammation, acid blockade is effective in improving patient's symptoms. Recent adult literature suggests that proton pump inhibitor therapy may be associated with a significantly increased risk of hip fractures if used for more than 1 year [36]. Further research into the safety of long-term proton pump inhibition therapy in adults and children is needed, and the risk–benefit ratio of any medication should always be evaluated in the individual patient clinical context. Topical, swallowed fluticasone has been shown to be an effective treatment for EoE [28,30]. Unfortunately, when therapy is discontinued, EoE almost always recurs. While the long-term use of topical steroids appears reasonably safe, several side effects have been reported which include esophageal candidiasis, epistaxis, and dry mouth. In addition, long-term effects on growth, bone health, and esophageal fibrosis are currently not known. Finally, in the future, biologic therapy utilizing monoclonal antibodies such as anti-IL-5 shows promising results for both initial and maintenance therapy for patients with moderate to severe EoE. These agents are currently undergoing clinical trials [34].

Eosinophilic gastroenteritis (gastroenterocolitis)

Introduction

Eosinophilic gastroenteritis or gastroenterocolitis (EoG) is a general term that describes a constellation of symptoms and a pathologic infiltration of the GI tract by eosinophils. EoG was originally described by Kaijser in 1937 [37]. It is a disorder characterized by tissue eosinophilia that can affect different layers of the bowel wall, anywhere from the mouth to the anus. In 1970, Klein classified EoG into three categories: mucosal, muscular, and serosal [38].

Definition

There are no strict diagnostic criteria for EoG, and its definition has been largely shaped by multiple case reports and case series. A combination of GI complaints with supportive histologic findings is sufficient to make the diagnosis of EoG and investigate the differential diagnosis (Table 15.4).

Prevalence

Currently, the prevalence of EoG is not known. Our clinical experience is that EoG occurs less frequently than inflammatory bowel disease in children (7 per 100,000 children) [39].

Table 15.4 Differential diagnosis of eosinophilic gastroenteritis

Celiac disease	
Chronic granulomatous disease	Infectious
	Ancylostoma caninium (hookworm)
Connective tissue	*Anisakis*
diseases/vasculitis	*Ascaris*
Systemic lupus erythematosus	EBV
Scleroderma	*Enterobius vermicularis* (pinworm)
Dermatomyositis	*Eustoma rotundatum*
Polymyositis	*Giardia lambila*
Churg–Strauss syndrome	*Helicobacter pylori*
Polyarteritis nodosa	Schistosomiasis trichus
Others	Stercoalis
	Strongyloides
Food allergies	Toxocara canis
	Trichinella spiralis
Hypereosinophilic syndrome	Others
	Inflammatory bowel disease*
	Inflammatory fibroid polyp
	Malignancy
	Medications
	Azathioprine
	Carbamazepine
	Clofazimine
	Enalapril
	Gemfibrozil
	Gold
	Others [40,41]

Note this list is not exhaustive – case reports of other etiologies have been reported.
*In our experience, inflammatory bowel disease (often in young children) can initially manifest histologically as eosinophilia.

Etiology

The exact etiology of EoG remains unknown, although it is now recognized to occur as a result of both IgE- and non-IgE-mediated sensitivity [42]. The association between IgE-mediated inflammatory response (typical allergy) and EoG is supported by the increased likelihood of other allergic disorders such as atopic disease, food allergies, and seasonal allergies [43,44]. Specific foods have been implicated in the cause of EoG [45,46]. In contrast, the role of non-IgE-mediated immune dysfunction, in particular the interplay between lymphocyte-produced cytokines and eosinophils, has also received attention. IL-5 is a chemoattractant responsible for tissue eosinophilia [47]. Desreumaux *et al.* found that among patients with EoG, the levels of IL-3, IL-5, and granulocyte–macrophage colony stimulating factor (GM-CSF) were significantly increased as compared to control patients [48]. Once recruited to the tissue, eosinophils may further recruit similar cells through their own production of IL-3 and IL-5, as well as production of leukotrienes [49]. This mixed type of immune dysregulation in EoG has implications in the way this disorder is diagnosed, as well as in the way it is treated [50].

Clinical features

EoG affects patients of all ages, with a slight male predominance. Most commonly, eosinophils infiltrate only the mucosa, leading to symptoms associated with malabsorption, such as growth failure, weight loss, diarrhea, and hypoalbuminemia. Additional symptoms of EoG include colicky abdominal pain, bloating, dysphagia, and vomiting [51–53]. Other features of severe disease include GI bleeding, iron deficiency anemia, protein losing enteropathy (hypoalbuminemia), and growth failure [51]. Approximately 75% of affected patients have an elevated blood eosinophil levels [51]. Rarely, ascites can occur [54,55]. In addition, up to 50% of patients have a past or family history of atopy [56].

In an infant, EoG may present in a manner similar to hypertrophic pyloric stenosis, with progressive vomiting, dehydration, electrolyte abnormalities, and thickening of the gastric outlet [57,58]. When an infant presents with this constellation of symptoms, in addition to atopic symptoms such as eczema and reactive airway disease, an elevated eosinophil count, or a strong family history of atopic disease, then EoG should be considered before surgical intervention.

Uncommon presentations of EoG include an acute abdomen (even mimicking acute appendicitis), isolated ulceration, obstruction, or mass lesions [59–63]. There also have been reports of serosal infiltration with eosinophils, with associated abdominal distention, eosinophilic ascites, and bowel perforation [55,61,64–67].

Diagnosis

EoG should be considered in any patient with a history of chronic symptoms including vomiting, abdominal pain, diarrhea, anemia, hypoalbuminemia, or poor weight gain in combination with the presence of eosinophils in the GI tract. The number of eosinophils that are defined as abnormal depends on the location in the GI tract, and has geographic variability [68,69].

A number of tests may aid in the diagnosis of EoG, however no single test is pathognomonic and there are no standards for diagnosis. Eosinophils in the GI tract must be documented before EoG can be truly entertained as a diagnosis. This is most readily done with biopsies of the upper GI tract through esophagogastroduodenoscopy and the lower tract through colonoscopy with terminal ileal intubation. In our experience, inflammatory bowel disease is an important entity in the differential diagnosis, and eosinophilia can be the initial presentation especially in young children. Mucosal EoG may affect any portion of the GI tract. A review of the biopsy findings in 38 children with EoG revealed that all patients examined had mucosal eosinophilia of the gastric antrum [56]. Seventy-nine percent of the patients also demonstrated eosinophilia of the proximal small intestine, with 60% having esophageal involvement, and 52% having involvement of the gastric corpus. Those with colonic involvement tended to be under 6 months of age and were ultimately classified as having allergic colitis.

Radiographic contrast studies may demonstrate mucosal irregularities or edema, wall thickening, ulceration, or luminal narrowing. A lacy mucosal pattern of the gastric antrum known as *areae gastricae* is a unique finding that may be present in patients with EoG [70].

Evaluation of other causes of eosinophilia should be undertaken that include parasitic infection, inflammatory bowel disease, neoplasm, chronic granulomatous disease, collagen vascular disease, and the hypereosinophilic syndrome [71–75] (Table 15.4). Specifically, consultations with an allergist, gastroenterologist, infectious disease specialist, and rheumatologist should be obtained. Signs of intestinal obstruction warrant abdominal imaging and surgical consultation.

Laboratory evaluation

In contrast to EoE, peripheral eosinophilia or an elevated IgE level occurs in approximately 70% of affected individuals [76]. Allergic investigation is the same as for patients with EoE, however it is less often revealing. Infectious work-up should include stool ova and parasite testing on three separate stool samples, serum (and possibly tissue) EBV PCR, giardia antigen, and *Helicobacter pylori* testing [77–82]. Rheumatologic testing should be considered in the appropriate clinical context [83,84]. Measures of absorptive activity such as the D-xylose absorption test and lactose hydrogen breath testing may reveal evidence of malabsorption, reflecting small intestinal damage. Inflammatory bowel disease serologies may also be considered, but with the recognition that they have limited sensitivity especially

in younger children [85,86]. Negative anti-Saccharomyces cerevisiae (ASCA) and perinuclear antineutrophil cytoplasmic antibodies (pANCA) do not exclude the diagnosis of inflammatory bowel disease.

Treatment
Acute management

Since EoG is a rare and difficult disease to diagnose, randomized trials for its treatment are lacking and there is considerable debate as to which treatment is best.

Food allergy is considered one of the underlying causes of EoG, and its management is the same as described previously for EoE. In some cases, the administration of a strict diet, utilizing an elemental formula, has been shown to be successful [44,87,88]. Unfortunately, unlike EoE, elemental diets are not uniformly successful for patients with EoG.

When the use of a restricted diet fails, corticosteroids are often employed due to their high likelihood of success in attaining remission [52]. However, when weaned, the duration of remission is variable and can be short-lived, leading to the need for repeated courses or continuous low doses of steroids [89]. In addition, the chronic use of corticosteroids carries an increased likelihood of undesirable side effects, including cosmetic problems (cushingoid facies, hirsutism, acne), decreased bone density, impaired growth, and personality changes. A response to these side effects has been to look for substitutes that may act as steroid-sparing agents, while still allowing for control of symptoms. Budesonide (Entocort®) is a steroid formulation with less systemic toxicity that has been successful for some patients with EoG [90,91].

Orally administered cromolyn sodium has been used with some success [51,91–94], and recent reports have detailed the efficacy of other oral anti-inflammatory medications. Montelukast, a selective leukotriene receptor antagonist used to treat asthma, has been reported to be successful in the treatment of two patients with EoG [95–97]. Treatment of EoG with inhibition of leukotriene D4, a potent chemotactic factor for eosinophils, relies on the theory that the inflammatory response in EoG is perpetuated by the presence of eosinophils already present in the mucosa. Suplatast tosilate and ketotifen have also been reported as treatments for EoG [98,99]. Anti-IL-5 therapy for EoG is also being investigated.

Long-term management

As with EoE, every attempt should be made to identify and restrict potential food allergens in a stepwise approach. Given the limited possibilities for treatment of EoG, the combination of therapies incorporating the best chance of success with the smallest likelihood of side effects should be employed.

When other treatments fail, corticosteroids remain a reliable treatment for EoG, with attempts at limiting the total dose, or the number of treatment courses where possible. Due to the diffused and inconsistent nature of symptoms in this disease, serial endoscopy with biopsy is a useful and important modality for monitoring disease progression. Particularly in younger children, protean manifestations of inflammatory bowel disease should be considered with every endoscopy.

Eosinophilic proctocolitis

Introduction

Eosinophilic proctocolitis (EoP), also known as allergic proctocolitis or milk-protein proctocolitis, has been recognized as one of the most common etiologies of rectal bleeding in infants [56,100]. This disorder is characterized by the onset of rectal bleeding, generally in children less than 2 months of age.

Definition

EoP is strictly defined as an abnormal number of eosinophils confined to the colon. However, in clinical practice, endoscopy is usually not performed. The diagnosis is established when infants present with rectal bleeding that resolves when placed on a protein hydrolysate formula.

Prevalence

It is felt that up to 7.5% of the population in developed countries exhibit cow's milk allergy, although there is wide variation in the reported data [101–103]. Soy-protein allergy is felt to be less common than cow's milk allergy, with a reported prevalence of approximately 0.5% [103]. However, soy-protein intolerance becomes more prominent in individuals who have developed milk-protein-induced proctocolitis, with a prevalence from 15% to 50% or more in milk-protein-sensitized individuals [105].

Etiology

The GI tract plays a major role in the development of oral tolerance to foods. Through the process of endocytosis by the enterocytes, food antigens are generally degraded into non-antigenic proteins [106,107]. Although the GI tract serves as an efficient barrier to ingested food antigens, this barrier may not be mature for the first few months of life [108]. As a result, ingested antigens may have an increased propensity for being presented intact to the immune system. These intact antigens have the potential for stimulating the immune system, and driving an inappropriate response directed at the GI tract. Because the major component of the young infant's diet is milk or formula, it stands to reason that the inciting antigens in EoP are derived from the proteins found in them. Cow's milk and soy proteins are the foods most frequently implicated in EoP.

Commercially available infant formulas most commonly utilize cow's milk as the protein source. There are at least 25 known immunogenic proteins within cow's milk, with the caseins and β-lactoglobulin serving as the most antigenic [104]. For this reason, substitution of a soy-protein-based formula for a milk-protein-based formula in patients with suspected milk-protein proctocolitis is often unsuccessful. However, because of the expense of protein hydrolysate formulas, practitioners may attempt to use soy formulas initially.

Maternal breast milk represents a different challenge to the immune system. Up to 50% of the cases of EoP occur in breast-fed infants; but, rather than developing an allergy to human milk protein, it is felt that the infants are manifesting allergy to antigens ingested by the mother and transferred via the breast milk. The transfer of maternal dietary protein via breast milk was first demonstrated in 1921 [109]. More recently, the presence of cow's milk antigens in breast milk has been established [110–112].

When a problem with antigen handling occurs, whether secondary to increased absorption through an immature GI tract or through a damaged epithelium secondary to gastroenteritis, sensitization of the immune system results. Once sensitized, the inflammatory response is perpetuated with continued exposure to the inciting antigen. This may explain the reported relationship between early exposures to cow's milk protein or viral gastroenteritis and the development of allergy [113–115].

Clinical manifestations

Diarrhea, rectal bleeding, and increased mucus production are the typical symptoms seen in patients who present with EoP [56,116]. There is a bimodal age distribution with the majority of patients presenting in infancy (mean age at diagnosis of 60 days) and the other group presenting in adolescence and early adulthood [117].

The typical infant with EoP is well appearing with no constitutional symptoms. Rectal bleeding begins gradually, initially appearing as small flecks of blood. Usually, increased stool frequency occurs accompanied by water loss or mucus streaks. The development of irritability or straining with stools is also common and can falsely lead to the initial diagnosis of anal fissuring. Atopic symptoms such as eczema and reactive airway disease may be associated. Continued exposure to the inciting antigen causes increased bleeding and may, on rare occasions, cause anemia or poor weight gain. Despite the progression of symptoms, the infants are generally well appearing. Other manifestations of GI tract inflammation such as vomiting, abdominal distention, or weight loss almost never occur (Table 15.5).

Diagnosis

EoP is primarily a clinical diagnosis, although several laboratory parameters and diagnostic procedures may be useful. Initial assessment should be directed at the overall health of the child. A toxic appearing infant is not consistent with

Table 15.5 Characteristics of eosinophilic proctocolitis

- Clinical symptoms
  - Blood streaked stools
  - Diarrhea
  - Mild abdominal pain
  - <3 months of age
  - Usually normal weight gain
  - Well appearing
  - Eczema, atopy – rare
- Laboratory features
  - Fecal leukocytes, eosinophils
  - Mild peripheral eosinophilia
  - Rarely
    - Hypoalbuminemia
    - Anemia
  - Pin prick, RAST testing negative (usually not needed)

the diagnosis of EoP and should prompt evaluation for other causes of GI bleeding. Stool studies for bacterial pathogens, such as *Salmonella* and *Shigella*, should be performed in the setting of rectal bleeding. In particular, an assay for *Clostridium difficile* toxins A and B should also be considered. While *C. difficile* may cause colitis, infants may be asymptomatically colonized with this organism [118,119]. A stool specimen may be analyzed for the presence of white blood cells, and specifically for eosinophils. The sensitivity of these tests is not well documented, and the absence of a positive finding on these tests does not exclude the diagnosis [120]. Eosinophils can also accumulate in the colon in other conditions such as pin and hookworm infections, drug reactions, vasculitis, and inflammatory bowel disease. Depending on the clinical situation, it may be important to exclude these diagnoses especially in older children.

Although not always necessary, flexible sigmoidoscopy may be useful to demonstrate the presence of colitis. Visually, one may find erythema, friability, or frank ulceration of the colonic mucosa. Alternatively, the mucosa may appear normal, or show evidence of lymphoid hyperplasia [121,122]. Histologic findings typically include increased eosinophils in focal aggregates within the lamina propria, with generally preserved crypt architecture. Findings may be patchy, so that care should be taken to examine many levels of each specimen if necessary [123,124].

Laboratory evaluation

A complete blood count is useful, as the majority of infants with EoP have a normal or borderline low hemoglobin. An elevated serum eosinophil count may be present. A stool smear for eosinophils (Wright stain) may also support the diagnosis. Stool cultures for ova and parasites, bacteria, and *Clostridium difficile* toxins should be obtained in the appropriate clinical setting.

Treatment
Acute management

In a well-appearing patient with a history consistent with EoP, it is acceptable to make an empiric formula change. Given the high degree of reactivity to both milk and soy protein in sensitized individuals, a protein hydrolysate formula is often the best choice [114]. However, in mild cases, soy formulas may be attempted initially given the expense of protein hydrolysate formulas. Resolution of symptoms begins almost immediately after the elimination of the problematic food. Although symptoms may linger for several days to weeks, continued improvement is the rule. If symptoms do not quickly improve or persist beyond 4–6 weeks, other antigens should be considered, as well as other potential causes of rectal bleeding. In breast-fed infants, dietary restriction of milk and soy-containing products for the mother may result in improvement; however, care should be taken to ensure that the mother maintains adequate protein and calcium intake from other sources.

Long-term management

EoP in infancy is generally benign and withdrawing the milk-protein trigger resolves the condition. Though gross blood in the stool usually disappears within 72 hours, occult blood loss may persist for longer [117]. The prognosis is excellent and the majority of patients are able to tolerate the introduction of the responsible milk protein by 1–3 years of age. Given the unlikely possibility of an allergic reaction following milk reintroduction, milk challenges should be performed in a physician's office at 1 year of age. If a reaction does occur, infants are typically rechallenged at 15 months of age and then referred to an allergist. The prognosis for older onset EoP is less favorable than the infant presentation and is typically chronic and relapsing.

References

1 Noel RJ, Putnam PE, Rothenberg ME. Eosinophilic esophagitis. *N Engl J Med* 2004;351:940–1.

2 Cherian S, Smith NM, Forbes DA. Rapidly increasing prevalence of eosinophilic oesophagitis in Western Australia. *Arch Dis Child* 2006;91:1000–4.

3 Ronkainen J, Talley NJ, Aro P, et al. Prevalence of oesophageal eosinophils and eosinophilic oesophagitis in adults: the population-based Kalixanda study. *Gut* 2006;56:615–20.

4 Spergel JM, Beausoleil JL, Mascarenhas M, Liacouras CA. The use of skin prick tests and patch tests to identify causative foods in eosinophilic esophagitis. *J Allergy Clin Immunol* 2002;109:363–8.

5 Mishra A, Rothenberg ME. Intratracheal IL-13 induces eosinophilic esophagitis by an IL-5, eotaxin-1, and STAT6-dependent mechanism. *Gastroenterology* 2003;125:1419–27.

6 Kelly KJ, Lazenby AJ, Rowe PC, et al. Eosinophilic esophagitis attributed to gastroesophageal reflux: improvement with an amino acid-based formula. *Gastroenterology* 1995;109:1503–12.

7 Mishra A, Hogan SP, Brandt EB, Rothenberg ME. An etiological role for aeroallergens and eosinophils in experimental esophagitis. *J Clin Invest* 2001;107:83–90.

8 Fogg MI, Ruchelli E, Spergel JM. Pollen and eosinophilic esophagitis. *J Allergy Clin Immunol* 2003;112:796–7.

9 Liacouras CA, Markowitz JE. Eosinophilic esophagitis: a subset of eosinophilic gastroenteritis. *Curr Gastroenterol Rep* 1999;1:253–8.

10 Liacouras CA. Failed Nissen fundoplication in two patients who had persistent vomiting and eosinophilic esophagitis. *J Pediatr Surg* 1997;32:1504–6.

11 Ruchelli E, Wenner W, Voytek T, *et al*. Severity of esophageal eosinophilia predicts response to conventional gastroesophageal reflux therapy. *Pediatr Dev Pathol* 1999;2:15–18.

12 Steiner SJ, Gupta SK, Croffie JM, Fitzgerald JF. Correlation between number of eosinophils and reflux index on same day esophageal biopsy and 24 hour esophageal pH monitoring. *Am J Gastroenterol* 2004;99:801–5.

13 Straumann A, Spichtin HP, Grize L, *et al*. Natural history of primary eosinophilic esophagitis: a follow-up of 30 adult patients for up to 11.5 years. *Gastroenterology* 2003;125:1660–9.

14 Katzka DA. Eosinophilic esophagitis. *Curr Treat Options Gastroenterol* 2003;6:49–54.

15 Orenstein SR, Shalaby TM, Di Lorenzo C, *et al*. The spectrum of pediatric eosinophilic esophagitis beyond infancy: a clinical series of 30 children. *Am J Gastroenterol* 2000;95:1422–30.

16 Fox VL, Nurko S, Teitelbaum JE, *et al*. High-resolution EUS in children with eosinophilic "allergic" esophagitis. *Gastrointest Endosc* 2003;57:30–6.

17 Konikoff MR, Blanchard C, Kirby C, *et al*. Potential of blood eosinophils, eosinophil-derived neurotoxin, and eotaxin-3 as biomarkers of eosinophilic esophagitis. *Clin Gastroenterol Hepatol* 2006;4:1328–36.

18 Spergel JM, Brown-Whitehorn T, Beausoleil JL, *et al*. Predictive values for skin prick test and atopy patch test for eosinophilic esophagitis. *J Allergy Clin Immunol* 2007;119:509–11.

19 Ngo P, Furuta GT, Antonioli DA, Fox VL. Eosinophils in the esophagus – peptic or allergic eosinophilic esophagitis? Case series of three patients with esophageal eosinophilia. *Am J Gastroenterol* 2006;101:1666–70.

20 Straumann A, Rossi L, Simon HU, *et al*. Fragility of the esophageal mucosa: a pathognomonic endoscopic sign of primary eosinophilic esophagitis? *Gastrointest Endosc* 2003;57:407–12.

21 Kaplan M, Mutlu EA, Jakate S, *et al*. Endoscopy in eosinophilic esophagitis: "feline" esophagus and perforation risk. *Clin Gastroenterol Hepatol* 2003;1:433–7.

22 Croese J, Fairley SK, Masson JW, *et al*. Clinical and endoscopic features of eosinophilic esophagitis in adults. *Gastrointest Endosc* 2003;58:516–22.

23 Lucendo AJ, De Rezende L. Endoscopic dilation in eosinophilic esophagitis: a treatment strategy associated with a high risk of perforation. *Endoscopy* 2007;39:376;author reply 7.

24 Eisenbach C, Merle U, Schirmacher P, *et al*. Perforation of the esophagus after dilation treatment for dysphagia in a patient with eosinophilic esophagitis. *Endoscopy* 2006;38:E43–4.

25 Liacouras CA, Wenner WJ, Brown K, Ruchelli E. Primary eosinophilic esophagitis in children: successful treatment with oral corticosteroids. *J Pediatr Gastroenterol Nutr* 1998;26:380–5.

26 Faubion Jr WA, Perrault J, Burgart LJ, *et al*. Treatment of eosinophilic esophagitis with inhaled corticosteroids. *J Pediatr Gastroenterol Nutr* 1998;27:90–3.

27 Arora AS, Perrault J, Smyrk TC. Topical corticosteroid treatment of dysphagia due to eosinophilic esophagitis in adults. *Mayo Clin Proc* 2003;78:830–5.

28 Noel RJ, Putnam PE, Collins MH, *et al*. Clinical and immunopathologic effects of swallowed fluticasone for eosinophilic esophagitis. *Clin Gastroenterol Hepatol* 2004;2:568–75.

29 Remedios M, Campbell C, Jones DM, Kerlin P. Eosinophilic esophagitis in adults: clinical, endoscopic, histologic findings, and response to treatment with fluticasone propionate. *Gastrointest Endosc* 2006;63:3–12.

30 Konikoff MR, Noel RJ, Blanchard C, *et al*. A randomized, double-blind, placebo-controlled trial of fluticasone propionate for pediatric eosinophilic esophagitis. *Gastroenterology* 2006;131:1381–91.

31 Aceves SS, Dohil R, Newbury RO, Bastian JF. Topical viscous budesonide suspension for treatment of eosinophilic esophagitis. *J Allergy Clin Immunol* 2005;116:705–6.

32 Liacouras CA, Spergel JM, Ruchelli E, *et al*. Eosinophilic esophagitis: a 10-year experience in 381 children. *Clin Gastroenterol Hepatol* 2005;3:1198–206.

33 Spergel JM, Andrews T, Brown-Whitehorn TF, *et al*. Treatment of eosinophilic esophagitis with specific food elimination diet directed by a combination of skin prick and patch tests. *Ann Allergy Asthma Immunol* 2005;95:336–43.

34 Stein ML, Collins MH, Villanueva JM, *et al*. Anti-IL-5 (mepolizumab) therapy for eosinophilic esophagitis. *J Allergy Clin Immunol* 2006;118:1312–19.

35 Liacouras CA. Eosinophilic esophagitis: treatment in 2005. *Curr Opin Gastroenterol* 2006;22:147–52.

36 Yang YX, Lewis JD, Epstein S, Metz DC. Long-term proton pump inhibitor therapy and risk of hip fracture. *JAMA* 2006;296:2947–53.

37 Kaijser R. Zur Kenntnis der allergischen Affektioner desima Verdeanungaskanal von Standpunkt desmia Chirurgen aus. *Arch Klin Chir* 1937;188:36–64.

38 Klein NC, Hargrove RL, Sleisenger MH, Jeffries GH. Eosinophilic gastroenteritis. *Medicine (Baltimore)* 1970;49:299–319.

39 Kugathasan S, Judd RH, Hoffmann RG, *et al*. Epidemiologic and clinical characteristics of children with newly diagnosed inflammatory bowel disease in Wisconsin: a statewide population-based study. *J Pediatr* 2003;143:525–31.

40 Barak N, Hart J, Sitrin MD. Enalapril-induced eosinophilic gastroenteritis. J Clin Gastroenterol 2001;33:157–8.

41 Kakumitsu S, Shijo H, Akiyoshi N, ct al. Eosinophilic enteritis observed during alpha-interferon therapy for chronic hepatitis C. J Gastroenterol 2000;35:548–51.

42 Spergel JM, Pawlowski NA. Food allergy. Mechanisms, diagnosis, and management in children. *Pediatr Clin North Am* 2002;49:73–96, vi.

43 Park HS, Kim HS, Jang HJ. Eosinophilic gastroenteritis associated with food allergy and bronchial asthma. *J Korean Med Sci* 1995;10:216–19.

44 Justinich C, Katz A, Gurbindo C, *et al.* Elemental diet improves steroid-dependent eosinophilic gastroenteritis and reverses growth failure. *J Pediatr Gastroenterol Nutr* 1996;23:81–5.

45 Leinbach GE, Rubin CE. Eosinophilic gastroenteritis: a simple reaction to food allergens? *Gastroenterology* 1970;59:874–89.

46 Caldwell JH, Sharma HM, Hurtubise PE, Colwell DL. Eosinophilic gastroenteritis in extreme allergy. Immunopathological comparison with nonallergic gastrointestinal disease. *Gastroenterology* 1979;77:560–4.

47 Kelso A. Cytokines: structure, function and synthesis. *Curr Opin Immunol* 1989;2:215–25.

48 Desreumaux P, Bloget F, Seguy D, *et al.* Interleukin 3, granulocyte-macrophage colony-stimulating factor, and interleukin 5 in eosinophilic gastroenteritis. *Gastroenterology* 1996;110:768–74.

49 Takafuji S, Bischoff SC, De Weck AL, Dahinden CA. IL-3 and IL-5 prime normal human eosinophils to produce leukotriene C4 in response to soluble agonists. *J Immunol* 1991;147:3855–61.

50 Kweon MN, Kiyono H. Eosinophilic gastroenteritis: a problem of the mucosal immune system? *Curr Allergy Asthma Rep* 2003;3:79–85.

51 Kelly KJ. Eosinophilic gastroenteritis. *J Pediatr Gastroenterol Nutr* 2000;30:S28–35.

52 Whitington PF, Whitington GL. Eosinophilic gastroenteropathy in childhood. *J Pediatr Gastroenterol Nutr* 1988;7:379–85.

53 Khan S. Eosinophilic gastroenteritis. *Best Pract Res Clin Gastroenterol* 2005;19:177–98.

54 Talley NJ, Shorter RG, Phillips SF, Zinsmeister AR. Eosinophilic gastroenteritis: a clinicopathological study of patients with disease of the mucosa, muscle layer, and subserosal tissues. *Gut* 1990;31:54–8.

55 Santos J, Junquera F, de Torres I, *et al.* Eosinophilic gastroenteritis presenting as ascites and splenomegaly. *Eur J Gastroenterol Hepatol* 1995;7:675–8.

56 Goldman H, Proujansky R. Allergic proctitis and gastroenteritis in children. Clinical and mucosal biopsy features in 53 cases. *Am J Surg Pathol* 1986;10:75–86.

57 Aquino A, Domini M, Rossi C, *et al.* Pyloric stenosis due to eosinophilic gastroenteritis: presentation of two cases in mono-ovular twins. *Eur J Pediatr* 1999;158:172–3.

58 Khan S, Orenstein SR. Eosinophilic gastroenteritis masquerading as pyloric stenosis. *Clin Pediatr (Phila)* 2000;39:55–7.

59 Redondo-Cerezo E, Cabello MJ, Gonzalez Y, *et al.* Eosinophilic gastroenteritis: our recent experience: one-year experience of atypical onset of an uncommon disease. *Scand J Gastroenterol* 2001;36:1358–60.

60 Shweiki E, West JC, Klena JW, *et al.* Eosinophilic gastroenteritis presenting as an obstructing cecal mass – a case report and review of the literature. *Am J Gastroenterol* 1999;94:3644–5.

61 Huang FC, Ko SF, Huang SC, Lee SY. Eosinophilic gastroenteritis with perforation mimicking intussusception. *J Pediatr Gastroenterol Nutr* 2001;33:613–15.

62 Siahanidou T, Mandyla H, Dimitriadis D, *et al.* Eosinophilic gastroenteritis complicated with perforation and intussusception in a neonate. *J Pediatr Gastroenterol Nutr* 2001;32:335–7.

63 Markowitz JE, Russo P, Liacouras CA. Solitary duodenal ulcer: a new presentation of eosinophilic gastroenteritis. *Gastrointest Endosc* 2000;52:673–6.

64 Deslandres C, Russo P, Gould P, Hardy P. Perforated duodenal ulcer in a pediatric patient with eosinophilic gastroenteritis. *Can J Gastroenterol* 1997;11:208–12.

65 Wang CS, Hsueh S, Shih LY, Chen MF. Repeated bowel resections for eosinophilic gastroenteritis with obstruction and perforation. Case report. *Acta Chir Scand* 1990;156:333–6.

66 Hoefer RA, Ziegler MM, Koop CE, Schnaufer L. Surgical manifestations of eosinophilic gastroenteritis in the pediatric patient. *J Pediatr Surg* 1977;12:955–62.

67 Lerza P. A further case of eosinophilic gastroenteritis with ascites. *Eur J Gastroenterol Hepatol* 1996;8:407.

68 Lowichik A, Weinberg AG. A quantitative evaluation of mucosal eosinophils in the pediatric gastrointestinal tract. *Mod Pathol* 1996;9:110–14.

69 Pascal RR, Gramlich TL, Parker KM, Gansler TS. Geographic variations in eosinophil concentration in normal colonic mucosa. *Mod Pathol* 1997;10:363–5.

70 Teele RL, Katz AJ, Goldman H, Kettell RM. Radiographic features of eosinophilic gastroenteritis (allergic gastroenteropathy) of childhood. *Am J Roentgenol* 1979;132:575–80.

71 DeSchryver-Kecskemeti K, Clouse RE. A previously unrecognized subgroup of "eosinophilic gastroenteritis". Association with connective tissue diseases. *Am J Surg Pathol* 1984;8:171–80.

72 Dubucquoi S, Janin A, Klein O, *et al.* Activated eosinophils and interleukin 5 expression in early recurrence of Crohn's disease. *Gut* 1995;37:242–6.

73 Levy AM, Yamazaki K, Van Keulen VP, *et al.* Increased eosinophil infiltration and degranulation in colonic tissue from patients with collagenous colitis. *Am J Gastroenterol* 2001;96:1522–8.

74 Griscom NT, Kirkpatrick Jr JA, Girdany BR, *et al.* Gastric antral narrowing in chronic granulomatous disease of childhood. *Pediatrics* 1974;54:456–60.

75 Harris BH, Boles Jr ET. Intestinal lesions in chronic granulomatous disease of childhood. *J Pediatr Surg* 1973;8:955–6.

76 Caldwell JH, Tennenbaum JI, Bronstein HA. Serum IgE in eosinophilic gastroenteritis. Response to intestinal challenge in two cases. *N Engl J Med* 1975;292:1388–90.

77 Tsibouris P, Galeas T, Moussia M, *et al.* Two cases of eosinophilic gastroenteritis and malabsorption due to *Enterobious vermicularis*. *Dig Dis Sci* 2005;50:2389–92.

78 Chira O, Badea R, Dumitrascu D, *et al.* Eosinophilic ascites in a patient with toxocara canis infection. A case report. *Rom J Gastroenterol* 2005;14:397–400.

79 Van Laethem JL, Jacobs F, Braude P, *et al.* Toxocara canis infection presenting as eosinophilic ascites and gastroenteritis. *Dig Dis Sci* 1994;39:1370–2.

80 Papadopoulos AA, Tzathas C, Polymeros D, Ladas SD. Symptomatic eosinophilic gastritis cured with *Helicobacter pylori* eradication. *Gut* 2005;54:1822.

81 Montalto M, Miele L, Marcheggiano A, et al. Anisakis infestation: a case of acute abdomen mimicking Crohn's disease and eosinophilic gastroenteritis. *Dig Liver Dis* 2005;37:62–4.

82 Koga M, Fujiwara M, Hotta N, et al. Eosinophilic gastroenteritis associated with Epstein–Barr virus infection in a young boy. *J Pediatr Gastroenterol Nutr* 2001;33:610–12.

83 Sunkureddi PR, Baethge BA. Eosinophilic gastroenteritis associated with systemic lupus erythematosus. *J Clin Gastroenterol* 2005;39:838–9.

84 Schwake L, Stremmel W, Sergi C. Eosinophilic enterocolitis in a patient with rheumatoid arthritis. *J Clin Gastroenterol* 2002;34:487–8.

85 Reese GE, Constantinides VA, Simillis C, et al. Diagnostic precision of anti-Saccharomyces cerevisiae antibodies and perinuclear antineutrophil cytoplasmic antibodies in inflammatory bowel disease. *Am J Gastroenterol* 2006;101:2410–22.

86 Mamula P, Telega GW, Markowitz JE, et al. Inflammatory bowel disease in children 5 years of age and younger. *Am J Gastroenterol* 2002;97:2005–10.

87 Vandenplas Y, Quenon M, Renders F, et al. Milk-sensitive eosinophilic gastroenteritis in a 10-day-old boy. *Eur J Pediatr* 1990;149:244–5.

88 Chehade M, Magid MS, Mofidi S, et al. Allergic eosinophilic gastroenteritis with protein-losing enteropathy: intestinal pathology, clinical course, and long-term follow-up. *J Pediatr Gastroenterol Nutr* 2006;42:516–21.

89 Chen MJ, Chu CH, Lin SC, et al. Eosinophilic gastroenteritis: clinical experience with 15 patients. *World J Gastroenterol* 2003; 9:2813–16.

90 Siewert E, Lammert F, Koppitz P, et al. Eosinophilic gastroenteritis with severe protein-losing enteropathy: successful treatment with budesonide. *Dig Liver Dis* 2006;38:55–9.

91 Tan AC, Kruimel JW, Naber TH. Eosinophilic gastroenteritis treated with non-enteric-coated budesonide tablets. *Eur J Gastroenterol Hepatol* 2001;13:425–7.

92 Van Dellen RG, Lewis JC. Oral administration of cromolyn in a patient with protein-losing enteropathy, food allergy, and eosinophilic gastroenteritis. *Mayo Clin Proc* 1994;69:441–4.

93 Moots RJ, Prouse P, Gumpel JM. Near fatal eosinophilic gastroenteritis responding to oral sodium chromoglycate. *Gut* 1988;29:1282–5.

94 Di Gioacchino M, Pizzicannella G, Fini N, et al. Sodium cromoglycate in the treatment of eosinophilic gastroenteritis. *Allergy* 1990;45:161–6.

95 Schwartz DA, Pardi DS, Murray JA. Use of montelukast as steroid-sparing agent for recurrent eosinophilic gastroenteritis. *Dig Dis Sci* 2001;46:1787–90.

96 Neustrom MR, Friesen C. Treatment of eosinophilic gastroenteritis with montelukast. *J Allergy Clin Immunol* 1999; 104:506.

97 Urek MC, Kujundzic M, Banic M, *et al.* Leukotriene receptor antagonists as potential steroid sparing agents in a patient with serosal eosinophilic gastroenteritis. *Gut* 2006;55: 1363–4.

98 Shirai T, Hashimoto D, Suzuki K, *et al.* Successful treatment of eosinophilic gastroenteritis with suplatast tosilate. *J Allergy Clin Immunol* 2001;107:924–5.

99 Katsinelos P, Pilpilidis I, Xiarchos P, *et al.* Oral administration of ketotifen in a patient with eosinophilic colitis and severe osteoporosis. *Am J Gastroenterol* 2002;97:1072–4.

100 Jenkins HR, Pincott JR, Soothill JF, *et al.* Food allergy: the major cause of infantile colitis. *Arch Dis Child* 1984;59:326–9.

101 Gerrard JW, MacKenzie JW, Goluboff N, *et al.* Cow's milk allergy: prevalence and manifestations in an unselected series of newborns. *Acta Paediatr Scand Suppl* 1973;234:1–21.

102 Host A, Halken S. A prospective study of cow milk allergy in Danish infants during the first 3 years of life. Clinical course in relation to clinical and immunological type of hypersensitivity reaction. *Allergy* 1990;45:587–96.

103 Strobel S. Epidemiology of food sensitivity in childhood – with special reference to cow's milk allergy in infancy. *Monogr Allergy* 1993;31:119–30.

104 Simpser E. Gastrointestinal allergy. In: Altschuler SM, Liacouras CA (eds.) *Clinical Pediatric Gastroenterology.* Philadelphia, PA: Churchill Livingstone, 1998:113–18.

105 Eastham EJ. Soy protein allergy. In: Hamburger RN (ed.) *Allergology, Immunology, and Gastroenterology.* New York: Raven Press, 1989:223–36.

106 Heyman M, Grasset E, Ducroc R, Desjeux JF. Antigen absorption by the jejunal epithelium of children with cow's milk allergy. *Pediatr Res* 1988;24:197–202.

107 Husby S, Host A, Teisner B, Svehag SE. Infants and children with cow milk allergy/intolerance. Investigation of the uptake of cow milk protein and activation of the complement system. *Allergy* 1990;45:547–51.

108 Kerner Jr JA. Formula allergy and intolerance. *Gastroenterol Clin North Am* 1995;24:1–25.

109 Shannon WR. Demonstration of food proteins in human breast milk by anaphylactic experiments in guinea pig. *Am J Dis Child* 1921;22:223–5.

110 Makinen-Kiljunen S, Palosuo T. A sensitive enzyme-linked immunosorbent assay for determination of bovine beta-lactoglobulin in infant feeding formulas and in human milk. *Allergy* 1992;47:347–52.

111 Axelsson I, Jakobsson I, Lindberg T, Benediktsson B. Bovine beta-lactoglobulin in the human milk. A longitudinal study during the whole lactation period. *Acta Paediatr Scand* 1986;75:702–7.

112 Pittschieler K. Cow's milk protein-induced colitis in the breast-fed infant. *J Pediatr Gastroenterol Nutr* 1990;10:548–9.

50 Van Sickle GJ, Powell GK, McDonald PJ, Goldblum RM. Milk and soy protein-induced enterocitis: evidence for lymphocyte sensitization to specific food proteins. *Gastroenterology* 1985;88:1915–21.

51 Hoffman KM, Ho DG, Sampson HA. Evaluation of the usefullness of lymphocyte proliferation assays in the diagnosis of cow's milk allergy. *J Allergy Clin Immunol* 1997;99:360–6.

52 Shek LP, Soderstrom L, Ahlstedt S, *et al.* Determination of food specific IgE levels over time can predict the development of tolerance in cow's milk and hen's egg allergy. *J Allergy Clin Immunol* 2004;114:387–91.

53 Rodriguez P, Heyman M, Candalh C, *et al.* Tumour necrosis factor-alpha induces morphological and functional alterations of intestinal HT29 cl.19A cell monolayers. *Cytokine* 1995;7:441–8.

54 Heyman M, Darmon N, Dupont C, *et al.* Mononuclear cells from infants allergic to cow's milk secrete tumor necrosis factor alpha, altering intestinal function. *Gastroenterology* 1994;106:1514–23.

55 Benlounes N, Candalh C, Matarazzo P, *et al.* The time-course of milk antigen-induced TNF-alpha secretion differs according to the clinical symptoms in children with cow's milk allergy. *J Allergy Clin Immunol* 1999;104:863–9.

56 Chung HL, Hwang JB, Park JJ, Kim SG. Expression of transforming growth factor beta1, transforming growth factor type I and II receptors, and TNF-alpha in the mucosa of the small intestine in infants with food protein-induced enterocolitis syndrome. *J Allergy Clin Immunol* 2002;109:150–4.

57 McDonald PJ, Goldblum RM, Van Sickle GJ, Powell GK. Food protein-induced enterocolitis: altered antibody response to ingested antigen. *Pediatr Res* 1984;18:751–5.

58 Schlossmann NA. Uber die giftwirkung des artfremden eiweisses in der milch auf den organismus des sauglings. *Arch Kinderheilkunde* 1905;41:99–103.

59 Lamy M, Nezelof C, Jos J, *et al.* Biopsy of intestinal mucosa in children: first results of study of malabsorption syndromes. *Presse Med* 1963;71:1267–70.

60 Davidson M, Burnstine MC, Kugler MM, Baure CH. Malabsorption defect induced by ingestion of lactoglobulin. *J Pediatr* 1965;66:545–54.

61 Kuitunen P. Duodeno-jejunal histology in the malabsorption syndrome in infants. *Ann Paediatr Fenn* 1966;12:101–32.

62 Visakorpi JK, Immonen P. Intolerance to cow's milk and wheat gluten in the primary malabsorption syndrome in infancy. *Acta Pediatr Scand* 1967;56:49–56.

63 Liu H-Y, Tsao MU, Moore B, Giday Z. Bovine milk-protein-induced intestinal malabsorption syndrome in infancy. *Gastroenterology* 1967;54:27–34.

64 Harrison M, Kilby A, Walker-Smith JA, *et al.* Cow's milk protein intolerance: A possible association with gastroenteritis, lactose intolerance, and IgA deficiency. *BMJ* 1976;1:1501–4.

65 Kuitunen P, Visakorpi JK, Savilahti E, Pelkonem P. Malabsorption syndrome with cow's milk intolerance: clinical findings and course in 54 cases. *Arch Dis Child* 1975;50:251–6.

66 Savilahti E. Food-induced malabsorption syndromes. *J Pediatr Gastroenterol Nutr* 2000;30:S61–6.

67 Saarinen K, Juntunen-Backman K, Jarvenpaa A-L, *et al.* Supplementary feeding in maternity hospitals and the risk of cow's milk allergy: a prospective study of 6209 infants. *J Allergy Clin Immunol* 1999;104:457–61.

68 Verkasalo M, Kuitunen P, Savilahti E. Changing pattern of cow's milk intolerance. *Acta Pediatr Scand* 1981;70:289–95.

69 Vitoria JC, Sojo A, Rodriguez-Soriano J. Changing pattern of cow's milk protein intolerance. *Acta Pediatr Scand* 1990; 79:566–7.

70 Kokkonen J, Haapalahti M, Laurila K, *et al.* Cow's milk protein-sensitive enteropathy at school age. *J Pediatr* 2001;139: 797–803.

71 Veres G, Westerholm-Ormio M, Kokkonen J, *et al.* Cytokines and adhesion molecules in duodenal mucosa of children with delayed-type food allergy. *J Pediatr Gastroenterol Nutr* 2003; 37:27–34.

72 Latcham F, Merino F, Lang A, *et al.* A consistent pattern of minor immunodeficiency and subtle enteropathy in children with multiple food allergy. *J Pediatr* 2003;143:39–47.

73 Ament ME, Rubin CE. Soy protein – another cause of the flat intestinal lesion. *Gastroenterology* 1972;62:227–34.

74 Iyngkaran N, Abdin Z, Davis K, *et al.* Acquired carbohydrate intolerance and cow milk protein-sensitive enteropathy in young infants. *J Pediatr* 1979;95:373–8.

75 Iyngkaran N, Yadav M, Boey CG, *et al.* Causative effect of cow's milk protein and soy protein on progressive small bowel mucosal damage. *J Gastroenterol Hepatol* 1989;4:127–36.

76 Walker-Smith JA. Cow's milk intolerance as a cause of postenteritis diarrhea. *J Pediatr Gastroenterol Nutr* 1982;1:163–75.

77 Walker-Smith JA. Transient gluten intolerance. *Arch Dis Child* 1970;45:523–6.

78 Iyngkaran N, Robinson NJ, Sumithran E, *et al.* Cow's milk protein-sensitive enteropathy. An important factor in prolonging diarrhoea in acute infective enteritis in early infancy. *Arch Dis Child* 1978;53:150–3.

79 Lake AM. Food protein-induced colitis and gastroenteropathy in infants and children. In: Metcalfe DD SHSR (ed.) *Food Allergy: Adverse Reactions to Foods and Food Additives*. Cambridge, MA: Blackwell Scientific Publications, 1997:277–86.

80 Iyngkaran N, Abidin Z. One hour D-xylose in the diagnosis of cow's milk protein sensitive enteropathy. *Arch Dis Child* 1982;57:40–3.

81 Paajanen L, Vaarala O, Karttunen R, *et al.* Increased IFN-gamma secretion from duodenal biopsy samples in delayed-type cow's milk allergy. *Pediatr Allergy Immunol* 2005;16:439–44.

82 Iyngkaran N, Yadav M, Boey CG, Lam KL. Effect of continued feeding of cow's milk on asymptomatic infants with milk protein sensitive enteropathy. *Arch Dis Child* 1988;63:911–15.

83 Kuitunen P, Rapola J, Savilahti E, Visakorpi JK. Response of the mucosa to cow's milk in the malabsorption syndrome with cow's milk intolerance. *Acta Pediatr Scand* 1973;62:585–95.

84 Shiner M, Ballard J, Brook CGD, Herman S. Intestinal biopsy in the diagnosis of cow's milk protein intolerance without acute symptoms. *Lancet* 1979;29:1060–3.

85 Baehler P, Chad Z, Gurbindo C, *et al.* Distinct patterns of cow's milk allergy in infancy defined by prolonged, two stage double-blind, placebo-controlled food challenges. *Clin Exp Allergy* 1996; 26:254–61.

86 Augustin M, Karttunen TJ, Kokkonen J. TIA1 and mast cell tryptase in food allergy of children: increase of intraepithelial lymphocytes expressing TIA1 associates with allergy. *J Pediatr Gastroenterol Nutr* 2001;32:11–18.

87 Hankard GF, Matarazzo P, Duong JP, *et al.* Increased TIA1-expressing intraepithelial lymphocytes in cow's milk protein intolerance. *J Pediatr Gastroenterol Nutr* 1997;25:79–83.

88 Augustin MT, Kokkonen J, Karttunen TJ. Duodenal cytotoxic lymphocytes in cow's milk protein sensitive enteropathy and coeliac disease. *Scand J Gastroenterol* 2005;40:1398–406.

89 Burgin-Wolff A, Gaze H, Hadziselimovic F, *et al.* Antigliadin and antiendomysium antibody determination for coeliac disease. *Arch Dis Child* 1991;66:941–7.

90 Meuli R, Pichler WJ, Gaze H, Lentze MJ. Genetic difference in HLA-DR phenotypes between coeliac disease and transitory gluten intolerance. *Arch Dis Child* 1995;72:29–32.

91 McNeish AS, Rolles CJ, Arthur LJ. Criteria for diagnosis of temporary gluten intolerance. *Arch Dis Child* 1976;51:275–8.

92 Maluenda C, Philips AD, Briddon A, Walker-Smith JA. Quantitative analysis of small intestinal mucosa in cow's milk-sensitive enteropathy. *J Pediatr Gastroenterol Nutr* 1984; 3:349–56.

93 Kuitunen P, Kosnai I, Savilahti E. Morphometric study of the jejunal mucosa in various childhood enteropathies with special reference to intraepithelial lymphocytes. *J Pediatr Gastroenterol Nutr* 1982;1:525–31.

94 Kosnai I, Kuitunen P, Savilahti E, Sipponen P. Mast cells and eosinophils in the jejunal mucosa of patients with intestinal cow's milk allergy and celiac disease. *J Pediatr Gastroenterol Nutr* 1984;3:368–72.

95 Augustin MT, Kokkonen J, Karttunen TJ. Evidence for increased apoptosis of duodenal intraepithelial lymphocytes in cow's milk sensitive enteropathy. *J Pediatr Gastroenterol Nutr* 2005;40:352–8.

96 Variend S, Placzek M, Raafat F, Walker-Smith JA. Small intestinal mucosal fat in childhood enteropathies. *J Clin Pathol* 1984;37:373–7.

97 Kosnai I, Kuitunen P, Savilahti E, *et al.* Cell kinetics in the jejunal epithelium in malabsorption syndrome with cow's milk protein intolerance and coeliac disease of childhood. *Gut* 1980;21:1046.

98 Savidge TC, Shmakov AN, Walker-Smith JA, Phillips AD. Epithelial cell proliferation in childhood enteropathies. *Gut* 1996;39:185–93.

99 Stern M, Dietrich R, Muller J. Small intestinal mucosa in coeliac disease and cow's milk protein intolerance: morphometric and immunofluorescent studies. *Eur J Pediatr* 1982;139:101–5.

100 Rosekrans PCM, Meijer CJLM, Cornelise CJ, *et al.* Use of morphometry and immunohistochemistry of small intestinal biopsy specimens in the diagnosis of food allergy. *J Clin Pathol* 1980;33:125–30.

101 Perkkio M, Savilahti E, Kuitunen P. Morphometric and immunohistochemical study of jejunal biopsies from children with intestinal soy allergy. *Eur J Pediatr* 1981;137:63–9.

102 Poley JR, Klein AW. Scanning electron microscopy of soy protein-induced damage of small bowel mucosa in infants. *J Pediatr Gastroenterol Nutr* 1983;2:271–87.

103 da Cunha Ferreira R, Forsyth LE, Richman PI, *et al.* Changes in the rate of crypt epithelial cell proliferation and mucosal morphology induced by a T-cell-mediated response in human small intestine. *Gastroenterology* 1990;98:1255–63.

104 MacDonald TT, Spencer J. Evidence that activated mucosal T cells play a role in the pathogenesis of enteropathy in human small intestine. *J Exp Med* 1988;167:1341–9.

105 Nagata S, Yamashiro Y, Ohtsuka Y, *et al.* Quantitative analysis and immunohistochemical studies on small intestinal mucosa of food-sensitive enteropathy. *J Pediatr Gastroenterol Nutr* 1995;20:44–8.

106 Chan K, Phillips AD, Walker-Smith JA, *et al.* Density of gamma/delta T cells in small bowel mucosa related to HLA-DQ status without celiac disease. *Lancet* 1993;342:492–3.

107 Pesce G, Pesce F, Fiorino N, *et al.* Intraepithelial gamma/delta-positive T lymphocytes and intestinal villous atrophy. *Int Arch Allergy Immunol* 1996;110:233–7.

108 Augustin MT, Kokkonen J, Karttunen R, Karttunen TJ. Serum granzymes and CD30 are increased in children's milk protein sensitive enteropathy and celiac disease. *J Allergy Clin Immunol* 2005;115:157–62.

109 Kokkonen J, Holm K, Karttunen TJ, Maki M. Enhanced local immune response in children with prolonged gastrointestinal symptoms. *Acta Paediatr* 2004;93:1601–7.

110 Veres G, Helin T, Arato A, *et al.* Increased expression of intercellular adhesion molecule-1 and mucosal adhesion molecule alpha4beta7 integrin in small intestinal mucosa of adult patients with food allergy. *Clin Immunol* 2001;99:353–9.

111 Raithel M, Matek M, Baenkler HW, *et al.* Mucosal histamine content and histamine secretion in Crohn's disease, ulcerative colitis and allergic enteropathy. *Int Arch Allergy Immunol* 1995;108:127–33.

112 Savilahti E. Immunochemical study of the malabsorption syndrome with cow's milk intolerance. *Gut* 1973;14:491–501.

113 Van Spreeuwel JP, Lindenman J, Van Maanen J, Meyer CJLM. Increased numbers of IgE-containing cells in gastric and duodenal biopsies: an expression of food allergy secondary to chronic inflammation? *J Clin Pathol* 1984;37:601–6.

114 Nakajima-Adachi H, Ebihara A, Kikuchi A, *et al.* Food antigen causes TH2-dependent enteropathy followed by tissue repair in T-cell receptor transgenic mice. *J Allergy Clin Immunol* 2006;117:1125–32.

115 Hauer AC, Breese EJ, Walker-Smith JA, MacDonald TT. The frequency of cells secreting interferon gamma and interleukin-4,-5,

Table 17.2 Presentations of CD (partial list)

Gastrointestinal	Non-gastrointestinal
Steatorrhea	Dermatitis herpetiformis
Chronic diarrhea	Infertility
Weight loss	Anemia
Elevated transaminases	Dementia
Recurrent pancreatitis	Osteoporosis
Bloating, abdominal pain	Neuropathy
Failure to thrive	Dental enamel defects
Enteropathy-associated T-cell lymphoma	Ataxia
Vomiting	Osteomalacia
Duodenal obstruction	Tetany

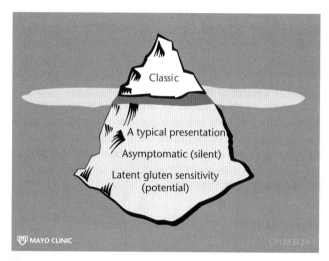

Figure 17.5 The celiac iceberg (see text) (copyright The Mayo Foundation).

(CD is considered the "modern impostor") including irritable bowel syndrome, deficiencies of single micronutrients, especially iron, folate, B12, and the fat-soluble vitamins. Other "atypical" presentations are secondary osteoporosis, osteomalacia, ataxia, dementia, fatigue, neuropathy, and chorea.

The presentation of CD in children similarly can result in stunting of growth and intellectual development, epilepsy, and dental abnormalities as single symptoms without the more classic malabsorption symptoms of malnourished pot-bellied infant with steatorrhea [45].

CD is defined according to the clinical presentation and has been likened to an iceberg, "the celiac iceberg" (Fig. 17.5).

The tip of the iceberg represents the most obvious part of the clinical spectra (classic malabsorption). If the patient's symptoms are characteristic of the malabsorption syndrome (diarrhea, steatorrhea, weight loss, fatigue); then the adjective "classical" is used. Then there is the "non-classical" CD, adjective applied when patients have non-specific symptoms such as abdominal discomfort, bloating, indigestion, or non-gastrointestinal (GI) symptoms (microcytic anemia).

Thus, this group of patients had minimal symptoms but can be detected clinically if there is a high suspicion for the diagnosis. Paradoxically, the "non-classical" is now the most frequent presentation of CD in the United States. Finally, there is the submerged part of the iceberg where patients have histologic evidence of CD but remain undetected. Some of that portion consists of identifiable at-risk groups such as families of people with CD and subjects with CD-associated diseases. In "silent" CD, intestinal biopsies show the characteristic morphologic changes in an asymptomatic patient. Autoantibodies may or may not be present. "Latent" disease refers to genetically susceptible persons, without symptoms or histologic evidence of CD who will ultimately go on to develop CD. These cases are found by following up persistently positive autoantibodies such as endomysial or tTG antibodies, in patients with DH who initially have an apparently normal small intestine who then develop CD while on a gluten-containing diet, or occasionally in asymptomatic family members of an index case.

Diagnostic tests for celiac disease

An important consideration is whether the patient has been on a GFD prior to the testing. All of the tests, including the intestinal biopsies, may have returned to normal, making confirmation difficult without reintroducing gluten into the diet.

The pre-modern diagnosis of CD was based on the constellation of features, especially steatorrhea and weight loss or failure to thrive, that are hallmarks of frank malabsorption. Almost simultaneously in the 1950s, advances in understanding of the specific pathologic lesion in the small intestinal mucosa and its gluten-induced etiology enhanced the precision with which the disease could be diagnosed; diagnosis included the response to therapy (GFD). Current guidelines require histologic evidence of enteropathy and a positive response of symptoms or signs to a GFD. The earlier requirement for three sets of biopsies (one at diagnosis, after treatment with GFD, and after gluten challenge) was both cumbersome and, in most cases, unnecessary to establish and confirm a diagnosis of CD. Three biopsies may be needed in individuals diagnosed at less than 3 years of age, when the population from which the individual comes is subject to common alternative diagnoses, and when the original diagnosis is uncertain or is challenged later [46].

Serologic testing has greatly facilitated the identification of CD in people with clinical presentations too mild to justify the invasiveness of a biopsy as the initial diagnostic test. The ready availability of serology has made detection accessible to primary-care doctors and their patients in primary care. Not only are more people being diagnosed, but many other issues have arisen about the accuracy of the diagnosis and how to incorporate serologic testing into the diagnostic approach (Fig. 17.6).

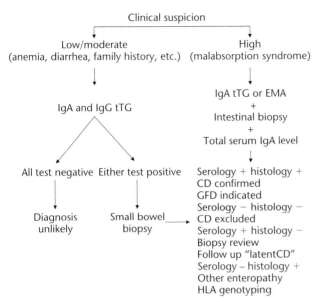

Figure 17.6 Approach to the diagnosis of CD. EMA, endomysial antibodies; positive +; negative −.

Table 17.3 Serologic tests for CD

Substrate/antigen	Antibody isotype	Test type	Sensitivity (%)	Specificity (%)
Gliadin	IgA	ELISA	31–100	85–100
Gliadin	IgG	ELISA	46–100	67–100
Endomysium	IgA	IFA	57–100	95–100
Tissue transglutaminase	IgA	ELISA	92–98	98

IFA, immunofluorescence assay.

Serology

A summary of serologic tests available for CD diagnosis is shown in Table 17.3.

Intestinal biopsies

Intestinal biopsy is always necessary to confirm the diagnosis of CD, except in the case of patients with biopsy-proven DH and positive celiac serology. The biopsy must be interpreted by an expert pathologist with recognition of the whole spectrum of the histologic lesion in CD. The most used histologic classification is that described by Marsh [47]. Briefly, Marsh type 0 is a normal mucosa. Marsh type I or "infiltrative" lesion is characterized by intra-epithelial lymphocytosis in the absence of other abnormality but is not specific for CD. Marsh type II or "hyperplastic" lesion is characterized by intra-epithelial lymphocytosis with crypt hyperplasia. Marsh type III or "atrophic" lesion is characterized by partial atrophy (3a), sub-total atrophy (3b), and total atrophy (3c) [48]. Marsh type IV refers to the most severe "hypoplastic" lesion.

Gluten challenge

It is no longer necessary to re-challenge most patients who have a well-established diagnosis of CD. However, in patients first diagnosed under the age of 3 years or those who have already embarked on a GFD and are seeking a confirmation of the diagnosis, a formal gluten challenge may be desirable [49]. This is not usually needed if the patient had a biopsy while on gluten-containing diet. Review of the original histology slides, if available, may suffice to confirm the diagnosis.

The length of time it takes to relapse with gluten challenge is quite variable [50]. The gluten in three to four slices of whole wheat bread daily should be sufficient to produce damage in 2–4 weeks, although it can take longer for the full pattern of injury to occur. Some very sensitive patients may need a reduction of this dose to prevent severe symptoms. Most patients relapse within 6 months although, in rare cases, it may take years to relapse.

Celiac crisis

A life-threatening presentation of CD has been reported in children and less frequently in adults [51,52]. Profuse acute diarrhea, dehydratation, hypokalemia, and severe metabolic acidosis, the so-called "celiac crisis," need emergent life-saving therapy. This dramatic clinical scenario can be a spontaneous clinical presentation or precipitated by the gluten challenge in patients very sensitive to the gluten.

Dermatitis herpetiformis

DH is characterized by chronic, intensely pruritic, polymorphic rash that causes vesicles–bullae on extensor surfaces of the elbows, knees, buttocks, and scalp [53]. There is a slight male preponderance of DH [54]. It is a skin manifestation of the intestinal immune response to ingested gluten that is characterized by the deposition of IgA granules at the dermoepidermal junction. The source of these IgA deposits in the skin is unknown, but they may be produced in the intestinal mucosa and are likely cross-reactive with the closely related skin-based autoantigen epidermal transglutaminase, which is similar to tTG (the primary autoantigen in the gut) [55]. The intestinal damage may be asymptomatic at the time of presentation of the skin rash, but it is indistinguishable from that seen in CD. A positive serologic test strengthens the certainty of the skin diagnosis, and would also mandate examination of the patient for consequences of malabsorption. However, it is not necessary to perform these antibody tests or even an intestinal biopsy to establish the etiologic role of intestinal gluten exposure in DH. That can be reliably inferred by the demonstration of the granular IgA deposits in the skin (Fig. 17.4). The serology test may be useful in cases in which there remains some doubt, for example, in distinguishing it from bullous linear IgA disease, which is not a gluten sensitive disorder. Gliadin antibodies may be seen in other bullous skin disorders and are not particularly helpful in this setting [56].

62 Pietzak MM. Follow-up of patients with celiac disease: achieving compliance with treatment. *Gastroenterology* 2005;128:S135–41.

63 Ivarsson A, Persson LA, Nystrom L, *et al.* Epidemic of celiac disease in Swedish children. *Acta Paediatr* 2000;89:165–71.

64 Ivarsson A, Hernell O, Stenlund H, Persson LA. Breast-feeding protects against celiac disease. *Am J Clin Nutr* 2002;75:914–21.

65 Johnston SD, Robinson J. Fatal pneumococcal septicemia in a celiac patient. *Eur J Gastroenterol Hepatol* 1998;10:353–4.

66 McKinley M, Leibowitz S, Bronzo R, *et al.* Appropriate response to pneumococcal vaccine in celiac sprue. *J Clin Gastroenterol* 1995;20:113–16.

67 Noh KW, Poland GA, Murray JA. Hepatitis B vaccine nonresponse and celiac disease. *Am J Gastroenterol* 2003;98:2289–92.

68 Krauss N, Schuppan D. Monitoring nonresponsive patients who have celiac disease. *Gastrointest Endosc Clin North Am* 2006;16:317–27.

69 Abdulkarim AS, Burgart LJ, See J, Murray JA. Etiology of nonresponsive celiac disease: results of a systematic approach. *Am J Gastroenterol* 2002;97:2016–21.

70 Trier JS, Falchuk Z, Carey M, Schreiber D. Celiac sprue and refractory sprue. *Gastroenterology* 1978;75:307–16.

71 Elsing C, Placke J, Gross-Weege W. Ulcerative jejunoileitis and enteropathy-associated T-cell lymphoma. *Eur J Gastroenterol Hepatol* 2005;17:1401–5.

72 Cellier C, Delabesse E, Helmer C, *et al.* Refractory sprue, celiac disease, and enteropathy-associated T-cell lymphoma. *Lancet* 2000;356:203–8.

73 Al-Toma A, Goerres MS, Meijer JW, *et al.* Cladribine therapy in refractory celiac disease with aberrant T cells. *Clin Gastroenterol Hepatol* 2006;4:1322–7.

74 Vivas S, Ruiz de Morales JM, Ramos F, Suarez-Vilela D. Alemtuzumab for refractory celiac disease in a patient at risk for enteropathy-associated T-cell lymphoma. *N Engl J Med* 2006;354:2514–15.

75 Rongey C, Micallef I, Smyrik T, Murray J. Successful treatment of enteropathy-associated T cell lymphoma with autologous stem cell transplant. *Dig Dis Sci* 2006;51:1082–6.

76 Cellier C, Cerf-Bensussan N. Treatment of clonal refractory celiac disease or cryptic intraepithelial lymphoma: a long road from bench to bedside. *Clin Gastroenterol Hepatol* 2006;4:1320–1.

77 Viljamaa M, Kaukinen K, Pukkala E, *et al.* Malignancies and mortality in patients with celiac disease and dermatitis herpetiformis: 30-year population-based study. *Dig Liver Dis* 2006;38:374–80.

78 West J, Logan RF, Smith CJ, *et al.* Malignancy and mortality in people with celiac disease: population based cohort study. *BMJ* 2004;329:716–9.

79 Halfdanarson TR, Litzow MR, Murray JA. Hematologic manifestations of celiac disease. *Blood* 2007;109:412–21.

80 Green PH, Fleischauer AT, Bhagat G, *et al.* Risk of malignancy in patients with celiac disease. *Am J Med* 2003;115:191–5.

81 Parnell N, Thomas P. Fatal pneumococcal septicemia in a celiac patient. *Eur J Gastroenterol Hepatol* 1998;10:899–900.

82 Fraser JS, King AL, Ellis HJ, *et al.* An algorithm for family screening for celiac disease. *World J Gastroenterol* 2006;12:7805–9.

18 CHAPTER 18

Occupational Reactions to Food Allergens

Maxcie Sikora, André Cartier, Matthew Aresery, Laurianne Wild, and Samuel B. Lehrer

---

KEY CONCEPTS

- Occupational diseases have significant social and economic impact on workers and society as a whole.

- Workers in the food industry, an industry that employs 10 million people in the United States, are exposed to a variety of food and non-food materials that can cause a wide range of dermatologic and respiratory illnesses.

- Rhinitis, conjunctivitis, asthma, hypersensitivity pneumonitis, and dermatitis are common manifestations associated with occupational exposure to food allergens/antigens.

- Early diagnosis and removal from the exposure environment result in the best prognosis for occupational disease in the food industry.

- Since the removal from the exposure environment is not always possible, especially when this may be a family's sole source of income, improvement of environmental conditions and use of protective devices are warranted.

Introduction

The United States Bureau of Labor Statistics has reported that in 2005 there were 145 million employed civilian individuals of which approximately 10 million work in some aspect of the food preparation and service industry. In addition, the USDA estimates there are up to 3 million Americans employed in the farming sector [1]. These workers can be exposed to a wide variety of substances that potentially may lead to hypersensitivity diseases. Most sensitizing materials are food-derived protein allergens, such as flour and shellfish. Non-food agents may also induce allergic or immunologic diseases (e.g. honey bees, grain storage mites, antibiotics, thermophilic actinomycetes, and even rubber boots). It is well established that these materials can affect the skin, gastrointestinal tract, and respiratory system. In occupational exposure to food allergens/antigens, the routes of exposure are primarily through inhalation and contact, and vary depending on agents and industries. The ensuing diseases include occupational rhinitis (OR), conjunctivitis, asthma, hypersensitivity pneumonitis (HP) (extrinsic allergic alveolitis), and occupational dermatitis.

Making a diagnosis of one of these occupational diseases can have significant social and economic impact on both the individual and the society as a whole. Diagnosing an occupational disease requires confirmation of the causal relationship between exposure at work and disease; although most cases have new onset disease, this is not exclusive, for example, the history of previous asthma does not exclude occupational asthma (OA). In the case of occupational dermatitis, the skin inflammation should improve while away from the workplace. In occupational lung diseases, unfortunately, the symptoms may be slow to resolve or still remain long after removal from the workplace. Each of these types of reactions will be discussed in greater detail. Several pertinent examples of each of the aforementioned diseases in occupational settings have been chosen to illustrate important points.

Definitions

The diagnosis of OA involves demonstrating asthma which can be attributed to work. Criteria have been established by numerous groups for the purpose of epidemiology and clinical evaluation. For example, the American College of Chest Physicians established criteria which include a compatible history, reversible airflow limitation, and airway hyperresponsiveness in the absence of airflow limitation, and objective demonstration of work relatedness [2].

Food Allergy: Adverse Reactions to Foods and Food Additives, 4th edition.
Edited by Dean D. Metcalfe, Hugh A. Sampson, and Ronald A. Simon.
© 2008 Blackwell Publishing. ISBN: 978-1-4501-5129-0.

A similar definition from Bernstein *et al.* is variable air-flow limitation and airway hyperresponsiveness due to causes and conditions that are attributable to a particular occupational environment and not to stimuli encountered outside the workplace [3]. Asthma occurring at the workplace is not necessarily OA, and it is important, for medico-legal reasons, to draw this distinction. Asthma can be exacerbated at work by exercise or by exposure to irritants such as cold air, dust, or fumes in excessive quantity.

Reactive airways dysfunction syndrome (RADS) or irritant-induced asthma is an occupational lung disease which occurs after acute high-level exposure to irritant gas, smoke, fumes, or vapors [4,5]. Unlike OA which results from a previous sensitization to a substance, there is no latent period in RADS. RADS will not be discussed further in the context of food-induced occupational reactions, although it may be seen in this industry due to accidental exposure, such as ammonia spills from refrigeration systems.

OR has been defined as the episodic work-related occurrence of sneezing, nasal discharge, pruritus, and congestion which contribute to distress, discomfort, and work inefficiency [6]. OR is 2–3 times more frequent than OA. It often coexists with OA. Rhinitis symptoms frequently precede the development of asthma in the work environment [7]. In 59 workers with laboratory animal allergy, Gross *et al.* reported that OR preceded the development of OA in 45% of subjects and occurred at the same time in 55%, but OR did not develop subsequently [8].

HP or extrinsic allergic alveolitis is an immunologically mediated inflammatory disease involving the terminal airways of the lung associated with intense or repeated exposure to various inhaled allergens. The result of this exposure is initially a lymphocytic alveolitis followed by granuloma formation and eventually irreversible pulmonary fibrosis in the untreated patient [9–10].

Traditionally, the term "contact dermatitis" has been used to describe any rash resulting from a substance touching the skin. Cutaneous manifestations of occupational exposure are generally divided into irritant contact dermatitis (ICD) and allergic contact dermatitis (ACD) or a combination of ICD and ACD. ICD is diagnosed based on the history and the clinical appearance. It is a non-immunologic form of dermatitis that, like RADS in the airways, does not require previous sensitization. On the other hand, ACD represents an immunologically mediated disorder that represents a form of type IV delayed hypersensitivity and thus occurs following an acquired sensitivity to a given substance.

Occupational contact urticaria is an occupational skin disorder of importance in the food industry, particularly among cooks, bakers, caterers, and food handlers. Morphologically, one sees an erythematous, papular, pruritic rash seen in classic hives; however, in this case it is associated with a specific occupational exposure. The mechanism is usually an immunoglobulin E (IgE)-mediated process.

Prevalence and incidence

Generally, of all the occupational lung diseases in an industrialized nation, OA is the most common. The overall frequency of OA, according to numerous sources of data, has remained stable in the last 10 years, although the causative agents may vary in frequency [11].

Determining prevalence or incidence of occupational diseases with any certainty is difficult, particularly in the food industries. Both employees and physicians tend to under-report health problems, and epidemiologic data on agriculture workers and food handlers remain scanty. However, as the importance of occupational lung disease has become more recognized, national databases have been established to monitor this data, including the SWORD and SHIELD in the United Kingdom, PROPULSE in Canada, and SENSOR in the United States.

According to the World Health Organization, worldwide as many as 300 million people of all ages and ethnicities suffer from asthma [12]. In the United States it is estimated that 21 million people have asthma, based on the US Centers for Disease Control and Prevention Behavioral Risk Factor Surveillance System [13]. According to the CDC's National Center for Health Statistics in 2002, 11.8 million people had experienced an asthma attack or episode in the previous 12 months in the United States, of which 4269 died [14]. The exact prevalence of OA is unknown but epidemiologic studies suggest that 9–15% of all cases of adult onset asthma are attributable to occupational exposure [15,16].

In those food-related industries in which prevalence of OA is available, rates do not significantly differ from those found in non-food industries. For example, OA occurs in 3% [17] to 10% [18] of workers exposed to green coffee beans, 9% to as many as 50% of snow-crab-processing workers [19,20], and 10% to 30% of bakers [21–24].

OR occurs 3 times more frequently than asthma in the occupational setting. Its prevalence in subjects with OA is 76–92% [7,19]. The prevalence of OR has been reported to be between 3% and 87% depending on the exposure environment [25,26]. In health care workers exposed to latex gloves, sensitization has been reported as high as 20% with OR occurring in 9–12% [26,27]. In seafood-processing workers, the prevalence of OR ranges from 5% to 22% [28] and nasal symptoms were reported by 24% of fish-food factory workers [29].

The incidence of HP is more difficult to determine because of the disease's generally low occurrence, problems with differential diagnosis, and the lack of prospective epidemiologic studies. Incidence also depends on exposure levels of the offending antigen and varies widely in different industries or even in areas of the same plant. For example, in one study it was estimated that farmer's lung affects less than 1–6% of farmers [30]. However, in a survey among 1054 farmers who grind moldy hay, the prevalence of farmer's lung was reported at 8.3–11.4% [31]. Farmer's lung on dairy farms in Wisconsin has been calculated to be 4.2 per 1000 farmers [32]. Other studies have noted incidence rates for farmer's lung between 2.5 and 153.1 per 1000 farmers. In a survey of 200 pigeon breeders, it has been estimated that 5% of breeders have findings consistent with bird fancier's lung [33].

Most epidemiologic studies of dermatologic reactions in food-industry workers have included only subjects already diagnosed with occupational skin disease. Consequently, although types of skin reactions can be distinguished and many of the important etiologic agents can be identified, the true prevalence of disease remains difficult to determine. In a study of 1052 workers in the Finnish food industry, 17% were identified as having a skin disease [34]. In that study, 8.5% of 541 female workers had occupational dermatitis, most commonly caused by fish, meat, and vegetables. Of the 196 workers handling food, hand dermatitis was present in 15%. In a 5-year retrospective study, 3662 consecutive patients, including 180 food handlers, were patch tested [35]. In 91 of 180 subjects (50.5%) dermatitis resulted from an occupational exposure of which 25 of 180 (13.8%) were from exposure to meats or vegetables. Patch tests were positive in 59 of 180 patients (32.7%). Another study involving 5285 patients in northern Bavaria found the incidence of occupational dermatitis was highest in pastry cooks (76%), cooks (69%), followed closely by food-processing industry workers and butchers (63%) [36]. Hjorth and Roed-Peterson evaluated 33 cases of occupational dermatitis occurring in restaurant kitchen workers [37]. Metals, onions, and garlic were implicated most frequently in contact dermatitis; fish and shellfish were the major agents responsible for provoking contact urticaria. The same food allergens were also identified as the most important in a study of caterers [38]. Table 18.1 represents allergens or irritants that may cause reactions in food handlers.

Using questionnaires, Smith estimated the mean annual incidence of skin conditions in the food manufacturing industry to be 2103 per million employees per year and 1414 per million employees per year in the retail/catering industry [39]. Other data on occupational dermatitis come from the EPIDERM and OPRA (Occupational Physicians Reporting Activity) surveillance plan which have been collecting data on occupational skin diseases in the United Kingdom since 1993. The dermatologists and occupational physicians that provided data for these studies report an annual incidence of occupational contact dermatitis of 12.9 per 100,000 [40].

Risk factors

Both industrial and individual factors are associated with an increased risk of developing occupational hypersensitivity. The best studies have been done in OA and rhinitis.

Table 18.1 Examples of substances that act as irritants and/or allergens in causing contact dermatitis in food preparation workers

Irritants	Irritants or allergens	
Vegetables and fruit juices (contact urticaria)	Basil	Mugwort
Raw fish	Bay leaf	Mustard
Raw meats (benzylpenicilloyl polylysine)	Capers	Nutmeg, mace
Garlic	Caraway	Oregano
Onion	Cardamom	Paprika
Leeks, chives, shallots	Cayenne, chili pepper	Parsley
Spices	Cinnamon	Parsnip
Moisture	Clove	Pepper
Sugar	Coriander	Rosemary
Flour	Curry	Sage
Heat	Dill	Sesame
Soaps and detergents	Fennel	Star anise
Scouring pads	Ginger	Tarragon
	Laurus nobilis	Thyme
	Lovage	Turmeric
	Mint, peppermint	

Adapted from Marks *et al.* [41], with permission from Elsevier.

Physicochemical properties of occupational agents, as well as dose, duration, and route of exposure, allergenic potency, and industrial hygiene and engineering practices influence the potential of occupational agents to induce allergic disease. The level of exposure in different settings is clearly a major determinant for many occupational agents [23,42–44].

As only a small proportion of exposed workers develop occupational reactions, host factors clearly play an important role in disease development. These factors may include atopy, genetic predisposition, cigarette smoking, and possibly pre-existing increased non-specific bronchial responsiveness (NSBR).

Atopy

Atopic individuals have a personal or family history of hay fever, asthma, or atopic dermatitis and exhibit a greater tendency to develop sensitivity to environmental agents than do normal subjects. Atopic individuals frequently show elevated total IgE levels. Nevertheless, history alone is not sufficient for the diagnosis of atopy, as identical symptoms can arise from allergic and non-allergic mechanisms. Prick skin testing or radioallergosorbent testing (RAST) is often used along with suggestive history to establish a diagnosis.

Although OA is frequently associated with increased production of specific IgE antibodies, atopy *per se* is not always associated with an increased incidence of OA. In general, the association between atopy and OA is found consistently in OA caused by high molecular weight (HMW) agents.

However, the association is not high and other factors are equally likely to be important in the ultimate development of disease such as the degree of exposure and concentration of the suspected agent. Atopy appears to be an important factor in some occupational exposures such as workers sensitized to papain [45], flour [21], and green coffee beans [17], while data on bakers are controversial [46–48]. In some instances where the incidence of OA might be expected to be influenced by a worker's atopic status, such as in snow-crab-processing workers [19,20] and grain handlers [49], no relationship between atopy and development of disease has been discerned although sensitization, as assessed by skin test. Although an association between sensitization to HMW agents and atopy has been observed in many food-related work environments, atopy and the development of OR have not been linked. Unlike OA, there is no higher incidence of HP disease in atopic subjects.

The role of atopy has not been clearly defined in the pathophysiology of occupational dermatoses. Atopic dermatitis in particular may predispose workers to develop ICD; however, it does not appear to predispose to ACD. In a prospective follow-up study evaluating hand dermatitis in bakers, confectioners, and bakery shop assistants in order to determine risk factors, Bauer *et al.* noted that mild to moderate ICD was the most frequent finding. Atopic individuals had a 3.9-fold relative risk of developing hand dermatitis. Total serum IgE was quantified but does not correlate with disease [50].

Genetics

Almost no information has been gathered on human leukocyte antigen (HLA) type and its relationship to the development of OA, OR, HP, or occupational dermatitis, particularly resulting from exposure to allergens in the food industry. With the results of the human genome project and interest in discovering the potential genetic basis of disease, it is anticipated that more data should become available with respect to OA.

As with OA, no specific genetic basis has been clearly identified for HP. The nature of the antigen, the quantity of antigen inhaled and frequency of exposure, and finally host susceptibility are important. A study by Camarena *et al.* in 44 patients with pigeon breeders' disease, a form of HP, looked at polymorphisms of the major histocompatibility complex (MHC) class II alleles. An increase of one HLA-DRB1 allele and one HLA-DQB1 allele was noted when MHC typing was performed by PCR-specific sequence oligonucleotide analysis. However, there is not a specific association between the alleles in question and the development of HP [51].

Very little data exists for the genetic basis of occupational dermatitis. Holst studied ICD in monozygotic and dizygotic twins and found a high degree of concordance among monozygotic twins [52].

Smoking

The role of cigarette smoke, including exposure to secondhand smoke, in development, exacerbation, or pathogenesis of OA is not clear. Exposure to cigarette smoke increases bronchial epithelial permeability [53], which might potentially allow inhaled antigens increased access to immunocompetent cells and evoke an immune response. A potential relationship between asthma, cigarette smoke, dust, aerosol, or vapor exposure appears intriguing, but epidemiologic studies in this area are limited. Smoking seems to be a risk factor for developing OA in several cases such as crab-processing workers [19], workers exposed to green coffee beans or castor beans and grain dust.

Smokers exposed occupationally to green coffee bean or castor bean dust appear to be at higher risk for the development of occupationally induced allergies than similarly exposed non-smokers [54]. Furthermore, a significantly higher proportion of smokers appear among "sensitized" than "non-sensitized" coffee factory workers, and sensitization appears to progress more rapidly in smokers [55]. Pulmonary effects of smoking and grain dust exposure are additive [56]. These findings underscore the importance of imposing controls for smoking during data analysis.

HP is uncommon in smokers, unlike other pulmonary disease in which smoking increases frequency of disease. Several studies have shown an underrepresentation of smokers among patients with HP. The mechanism by which smoking seems to prevent the development of HP is not known. It may be through an impairment of immune cellular function induced by smoking [57–59]. However, Dangman *et al.* reported that smoking affects the laboratory and clinical findings used in the diagnosis of HP, making the confirmation of HP difficult, which may contribute to the apparent protective effect of smoking [60]. More studies are needed to confirm the role that smoking plays in the development of HP. Nevertheless, once HP has started, smoking does not appear to be protective [61].

Bronchial responsiveness

OA, at least in a worker still exposed and symptomatic, is usually associated with increased NSBR, as demonstrated by histamine or methacholine inhalation challenges. There is no evidence that increased NSBR is a risk factor for the development of OA [62].

Agents associated with allergic occupational diseases of food workers

Hundreds of agents are known to cause occupational rhinoconjunctivitis and asthma. Most of these substances are chemicals, pharmaceuticals, wood dusts, and metals [63,64]; in addition more than 50 agents encountered in food or food-related industry are known to induce OR and OA. In fact, the food industry accounts for the largest number of cases of OR [65]. In some industries, such as coffee factories, OA is a well-recognized problem; in other types of workplaces, only individual case reports have been reported. Agents encountered in food industries that are known to cause OR and OA are listed in Table 18.2. A more wide-ranging

list of airway sensitizing agents can be found in a review by van Kampen [66]. Additionally, Siracusa *et al.* have a comprehensive list of agents specifically for OR [67].

Organic dust derived from bacteria, fungi, protozoa, plant and animal products, and simple chemicals can induce HP.

Table 18.2 Materials used in food or food-related industries that are known to induce OA or rhinitis

Agents	Occupational exposure	References	Agents	Occupational exposure	References
Animal products			Soybeans, soybean lecithin	Agricultural workers	[137,138]
Sea animals			Grain dust	Grain handlers	[139–142]
Prawn, crab, king crab, snow crab, lobster, oyster, clams	Seafood processing	[19,28, 68–79]			
			Spices/herbs		
			Garlic	Factory workers, farmers	[143–146]
Shrimp meal	Aquaculture	[80]	Coriander, mace, ginger, paprika	Factory workers	[147,148]
Fish meal, fish flour	Factory workers	[81–83]			
Mother of pearl	Button factory workers	[84]	Cinnamon	Spice workers	[149]
Sea squirt	Oyster shuckers	[85,86]	Paprika plants	Greenhouse workers	[150]
Seashells	Shell grinders	[87]	Aromatic herbs	Butcher	[151,152]
Trout	Processing workers	[88]	Ginseng	Cook	[153]
Farm products			*Vegetables/fruits*		
Cows	Dairy farmers	[89–91]	Green beans	Homemaker	[154]
Milk	Factory worker	[92]	Okra	Homemaker	[155]
Hogs, swine food	Hog farmers	[93–96]	Raspberry		[156]
Poultry	Poultry workers	[97]	Carrots	Cook	[157]
Pheasants, quail, doves	Breeders	[98]	Bell pepper	Cook	[158]
Eggs, egg lysozyme	Egg processor, bakery workers	[99–105]	Brocolli/cauliflower	Cook	[159]
			Cabbage	Cook	[160]
			Leek	Cook	[161]
Insects			Asparagus	Cook	[162]
Poultry mites (*Ornithonyssus sylviarum*)	Poultry workers	[106,107]	Spinach	Field workers	[163]
Grain storage mites (*Glycyphagus destructor*)	Grain workers	[108–111]	*Enzymes*		
			Fungal amylase, xylanase	Bakers	[164–166]
Honey bees	Bee-keepers, honey processors	[112–114]	Bromelain, papain	Factory workers	[167–173]
Bee moth	Fish-bait breekers	[115]	*Miscellaneous*		
Rice flower beetle	Rice flower workers	[116]	Castor beans	Factory workers, dock workers	[174]
Enzymes			Tea, herbal tea	Tea factory workers, tea garden workers	[175–180]
Pepsin, trypsin, pancreatic enzymes	Pharmaceutical workers	[117–120]			
			Pollens	Sugarbeet workers	[181]
Miscellaneous				Sunflower workers	[182]
Spiramycin	Chick breeders	[121]		Grape growers	[183]
Pyrolysis products of polyvinyl chloride or label adhesives	Meat wrappers	[122–128]	Pectin	Candy or jam makers	[184,185]
			Alkaline hydrolysis derivative of gluten	Bakers	[186]
Plant/fungi			*Alternaria/Aspergillus*	Bakers	[187]
Grains/flours			Colophony	Poultry venders	[188]
Coffee	Coffee factory workers	[106]	Hops	Brewery chemists	[189]
Flour (wheat, rye)	Bakers, millers	[129–132]	Devil's tongue (*Amorphophallus konjac*)	Food workers	[190]
Buckwheat, carob bean flour	Food workers	[133–135]	Mushrooms	Soup manufacturers	[191]
				Growers	[192,193]
Rice	Rice millers	[136]	*Verticillium albo-atrum*	Greenhouse workers	[194]

Table 18.3 Etiology of HP occurring in food and food-related industries

Agent	Source/exposure	Disorders	References
Thermophilic actinomycetes			
Faenia rectivirgula	Moldy hay	Farmer's lung	[195,196]
Micropolyspora faeni	Moldy compost	Mushroom workers' lung	[197]
Thermoactinomyces sacchari	Moldy sugar cane	Bagassosis	[198]
T. vulgaris	Moldy compost	Mushroom workers' lung	[192]
	Moldy hay	Farmer's lung	[199]
T. viridis	Vineyards	Vineyard sprayers' lung	[200]
Fungi			
Aspergillus clavatus	Moldy barley/malt	Malt workers' lung	[201–203]
A. clavatus	Moldy cheese	Cheese workers' lung	[204]
A. flavus	Moldy corn	Farmer's lung	[205]
A. fumigatus	Vegetable compost		[206]
A. oryzae	Soy sauce brewer		[207]
Cladosporium	Moldy hay	Farmer's lung	[199]
Mucor stolonifer	Moldy paprika pods	Paprika slicers' disease	[208]
Penicillium sp.	Moldy hay	Farmer's lung	[199]
P. caseii, P. roqueforti	Cheese	Cheese workers' lung	[209–211]
Botrytis cinerea	Moldy grapes	Wine growers' lung	[212]
Insects			
Grain weevil (*Sitophilus grainarius*)	Infested wheat	Millers' lung	[213,214]
Cheese mites (*Acarus siro*)	Cheese	Cheese workers' lung	[215]
Animal products			
Duck proteins	Feathers	Duckfever	[216]
Chicken proteins	Chicken products	Feather pluckers' disease	[217,218]
	Hen litter		[219]
Turkey proteins	Turkey products	Turkey handlers' disease	[220]
Goose proteins	Feathers		[221]
Bird proteins	Fishermen		[222]
Fish meal	Fishmeal workers		[222]
Plant products			
Miscellaneous			
Mushrooms	Spores	Mushroom workers' disease	[223,224]
Erwina herbicoa (Enterobacter agglomerans)	Contaminated grain	Grain workers' lung	[225]
Tea plants		Tea growers' lung	[226]
Oyster shells	Oyster shell dust		[227]
Cork	Cork dust from wine bottles		[228]
Prawn	Factory workers	Prawn-processing workers	[229]

A list of agents encountered in food industries that are known to induce HP are given in Table 18.3. Many of these materials are of fungal origin. Coffee dust has been omitted from this list because the single case of "coffee worker's lung" [230] was subsequently redescribed as cryptogenic fibrosing alveolitis associated with rheumatoid arthritis [231].

A wide variety of foods, additives, and flavorings, as well as materials used in food preparation, are known to induce several types of occupational skin disease. Table 18.4 lists etiologic agents, along with diagnoses. Some materials, such

as seafood and garlic, commonly induce dermatitis, whereas others, including non-food items such as betadine, are seldom reported to cause occupational skin disease.

Relationship of sensitization routes: inhalation at the workplace versus ingestion at home

The relationship between sensitization by inhalation and symptoms following inhalation or ingestion of the same or a related antigen is intriguing. Exposure to food allergens

Table 18.4 Dermatitis in food-processing and food service workers

Industry	Exposure	Diagnosis	References
Agriculture			
Milk controllers, milk recorders, milkers	Bronopol, Kathon CG	Dermatitis	[232–234]
Milk testers	Chrome, dichromate		[235,236]
Milk analyzers	Dichromate	Allergic contact dermatitis	[237]
Ewe milker		Dermatitis	[238]
Celery harvesters	Celery fungus (*Sclerotinia sclerotiorum*)	Phototoxic dermatitis	[239,240]
Apple packers	Apples sprayed with ethoxyquin	ACD	[241]
Orange pickers	Omite-CR	Dermatitis	[242]
Coconut pickers		Conjunctivitis	[243]
Grocery workers	Celery (furocoumarins)		[244,245]
Mushroom harvesters		Dermatitis	[246]
Food preparation			
Fish factory workers	Fish, mustard	Dermatitis, contact urticaria	[247]
Cooks	Mustard, rape	Dermatitis	[248]
Cooks	Garlic/onions	Dermatitis	[249]
Cooks	Paprika, curry	Contact dermatitis	[250]
Salad makers	Mustard	Dermatitis	[251]
Food workers	Cashew nuts (cardol)	Dermatitis	[252]
Sandwich makers	Codfish, plaice, chicken, onion, garlic	Dermatitis	[37]
Food workers	Lettuce	Dermatitis	[253]
Food workers	Lettuce, chickory, endive	Contact dermatitis	[254]
Bakers	Sodium metabisulfite	Contact dermatitis	[255]
	Persulfate	Contact dermatitis	[250]
	Cinnamon	Dermatitis	[256]
	Sorbic acid	Dermatitis	[257]
	Propyl gallate	Allergic contact dermatitis, dermatitis	[258]
	Dodecyl gallate	Dermatitis	[259]
	Chromium	Dermatitis	[260]
	Flour mite	Dermatitis	[261]
	Sugar mite	Dermatitis	[262]
	Karaya gum	Dermatitis	[263]
	Flour	Contact urticaria	[261]
Butchers/poultry processors			
Butchers	Rubber boots	Allergic contact dermatitis	[264]
Butchers	Knife handle	Dermatitis	[265,266]
Butchers	Povidone iodine	Allergic contact dermatitis	[267]
Slaughtermen	Blood (cow and pig), gut casings	Contact urticaria, eczema	[268,269]
Butchers	Calf's liver, pig's gut, beef	Urticaria	[270–272]
Poultry workers	Various	Irritant allergic dermatitis, eczema	[273]
Chicken vaccinators	Antibiotics	Contact dermatitis	[274]
Seafood			
Fishmarket workers	Shrimp	Allergic contact urticaria	[275]
Caterers	Shrimp	Contact urticaria	[276]
Seafood processors	Prawns	Dermatitis	[68]
Crabs processors	Crabs	Urticaria, dermatitis	[277]
Oyster shuckers	Oysters	Dermatitis	[278]
Mussel processors	Mussels	Dermatitis	[279]
Food handlers	Fish and shellfish	Contact dermatitis	[280,281]
Food handlers	Cuttlefish	Contact dermatitis	[282]
Fishermen	Fish	Dermatitis	[283]
Fish workers	Fish	Contact urticaria	[284]

(Continued)

Table 18.4 (*Continued*)

Industry	Exposure	Diagnosis	References
Cooks	Fish	Contact urticaria	[285]
Fishermen	Fish	Dermatoses	[286]
Caterers	Fish	Dermatitis	
Trawlermen	Bryozoa	Dermatitis, eczema	[287,288]
Fishermen	Rubber boots	Dermatitis	[289]
Fishnet repairers	Fishnets	Dermatitis	[290]
Miscellaneous			
Snackbar meat prod	Penicillin residues	Dermatitis	[291]
Spice workers	Turmeric, cinnamon, cinnamic aldehyde	Allergic contact dermatitis	[292,293]
Margarine manufacturers, workers	Octyl gallate	Eczema, dermatitis	[294]
Peanut butter manufacturers	Octyl gallate	Dermatitis	[294]
Processing plant workers	Green coffee beans	Dermatitis	[295]
Food workers	Sesame oil	Contact sensitivity	[296]
Food workers	Artichokes	Eczema	[297]
Confectioners	Cardamom	Allergic contact dermatitis	[298]
Cookie workers	"Thin mint" cookies	Eczema	[299]
Bee-keepers	Propolis	Dermatitis	[300,301]
Bee-keepers	Beeswax (poplar resin)	Dermatitis	[302]
Coconut climber	Coconut trees/coconuts	Dermatitis	[303]
Bartender	Citrus peel, geraniol citral	Allergic contact dermatitis	[304]

typically occurs only via ingestion. Having subjects sensitized to traditional food allergens by inhalation presents an opportunity to compare elements of the two exposure routes. Most food-related occupational allergens have not been shown to induce symptoms following ingestion by workers sensitized by inhalation. In some individuals, certain allergens can elicit symptoms following inhalation and ingestion: a spice factory worker who developed asthma following inhalation of garlic dust noted the immediate onset of wheezing after eating garlic-containing foods [143]. A provocative challenge with garlic aerosol produced an immediate 35% reduction in forced expiratory volume in 1 second (FEV1). An oral challenge with 1600 mg of garlic (in capsules) induced apprehension, flushing, and nausea within 10 minutes. Diarrhea, increased pulse rate, and a 21% reduction in FEV1 appeared within 2 hours. In contrast to the immediate response to inhalation challenge and natural ingestion of garlic-containing foods, maximal symptoms were noted 2 hours after laboratory challenge, suggesting that inhalation of garlic vapors or absorption through the oral mucosa was necessary to produce an immediate response. Buckwheat [305], pineapple protease [167], snow crab [19], and honey/pollen [182,306] have also been shown to produce allergic reactions following inhalation and ingestion by sensitive subjects.

Some individuals sensitized by inhalation to one occupational agent report symptoms following ingestion of a related antigen. A bird breeder developed OA following exposure to birds concomitant with an exquisite gastrointestinal sensitivity to ingested chicken eggs. Her primary sensitization involved bird serum antigens, which cross-reacted with ingested egg yolk proteins [98]. Butcher and colleagues [307] described an individual who developed and lost sensitivity to TDI vapor and ingested radishes, which contain isothiocyanates. Similarly, several crab-processing workers with OA developed allergy to ingested crab as reported by Cartier *et al.* [19].

Pathophysiology of occupational allergies

Occupational rhinitis

OR has been classified by Bardana [308] as annoyance, irritational, corrosive, or immunologic. Annoyance, irritational, and corrosive rhinitis have no immunologic or allergic basis. Immunologic or allergic rhinitis is usually IgE-mediated although the exact mechanism is unknown for most low molecular weight (LMW) agents. Annoyance reactions occur from exposure to mild workplace irritants. These reactions are triggered by exposure to perfumes, air fresheners, and cooking odors. Irritational rhinitis is caused by inhalation of high concentrations of airborne chemicals. This reaction is often associated with a burning sensation. The proposed mechanism for this reaction is release of substance P and neuropeptides from nasal sensory nerves. Vasodilation and neurogenic inflammation result from substance P [65,308,309]. Corrosive rhinitis occurs after exposure to high concentrations of chemical gases, like ammonia, chlorine, and organophosphides. Signs of systemic intoxication may also be present.

Immunologic or allergic OR can result from HMW or LMW allergens. HMW allergens are more sensitizing, especially in atopic workers. The majority of allergens in the food industry are of HMW. Examples include flour, soybean dust, vegetable gums, and animal proteins. Guar gum is a common cause of OR in the food industry being used as a thickener and gelling agent.

Occupational asthma

The characteristic bronchial reaction observed in OA may result from pharmacologic, or type I, IgE-mediated mechanisms [310]. Complex organic mixtures, such as grain dust, have numerous biologic actions, which may or may not be pathogenic. Other agents induce OA by an as-yet undefined mechanism.

Pharmacologic mechanism

The classic example of acute asthma caused by a pharmacologic mechanism occurs in farm workers exposed to organophosphate insecticides [311,312]. These chemicals irreversibly inactivate cholinesterase, which causes an accumulation of acetylcholine, with subsequent bronchospasm.

Immune mechanisms

Many agents encountered in the workplace are antigenic or allergenic and elicit type I, IgE-mediated reactions in sensitized individuals. As with other agents inducing IgE-mediated OA, only a small proportion of exposed workers develop disease. A latent period, ranging from several weeks to years, precedes development of symptoms [313]. A common classification system is to divide the agents into HMW and LMW agents. In general, HMW agents act through an IgE-mediated mechanism. Certain LMW agents cause production of IgE antibodies; others act as haptens that must be conjugated to a carrier protein to be allergenic. LMW allergens cause disease through largely unknown mechanisms, though non-IgE-mediated and cell-dependent immunologic mechanisms appear to be important.

Asthma in seafood workers

The seafood industry is an example of a sector of the food industry that has continued to grow to meet world demands and consequently has had greater exposures and corresponding disease. In 2005, the world's production of fish, crustaceans, and mollusks reached 140.5 million tons. Of this amount, 95 million tons were derived from capture fisheries and 45.5 million tons were from aquaculture [314]. This makes seafood one of the most highly traded commodities in the world market [315]. With this increase in the production and consumption of seafood have come more allergic reactions occurring in the occupational setting [316]. The reported prevalence of OA due to seafood alone varies from 7% to 36% [317]. In a recent study of seafood-industry workers from Norway, the 1-year prevalence of work-related upper and lower respiratory symptoms was 42.8% and 25% between production workers and administrative workers, respectively. The study also stated that specific IgE to shrimp antigen was found in 20% of production workers in shrimp factories in Norway [318,319].

Besche [320] published the first report of occupational allergy from seafood in a 1937 paper describing a fisherman with asthma, angioedema, and conjunctivitis. Since Besche's time, seafood-processing plants have become technologically advanced with varying processing procedures. Crab, fish, mussel, and prawn processing cause an aerosolized protein exposure to which workers can become sensitized by inhalation [321]. Table 18.5 lists possible exposures in the seafood industry. Sensitization by inhalation frequently makes the respiratory tract a primary route of occupational exposure during seafood processing [322]. Occupational exposure to crab has been extensively studied, with a range of allergic diseases including asthma being characterized. A 1982 National Institute for Occupational Safety and Health (NIOSHA) investigation concluded that during the crab-processing season in Alaska, the monthly incidence of new cases of asthma was 80 times that reported for the general population, controlling for age [323].

A 1998 survey was conducted with symptom questionnaires, spirometry, and serologic testing on 107 workers in a crab-processing facility. In this study the incidence of asthma-like symptoms was 26%. The prevalence of asthma-like symptoms was noted to be 14% early in the crab season and 32% late in the season. At the end of the season, 4% met the criteria for an obstructive pattern by spirometry. Only 9% of the workers with asthma-like symptoms had elevated IgE antibody to crab [324]. Small study group size and short duration of follow-up may have limited the study, but the observations are interesting. Further investigation into occupational exposure to seafood agents is necessary to better understand the health effects for seafood workers. These investigations should include characterization of aerosolized protein antigen, dose–response relations, exposure routes, temporal component to exposure, extent of antigen cross-reactivity, and host factors [325].

Hypersensitivity pneumonitis

Occupations at risk of developing disease that are commonly cited in the literature include farmers, sugarcane harvesting, and mushroom packing. Mushroom worker's lung (MWL) represents a good example of this disease.

Pathogenesis

The complete relationships between the immunologic response and environmental factors that lead to the development of hypersensitivity pheumonitis (HP) have not been fully elucidated. One of the questions that remains unanswered is why only certain subjects in a group of similarly exposed subjects go on to develop HP. The mechanisms

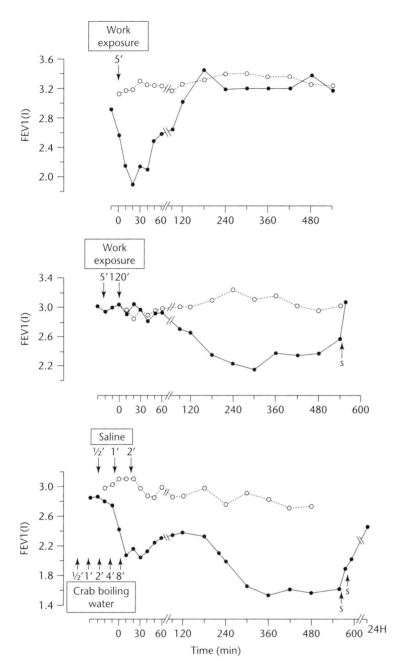

Figure 18.4 Specific inhalation challenges in crab-processing workers. The upper panel illustrates the change in FEV1 in a worker presenting an immediate type of asthmatic reaction, after a 5 minutes exposure in the workplace. The middle panel illustrates a late asthmatic reaction occurring about 2 hours after the 125 minutes of exposure in the workplace with full recovery at the end of the day post-albuterol (S). The lower panel illustrates a dual asthmatic response following the inhalation of crab boiling water in the laboratory. (Adapted from Cartier A *et al.* [19], with permission from the American Academy of Allergy, Asthma, and Immunology.)

the best prognosis results when there is early diagnosis and early removal from the exposure environment [308].

In other types of OA, a similar pattern of improvement has been shown [375]. Individuals who continue to work are thus at risk to develop irreversible disease, stressing the importance of early removal from exposure. While NSBR usually improves with work withdrawal, most workers will still exhibit persistent specific bronchial responsiveness if re-challenged with the agent responsible for their OA, after several years off work [381].

The socio-economic consequences of OA are not negligible [382–384] and vary between countries according to the compensation systems and retraining programs. This stresses the importance of making a proper diagnosis. In Quebec, where workers are no longer exposed to their offending agent once the diagnosis is made, about one-third of subjects find an adequate job with the same employer while one-third find a different job with another employer. Only 8% of subjects remain unemployed after 2 years of follow-up. Quality of life of subjects with OA in the same province is slightly though significantly less satisfactory than subjects with common asthma of comparable severity. In other countries, the situation is less favorable, the number of subjects still unemployed varying between 25% and 69%

[385,386]. In many situations, workers have to stay in the same environment, which may be associated with deterioration in their asthma. Moscato *et al.* showed that subjects with OA who stayed at work needed more medication than those who ceased to be exposed [376]. Although much work has been put into prognostic indicators for OA, the prognosis of OR has not been well studied.

The clinical prognosis for individuals with HP depends primarily on the amount of damage at the time of diagnosis and the ability of the individual to avoid contact with the etiologic agent, although this may not affect PFTs and chest radiographs [387,388]. When HP is diagnosed early and ongoing exposure with the antigen is avoided, the outcomes are generally good and clinical, radiographic and pulmonary function return to baseline. Most of the recovery should occur within several months. If the patient still has changes after 6 months away from the exposure, the changes are likely to be permanent. With delays in diagnosis and treatment, subjects may progress to the chronic form of the disease which may lead to irreversible changes as well. Patients may also go on to develop symptoms of asthma or emphysema. As with diagnosis, there are also no pathognomonic prognostic markers for HP. There have also been reports of continued decline in lung function despite removal from the inciting agent at the acute stage. In particular, there was continued decline in DLCO and TLC over several years. If the subject does progress to the chronic fibrosis stage, they may go on to respiratory failure and death or right-sided heart failure.

The majority of individuals with contact dermatitis have an excellent prognosis, provided that exposure to the allergen is eliminated. If an employee cannot change jobs, dermatitis can become chronic. Chronic dermatitis can also occur in some subjects despite the apparent elimination of allergen exposure. This condition is particularly troublesome in industrial settings and may reflect complex exposures or mixed disease, endogenous or irritant dermatitis.

Prevention and treatment

The best "treatment" of allergic occupational disease is prevention [389]. Reduction of exposure levels is the only way to reduce significantly the incidence of respiratory symptoms among workers, although some individuals may still be sensitized at very low levels. This may be achieved, for example, by enclosing the responsible process, improving ventilation and personal protection devices, and modifying the process by encapsulating the agent. While threshold limit values have been established to prevent exposure to irritant levels of various agents, limit values to prevent sensitization are not known for most agents [44,390]. However, once an individual has developed clinical evidence of OA, asthmatic responses will occur at minute exposure levels, usually less than any industrial plant can maintain.

Pre-employment screening and periodic health monitoring with education of workers about risk of disease and means to reduce exposure have been suggested as ways to prevent development of allergic respiratory disease. Questions arise over which tests are appropriate. Skin prick testing with specific allergens may prove useful for monitoring, although positive responses do not necessarily correlate with disease and, as for atopy, do not predict adequately who will develop OA [387,391]. Furthermore, human rights laws would not allow using pre-screening to exclude subjects from being hired. However, monitoring of skin prick tests for specific allergens during work in high-risk industries may be useful and allow reallocation of sensitized individuals to low exposure environment and thus less risk of developing clinical diseases [388].

Once OA or HP has been diagnosed, the worker should be removed permanently from further exposure to the offending agent in order to prevent further deterioration and improve the prognosis [391]. Although OR and/or conjunctivitis may precede OA [7], there is little information on the level of risk to develop OA in workers with OR [392]. In such subjects, removal of exposure will improve the symptoms but simple treatment with H1-antagonists or inhaled corticosteroids may be enough to control the symptoms and allow the worker to continue his job, preferably in a much lower exposure environment.

Furthermore, when cases of HP are discovered in an occupational environment, it will be important to follow non-affected workers as well, since they may eventually develop symptoms or disease. For example, when HP caused by inhalation of mollusc shell dust was discovered among employees in a factory, evaluation of the health status of the other factory employees was undertaken. This revealed functional decline in the subjects originally unaffected, despite attempts at improving the occupational environment [393].

The specific treatment of OA, aside from removal of the inciting agent, is the same as non-OA. In more severe cases of HP, systemic corticosteroids may be needed. When this approach is used, it should be with careful monitoring of X-ray, PFT, and clinical symptoms. The subject should have slow tapering of the steroids after clinical improvement, as rapid tapering may cause relapse. Although steroids will improve the acute symptoms, there is concern that steroid-treated patients may potentially be at higher risk of disease relapse [394].

As with respiratory disease, drug treatment of occupational dermatoses produce only temporary benefit unless the individual receives no further exposure. Specifically, workers with less than 10% skin involvement are treated with topical steroids and those with more extensive involvement may be treated with oral steroids. The steroids should be tapered and not stopped abruptly, as prematurely stopping steroids can cause a flare of skin symptoms. Protective measures that reduce skin contact, such as appropriate clothing and gloves, may be used if avoidance is impossible. It should not be automatically assumed that such devices are impervious to all materials. Workers have had better outcomes of their occupational dermatitis when they have received hands-on instructions on the measures needed to improve the dermatitis. However, if these measures do not improve or resolve the dermatitis, the worker should be withdrawn from exposure.

Conclusion

Exposure to a wide variety of food-derived and food-associated materials encountered in the workplace is associated with development of OA, HP, rhinitis/conjunctivits, and dermatitis in sensitized individuals. The number of causative agents will undoubtedly continue to rise as new agents are introduced into the workplace and as physician awareness of these conditions continues to grow. Little is known about the prevalence and incidence, importance of host factors, treatment, or prognosis of the occupational diseases resulting from exposure to these antigens. As the number of individuals employed in the food industry grows, the need for this type of information will increase significantly.

The examples described in this chapter are but a few of the wide array of food-associated occupational hypersensitivity reactions. New agents causing occupational allergies are being reported. With globalization of world markets and a continuing increase of individuals employed in the food industry, it is essential for the clinician to keep abreast of any new reactions when diagnosing a new or unusual occupational reaction. For example, a particular interest is the development of genetically modified (GM) crops that may contain novel proteins to which no prior human exposure has occurred. Although most efforts at food safety analysis are directed at ingestion of foods developed through biotechnology, by consumers, it is possible that such novel proteins could also cause occupationally related allergic reactions in food workers. Although this is unlikely to occur due to the low expression levels of such proteins, such a possibility should be considered whenever occupational reactions occur in industries' growing/processing foods developed by biotechnology or using ingredients that have been similarly altered [395].

References

1 US Bureau of Labor Statistics. http://www.bls.gov/

2 Chan-Yeung M, Brooks S, Alberts WM, *et al.* Assessment of asthma in the workplace. ACCP consensus statement. American College of Chest Physicians. *Chest* 1995;108:1084–117.

3 Bernstein IL, Bernstein DI, Chan-Yeung M, Malo JL. Definition and classification of asthma in the workplace. In: Bernstein IL, Chan-Yeung M, Malo JL, Bernstein DI (eds.) *Asthma in the Workplace and Related Conditions*. New York: Taylor & Francis Group, 2006:1–8.

4 Brooks S, Weiss M, Bernstein I. Reactive airways dysfunction syndrome (RADS): persistent asthma syndrome after high level irritant exposures. *Chest* 1985;88:376–84.

5 Tarlo SM, Broder I. Irritant-induced occupational asthma. *Chest* 1989;96:297–300.

6 Salvaggio JE, Taylor G, Weill H. Occupational asthma and rhinitis. In: Merchant JA, ed. Occupational respiratory disease. Cincinnati: US Department of Health and Human Services, Public Health Service, CDC, 1986; DHHS Publication no. (NIOSH) 86–102.

7 Malo JL, Lemière C, Desjardins A, Cartier A. Prevalence and intensity of rhinoconjunctivitis in subjects with occupational asthma. *Eur Respir J* 1997;10:1513–15.

8 Gross N. Allergy to laboratory animals: epidemiologic, clinical, and physiologic aspects, and a trial of cromolyn in its management. *J Allergy Clin Immunol* 1980;66:158–65.

9 Patel AM, Ryu JH, Reed CE. Hypersensitivity pneumonitis: current concepts and future questions. *J Allergy Clin Immunol* 2001;108:661–70.

10 Pepys J. Hypersensitivity diseases of the lungs due to fungi and organic dusts. *Monogr Allergy* 1969;4:1–147.

11 McDonald JC, Keynes HL, Meredith SK. Reported incidence of occupational asthma in the United Kingdom, 1989–97. *Occup Environ Med* 2000;57:823–9.

12 Global Initiative for Asthma 2004. World Health Organization. http://www.who.int

13 Behavioral Risk Factor Surveillance System. US Centers for Disease Control and Prevention 2004. http://www.cdc.gov

14 National Center for Health Statistics. US Centers for Disease Control and Prevention 2002. http://www.cdc.gov

15 Blanc PD, Toren K. How much adult asthma can be attributed to occupational factors? *Am J Med* 1999;107:580–7.

16 Balmes J, Becklake M, Blanc P, *et al.* American Thoracic Society Statement: occupational contribution to the burden of airway disease. *Am J Respir Crit Care Med* 2003;167:787–97.

17 Jones R, Hughes J, Lehrer S, *et al.* Lung function consequences of exposure and hypersensitivity in workers who process green coffee beans. *Am Rev Respir Dis* 1982;125:199–202.

18 Kaye M, Freedman SO. Allergy to raw coffee – an occupational disease. *Can Med Assoc J* 1961;84:199–202.

19 Cartier A, Malo JL, Forest F, *et al.* Occupational asthma in snow crab-processing workers. *J Allergy Clin Immunol* 1984;74:261–9.

20 Cartier A, Lehrer SB, Horth-Susin L, *et al.* Prevalence of crab asthma in plant crab workers in Newfoundland and Labrador. *Int J Circumpolar Health* 2004;63:333–6.

21 Erxheimer H. The skin sensitivity to flour of baker's apprentices: a final report of long term investigation. *Acta Allergol* 1967;28:42–9.

22 Smith TA, Lumley KP. Work-related asthma in a population exposed to grain, flour and other ingredient dusts. *Occup Med* 1996;46:37–40.

23 Musk AW, Venables KM, Crook B, *et al.* Respiratory symptoms, lung function, and sensitisation to flour in a British bakery. *Br J Indust Med* 1989;46:636–42.

24 Talini D, Benvenuti A, Carrara M, *et al.* Diagnosis of occupational flour-induced asthma in a cross sectional study. *Respir Med* 2002;96:236–43.

25 Gautrin D, Desrosiers M, Castano R. Occupational rhinitis. *Curr Opin Allergy Clin Immunol* 2006;6:77–84.

26 Saary MJ, Kanani A, Alghadeer H, *et al*. Changes in rates of natural rubber latex sensitivity among dental school students and staff after changes in latex gloves. *J Allergy Clin Immunol* 2002;109:131–5.

27 Vandenplas O, Delwiche JP, Evrard G, *et al*. Prevalence of occupational asthma due to latex among hospital personnel. *Am J Respir Crit Care Med* 1995;151:54–60.

28 Desjardins A, Malo JL, L'Archevêque J, *et al*. Occupational IgE-mediated sensitization and asthma caused by clam and shrimp (abstract). *J Allergy Clin Immunol* 1995;96:608–17.

29 Liebers V, Hoernstein M, Baur X. Humoral immune response to the insect allergen Chi t I in aquarists and fish-food factory workers. *Allergy* 1993;48:236–9.

30 Grant IW, Blyth W, Wardrop VE, *et al*. Prevalence of farmer's lung in Scotland: a pilot survey. *BMJ* 1972;1:530–4.

31 Tao BG, Shen YE, Chen GX, *et al*. An epidemiological study on farmer's lung among hay grinders in Dafeng County. *Biomed Environ Sci* 1988;1:13–18.

32 Marx JJ, Guernsey J, Emanuel DA, *et al*. Cohort studies of immunologic lung disease among Wisconsin dairy farmers. *Am J Ind Med* 1990;18:263–8.

33 Fink JN, Schlueter DP, Sosman AJ, *et al*. Clinical survey of pigeon breeders. *Chest* 1972;62:277–81.

34 Peltonen L, Wickstrom G, Vaahtoranta M. Occupational dermatoses in the food industry. *Derm Beruf Umwelt* 1985;33:166–9.

35 Veien NK, Hattel T, Justesen O, Norholm A. Causes of eczema in the food industry. *Derm Beruf Umwelt* 1983;31:84–6.

36 Dickel H, Kuss O, Schmidt A, *et al*. Importance of irritant contact dermatitis in occupational skin disease. *Am J Clin Dermatol* 2002;3:283–9.

37 Hjorth N, Roed-Petersen J. Occupational protein contact dermatitis in food handlers. *Contact Dermatitis* 1976;2:28–42.

38 Cronin E. Dermatitis of the hands in caterers. *Contact Dermatitis* 1987;17:265–9.

39 Smith TA. Occupational skin conditions in the food industry. *Occup Med (Lond)* 2000;50:597–8.

40 Cherry N, Meyer JD, Adisesh A, *et al*. Surveillance of occupational skin disease: EPIDERM and OPRA. *Br J Dermatol* 2000;142:1128–34.

41 Marks Jr JG, DeLeo VA. Occupational skin disease. In: Marks Jr JG, Elsner P, DeLeo VA (eds.) *Contact and Occupational Dermatology*. St. Louis, MO: Mosby-Year Book, 2002:239–303.

42 Houba R, Heederik D, Doekes G. Wheat sensitization and work-related symptoms in the baking industry are preventable. An epidemiologic study. *Am J Respir Crit Care Med* 1998;158:1499–503.

43 Cullinan P, Lowson D, Nieuwenhuijsen MJ, *et al*. Work related symptoms, sensitisation, and estimated exposure in workers not previously exposed to flour. *Occup Environ Med* 1994;51:579–83.

44 Baur X, Chen Z, Liebers V. Exposure–response relationships of occupational inhalative allergens. *Clin Exp Allergy* 1998;28:537–44.

45 Novey HS, Keenan WJ, Fairshter RD, *et al*. Pulmonary disease in workers exposed to papain: clinico-physiological and immunological studies. *Clin Allergy* 1980;10:721–31.

46 De Zotti R, Bovenzi M. Prospective study of work related respiratory symptoms in trainee bakers. *Occup Environ Med* 2000;57:58–61.

47 Anton M, Bataille A, Mollat F, *et al*. Allergies respiratoires des boulangers et des pâtissiers: enquête épidémiologique réalisée en 1991 par des médecins du travail de Loire-Atlantique. *Allerg Immunol (Paris)* 1995;27:12–15.

48 Gautrin D, Infante-Rivard C, Dao TV, *et al*. Specific IgE-dependent sensitization, atopy, and bronchial hyperresponsiveness in apprentices starting exposure to protein-derived agents. *Am J Respir Crit Care Med* 1997;155:1841–7.

49 Mink JT, Gerrard JW, Cockcroft DW, *et al*. Increased bronchial reactivity to inhaled histamine in nonsmoking grain workers with normal lung function. *Chest* 1980;77:28–31.

50 Bauer A, Bartsch R, Hersmann C, *et al*. Occupational hand dermatitis in food industry apprentices: results of a 3-year follow-up cohort study. *Int Arch Occup Environ Health* 2001;74:437–42.

51 Camarena A, Juarez A, Mejia M, *et al*. Major histocompatibility complex and tumor necrosis factor-alpha polymorphisms in pigeon breeder's disease. *Am J Respir Crit Care Med* 2001;163:1528–33.

52 Holst R, Moller H. One hundred twin pairs patch tested with primary irritants. *Br J Dermatol* 1975;93:145–9.

53 Hulbert WC, Walker DC, Jackson A, Hogg JC. Airway permeability to horseradish peroxidase in guinea pigs: the repair phase after injury by cigarette smoke. *Am Rev Respir Dis* 1981;123:320–6.

54 Zetterström O, Osterman K, Machado L, Johansson S. Another smoking hazard: raised serum IgE concentration and increased risk of occupational allergy. *BMJ* 1981;283:1215–17.

55 Osterman, K. Coffee worker's allergy. A clinical and immunological study. PhD dissertation, 1984:1–48.

56 Cotton DJ, Graham BL, Li KY, *et al*. Effects of grain dust exposure and smoking on respiratory symptoms and lung function. *J Occup Med* 1983;25:131–41.

57 Holt P. Immune and inflammatory function in cigarette smokers. *Thorax* 1987;42:241–9.

58 Murin S, Bilello KS, Matthay R. Other smoking-affected pulmonary diseases. *Clin Chest Med* 2000;21:121–37, ix.

59 Hagiwara E, Takahashi KI, Okubo T, *et al*. Cigarette smoking depletes cells spontaneously secreting Th(1) cytokines in the human airway. *Cytokine* 2001;14:121–6.

60 Dangman KH, Storey E, Schenck P, Hodgson MJ. Effects of cigarette smoking on diagnostic tests for work-related hypersensitivity pneumonitis: data from an outbreak of lung disease in metalworkers. *Am J Ind Med* 2004;45:455–67.

61 Arima K, Ando M, Ito K, *et al*. Effect of cigarette smoking on prevalence of summer-type hypersensitivity pneumonitis caused by *Trichosporon cutaneum. Arch Environ Health* 1992;47:274–8.

62 Renstrom A, Malmberg P, Larsson K, *et al*. Allergic sensitization is associated with increased bronchial responsiveness: a prospective study of allergy to laboratory animals. *Eur Respir J* 1995;8:1514–19.

63 Chan-Yeung M, Lam S. Occupational asthma. *Am Rev Respir Dis* 1986;133:686–703.

64 O'Neil CE, Salvaggio JE. The pathogenesis of occupational asthma. In: Kay AB (ed.) *Ballieres Clinical Immunology and Allergy. The Allergic Basis of Asthma.* PA: WB Saunders Co., 1988:143–75.

65 Meggs WJ. RADS and RUDS – the toxic induction of asthma and rhinitis. *J Toxicol Clin Toxicol* 1994;32:487–501.

66 van Kampen V, Merget R, Baur X. Occupational airway sensitizers: an overview on the respective literature. *Am J Ind Med* 2000;38:164–218.

67 Siracusa A, Desrosiers M, Marabini A. Epidemiology of occupational rhinitis: prevalence, aetiology and determinants. *Clin Exp Allergy* 2000;30:1519–34.

68 McSharry C, Wilkinson PC. Serum IgG and IgE antibody against aerosolised antigens from *Nephrops norvegicus* among seafood process workers. *Adv Exp Med Biol* 1987;216A:865–8.

69 Orford RR, Wilson JT. Epidemiologic and immunologic studies in processors of the king crab. *Am J Ind Med* 1985;7:155–69.

70 Lemière C, Desjardins A, Lehrer S, Malo JL. Occupational asthma to lobster and shrimp. *Allergy* 1996;51:272–3.

71 Patel PC, Cockcroft DW. Occupational asthma caused by exposure to cooking lobster in the work environment: a case report. *Ann Allergy* 1992;68:360–1.

72 Nakashima T. Studies of bronchial asthma observed in culture oyster workers. *Hiroshima J Med Sci* 1969;3:141–84.

73 Wada S, Nishimoto Y, Nakashima T, *et al.* Clinical observation of bronchial asthma in workers who culture oysters. *Hiroshima J Med Sci* 1967;16:255–66.

74 Beudet N, Brodkin CA, Stover B, *et al.* Crab allergen exposures aboard five crab-processing vessels. *AIHA J* 2002;63:605–9.

75 Barraclough RM, Walker J, Hamilton N, *et al.* Sensitization to king scallop (*Pectin maximus*) and queen scallop (*Chlamys opercularis*) proteins. *Occup Med* 2006;56:63–6.

76 Madsen J, Sherson D, Kjoller H, *et al.* Occupational asthma caused by sodium disulphite in Norwegian lobster fishing. *Occup Environ Med* 2004;61:873–4.

77 Baur X, Huber H, Chen Z. Asthma to Gammarus shrimp. *Allergy* 2000;55:96–7.

78 Goetz DW, Whisman BA. Occupational asthma in a seafood restaurant worker: cross-reactivity of shrimp and scallops. *Ann Allergy Asthma Immunol* 2000;85: 461–6.

79 Fontan M, Anibarro B, Postigo I, Martinez J. Allergy to freshwater shrimp (*Gammarus*). *J Investig Allergol Clin Immunol* 2005; 15:150–2.

80 Carino M, Elia G, Molinini R, *et al.* Shrimpmeal asthma in the aquaculture industry. *Med Lav* 1985;76:471–5.

81 Droszcz W, Kowalski J, Piotrowska B, *et al.* Allergy to fish in fish meal factory workers. *Int Arch Occup Environ Health* 1981;49:13–19.

82 Zuskin E, Kanceljak B, Schachter EN, *et al.* Immunological and respiratory changes in animal food processing workers. *Am J Ind Med* 1992;21:177–91.

83 Nieuwenhuizen N, Lopata AL, Jeebhay MF, *et al.* Exposure to the fish parasite *Anisakis* causes alleric airway hyperreactivity and dermatitis. *J Allergy Clin Immunol* 2006;117:1098–105.

84 Tas J. Respiratory allergy caused by mother-of-pearl. *Isr J Med Sci* 1972;81:630.

85 Jyo T, Katsutani T, Otsuka T. Studies on asthma caused by sea-squirts. (7). Clinical examination of the sea-squirt antigen. *Arerugi* 1967;16:509–11.

86 Tanifuji K, Daibo A, Sudo M, *et al.* The correlation between crude and purified sea-squirt antigens and histamine release in sea-squirt asthma. *Arerugi* 1984;33:78–82.

87 Kim WH, Lee SK, Lee HC, *et al.* Shell – grinder's asthma. *Yonsei Med J* 1982;23:123–30.

88 Sherson D, Hansen I, Sigsgaard T. Occupationally related respiratory symptoms in trout-processing workers. *Allergy* 1989;44:336–41.

89 Rautalahti M, Terho EO, Vohlonen I, Husman K. Atopic sensitization of dairy farmers to work-related and common allergens. *Eur J Respir Dis Suppl* 1987;152:155–64.

90 Terho EO, Husman K, Vohlonen I, *et al.* Allergy to storage mites or cow dander as a cause of rhinitis among Finnish dairy farmers. *Allergy* 1985;40:23–6.

91 Virtanen T, Vilhunen P, Husman K, Mantyjarvi R. Sensitization of dairy farmers to bovine antigens and effects of exposure on specific IgG and IgE titers. *Int Arch Allergy Appl Immunol* 1988;87:171–7.

92 Bernaola G, Echechipia S, Urrutia I, *et al.* Occupational asthma and rhinoconjunctivitis from inhalation of dried cow's milk caused by sensitization to alpha-lactalbumin. *Allergy* 1994;49:189–91.

93 Harries M, Cromwell O. Occupational asthma caused by allergy to pigs' urine. *BMJ (Clin Res Ed)* 1982;284:867.

94 Matson SC, Swanson MC, Reed CE, Yuninger JW. IgE and IgG-immune mechanisms do not mediate occupation-related respiratory or systemic symptoms in hog farmers. *J Allergy Clin Immunol* 1983;72:299–304.

95 Zuskin E, Kanceljak B, Schachter EN, *et al.* Immunological and respiratory findings in swine farmers. *Environ Res* 1991;56:120–30.

96 Donnay C, Barderas R, Kopferschmitt-Kubler MC, *et al.* Sensitization to pig albumin and gamma-globulin responsible for occupational respiratory allergy. *Allergy* 2006;61:143–4.

97 Bar-Sela S, Teichtahl H, Lutsky I. Occupational asthma in poultry workers. *J Allergy Clin Immunol* 1984;73:271–5.

98 Hoffman DR, Guenther DM. Occupational allergy to avian proteins presenting as allergy to ingestion of egg yolk. *J Allergy Clin Immunol* 1988;81:484–8.

99 Smith A, Bernstein D, Aw TC, *et al.* Occupational asthma from inhaled egg protein. *Am J Ind Med* 1987;12:205–18.

100 Edwards JH, McConnochie K, Trotman DM, *et al.* Allergy to inhaled egg material. *Clin Allergy* 1983;13:427–32.

101 Bernstein JA, Kraut A, Bernstein DI, *et al.* Occupational asthma induced by inhaled egg lysozyme. *Chest* 1993;103:532–5.

102 Bernstein DI, Smith AB, Moller DR, *et al*. Clinical and immuno-logic studies among egg-processing workers with occupational asthma. *J Allergy Clin Immunol* 1987;80:791–7.

103 Smith AB, Bernstein DI, London MA, *et al*. Evaluation of occu-pational asthma from airborne egg protein exposure in multiple settings. *Chest* 1990;98:398–404.

104 Blanco Carmona JG, Juste Picon S, Garces Sotillos M, Rodriguez Gaston P. Occupational asthma in the confectionary industry caused by sensitivity to egg. *Allergy* 1992;47:190–1.

105 Escudero C, Quirce S, Fernandez-Nieto M, *et al*. Egg white protein as inhalant allergens associated with baker's asthma. *Allergy* 2003;58:616–20.

106 Lutsky I, Bar-Sela S. Northern fowl mite (*Ornithonyssus sylviarum*) in occupational asthma of poultry workers. *Lancet* 1982; 2:874–85.

107 Lutsky I, Teichtahl H, Bar-Sela S. Occupational asthma due to poultry mites. *J Allergy Clin Immunol* 1984;73:56–60.

108 Cuthbert OD, Brostoff J, Wraith DG, Brighton WD. "Barn allergy": asthma and rhinitis due to storage mites. *Clin Allergy* 1979;9:229–36.

109 Cuthbert OD, Jeffrey IG, McNeill HB, *et al*. Barn allergy among Scottish farmers. *Clin Allergy* 1984;14:197–206.

110 Ingram CG, Jeffrey IG, Symington IS, Cuthbert OD. Bronchial provocation studies in farmers allergic to storage mites. *Lancet* 1979;2:1330–2.

111 Alvarez MJ, Castillo R, Rey A, *et al*. Occupational asthma in a grain worker due to *Lepidoglyphus destructor*, assessed by bronchial provocation test and induced sputum. *Allergy* 1999;54:884–9.

112 Ostrom NK, Swanson MC, Agarwal MK, Yunginger JW. Occupational allergy to honeybee-body dust in a honey-processing plant. *J Allergy Clin Immunol* 1986;77:736–40.

113 Reisman RE, Hale R, Wypych JI. Allergy to honeybee body components: distinction from bee venom sensitivity. *J Allergy Clin Immunol* 1983;71:18–20.

114 Yunginger JW, Jones RT, Leiferman KM, *et al*. Immunological and biochemical studies in beekeepers and their family members. *J Allergy Clin Immunol* 1978;61:93–101.

115 Randolph J. Allergic response to dust of insect origin. *JAMA* 1934;103:560–2.

116 Schultze-Werninghaus G, Zachgo W, Rotermund H, *et al*. *Tribolium confusum* (confused flour beetle, rice flour beetle) – an occupational allergen in bakers: demonstration of IgE anti-bodies. *Int Arch Allergy Appl Immunol* 1991;94:371–2.

117 Cartier A, Malo JL, Pineau L, Dolovich J. Occupational asthma due to pepsin. *J Allergy Clin Immunol* 1984;73:574–7.

118 Colten HR, Polakoff PL, Weinstein SF, Strieder DJ. Immediate hypersensitivity to hog trypsin resulting from industrial expo-sure. *N Engl J Med* 1975;292:1050–3.

119 Pilat L, Teculescu D. Bronchial asthma and allergic rhinitis associated with inhalation of pancreatic extracts. *Am Rev Respir Dis* 1975;112:275.

120 Hill D. Pancreatic extract lung sensitivity. *Med J Aust* 1975;2:553–5.

121 Paggiaro P, Loi A, Toma G. Bronchial asthma and dermatitis due to spiramycin in a chick breeder. *Clin Allergy* 1979;9:571–4.

122 Andrasch RH, Bardana Jr EJ, Koster F, Pirofsky B. Clinical and bronchial provocation studies in patients with meatwrapper's asthma. *J Allergy Clin Immunol* 1976;58:291–8.

123 Eisen E, Wegman D, Smith T. Across-shift changes in the pulmonary function of meat-wrappers and other workers in the retail food industry. *Scand J Work Environ Health* 1985; 11:21–6.

124 Pauli G, Bessot JC, Kopferschmitt-Kubler MC, *et al*. Meat wrapper's asthma: identification of the causal agent. *Clin Allergy* 1980;10:263–9.

125 Polakoff PL, Lapp NL, Reger R. Polyvinyl chloride pyrolysis products. A potential cause for respiratory impairment. *Arch Environ Health* 1975;30:269–71.

126 Butler J, Culver BH, Robertson HT. Meat wrappers' asthma. *Chest* 1981;80:71–3.

127 Aelony Y. "Meat-wrappers' asthma". *JAMA* 1976;236:1117–18.

128 Andrasch RH, Bardana Jr EJ. Thermoactivated price-label fume intolerance. A cause of meat-wrapper's asthma. *JAMA* 1976;235:937.

129 Block G, Tse KS, Kijek K, *et al*. Baker's asthma. Clinical and immunological studies. *Clin Allergy* 1983;13:359–70.

130 Wilbur RD, Ward Jr GW. Immunologic studies in a case of bak-er's asthma. *J Allergy Clin Immunol* 1976;58:366–72.

131 Hendrick DJ, Davies RJ, Pepys J. Bakers' asthma. *Clin Allergy* 1976;6:241–50.

132 Ehrlich R, Prescott R. Baker's asthma with a predominant clinical response to rye flour. *Am J Ind Med* 2005;48:153–5.

133 Gohte CJ, Wieslander G, Ancker K, Forsbeck M. Buckwheat allergy: health food, an inhalation health risk. *Allergy* 1983;38:155–9.

134 Valdivieso R, Moneo I, Pola J, *et al*. Occupational asthma and contact urticaria caused by buckwheat flour. *Ann Allergy* 1989;63:149–52.

135 Van der Brempt X, Ledent C, Mairesse M. Rhinitis and asthma caused by occupational exposure to carob bean flour. *J Allergy Clin Immunol* 1992;90:1008–10.

136 Lim HH, Domala Z, Joginder S, *et al*. Rice millers' syndrome: a preliminary report. *Br J Indust Med* 1984;41:445–9.

137 Bush R, Cohen M. Immediate and late onset asthma from occupational exposure to soybean dust. *Clin Allergy* 1977;7:369–73.

138 Lavaud F, Perdu D, Prevost A, *et al*. Baker's asthma related to soybean lecithin exposure. *Allergy* 1994;49:159–62.

139 Cockcroft AE, McDermott M, Edwards JH, McCarthy P. Grain exposure – symptoms and lung function. *Eur J Respir Dis* 1983;64:189–96.

140 Darke CS, Knowelden J, Lacey J, Milford WA. Respiratory dis-ease of workers harvesting grain. *Thorax* 1976;31:294–302.

141 doPico GA, Reddan W, Flaherty D, *et al*. Respiratory abnormal-ities among grain handlers: a clinical, physiologic, and immu-nologic study. *Am Rev Respir Dis* 1977;115:915–27.

142 Park HS, Nahm DH, Suh CH, *et al*. Occupational asthma and IgE sensitization to grain dust. *J Korean Med Sci* 1998;13:275–80.

143 Lybarger JA, Gallagher JS, Pulver DW, *et al*. Occupational asthma induced by inhalation and ingestion of garlic. *J Allergy Clin Immunol* 1982;69:448–54.

144 Falleroni AE, Zeiss CR, Levitz D. Occupational asthma secondary to inhalation of garlic dust. *J Allergy Clin Immunol* 1981;68:156–60.

145 Henson GE. Garlic: an occupational factor in the etiology of bronchial asthma. *J Fla Med Assoc* 1940;27:86.

146 Couturier P, Bousquet J. Occupational allergy secondary inhalation of garlic dust. *J Allergy Clin Immunol* 1982;70:145.

147 van Toorenenbergen AW, Dieges PH. Immunoglobulin E antibodies against coriander and other spices. *J Allergy Clin Immunol* 1985;76:477–81.

148 Zuskin E, Kanceljak B, Skuric Z, *et al*. Immunological and respiratory findings in spice-factory workers. *Environ Res* 1988;47:95–108.

149 Uragoda CG. Asthma and other symptoms in cinnamon workers. *Br J Ind Med* 1984;41:224–7.

150 van Toorenenbergen AW, Dieges PH. Occupational allergy in horticulture: demonstration of immediate-type allergic reactivity to freesia and paprika plants. *Int Arch Allergy Appl Immunol* 1984;75:44–7.

151 Lemière C, Cartier A, Lehrer SB, Malo JL. Occupational asthma caused by aromatic herbs. *Allergy* 1996;51:647–9.

152 Ferrer A, Marco FM, Andreu C, Sempere JM. Occupational asthma to carmine in a butcher. *Int Arch Allergy Immunol* 2005:138:243–50.

153 Lee JY, Lee YD, Bahn JW, Park HS. A case of occupational asthma and rhinitis caused by Sanyak and Korean ginseng dusts. *Allergy* 2006;61:392–3.

154 Igea JM, Fernandez M, Quirce S, *et al*. Green bean hypersensitivity: an occupational allergy in a homemaker. *J Allergy Clin Immunol* 1994;94:33–5.

155 Ueda A, Manda F, Aoyama K, *et al*. Immediate-type allergy related to okra (*Hibiscus esculentus* Linn) picking and packing. *Environ Res* 1993;62:189–99.

156 Sherson D, Andersen B, Hansen I, Kjoller H. Occupational asthma due to freeze-dried raspberry. *Ann Allergy Asthma Immunol* 2003;90:660–3.

157 Moreno-Ancillo A, Gil-Adrados AC, Dominguez-Noche C, *et al*. Occupational asthma due to carrot in a cook. *Allergol Immunopathol (Madr)* 2005;33:288–90.

158 Vermeulen AM, Groenewoud GC, de Jong NW, *et al*. Primary senstitization to sweet bell pepper pollen in greenhouse workers with occupational allergy. *Clin Exp Allergy* 2003;33:1439–42.

159 Hermanides HK, Lahey-de Boer AM, Zuimeer L, *et al*. *Brassica oleracea* pollen, a new source of occupational allergens. *Allergy* 2006;61:498–502.

160 Quirce S, Madero MF, Fernandez-Nieto M, *et al*. Occupational asthma due to the inhalation of cauliflower and cabbage vapors. *Allergy* 2005;60:969–70.

161 Armentia A, Lombardero M, Fernandez S, *et al*. Occupational rhinitis to leek (*Allium porrum*). *Allergy* 2005;60:132–3.

162 Tabar AI, Alvarez-Puebla MJ, Gomez B, *et al*. Diversity of asparagus allergy: clinical and immunological features. *Clin Exp Allergy* 2004;34:131–6.

163 Schuller A, Morisset M, Maadi F, *et al*. Occupational asthma due to allergy to spinach powder in a pasta factory. *Allergy* 2005;60:408–9.

164 Flindt ML. Allergy to alpha-amylase and papain. *Lancet* 1979;1:1407–8.

165 Blanco Carmona JG, Juste Picón S, Garcés Sotillos M. Occupational asthma in bakeries caused by sensitivity to alpha-amylase. *Allergy* 1991;46:274–6.

166 Baur X, Sander I, Posch A, Raulf-Heimsoth M. Baker's asthma due to the enzyme xylanase – a new occupational allergen. *Clin Exp Allergy* 1998;28:1591–3.

167 Baur X, Fruhmann G. Allergic reactions, including asthma, to the pineapple protease bromelain following occupational exposure. *Clin Allergy* 1979;9:443–50.

168 Lemière C, Pizzichini MM, Balkissoon R, *et al*. Diagnosing occupational asthma: use of induced sputum. *Eur Respir J* 1999;13:482–8.

169 Galleguillos F, Rodriguez JC. Asthma caused by bromelin inhalation. *Clin Allergy* 1978;8:21–4.

170 Milne J, Brand S. Occupational asthma after inhalation of dust of the proteolytic enzyme, papain. *Br J Indust Med* 1975;32:302–7.

171 Baur X, Konig G, Bencze K, Fruhmann G. Clinical symptoms and results of skin test, RAST and bronchial provocation test in thirty-three papain workers: evidence for strong immunogenic potency and clinically relevant "proteolytic effects of airborne papain". *Clin Allergy* 1982;12:9–17.

172 Flindt ML. Respiratory hazards from papain. *Lancet* 1978;1:430–2.

173 Baur X, Fruhmann G. Papain-induced asthma: diagnosis by skin test, RAST and bronchial provocation test. *Clin Allergy* 1979;9:75–81.

174 Patussi V, De Zotti R, Riva G, *et al*. Allergic manifestations due to castor beans: an undue risk for the dock workers handling green coffee beans. *Med Lav* 1990;81:301–7.

175 Castellan RM, Boehlecke BA, Petersen MR, *et al*. Pulmonary function and symptoms in herbal tea workers. *Chest* 1981;79:81S–5S.

176 Zuskin E, Skuric Z. Respiratory function in tea workers. *Br J Ind Med* 1984;41:88–93.

177 MacKay DM. Disease patterns in tea garden workers in Bangladesh. *J Occup Med* 1975;19:469–71.

178 Uragoda CG. Tea maker's asthma. *Br J Indust Med* 1970;27:181–2.

179 Blanc PD, Trainor WD, Lim DT. Herbal tea asthma. *Br J Indust Med* 1986;43:137–8.

180 Shirai T, Reshad K, Yoshitomi A, *et al*. Green tea-induced asthma: relationship between immunological reactivity, specific and non-specific bronchial responsiveness. *Clin Exp Allergy* 2003;33:1252–5.

181 Dulton LO. Beet pollen and beet sugar seed dust causing hay-fever and asthma. *Allergy* 1938;9:607–9.

182 Bousquet J, Dhivert H, Clauzel AM, *et al*. Occupational allergy to sunflower pollen. *J Allergy Clin Immunol* 1985;75:70–4.

183 Tsukioka K, Hirono S, Ishikawa K. A case of occupational grape pollinosis. *Arerugi* 1984;33:247–50.

184 Cohen AJ, Forse MS, Tarlo SM. Occupational asthma caused by pectin inhalation during the manufacture of jam. *Chest* 1993;103:309–11.

185 Kraut A, Peng Z, Becker AB, Warren CP. Christmas candy maker's asthma. IgG4-mediated pectin allergy. *Chest* 1992;102:1605–7.

186 Lachance P, Cartier A, Dolovich J, Malo JL. Occupational asthma from reactivity to an alkaline hydrolysis derivative of gluten. *J Allergy Clin Immunol* 1988;81:385–90.

187 Klaustermeyer W, Bardana E, Hale F. Pulmonary hypersensitivity to *Alternaria* and *Aspergillus* in baker's asthma. *Clin Allergy* 1977;7:227–33.

188 So SY, Lam WK, Yu D. Colophony-induced asthma in a poultry vender. *Clin Allergy* 1981;11:395–9.

189 Newmark F. Hops allergy and terpene sensitivity: an occupational disease. *Ann Allergy* 1978;41:311–12.

190 Kobayashi S. Occupational asthma due to inhalation of pharmacological dusts and other chemical agents with some reference to other occupational asthmas in Japan. *Allergology Proceedings of the VIII International Congress of Allergology*, Tokyo, 1974; Amsterdam: Excerpta Medica, 124–32.

191 Symington IS, Kerr JW, McLean DA. Type I allergy in mushroom soup processors. *Clin Allergy* 1981;11:43–7.

192 Tanaka H, Saikai T, Sugawara H, *et al*. Workplace-related chronic cough on a mushroom farm. *Chest* 2002;122:1080–5.

193 Shichijo K, Kondo T, Yamada M, *et al*. A case of bronchial asthma caused by spore of lentinus edodes (Berk) sing. *Nippon Naika Gakkai Zasshi* 1969;58:405–9.

194 Davies PD, Jacobs R, Mullins J, Davies BH. Occupational asthma in tomato growers following an outbreak of the fungus *Verticillium albo-atrum* in the crop. *J Soc Occup Med* 1988;38:13–17.

195 Cross T, Maciver AM, Lacey J. The thermophilic actinomycetes in mouldy hay: *Micropolyspora faeni* sp.nov. *J Gen Microbiol* 1968;50:351–9.

196 Gaur SN, Gangwar M, Khan ZU, *et al*. Farmer's lung disease in north-western India – a preliminary report. *Indian J Chest Dis Allied Sci* 1992;34:49–56.

197 Sanderson W, Kullman G, Sastre J, *et al*. Outbreak of hypersensitivity pneumonitis among mushroom farm workers. *Am J Ind Med* 1992;22:859–72.

198 Seabury J, Salvaggio J, Buechner H, Kundur VG. Bagassosis. 3. Isolation of thermophilic and mesophilic actinomycetes and fungi from moldy bagasse. *Proc Soc Exp Biol Med* 1968;129:351–60.

199 Belin L. Health problems caused by actinomycetes and moulds in the industrial environment. *Allergy*. 1985;40:24–9.

200 Salvaggio JE. Diagnosis and management of hypersensitivity pneumonitis. *Hosp Pract* 1980;15:93.

201 Channell S, Blyth W, Lloyd M, *et al*. Allergic alveolitis in malt-workers. A clinical, mycological, and immunological study. *Q J Med* 1969;38:351–76.

202 Grant IW, Blackadder ES, Greenberg M, Blyth W. Extrinsic allergic alveolitis in Scottish maltworkers. *BMJ* 1976;1:490–3.

203 Riddle HF, Channell S, Blyth W, *et al*. Allergic alveolitis in a maltworker. *Thorax* 1968;23:271–80.

204 Fink JN. Hypersensitivity pneumonitis. *J Allergy Clin Immunol* 1984;74:1–10.

205 Patterson R, Sommers H, Fink JN. Farmer's lung following inhalation of *Aspergillus flavus* growing in mouldy corn. *Clin Allergy* 1974;4:79–86.

206 Vincken W, Roels P. Hypersensitivity pneumonitis due to *Aspergillus fumigatus* in compost. *Thorax* 1984;39:74–5.

207 Tsuchiya Y, Shimokata K, Ohara H, *et al*. Hypersensitivity pneumonitis in a soy sauce brewer caused by *Aspergillus oryzae*. *J Allergy Clin Immunol* 1993;91:688–9.

208 Hunter D. *The Diseases of Occupations*. London: The English Universities Press, 1959.

209 Campbell JA, Kryda MJ, Treuhaft MW, *et al*. Cheese worker's hypersensitivity pneumonitis. *Am Rev Respir Dis* 1983;127:495–6.

210 Minnig H, De Weck AL. Cheesewasher's disease. Immunologic and epidemiologic study. *Schweiz Med Wochenschr* 1972;102:1205–12.

211 De Weck AL, Gutersohn J, Butikofer E. Cheese washer's disease ("Kaesewascherkrankheit"), a special form of farmer's lung syndrome. *Schweiz Med Wochenschr* 1969;99:872–6.

212 Popp W, Ritschka L, Zwick H, Rauscher H. "Berry sorter's lung" or wine grower's lung – an exogenous allergic alveolitis caused by *Botrytis cinerea* spores. *Prax Klin Pneumol* 1987;41:165–9.

213 Lunn JA. Millworkers' asthma: allergic responses to the grain weevil (*Sitophilus granarius*). *Br J Ind Med* 1966;23:149–52.

214 Lunn JA, Hughes DT. Pulmonary hypersensitivity to the grain weevil. *Br J Ind Med* 1967;24:158–61.

215 Pepys J. Occupational allergic lung disease caused by organic agents. *J Allergy Clin Immunol* 1986;78:1058–62.

216 Plessner MM. Une maladie des trieurs de plumes: la fièvre de canard. *Arch Mal Prof* 1960;21:67–9.

217 Warren CP, Tse KS. Extrinsic allergic alveolitis owing to hypersensitivity to chickens-significance of sputum precipitins. *Am Rev Respir Dis* 1974;109:672–7.

218 Elman AJ, Tebo T, Fink JN, Barboriak JJ. Reactions of poultry farmers against chicken antigens. *Arch Environ Health* 1968;17:98–100.

219 Korn DS, Florman AL, Gribetz I. Recurrent pneumonitis with hypersensitivity to hen litter. *JAMA* 1968;205:114–15.

220 Boyer RS, Klock LE, Schmidt CD, *et al*. Hypersensitivity lung disease in the turkey raising industry. *Am Rev Respir Dis* 1974;109:630–5.

221 Luksza AR, Bennett P, Earis JE. Bird fancier's lung: hazard of the fishing industry. *BMJ (Clin Res Ed)* 1985;291:1766.

222 Avila R. Extrinsic allergic alveolitis in workers exposed to fish meal and poultry. *Clin Allergy* 1971;1:343–6.

223 Cox A, Folgering HT, van Griensven LJ. Extrinsic allergic alveolitis caused by spores of the oyster mushroom *Pleurotus ostreatus*. *Eur Respir J* 1988;1:466–8.

224 Tsushima K, Fujimoto K, Yoshikawa S, *et al*. Hypersensitivity pneumonitis due to Bunashimeji mushrooms in the mushroom industry. *Int Arch Allergy Immunol* 2005;137:241–8.

225 Dutkiewicz J, Kus L, Dutkiewicz E, Warren CP. Hypersensitivity pneumonitis in grain farmers due to sensitization to *Erwinia herbicola*. *Ann Allergy* 1985;54:65–8.

226 Hammar S. Hypersensitivity pneumonitis. *Pathol Annu* 1988;23:195–215.

227 Weiss W, Baur X. Antigens of powdered pearl-oyster shell causing hypersensitivity pneumonitis. *Chest* 1987;91:146–8.

228 Deschamps F, Foudrinier F, Dherbecourt V, *et al*. Respiratory diseases in French cork workers. *Inhal Toxicol* 2003;15:1479–86.

229 Gaddie J, Legge JS, Friend JA, Reid TM. Pulmonary hypersensitivity in prawn workers. *Lancet* 1980;2:1350–3.

230 van Toorn DW. Coffee worker's lung. A new example of extrinsic allergic alveolitis. *Thorax* 1970;25:399–405.

231 van den Bosch JM, van Toorn DW, Wagenaar SS. Coffee worker's lung: reconsideration of a case report. *Thorax* 1983;38:720.

232 Grattan CE, Harman RR, Tan RS. Milk recorder dermatitis. *Contact Dermatitis* 1986;14:217–20.

233 Crippa M, Sala E, Alessio L. Occupational protein contact dermatitis from milk proteins. *Contact Dermatitis* 2004;51:42.

234 Sell L, Flyyholm MA, Lindhard G, Mygind K. Implementation of an occupational skin disease prevention programme in Danish cheese dairies. *Contact Dermatitis* 2005;53:155–61.

235 Rudski E, Czerwinska-Dihnz I. Sensitivity to dichromate in milk testers. *Contact Dermatitis* 1977;3:107.

236 Rogers S, Burrows D. Contact dermatitis to chrome in milk testers. *Contact Dermatitis* 1975;1:387–8.

237 Huriez C, Martin P, Lefebvre M. Sensitivity to dichromate in a milk analysis laboratory. *Contact Dermatitis* 1975;1:247–8.

238 Quirce S, Olaguibel JM, Muro MD, Tabar AI. Occupational dermatitis in a ewe milker. *Contact Dermatitis* 1992;27:56.

239 Birmingham DJ, Key MM, Tubich GE, Perone VB. Phototoxic bullae among celery harvesters. *Arch Dermatol* 1961;83:73–87.

240 Austad J, Kavli G. Phototoxic dermatitis caused by celery infected by *Sclerotinia sclerotiorum*. *Contact Dermatitis* 1983;9:448–51.

241 Wood W, Fulton R. Allergic contact dermatitis from ethoxyquin in apple packers. *J Occup Med* 1972;11:295.

242 Saunders LD, Ames RG, Knaak JB, Jackson RJ. Outbreak of Omite-CR-induced dermatitis among orange pickers in Tulare County, California. *J Occup Med* 1987;29:409–13.

243 Wittczak T, Pas-Wyroslak A, Palczynski C. Occupational allergic conjunctivitis due to coconut fibre dust. *Allergy* 2005;60:970–1.

244 Seligman PJ, Mathias CG, O'Malley MA, *et al*. Phytophotodermatitis from celery among grocery store workers. *Arch Dermatol* 1987;123:1478–82.

245 Berkley SF, Hightower AW, Beier RC, *et al*. Dermatitis in grocery workers associated with high natural concentrations of furanocoumarins in celery. *Ann Int Med* 1986;105:351–5.

246 Aalto-Korte K, Susitaival P, Kaminska R, Makinen-Kiljunen S. Occupational protein contact dermatitis from shitake mushroom and demonstration of shiitake-specific immunoglobulin E. *Contact Dermatitis* 2005;53:211–13.

247 Kavli G, Moseng D. Contact urticaria from mustard in fish-stick production. *Contact Dermatitis* 1987;17:153–5.

248 Meding B. Immediate hypersensitivity to mustard and rape. *Contact Dermatitis* 1985;13:121–2.

249 van Ketel WG, de Haan P. Occupational eczema from garlic and onion. *Contact Dermatitis* 1978;4:53–4.

250 Hafner J, Riess CE, Wuthrich B. Protein contact dermatitis from paprika and curry in a cook. *Contact Dermatitis* 1992;26:51–2.

251 Dannaker CJ, White IR. Cutaneous allergy to mustard in a salad maker. *Contact Dermatitis* 1987;16:212–14.

252 Marks Jr JG, DeMelfi T, McCarthy MA, *et al*. Dermatitis from cashew nuts. *J Am Acad Dermatol* 984;10:627–31.

253 Binkel HJ, Bayleat RM. Occupational dermatitis due to lettuce. *JAMA* 1932;98:137–8.

254 Apetato M, Marques MS. Contact dermatitis caused by sodium metabisulphite. *Contact Dermatitis* 1986;14:194.

255 White IR, Catchpole HE, Rycroft RJ. Rashes amongst persulphate workers. *Contact Dermatitis* 1982;8:168–72.

256 Malten KE. Four bakers showing positive patch-tests to a number of fragrance materials, which can also be used as flavors. *Acta Derm Venereol Suppl (Stockh)* 1979;59:117–21.

257 Fisher AA. Cutaneous reactions to sorbic acid and potassium sorbate. *Cutis* 1980;25:350, 352, 423.

258 Bojs G, Nicklasson B, Svensson A. Allergic contact dermatitis to propyl gallate. *Contact Dermatitis* 1987;17:294–8.

259 Brun R. Kontakekzem auf Laurylgallat und *p*-hydroxy-benzoate saureester. *Berufsdermatosen* 1964;12:281–4.

260 Heine A, Fox G. Baker's eczema through chromium compound in flour. *Derm Beruf Umwelt* 1980;28:113–15.

261 Fisher AA. Hand dermatitis – a "baker's dozen". *Cutis* 1982;29:214, 217–18, 221.

262 Baker EW, Wharton GW. *Acarology*. New York: Macmillan, 1952.

263 Figley KD. Karaya gum hypersensitivity. *JAMA* 1940; 114:747–8.

264 Ho VC, Mitchell JC. Allergic contact dermatitis from rubber boots. *Contact Dermatitis* 1985;12:110–11.

265 Cronin E, Calnan CD. Rosewood knife handle. *Contact Dermatitis* 1975;1:121.

266 Fancalanci S, Giorgini S, Gola M, Sertoli A. Occupational dermatitis in a butcher. *Contact Dermatitis* 1984;11:320–1.

267 Lachapelle JM. Occupational allergic contact dermatitis to povidone-iodine. *Contact Dermatitis* 1984;11:189–90.

268 Hjorth N. Gut eczema in slaughterhouse workers. *Contact Dermatitis* 1978;4:49–52.

269 Goransson K. Occupational contact urticaria to fresh cow and pig blood in slaughtermen. *Contact Dermatitis* 1981; 7:281–2.

270 Moseng D. Urticaria from pig's gut. *Contact Dermatitis* 1982;8:135–6.

271 Jovanovic M, Oliwiecki S, Beck MH. Occupational contact urticaria from beef associated with hand eczema. *Contact Dermatitis* 1992;27:188–9.

272 Fisher AA, Stengel F. Allergic occupational hand dermatitis due to calf's liver. An urticarial "immediate" type hypersensitivity. *Cutis* 1977;19:561–5.

273 Marks Jr JG, Rainey CM, Rainey MA, Andreozzi RJ. Dermatoses among poultry workers: "chicken poison disease". *J Am Acad Dermatol* 1983;9:852–7.

274 Vilaplana J, Romaguera C, Grimalt F. Contact dermatitis from lincomycin and spectinomycin in chicken vaccinators. *Contact Dermatitis* 1991;24:225–6.

275 Fisher AA. Allergic contact urticaria of the hands due to seafood in food handlers. *Cutis* 1988;42:388–9.

276 Maibach HI. Regional variation in elicitation of contact urticaria syndrome (immediate hypersensitivity syndrome): shrimp. *Contact Dermatitis* 1986;15:100.

277 Castillo R, Carrilo T, Blanco C, *et al*. Shellfish hypersensitivity: clinical and immunological characteristics. *Allergol Immunopathol (Madr)* 1994;22:83–7.

278 Yamura T, Kurose H. Oyster-shucker's dermatitis. *Arerugi* 1966;15:813.

279 Zhovtyi VR, Borzov MV. Dermatitis in workers processing mussels. *Vestn Dermatol Venerol* 1973;47:71–3.

280 Asmoe L, Bang B, Andorsen GS, *et al*. Skin symptoms in the seafood-processing industry in north Norway. *Contact Dermatitis* 2005;52:102–7.

281 Lopata AL, Baatjies R, Thrower SJ, Jeebhay MF. Occupational allergies in the seafood industry – a comparative study of Australian and South African workplaces. *Int Marit Health* 2004;55:61–73.

282 Burches E, Morales C, Pelaez A. Contact dermatitis from cuttlefish. *Contact Dermatitis* 1992;26:277.

283 Raszeja-Kotelba B, Khoetska A, Karas Z, Preisler A. Skin diseases in fisherman. *Vestn Dermatol Venerol* 1979;5:46–7.

284 Beck HI, Nissen BK. Contact urticaria to commercial fish in atopic persons. *Acta Derm Venereol* 1983;63:257–60.

285 Goransson K. Contact urticaria to fish. *Contact Dermatitis* 1981;7:282–3.

286 Sabatini C. Fisherman's dermatoses. *Folia Med (Napoli)* 1969;52:109–17.

287 Audebert C, Lamoureux P. [Professional eczema of trawlermen by contact with bryozoaires in the "baie de scine" (first French cases 1975–1977) (author's transl)]. *Ann Dermatol Venereol* 1978;105:187–92.

288 Newhouse ML. Dogger Bank itch among Lowestoft trawlermen. *Proc Roy Soc Med* 1966;59:1119–20.

289 Ross JB. Rubber boot dermatitis in Newfoundland: a survey of 30 patients. *Can Med Assoc J* 1969;100:13–19.

290 Raszeja-Kotelba B, Chojecka A, Flieger M, Karas Z. Occupational dermatitis and skin changes in workers manufacturing and repairing fishing nets. *Przegl Dermatol* 1979;66:367–74.

291 de Boer EM, van Ketel WG. Occupational dermatitis caused by snackbar meat products. *Contact Dermatitis* 1984;11:322.

292 Meding B. Skin symptoms among workers in a spice factory. *Contact Dermatitis* 1993;29:202–5.

293 Goh CL, Ng SK. Allergic contact dermatitis to *Curcuma longa* (turmeric). *Contact Dermatitis* 1987;17:186.

294 van Ketel WG. Dermatitis from octyl gallate in peanut butter. *Contact Dermatitis* 1978;4:60–1.

295 Diba VC, English JS. Contact allergy to green coffee bean dust in a coffee processing plant worker. *Contact Dermatitis* 2002;47:56.

296 Kubo Y, Nonaka S, Yoshida H. Contact sensitivity to unsaponifiable substances in sesame oil. *Contact Dermatitis* 1986;15:215–17.

297 Gougerot S. Occupational eczema due to artichokes. *Bull Soc Fr Dermatol Syph* 1926;43:1463–7.

298 Mobacken H, Fregert S. Allergic contact dermatitis from cardamom. *Contact Dermatitis* 1975;1:175–6.

299 Spencer LV, Fowler Jr JF. "Thin mint" cookie dermatitis. *Contact Dermatitis* 1988;18:185–6.

300 Bunney MH. Contact dermatitis in beekeepers due to propolis (bee glue). *Br J Dermatol* 1968;80:17–23.

301 Melli MC, Giorgini S, Sertoli A. Occupational dermatitis in a bee-keeper. *Contact Dermatitis* 1983;9:427–8.

302 Rothenborg HW. Occupational dermatitis in beekeeper due to poplar resins in beeswax. *Arch Dermatol* 1967;95:381–4.

303 Balachandran C, Srinivas CR, Shenoy SD, Edison KP. Occupational dermatosis in coconut palm climbers. *Contact Dermatitis* 1992;26:143.

304 Cardullo AC, Ruszkowski AM, DeLeo VA. Allergic contact dermatitis resulting from sensitivity to citrus peel, geraniol, and citral. *J Am Acad Dermatol* 1989;21:395–7.

305 Nakamura S, Yamaguchi M, Oishi M, Hayama T. Studies on the buckwheat allergose report 1: on the cases with the buckwheat allergose. *Allerg Immunol (Leipz)* 1974;20–21:449–56.

306 Bousquet J, Campos J, Michel FB. Food intolerance to honey. *Allergy* 1984;39:73–5.

307 Butcher BT, O'Neil CE, Reed MA, *et al*. Development and loss of toluene diisocyanate reactivity: immunologic, pharmacologic, and provocative challenge studies. *J Allergy Clin Immunol* 1982;70:231–5.

308 Bardana EJJ. Occupational asthma and related respiratory disorders. *Dis Mon* 1995;41:143–99.

309 Slavin RG. Occupational and allergic rhinitis: impact on worker productivity and safety. *Allergy Asthma Proc* 1998;19:277–84.

310 Frew A, Chan H, Dryden P, *et al*. Immunologic studies of the mechanisms of occupational asthma caused by western red cedar. *J Allergy Clin Immunol* 1993;92:466–78.

311 Weiner A. Bronchial asthma due to organic phosphate insecticide. *Ann Allergy* 1961;19:397–401.

312 O'Malley M. Clinical evaluation of pesticide exposure and poisonings. *Lancet* 1997;349:1161–6.

313 Malo JL, Ghezzo H, D'Aquino C, *et al*. Natural history of occupational asthma: relevance of type of agent and other factors in the rate of development of symptoms in affected subjects. *J Allergy Clin Immunol* 1992;90:937–44.

314 2006 Annual Report on United States Seafood Industry. H.M. Johnson and Associates. http://www.hmj.com

315 Choo, PS. Seafood production and trade in various APEC economies: the need for harmful biotoxin regulatory mechanisms. *Second International Conference on Harmful Algae Management and Mitigation*, 12–16 November 2001, Qingdao, China.

316 Lehrer SB. Seafood allergy. Introduction. *Clin Rev Allergy* 1993;11:155–7.

317 Quirce S, Bernstein DI, Malo JL. High-molecular-weight protein agents. In: Bernstein IL, Chan-Yeung M, Malo JL, Bernstein DI (eds.) *Asthma in the Workplace and Related Conditions*. New York: Taylor & Francis Group, 2006:463–79.

318 Boulet L, Lemiere C, Gautrin D, Cartier A. New insights into occupational asthma. *Curr Opin Allergy Clin Immunol* 2007;7:96–101.

319 Bang B, Aasmoe L, Aamodt BH, *et al*. Exposure and airway effects of seafood industry workers in northern Norway. *J Occup Environ Med* 2005;47:482–92.

320 De Besche A. On asthma bronchiale in man provoked by cat, dog, and different other animals. *Acta Medica Scandinavica* 1937;42:237–55.

321 Weytjens K, Cartier A, Malo JL, *et al*. Aerosolized snow-crab allergens in a processing facility. *Allergy* 1999;54:892–3.

322 Malo JL, Cartier A. Occupational reactions in the seafood industry. *Clin Rev Allergy* 1993;11:223–40.

323 Ortega HG, Daroowalla F, Petsonk EL, *et al*. Asthma-like illness among crab-processing workers-Alaska. *MMWR* 1982;31:95–6.

324 Ortega HG, Daroowalla F, Petsonk EL, *et al*. Respiratory symptoms among crab processing workers in Alaska: epidemiological and environmental assessment. *Am J Ind Med* 2001;39:598–607.

325 Jeebhay MF, Robins TG, Lehrer SB, Lopata AL. Occupational seafood allergy: a review. *Occup Environ Med* 2001;58:553–62.

326 Pardo A, Barrios R, Gaxiola M, *et al*. Increase of lung neutrophils in hypersensitivity pneumonitis is associated with lung fibrosis. *Am J Respir Crit Care Med* 2000;161:1698–704.

327 Berger I, Schierl R, Ochmann U, *et al*. Concentrations of dust, allergens and endotoxins in stables, living rooms and mattresses from cattle farmers in southern Bavaria. *Ann Agric Environ Med* 2005;12:101–7.

328 Fujishima S, Nakamura M, Nakamura H, *et al*. Flow cytometric detection of cell-associated interleukin-8 alveolar macrophages *in vivo* from patients with hypersensitivity pneumonitis and sarcoidosis. *Scand J Clin Lab Invest* 2004;64:237–43.

329 Trentin L, Migone N, Zambello R, *et al*. Mechanisms accounting for lymphocytic alveolitis in hypersensitivity pneumonitis. *J Immunol* 1990;145:2147–54.

330 Semenzato G, Trentin L, Zambello R, *et al*. Different types of cytotoxic lymphocytes recovered from the lungs of patients with hypersensitivity pneumonitis. *Am Rev Respir Dis* 1988;137:70–4.

331 Denis M. Proinflammatory cytokines in hypersensitivity pneumonitis. *Am J Respir Crit Care Med* 1995;151:164–9.

332 US Mushroom Production. http://www.nass.usda.gov/ut/Pdf/semimonthly/semi0177,pdf

333 Bringhurst LS, Byrne RN, Gershon-Cohen J. Respiratory disease of mushroom workers. *JAMA* 1959;171:15–18.

334 Sakula A. Mushroom-worker's lung. *BMJ* 1967;3:708–10.

335 Lacey J. Allergy in mushroom workers. *Lancet* 1974;1:366.

336 Michils A, De Vuyst P, Nolard N, *et al*. Occupational asthma to spores of *Pleurotus cornucopiae*. *Eur Respir J* 1991;4:1143–7.

337 Tarvainen K, Salonen JP, Kanerva L, *et al*. Allergy and toxicodermia from shiitake mushrooms. *J Am Acad Dermatol* 1991;24:64–6.

338 Vandenplas O, Ghezzo H, Munoz X, *et al*. What are the questionnaire items most useful in identifying subjects with occupational asthma? *Eur Respir J* 2005;26:1056–63.

339 Malo JL, Ghezzo H, L'Archevêque J, *et al*. Is the clinical history a satisfactory means of diagnosing occupational asthma? *Am Rev Respir Dis* 1991;143:528–32.

340 Emmett EA. Occupational skin disease. *J Allergy Clin Immunol* 1983;72:649–56.

341 Hargreave FE, Ramsdale EH, Pugsley SO. Occupational asthma without bronchial hyperresponsiveness. *Am Rev Respir Dis* 1984;130:513–15.

342 Vandenplas O, Delwiche JP, Jamart J, Vandeweyer R. Increase in non-specific bronchial hyperresponsiveness as an early marker of bronchial response to occupational agents during specific inhalation challenges. *Thorax* 1996;51:472–8.

343 Baur X, Huber H, Degens PO, *et al*. Relation between occupational asthma case history, bronchial methacholine challenge, and specific challenge test in patients with suspected occupational asthma. *Am J Ind Med* 1998;33:114–22.

344 Gailhofer G, Wilders-Truschnig M, Smolle J, Ludvan M. Asthma caused by bromelain: an occupational allergy. *Clin Allergy* 1988;18:445–50.

345 Thorpe SC, Kemeny DM, Panzani R, Lessof MH. Allergy to castor bean. I. Its relationship to sensitization to common inhalant allergens (atopy). *J Allergy Clin Immunol* 1988;82:62–6.

346 Di Franco A, Vagaggini B, Bacci E, *et al*. Leukocyte counts in hypertonic saline-induced sputum in subjects with occupational asthma. *Respir Med* 1998;92:550–7.

347 Chmelik F, doPico G, Reed CE, Dickie H. Farmer's lung. *J Allergy Clin Immunol* 1974;54:180–8.

348 Akira M. High-resolution CT in the evaluation of occupational and environmental disease. *Radiol Clin North Am* 2002;40:43–59.

349 Selman, M. Hypersensitivity pneumonitis: a multifaceted deceiving disorder. *Clin Chest Med* 2004;25:531–47.

350 Yoshizawa Y, Ohtani Y, Hayakawa H, *et al*. Chronic hypersensitivity pneumonitis in Japan: a nationwide epidemiologic survey. *J Allergy Clin Immunol* 1999;103:315–20.

351 Grubek-Jaworska H, Hoser G, Droszcz P, Chazan R. CD4/CD8 lymphocytes in BALF during the efferent phase of lung delayed-type hypersensitivity reaction induced by single antigen inhalation. *Med Sci Monit* 2001;7:878–83.

352 Popper HH. Which biopsies in diffuse infiltrative lung diseases and when are these necessary? *Monaldi Arch Chest Dis* 2001;56:446–52.

353 Gawkrodger DJ. Patch testing in occupational dermatology. *Occup Environ Med* 2001;58:823–8.

354 Adams RM. *Occupational Skin Disease*, 3rd edn. Philadelphia, PA: WB Saunders, 1999.

355 Rietschel RL, Fowler Jr JF. *Fisher's Contact Dermatitis*, 5th ed. Lippincott, PA: Williams & Wilkins,2000.

356 Beltrani VS, Bernstein L, Cohen DE, Fonacier L. Contact dermatitis: a practice parameter. *Ann.Allergy Asthma Immunol* 2006;97:S1–17.

357 Perrin B, Lagier F, L'Archevêque J, *et al*. Occupational asthma: validity of monitoring of peak expiratory flow rates and nonallergic bronchial responsiveness as compared to specific inhalation challenge. *Eur Respir J* 1992;5:40–8.

358 Burge PS, O'Brien I, Harries M. Peak flow rate records in the diagnosis of occupational asthma due to isocyanates. *Thorax* 1979;34:317–23.

359 Côtè J, Kennedy S, Chan-Yeung M. Sensitivity and specificity of PC20 and peak expiratory flow rate in cedar asthma. *J Allergy Clin Immunol* 1990;85:592–8.

360 Malo JL, Trudeau C, Ghezzo H, *et al*. Do subjects investigated for occupational asthma through serial peak expiratory flow measurements falsify their results. *J Allergy Clin Immunol* 1995;96:601–7.

361 Quirce S, Contreras G, Dybuncio A, Chan-Yeung M. Peak expiratory flow monitoring is not a reliable method for establishing the diagnosis of occupational asthma. *Am J Respir Crit Care Med* 1995;152:1100–2.

362 Leroyer C, Perfetti L, Trudeau C, *et al*. Comparison of PEF and FEV$_1$ monitoring with specific inhalation challenge in the diagnosis of occupational asthma (abstract). *Am J Respir Crit Care Med* 1997;155:A137.

363 Moscato G, Godnic-Cvar J, Maestrelli P. Statement on self-monitoring of peak expiratory flows in the investigation of occupational asthma. Subcommittee on Occupational Allergy of European Academy of Allergy and Clinical Immunology. *J Allergy Clin Immunol* 1995;96:295–301.

364 Bright P, Burge PS. Occupational lung disease. 8. The diagnosis of occupational asthma from serial measurements of lung function at and away from work. *Thorax* 1996;51:857–63.

365 Tarlo SM, Boulet LP, Cartier A, *et al*. Canadian Thoracic Society. Guidelines for occupational asthma. *Can Respir J* 1998;5:289–300.

366 Cartier A, Bernstein IL, Burge PS, *et al*. Guidelines for bronchoprovocation on the investigation of occupational asthma. *Report of the Subcommittee on Bronchoprovocation for Occupational Asthma. J Allergy Clin Immunol* 1989;84:823–9.

367 Weytjens K, Malo JL, Cartier A, *et al*. Comparison of peak expiratory flows and FEV1 in assessing immediate asthmatic reactions due to occupational agents. *Allergy* 1999;54:621–5.

368 Bérubé D, Cartier A, L'Archevêque J, *et al*. Comparison of peak expiratory flow rate and FEV1 in assessing bronchomotor tone after challenges with occupational sensitizers. *Chest* 1991;99:831–6.

369 Uzzaman A, Metcalfe D, Komarow HD. Acoustic rhinometry in the practice of allergy. *Ann Allergy Asthma Immunol* 2006;97:745–51.

370 Hytonen ML, Sala EL, Malmberg HO, Nordman H. Acoustic rhinometry in the diagnosis of occupational rhinitis. *Am J Rhinol* 1996;10:393–7.

371 Perrin B, Cartier A, Ghezzo H, *et al*. Reassessment of the temporal patterns of bronchial obstruction after exposure to occupational sensitizing agents. *J Allergy Clin Immunol* 1991;87:630–9.

372 Davies R, Green M, Schoefield N. Recurrent nocturnal asthma after exposure to grain dust. *Am Rev Respir Dis* 1976; 114:1011–19.

373 Bourke SJ, Dalphin JC, Boyd G, *et al*. Hypersensitivity pneumonitis: current concepts. *Eur Respir J* 2001;32:81s–92s.

374 Ameille J, Descatha A. Outcome of occupational asthma. *Curr Opin Allergy Clin Immunol* 2005;5:125–8.

375 Chan-Yeung M, Malo JL. Natural history of occupational asthma. In: Bernstein IL, Chan-Yeung M, Malo JL, Bernstein DI (eds.) *Asthma in the Workplace*. New York: Marcel Decker Inc., 1999:129–43.

376 Moscato G, Dellabianca A, Perfetti L, *et al*. Occupational asthma: a longitudinal study on the clinical and socioeconomic outcome after diagnosis. *Chest* 1999;115:249–56.

377 Hudson P, Cartier A, Pineau L, *et al*. Follow-up of occupational asthma caused by crab and various agents. *J Allergy Clin Immunol* 1985;76:682–8.

378 Malo JL, Cartier A, Ghezzo H, *et al*. Patterns of improvement in spirometry, bronchial hyperresponsiveness, and specific IgE antibody levels after cessation of exposure in occupational asthma caused by snow-crab-processing. *Am Rev Respir Dis* 1988;138:807–12.

379 Lemière C, Cartier A, Malo JL, Lehrer SB. Persistent specific bronchial reactivity to occupational agents in workers with normal nonspecific bronchial reactivity. *Am J Respir Crit Care Med* 2000;162:976–80.

380 Dewitte JD, Chan-Yeung M, Malo JL. Medicolegal and compensation aspects of occupational asthma. *Eur Respir J* 1994;7:969–80.

381 Ameille J, Pairon JC, Bayeux MC, *et al*. Consequences of occupational asthma on employment and financial status: a follow-up study. *Eur Respir J* 1997;10:55–8.

382 Gassert TH, Hu H, Kelsey KT, Christiani DC. Long-term health and employment outcomes of occupational asthma and their determinants. *J Occup Environ Med* 1998;40:481–91.

383 Piirila PL, Keskinen HM, Luukkonen R, *et al.* Work, unemployment and life satisfaction among patients with diisocyanate induced asthma – a prospective study. *J Occup Health* 2005;47:112–18.

384 Leigh JP, Romano PS, Schenker MB, Kreiss K. Costs of occupational COPD and asthma. *Chest* 2002;121:264–72.

385 Braun SR, doPico GA, Tsiatis A, *et al.* Farmer's lung disease: long-term clinical and physiologic outcome. *Am Rev Respir Dis* 1979;119:185–91.

386 Zacharisen MC, Schlueter DP, Kurup VP, Fink JN. The long-term outcome in acute, subacute, and chronic forms of pigeon breeder's disease hypersensitivity pneumonitis. *Ann Allergy Asthma Immunol* 2002;88:175–82.

387 Hendrick DJ. Management of occupational asthma. *Eur Respir J* 1994;7:961–8.

388 Nicholson PJ, Newman Taylor AJ, Oliver P, Cathcart M. Current best practice for the health surveillance of enzyme workers in the soap and detergent industry. *Occup Med (Lond)* 2001;51:81–92.

389 Tarlo SM, Liss GM. Prevention of occupational asthma-practical implications for occupational physicians. *Occup Med (Lond)* 2005;55:588–94.

390 Baur X. Are we closer to developing threshold limit values for allergens in the workplace? *Ann Allergy Asthma Immunol* 2003;90:11–18.

391 Nicholson PJ, Cullinan P, Taylor AJ, *et al.* Evidence based guidelines for the prevention, identification, and management of occupational asthma. *Occup Environ Med* 2005;62:290–9.

392 Karjalainen A, Martikainen R, Klaukka T, *et al.* Risk of asthma among Finnish patients with occupational rhinitis. *Chest* 2003;123:283–8.

393 Orriols R, Aliaga JL, Anto JM, *et al.* High prevalence of mollusc shell hypersensitivity pneumonitis in nacre factory workers. *Eur Respir J* 1997;10:780–6.

394 Kokkarinen JI, Tukiainen HO, Terho EO. Effect of corticosteroid treatment on the recovery of pulmonary function in farmer's lung. *Am Rev Respir Dis* 1992;145:3–5.

395 Bernstein JA, Bernstein L, Bucchini L, *et al.* Clinical and laboratory investigation of allergy to genetically modified foods. *Environ Health Perspect* 2003;111:1114–21.

PART 3

Adverse Reactions to Foods: Diagnosis

19

CHAPTER 19

In Vitro Diagnostic Methods in the Evaluation of Food Hypersensitivity

Staffan Ahlstedt, Lars Söderström, and Anita Kober

KEY CONCEPTS

- There are validated *in vitro* markers for food allergy diagnosis.
  - Specific IgE antibodies in case of IgE-mediated allergy.
  - Specific IgA/IgG antibodies to gliadin and endomysium in case of celiac disease.
- More information is obtained if markers are evaluated quantitatively.
  - Information both regarding the risk of a reaction and of possible outgrowth can be achieved.
- Cross-reactivity between different allergens needs to be taken into account.
- Evaluation of allergen components, epitopes, and genetic markers are promising for providing increased information in the future.
- It is important to use a technically well-validated and clinically evaluated laboratory system to achieve useful information.

Introduction

The technical feasibility and clinical utility of *in vitro* determinations of antibodies and other markers will be discussed with specific emphasis on food allergy. Allergic diseases including reactions to foods represent an increasing problem in the Western world, with symptoms that may not be easily distinguished from other disorders. In this chapter, the term "hypersensitivity" is defined as something that induces objectively reproducible symptoms or signs initiated by exposure to a defined stimulus at a dose tolerated by normal subjects [1]. Hypersensitivity can be differentiated into allergic hypersensitivity which involves an immune mechanism and non-allergic hypersensitivity where immune mechanisms are excluded. Different tests must be applied to distinguish between such conditions. An allergic hypersensitivity can be either IgE mediated or non-IgE mediated; an example of non-IgE-mediated hypersensitivity is celiac disease (CD), which involves immune cells and antibodies of IgG and IgA isotypes. In distinguishing between the two types of allergic hypersensitivity, a given test should identify the IgE- or IgG/IgA-related allergic mechanisms in allergic patients from those of other patients suffering from similar symptoms.

When suffering from allergy, most patients are sensitized to more than one allergen that may trigger their clinical symptoms. It is often difficult to distinguish which is the clinically responsible allergen. Furthermore, allergic symptoms related to IgE antibodies depend not only on those IgE antibodies, but also on a number of related and unrelated confounding factors. These factors include inflammation, organ function, presence of infection, physical and psychological stress, and hormonal influences and the IgE antibody results must always be interpreted in context of these confounding factors. For patients with food allergy and intolerance, the double-blind, placebo-controlled food challenge (DBPCFC) is considered the gold standard [2,3]. However, this technique does not distinguish among allergic hypersensitivity involving IgE antibodies, antibodies of IgG/IgA isotypes, and cellular immune mechanisms, and those of intolerance, including enzyme deficiencies or other unknown mechanisms exhibiting similar degree of hypersensitivity.

A clinical diagnosis of IgE-mediated allergy should be based on the patient's history, symptoms, findings on physical examination, together with laboratory test results. Diagnosing patients with IgE-mediated allergy would differentiate them

Food Allergy: Adverse Reactions to Foods and Food Additives, 4th edition.
Edited by Dean D. Metcalfe, Hugh A. Sampson, and Ronald A. Simon.
© 2008 Blackwell Publishing, ISBN: 978-1-4501-5129-0.

from those having several other disease etiologies presenting with similar symptom profiles. Because there is no working gold standard for true allergy diagnosis, only one for food hypersensitivity and CD, such diagnosis is complicated. With the recognition that the prevalence of allergic problems is increasing and differential diagnosis by history and physical examination is difficult, tools should be used to differentiate the mechanisms behind the symptoms. The present communication discusses well-defined blood tests for specific IgE or IgG/IgA antibodies and other markers, representing objective means to identify food-specific allergies in individual patients. The presence or absence of such antibodies or markers can be determined with high sensitivity and precision. Such information represents one piece of information among others that must be used to compile a definitive clinical diagnosis.

Antibodies to various allergens may be present without obvious clinical disease. Nevertheless, the presence in a very young child of minute levels of specific IgE antibodies, especially to hen's egg white and, to a lesser extent, cow's milk, can be used as a predictor of evolving sensitization to inhalant allergens and allergic disease [4]. In contrast, the presence of IgG/IgA antibodies to a specific food may just be the result of exposure to the substance or allergen, sometimes associated with increased permeability of the gastrointestinal mucosa, but without an obvious link to a clinical disorder [5–7]. Exceptions are the IgG/IgA antibodies to gliadin as well as tissue transglutaminase (tTG) in CD [8] (Box 19.1).

For markers of inflammation, the situation is less consistent and sampling is often problematic. However, there are methods for determining markers from (1) mast cells, for example histamine, tryptase, prostaglandins, and leukotrienes [9–11]; (2) eosinophils, for example the eosinophil granular constituents such as eosinophil cationic protein (ECP), eosinophil protein X (EPX), eosinophilic peroxidase (EPO), major basic protein (MBP), and leukotrienes [9–11]; (3) basophils, for example histamine and leukotrienes [9,10]; and (4) neutrophils, for example myeloperoxidase (MPO), human neutrophil lipocalin (HNL), lactoferrin, and lysozyme [11], although these are often not well established as clinical diagnostic methods but are to be considered more as research tools [9–11].

Box 19.1

Case history, physical examination + laboratory tests = clinical diagnosis

Presence of markers + clinical symptoms = possible clinical disease

Presence of markers + no clinical symptoms = may suggest ongoing disease or outgrowth of disease

For conditions due to enzyme deficiencies, the situation is even worse, except for lactose intolerance, most tests to determine enzyme deficiency are less well proven. For example, in histamine intolerance mediated by a deficient diamine oxidase system [12], standardized methods have not been established, despite the fact that the clinical condition is recognized and often presents as headache after ingestion of certain histamine-, phenyl ethylamine-, or serotonin-containing foods such as red wine. Since the enzyme is located primarily in the jejunal mucosa, the problems are induced by gastrointestinal exposure. The diagnostic tests for this condition are of a research nature and are difficult to use in clinical practice [12]. However, recently there have been promising reports suggesting new methods to diagnose such conditions as irritable bowel syndrome by ultrasonic sound, focusing on local edema in the intestinal tract [13,14], so new diagnostic methods for other disorders are likely to be developed.

Markers and methods with confirmed value

IgE antibodies

It is well known that the presence of IgE antibodies to a specific food indicates a certain probability of a clinical reaction to that food, although the risk levels are unique in each patient. Virtually any food may lead to a reaction, although only a small number of foods, such as in children where hen's egg, cow's milk, peanuts, soy, wheat, tree nuts, and fish account for about 90% of the reactions [15–17]. In adults, peanuts, tree nuts, fish, and shellfish are the most common, although sensitivity to other allergens may be present and must be identified by case history together with allergy testing [18–20]. Negative results obtained with *in vivo* tests and skin prick tests (SPTs) are informative with a very high negative predictive value (NPV) (>95%) [21,22]. When interpreted as a positive result, allergy tests show great variations in clinical specificity for different allergens in different patient groups. Evaluating the quantity of IgE antibodies, rather than using results in a simple dichotomous manner, has been shown to provide more information. The correlation of the quantity of allergen-specific IgE and the probability of clinical reactivity were first demonstrated by Sampson and co-workers [23,24] and later confirmed by other investigators [25–32]. However, it is important to emphasize that the age of the food-allergic patient affects the interpretation of the level of the IgE antibodies [25,26,29,33]. Utilizing the fine-tuning of IgE antibody specificities to different epitopes may in the future provide an even better predictor of which patients will experience allergic reactions when eating a food, rather than just being sensitized [34] (Box 19.2).

Monitoring IgE levels also may be clinically important in the follow-up of patients with allergy to food. For example, in patients destined to "outgrow" their allergies to cow's milk protein, the levels of IgE antibodies to cow's milk proteins were found to be lower than in those patients with persistent allergy [35–37]. The antibody specificity and especially the diversity of antibody specificities also seem to impact the patient outcome [38,39].

IgG/IgA antibodies in celiac disease

The etiology of CD is yet to be fully resolved. It involves an autoimmune enteropathy triggered by the ingestion of gluten in susceptible individuals. Even though CD is usually considered to present in early childhood, only a minority of patients are diagnosed during this time, while the vast majority of CD patients are diagnosed much later or not at all. The typical intestinal damage, such as loss of villi and hyperplasia of crypts, resolves completely upon elimination of gluten from the diet. Besides failure-to-thrive, a large proportion of CD patients present with atypical symptoms such as general weakness, bad temper, anemia, menstruation disturbance, or even depression.

Historically the diagnosis of CD has included the need for several intestinal biopsies as outlined in the first European Society of Pediatric Gastroenterology, Hepatology, and Nutrition guidelines [40]. Since the development of more sensitive and specific *in vitro* tests for specific IgA and IgG antibodies to gliadin, endomysium, and tTG, the guidelines have been revised and the number of biopsies needed to ascertain a valid diagnosis has been reduced [41]. The combined use of IgA and IgG anti-gliadin antibodies (AGA) measurements available in different *in vitro* assay formats (e.g. enzyme-linked immunosorbent assay, ELISA; ImmunoCAP) has been shown to be sensitive and specific in relation to the presence of clinical disease [8].

Histochemical staining methods used to detect IgA antibodies to endomysium have been considered more specific and sensitive, but also more difficult to perform in a standardized manner. The demonstration that tissue tTG is the main target of the autoimmune response [42] has led to the development of several specific IgA assays based on guinea pig or, preferably, human tTG, giving very high sensitivities and specificities. Tests with recombinant human tTG seem to perform the best and are a useful tool in both small children and adults [8,43–46]. In the cases of IgA deficiency, specific IgG antibodies to gliadin and tTG are of special value [47,48].

The presence of serum tissue tTG and endomysial autoantibodies is predictive of small-bowel abnormalities indicative of CD. There is a good correlation between autoantibody positivity and specific human leukocyte antigen (HLA) haplotypes. Although population screening for CD using serological tests is still a controversial topic, screening of high-risk groups, such as first-degree relatives of CD patients, patients suffering from osteoporosis, anemia, type I diabetes, thyroiditis, IgA deficiency, or other autoimmune diseases, is strongly recommended [49–51] (Box 19.3).

Allergen and antigen properties in the *in vitro* diagnosis

Allergen sources

The ability of a test to detect specific IgE and other antibodies depends on the presence of all relevant allergen components in the test system. Food is prepared from both animal and plant origin and the antibody patterns of patients sensitized to food are often even more complex than those seen for inhalant allergens. The use of native allergen source material of the highest quality and containing all relevant allergen components is of primary importance. The mode of preparation of extracts for preservation of allergenic potency during processing is vital [52–54].

Intact macromolecules from the partly digested food may pass through the intestinal mucosa into the circulation and act as allergens [5–7]. Attention has also been drawn to the possible creation of neo-allergens during processing and digestion of food; for example, the allergenic determinants are enhanced and/or formed by roasting peanuts [55,56]. In some cases, food allergens are destroyed during processing, as exemplified by the fact that some patients may tolerate the cooked food, but not its raw counterpart [57,58]. To be able to detect all patients with differing antibody specificities, a native food source material that is representative of the natural exposure should be used. Fermented food may have a lower content of effective allergens or exposure of such allergens to the gastrointestinal tract [59,60].

IgE antibodies are produced as a consequence of exposure to allergens in the diet and environment. Regional differences in food habits may result in different patterns of IgE antibody specificity [53,61–64]. However, increasing international trade, and use of tropical food, ornamental plants, and herbs widen possible exposure far from what is common in the local environment.

Currently, considerable research efforts are directed at characterization of individual food allergen components. Today more than 70 food allergen components are listed by the International Union of Immunological Societies (IUIS) (http://www.allergen.org) and many more components are described in the Allergome database (www.allergome.org) Many of these components have been cloned and may in the future be available as recombinant proteins [65]. The use of separate components or combinations of components may lead to new and better tools in the diagnosis of food allergy in the future and already today the increasing knowledge of reactivity patterns to different components can be useful in clinical practice [66,67] (Box 19.4).

Epitopes

Clinical sensitivity to a certain food allergen often changes over time. It is estimated that about 80% of children outgrow their cow's milk allergy [18], although only 20% outgrow their peanut allergy [68]. Some results suggest that IgE antibodies from individuals with persistent allergy may be directed against different epitopes than those in patients with transient allergy [34,38,39,69]. Epitopes may be continuous (linear or sequential) or conformational (involving different parts of peptide chains due to folding on the peptide chain), and the specificity of an antibody depends on the uniqueness of the epitope. The measurement of specific IgE to single epitopes may provide a new way of not only diagnosing, but also predicting allergic reactions in food-allergic children. In the future we may see tests identifying antibodies to different epitopes and then predicting whether the allergy is transient or persistent. Newer information also suggests a possibility to reveal the risk for anaphylaxis by utilizing the spectrum of IgE specificities to different epitopes on the same allergen molecule [38]. To obtain

such information by monitoring epitope-specific IgE antibodies over time, the test system needs to be quantitative and give correct results over the whole measuring range. The development of the multiplex technology platform would facilitate the use and interpretation of IgE antibody-binding patterns to define multiple components and epitopes [38,70,71].

Antigen sources

Gliadin, tTG: The common antigen source for determination of gliadin-specific IgA and IgG antibodies is crude or purified fractions of wheat gliadin. Gliadin is obtained as the alcohol-soluble fraction from wheat gluten prolamins. Prolamins from other closely related cereals such as rye, barley, and oats show some degree of cross-reactivity but are not commonly used for CD diagnostics [72,73]. For measurements of IgA and IgG antibodies to tTG, guinea pig-derived antigen was used initially, but human tTG has been shown to give higher sensitivity and specificity [8,44,73,74].

Cross-reactivity

Cross-reactivity between allergen-specific IgE and related allergens *in vitro* is also seen with SPTs. Consequently, the clinical relevance between different allergens must be determined individually for each patient, taking the clinical history and provocation/elimination diet results into account. Proteins with similar functions in different plant species may have a similar structure [75]. The IgE antibodies may detect such similarities between allergens from different sources as a function of biology and chemistry resulting in allergic reactions despite the fact that no apparent exposure to the allergen can be identified. Among foods there are several groups of cross-reactive allergens. The pollen-related food allergies to fruit and vegetables are well known, but cross-reactions have also been demonstrated between shellfish and other animals, between fruit and latex, and between different fruits [19,65,76–79]. The knowledge of cross-reactivities can be used for better assessment and thereby clinical management of the patients [67].

As discussed in Chapter 3, many food allergens from plant sources are proteins belonging to the "pathogenesis-related" (PR) protein family, for example, Bet v 1 homologs that have been identified in a great number of pollens and fruits [80,81]. Another group of PR proteins include the chitinases that are present in latex and fruits [80]. Other allergens known to induce cross-reactivity between pollens and fruits are profilins with highly preserved protein structures [82]. Lipid-transfer proteins (LTPs) compose another group of very stable proteins present in fruits and vegetables and cause cross-reactions both *in vitro* and *in vivo* [61,83–85]. In foods of animal origin, tropomyosins and serum proteins are known to be cross-reactive [76]. Future research on the basis of recombinant (or purified native) components

Table 19.1 Examples of common food allergens

Protein classification	Property	Allergen source (allergen)
PR-2	β-1-3-glucanases	Fruits, banana, latex (Hev b 2)
PR-3	Type 1 (basic) and Type II (acidic) chitinases	Avocado (Pers a 1), banana, chestnut
PR-4	Chitinases	Turnip, elderberry
PR-5	Thaumatin- and osmotin-like proteins (antifungal)	Cherry (Pru av 2), apple (Mal d 2), bell pepper
PR-6	Protease and amylase inhibitors	Soy, wheat, barley, rye, rice
PR-9	Peroxidase	Wheat, barley
PR-10	Bet v 1 homologs similar to ribonucleases	Apple (Mal d 1), pear (Pyr c 1), cherry (Pru av 1), apricot (Pru ar1), hazelnut (Cor a 1.04), carrot (Dau c 1), celery (Api g 1), soy (Gly m 4), peanut (Ara h 8)
PR-14	non-specific lipid-transfer proteins (nsLTP), lipid metabolism	Peach (Pru p 3), apricot, plum, cherry (Pru av 3), apple (Mal d3), hazelnut (Cor a 8), maize, broccoli, carrot, rapeseed
Profilin	Actin binding, signal transduction	Celery (Api g 4), potato, hazelnut, apple (Mal d 4), pear (Pyr c 4), tomato, cherry (Pru av 4), soybean (Gly m 3), peanut (Ara h 5)
Parvalbumin	Ca^{2+}-binding proteins	For example, cod (Gad c 1), carp (Cyp c 1), calmon (Sal s 1)
Tropomyosin	Muscle protein	For example, shrimp (Met e 1, Pen a 1, Pen i 1), lobster (Hom a 1), squid (Tod p 1), abalone (Hal m 1), scallop, crab (Cha f 1)
Seed storage proteins	Prolamin superfamily; 2S albumins, prolamins	Brazil nut (Ber e 1), walnut (Jug r 1), sesame (Ses i 1–2), cashew (Ana o 3), mustard (Sin a 1), rapeseed (Bra r 1), castor bean (Ric c 1), peanut (Ara h 2, Ara h 6–7), wheat (Tri a 19), rye (Sec c 20)
Seed storage proteins	Cupin superfamily; vicilins, legumins	Peanut (Ara h 1, Ara h 3, Ara h 4), soy, walnut (Jug r 2, Jug r 4), hazelnut (Cor a 9), vashew (Ana o 1–2), sesame (Ses i 3)
Protease	Proteolysis	Papaya (papain), pineapple (bromelain), fig (ficin), kiwi (Act c 1), soy (Gly m 1)

is needed to provide further information about correlations between structure and allergenic reactivity, and ideally will lead to the development of more specific tools for diagnosis. Table 19.1 shows some common food allergens.

Carbohydrate structures on glycoproteins may be involved in cross-reactivity between foods and pollens (cross-reactive carbohydrate determinants, CCD) [77,86,87]. Some of these carbohydrates have been identified and at least two important epitopes have been described that contain xylose and fucose [87]. An important and widely discussed issue is that IgE antibodies in a blood test may be bound to a univalent structure such as a carbohydrate, whereas biological activity, such as that shown in a skin test, may be negative because of the univalency of the test material [88]. However, this does not prove that clinical reactions will not occur when the individual is exposed to allergenic material containing the carbohydrates in a different multivalent conformation that can induce the biological activation of cells and mediators, triggering clinical reactions. Proteins carrying multivalent carbohydrate epitopes can induce histamine release [89], and these kinds of structures in some foods may be important in the clinical response [90]. Thus, it cannot be concluded that the IgE antibodies directed at carbohydrate structures are without biological and clinical significance [91,92] (Box 19.5).

Box 19.5

Common cross-reactivities

Plant	Animals
Pollen – food	
Bet v 1 homologs	Serum proteins
LTPs	Tropomyosin
Profilin	
Ca^{2+}-binding proteins	
CCD (cross-reactive carbohydrate determinants)	

Performance characteristics of laboratory tests

Standardization of allergen and antigen extract in antibody tests

Extracts of allergen, antigen, or other markers of the inflammatory process used in allergy tests need to be standardized. These markers can be assessed with biochemical methods and/or by demonstrating antibodies in sera from known allergic individuals. Common methods include immunoblotting and inhibition of binding to the solid phase. It is of utmost importance to verify the reproducibility of different allergen batches produced. In particular, because the antibody specificities in different patients are unique to various allergen components [93], the reproducible presence of all components on the solid phase of the assay system must be assured in order to obtain results relevant for a clinical interpretation.

Interactions between antibody and antigen

The immunological methods used to determine the presence and levels of antibodies and antigens in solution and on a solid phase matrix follow simple chemical rules. Many assays today utilize a solid phase for easy separation of reacted and non-reacted reagents. Similar chemical rules regulate the interactions between receptors on cells and their ligands. From the law of mass action applied to a heterogeneous solid phase immunoassay, it can be concluded that when the value of the allergen concentration multiplied by the equilibrium constant exceeds 10, more than 90% of the antibodies are bound and the reaction becomes antibody affinity independent [63]. Therefore, all allergen components in an allergen extract used in the method need to be in large excess to provide such high binding capacity for all antibodies regardless of antibody affinity and antibody class. A few commercial assay systems fulfill these criteria [94], which enable them to quantitatively measure all IgE antibodies present in serum samples without being distorted by background noise or inhibited by simultaneously binding IgG antibodies [95]. For instance, in two of the most extensively studied systems for IgE antibody determination, it was shown that 85–100% of the allergen-specific IgE antibodies present in allergic serum samples were bound to the solid phase surface [96]. Furthermore, using the same two systems, immunoblotting experiments revealed that all IgE antibody specificities present in a serum sample are similarly bound to the allergens on the solid phase, giving a representative quantitative result [96]. It is important to emphasize that such efficient binding of all relevant antibodies indeed is not true for all assay systems in use today [94,97]. In contrast, other systems have been proven to only determine antibodies of high affinity and failing to detect those with low affinity [98]. The consequences of such measurements are still unknown, however, and further studies are warranted before any conclusions can be made.

The test construction may impact this as was clearly demonstrated recently using chimeric antibodies [97]. In particular it has been demonstrated that the relative binding efficiency of the surface of a microwell used in many ELISA systems is too low to be able to pick up all antibodies. The reaction becomes affinity dependent, resulting in dilution curves that are not parallel; a true quantification is therefore impossible and gives results difficult to interpret [99]. Therefore, serum samples must always be diluted to reach optimal concentration conditions in such systems. For instance, IgA and IgG antibodies to gliadin and tTG can be accurately quantified in such systems after 100-fold dilutions. Table 19.2 shows examples of some test principles.

Calibration

Much effort has been focused on assays that can identify allergen-specific IgE antibodies because of their clinical importance in mediating immediate hypersensitivity reactions, including anaphylactic reactions, and their low levels in patients' sera. Since the first test for IgE antibody determination became available, there has been considerable development in the field. The original radio allergosorbent test (RAST), which became available in 1974, included a calibrator consisting of serial dilutions of a serum sample containing IgE antibodies to birch pollen. This was used to construct a calibration curve providing results in arbitrary units (Phadebas RAST unit/ml) and internally calibrated against the World Health Organization (WHO) International Reference Preparation for Human IgE 69/204 [100]. Newer generations of test systems usually replace the allergen-specific IgE antibody reference with a calibrator directly traceable to the WHO International Reference Preparation for Human IgE 75/502, which is one prerequisite for quantitative measurements of IgE antibodies [93]. In addition, specific absorption of antibodies should result in a parallel decrease of the content of total IgE [93,96,101]. The newer test technologies enable IgE detection at $0.1\,kU_A/l$, without jeopardizing the specificity of the test [102]. All test systems do not meet requirements for such sensitivity, however. The clinical relevance of detecting antibodies in such low range remains to be established, however.

For tests measuring IgG and IgA antibodies and other markers, development of calibration has been studied less extensively. However, several systems have applied calibration curves that provide determinations in relative units in a semi-quantitative manner and allow the comparison of results from time to time. Because there are no international reference preparations for allergen-specific IgG or IgA antibodies, the same concept used for specific IgE has also been used in some systems, that is, the use of a calibration curve consisting of total IgG or IgA for which there are WHO reference preparations available. The prerequisite for using this kind of calibration is that dilutions of samples are parallel to the calibrator curve in the system used. This approach can ensure stability and reproducibility over time.

Validation

For IgE antibody determinations, specific recommendations for performing tests have been published by the Clinical and Laboratory Standards Institute (CLSI) [103]. The recommendations include procedures for quality control for daily performance in clinical laboratory setting, and minimal performance targets of 15% coefficient of variation of IgE antibody assays. The College of American Pathologists has similar recommendations for IgG and IgA antibody determinations, as well as for determinations of other markers [101]. According to the guidelines by CLSI, a quantitative assay should meet criteria that include recovery of antibodies, precision, linearity and parallelism of dilution curves,

Table 19.2 Tests for discriminating the presence of allergy and tests for the identification of the offending allergen

Aim of the test to identify	Principle of the test	Basic technology	Major test system	Allergen coupling	Detection system
Presence of atopic condition	Multi-IgE antibody tests; for example, Phadiatop, including allergens from several different sources	Heterogeneous assay using a solid phase for separation of allergen-bound-specific IgE antibodies, labeled anti-IgE reagents	Phadiatop AlaTOP Allergy screen Multiscreen	Cellulose foam Soluble polymer Biotin-labeled allergen in solution Paper disk	Enzyme/fluorescence Enzyme/chemiluminescence Chemiluminescence Enzyme/absorbance
Presence of sensitization to specific allergens	IgE antibody tests to allergens from one source material	As above	ImmunoCAP Immulite 2000 Advia Centaur HY-TEC CLA-MAST	Cellulose foam Soluble polymer Biotin-labeled allergen in solution Paper disk Cellulose threads	Enzyme/fluorescence Enzyme/chemiluminescence Chemiluminescence Enzyme/absorbance Enzyme/luminescence
Presence of sensitization to specific allergen component	IgE antibody tests to one single allergen component	As above	ImmunoCAP ISAC	Cellulose foam Glass slide μ-array	Enzyme/fluorescence Fluroscence
Presence of antibodies to specific antigens	IgA/IgG/IgG4 antibody tests to single antigens	Heterogeneous assay using a solid phase for separation of antigen-bound-specific Ig antibodies, labeled anti-Ig reagents	ELISA tests ImmunoCAP	Polystyrene Cellulose foam	Enzyme/absorbance/ fluorescence Enzyme/fluorescence
Presence of inflammation mediators from different cells	Histamine from basophils and mast cells	Solid phase with catching antibody, labeled anti-mediator reagents	RIA ELISA tests	Microparticles Polystyrene	Radioactivity Enzyme/absorbance/ fluorescence
	Tryptase from mast cells		ImmunoCAP RIA	Cellulose foam Microparticles	Enzyme/fluorescence Radioactivity
	Lipid mediators like leukotrienes and prostaglandins		CAST-ELISA ELISA tests	Polystyrene Polystyrene	Enzyme/absorbance Enzyme/absorbance/ fluorescence
	Eosinophil mediators like ECP, EPX, EPO Neutrophil mediators like MPO, HNL		ImmunoCAP RIA RIA	Cellulose foam Microparticles Microplates	Enzyme/fluorescence Radioactivity Radioactivity
	Lymphocyte mediators like cytokines		ELISA tests	Polystyrene	Enzyme/absorbance/ fluorescence
Cellular immune response	T-cell proliferation	Cell cultivation with specific allergen/antigen stimulation and analysis of cell proliferation			

and calibrators over the measuring range. It states that all assay designs at the present time include a solid phase for separation of bound and unbound IgE antibodies, and all allergen components used must be in excess.

The question of whether different specific IgE antibody blood tests really give interchangeable results has been addressed. Proficiency testing is being undertaken in the United States by the College of American Pathologists, but is not being published and may be difficult to gain access to.

However, results from similar proficiency testing programs in Europe have been published. Those programs assess the performance of several commercial systems for the measurement of IgE antibodies specific to different allergens [104]. The testing indicated that the results from different assay systems are often not equivalent or interchangeable, although it has been demonstrated that some systems possess good performance characteristics [94,97,105]. In contrast, several other systems and assays do not meet

acceptable standards. However, such proficiency testing is more common for inhalant allergens than for food
allergens.

Other tests of IgG and IgA antibodies and inflammation
markers have been much less standardized. This makes
comparisons between results obtained with different tests
and methods more difficult.

Qualitative assessment

The qualitative performance of a particular test is usually
evaluated in a clinical setting with a known population of
individuals with and without disease and presented as the
tests sensitivity and specificity. In such defined population, sensitivity is defined as the proportion of test-positive
patients in relation to the total number of patients with the
disease, whereas specificity is the proportion of test-negative
persons in relation to the total number of individuals without disease. It is also common that the same known population and set-up is used to estimate the tests predictive
value, that is, the proportion of test-positive patients in
relation to the total number of patients positive by the test
(Table 19.3) [106].

There is a considerable documentation for the presence of
IgE antibodies in allergic disease, more than for many other
test systems, and IgE antibody tests may therefore be taken
as an example for the discussion. Thus, for IgE antibody
tests, very good results of sensitivity and specificity have
been documented for a variety of allergens [107]. Even
for the early tests that were developed and marketed, data
showed a good correlation between the levels of specific IgE
antibodies and skin test reactivity or symptom scores [108].

IgE antibody test values of more than 90% for sensitivity, specificity, and predictive values have been obtained
for certain test systems documented with several hundred
patients [109]. However, it is difficult to relate the presence or absence of IgE antibodies exactly to the presence of
clinical disease in an individual patient, especially because
there is no absolute gold standard for IgE-mediated clinical
food-allergic disease. Studies have confirmed the association between the levels of specific IgE antibodies and the
degree of allergen exposure and development of symptoms [25–27,101,108–111]. Furthermore, in adults there
may be clear-cut clinical evidence of food allergy without
any detectable IgE antibodies [112]. In other situations, low
levels of antibodies cannot easily be associated with clinical
disease [23,24]. In CD, the gold standard is biopsy and clinical improvement with gluten-free diet [41].

When interpreting results from a dichotomized evaluation,
it is crucial to carefully examine all conditions that the results
are based on: the population used in the study, the number
of subjects, etc. For all studies involving specific markers such
as antigen-specific IgE, IgG, or IgA antibodies, it is also mandatory to specify the basis for defining a truly positive individual (Box 19.6), that is, to define the "gold standard."

Table 19.3 Concepts in clinical validation of a test

		Test status +	−	
Gold	+	A	B	A + B
standard	−	C	D	C + D
		A + C	B + D	A + B + C + D

True positive: A   False positive: C
True negative: D   False negative: B
Clinical sensitivity: A/(A + B)   Clinical sensitivity: D/(C + D)
Positive predictive value: A/(A + C)   Negative predictive value: D/(B + D)
Prevalence – Prior probability:
  (A + B)/(A + B + C + D)
Efficiency – Concordance:
  (A + D)/(A + B + C + D)

Quantitative assessment

Performance characteristics, like sensitivity and specificity,
are necessary measures to demonstrate that a diagnostic test has the ability to discriminate between individuals
with and without disease in a known population. However,
when a quantitative marker is used, a dichotomization of
the test result is a great over simplification. With the aim
to decrease the number of time-consuming DBPCFCs for
diagnosing patients with food allergy, Sampson [21,22]
described the use of clinical "decision points" in a given food.
He also applied a probability model for the same data, giving
information regarding the decision points, and the important information indicating that even a low concentration
of food-specific IgE antibodies may be associated with a
certain – albeit low – risk of clinical reactivity.

The probability model is based on a logistic regression
model relating the quantitative test result with the clinical outcome. The estimated relationship can be interpreted
as the probability that a patient will react to an allergen as
a function of the level of the specific marker, that is, the
quantitative correspondence to the dichotomous positive
predictive value. A low level will give a low probability for
a patient to react and a high concentration will give a high
probability for a patient to react (Fig. 19.1).

Different shapes of the relationship will indicate different identification patterns of symptoms; a steep curve indicates identification of symptoms even with low levels of the
marker, whereas a flatter curve usually indicates that higher

Box 19.6

Qualitative approach   **Quantitative approach**
Dichotomous
Yes = presence; no = absence   Concentration of markers =
of marker disease   risk of disease

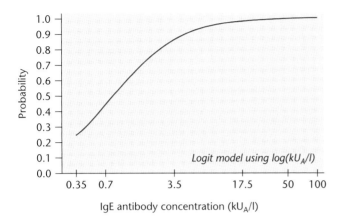

Figure 19.1 Representative logistic relationship between antibody concentration and the probability of reaction or obvious symptoms.

levels of the marker are required to make a diagnosis, or that no clear identification of the disorder can be attained with the test. Similar arguments can be made for IgA and, to a lesser extent, for IgG antibodies to gliadin and tTG and for other markers in which different concentrations result in different likelihoods of disease. The actual shape of these relationships must be studied for each individual marker.

Quantification of the marker and the use of logistic regression models can also be used for prediction of a likelihood that an event will occur. Shek *et al.* [36] used the decrease in specific IgE for hen's egg and cow's milk to predict the probability for a child to develop clinical tolerance. Their model would further improve if the time until clinical tolerance was included in the model, resulting in a higher probability for clinical tolerance if the decrease in specific IgE took place in a rather short time.

Compared with a dichotomous use of the decision points, quantification of the marker and the use probability models give more information about how the levels of antibodies are related to the likelihood of reactivity to food hypersensitivity.

Markers and methods with no confirmed value

Total serum IgE

Measurements of total serum IgE are used to give a very rough indication of whether there are any prerequisites of IgE-mediated disease in a patient. Given the considerable overlap between IgE levels in allergic patients and normal controls, and those with other disorders that may increase serum IgE (e.g. parasite infections), total serum IgE does not add considerable insight into the diagnosis of food allergy.

IgG/IgA antibodies in atopic allergy

There is no firm evidence that tests of IgG and IgG4 antibodies give any indication of the causes of clinical symptoms

in cases of immediate IgE-mediated reactions. Thus, IgG and IgA antibodies to foods are commonly found in both food-allergic patients and healthy persons. Such antibodies appear to be secondary to exposure to the food antigens/allergens and have not been shown to have any clinical value in the diagnosis of food allergy [113–117]. As an example, patients with CD often have high levels of IgG antibodies to cow's milk proteins. During the acute phase of the disease, they may have high levels of milk-specific IgG, and when the patient is in remission (after implementation of a gluten-free diet), levels decline [5,7]. However, recently there have been reports suggesting that IgG4 antibodies can have some association to delayed, non-IgE-mediated cow's milk allergy and in cow's milk-sensitive allergic eosinophilic gastroenteritis in children and young adults [118,119]. These studies were performed in patient groups rather than on an individual level and neither sensitivity and specificity nor probability for disease was given. Hence, it is too early to give any recommendation regarding such determination in the diagnosis of food allergy and more studies are warranted.

Histamine and basophil histamine test

Histamine released into the tissue and blood is gradually inactivated to methyl histamine. The relative amount of histamine and its metabolites over time following a clinical reaction is difficult to establish. Methyl histamine, which cross-reacts with histamine to some extent, can be determined by radioimmunoassay, although the half-life of both species is in minutes [120]. In the urine, histamine is not present, and methyl histamine or some other metabolite must be determined.

The basophil histamine test determines the release of histamine from peripheral blood basophils induced by cross-linking IgE antibodies bound to their specific cell receptors [121]. Also, complement activation and direct activation in some cases of idiosyncratic reactions to aspirin can release histamine. Given the difficulty of establishing optimum doses of allergens for release of histamine, and the difficulty of obtaining fresh blood cells, the test has been limited to academic and research settings. Development of whole blood semi-automated systems may, to some degree, circumvent the problem with high "spontaneous" basophil histamine release seen in food-allergic individuals who frequently ingest small amounts of the offending allergenic food [122]. A good correlation of this test method has been demonstrated compared to IgE antibody determinations in serum and to food challenges, although the results were never more predictive than IgE antibody determinations in blood or than SPTs [123]. When patients were compliant with diets excluding their offending allergenic food for several months, "spontaneous histamine release" decreases considerably [124]. In cases of *in vitro* challenges of peripheral blood cells with allergen, the results have been less conclusive. Furthermore, about 10% of the population have non-responsive basophils that fail to release their histamine following allergen challenge *in vitro* [125]. The utility as well as the pitfalls of this test was recently reviewed [126]. Regardless of the difficulty in standardizing this test, the use of basophil histamine release may be warranted in particular situations using very well-controlled allergen components, for instance when anaphylaxis is suspected [126,127].

Tryptase, eosinophil cationic protein, and eosinophil protein X

Tryptase is found almost exclusively in mast cells. It has a much longer half-life in peripheral blood than histamine or histamine metabolites [128]. Unfortunately, in food-allergic reactions, the only situation in which tryptase determinations have been useful has been in some forms of anaphylactic reactions, where elevated levels have been documented in a minority of patients in both research and clinical practice settings [128,129]. However, the majority of fatal food-induced anaphylactic reactions where the tryptase level was measured in the peripheral blood demonstrated no elevation of plasma tryptase [130].

Eosinophil markers such as ECP and EPX in peripheral blood have also been used as research tools following food challenges in allergic individuals. Increased levels of these markers have been reported after positive challenges, sometimes in connection with decreased numbers of total eosinophils [131]. Recently, some investigators have been evaluating levels of EPX in the feces of patients undergoing challenges with suspected foods. It is still too early to determine the clinical usefulness of this procedure [132].

Granular constituents from eosinophils (ECP, EPX, EPO, MBP), neutrophils (MPO, HNL, lactoferrin), monocytes (lysozyme), and mast cells (tryptase) need to be isolated or cloned from human cells, because there is limited cross-reactivity between species [133].

Leukotrienes

Leukotrienes and, to some extent, prostaglandins have been used to monitor inflammation in allergic situations, mostly in patients with rhinitis, asthma, and drug allergy. Both LTE4 and the PGD2 metabolite 9α,11β-PGF2 can be determined in the urine, although there is rather limited information on this in relation to food-allergic reactions [134]. A specific test, CAST-ELISA, has been developed to measure the leukotrienes LTC4, LTD4, and LTE4 released from peripheral blood cells [9–11,135]. Even if results have been reported from applications in food allergy, all these methods need further documentation of clinical correlations before they become widely applied in routine clinical evaluation. In particular, when allergens are applied to peripheral blood cells, care must be taken to avoid endotoxin contamination, which may give false-positive results [135].

Box 19.7

Clinically confirmed markers	*Clinically non-confirmed markers*
IgE antibodies in atopy	Total IgE
	IgG/IgA antibodies in atopy
IgG/IgA antibodies in CD	Histamine/basophil histamine test
	Tryptase, ECP, EPX
	Leukotrienes
	Cytokines

Cytokines

Serum cytokines have not yet proven useful in the clinical setting. This may be due to complexities related to the time they are obtained in relationship to the reactions and the different cells being activated [112]. Some studies have reported an imbalance of interleukin-4 (IL-4) and interferon-γ (IFN-γ) in children [136] and adults [137] suffering from allergic disorders. In infants with atopic dermatitis and cow's milk allergy, lymphocytes stimulated with allergen secreted high levels of IL-4, IL-5, and IL-13, in contrast to those tolerating milk who produced high levels of IFN-γ and very low levels of IL-4, IL-5, and IL-13 [138]. Other investigatators have demonstrated that it may be of importance also to determine what cell population is producing the cytokines in the different conditions [139]. However, much more information is needed before such assays can be used in routine clinical evaluations. Table 19.2 shows various antibody and inflammation marker tests.

Tests to determine the T-cell response to gliadin in celiac patients expressing the genetic heterodimers of HLA-DQ2 or HLA-DQ8 may also be developed in the future [51] (Box 19.7).

References

1 Johansson SG, Hourihane JO, Bousquet J, *et al*. EAACI (the European Academy of Allergology and Clinical Immunology) nomenclature task force. A revised nomenclature for allergy. An EAACI position statement from the EAACI nomenclature task force. *Allergy* 2001;56:813–24.

2 Bruijnzeel-Koomen C, Ortolani C, Aas K, *et al*. Adverse reactions to food. European Academy of Allergology and Clinical Immunology Subcommittee. *Allergy* 1995;50:623–35.

3 Bock SA, Sampson HA, Atkins FM, *et al*. Double-blind, placebo-controlled food challenge (DBPCFC) as an office procedure: a manual. *J Allergy Clin Immunol* 1988;82:986–97.

4 Wahn U, Von Mutius E. Childhood risk factors for atopy and the importance of early intervention. *J Allergy Clin Immunol* 2001;107:567–74.

5 Husby S, Jensenius JC, Svehag SE. Passage of undegraded dietary antigen in the blood of healthy adults. Quantification, estimation of size distribution, and relation to uptake to levels of specific antibodies. *Scand J Immunol* 1985;22:83–92.

6 Udall J, Pang K, Fritze L, *et al*. Development of gastrointestinal mucosal barrier. I. The effect of age on intestinal permeability to macromolecules. *Pediatr Res* 1981;15:241–4.

7 Heyman M, Grasset E, Ducroc R, Desjeux JF. Antigen absorption by the jejunal epithelium of children with cow's milk allergy. *Pediatr Res* 1988;24:197–202.

8 Fasano A, Catassi C. Current approaches to diagnosis and treatment of CD: an evolving spectrum. *Gastroenterology* 2001; 120:636–51.

9 Moneret-Vautrin DA, Sainte-Laudy J, Kanny G, Fremont S. Human basophil activation measured by CD63 expression and LTC4 release in IgE-mediated food allergy. *Ann Allergy Asthma Immunol* 1999;82:33–40.

10 Gietkiewicz K, Wrzyszcz M. Comparative study between skin prick tests and TOP-CAST allergen leukocyte stimulation in diagnosis of allergic status. *J Invest Allergol Clin Immunol* 1997; 7:115–18.

11 Ahlstedt S. Mediators in allergy diagnosis. *ACI International* 1998;10:37–44.

12 Jarisch R, Wantke F. Wine and headache. *Int Arch Allergy Immunol* 1996;110:7–12.

13 Arslan G, Gilja OH, Lind R, *et al*. Response to intestinal provocation monitored by transabdominal ultrasound in patients with food hypersensitivity. *Scand J Gastroenterol* 2005;40:386–94.

14 Arslan G, Lillestol K, Mulahasanovic A, *et al*. Food hypersensitivity reactions visualised by ultrasonography and magnetic resonance imaging in a patient lacking systemic food-specific IgE. *Digestion* 2006;73:111–15.

15 Sampson HA, McCaskin CC. Food hypersensitivity and atopic dermatitis: evaluation of 113 patients. *J Pediatr* 1985;107:669–75.

16 Burks AW, James JM, Hiegel A, *et al*. Atopic dermatitis and food hypersensitivity reactions. *J Pediatr* 1998;132:132–6.

17 Bock SA, Atkins FM. Patterns of food hypersensitivity during sixteen years of double-blind, placebo-controlled food challenges. *J Pediatr* 1990;117:561–7.

18 Sicherer SH, Sampson HA. Food hypersensitivity and atopic dermatitis: pathophysiology, epidemiology, diagnosis, and management. *J Allergy Clin Immunol* 1999;104:S114–22.

19 Ring J, Brockow K, Behrendt H. Adverse reactions to foods. *J Chromatogr B Biomed Sci Appl* 2001;756:3–10.

20 Yman L. Standardization of *in vitro* methods. *Allergy* 2001;56:70–4.

21 Sampson HA, Albergo R. Comparison of results of skin tests, RAST, and double-blind, placebo-controlled food challenges in children with atopic dermatitis. *J Allergy Clin Immunol* 1984; 74:26–33.

22 Bock SA, Buckley J, Holst A, May CD. Proper use of skin tests with food extracts in diagnosis of hypersensitivity to food in children. *Clin Allergy* 1977;7:375–83.

23 Sampson HA, Ho DG. Relationship between food-specific IgE concentrations and the risk of positive food challenges in children and adolescents. *J Allergy Clin Immunol* 1997;100:444–51.

24 Sampson HA. Utility of food-specific IgE concentrations in predicting symtomatic food allergy. *J Allergy Clin Immunol* 2001;107:891–6.

25 Garcia-Ara C, Boyano-Martinez T, Diaz-Pena JM, *et al*. Specific IgE levels in the diagnosis of immediate hypersensitivity to cows' milk protein in the infant. *J Allergy Clin Immunol* 2001;107:185–90.

26 Boyano-Martinez T, Garcia-Ara C, Diaz-Pena JM, *et al*. Validity of specific IgE antibodies in children with egg allergy. *Clin Exp Allergy* 2001;31:1464–9.

27 Crespo JF, Pascual C, Ferrer A, *et al*. Egg white-specific IgE level as a tolerance marker in the follow up of egg allergy. *Allergy Proc* 1994;15:73–6.

28 Soderstrom L, Kober A, Ahlstedt S, *et al*. A new approach to the evaluation and clinical use of specific IgE antibody testing in allergic diseases. *Allergy* 2003;58:921–8.

29 Celik-Bilgili S, Mehl A, Verstege A, *et al*. The predictive value of specific immunoglobulin E levels in serum for the outcome of oral food challenges. *Clin Exp Allergy* 2005;35:268–73.

30 Clark AT, Ewan PW. Interpretation of tests for nut allergy in one thousand patients, in relation to allergy or tolerance. *Clin Exp Allergy* 2003;33:1041–5.

31 Fleischer DM, Conover-Walker MK, Matsui EC, Wood RA. The natural history of tree nut allergy. *J Allergy Clin Immunol* 2005;116:1087–93.

32 Roberts G, Lack G. Avon longitudinal study of parents and children study team. Diagnosing peanut allergy with skin prick and specific IgE testing. *J Allergy Clin Immunol* 2005;115:1291–6.

33 Osterballe M, Binslev-Jensen C. Threshold levels in food challenge and specific IgE in patients with egg allergy: is there a relationship? *J Allergy Clin Immunol* 2003;112:196–201.

34 Beyer K, Ellman-Grunther L, Jarvinen KM, *et al*. Measurement of peptide-specific IgE as an additional tool in identifying patients with clinical reactivity to peanuts. *J Allergy Clin Immunol* 2003;112:202–7.

35 Sicherer SH, Sampson HA. Cow's milk protein-specific IgE concentrations in two age groups of milk-allergic children and in children achieving clinical tolerance. *Clin Exp Allergy* 1999;29:507–12.

36 Shek LP, Soderstrom L, Ahlstedt S, *et al*. Determination of food specific IgE levels over time can predict the development of tolerance in cow's milk and hen's egg allergy. *J Allergy Clin Immunol* 2004;114:387–91.

37 Boyano-Martinez T, Garcia-Ara C, Diaz-Pena JM, Martin-Esteban M. Prediction of tolerance on the basis of quantification of egg white-specific IgE antibodies in children with egg allergy. *J Allergy Clin Immunol* 2002;110:304–9.

38 Shreffler WG, Beyer K, Chu TH, *et al*. Microarray immunoassay: association of clinical history, *in vitro* IgE function, and heterogeneity of allergenic peanut epitopes. *J Allergy Clin Immunol* 2004;113:776–82.

39 Shreffler WG, Lencer DA, Bardina L, Sampson HA. IgE and IgG4 epitope mapping by microarray immunoassay reveals the diversity of immune response to the peanut allergen, Ara h 2. *J Allergy Clin Immunol* 2005;116:893–9.

40 Meeuwisse GW. Diagnostic criteria in celiac disease. *Acta Paediatr Scand* 1970;59:461–3.

41 Walker-Smith JA, Guandalini S, Scgmitz J, *et al*. Revised criteria for diagnosis of coeliac disease. Report of Working Group of

European Society of Paediatric Gastroenterology and Nutrition. *Arch Dis Child* 1990;65:909–11.

42 Dieterich W, Ehnis T, Bauer M, *et al.* Identification of tissue transglutaminase as the autoantigen of celiac disease. *Nat Med* 1997;3:797–801.

43 Hansson T, Dahlbom I, Rogberg S, *et al.* Recombinant human tissue transglutaminase for diagnosis and follow-up of childhood disease. *Pediatr Res* 2002;51:700–5.

44 Wolters V, Vooijs-Moulaert A-F, Burger H, *et al.* Human tissue transglutaminase enzyme linked immunosorbent assay outperforms both the guinea pig based tissue transglutaminase assay and anti-endomysium antibodies when screening for coeliac disease. *Eur J Pediatr* 2002;161:284–7.

45 Hill PG, Forsyth JM, Semeraro D, Holmes GKT. IgA antibodies to human tissue transglutaminase: audit of routine practice confirms high diagnostic accuracy. *Scand J Gastroenterol* 2004;39:1078–82.

46 Collin P, Kaukinen K, Vogelsang H, *et al.* Antiendomysial and antihuman recombinant tissue transglutaminase antibodies in the diagnosis of coeliac disease: a biopsy-proven European multicentre study. *Eur J Gastroenterol Hepatol* 2005;17:85–91.

47 Cataldo F, Lio D, Marino V, *et al.* IgG(l) antiendomysium and IgG antitissue transglutaminase (anti-tTG) antibodies in coeliac patients with selective IgA deficiency. Working Groups on Celiac Disease of SIGEP and Club del Tenue. *Gut* 2000;47:366–9.

48 Korponay-Szabó IR, Dahlbom I, Laurila K, *et al.* Elevation of IgG antibodies against tissue transglutaminase as a diagnostic tool for coeliac disease in selective IgA deficiency. *Gut* 2003;52:1567–71.

49 Mäki M, Mustalahti K, Kokkonen J, *et al.* Prevalence of celiac disease among children in Finland. *N Engl J Med* 2003; 348:2517–24.

50 Sollid LM. Coeliac disease: dissecting a complex inflammatory disorder. *Nat Rev* 2002;2:647–54.

51 Sollid L, Lie BA. Celiac disease genetics: current concepts and practical applications. *Clin Gastroenterol Hepatol* 2005;3:843–51.

52 Vieths S, Hoffman A, Holzhauser T, *et al.* Factors influencing the quality of food extracts for *in vitro* and *in vivo* diagnosis. *Allergy* 1998;53:65–71.

53 Vieths S, Scheurer S, Reindl J, *et al.* Optimized allergen extracts and recombinant allergens in diagnostic applications. *Allergy* 2001;56:78–82.

54 Becker WM, Reese G. Immunological identification and characterization of individual food allergens. *J Chromatogr B Biomed Sci Appl* 2001;756:131–40.

55 Maleki SJ, Chung SY, Champagne ET, Raufman JP. The effects of roasting on the allergenic properties of peanut proteins. *J Allergy Clin Immunol* 2000;106:763–8.

56 Fiocchi A, Bouygue GR, Sarratud T, *et al.* Clinical tolerance of processed foods. *Ann Allergy Asthma Immunol* 2004;93:S38–46.

57 Ballmer-Weber BK, Hoffmann A, Wuthrich B, *et al.* Influence of food processing on the allergenicity of celery: DBPCFC with celery spice and cooked celery in patients with celery allergy. *Allergy* 2002;57:228–35.

58 Cooke SK, Sampson HA. Allergenic properties of ovomucoid in man. *J Immunol* 1997;159:2026–32.

59 Ehn BM, Ekstrand B, Bengtsson U, Ahlstedt S. Modification of IgE binding during heat processing of the cow's milk allergen beta-lactoglobulin. *J Agric Food Chem* 2004;52:1398–403.

60 Wal JM. Thermal processing and allergenicity of foods. *Allergy* 2003;58:727–9.

61 Scheurer S, Pastorello EA, Wangorsch A, *et al.* Recombinant allergens Pm av 1 and Pm av 4 and a newly identified lipid transfer protein in the *in vitro* diagnosis of cherry allergy. *J Allergy Clin Immunol* 2001;107:724–31.

62 Fernandez-Rivas M, van Ree R, Cuevas M. Allergy to Rosaceae fruits without related pollinosis. *J Allergy Clin lmmunol* 1997; 100:728–33.

63 Fernandez-Rivas M, Bolhaar S, Gonzalez-Mancebo E, *et al.* Apple allergy across Europe: how allergen sensitization profiles determine the clinical expression of allergies to plant foods. *J Allergy Clin Immunol* 2006;118:481–8.

64 Shek LPC, Lee BW. Food allergy in Asia. *Curr Opin Allergy Clin Immunol* 2006;6:197–201.

65 Lorenz AR, Schemer S, Haustein D, Vieths S. Recombinant food allergens. *J Chromatogr B Biomed Sci Appl* 2001;756:255–79.

66 Lidholm J, Barbara K, Ballmer-Weberb, *et al.* Component-resolved diagnostics in food allergy. *Curr Opin Allergy Clin Immunol* 2006;6:234–40.

67 Asero R. Plant food allergies: a suggested approach to allergen-resolved diagnosis in the clinical practice by identifying easily available sensitization markers. *Int Arch Allergy Immunol* 2005;138:1–11.

68 Hourihane JO, Roberts SA, Warner JO. Resolution of peanut allergy: case-control study. *BMJ* 1998;316:1271–5.

69 Vila L, Beyer K, Jarvinen KM, *et al.* Role of conformational and linear epitopes in the achievement of tolerance in cow's milk allergy. *Clin Exp Allergy* 2001;31:1599–606.

70 Harwanegg C, Hiller R. Protein microarrays for the diagnosis of allergic diseases: state-of-the-art and future development. *Clin Chem Lab Med* 2005;43:1321–6.

71 Templin MF, Stoll D, Bachmann J, *et al.* Protein microarrays and multiplexed sandwich immunoassays: what beats the beads? *Comb Chem High Throughput Screen* 2004;7:223–9.

72 Kasarda DD. Gluten and gliadin: precipitating factors in celiac disease. In: Mäki M, Collin P, Visakorpi J (eds.) *Proceedings of the 7th International Symposium on Coeliac Disease,* 1996:195–212.

73 Ribes-Koninckx C, Alfonso P, Ortigosa L, *et al.* Beta-turn rich oats peptide as an antigen in an ELISA method for the screening of coeliac disease in a paediatric population. *Eur J Clin Invest* 2000;30:702–8.

74 Hansson T, Dahlbom I, Hall J, *et al.* Antibody reactivity against human and guinea pig tissue transglutaminase in children with celiac disease. *J Pediatr Gastroenterol Nutr* 2000;30:379–84.

75 Aalberse RC. Structural biology of allergens. *J Allergy Clin Immunol* 2000;106:228–38.

76 Sicherer SH. Clinical implications of cross-reactive food allergens. *J Allergy Clin Immunol* 2001;108:881–90.

77 Aalberse RC, Akkerdaas J, van Ree R. Cross-reactivity of IgE antibodies to allergens. *Allergy* 2001;56:478–90.

78 Breiteneder H, Ebner C. Molecular and biochemical classification of plant-derived food allergens. *J Allergy Clin Immunol* 2000;106:27–36.

79 Caballero T, Martin-Esteban M. Association between pollen hypersensitivity and edible vegetable allergy: a review. *J Invest Allergol Clin Immunol* 1998;8:6–16.

80 Ebner C, Hofflnann-Sommergruber K, Breiterleder H. Plant food allergens homologous to pathogenes-related proteins. *Allergy* 2001;56:43–4.

81 Hoffmann-Sommergruber K. The SAFE project: "plant food allergies: field to table strategies for reducing their incidence in Europe" an EC-funded study. *Allergy* 2005;60:436–42.

82 Schemer S, Wangorsch A, Nerkamp J, *et al.* Cross-reactivity within the profilin panallergen family investigated by comparison of recombinant profilins from pear (Pyr c 4), cherry (Fru av 4) and celery (Api g 4) with birch pollen profilin Bet v 2. *J Chromatogr B Biomed Sci Appl* 2001;756:315–25.

83 Pastorello EA, Pompei C, Pravettoni V, *et al.* Lipid transfer proteins and 2S albumins as allergens. *Allergy* 2001;56:45–7.

84 Asero R, Mistrello G, Roncarolo D, *et al.* Lipid transfer protein: a pan-allergen in plant-derived foods that is highly resistant to pepsin digestion. *Int Arch Allergy Immunol* 2000;122:20–32.

85 Scheurer S, Lauer I, Foetisch K, *et al.* Strong allergenicity of Pru av 3, the lipid transfer protein from cherry, is related to high stability against thermal processing and digestion. *J Allergy Clin Immunol* 2004;114:900–7.

86 Aalberse RC, van Ree R. Crossreactive carbohydrate determinants. *Clin Rev Allergy Immunol* 1997;15:375–87.

87 Wilson IB, Zeleny R, Kolarich D, *et al.* Analysis of Asn-linked glycans from vegetable foodstuffs: widespread occurrence of Lewis a, core alpha 1,3-linked fucose and xylose substitutions. *Glycobiology* 2001;11:261–74.

88 Mari A, Iacovacci P, Afferni C, *et al.* Specific IgE to cross-reactive carbohydrate determinants strongly affect the *in vitro* diagnosis of allergic diseases. *J Allergy Clin Immunol* 1999;103:1005–11.

89 Fotisch K, Altmann F, Haustein D, Vieths S. Involvement of carbohydrate epitopes in the IgE response of celery-allergic patients. *Int Arch Allergy lmmunol* 1999;120:30–42.

90 Lüttkopf D, Ballmer-Weber BK, Wütrich B, Vieths S. Celery allergens in patients with positive double-blind placebo controlled food challenge. *J Allergy Clin Immunol* 2000;106:390–9.

91 Fötisch KS, Westphal I, Lauer M, *et al.* Biological activity of IgE specific for cross-reactive carbohydrate determinants. *J Allergy Clin Immunol* 2003;111:889–96.

92 Wicklein DB, Lindner H, Moll D, *et al.* Carbohydrate moieties can induce mediator release: a detailed characterization of two major timothy grass pollen allergens. *Biol Chem* 2004; 385:397–407.

93 Yman L. Allergy. In: Wild D, editor. *The Immunoassay Handbook.* 2:nd col. London: Nature publishing Group; 2001. P. 664-80.

94 Williams PB, Barnes JH, Szeinbach SL, *et al.* Analytic precision and accuracy of commercial immunoassays for specific

IgE: establishing a standard. *J Allergy Clin Immunol* 2000; 105:1221–30.

95 Costongs GMPJ, Janson PCW, Hermans WTJA, *et al.* Evaluation of performance characteristics of automated measurement systems for allergy testing. *Eur J Clin Chem Clin Biochem* 1995;33:295–305.

96 Lindquist A, Maaninen E. Zimmerman, K, *et al.* Quantitative measurement of allergen-specific IgE antibodies applied in a new assay system, UniCAP™. In: Basomba A, Hernandez FdR (eds.) *XVI European Congress of Allergology and Clinical Immunology ECACI '95.* Bologna, Italy: Monduzzi Editore, 1995:195–200.

97 Wood RA, Segall N, Ahlstedt S, Williams PB. Not all IgE antibody laboratory results provide accurate information for clinical judgement. *Ann Allergy Asthma Immunol,* 2007; 99:34-41.

98 Fromberg P. IgE as a marker in allergy and the role of IgE affinity. *Allergy* 2006;61:1234.

99 Lehtonen O-P, Eerola E. The effect of different antibody affinities on ELISA absorbance and titer. *J Immunol Meth* 1982;54:233–40.

100 Lundquist U. Research and development of the RAST technology. In: Evans R (ed.) *Advances in Diagnosis of Allergy: RAST.* Miami, FL: Symposia Specialists, 1975:85–99.

101 Yunginger JW, Ahlstedt S, Eggleston PA, *et al.* Quantitative IgE antibody assays in allergic diseases. *J Allergy Clin Immunol* 2000;105:1077–84.

102 Forkman J, Söderström L, Kober A. A new method for quantitative measurments of low levels of allergen specific IgE antobodies: ImmunoCAP Specific IgE 0-100. *Allergy Clin Immunol Int J World Allergy Org* 2005:193.

103 *Review Criteria for the Assessment of Allergen-Specific Immunoglobulin E (IgE) In Vitro Diagnostic Devices Using Immunological Methods.* Washington, DC: Public Health Service, Division of Clinical Laboratory Devices, Office of Device Evaluation, 2000:1–18.

104 Gausset P. Tests biologiques en allergologie: le controle de qualite national de l'agence du medicament consequences practiques. *Rev Int Ped* 1997;28:33–6.

105 Szeinbach SL, Barnes JH, Sullivan TJ, *et al.* Precision and accuracy of commercial laboratories' ability to classify positive and/ or negative allergen-specific IgE results. *Ann Allergy Asthma Immunol* 2001;86:373–81.

106 Rossner B. *Fundamentals of Biostatistics.* Boston, MA: PWS-Kent Publishing Company, 1990.

107 Yman L. Die neue Generation der Allergie-Testung: Pharmiacia CAP System *in-vitro* Diagnostica Special. *Das wissenschaftliche Magazin zum Thema* 1990;1:18–22.

108 Williams PB, Dolen WK, Koepke JW, *et al.* Comparison of skin prick testing and three *in vitro* assays for specific IgE in the clinical evaluation of immediate hypersensitivity. *Ann Allergy* 1992;68:35–45.

109 Paganelli R, Quinti I, D'Offizi GP, *et al.* Studies on the *in vitro* effects of auto-anti-IgE. Inhibition of total and specific serum IgE detection by a human IgG autoantibody to IgE. *J Clin Lab Immunol* 1988;26:153–7.

110 Wood RA, Phipatanakul W, Hamilton RG, Eggleston PA. A comparison of skin prick tests, intradermal skin tests, and

RASTs in the diagnosis of cat allergy. *J Allergy Clin Immunol* 1999;103:773–9.

111 Pastorello EA, Incorvaia C, Ortolani C, *et al.* Studies on the relationship between the level of specific IgE antibodies and the clinical expression of allergy. I. Definition of levels distinguishing patients with symptomatic from patients with asymptomatic allergy to common aeroallergens. *J Allergy Clin Immunol* 1995;96:580–7.

112 Lin XP, Magnusson J, Ahlstedt S, *et al.* Local allergic reaction in food hypersensitive adults despite lack of systemic food-specific IgE. *J Allergy Clin Immunol* 2002;109:879–87.

113 Host A. Cow's milk protein allergy and intolerance in infancy. Some clinical, epidemiological and immunological aspects. *Pediatr Allergy Immunol* 1994;5:1–36.

114 Lilja G, Magnusson CG, Oman H, Johansson SG. Serum levels of IgG subclasses in relation to IgE and atopic disease in early infancy. *Clin Exp Allergy* 1990;20:407–13.

115 Morgan JE, Daul CB, Lehrer SB. The relationships among shrimp-specific IgG subclass antibodies and immediate adverse reactions to shrimp challenge. *J Allergy Clin Immunol* 1990;86:387–92.

116 Tainio VM, Savilahti E. Value of immunologic tests in cow milk allergy. *Allergy* 1990;45:189–96.

117 Barnes RM. IgG and IgA antibodies to dietary antigens in food allergy and intolerance. *Clin Exp Allergy* 1995;25:7–9.

118 Sletten GB, Halvorsen R, Egaas E, Halstensen TS. Changes in humoral responses to beta-lactoglobulin in tolerant patients suggest a particular role for IgG(4) in delayed, non-IgE-mediated cow's milk allergy. *Pediatr Allergy Immunol* 2006;17:435–43.

119 Shek LP, Bardina L, Castro R, *et al.* Humoral and cellular responses to cow milk proteins in patients with milk-induced IgE-mediated and non-IgE-mediated disorders. *Allergy* 2005;60:912–19.

120 Yamauchi K, Sekizawa K, Suzuki H, *et al.* Structure and function of human *N*-methyltransferase: critical enzyme in histamine metabolism in airway. *Am J Physiol* 1994;267:L342–9.

121 James IM, Burks Jr AW. Food allergy: current diagnostic methods and interpretation of results. *Clin Allergy Immunol* 2000;15:199–215.

122 May CD, Remigio L. Observations of high spontaneous release of histamine from leukocytes *in vitro. Clin Allergy* 1982;12:229–41.

123 Nolte H, Schiotz PO, Kruse A, Skov S. Comparison of intestinal mast cell and basophil histamine release in children with food allergic reactions. *Allergy* 1989;44:554–65.

124 Sampson HA, Broadbent KR, Bernhisel-Broadbent J. Spontaneous release of histamine from basophils and histamine-releasing factor in patients with atopic dermatitis and food, hypersensitivity. *N Engl J Med* 1989;321:228–32.

125 Bindslev-Jensen C, Poulsen LK. *In vitro* diagnostic methods in the evaluation of food hypersensitivity. In: Metcalfe W, Sampson HA, Simon RA (eds.) *Food Allergy: Adverse Reactions to Foods and Food Additives*, 2nd edn. Boston, MA: Blackwell Science, 1997:137–50.

126 Kleine-Tebbe J, Erdmann S, Knol EF, *et al.* Diagnostic tests based on human basophils: potentials, pitfalls and perspectives. *Int Arch Allergy Immunol* 2006;141:79–90.

127 Shreffler WG. Evaluation of basophil activation in food allergy: present and future applications. *Curr Opin Allergy Clin Immunol* 2006;6:226–33.

128 Kanthawatana S, Carias K, Anaout R, *et al.* The potential clinical utility of serum alfa-protryptase levels. *J Allergy Clin Immunol* 1999;103:1092–9.

129 Beyer K, Niggemann B, Schultze S, Wahn U. Serum tryptase and urinary 1-methylhistamine as parameters for monitoring oral food challenges in children. *Int Arch Allergy Immunol* 1994;104:348–51.

130 Yuninger JW, Nelson DR, Squillace DL, *et al.* Laboratory investigation of deaths due to anaphylaxis. *J Forensic Sci* 1991;36:857–65.

131 Niggemann B, Beyer K, Wahn U. The role of eosinophils and eosinophil cationic protein in monitoring oral challenge tests in children food-sensitive atopic dermatitis. *J Allergy Clin Immunol* 1994;94:963–71.

132 Magnusson J, Gellerstedt M, Ahlstedt S, *et al.* A kinetic study in adults with food hypersensitivity assessed as eosinophil activation in faecal samples. *Clin Exp Allergy* 2003;33:1052–9.

133 Venge P, Bergstrand H, Håkansson L. Neutrophils and eosinophils. In: Kelly WN, Harris ED, Ruddy S, Sledge CB (eds.) *Textbook of Rheumatology*, 4th edn. Philadelphia, PA: WB Saunders Company, 1993:269–78.

134 Kumlin M. Measurement of leukotrienes in humans. *Am J Respir Crit Care Med* 2000;161:S102–6.

135 Van Rooyen C, Anderson R. Assessment of determinants of optimum performance of the CAST-2000 ELISA procedure. *J Immunol Methods* 2004;288:1–7.

136 Hauer AC, Breese EJ, Walker-Smith JA, MacDonald TT. The frequency of cells secreting interferon-gamma and interleukin-4, -5, and -10 in the blood and duodenal mucosa of children with cow's milk hypersensitivity. *Pediatr Res* 1997;42:629–38.

137 Andre F, Pene J, Andre C. Interleukin-4 and interferon-gamma production by peripheral blood mononuclear cells from food-allergic patients. *Allergy* 1996;51:350–5.

138 Schade RP, Van Ieperen-Van Dijk AG, Van Reijsen FC, *et al.* Differences in antigen-specific T-cell responses between infants with atopic dermatitis with and without cow's milk allergy: relevance of TH2 cytokines. *J Allergy Clin Immunol* 2000;106:1155–62.

139 Scott-Taylor TH, Hourihane JB, Harper J, Strobel S. Patterns of food allergen-specific cytokine production by T lymphocytes of children with multiple allergies. *Clin Exp Allergy* 2005;35:1473–80.

CHAPTER 20

In Vivo Diagnosis: Skin Testing and Challenge Procedures

Scott H. Sicherer

KEY CONCEPTS

- The medical history is the cornerstone for establishing an accurate diagnosis of food allergy.

- Prick skin tests determine sensitization (presence of food-specific IgE) and provide significant diagnostic value when considered in the context of the medical history.

- Increasingly larger skin test wheals are associated with increasing risks for clinical reactions.

- Response to elimination diets may provide presumptive evidence of food-related disease.

- The oral food challenge, in particular when double-blind and placebo-controlled, is the most definitive modality available to diagnose a food-related illness.

Introduction

This chapter focuses on food allergen skin tests, obtaining an informative medical history, and decision making in regard to undertaking physician-supervised oral food challenges (OFCs). These *in vivo* modalities provide immediate diagnostic information that is crucial in the evaluation of an individual with suspected food allergy. The OFC is the tool at the physician's disposal that can most definitively diagnose an adverse reaction to food. The results of an OFC are informative and do not depend on the specific etiology or immunopathology of an adverse reaction to a food, whether the problem is due to intolerance, a pharmacologic response, an allergic (immunologic) reaction, or a psychological one. While potentially definitive, OFCs carry risks because severe reactions may be induced. The clinician, therefore, must also rely upon patient histories and a number of additional tests to help determine the likelihood of a true allergy or adverse reaction to food prior to, and sometimes in place of, undertaking an OFC. For allergic reactions that are mediated by IgE antibody, the tests most familiar to the allergist are the prick skin test (PST), a focus of this chapter, and the determination of serum food-specific IgE antibodies (Chapters 19 and 21), and possibly patch tests (Chapter 22). Numerous additional tests

may be needed in various clinical scenarios (e.g. stool culture, endoscopy with biopsy, pH probe, breath hydrogen) to assist in determining if an adverse reaction to food is the cause of a clinical problem. In addition, refinements on currently available tests, clinical evaluations of proposed tests (e.g. patch tests with food), and additional novel tests are under investigation to improve and expand the diagnostic armamentarium. Despite the potential for inaccurate histories and various limitations of *in vitro* and *in vivo* tests, the OFC can provide a final diagnostic answer. Oral challenges designed to be double-blind and placebo-controlled so as to reduce subject and observer bias are considered the "gold standard" for the diagnosis of food hypersensitivity.

Historical background

The typical diet includes several meals and snacks distributed throughout the day. Since the frequency of food intake is high, any sudden adverse physiologic event or chronic illness could incorrectly be ascribed to food. Once a patient makes an erroneous association between a food and a symptom, it may be difficult to dissuade the patient from their notion of cause and effect. In a paper published in 1950, Graham and colleagues [1] performed experiments that would be difficult to undertake today for ethical reasons. Subjects with strong beliefs regarding their reactions to foods were given water by nasogastric tube and told they were receiving the test food and were given the test food and advised that the water was being instilled. Reactions to the tests

---

Food Allergy: Adverse Reactions to Foods and Food Additives, 4th edition.
Edited by Dean D. Metcalfe, Hugh A. Sampson, and Ronald A. Simon.
© 2008 Blackwell Publishing, ISBN: 978-1-4501-5129-0.

correlated with suggestion. To address the evident subject bias, masked ingestions were introduced by Loveless in several studies in the 1950s [2,3]. In an accompanying editorial, Lowell [4] emphasized the need for blinded challenges to demonstrate cause–effect relationships in the evaluation of adverse reactions to foods. Charles May is credited with bringing double-blind, placebo-controlled oral food challenges (DBPCFCs) into routine clinical practice and research use [5].

By the late 1980s, a number of seminal points concerning the epidemiology of food hypersensitivity were confirmed and refined through the use of masked and placebo-controlled OFCs. Challenges confirmed the role of food allergy in chronic disease such as childhood atopic dermatitis [6] and in immediate reactions [7], and determined that 6–8% of young children experience genuine adverse reactions to foods, but that most of the sensitivities resolved in early childhood [8]. The types of symptoms elicited by foods were confirmed to be most commonly associated with the skin (hives, atopic dermatitis), gut, and respiratory tract, and not commonly with behavioral problems [6–11].

The foods involved were generally confined to a rather limited number with children affected by allergy to cow's milk, egg, soy, wheat, peanut, and tree nuts, and older individuals to peanut, nuts, and seafood. The inaccuracy of the patient's history in regard to the relationship of food allergy to chronic disease was also underscored by several studies with an accuracy generally under 40% when compared to blinded food challenges [7,12–14]. In addition, food additives/preservatives were not a frequent cause of problems [11].

DBPCFCs are now a fundamental tool for scientifically establishing a number of important features of food hypersensitivity reactions. Studies have broadened our understanding of the spectrum of food hypersensitivity disorders. A growing number of studies point out the role of food hypersensitivity in isolated gastrointestinal disorders [15]; however, food allergy is not a frequent cause of isolated chronic respiratory disease [16]. The number of foods proven to cause reactions is ever expanding and includes seeds, fruits, vegetables, meats, and virtually every type of spice [17,18]. Despite advances in *in vitro* and *in vivo* diagnostic tests, the OFC has remained the final endpoint ("gold standard") to determine clinical tolerance or reactivity to food. Table 20.1 summarizes the early and recent advances in our understanding of food hypersensitivity obtained through OFCs.

Prick skin tests

Tests to detect food-specific IgE antibody are central to identify or exclude foods responsible for immediate type, and some chronic disease-inducing food-allergic reactions (e.g. atopic dermatitis and eosinophilic gastroenteropathies). The most familiar, convenient, and commonly used method is prick/puncture skin testing (PST). The intradermal form

Table 20.1 Features about adverse reactions to foods determined through studies using OFCs

Epidemiology	6–8% of children
	1–2% of adults
	Most common foods: egg, milk, peanut, tree nut, seafood, soy, wheat
	Increasingly wide variety of foods
Associated disorders	Anaphylaxis (acute skin, gut, respiratory and cardiovascular reactions)
	Atopic dermatitis (~35% with moderate skin disease)
	Numerous gastrointestinal disorders
Infrequently associated disorders (2–5%)	Isolated chronic respiratory disease
	Chronic urticaria
Clinical symptoms only rarely, or possibly not associated	Behavioral disorders
	Neurologic disorders

of allergen skin testing was introduced by Blackley [19] over 100 years ago, and the prick test was described by Lewis and Grant in 1924 [20]. The technique of PST is simple, but specific variations exist. While the patient is off antihistamines for an appropriate length of time, a device such as a needle, bifurcated needle, probe, or lancet is used to puncture the epidermis through an extract of a food. Appropriate positive (histamine) and negative (saline–glycerine) controls are also placed. The test site is examined 10–20 minutes later. A local wheal and flare response indicate the presence of food-specific IgE antibody. A mean wheal diameter 3 mm or greater compared to a saline control is generally considered positive [21,22], but interpretation will be discussed in more detail below. Of course, the test would not be expected to be positive for food reactions that are not mediated by IgE antibodies, such as several of the infantile gastrointestinal disorders including food-protein-induced enterocolitis syndrome and proctocolitis. Clearly, the PST is an invaluable screening tool for the allergist. However, the clinician using PSTs for the diagnosis of food hypersensitivity must be aware of the utility and limitations of the test in order to use it to the best advantage for clinical and research purposes.

Technical considerations

Skin test results are influenced by variables such as test reagents, type of skin test device, location of test placement, patient factors, and methods of measuring results. The selection of skin test reagent is of primary importance. Unfortunately, standardized food extracts are not currently available despite a clear, long-standing recognition for the need [21,22]. Commercial extracts are usually prepared as glycerinated extracts of 1:10 or 1:20 dilution. With the lack of standardized extracts, it is well recognized that variations exist in allergen distribution and concentration between lots and manufacturers [23,24]. The problem of protein stability must also be considered. An example demonstrating the liability of certain food extracts is the evaluation of food allergy in pollen–food syndrome (oral allergy syndrome to fresh fruits and vegetables). Patients may react to the uncooked, but not the cooked form of the food and this may similarly be reflected in skin test results as commercial extracts may lack the ability to display the labile proteins involved [25]. For the evaluation of allergy to fresh fruits and vegetables, and possibly other foods, many authorities have suggested the use of fresh foods (e.g. fresh milk, egg white, fruits, and vegetables) [26]. The PST can be performed using liquid foods, by creating an in-house extract, or using a prick–prick technique (pricking the fruit and then the patient, thereby transferring the juice) [27]. Presumably, such in-house reagents are more concentrated and this may increase sensitivity, a possible deficit in some circumstances, and may increase the risk for side effects from the test itself. The impact of allergen concentration on wheal size is somewhat tempered by the fact that wheal size increases by a factor of ~1.5 for each logarithmic increase in concentration [28].

The device used for pricking the skin, and the technique used with any given device, may also influence the results. A variety of devices are on the market for introducing the allergen into the epidermis. As may be imagined, the more penetration, the more likely there will be a response and so the area and depth to which the allergen is introduced is pertinent. Therefore, the configuration of the device, the pressure applied by the operator, and the time over which pressure is applied must be considered [29]. Test results also vary according to the location on the body on which they are placed. For example, the back is ~20% more reactive than the arm [30]. Studies that evaluate histamine reactivity indicate that wheals become detectable in early infancy and increase in size with age until adulthood [31,32]. These physical and patient variables become relevant when comparing study results, and for clinical decision making. In practice, consistency of materials and procedures, and review of precision (coefficient of variation should be <20% for wheal diameter) should be undertaken by comparing repeated tests by personnel administering them. Various single- and multi-headed devices are available, with significant differences in all areas of device performance among all devices examined. In one study, multi-headed devices were judged more painful than single devices and had larger reactions on the back, whereas single devices had larger reactions on the arms [33].

Additional variations concerning PSTs are the timing at which they are read and the manner in which they are measured and reported. The histamine test peaks at 10 minutes while allergen wheal size generally peaks at 15–20 minutes [34]. One suggested method of measurement is to determine the greatest wheal (or flare) diameter, its perpendicular maximum diameter, and to determine the mean of these

Table 20.2 Aspects that impact sensitivity of PSTs

Feature	Correlation with sensitivity
Extract concentration	Direct
Device used	Variable
Pressure applied during application	Direct
Location	Back > volar aspect arm
Reporting progressively larger reaction sizes (e.g. wheal 4 mm instead of 3 mm) as categorically positive	Inverse

two measurements [34]. However, many researchers report the longest diameter, which is less time consuming to measure but presents, on average, a higher value than the mean diameter. Presenting the result in millimeters is preferred, with additional presentation of the size of the histamine and saline controls for comparison. The measurement of the saline control is typically subtracted from the allergen and histamine results to account for dermographism. Thus, a positive test (reflecting IgE) is generally regarded as one with a mean wheal diameter at least 3 mm greater than the saline control. In practice, reporting of results often varies by investigator and may be reported as mean diameter, mean diameter compared to histamine control categorically (e.g. 1+, 2+, etc.), or as a calculated area. Studies must be evaluated carefully because individual investigators may be reporting data based on a variety of methods that may not be directly comparable (e.g. mean wheal diameter versus largest diameter). Despite the numerous potential confounding variables involved in the PST procedure, the clinical utility is excellent. Technical issues that can impact PST sensitivity are summarized in Table 20.2.

Diagnostic value

The ability of a test to indicate the presence or absence of disease depends on intrinsic characteristics of the test itself and also features of the population on which it is being applied. The PST is excellent for detecting food-specific IgE antibody and when it is negative, it is highly likely that there is none, and that no IgE antibody-mediated allergic reaction would occur to the tested food (excellent negative predictive accuracy, NPA). However, this conclusion, when considering the individual patient, depends strongly on the prior probability of true allergy, a concept discussed further below. Obviously, a negative result does not exclude the possibility of cell-mediated allergic reactions or intolerance. To complicate matters for the allergist and patient, the presence of IgE to a food often does not equate with clinical reactions; that is, there is often (~50%) clinically inconsequential sensitization. Again, this statement depends on the prior probability of risk of true allergy in the study population. For example, skin testing to peanut in the general population (no selection for allergy) performed in the United States showed 8% had a positive PST [35], yet population-based studies of true allergy to peanut show that only 0.6% are allergic [36]. Therefore, in unselected patients, one could conclude that nearly 93% of positive tests are "false positive."

The sensitivity and specificity of a test provide information about its ability to identify a known condition. Sensitivity refers to the proportion of patients with an illness who test positive, and for IgE-mediated food allergy, the sensitivity of the PST is usually high (>80%). Specificity refers to the proportion of individuals without the disorder who test negative, and for IgE antibody-mediated food allergy, specificity of the PST is usually lower than the sensitivity but usually better than 50% [26,37,38]. Sensitivity and specificity are impacted by intrinsic properties of the test (Table 20.2), but the clinical question of import to the physician concerns the probability that a patient has food allergy if the test is positive (positive predictive accuracy, PPA) or does not have food allergy if the test is negative (negative predictive accuracy, NPA). The predictive accuracy is impacted by the prevalence of the disorder in the population being tested (or as applied to the individual, the prior probability that the person being tested has the disorder). In studies using referred patients with an increased probability of disease, and a definition of positive PST as one with a mean wheal diameter of ≥3 mm, PSTs have an excellent NPA (~90%) but the PPA is on the order of only 50% [26,37,38].

The definition used to indicate a positive test (or degree of positive) will additionally impact the PPA and NPA. For example, increasing skin test size correlates directly with increasing IgE antibody and the risk of clinical reactions. Therefore, if one were to analyze skin test sizes (rather than just labeling them categorically as positive or negative at a mean wheal size of 3 mm), there would be variation in sensitivity and specificity with each incremental change in size. In general, as the definition of a positive test requires a larger wheal, specificity increases and sensitivity decreases. Receiver operator curves are used to display the association of test size defined as positive with sensitivity and specificity that must be determined experimentally (Fig. 20.1). The uppermost left quadrant on the curve would be the point where combined maximum sensitivity and specificity could be achieved. Similarly, as "cut-off" for positive increases, so does PPA while the NPA simultaneously decreases. Since these indices of predictive value are population dependant, the predictive value drops (illness is overestimated) when results obtained in a referral center (high prevalence) are applied to unselected individuals.

An additional way of considering the meaning of a test is to consider the chance that a person with food allergy would have a positive test compared to the chance that one without food allergy would have a negative test. This ratio

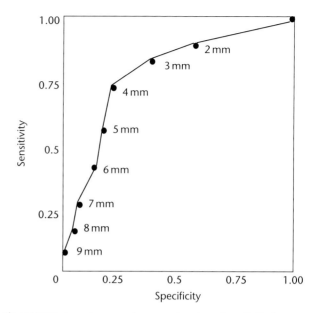

Figure 20.1 A receiver operator curve showing a hypothetical experiment in which PST sensitivity and specificity were determined for various wheal sizes. When different skin test sizes are considered as a positive "cut-off," there is a trade-off between sensitivity and specificity. The single point at which sensitivity and specificity is maximized is the one closest to the upper left corner (4 mm in this example). When the skin test size meets and exceeds 9 mm in this example, there is 100% specificity and all patients would be expected to react to this food.

is termed a likelihood ratio. This ratio is independent of population prevalence, but in order to use it for predicting food allergy, one must have a sense for pre-test probability in the individual tested (i.e. the impact is similar to population prevalence of disease on PPA and NPA). If one knows the likelihood ratio of a skin test and the pre-test probability of food allergy, it is possible to calculate a post-test probability by multiplying the likelihood ratio by the pre-test probability [39]. While the specific data is not worked out for most foods, the concept is clinically vital to appreciate and underscores the importance of a careful history. Consider, for example, three individuals: one had three severe allergic reactions to egg requiring epinephrine, another has atopic dermatitis and no history of a reaction to egg, and a third sometimes has headaches when he eats egg. Each patient is tested by PST to egg white and has a 4-mm wheal. The meaning of a 4-mm wheal to egg when there has been recurrent anaphylaxis to egg is that it confirms reactivity because the pre-test probability is high. In a chronic condition like atopic dermatitis, a modest size skin test may reflect clinical reactivity in only about half of patients (depending also on age) and may be a relevant positive in this scenario needing confirmation by other means. The test result in the situation of isolated headaches is most likely of no clinical concern as the pre-test probability is essentially zero. Considering again the patient with multiple episodes of egg-related anaphylaxis, if there were no wheal to egg the clinician would not be likely to trust the result because the pre-test probability is so high and the correct course of action would be to repeat the test and consider a supervised OFC if the test were negative. These features underscore the importance of considering the medical history when evaluating test results. Likelihood ratios can be calculated for increasing skin test wheal sizes which in turn can assist in broadening the ability to predict reactions in various clinical scenarios, but more studies are needed to provide reliable data for a large number of foods [40]. Such data would be particularly helpful for the interpretation of skin tests performed to foods with homologous proteins (see Chapters 4 and 25) in persons who have a bona fide allergy to one of a group of related foods.

It has been observed by some investigators that particularly large PSTs may have 100% positive predictive value. This concept was demonstrated in a study [40] showing that for young infants, reactions to egg, milk, and peanut were certain to occur if the skin test wheal was ≥8 mm for cow's milk and peanut and ≥7 mm for egg. The scenario reflects increasing likelihood ratio with increasing sizes of skin tests (likelihood ratios over 12.5 for all three allergens with wheals ≥6 mm in the referral population). This result requires replication in further studies. These investigators [41] also evaluated children of 4 months to 19 years of age referred for suspected nut allergy with a single lancet technique and commercial extracts (except whole food for sesame and pistachio) and compared skin test sizes to food challenge outcomes. Positive challenges were associated (>95% accuracy) with wheal sizes ≥8 mm for cashew, hazel, walnut, and sesame. Correlation was poor for almond, pistachio, pecan, and brazil nut though fewer subjects were tested.

When considering the clinical use of such study results, it is also important to consider the variables mentioned previously concerning method of interpretation, skin test device, reagents, study population, etc. Table 20.3 summarizes predictive values of skin tests from representative international studies [40,42–44]. As indicated in the table, the populations differed but included various groups with an elevated prior probability of allergy. It is important to recognize that skin test sizes reflecting "100% specificity," or diagnostic value, varied by the study. The clinical utility of PSTs is maximized when two decision point wheal sizes are considered in the interpretation: one with high NPA and another with high PPA. When considered together, this may reduce the need for further evaluations (e.g. OFCs).

Risks of prick skin tests

PSTs are typically considered of low risk because allergen exposure is minute and a generalized systemic allergic reaction is rare. In a review of a database of 34,905 skin tests to foods in 1138 patients, the systemic reaction rate was 0.008% and there were no severe reactions [45]. Devenney

et al. [46] identified six infants with generalized reactions representing a rate of 521 per 100,000 tested children or 6522 per 100,000 tested infants. All of the reactions identified were in infants under 6 months of age and they were tested with fresh foods rather than extracts. There is one fatality associated with PST; an adult with food allergy and asthma with a recent exacerbation was tested to 90 foods at one time and experienced a fatal respiratory arrest [47]. In general, these studies support the notion that PSTs are low risk, but caution is needed for infants, use of undiluted extracts, and application of excessive numbers of tests. The physician performing allergy tests should appreciate the low but possible risk of anaphylaxis and be prepared to identify and treat reactions. Intradermal allergy skin tests with food extracts give an unacceptably high false-positive rate, have been associated with systemic reactions including fatal anaphylactic reactions, and should not be used [48].

Pitfalls of skin tests and future diagnostic possibilities

It is not clear why PSTs are occasionally negative despite apparent acute allergic reactions during a food challenge. As has been indicated for venom testing [49], it may be prudent to perform both serum IgE and PST to a food to improve sensitivity when suspicion of reactions are high based on history. In addition, it has been suggested, when suspicion of allergy is high and before proceeding to OFC, to follow a negative PST performed with a commercial extract with a fresh extract of the same food. Presumably this procedure is more sensitive because labile proteins are displayed, compared to commercial extracts, and proteins that may not have been represented during aqueous extraction in creating a commercial extract may be presented as well [50]. For example, Hauswirth and Burks [51] described a patient with systemic anaphylaxis to banana whose commercial, but not fresh extract, skin testing was positive. The *in vitro* tests for detection of serum food-specific IgE antibodies are also very sensitive and specific, but may not display the very same allergen profile as the skin tests. The tests can therefore be used in a complementary fashion when needed. For example, Knight *et al.* [43] challenged children to egg when their serum IgE concentrations to egg white was favorable, approximately 50%, to pass an OFC, for example around 2 kU$_A$/l. The size of the wheal to a commercial egg extract PST correlated with the outcome of the food challenges: 20% of those with a negative skin test reacted to OFC while 90% with a wheal size of 9 mm reacted.

Improvement in the diagnostic accuracy of PSTs for the future will require additional studies to better characterize the test utility over a broad spectrum of disease, patient age, and types of foods. Standardization of commercial extracts is needed, but development of extracts using bioengineered, well-characterized proteins may also prove beneficial. Test results currently do not correlate well with

Table 20.3 Predictive values of skin tests from various studies

Allergen	Age	Skin test wheal	Probability of reaction/ reaction rates	Comments	Reference
Milk	Median 3 years	8 mm	~100%	Australia, referred for suspected allergy, lancet technique, commercial extracts, wheal diameter, open OFC	[40]
	<2 years	6 mm	~100%	Same as above	
	Median 3 years	0 mm	~15%	Same as above	
	Median 22 months	12.5 mm	95%	Germany, all OFC, suspected allergy, 87% atopic dermatitis, fresh foods, mean wheal diameter, lancet technique	[42]
Egg	Mean 5 years	0 mm	20%	United States, children without recent egg reaction and serum IgE typically below 2.5 kU$_A$/l, bifurcated needle, commercial extract, mean wheal diameter	[43]
		3 mm	50%	As above	
		9 mm	90%	As above	
	Median 3 years	7 mm	~100%	Australia, referred for suspected allergy, lancet technique, commercial extracts, wheal diameter, open OFC	[40]
	<2 years	5 mm	~100%	Same as above	
	Median 22 months	13 mm	95%	Germany, all OFC, suspected allergy, fresh foods, mean wheal diameter, lancet technique	[42]
Peanut	Median 3 years	8 mm	~100%	Australia, referred for suspected allergy, lancet technique, commercial extracts, wheal diameter, open OFC	[40]
	<2 years	4 mm	~100%	Same as above	
	Mean 7 years	8 mm	~95%	United Kingdom, mixed suspected allergy, ages 1–16 years, lancet technique, extract, longest diameter	[44]
		3 mm	~50%	As above	
		0 mm	~13%	As above	
			~28%	As above	
			92%	As above	

severity of a reaction or level of patient sensitivity, but diagnosis using specific proteins to which IgE binding is associated with severe reactions may allow future diagnosis that is more sensitive and specific with additional predictive value in regard to severity [52–54].

Additional diagnostic steps prior to oral food challenges

An OFC can determine whether a specific food triggers disease, but it is time consuming and carries risk. Therefore, additional diagnostic steps are taken to determine if an OFC would be of utility and, if so, additional consideration about risks/benefits are considered prior to proceeding. To determine a diagnosis and to determine whether an OFC is needed for a diagnosis requires consideration of patient history, test results, the immunopathology of the disorder under consideration, the physical examination, and the results of elimination

diets. These diagnostic steps are considered in more detail in Chapter 24. Specific information about diagnostic tests such as determination and interpretation of serum IgE (Chapters 19 and 21), and the atopy patch test (Chapter 20) are described elsewhere. Here, the specific components of the history and physical examination that are of import for diagnosing food allergy will be described. The value and limitations of diet diaries and elimination diets will be explained. Lastly, decisions about undertaking an OFC and the type of OFC will be reviewed. Specific details about undertaking an elimination diet and performing an OFC will be described in Chapter 23.

The history and physical examination

The history and physical examination are undertaken prior to the selection of any diagnostic tests. The clinician must consider from the history whether the complaints are likely to be associated with food allergy, intolerance or toxic effects, or not related to foods whatsoever. Furthermore, the physician is interested in constructing *a priori* assessments of the chance that foods are playing a role, which foods may be involved and whether the pathophysiology, if it is related to a hypersensitivity reaction, is IgE antibody mediated, cell mediated, or a combination. The physical examination may confirm atopic dermatitis, growth problems, urticaria, and other symptoms of atopic disease, or may exclude them. A careful history should focus upon: the symptoms attributed to food ingestion (type, acute versus chronic), the food(s) involved, consistency of reactions, the quantity of food required to elicit symptoms, the timing between ingestion and onset of symptoms, the most recent reaction/patterns of reactivity, the manner in which the food was prepared (raw, cooked), potential contamination with known allergens, and any ancillary associated activity that may play a role (i.e. exercise, alcohol ingestion). The importance of these queries, many of which are self-evident, derive from various observations about food-allergic reactions. For example, consistent reactions raise prior probability that a suspect food is causal. If a food is an infrequent part of the diet, it is more likely a culprit than a food eaten often. Proteins may be altered through cooking resulting in variations in reaction. Sometimes a rather large amount of a food needs to be ingested for a reaction to occur, or ancillary activities such as exercise or ingestion of medications is required [55]. A person with a prior known allergy may have reacted to contamination of their food with a known allergen, rather than have developed a new allergy, so careful discussion is required. Details about the meal may disclose nuances of note. Consider, for example, an allergic reaction to ingestion of fish in a person where fish-allergic reactions have not been consistent. Canned tuna and salmon are typically tolerated by those who react to fish that is not canned, though allergy to canned tuna is also described [56]. Various fish preparation methods (e.g. boiling versus frying versus eating raw) may have different outcomes on protein allergenicity for different types of fish [57]. Use of antacids (concomitant medications) may reduce digestion and may result in reactions despite prior tolerance [58–60]. The part of the fish ingested can have different levels of the major allergen, such that dark or red muscle may lack the allergen compared to white muscle [61,62]. Lastly, allergy to parasites in fish, specifically to anisakis simplex, represents another potential confounding diagnostic issue [63–66]. A thorough history is needed to appropriately address these possibilities.

It is convenient, and possibly quite illuminating, to have patients keep a symptom diary and chart the foods they consume with and without symptoms and also to collect ingredient labels from the foods they eat. For example, they may chart 3–7 days of meals and snacks, showing the time of ingestions, the amount eaten, brands, preparation methods, and any symptoms. The accuracy and diagnostic utility of such records have not been evaluated. To improve the quality of the information, patients/families should be reminded to record all foods and medications ingested, as they may be prone to neglect beverages, snacks, medications, and condiments. The information gathered from the general history, physical examination, and diet records are used to determine the best mode of diagnosis or may lead to dismissal of the problem from the history alone.

In the case of acute reactions following the isolated ingestion of a particular food with classical food-allergic symptoms, such as acute urticaria or anaphylaxis, the history may clearly implicate a particular food and a positive test for specific IgE antibody (PST/RAST) would be confirmatory and exclude the need for OFC. In the context of an acute reaction to a food to which IgE has been detected, elimination is not considered diagnostic, but rather for purposes of treatment. If the ingestion was of mixed foods and the causal food was uncertain (i.e. a meal with five ingredients), the history may help to eliminate some of the foods. For example, foods frequently ingested without symptoms are generally excluded as potential triggers when evaluating symptoms associated with acute reactions. Tests for food-specific IgE antibodies may help to further narrow the possibilities.

Diagnostic elimination diets

In chronic disorders such as atopic dermatitis, eosinophilic gastroenteropathies, or asthma, it is more difficult to pinpoint causal food(s) [67]. The history is helpful, but since these disorders have a waxing and waning course, and considering limitations in diagnostic laboratory tests, false associations to food ingestions are common. The evaluation of these disorders may require a period of dietary elimination to observe for symptom resolution. This period of trial diet requires selection of foods to be eliminated (based usually on history, test results, epidemiology of the disorder, etc.). The diet trial could be confounded if additional therapies are simultaneously undertaken (e.g. steroids for eosinophilic gastrointestinal disorders, an improved skin care regiment for atopic dermatitis, etc.). Therefore, it is usually prudent to alter one variable at a time. Chronic symptoms should resolve during a period of elimination and if they do, OFCs may be needed to determine which food(s) were causing the chronic symptoms. If symptoms do not resolve, then the eliminated foods are not causal. Elimination of foods to which IgE antibodies are demonstrable, but to which acute reactions are not observed, may carry a risk of loss of a desensitized state, where reintroduction later can trigger more evident acute reactions (e.g. urticaria, anaphylaxis) [68,69]. The frequency of this occurrence is unknown and the length of time for elimination to warrant this concern is currently unclear, but the risk should be considered in decisions to begin dietary trials. Additional details about elimination diets are provided in Chapter 23.

Oral food challenges

OFCs are typically undertaken to identify a causal food when allergy is otherwise unclear (e.g. tests are equivocal or irrelevant), or to monitor for resolution of an allergy. The specific routine for deciding upon OFC and undertaking them is described in Chapter 23. OFC is usually the only means to evaluate disorders or complaints where ancillary tests are irrelevant. For example, the evaluation of reactions to food dyes and preservatives usually requires OFCs. Similarly, patients may attribute a host of medical complaints to food ingestion in disorders that are not proven to be pathophysiologically linked to food allergy (e.g. arthritis, fatigue, behavioral problems, etc.). In all of the circumstances where chronic complaints are involved, the OFC is capable of revealing or excluding relationships to foods. Such determinations are crucial because patients may undertake unnecessary dietary alterations that can have nutritional and social consequences [70,71]. Overall, the approach to diagnosis in chronic disorders, where most readily available diagnostic tests are of limited value, requires elimination diets and OFC to confirm suspected associations.

In regard to undertaking an OFC when there is supporting evidence of allergy, the decision requires consideration of risk, nutritional need, social need, and other factors. The issues to consider when deciding whether to undertake an oral challenge and what challenge setting (e.g. open, single, or double masked) are summarized in Table 20.4. Diagnostic tests considered in this chapter and elsewhere, results of elimination diets, and historical points are central to decision making. There are settings in which oral challenges may be optional or contraindicated. Severe anaphylaxis to an isolated ingestion, with a positive test for specific IgE antibody to the causal food, is one example of a relative contraindication for oral challenge. On the other hand, in some circumstances even a patient with this convincing history may require a challenge; for example, if enough time has passed and laboratory indices are favorable for the possibility that tolerance has developed. If the food being eliminated is not nutritionally or socially important (e.g. star fruit), then challenge may be unwarranted. These same rules may apply if several members of a food family are being eliminated, but the food family is not a major part of the diet (e.g. elimination of all tree nuts when an allergy to one is certain). An evaluation of the history and test results may allow an assessment of a probability that a challenge would be tolerated. Depending on patient preferences and physician judgment, the decision to proceed may vary. For example, an estimation of an 80% risk of a reaction to peanut for a 2 year old is not as likely to result in a decision to challenge as it might be for a 16 year old. Overall, a variety of safety and social issues should be considered.

There are three general modalities to perform OFC and their selection depends on various considerations [12,72–74]. Challenges can be done "openly" with the patient ingesting the food in its natural form, "single-blind" with the food masked and the patient unaware if the test substance contains the target food or double-blind and placebo-controlled (DBPCFC) where neither patient nor physician knows which challenges contain the food being tested. In the latter two formats, the food must be hidden in some way, such as in another food or opaque capsules. When challenges are undertaken for research purposes, the DBPCFC is the preferred format because there is the least chance for bias from either the patient or physician who must monitor for symptoms. The false-positive and false-negative rate for the DBPCFC, based primarily on studies in children with atopic dermatitis, is 0.7% and 3.2%, respectively [75,76]. Because the food is masked, it is sometimes difficult to provide meal sized portions in a foods' natural state. To help exclude false

Table 20.4 Issues to consider for undertaking an OFC

Category	Variables	Factors
Indication to challenge	Probability to pass (risks)	History, physical examination, test results, nature of allergen, natural history of disease
	Needs (benefits)	Social
		Nutritional
Challenge type	Open	Numerous foods to screen, disorder with objective symptoms, allowance for bias
	Single-blind	Less prone to bias than open
	DBPCFC	Least prone to bias, most definitive approach for subjective symptoms
Challenge location	Home	Adding foods in chronic or behavioral disorders with no risk of acute/severe reactions
	Office	Challenges at low risk for severe reaction
	Hospital/ICU	Challenges that are more likely to elicit reactions requiring medical intervention

negatives, it has long been suggested to include an open feeding under supervision of a meal size portion of the tested food prepared in its usual manner as a follow-up to any negative DBPCFC [76]. Increasing the number of challenges (additional placebo and true foods) helps to diminish the possibility of a random association, but this can be a very labor-intensive approach [77,78].

There are several factors that weigh in deciding which type of challenge to use, and DBPCFC, a labor-intensive format, may not be the initial choice. Although the open challenge is most prone to bias, it is easy to perform since no special preparation is needed to mask the food. Indeed, if the patient tolerates the ingestion of the food, there is little concern about bias. It is only when symptoms, especially subjective ones, arise that the issue of bias come into play. Therefore, open challenges are a good option for screening when several foods are under consideration and if a food is tolerated, nothing further is needed. If there is a reaction to an open challenge used in the clinical setting, and there is concern that the reaction may have been psychological, the format could be altered to include blinding and controls. Single-blind challenges help to alleviate patient bias and may be an option to increase efficiency (since a second placebo arm is not always needed). Additional information about undertaking OFC is presented in Chapter 23.

Summary

In vivo tests are primary tools among the armamentarium available to the clinician for the diagnosis of adverse reactions to foods. The medical history, perhaps supplemented with diet records, is the cornerstone of diagnosis. Skin testing is safe, cost effective, and when properly performed and interpreted, highly informative for the diagnosis of IgE antibody-mediated disorders. Elimination diets may provide presumptive evidence of a food-responsive disease. OFCs are the most definitive test available for the final confirmation of these disorders. While oral challenges are time consuming and may elicit severe reactions, they can be safely and efficiently performed with the proper preparation and remain the mainstay of diagnosis for clinical and research settings.

References

1 Graham DT, Wolf S, Wolff HG. Changes in tissue sensitivity associated with varying life situations and emotions; their relevance to allergy. *J Allergy* 1950;21:478–86.

2 Loveless MH. Milk allergy: a survey of its incidence; experiments with a masked ingestion test. *J Allergy* 1950;21:489–99.

3 Loveless MH. Allergy for corn and its derivatives: experiments with a masked ingestion test for its diagnosis. *J Allergy* 1950;21:500–9.

4 Ingelfinger FJ, Lowell FC, Franklin W. Gastrointestinal allergy. *N Engl J Med* 1949;241:303.

5 May CD. Objective clinical and laboratory studies of immediate hypersensitivity reactions to food in asthmatic children. *J Allergy Clin Immunol* 1976;58:500–15.

6 Sampson HA, McCaskill CC. Food hypersensitivity and atopic dermatitis: evaluation of 113 patients. *J Pediatr* 1985;107:669–75.

7 Atkins FM, Steinberg SS, Metcalfe DD. Evaluation of immediate adverse reactions to foods in adult patients. II. A detailed analysis of reaction patterns during oral food challenge. *J Allergy Clin Immunol* 1985;75:356–63.

8 Bock SA. Prospective appraisal of complaints of adverse reactions to foods in children during the first 3 years of life. *Pediatrics* 1987;79:683–8.

9 Wolraich ML, Lindgren SD, Stumbo PJ, *et al*. Effects of diets high in sucrose or aspartame on the behavior and cognitive performance of children. *N Engl J Med* 1994;330:301–7.

10 Onorato J, Merland N, Terral C, *et al*. Placebo-controlled double-blind food challenge in asthma. *J Allergy Clin Immunol* 1986;78:1139–46.

11 National Institutes of Health Consensus Development Panel. Conference statement: defined diets and hyperactivity. *Am J Clin Nutr* 1983;37:161–5.

12 Bock SA, Sampson HA, Atkins FM, *et al*. Double-blind, placebo-controlled food challenge (DBPCFC) as an office procedure: a manual. *J Allergy Clin Immunol* 1988;82:986–97.

13 Bernstein M, Day J, Welsh A. Double-blind food challenge in the diagnosis of food sensitivity in the adult. *J Allergy Clin Immunol* 1982;70:205–10.

14 Bock S, Lee W, Remigio L, May C. Studies of hypersensitivity reactions to food in infants and children. *J Allergy Clin Immunol* 1978;62:3327–34.

15 Sampson HA, Anderson JA. Summary and recommendations: classification of gastrointestinal manifestations due to immunologic reactions to foods in infants and young children. *J Pediatr Gastroenterol Nutr* 2000;30:S87–94.

16 Sicherer SH, Sampson HA. The role of food allergy in childhood asthma. *Immunol Allergy Clin North Am* 1998;18:49–60.

17 Hefle SL, Nordlee JA, Taylor SL. Allergenic foods. *Crit Rev Food Sci Nutr* 1996;36:S69–89.

18 Scholl I, Jensen-Jarolim E. Allergenic potency of spices: hot, medium hot, or very hot. *Int Arch Allergy Immunol* 2004; 135:247–61.

19 Blackley C. *Hay Fever: Its Causes, Treatment and Effective Prevention, Experimental Researches*, 2nd edn. London, Bailliere, Tindall & Cox 1880.

20 Lewis T, Grant R. Vascular reactions of the skin to injury. *Heart* 1924;209:1924.

21 The use of standardized allergen extracts. American Academy of Allergy, Asthma and Immunology (AAAAI). *J Allergy Clin Immunol* 1997;99:583–6.

22 Position paper: Allergen standardization and skin tests. The European Academy of Allergology and Clinical Immunology. *Allergy* 1993;48:48–82.

23 Hefle SL, Helm RM, Burks AW, Bush RK. Comparison of commercial peanut skin test extracts. *J Allergy Clin Immunol* 1995;95:837–42.

24 Herian AM, Bush RK, Taylor SL. Protein and allergen content of commercial skin test extracts for soybeans. *Clin Exp Allergy* 1992;22:461–8.

25 Asero R. Detection and clinical characterization of patients with oral allergy syndrome caused by stable allergens in Rosaceae and nuts. *Ann Allergy Asthma Immunol* 1999; 83:377–83.

26 Ortolani C, Ispano M, Pastorello EA, *et al.* Comparison of results of skin prick tests (with fresh foods and commercial food extracts) and RAST in 100 patients with oral allergy syndrome. *J Allergy Clin Immunol* 1989;83:683–90.

27 Dreborg S. Skin tests in the diagnosis of food allergy. *Pediatr Allergy Immunol* 1995;6:38–43.

28 Dreborg S. Diagnosis of food allergy: tests *in vivo* and *in vitro*. *Pediatr Allergy Immunol* 2001;12:24–30.

29 Nelson HS, Rosloniec DM, McCall LI, Ikle D. Comparative performance of five commercial prick skin test devices. *J Allergy Clin Immunol* 1993;92:750–6.

30 Nelson HS, Knoetzer J, Bucher B. Effect of distance between sites and region of the body on results of skin prick tests. *J Allergy Clin Immunol* 1996;97:596–601.

31 Menardo JL, Bousquet J, Rodiere M, *et al.* Skin test reactivity in infancy. *J Allergy Clin Immunol* 1985;75:646–51.

32 Skassa-Brociek W, Manderscheid JC, Michel FB, Bousquet J. Skin test reactivity to histamine from infancy to old age. *J Allergy Clin Immunol* 1987;80:711–6.

33 Carr WW, Martin B, Howard RS, *et al.* Comparison of test devices for skin prick testing. *J Allergy Clin Immunol* 2005;116:341–6.

34 Bernstein IL, Storms WW. Practice parameters for allergy diagnostic testing. Joint Task Force on Practice Parameters for the Diagnosis and Treatment of Asthma. The American Academy of Allergy, Asthma and Immunology and the American College of Allergy, Asthma and Immunology. *Ann Allergy Asthma Immunol* 1995;75:543–625.

35 Arbes Jr SJ, Gergen PJ, Elliott L, Zeldin DC. Prevalences of positive skin test responses to 10 common allergens in the US population: results from the third National Health and Nutrition Examination Survey. *J Allergy Clin Immunol* 2005;116: 377–83.

36 Sicherer SH, Muñoz-Furlong A, Sampson HA. Prevalence of peanut and tree nut allergy in the United States determined by means of a random digit dial telephone survey: a 5-year follow-up study. *J Allergy Clin Immunol* 2003;112:1203–7.

37 Eigenmann PA, Sampson HA. Interpreting skin prick tests in the evaluation of food allergy in children. *Pediatr Allergy Immunol* 1998;9:186–91.

38 Majamaa H, Moisio P, Holm K, *et al.* Cow's milk allergy: diagnostic accuracy of skin prick and patch tests and specific IgE. *Allergy* 1999;54:346–51.

39 Fagan TJ. Letter: nomogram for Bayes theorem. *N Engl J Med* 1975;293:257.

40 Sporik R, Hill DJ, Hosking CS. Specificity of allergen skin testing in predicting positive open food challenges to milk, egg and peanut in children. *Clin Exp Allergy* 2000;30:1541–6.

41 Ho MH, Heine RG, Wong W, Hill DJ. Diagnostic accuracy of skin prick testing in children with tree nut allergy. *J Allergy Clin Immunol* 2006;117:1506–8.

42 Verstege A, Mehl A, Rolinck-Werninghaus C, *et al.* The predictive value of the skin prick test weal size for the outcome of oral food challenges. *Clin Exp Allergy* 2005;35:1220–6.

43 Knight AK, Shreffler WG, Sampson HA, *et al.* Skin prick test to egg white provides additional diagnostic utility to serum egg white-specific IgE antibody concentration in children. *J Allergy Clin Immunol* 2006;117:842–7.

44 Roberts G, Lack G. Diagnosing peanut allergy with skin prick and specific IgE testing. *J Allergy Clin Immunol* 2005;115: 1291–6.

45 Codreanu F, Moneret-Vautrin DA, Morisset M, *et al.* The risk of systemic reactions to skin prick-tests using food allergens: CICBAA data and literature review. *Allerg Immunol (Paris)* 2006;38:52–4.

46 Devenney I, Falth-Magnusson K. Skin prick tests may give generalized allergic reactions in infants. *Ann Allergy Asthma Immunol* 2000;85:457–60.

47 Bernstein DI, Wanner M, Borish L, Liss GM. Twelve-year survey of fatal reactions to allergen injections and skin testing: 1990–2001. *J Allergy Clin Immunol* 2004;113:1129–36.

48 Sampson HA, Rosen JP, Selcow JE, *et al.* Intradermal skin tests in the diagnostic evaluation of food allergy. *J Allergy Clin Immunol* 1996;98:714–15.

49 Moffitt JE, Golden DB, Reisman RE, *et al.* Stinging insect hypersensitivity: a practice parameter update. *J Allergy Clin Immunol* 2004;114:869–86.

50 Leduc V, Moneret-Vautrin DA, Tzen JT, *et al.* Identification of oleosins as major allergens in sesame seed allergic patients. *Allergy* 2006;61:349–56.

51 Hauswirth DW, Burks AW. Banana anaphylaxis with a negative commercial skin test. *J Allergy Clin Immunol* 2005;115:632–3.

52 Shreffler WG, Beyer K, Chu TH, *et al.* Microarray immunoassay: association of clinical history, *in vitro* IgE function, and heterogeneity of allergenic peanut epitopes. *J Allergy Clin Immunol* 2004;113:776–82.

53 Astier C, Morisset M, Roitel O, *et al.* Predictive value of skin prick tests using recombinant allergens for diagnosis of peanut allergy. *J Allergy Clin Immunol* 2006;118:250–6.

54 Schocker F, Luttkopf D, Scheurer S, *et al.* Recombinant lipid transfer protein Cor a 8 from hazelnut: a new tool for *in vitro* diagnosis of potentially severe hazelnut allergy. *J Allergy Clin Immunol* 2004;113:141–7.

55 Rubio M, Tornero P, de Barrio M, *et al.* Food allergy: a practice parameter. *Ann Allergy Asthma Immunol* 2006;96:S1–68.

56 Kelso JM, Bardina L, Beyer K. Allergy to canned tuna. *J Allergy Clin Immunol* 2003;111:901.

57 Chatterjee U, Mondal G, Chakraborti P, *et al.* Changes in the allergenicity during different preparations of pomfret, hilsa, bhetki and mackerel fish as illustrated by enzyme-linked immunosorbent assay and immunoblotting. *Int Arch Allergy Immunol* 2006;141:1–10.

58 Untersmayr E, Scholl I, Swoboda I, *et al.* Antacid medication inhibits digestion of dietary proteins and causes food allergy: a fish allergy model in BALB/c mice. *J Allergy Clin Immunol* 2003;112:616–23.

59 Untersmayr E, Poulsen LK, Platzer MH, *et al.* The effects of gastric digestion on codfish allergenicity. *J Allergy Clin Immunol* 2005;115:377–82.

60 Untersmayr E, Bakos N, Scholl I, *et al.* Anti-ulcer drugs promote IgE formation toward dietary antigens in adult patients. *FASEB J* 2005;19:656–8.

61 Lim DL, Neo KH, Goh DL, *et al.* Missing parvalbumin: implications in diagnostic testing for tuna allergy. *J Allergy Clin Immunol* 2005;115:874–5.

62 Kobayashi A, Tanaka H, Hamada Y, *et al.* Comparison of allergenicity and allergens between fish white and dark muscles. *Allergy* 2006;61:357–63.

63 Asturias JA, Eraso E, Moneo I, Martinez A. Is tropomyosin an allergen in Anisakis? *Allergy* 2000;55:898–9.

64 Sastre J, Lluch-Bernal M, Quirce S, *et al.* A double-blind, placebo-controlled oral challenge study with lyophilized larvae and antigen of the fish parasite, Anisakis simplex. *Allergy* 2000; 55:560–4.

65 Baeza ML, Rodriguez A, Matheu V, *et al.* Characterization of allergens secreted by Anisakis simplex parasite: clinical relevance in comparison with somatic allergens. *Clin Exp Allergy* 2004;34:296–302.

66 Daschner A, Pascual CY. Anisakis simplex: sensitization and clinical allergy. *Curr Opin Allergy Clin Immunol* 2005;5:281–5.

67 Sicherer SH, Sampson HA. Food hypersensitivity and atopic dermatitis: pathophysiology, epidemiology, diagnosis, and management. *J Allergy Clin Immunol* 1999;104:S114–22.

68 Flinterman AE, Knulst AC, Meijer Y, *et al.* Acute allergic reactions in children with AEDS after prolonged cow's milk elimination diets. *Allergy* 2006;61:370–4.

69 David TJ. Anaphylactic shock during elimination diets for severe atopic dermatitis. *Arch Dis Child* 1984;59:983–6.

70 Roesler TA, Barry PC, Bock SA. Factitious food allergy and failure to thrive. *Arch Pediatr Adolesc Med* 1994;148:1150–5.

71 Sicherer SH, Noone SA, Muñoz-Furlong A. The impact of childhood food allergy on quality of life. *Ann Allergy Asthma Immunol* 2001;87:461–4.

72 Sicherer SH. Food allergy: when and how to perform oral food challenges. *Pediatr Allergy Immunol* 1999;10:226–34.

73 Niggemann B, Rolinck-Werninghaus C, Mehl A, *et al.* Controlled oral food challenges in children – when indicated, when superfluous? *Allergy* 2005;60:865–70.

74 Bindslev-Jensen C. Standardization of double-blind, placebo-controlled food challenges. *Allergy* 2001;56:75–7.

75 Caffarelli C, Petroccione T. False-negative food challenges in children with suspected food allergy. *Lancet* 2001;358:1871–2.

76 Sampson HA. Use of food-challenge tests in children. *Lancet* 2001; 358:1832–3.

77 Briggs D, Aspinall L, Dickens A, Bindslev-Jensen C. Statistical model for assessing the proportion of subjects with subjective sensitisations in adverse reactions to foods. *Allergy* 2001; 56:83–5.

78 Chinchilli VM, Fisher L, Craig TJ. Statistical issues in clinical trials that involve the double-blind, placebo-controlled food challenge. *J Allergy Clin Immunol* 2005;115:592–7.

CHAPTER 23

Elimination Diets and Oral Food Challenges

Scott H. Sicherer

KEY CONCEPTS

- Diagnostic elimination diets are undertaken to provide presumptive evidence that a disorder or symptoms are food responsive.

- Prolonged diagnostic elimination diets may carry risks of nutritional deficiencies or loss of a state of desensitization.

- The oral food challenge (OFC), in particular when double-blind and placebo-controlled, is the most definitive modality available to diagnose a food-related illness.

- An OFC may induce anaphylaxis.

- Decisions about when and how to undertake an OFC require consideration of benefits (nutritional, social) and risks.

- Performance of an OFC requires preparation and consideration about dosing, understanding when to stop a challenge and treat a reaction, and how to instruct patients about introducing or avoiding a food following a challenge.

Introduction

The oral food challenge (OFC) is a definitive diagnostic test used to determine if a food is tolerated. The double-blind, placebo-controlled oral food challenge (DBPCFC) is considered the "gold standard" of diagnosis [1]. The test does not depend on the pathophysiology of an adverse reaction, and so it is valid for determination of food allergy, intolerance, and for pharmacologic reactions to foods. Steps taken to determine the need for an OFC, and deciding upon masking and placebo controls, are explained in Chapters 20 and 24. Here, the technique of performing an OFC will be described, including a review of risks and benefits, selection of challenge location, challenge procedures, dosing, monitoring, and challenge preparation and aftercare. OFCs typically follow a period of dietary elimination undertaken either as treatment of a known or likely allergy, or as a diagnostic trial to determine if a condition is food responsive. Procedural issues in undertaking a diagnostic elimination diets will be described here as well.

Food Allergy: Adverse Reactions to Foods and Food Additives, 4th edition.
Edited by Dean D. Metcalfe, Hugh A. Sampson, and Ronald A. Simon.
© 2008 Blackwell Publishing, ISBN: 978-1-4501-5129-0.

Food elimination diets

When food hypersensitivity is under consideration as a cause for a chronic disease such as atopic dermatitis or eosinophilic gastroenteropathy, a diagnostic elimination diet is often required prior to undertaking OFCs [2]. Another reason for dietary elimination prior to a food challenge may be to avoid a suspected or known trigger of reactions. There are three types of elimination diets (Table 23.1) and the type selected for a particular patient will depend on the clinical scenario being evaluated and the results of tests for IgE antibody. The first type involves the elimination of one or several foods from the diet. This may be the obvious course of action when an isolated food ingestion (i.e. peanut) causes a sudden acute reaction and there is a positive test for IgE to the food. This would represent a therapeutic intervention, rather than a diagnostic one. However, eliminating one or a few suspected foods from the diet when the diagnosis is not so clear (asthma, atopic dermatitis, chronic urticaria) can be a crucial step in determining if food is causal in the disease process. If symptoms persist, the eliminated food(s) is (are) excluded as a cause of symptoms. The length of trial depends on the type of symptoms, but 1–6 weeks is usually the time interval required. A brief dietary trial should suffice for disorders with frequent acute reactions while longer trials may be required to allow chronic inflammation to subside.

Table 23.1 Types of elimination diets used to evaluate the role of adverse food reactions in chronic disease

Diet	Description/target	Example
Specific Food(s)	Targeted diet to one or several suspected foods; may be therapeutically necessary as final treatment	Elimination of egg in toddler with atopic dermatitis; elimination of food dyes and preservatives in child with chronic urticaria
Oligoantigenic	Palatable, balanced diet devised according to patient preferences, but eliminating a large group of common or suspected allergens (e.g. egg, milk, peanut, seafood, etc.)	Allow lamb, broccoli, squash, sweet potato, rice, corn, beets, cooked apple and pear, sugar, salt, and vegetable oil for 6 weeks in patient with reflux and atopic dermatitis
Elemental	Amino-acid-based formula (or, less ideally, an extensive hydrolysate) as sole nutrition	Used for 8 weeks to evaluate severe eosinophilic gastroenteropathy in a 3-year old with failure to thrive

Table 23.2 Example of elimination diet (*see text*)

Pick one meat	Chicken or lamb
Pick one grain substitute*	Corn or rice
Pick three vegetables (cooked)	Broccoli, sweet potato*, carrot, squash, string bean
Pick three fruits	Apple, pear, peach, plum, banana
Consider supplement	"Complete" hypoallergenic formula

*Allows for variety of textures (breads, pastas, sweet potato chips/mashed, pancakes).

The second type of diet consists of eliminating a large number of foods suspected to cause a chronic problem (usually including those that are common epidemiologically as causes of food-allergic reactions as described above) and giving a list of "allowed foods." This "oligoantigenic" diet is useful for evaluation of chronic disorders when a larger number of foods are suspected. In most cases, this is the situation with atopic dermatitis, eosinophilic gastroenteropathies, or chronic urticaria. An example of such a diet is given in Table 23.2, but individualization is almost always needed. The advantage of this diet is that a nutritionally balanced, palatable diet is maintained while most possible causal foods are removed. The primary disadvantage is that, if symptoms persist, the cause could still be attributed to foods left in the diet. For finicky eaters, it may be helpful to assess exactly what foods are favorites and try to allow foods of low risk that are enjoyed by the patient and can be used for meals and snacks.

The most limited type of diet is an elemental diet in which calories are obtained from an extensively hydrolyzed formula or from an amino-acid-based formula. A subset of milk-allergic children react to extensively hydrolyzed casein-based infant formulas but tolerate amino-acid-based ones [3]. A variation is to include a few foods likely to be tolerated (however, this adds the possibility that persistent symptoms are caused by these foods). Unfortunately, except for the most severe disorders that warrant its use, this is a severe diet to impose and is extremely difficult to maintain in patients beyond infancy. In extreme cases, nasogastric feeding of the amino-acid-based formula can be achieved, although most patients can tolerate the taste of these

formulas with gradual introduction or the use of flavoring agents provided by the manufacturers. This diet may be required when the diets mentioned above fail to resolve symptoms, but suspicion for food-related illness remains high. It is also often required in disorders associated with multiple food allergies such as the allergic gastroenteropathies [4–6].

Information concerning strict adherence to the diet must be carefully reviewed. Errors are common [7]. Patients and families must be educated about label reading, cross-contamination, and the fact that the food protein, as opposed to sugar or fat, is the ingredient being eliminated (e.g. lactose-free milk contains cow's milk protein). If there is no improvement with elimination, then the foods eliminated are not likely to be a cause of the complaints. However, it is crucial to ensure that the diet was followed as prescribed before concluding that the result was negative. If resolution of symptoms is achieved, OFCs may be warranted as a next step in identifying which foods from among those eliminated are or are not tolerated.

There are potential risks when undertaking elimination diets. Elimination diets are usually required for just a few weeks and so nutritional deficiencies are not likely but must be considered if elimination is prolonged [8]. If multiple foods were eliminated and symptoms resolved, a patient or family may wish to maintain the prescribed diet. In this case, the nutritional adequacy of the diet, now being followed long term for treatment rather than diagnosis, should be assessed (see Chapter 38). An additional risk is that elimination of foods to which IgE antibodies were identified and which were associated with chronic inflammatory disease may result in loss of a desensitized state, leading to an acute reaction such as anaphylaxis or urticaria when the food is reintroduced [9,10]. The frequency of this occurrence and the length of time of elimination associated with loss of the desensitized state is unknown. However, the risk should be considered when undertaking prolonged elimination trials.

Oral food challenges

Chapter 20 defines the parameters under which an OFC is typically undertaken, and the factors that may be considered in deciding to utilize open, single, or double-blind, placebo-controlled challenges. Briefly, this process requires consideration of the likelihood that a food will be tolerated, which typically derives from the past history and test results. Additional consideration includes assessment of nutritional, social, and emotional factors that may indicate the need for, or deferral of an oral challenge. The DBPCFC is considered the "gold standard" for diagnosing food allergy [11,12]. Any test, however, can have limitations. The false positive and false negative rate for the DBPCFC based primarily on studies in children with atopic dermatitis is 0.7% and 3.2%, respectively [13,14]. To help exclude false negatives, it has long been suggested to include an open feeding under supervision of a meal size portion of the tested food prepared in its usual manner as a follow-up to any negative DBPCFC [15–17]. When one is evaluating subjective symptoms, there is a greater likelihood that false positive or negative determinations would occur. Increasing the number of challenges (additional placebo and true foods) helps to diminish the possibility of a random association, but this can be a very labor intensive approach [18,19]. While the DBPCFC can elucidate the relationship of symptoms to foods, it is not specific for food hypersensitivity. Any adverse reaction to food (intolerance, pharmacologic effect) can potentially be evaluated, so demonstration of an immunological explanation is still needed to label a reaction as a food allergy [1]. Oral challenges are almost the only methodology to adequately evaluate reactions to food additives (coloring and flavoring agents and preservatives) [20,21]. The same can be said for symptoms not likely to be associated with food allergy (behavior, etc.). This chapter focuses upon factors pertinent to undertaking the OFC including presenting the concept to a patient/family and considering risks/benefits, making a risk assessment for choosing an appropriate location for a challenge and selecting a dosing schedule, preparing challenge materials, preparing to treat a reaction, how to monitor for symptoms and to decide when to discontinue a challenge and treat symptoms, and how to instruct families following a successful or failed procedure.

Discussing the procedure with a patient

The challenge procedure, its risks, and benefits must be discussed with the family/patient. As described in Chapter 20, numerous factors are considered including the assessment of the odds for passing, the nutritional/social need for the food, and ability of the patient to cooperate with the challenge. Patients should understand that the test is being done to determine if the food is safe for them to ingest, but also that should they tolerate the food, it should be added to the diet following a successful challenge. Persons who passed a food challenge to peanut, for example, but do not incorporate the food into the diet may be at risk to redevelop reactions [22,23]. Although OFCs may be used to determine thresholds of reactivity, challenges are not routinely performed for clinical purposes in persons who are expected to react simply for the purpose of defining a safe threshold. In addition, since challenges are stopped when symptoms develop, they may not reflect severity of reactions from exposures due to accidental ingestion. Risks include anaphylaxis, though no deaths have been reported from physician-supervised OFCs. Risks may also include emotional ones from failed challenges. Following review of risks and benefits, informed consent should be documented.

Deciding upon a challenge location

If a challenge is undertaken, a risk assessment is needed to determine a safe location/setting in which to undertake the challenge. In rare circumstances, the food may be administered without physician supervision at home. For example, if vague complaints or ones not usually associated with food allergy (headache, behavioral issues) are being evaluated and there is no risk of an acute anaphylactic reaction, and especially when symptom onset is perceived to be delayed, foods (even in a double-blind, placebo-controlled structure) could be added at home. Similarly, if many foods were eliminated for a chronic, non-IgE-mediated disease and acute reactions are not a concern, adding the previously tolerated foods back into the diet at home for observation of recurrence of chronic symptoms is reasonable because doing so would not likely cause a severe reaction. On the other hand, whenever there is an even remote potential for an acute and/or severe reaction, physician supervision is mandatory.

Except in the uncommon circumstances described previously, OFCs are undertaken under direct medical supervision. A physician or trained health care worker evaluates symptoms during a challenge. The decision to undertake a supervised challenge includes, but is not limited to, the evaluation of disorders that include a potential for severe reactions. The next issue at hand is whether the challenge is considered of "low risk" and can be done in an office setting or should be conducted in a location with heightened capabilities for the management of severe anaphylaxis (e.g. hospital, intensive care unit). Whether intravenous access should be established prior to commencing the challenge must also be considered. The decisions about challenge location and whether to secure intravenous access prior to commencing a challenge are based on the same types of data evaluated for the consideration of food allergy in the early diagnostic process: the history (severity of prior reactions, history of reactions to the test food, etc.), prick skin test (PST) results, serum food-specific IgE tests. The higher the probability of a reaction the more likely a physician may wish to undertake the procedure in a more highly monitored (e.g. hospital) setting. Additional consideration is given to the potential severity of a reaction, should one occur. For consideration in this regard are co-morbid conditions (such as asthma), the type of food (e.g. risk of causing a severe reaction), severity of prior reactions, a history of reacting to small doses, etc. In any setting, it must be appreciated that oral challenges can elicit severe, anaphylactic reactions, so the physician must be comfortable with this potential and be prepared with emergency medications and equipment to promptly treat such a reaction no matter where the test is undertaken. In the office setting, such preparations are similar to those recommended in the context of offices that administer allergens by injection for immunotherapy [11,24].

If the challenge is considered "high risk" (e.g. positive test for IgE, previous severe reaction, asthmatic patient), then it is best to perform it in a very controlled setting (e.g. hospital). In high-risk challenges, it may also be prudent to have intravenous access prior to commencing challenges. One research group reviewed their record with 349 food challenges in children with atopic dermatitis and recommended intravenous access for challenges when the history indicated a prior need for medical intervention or when particular tests for IgE antibody indicated a fairly high risk for reactions [25]. A study by Perry *et al.* [26] reviewed risks of OFCs in children typically assessed to have a 50% risk or less of a reaction prior to challenge. Of the 584 challenges completed, 253 (43%) were positive to: milk (90), egg (56), peanut (71), soy (21), and wheat (15). Of patients who failed, there were 197 (78%) cutaneous, 108 (43%) gastrointestinal, 66 (26%) oral, 67 (26%) lower respiratory, and 62 (25%) upper respiratory reactions. Despite presumptions about certain foods causing more severe (e.g. peanut) reactions than others (e.g. egg, milk) there was no difference between foods in the severity of failed challenges or the type of treatment required to reverse symptoms. These observations underscore the need for preparation to treat severe reactions whenever undertaking an OFC.

Food protein-induced enterocolitis syndrome can result in hypotension and should be performed with intravenous access in a hospital setting [27]. This cell-mediated disorder results in a symptom complex of poor growth and profuse vomiting and diarrhea with or without microscopic blood in the stool while the causal food(s) are part of the diet [27]. When severe, particularly with re-feeding after a period of elimination as is the case during the OFC, reactions may include lethargy, dehydration, and hypotension, and may be complicated by acidosis and methemoglobinemia.

Preparing the patient for the challenge and baseline assessments

Patients must be given specific preparatory instruction prior to undertaking the challenge. Patients avoid the suspected food(s) for at least 2 weeks, antihistamines are discontinued according to their elimination half-life, and chronic asthma medications are reduced as much as possible prior to undertaking the challenge. β-agonists are eliminated for a relevant time period before challenges are undertaken. Medications such as β-blockers that may interfere with treatment should be substituted as possible. The patient should be examined

carefully prior to challenge to confirm that they are not already having chronic symptoms, and to determine their "baseline." It would not be prudent to undertake a challenge in an individual with, for example, mild wheezing for both the ability to judge a reaction and for safety concerns. Patients should be queried about any symptoms they have been experiencing that could confuse the interpretation of a food challenge, such as urticaria or rhinitis. It is prudent to avoid performing challenges if a patient recently had an exacerbation of asthma, particularly one requiring oral steroids. For some diseases (i.e. severe atopic dermatitis) hospitalization may be necessary to treat acute disease and establish a stable baseline prior to challenges. The patient should avoid food or drink for about 4 hours prior to challenge, although for young children or infants, clear fluids may be allowed.

Decisions on dosing

Despite attempts and discussions to make a uniform international protocol for performing OFCs, no consensus has been reached and many published studies use variations on a general theme [11,17,28]. In all challenges, the food is given in gradually increasing amounts. This is for safety reasons. For most IgE-mediated reactions, the author and colleagues [29] give a total of 8–10 g of the dry food or 100 ml of wet food (double amount for meat/fish) in gradually increasing doses at 10–15 minute intervals over about 90 minutes followed by a larger, meal size portion of food a few hours later. The doses may be distributed, for example, in portions such as (0.1%, 0.5%), 1%, 4%, 10%, 20%, 20%, 20%, 25%. However, researchers and clinicians have used a variety of other challenge regimens (lower starting doses, variations in the degree of dosing increases, different time intervals, etc.) with good success [28,30–32]. The dosing interval may be increased or doses repeated either because the observer is unsure of symptoms or to more closely mimic the history of reactions. In the latter situation, doses may be administered over days if the history indicates that several days of ingestion were required to trigger symptoms.

The starting dose to select varies among studies, but clinical correlation may be helpful. To place this in perspective, it is reported that highly sensitive cow's milk-allergic patients may react to trace milk contamination (e.g. 8.8–14 ppm) in commercial products, but these are generally not patients with a profile conducive to oral challenges [33,34]. In a study of adult peanut-allergic patients undergoing DBPCFCs, 50 mg of peanut was generally the lowest dose that elicited objective reactions (one patient experienced subjective symptoms at only 100 μg of peanut) [35]. We reviewed challenge data for 513 positive challenges to six common allergenic foods in children with atopic dermatitis [29]. Starting doses were usually 500 mg, but at the physician's discretion, starting doses were sometimes 100 or 250 mg. The percentage of children reacting at the first dose (500 mg or less) were as follows: egg 49%, milk 55%, soy 28%, wheat 25%, peanut 26%, and fish 17%. Twenty-six milk challenges and 22 egg challenges were positive at a first dose of 250 mg; 3 milk challenges and 7 egg challenges were positive at a first dose of 100 mg. Eleven percent of the reactions that occurred on first dose were judged severe. The dose to elicit a reaction was not predictable with PST size or IgE antibody concentration, as was also observed in the study by Perry [26]. Based on these results, starting doses of 100 mg or less were recommended. To be particularly cautious, one could argue for starting doses that begin under the thresholds reported to induce reactions. Unfortunately, the published thresholds vary by logarithmic differences among studies and data are not available for most foods. However, reactions are usually not reported under 0.25 mg of protein for peanut, 0.13 for egg, and 0.6 for milk (milligram of protein varies according to the form of the food) [36]. Some workers begin challenges by placing the food extract on the lower lip for 2 minutes (labial food challenge) and observing for local or systemic reactions in the ensuing 30 minutes [30]. The development of a contiguous rash of the cheek and chin, edema of the lip with conjunctivitis or rhinitis, or a systemic reaction is considered a positive test. Negative labial challenges are generally followed by an OFC. However, the validity of labial challenges has not been thoroughly investigated.

Dosing regimens for food protein-induced enterocolitis syndrome are slightly different [27,37]. Food challenges for this non-IgE-mediated syndrome are typically performed with 0.15–0.6 g/kg of the causal protein (usually cow's milk or soy), and reactions of profuse vomiting and diarrhea typically begin 2–4 hours after the ingestion and are accompanied by a rise in the absolute neutrophil count of over 3500 cells/mm^3.

Making and administering the challenge food

The successful administration of OFCs to young children requires a great deal of preparation, ingenuity, and patience. Young children may become stubborn and refuse to ingest the challenge food. Prior planning with the family to select palatable or familiar forms of challenge foods or vehicles to hide foods in, if the challenge is masked, can be helpful in improving the experience [38]. For example, milk protein may be mixed and hidden in soy frozen dessert products. Having additional challenge vehicles, for example liquid and solid forms of the challenge substance, readily at hand may prevent delays. Allowing the use of well-cleansed utensils and dinnerware that are familiar to the child (e.g. a favorite cup or plate) makes the challenge more natural appearing. Diversions such as toys, games, or videotapes are helpful. Since splattered or drooled food can elicit a local skin reaction from direct skin contact (but not necessarily from ingestion), it is helpful to have wet napkins on hand and straws for liquid challenges. Similarly, when performing OFCs with children, it is better to feed them rather than to let them feed themselves and risk splattering.

The set-up for a DBPCFC is more complicated than what is needed for open or single-blind challenges. Although the procedure is more labor intensive, it can be carried out in an office setting if the challenge is not high risk [12]. The procedure still introduces graded doses but in this case either a challenge food or a "placebo" food is administered. The aid of a "third party" is needed to prepare the challenges so that the observer and patient are kept unaware whether a true or placebo challenge is being undertaken. A "coin flip" can be used by the third party to randomize the order of administration. The food is hidden either in another food or in opaque capsules. Suggestions for materials to have on hand for creating masked challenges are shown in Table 23.3. It is beneficial to stretch the imagination in trying to best mask foods, especially foods with strong odors. Creating meals that definitively mask taste is often difficult and to do it well requires studies of successful test foods, by tasting panels [38,39]. This procedure may be warranted for challenges performed for research purposes. To prevent false associations, it has been calculated that multiple challenges may be needed, with several placebo and verum feedings, but this procedure has practical limitations [19].

It is easiest to use opaque capsules because bias, possible if masking of foods is done poorly, is eliminated. However, oral symptoms are then bypassed and some patients are unable to ingest enough capsules. Bypassing oral symptoms by using capsules could theoretically result in stronger reactions, should multiple capsules begin to discharge their contents more closely in time than expected. It is often easier to mask liquid into liquid and to use powder or dehydrated forms of foods that can be folded into solid vehicles. Certain flavoring agents such as mint can also help to mask odors. It is important to select vehicles that are clearly tolerated by the patient. If a gritty food is being hidden in a vehicle, then a similarly gritty food should be added as placebo to the carrier vehicle. For example, oat as an allergen mixed in apple sauce may be matched to corn meal in apple sauce. It is also important to appreciate that certain preparation methods (canning, dehydration) may alter the allergens, hence an open challenge with a meal size portion of the food prepared

Table 23.3 Equipment and common foods to stock for use in creating masked food challenges

Equipment	Common allergens	Useful carrier agents
Paper plates, cups utensils	Peanut flour, peanut butter	Proprietary formulas (hydrolyzed casein, amino acid)
Mixing bowls	Powdered egg white	
Scale	Powdered/fresh milk	Baby foods (squash, carrot, potato)
Mortar/pestle	Soy milk, soy flour	
Blender	Wheat breads, flour	Apple sauce
Microwave	Baby foods	Juices

in its natural state for consumption following a negative DBPCFC is essential. It is preferable not to use fatty foods as vehicles since they can delay gastric absorption [40,41].

Depending on the particular food hypersensitivity disorder under consideration, timing of dose administration can be adjusted. For example, when evaluating potentially IgE antibody-mediated reactions, two challenges may be performed on a single day with 2–4 hours between challenges (one is placebo, one is active – so one food is tested each day). The practice of interspersing placebo and active food proteins during a single challenge (i.e. random ordering of sequential doses that may or may not contain the causal protein) should be discouraged since it can be difficult to determine if a reaction shortly after a particular dose, possibly a placebo dose, was actually a delayed response from an active dose administered previously.

Open or single-blind food challenges are typically used clinically instead of DBPCFC to screen for reactions, unless bias is suspected or subjective symptoms are the expected outcome. These open challenges are less labor and time intensive than DBPCFC and objective reactions are usually reliable. Ambiguous results of open or single-blind challenges can be confirmed using a DBPCFC. A negative DBPCFC is followed, usually a few hours later, with a meal sized portion of the food prepared in its natural form to ensure it is tolerated.

Monitoring and stopping a challenge/treatment

Challenges should be performed with appropriate monitoring equipment and emergency treatment medications, equipment, and oxygen immediately available. Medication doses (e.g. epinephrine, steroids, antihistamines, H-2 blockers, glucagons, vasopressors, etc.) should be precalculated by patient weight. The physician or health care worker records the dose given, the time of administration, and any symptoms that arise during the challenge [11]. Forms for recording vital signs, skin, respiratory, gastrointestinal, and cardiovascular examinations have been published [11,12]. Frequent assessments are made for symptoms affecting the skin, gastrointestinal tract, and/or respiratory tract, for example prior to each dose. With children, early indications of a reaction can include subtle signs such as moving the tongue in the mouth to rub an itchy palate, or ear pulling due to referred pruritus. While some families believe increased physical activities (hyperactivity) are a sign of food allergy, a common early response for children as they begin to experience a reaction is that they become suddenly quiet or assume a fetal position as a prodrome to more objective symptoms. Children with atopic dermatitis may develop a maculopapular rash in predilection areas of eczema. Objective monitoring can be done with peak flow or spirometry. Challenges are terminated when a reaction becomes apparent and medications are given, as needed. Judgment is required to decide upon discontinuing a challenge, continuing or modifying the dose, or timing for

subjective symptoms. Generally, antihistamines are given at the earliest sign of a reaction with epinephrine and other treatments given if there is progression of symptoms or any potentially life-threatening symptoms, but this is open to the judgment of the supervising staff, who must take the patient's history into consideration. In some cases, families or individuals may question whether it is necessary to treat the symptoms at all, or may even ask to proceed with more doses to see "how bad" the reaction could be. This is not advisable for obvious safety reasons and also because the reactions are not likely to reflect what a subsequent exposure may cause in an uncontrolled setting.

Patients may be observed for 2 hours or longer as clinically indicated after a negative OFC. Though most reactions occur promptly, it is possible to have late onset symptoms. Observation may be longer if the history indicates prior delayed reactions or if prior reactions were severe. If a reaction was treated, the patient should be observed 2–4 hours or longer past resolution of symptoms depending on the features/severity of the symptoms. During that period, repeated assessments are made and additional therapies used as indicated.

Post-challenge care

There are several issues that need to be addressed when an OFC results in a reaction. The disappointment engendered should be openly discussed. Sometimes patients or families can be partly consoled to know that their hard work at avoidance was necessary and successful. Patients often wish to know if future reactions could be severe, a question whose answer may not be related to the result of the challenge because dosing is gradual rather than sudden and possibly high during accidental exposures. In some cases, it may be apparent that patients were not symptomatic with small exposures during the challenge and may have a margin for error in terms of potential accidental exposures. Patients and families may also inquire as to the possibility that the challenge could "boost" or prime their allergy. While there are no published data to clearly support or refute this concern, the OFC is ultimately the only way to know whether the food is tolerated and is performed clinically when risk assessments are favorable for passing, thus making this concern essentially moot. A plan for re-evaluation with laboratory tests and OFCs should be discussed depending on the usual natural course for the food in question and patient-specific determinants such as age and other food allergies. Review of food avoidance measures is also helpful, and a re-evaluation of any nutritional impact that avoidance may have engendered should be undertaken.

Patients who have passed a challenge often need additional counseling about how to introduce or reintroduce the food. In some cases, a remaining fear could result in continued avoidance. There may also be concerns about re-developing the food allergy, a situation that is quite rare. Patients with remaining food allergies must be cautioned specifically about any increased risk of exposure to an allergen that is commonly associated with the food that they are now able to ingest. For example, a patient with milk and egg allergy who passes an OFC to wheat must be warned to carefully check wheat products, now new to the patient, that may often also contain milk and egg. When there are no remaining food allergies, patients may be loathe to discontinue carrying epinephrine, and this should be discussed as well with consideration for a period of continued availability to reduce stress.

Summary

Elimination diets are used as treatment of a known food allergy or for diagnosis to provide presumptive evidence of causality. OFCs provide a definitive means to determine whether a food is causal of symptoms. The safety of the procedure is ensured by careful gradual dosing, close monitoring, promptly discontinuing administration and providing treatment in the event of symptoms, and providing continued monitoring and therapy as indicated until symptoms resolve. The DBPCFC is considered the "gold standard" for diagnosing a food allergy.

References

1 Sicherer SH, Teuber S. Current approach to the diagnosis and management of adverse reactions to foods. *J Allergy Clin Immunol* 2004;114:1146–50.

2 Sicherer SH. Food allergy: when and how to perform oral food challenges [In Process Citation]. *Pediatr Allergy Immunol* 1999;10:226–34.

3 Sicherer SH, Noone SA, Koerner CB, *et al.* Hypoallergenicity and efficacy of an amino acid-based formula in children with cow's milk and multiple food hypersensitivities. *J Pediatr* 2001;138:688–93.

4 Chehade M, Magid MS, Mofidi S, *et al.* Allergic eosinophilic gastroenteritis with protein-losing enteropathy: intestinal pathology, clinical course, and long-term follow-up. *J Pediatr Gastroenterol Nutr* 2006;42:516–21.

5 Spergel JM, Andrews T, Brown-Whitehorn TF, *et al.* Treatment of eosinophilic esophagitis with specific food elimination diet directed by a combination of skin prick and patch tests. *Ann Allergy Asthma Immunol* 2005;95:336–43.

6 Liacouras CA, Spergel JM, Ruchelli E, *et al.* Eosinophilic esophagitis: a 10-year experience in 381 children. *Clin Gastroenterol Hepatol* 2005;3:1198–206.

7 Joshi P, Mofidi S, Sicherer SH. Interpretation of commercial food ingredient labels by parents of food-allergic children. *J Allergy Clin Immunol* 2002;109:1019–21.

8 Isolauri E, Sutas Y, Salo MK, *et al.* Elimination diet in cow's milk allergy: risk for impaired growth in young children. *J Pediatr* 1998;132:1004–9.

9 David TJ. Anaphylactic shock during elimination diets for severe atopic dermatitis. *Arch Dis Child* 1984;59:983–6.

10 Flinterman AE, Knulst AC, Meijer Y, *et al.* Acute allergic reactions in children with AEDS after prolonged cow's milk elimination diets. *Allergy* 2006;61:370–4.

11 Bock SA, Sampson HA, Atkins FM, *et al.* Double-blind, placebo-controlled food challenge (DBPCFC) as an office procedure: a manual. *J Allergy Clin Immunol* 1988;82:986–97.

12 Food allergy: a practice parameter, American college of Allergy, Asthma and Immunology. *Ann Allergy Asthma Immunol* 2006; 96:S1–68.

13 Sampson HA. Food allergy. Part 2. Diagnosis and management [In Process Citation]. *J Allergy Clin Immunol* 1999;103:981–9.

14 Caffarelli C, Petroccione T. False-negative food challenges in children with suspected food allergy. *Lancet* 2001;358:1871–2.

15 May CD. Objective clinical and laboratory studies of immediate hypersensitivity reactions to food in asthmatic children. *J Allergy Clin Immunol* 1976;58:500–15.

16 Metcalfe D, Sampson H. Workshop on experimental methodology for clinical studies of adverse reactions to foods and food additives. *J Allergy Clin Immunol* 1990;86:421–42.

17 Niggemann B, Wahn U, Sampson HA. Proposals for standardization of oral food challenge tests in infants and children. *Pediatr Allergy Immunol* 1994;5:11–13.

18 Briggs D, Aspinall L, Dickens A, Bindslev-Jensen C. Statistical model for assessing the proportion of subjects with subjective sensitisations in adverse reactions to foods. *Allergy* 2001;56:83–5.

19 Chinchilli VM, Fisher L, Craig TJ. Statistical issues in clinical trials that involve the double-blind, placebo-controlled food challenge. *J Allergy Clin Immunol* 2005;115:592–7.

20 Wilson BG, Bahna SL. Adverse reactions to food additives. *Ann Allergy Asthma Immunol* 2005;95:499–507.

21 Simon RA. Adverse reactions to food additives. *Curr Allergy Asthma Rep* 2003;3:62–6.

22 Busse PJ, Nowak-Wegrzyn AH, Noone SA, *et al.* Recurrent peanut allergy. *N Engl J Med* 2002;347:1535–6.

23 Fleischer DM, Conover-Walker MK, Christie L, *et al.* Peanut allergy: recurrence and its management. *J Allergy Clin Immunol* 2004;114:1195–201.

24 American Academy of Allergy and Immunology. Personnel and equipment to treat systemic reactions caused by immunotherapy with allergenic extracts. *J Allergy Clin Immunol* 1986;77:271–3.

25 Reibel S, Rohr C, Ziegert M, *et al.* What safety measures need to be taken in oral food challenges in children? *Allergy* 2000;55:940–4.

26 Perry TT, Matsui EC, Conover-Walker MK, Wood RA. Risk of oral food challenges. *J Allergy Clin Immunol* 2004;114:1164–8.

27 Sicherer SH. Food protein-induced enterocolitis syndrome: case presentations and management lessons. *J Allergy Clin Immunol* 2005;115:149–56.

28 Bindslev-Jensen C. Standardization of double-blind, placebo-controlled food challenges. *Allergy* 2001;56:75–7.

29 Sicherer SH, Morrow EH, Sampson HA. Dose–response in double-blind, placebo-controlled oral food challenges in

children with atopic dermatitis. *J Allergy Clin Immunol* 2000; 105:582–6.

30 Rance F, Dutau G. Labial food challenge in children with food allergy. *Pediatr Allergy Immunol* 1997;8:41–4.

31 Taylor SL, Hefle SL, Bindslev-Jensen C, *et al*. A consensus protocol for the determination of the threshold doses for allergenic foods: how much is too much? *Clin Exp Allergy* 2004;34:689–95.

32 Skamstrup HK, Vestergaard H, Stahl SP, *et al*. Double-blind, placebo-controlled food challenge with apple. *Allergy* 2001;56:109–17.

33 Gern J, Yang E, Evrard H, Sampson H. Allergic reactions to milk-contaminated "non-dairy" products. *N Engl J Med* 1991;324:976–9.

34 Laoprasert N, Wallen ND, Jones RT, *et al*. Anaphylaxis in a milk-allergic child following ingestion of lemon sorbet containing trace quantities of milk. *J Food Prot* 1998;61:1522–4.

35 Hourihane JB, Kilburn SA, Nordlee JA, *et al*. An evaluation of the sensitivity of subjects with peanut allergy to very low doses of peanut protein: a randomized, double-blind, placebo-controlled food challenge study. *J Allergy Clin Immunol* 1997; 100:596–600.

36 Taylor SL, Hefle SL, Bindslev-Jensen C, *et al*. Factors affecting the determination of threshold doses for allergenic foods: how much is too much? *J Allergy Clin Immunol* 2002;109:24–30.

37 Powell G. Food protein-induced enterocolitis of infancy: differential diagnosis and management. *Compr Ther* 1986;12:28–37.

38 Huijbers GB, Colen AA, Jansen JJ, *et al*. Masking foods for food challenge: practical aspects of masking foods for a double-blind, placebo-controlled food challenge. *J Am Diet Assoc* 1994; 94:645–9.

39 Vlieg-Boerstra BJ, Bijleveld CM, Van Der HS, *et al*. Development and validation of challenge materials for double-blind, placebo-controlled food challenges in children. *J Allergy Clin Immunol* 2004;113:341–6.

40 Grimshaw KE, King RM, Nordlee JA, *et al*. Presentation of allergen in different food preparations affects the nature of the allergic reaction – a case series. *Clin Exp Allergy* 2003;33:1581–5.

41 Teuber SS. Hypothesis: the protein body effect and other aspects of food matrix effects. *Ann NY Acad Sci* 2002;964:111–16.

CHAPTER 24

General Approach to Diagnosis: IgE- and Non-IgE-Mediated Reactions

S. Allan Bock and Hugh A. Sampson

KEY CONCEPTS

- Thorough and complete history and physical examination are critical to the diagnosis of food allergy.

- It is important to review the possible diagnoses with the patient/parents.

- Appropriate *in vitro* and *in vivo* testing will often narrow or confirm the diagnosis.

- Educating patients/parents about how to strictly avoid particular food allergens and how to recognize early signs of an allergic reaction and to initiate emergency therapy is the only approved form of treatment at this time.

- Ongoing education especially for the management of life-threatening conditions is a critical part of patient care.

- Periodic re-evaluation is necessary to ensure that patients are maintaining appropriate allergen-avoidance diets and maintaining appropriate vigilance to prevent an accidental allergic reaction.

Introduction

Over the last three decades our understanding of adverse food reactions, known to have or likely to have an immunologic basis, has expanded significantly [1–4]. This has occurred as the incidence and prevalence of these conditions has also increased significantly [4–8]. The goal of this chapter is to present an overview of the approach to the evaluation and management of these conditions based on evidence acquired through basic and clinical studies into these illnesses. Immediate hypersensitivity, IgE-mediated conditions are understood the best at this time, from both a basic science and clinical point of view. As their frequency and perhaps severity have increased, our understanding of how to diagnose and manage them has improved as well to the point that a cogent approach may be recommended. By contrast the non-immediate, non-IgE-medicated group of conditions continues to present a challenge from both a diagnostic and a management standpoint (Fig. 24.1).

In understanding patients with complaints of adverse reactions to food that may have an immune basis, one may approach the evaluation by considering the group of symptoms and trying to categorize them, or by thinking in terms of possible immunologic mechanisms, or by a combination

of these approaches [3,4,9]. The combination approach is advocated in this discussion. Once a likely diagnosis is established, it is important to be able to communicate this to the patient/parents and to design a plan for ongoing care, education, and periodic re-evaluation. For those conditions that are less well defined, it is crucial to help families understand that the search for understanding of the condition is continuous and may be more of a process than a single interaction.

At this time there is also some controversy about definitions of the various categories of adverse food reactions. Therefore it is crucially important that authors define their terms carefully and completely. For this discussion the various conditions will be divided, as noted above, into IgE-mediated and non-IgE-mediated conditions with an additional discussion of those that seem to be overlap conditions with multiple immune mechanisms [3,4,10–12].

An important goal of this discussion is to outline an approach to patients with a history of adverse food reactions that can be applied in a timely and practical manner. It is important to be able to acquire a thorough and detailed history as concisely as possible and then to design an approach to each individual's problem. Once the diagnosis is made and the problem categorized, then an ongoing care plan may be designed. This involves the very important components of education concerning the relationship between a food and symptoms, and a plan for continuing education as well as longitudinal re-evaluation.

Food Allergy: Adverse Reactions to Foods and Food Additives, 4th edition.
Edited by Dean D. Metcalfe, Hugh A. Sampson, and Ronald A. Simon.
© 2008 Blackwell Publishing, ISBN: 978-1-4501-5129-0.

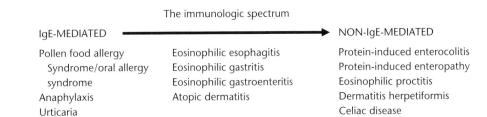

Figure 24.1 Adverse reactions to food.

Table 24.1 Historical features of importance (maybe used to design a challenge)

- Description of symptoms and signs, obtain all details for each food.
- Timing from ingestion to onset of symptoms.
- Frequency with which reactions have occurred.
- Time of most recent occurrence.
- Quantity of food required to evoke the reaction on each occasion.
- Associated factors (activity, medication, alcohol).

When the history is complex consider having the patient/parents list the details for each food on a worksheet that they take home.

IgE-mediated conditions

Most if not all of the IgE-mediated conditions have an immediate onset. The main *cutaneous* symptoms include an eczematous rash (atopic dermatitis), flushing, and urticaria/angioedema. One of the major characteristics of urticarial responses is that their duration is relatively short (minutes to hours). *Gastrointestinal* (GI) symptoms often begin with acute abdominal pain and then quickly progress to nausea and vomiting. However, vomiting may be delayed for several hours depending on the components of the meal. Some individuals will have diarrhea as part of the acute reaction and it may start a few hours after the ingestion and continue for several hours. *Respiratory* symptoms include both the upper and lower airway, and ocular symptoms are often included in this category. Sneezing, profuse rhinorrhea, nasal blockage, mouth and throat swelling, laryngeal edema and laryngospasm, cough (that may sound very harsh and staccato), wheezing, dyspnea, and chest tightness may all be seen in IgE-mediated reactions to food. They may occur singly or in combinations and may mimic other reactions such as acute aeroallergen exposure. The *ocular* symptoms of chemosis, scleral edema, and eyelid edema are often quite impressive and disabling. *Cardiovascular* signs may appear without any GI, respiratory, or cutaneous signs or symptoms. The blood pressure may drop precipitously, there may be palpitations and the peripheral vasodilation of an allergic reaction may fool observers. There may also be signs and symptoms that are less specific and harder to classify. For example patients may complain of feeling dizzy or light headed without other localizing symptoms. Another symptom that is often confusing is cramping lower abdominal pain in women.

The situation is clarified when the patient (often in embarrassment) says that she is feeling like she is going to have a baby. Indeed uterine pain and contractions may be the first or only symptom of an acute allergic reaction. These, then, are the signs and symptoms most commonly seen in IgE-mediated, immediate hypersensitivity reaction.

With these as a background, an experienced clinician will use the history to detect patterns of presentation that suggest IgE-mediated food reactions (Table 24.1). The history may begin with the patient giving a narrative but may be directed to obtain facts about the following issues. It is important and useful to encourage the patient to present the details of each food individually. What are the symptoms and, if possible, in what order did they occur and with what timing. When was the first reaction (at what age)? How many reactions have occurred and are the details of each recalled? Can the details of food preparation and quantity ingested be recalled? The details of the most recent reaction for each food should be elicited, as they are often the ones best recalled. Have any foods that contain the putative culprit been ingested recently without symptoms having occurred? What treatment was used if any? Was the individual seen in an ED or other medical facility and are records available that might give more details about the physical findings and treatment? At times the details recorded by the paramedics who transported the patient may also list information that is not otherwise recalled.

There are additional factors that should be included in the history including whether or not activity (exercise) was involved, a list of the patient's medication, and in situations where there is a known historical food culprit, but a recent event does not clearly incriminate the known culprit, then whether cross-contact or outright contamination (dust mites) could have occurred. In adults one should determine if there is non-steroidal anti-inflammatory usage or if alcohol accompanied the meal precipitating the reaction [13–17].

When the patient presents with a complaint of an adverse food reaction, the details are often elicited with some leading questions, but often the patient comes with a totally different complaint and the issue of food allergy is only determined by direct questioning. New patients, even those complaining of seasonal allergy symptoms will often neglect to mention the oral symptoms commonly present in oral allergy syndrome/pollen–food allergy syndrome (see Chapter 12) [18]. It is often surprising how long the list of avoided foods is without being mentioned in the absence of direct questioning. During the evaluation of this condition it is crucial to distinguish between true local non-life-threatening reactions and those that are potentially fatal [19].

Another omission is in the care of a long-standing patient who develops a new food allergy (a reaction to shellfish in an adult), and this is not mentioned unless the interim historical questions are directly concerned with food allergy. Sometimes these particular sets of facts are mentioned in passing as the patient is leaving the visit or to the nurse at some point in the appointment. This requires a pause while appropriate questions are asked and answers sought because some of these new "allergies" are life threatening and need full investigation, protective education, and a prescription of epinephrine [20].

The physical examination seeks stigmata of IgE-mediated reactions. Unless the examination occurs in immediate proximity to the reaction, there may be no significant findings. If urticaria is present, the duration should be queried. Urticaria persisting for several days to weeks makes IgE-mediated reaction less likely unless there is a food in the diet that is being consumed daily [21]. Extensive atopic dermatitis may indicate an allergy to a food in the diet that has not been identified and excluded.

Respiratory signs including chronic rhinorrhea, cough, wheezing, and chronic ear changes (serous otitis media, eustachian tube dysfunction) are often attributed to food allergy, but isolated respiratory symptoms, without GI or cutaneous symptoms, are unlikely to be due to food allergy, especially in children. (The issue of chronic rhinitis/congestion in adults remains an anecdotal observation that has been frequently reported but has not been confirmed by blinded food challenges.)

Testing for IgE-mediated food allergy has advanced significantly over the last three decades [3,4]. It is possible to use the history combined with skin testing for many foods and *in vitro* serum antibody measurements to refine the diagnosis and decrease the number of food challenges that may be required.

Skin testing for food allergy is best performed using the prick skin test and commercially available extracts for a number of foods. While it is still true that more highly standardized food allergen extracts need to be developed, those that are available may be quite useful. It remains the job of the practitioner to be certain that the extracts that are being used are "verified." This means that one has demonstrated that the material specified on the label actually detects antibody in sensitized subjects. It is not unheard of for a commercial extract to contain no detectable allergenic protein. It is also true that for most fruit and vegetable extracts, the commercial material may not be very potent because many of the allergenic proteins in these foods are unstable and breakdown during preparation. For these foods it is more useful to use the "prick and prick" method

employing fresh foods and vegetables [22]. However, it must be remembered that a negative skin test with a fresh fruit or vegetable may have a low predictive accuracy while a positive result may be more useful.

At this time there are a number of very useful studies of skin testing (see Chapter 21), especially in young children that predict the likelihood of a clinically significant reaction upon challenge, thus obviating the need for the challenge. In children the foods that have been best studied, with predictable results, are egg white, cow's milk, peanut, and many of the tree nuts, although additional studies of the tree nuts would be welcomed [23–28]. Another point to keep in mind is the fact that the negative predictive accuracy of the commonly used food skin tests is greater in older subjects and lower in younger ones. By contrast, the positive predictive accuracy for selected foods may be higher in younger subjects and lower in older individuals. For some of the most commonly incriminated foods, the skin test sensitivity and specificity are not very good, with wheat being perhaps the most notable example. There are also some useful studies for a limited list of foods in adults [29,30].

Advances in the use of *in vitro testing* have also been quite significant especially for the major food allergens (see Chapter 20). The development of "decision points" and predictive curves has been extremely helpful to the practitioner [29,30–39]. Skill in applying these values allows the prediction of a positive food challenge and will decrease the number of food challenges that may be needed in the clinical setting. Serial measurements over time have shown that for some foods in some individuals, the decrease in the measured level will predict when the food allergy is "outgrown" and when it is likely that the challenge will be negative. Comments regarding skin testing may also be applied to *in vitro* testing. The foods for which the most useful information is available are egg white, cow's milk, and peanut. Data for tree nut "cut-off" values is accumulating and further studies for both tree nuts and other foods should be forthcoming and helpful. As with skin testing, *in vitro* serum antibody measurements for wheat and for soy have not proven to have the hope for predictive accuracies. As with skin test studies, very little data exist on adults (Table 24.2).

Table 24.2 Practical use of testing: *in vivo/in vitro*

- Choose the tests that fit the history instead of using panels or lists.
- Use skin tests first in most situations.
- Use *in vitro* tests especially in situations where there is data to give predictive information on the likelihood of a reaction during challenge. This should increase the number of negative challenges.
- Use the data from both tests to decide on performance of a challenge.
- Always use the historical details and the context to interpret the results of testing.

The details of *food challenges* have been reviewed in Chapter 23. How do food challenges fit into the current scheme of the evaluation for IgE-mediated food allergy and what is their future? Food challenges became the "gold standard" for the confirmation or refutation of true adverse reactions to food beginning with Charles May's publication in 1976 [40]. The procedure has evolved over the last 30 years, especially as it may be applied in the clinical setting, be it a private office or hospital clinic [39–51]. The techniques used for research purposes may be modified for use in daily practice where open challenges are often utilized to demonstrate that certain foods are not currently causing symptoms (*see Algorithm 1 for IgE-mediated reactions*). The process begins with the elimination diet that is used to

determine whether the symptoms that have been reported will resolve with the removal of one or more foods from the diet. The elimination diet may be as simple as the removal of a single food or as complex as the provision of a "few food diet" that is maintained for several days to about 2 weeks. If the symptoms resolve, then either food challenges performed with the food or foods incriminated, or if a very limited diet is being used, a normal diet may be restarted to see if the symptoms return (this approach is not used when evaluating histories of anaphylaxis).

Oral food challenges may be performed openly, single blindly, or double blindly with placebo control. The particular technique depends on the history that is to be reproduced, the degree of subjectivity of the complaint, the goals

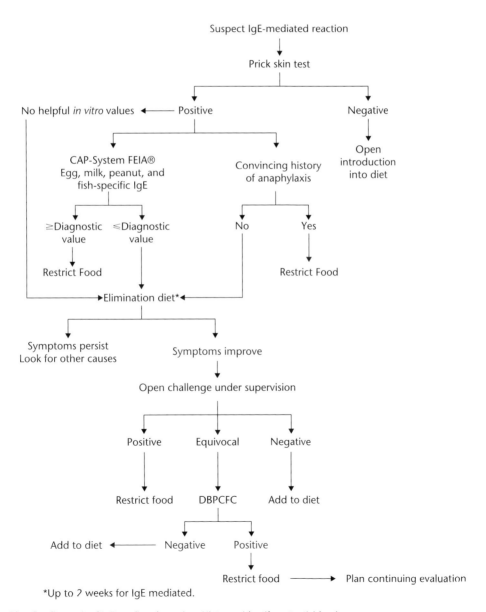

Algorithm 1 Algorithm for diagnosis of IgE-mediated reaction: History – identify potential foods.

of the patient, and the ability of the observers (including the patient/parents) to be objective. When challenge demonstrates that the food is tolerated it is added to the diet to be consumed in usual portions prepared by all the customary means. Once the food is in the diet, there must be some follow-up to be certain that the food is in fact tolerated over the long term. It has recently been recommended that negative peanut challenges (and probably nut challenges as well) be followed by regular consumption of the food to decrease the possible risk of redeveloping clinical reactivity [52]. This does not appear to be a risk for any of the other common (or uncommon) food culprits, especially egg, milk, and wheat.

When food challenges are positive, then one must consider whether the observations and reports of symptoms and signs are accurate. The more objective the symptoms and signs, the less likely that patient/parent/observer bias enters into the situation. However if the reported reaction is subjective (headache, abdominal pain, nausea without vomiting, oral pruritus, throat symptoms, or joint complaints), then a regular plan of follow-up and re-challenge must be arranged. All of the subsequent challenges of subjective symptoms should be arranged to be blinded.

Continuing evaluation and management

Once it has been determined that one or more foods should be eliminated from the diet, the practitioner in conjunction with the patient/family must outline a plan for ongoing care. This may be as simple as recommending a return for retesting in a year or a plan for more regular visits and challenges at regular intervals. The intervals are determined by the history, the most recent reaction, the results of *in vivo* and *in vitro* testing, and the family's wishes. It is a good idea to encourage the family to maintain a log of any reactions with as many details as possible so that these events may be used to modify the ongoing care plan. Suggested details in the log should include a brief description of the symptoms, the food consumed, the quantity consumed if it is known, the circumstances of preparation or accidental ingestion (milk poured into a milk allergic child's cup or drinking from the wrong cup), the treatment if any, and the duration of the symptoms.

Treatment of IgE-mediated immediate food reactions

When avoidance measures fail, the reactions usually involve the symptoms outlined above and in previous chapters, and the treatment is relatively straightforward with a number of caveats. For mild symptoms (skin, mild abdominal pain, nausea) no treatment may be necessary or perhaps oral antihistamines could be used to improve patient comfort. For more severe symptoms, especially anything threatening the airway or cardiovascular system,

epinephrine should be administered by injection and the Emergency Medical System (appropriate to the location) should be activated. The caveats involve issues of when to use antihistamines or epinephrine. There is no universal agreement on this subject, and even among nations there are differences of opinion among the medical communities. Two recent meetings of physicians from many nations have attempted to formulate some testable questions to address these issues [53,54]. For example, should epinephrine be given at the first sign of a reaction in a patient known to have ingested an allergen that has produced mild symptoms previously or systemic symptoms previously? Many practitioners would say maybe to the former and definitely to the latter. Some families would prefer to delay the administration of epinephrine and others would prefer to inject it promptly. These are issues that, while not having simple, universally agreed upon answers, need to be individualized for each patient with the problem. Eventually it is hoped that research will yield more concrete recommendations based on controlled observations; however, the chance of ever designing a true controlled trial of these difficult problems is unlikely for ethical reasons. Nevertheless, protocols that may serve as guidelines are likely to be forthcoming. Meanwhile clinicians can develop their own written plans that may be modified in each situation [55–64].

Education

As has been pointed out elsewhere, avoidance with proper education is the only currently recommended means of "treating" IgE-mediated food allergy. (There are new treatments on the horizon that we may hope will soon be available; see Chapter 47.) It must be made clear to patients/families that this is an ongoing process and not a single event (see Chapter 36). Once the diagnosis has been made and presented to families, there are a number of different reactions ranging from acceptance with many questions to denial and unwillingness to take the results seriously. In any case, there is a great deal of helpful information that must be presented in an efficient manner at the time of the initial diagnosis. Usually numerous questions are raised and will be raised over the ensuing weeks to months. Arrangements must be made to address these concerns in an ongoing manner. For these purposes there are excellent materials available especially from the Food Allergy and Anaphylaxis Network (www.foodallergy.org) [65,66].

Case examples

A few illustrative examples may be helpful. Case #1: A 2-year-old boy is brought to the allergist with moderate atopic dermatitis that has been difficult to control at times, but overall it seems to be slowly improving with consistent skin care measures. The mother is anxious for the problem to resolve completely and is resistant to using topical prescription medications. She has modified the child's diet both while nursing (up to 8 months of age when he was weaned) and since weaning by limiting his milk intake, but not using a dairy product-free diet. The child is also avoiding whole eggs but eats egg-containing foods. The skin tests detect antibody to egg with a 5 mm wheal and to milk with a 3 mm wheal. The histamine skin test is 3 mm and the negative control is negative. Skin testing for peanut, wheat, and soy do not detect antibody. The serum antibody level to milk is 5 kU/l and to egg it is 1.5 kU/l. A diet completely free of dairy and egg results in easier to manage atopic dermatitis but not complete resolution. Open food challenges are performed in the physician's office. The milk challenge is negative and dairy is introduced into the child's diet with no change in the eczema control. The egg challenge results in a few small hives on the child's face with a prompt increase in irritability and pruritus over the subsequent few hours. By late in the day there is an increase in erythema and papular dermatitis in the flexural areas where the child usually has atopic dermatitis lesions.

While this example is fairly straightforward, it does make some important points. Food elimination diets rarely eliminate eczematous lesions completely. While it could be argued that this child should have a more complete elimination diet, parents are often content to find that simple measures lead to improvement and easier management. As is often the case, antibodies are detected by both skin testing and *in vitro* measurement, but are not always predictive of a reaction. In this situation, there appears to be asymptomatic sensitization to milk and symptomatic sensitization to egg. In the end, only the challenge makes the situation clear. However, the ongoing evaluation and management is quite important and it was suggested that the egg-allergy status be re-evaluated in 6 months.

Case #2: A 28-year-old woman presents with concerns about reactions to tree nuts. She knows that she can eat peanuts and is certain that almond, walnut, and pecan can be ingested without a problem, although she has tended to minimize her nut consumption. Her last identifiable reaction occurred when she was eating nuts in the shell that she and her husband were cracking and eating. She is certain that hazelnuts, Brazil nuts, and almonds were in the bowl. The symptoms that developed were itching in the mouth and a feeling that her tongue and lips were swelling slightly. There may have been some difficulty swallowing but no problem breathing. There were no GI symptoms, no urticaria, and no definite respiratory symptoms. She is about to spend a month in Europe and would like the list narrowed as much as possible. She is very concerned about reacting to hazelnuts. Her skin tests detected antibody to walnut, almond, hazelnut, and Brazil nut, each being 3 mm. There was no detectable antibody to cashew,

pecan, and pistachio. The histamine skin test was 3 mm and the negative control was negative. Serum antibody levels were below the level of detection for all of the nuts. Challenges were performed openly and were negative to all but the Brazil nut, which reproduced the symptoms that she described. She was instructed to eat various tree nuts, except Brazil nuts, regularly before her trip, to carry self-injectable epinephrine on the trip, and to learn the words for each of the tree nuts in the languages of the countries to which she was traveling. As in the case of the 2-year-old boy above, the only definitive way to achieve her stated goals was with food challenges, but the *in vivo* and *in vitro* data allowed the challenges to be arranged with a feeling that they would be safe and useful. Some might argue that a completely different approach should be used, namely to have her avoid all tree nuts all the time. While this may be the correct advice in some situations and when the culprit is more commonly found in the diet and therefore more difficult to avoid, in this situation, the approach was guided by the patient's goals and wishes which were accomplished.

Non-IgE-mediated conditions

The main non-IgE-mediated food reactions that have data to support an immunologic basis occur in the GI tract and in the skin. Whether non-IgE-mediated immune reactions in the respiratory system are due to food remains the subject or research. Similarly neurologic symptoms due to immune reactions to food are likely to be the subject of future research as our ability to study the physiology of the central nervous system advances.

The non-IgE-mediated reactions involving the GI tract begin at the mouth and end in the colon. Some of them may actually be a spectrum that might involve IgE as well as being primarily a non-IgE-mediated condition (see next section). Involvement of the small intestine involves several conditions that may be overlapping. Cow's milk-protein enteropathy, soy-protein enteropathy, and probably other less well-defined food culprits produce changes in the intestinal mucosa that share a number of characteristic with celiac disease (gluten-sensitive enteropathy). The prototypic condition, celiac disease, results in an extreme alteration of the intestine with total villous atrophy in contrast to the more patchy lesions and less severe villous alterations in the other protein enteropathies. These conditions are usually found in young children and unlike celiac disease are almost always outgrown [67]. However, there are sporadic case reports of older children and adults whose condition does not remit. In young children, the usual presentation of these conditions occurs in the first few months of life and include protracted diarrhea (sometimes with steatorrhea) and failure to thrive [68]. One factor that may delay diagnosis is the finding that exclusively breast-fed children may have these conditions due to the proteins in their mother's diet crossing her intestinal barrier and then being excreted into her breast milk. (This is also true for IgE-mediated GI symptoms.) The proteins are intact enough from the mother's mouth to the infant's gut to trigger the pathologic changes.

Infantile cow's milk-induced colitis appears in the first few weeks to months of life and is characterized by visible blood in the stools (see Chapter 16). Removal of cow's milk from the infants diet (including the lactation diet if the mother is nursing) results in prompt resolution of the symptoms. In the earlier stages of this illness, when it is usually diagnosed by the primary care practitioner, there are rarely any other signs or symptoms. At this time the immune mechanism remains poorly defined.

A more severe condition is food-protein-induced entero-colitis syndrome (FPIES) in which the small and large intestines are involved (see Chapter 17). These infants may present when they are quite ill. They often have protracted vomiting and diarrhea with irritability and diarrhea that is severe enough to result in dehydration and require fluid resuscitation. They often present having had multiple episodes. While cow's milk and soy proteins are the most frequent cause of this condition, it is clear that other proteins including those in unsuspected solid foods may be responsible for this condition (e.g. rice, barley, beef, peanut). A high index of suspicion, familiarity with the syndrome, and careful

questioning will often lead to the diagnosis. This is the one condition in which it seems mandatory to undertake food challenges in the hospital with resuscitation equipment available. It is often recommended that food challenges be performed in these children with and indwelling catheter, since volume expansion is the mainstay of therapy [69–73].

As pointed out in several earlier chapters, the diagnosis of these conditions is likely to require a gastroenterologist for evaluation, endoscopy, and biopsy (optimal) to define the exact condition. Food challenges to confirm the exact foods require great care, especially with FPIES, and meticulous precautions. It is important to discourage families from reintroducing foods into the child's diet outside a medical setting. Close longitudinal care, often using a team approach, will ensure an optimal outcome for these youngsters whose condition usually resolves with time (see Algorithm 2 for non-IgE-mediated conditions).

Dermatitis herpetiformis is a skin condition that accompanies celiac disease in some individuals. It may be confused with and treated as atopic dermatitis, but when the GI condition is discovered and the diet altered, the skin lesions typically resolve.

There are a small group of young children who have been reported to have pulmonary hemosiderosis in association with the consumption of cow's milk, a condition termed

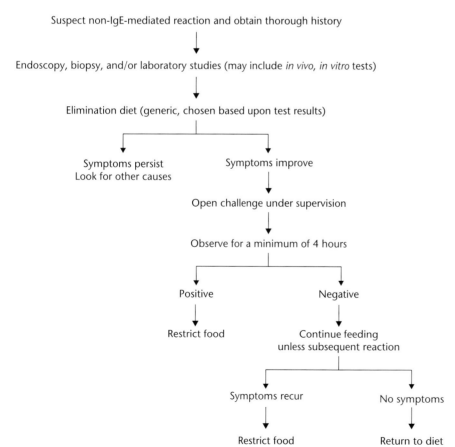

Algorithm 2 Algorithm for diagnosis of non-IgE-mediated immediate food hypersensitivity reactions.

Heiner's syndrome [74]. Removal of cow's milk from the diet brings about resolution of the pulmonary hemorrhages and the children begin to thrive. The mechanism of this condition has been thought to involve cell-mediated events, but this has not been proven. The exact pathophysiology, incidence, and natural history of this condition remain to be better defined.

A number of patients have incriminated food proteins in the exacerbation of their arthritis (see Chapter 45) [75]. There is one case of this being documented by blinded food challenge. At this time it seems inadvisable to recommend large numbers of arthritis sufferers removing foods from their diets. Additional studies in this area would be welcomed.

Combined or mixed conditions

The allergic eosinophilic conditions are illnesses that seem to be increasing in incidence and prevalence. Recent work has shed some light on the mechanism and genetics of eosinophilic esophagitis [7,8]. The symptoms that should call attention to the possibility of this condition may only be elicited by directed questioning. In older patients, asking about difficulty swallowing, substernal chest discomfort, food becoming lodged in the esophagus requiring visits for urgent care, and early satiety are often present either singly or in combination. As noted in an earlier chapter (see Chapter 16), there is general and growing consensus about the biopsy appearance and number of eosinophils present within the biopsy sample to make a diagnosis of eosinophilic esophagitis. Earlier referral for endoscopy will often decrease the duration of patient suffering [76]. The proper use of diagnostic tests to arrive at a practical food elimination program remains difficult. Prick skin testing and atopy patch testing remain under study as means to more accurately identify food culprits [77–79]. Clinicians must help patients determine just how strict a diet they can tolerate and the recommended duration of the dietary restriction, before embarking on a diet. A recent report in children indicated that a six-food elimination diet will result in marked improvement in the majority of patients [80]. Treatment with medication [81,82] and the provision of an allergen-avoidance diet could be recommended by GI and allergy specialists and individualized for patient preferences. One of the ongoing issues is having an endpoint to follow in order to determine the effectiveness of the diet and medication. While serial biopsies are optimal, it may be difficult to get patients to agree to this program.

Further down the intestine there are also eosinophilic infiltrative conditions in the stomach and intestines that currently seem to be somewhat less common. It is even harder to demonstrate immune reactions to foods for reasons similar to those mentioned above. Food challenges in these patients do not give immediate responses and

elimination diets and food reintroduction require meticulous observation over weeks, making the accurate diagnosis difficult.

Atopic dermatitis is another condition in which multiple immunologic mechanisms appear to be involved. The sequence of immune events that are now becoming better defined gives us insight into the extremely complex nature of this condition. It is clear from challenge studies that there are immediate changes in the skin following food allergen ingestion. These initial changes are then followed by a sequence of ongoing cellular events. Studies as outlined in Chapter 10 make it clear that there are many factors contributing to the chronic skin changes seen in these individuals. By extrapolation, one must wonder whether the GI conditions mentioned above will ultimately be found to have a similar process of initiation and then perpetuation. While IgE-mediated skin tests are often helpful in these individuals, the benefit of prolonged elimination diets must be clearly shown to be helpful. It is often useful to remind parents/patients that atopic dermatitis is a complex disease with multiple precipitating factors and that it is uncommon for food elimination to bring about complete resolution of the condition. There are times when skin symptoms seem to wax and wane, and parents may want to attribute this to new food allergies. However, this may be due to a variety of environmental factors or "unknown" factors, but it may be useful for families to maintain a food diary for a short period of time to determine if culprit foods are inadvertently being ingested as components of other foods.

Migraine headaches have been shown in a few patients to be triggered by apparent adverse food reactions (see Chapter 42). These studies seemed to show the relationship with the culprit food and the headache, but the number of patients reported has been small, and no subsequent systematic investigation confirming these observations has been reported [83].

Longitudinal evaluation, management, and the importance of education (Tables 24.3 and 24.4)

While we await treatments and a cure for food allergy, the longitudinal evaluation, management, and importance of family and community education cannot be overstated. It is generally acknowledged that there are numerous unreported deaths from food allergy. We certainly know of a number of these and they are almost all preventable tragedies [84–87]. Where are the problems? The current answers suggest that they fall into a few large categories. The ongoing evaluation of children with IgE-mediated food allergy will help determine which problems are going to be present for the long term and which have or are likely to resolve. Even young children with peanut and tree nut allergy experience remission of their allergic reactions in about 20% of cases [88–90].

Table 24.3 Education issues

- Educate the medical profession to ask about food allergy, and promptly diagnose it.
- Urge the patients to be evaluated by an allergist with knowledge in the identification of food allergen culprit(s) and the ability to educate patients and those around them.
- Prescribe epinephrine and insist that patients carry it, check periodically that patients are complying.
- Educate patients about the diagnosis, the importance of asking about ingredients, symptom recognition, and discrimination between asthma flares and anaphylaxis.
- Undertake age appropriate education of youngsters and use handouts that emphasize particular points.
- Check the availability of epinephrine to emergency medical services in local areas and urge prompt dispatch of paramedics or EMTs who can carry and administer epinephrine.
- Improve school personnel education including food preparation and staff training. Be certain that school plans are updated and understood.
- Educate the public about the potential fatal nature of food allergy and its recognition.
- Educate the restaurant industry concerning the full and complete disclosure of food ingredients and assisting patrons in identifying ingredients that could cause reactions.

Table 24.4 Practical approach to continuing evaluation

- Meet with patients regularly to review the history of accident ingestions and symptoms that may have occurred.
- Determine if repeated *in vivo/in vitro* testing is indicated.
- Use history and testing results to design and perform appropriate food challenges.
- Review educational and research information and long-term expectations.
- Help patients interpret information obtained from public sources.

Continuing research is seeking to determine the recurrence rate for these particular problems. The natural history of milk and egg allergy is much more encouraging since most children (i.e. about 80%) lose their clinical reactivity. The situation in older children and adults with food allergy that will not remit requires a different approach. These patients need regular contact with a physician to reinforce the serious nature of some IgE-mediated food allergies (peanut, tree nuts, fish, and shellfish most commonly). The annual review of checklists and handouts that include updates on the latest research will offer patients both education and hope for resolution of the problem. This review will reinforce the important specifics of avoidance, the availability of emergency medication, and the assistance and crucial importance of educating people around them (e.g. baby-sitters, teachers, coaches, friends). A number of the documented fatalities could have been prevented if the patient had inquired about

a meal's ingredients, but just as importantly, they could have been prevented if the people around them were watchful and protective. Fear of embarrassment often leads adolescents and young adults to hide their severe food allergy problems. Better education of the community about these conditions is an ongoing and important issue. Fortunately progress is being made in schools, restaurants, camps, and other public places. Unfortunately, interpersonal education continues to be inadequate and we need programs to improve this situation (one important program is the FAAN PAL program). Specific tools for patients and for the use of physicians are available and their dissemination is a continuing goal.

With respect to the non-IgE-mediated food reactions, the problems of ongoing care and management are somewhat different. While these conditions are very unlikely to be fatal, they can be extremely debilitating. Helping patients identify effective diets and then sustaining them for prolonged periods is particularly difficult and requires regular contact. The reward is that the patient begins to feel better. Fortunately there are support organizations for these conditions. American Partnership for Eosinophilic Disorders: www.apfed.org; Celiac Sprue Association: www.csaceliacs.org.

In conclusion, IgE-mediated and non-IgE-mediated conditions represent a spectrum of illness for which the molecular biology is being unraveled. Our diagnostic tools have improved, our ability to be helpful has increased, and the prospect for treatments and ultimately prevention look bright.

References

1 Sampson HA. Food allergy. Part 1. Immunopathogenesis and clinical disorders. *J Allergy Clin Immunol* 1999;103:717–29.

2 Sampson HA. Food allergy. Part 2. Diagnosis and management. *J Allergy Clin Immunol* 1999;103:981–9.

3 Sampson HA. Update on food allergy. *J Allergy Clin Immunol* 2004;113:805–19.

4 Sicherer SH, Sampson HA. Food allergy. *J Allergy Clin Immunol* 2006;117:S470–5.

5 Sicherer SH, Munoz-Furlong A, Burks AW, Sampson HA. Prevalence of peanut and tree nut allergy in the US determined by a random digit dial telephone survey. *J Allergy Clin Immunol* 1999;103:559–62.

6 Sicherer SH, Munoz-Furlong A, Sampson HA. Prevalence of peanut and tree nut allergy in the United States determined by means of a random digit dial telephone survey: a 5-year follow-up study. *J Allergy Clin Immunol* 2003;112:1203–7.

7 Guajardo JR, Plotnick LM, Fende JM, *et al.* Eosinophil-associated gastrointestinal disorders: a world-wide-web based registry. *J Pediatr* 2002;141:576–81.

8 Rothenberg ME. Eosinophilic gastrointestinal disorders EGID. *J Allergy Clin Immunol* 2004;113:11–28.

9 Bock SA. Diagnostic evaluation. *Pediatrics* 2003;111:1636–44.

10 Chapman JA, Bernstein IL, Lee RE, Oppenheimer JO (eds.). Food allergy: a practice parameter. *Ann Allergy Asthma Immunol* 2006;96:S1–68.

11 Bruijnzeel-Koomen C, Ortolani C, Aas K, *et al.* Adverse reactions to food (position paper). *Allergy* 1995;50:623–35.

12 Johansson SG, Bieber T, Dahl R, *et al.* Revised nomenclature for allergy for global use: *Report of the Nomenclature Review Committee of the World Allergy Organization*, October 2003. *J Allergy Clin Immunol* 2004;113:832–6.

13 Wen DC, Shyur SD, Ho CM, *et al.* Systemic anaphylaxis after the ingestion of pancake contaminate with the storage mite *Blomia freemani*. *Ann Allergy Asthma Immunol* 2005; 95:612–14.

14 Aihara M, Miyazawa M, Osuna H, *et al.* Food-dependent exercise induced anaphylaxis: influence of concurrent aspirin administration on skin testing and provocation. *Br J Derm* 2002;146:466–72. Some FDEIA pts should not take ASA, it may enhance the problem.

15 Aihara Y, Kotoyori T, Takahashi Y, *et al.* The necessity for dual food intake to provoke food-dependent exercise-induced anaphylaxis (FEIAn): a case report of FEIAn with simultaneous intake of wheat and umeboshi. *J Allergy Clin Immunol* 2001;107:1100–5.

16 Aihara Y, Takahashi Y, Kotoyori T, *et al.* Frequency of food-dependent, exercise induced anaphylaxis in Japanese high school students. *J Allergy Clin Immunol* 2001;108:1035–9.

17 Maulitz RM, Pratt DS, Schocket AL. Exercise-induced anaphylaxic reaction to shellfish. *J Allergy Clin Immunol* 1979; 63:433–4.

18 Osterballe M, Hansen TK, Mortz CG, Bindslev-Jensen C. The clinical relevance of sensitization to pollen-related fruits and vegetables in unselected pollen-sensitized adults. *Allergy* 2005;60:218–25.

19 Monserrat F-R, Bolhaar S, Gonzalez-Mancebo E, *et al.* Apple allergy across Europe: how allergen sensitization profiles determine the clinical expression of allergies to plant foods. *J Allergy Clin Immunol* 2006;118:481–8.

20 Sicherer SH, Munoz-Furlong A, Sampson HA. Prevalence of seafood allergy in the United States determined by a random telephone survey. *J Allergy Clin Immunol* 2004; 114:159–65.

21 Goodman DL, McDonnell JT, Nelson HS, *et al.* Chronic urticaria exacerbated by the antioxidant food preservatives, butylated hydroxyanisole (BHA) and butylated hydroxytoluene (BHT). *J Allergy Clin Immunol* 1990;86:570–5.

22 Rance F, Juchet A, Bremont F, Dutau G. Correlations between skin prick tests using commercial extracts and fresh foods, specific IgE, and food challenges. *Allergy* 1997;52: 1031–5.

23 Hill DJ, Hosking CS, Reyes-Benito LV. Reducing the need for food allergen challenges in young children: a comparison of *in vitro* with *in vivo* tests. *Clin Exp Allergy* 2001;31:1031–5.

24 Hill DJ, Heine RG, Hosking C. The diagnostic value of skin prick testing in children with food allergy. *Pediatr Allergy Immunol* 2004;15:435–41. Good review of all DJH studies.

25 Eigenmann PA, Sampson HA. Interpreting skin prick tests in the evaluation of food allergy in children. *Pediatr Allergy Immunol* 1998;9:186–91.

26 Knight AK, Shreffler WG, Sampson HA, *et al.* Skin prick test to egg white provides additional diagnostic utility to serum egg white-specific IgE antibody concentration in children. *J Allergy Clin Immunol* 2006;117:842–7.

27 Hansen TK, Host A, Bindslev-Jensen C. An evaluation of the diagnostic value of different skin tests with egg in clinically egg-allergic children having atopic dermatitis. *Pediatr Allergy Immunol* 2004;15:428–34.

28 Verstege A, Mehl A, Rolinck-Werninghaus C, *et al.* The predictive value of the skin prick test weal size for the outcome of oral food challenges. *Clin Exp Allergy* 2005;35:1220–6.

29 Bjornsson E, Janson C, Plaschke P, *et al.* Prevalence of sensitization to food allergens in adult Swedes. *Ann Allergy Asthma Immunol* 1996;77:327–32.

30 Norgaard A, Skov PS, Bindslev-Jensen C. Egg and milk allergy in adults: comparison between fresh foods and commercial allergen extracts in skin prick test and histamine release from basophils. *Clin Exp Allergy* 1992;22:940–7.

31 Sampson HA, Ho DG. Relationship between food-specific IgE concentrations and the risk of positive food challenges in children and adolescents. *JACI* 1997;100:444–51.

32 Sampson HA. Utility of food-specific IgE concentrations in predicting symptomatic food allergy. *J Allergy Clin Immunol* 2001;107:891–6.

33 Boyano-Martinez T, Garcia-Ara C, Diaz-Pena JM, *et al.* Validity of specific IgE antibodies in children with egg allergy. *CEA* 2001;31:1464–9.

34 Boyano-Martinez T, Garcia-Ara C, Diaz-Pena JM, Martin-Esteban M. Prediction of tolerance on the basis of quantification of egg white-specific IgE antibodies in children with egg allergy. *J Allergy Clin Immunol* 2002;110:304–9.

35 Garcia-Ara C, Boyano-Martinez T, Diaz-Pena JM, *et al.* Specific IgE levels in the diagnosis of immediate hypersensitivity to cows' milk protein in the infant. *J Allergy Clin Immunol* 2001;107: 185–90. CAP values for milk in infants.

36 Garcia-Ara MC, Boyano-Martinez MT, Diaz-Pena JM, *et al.* Cow's milk specific immunoglobulin E levels as predictors of clinical reactivity in the follow-up of the cow' milk allergy infants. *Clin Exp Allergy* 2004;34:866–70.

37 Perry TT, Matsui EC, Conover-Walker JK, Wood RA. The relationship of allergen specific IgE levels and oral food challenge outcome. *J Allergy Clin Immunol* 2004;113:144–9.

38 Norgaard A, Bindslev-Jensen C, Skov PS, Poulsen LK. Specific serum IgE in the diagnosis of egg and milk allergy in adults. *Allergy* 1995;50:636–47.

39 Sampson HA. Food allergy – accurately identifying clinical reactivity. *Allergy* 2005;60:19–24.

40 May CD. Objective clinical and laboratory studies of immediate hypersensitivity reactions to foods in children. *J Allergy Clin Immunol* 1976;58:500–15.

41 Bindslev-Jensen C, Ballmer-Weber BK, *et al.* Standardization of food challenges in patients with immediate reactions to

foods – position paper from the European Academy of Allergology and Clinical Immunology. *Allergy* 2004;59:690–97.

42 Sampson HA. Use of food-challenge tests in children. *Lancet* 2001;358:1832–3.

43 Bock SA, Sampson HA, Atkins FM, *et al*. Double-blind, placebo-controlled food challenge (DBPCFC) as an office procedure: a manual. *J Allergy Clin Immunol* 1988;82:986–97.

44 Sicherer SH. Food allergy: when and how to perform oral food challenges. *Pediatr Allergy Immunol* 1999;10:226–34.

45 Vlieg-Boerstra BJ, Bijleveld CMA, van der Heide S, *et al*. Development and validation of challenge materials for double-blind, placebo-controlled food challenges in children. *J Allergy Clin Immunol* 2004;113:341–6.

46 Chinchilli VM, Fisher L, Craig TJ. Statistical issues in clinical trials that involve the double-blind, placebo-controlled food challenge. *J Allergy Clin Immunol* 2005;115:592–7.

47 Gellerstedt M, Magnusson J, Grajo U, *et al*. Interpretation of subjective symptoms in double-blind placebo-controlled food challenges – interobserver reliability. *Allergy* 2004;59:354–56.

48 Niggemann B, Wahn U, Sampson HA. Proposals for standardization of oral food challenge test in infants and children. *Pediatr Allergy Immunol* 1994;5:11–14.

49 Niggemann B, Rolinck-Werninghaus A, Mehl A, *et al*. Controlled oral food challenges in children – when indicated, when superfluous. *Allergy* 2005;60:865–70.

50 Perry TT, Matsui EC, Conover-Walker MK, Wood RA. Risk of oral food challenges. *J Allergy Clin Immunol* 2004;114:1164–8.

51 Reibel S, Rohr C, Ziegert M, *et al*. What safety measures need to be taken in oral food challenges in children? *Allergy* 2000;55:940–44.

52 Fleischer DM, Conover-Walker MK, Christie L, *et al*. Peanut allergy: recurrence and its management. *J Allergy Clin Immunol* 2004;114:1195–210.

53 Sampson HA, Munoz-Furlong A, Bock SA, *et al*. Symposium on the definition and management of anaphylaxis: summary report. *J Allergy Clin Immunol* 2005;115:584–91.

54 Sampson HA, Munoz-Furlong A, Campbell RL, *et al*. Second symposium on the definition and management of anaphylaxis: summary report – *Second National Institute of Allergy and Infectious Disease/Food Allergy and Anaphylaxis Network Symposium. J Allergy Clin Immunol* 2006;117:391–7.

55 Brown AF, McKinnon D, Chu K. Emergency department anaphylaxis: a review of 142 patients in a single year. *J Allergy Clin Immunol* 2001;108:861–6.

56 Brown SGA. Clinical features an severity grading of anaphylaxis. *J Allergy Clin Immunol* 2004;114:371–6.

57 Haymore BR, Carr WW, Frank WT. Anaphylaxis and epinephrine prescribing patterns in a military hospital: underutilization of the intramuscular route. *Allergy Asthma Proc* 2005;26:361–5.

58 McIntyre CL, Sheetz AH, Carroll CR, Young MC. Administration of epinephrine for life-threatening allergic reactions in school setting. *Pediatrics* 2005;116:1134–40.

59 Krugman SD, Chiaramonte DR, Matsui EC. Diagnosis and Management of Food Induced Anaphylaxis: a national survey of pediatricians. *Pediatrics* 2006;118:e554–60. http://pediatrics. aappublications.org/cgi/content/full/118/3/e554 [last accessed 10/05/07].

60 Pumphrey RSH. Lessons for management of anaphylaxis from a study of fatal reactions. *Clin Exp Allergy* 2000;30:1144–50.

61 Pumphrey RSH, Nicholls JM. Epinephrine-resistant food anaphylaxis (Correspondence). *Lancet* 2000;355:1099.

62 Sicherer SH, Forman JA, Noone SA. Use assessment of self-administered epinephrine among food-allergic children and pediatricians. *Pediatrics* 2000;105:359–62.

63 Sicherer SH, Simons FER. Quandaries in prescribing an emergency action plan and self injectable epinephrine for the first-aid management of anaphylaxis in the community. *J Allergy Clin Immunol* 2005;115:575–83.

64 Simons FER. First aid treatment of anaphylaxis to food: focus on epinephrine. *J Allergy Clin Immunol* 2004;113:837–44.

65 Sicherer SH, Noone SA, Munoz-Furlong A. The impact of childhood food allergy on quality of life. *Ann Allergy Asthma Immunol* 2001;87:461–4.

66 Cohen BL, Noone S, Munoz-Furlong A, Sicherer SH. Development of a questionnaire to measure quality of life in families with a child with food allergy. *J Allergy Clin Immunol* 2004;114:1159–63.

67 Kokkonen J, Haapalahti M, Laurila K, *et al*. Cow's milk protein-sensitive enteropathy at school age. *J Pediatr* 2001;139: 797–803.

68 D'netto MA, Herson VC, Hussain N, *et al*. Allergic gastroenteropathy in preterm infants. *J Pediatr* 2000;137:480–6.

69 Nowak-Wegrzyn A, Sampson HA, Wood RA, Sicherer SH. Food protein-induced enterocolitis syndrome caused by solid food proteins. *Pediatrics* 2003;111:829–35.

70 Levy Y, Danon YL. Food protein-induced enterocolitis syndrome – not only due to cow's milk and soy. *Pediatr Allergy Immunol* 2003;14:325–9.

71 Shek LPC, Bardina L, Castro R, *et al*. Humoral and cellular responses to cow milk proteins in patients with milk-induced IgE-mediated and non-IgE-mediated disorders. *Allergy* 2004;60: 912–19.

72 Sicherer SH, Eigenmann PA, Sampson HA. Clinical features of food protein-induced enterocolitis syndrome. *J Pediatr* 1998; 133:214–19.

73 Sicherer SH. Food protein induced enterocolitis: case presentations and management lessons. *J Allergy Clin Immunol* 2005;115:149–56.

74 Moissidis I, Chaidaroon D, Vichyanond P, Bahna SL. Milk-induced pulmonary disease in infants (Heiner syndrome). *Pediatr Allergy Immunol* 2005;16:545–52.

75 Hvatum M, Kanerud L, Hallgren R, Brandtzaeg P. The gut-joint axis: cross reactive food antibodies in rheumatoid arthritis. *Gut* 2006;55:1240–7.

76 Liacouras CA, Spergel JM, Ruchelli E, *et al*. Eosinophilic esophagitis: a 10-year experience in 381 children. *Clin Gastroent Hepatol* 2005;3:1198–206.

77 Perackis K, Celik-Bilgili S, Staden U, *et al*. Influence of age on the outcome of the atopy patch test with food in children with atopic dermatitis. *J Allergy Clin Immunol* 2003;112:625–7.

78 Spergel JM, Beausoliel JL, Mascarenhas M, Liacouras CA. The use of skin prick tests and patch tests to identify causative foods in eosinophilic esophagitis. *J Allergy Clin Immunol* 2002;109:363–8.

79 Fogg MI, Brown-Whitehorm TA, Pawlowski NA, Spergel JM. Atopy patch test for the diagnosis of food protein-induced enterocolitis syndrome. *Pediatr Allergy Immunol* 2005;17:351–5.

80 Kagalwalla AF, Sentongo TA, Ritz S, *et al*. Effect of six-food elimination diet on clinical and histologic outcomes in eosinophilic esophagitis. *Clin Gastroent Hepatol* 2006;4: 1097–1102.

81 Faubion WA, Perrault J, Burgart LJ, *et al*. Treatment of eosinophilic esophagitis with inhaled corticosteroids. *J Pediatr Gastroen Nutri* 1998;27:90–3.

82 Liacouras CA. Eosinophilic esophagitis: treatment in 2005. *Curr Opin Gastroenterol* 2006;22:147–52.

83 Vaughan TR. The role of food in the pathogenesis of migraine headache. *Clin Rev Allergy* 1994;12:167–80.

84 Sampson HA, Mendelson L, Rosen JP. Fatal and near-fatal anaphylactic reaction to food in children and adolescents. *N Engl J Med* 1992;327:380–4.

85 Bock SA, Munoz-Furlong A, Sampson HA. Fatalities due to anaphylactic reactions to foods. *J Allergy Clin Immunol* 2001;107:101–3.

86 Bock SA, Muno-Furlong A, Sampson HA. Further fatalities caused by anaphylactic reactions to food 2001–2006. *J Allergy Clin Immunol* 2007;119:1016–18.

87 Pumphrey R. Further fatal allergic reactions to food in the United Kingdom 1999–2006. *J Allergy Clin Immunol* 119;1018–19.

88 Fleischer DM, Conover-Walker MK, Christie L, *et al*. The natural progression of peanut allergy resolution and the possibility of recurrence. *J Allergy Clin Immunol* 2003;112:183–9.

89 Fleischer DM, Conover-Walker MK, Matsui EC, Wood RA. The natural history of tree nut allergy. *J Allergy Clin Immunol* 2005;116:1087–93.

90 Vander Leek TK, Liu AH, Stefanski K, *et al*. The natural history of peanut allergy in young children and its association with serum peanut-specific IgE. *J Pediatr* 2000;137:749–55.

CHAPTER 25

Hidden and Cross-Reacting Food Allergens

Scott H. Sicherer

KEY CONCEPTS

- False assumptions of multiple food allergy may derive from reactions to hidden ingredients, or from positive allergy tests to cross-reactive foods.

- Hidden or unexpected exposure to food allergens may occur from undeclared ingredients, cross-contact with an allergen, or from exposures not expected to carry food proteins, such as kissing, from airborne proteins, or in medications and cosmetics.

- Among related foods, cross-sensitization (positive tests) is more common than clinical cross-reactivity.

- Clinical cross-reactivity is more common (>35%) among tree nuts, fish, shellfish, certain mammalian milks, and certain fruits, than among grains and legumes (<20%).

- Individualization by testing and oral food challenge may be needed to confirm tolerance of potentially cross-reactive foods.

Introduction

The physician is often challenged by the patient who experiences reactions to multiple foods that are sometimes phylogenetically related and sometimes apparently unrelated. The two topics discussed in this chapter, hidden and cross-reacting food allergens, are ones that may lead to a conclusion of multiple food allergies. Table 25.1 lists several of the considerations for evaluating multiple food hypersensitivity. For the two general categories presented here, hidden food allergens may lead to the false assumption of multiple food hypersensitivities, because one or more previously identified food allergens are responsible for reactions to seemingly diverse food products through exposure in an unexpected manner. On the other hand, cross-reactivity may account for reactions to a variety of related foods of plant or animal origin based on immune reactions toward homologous proteins shared among them. Topics concerning the specific food proteins that frequently account for cross-reactions, oral allergy syndrome, and diagnostic methods and management of food allergy will not be emphasized here; rather, this chapter will introduce concepts and provide information to enhance the evaluation of patients with

possible multiple food allergies, in regard to hidden and cross-reacting food allergens.

Hidden food allergens

For the purpose of this chapter, the term "hidden food allergens" will refer to a variety of unexpected ways in which an individual may be exposed to food allergens [1–3]. Of course, a "hidden" food allergen may only be unknown to the consumer, not necessarily to a manufacturer or chef who provided the food. The use of peanut flour to thicken and provide unique flavor to tomato sauce or chili is one such example that underscores the importance of maintaining a clear line of communication when an allergic individual is depending on food provided from a restaurant or other commercial source without ingredient labels. Food proteins can also turn up in many unexpected ways. For example, a teacher may use egg white to make finger paints smoother or wheat may be an ingredient in modeling clay. Table 25.2 lists the ways in which exposure may occur within the context of hidden food allergens.

Commercial food products: manufacturing and labeling issues

Consumers with a known food allergy depend on accurate food label ingredient lists to determine the safety of their food. Their safety is predicated both on the accuracy of the

Food Allergy: Adverse Reactions to Foods and Food Additives, 4th edition.
Edited by Dean D. Metcalfe, Hugh A. Sampson, and Ronald A. Simon.
© 2008 Blackwell Publishing, ISBN: 978-1-4501-5129-0.

Table 25.1 Considerations when evaluating patients with apparent MFA

Type	Cause	Example
True reactions to multiple food types		
True MFA	True allergic reactions to multiple, diverse food allergens. Usually in highly atopic patients	Reactions to egg, milk, wheat, and soy in one child
Intolerance	Non-immune-mediated conditions causing adverse reactions when various foods are ingested	Intolerance of fat resulting in gastrointestinal upset to fatty meats; lactase deficiency resulting in symptoms from milk; fructose/sorbitol intolerance resulting in "acidic" diarrhea from multiple fruits
Cross-reactivity	Homologous proteins among foods and between foods and environmental allergens	Pollen-allergy syndrome, latex–fruit syndrome, panallergens in related foods
False assumption of multiple food allergy		
Multiple positive prick skin tests/RAST	Multiple tests for IgE antibody are positive and reactions are assumed to be related without further evaluation (history, oral challenge)	Atopic individual inappropriately tested to a wide battery of allergens has numerous positive tests and told to avoid all of the foods
Hidden ingredients	Reactions to apparently diverse products because of exposure to a hidden/unexpected source of one or a few previously identified allergens	Milk-allergic child reacts to soy desserts and canned tuna because they contain casein
Unproven tests	Use of unproven/experimental tests that identify multiple problematic foods for potentially vague symptoms	IgG antibody tests identify 43 foods purported to cause weakness in an elderly patient
Psychological	Previous food-allergy-related traumatic event generalizes to increasing numbers of reactions that are based on psychological triggers	A severe peanut-allergic patient develops paleness and syncope when exposed to products that she thought contained peanut, but did not
Misperception	Chronic complaints attributed to adverse reactions to a variety of foods without a pathophysiological explanation	Patient with perception that his headaches are triggered by orange foods (carrot, sweet potato, squash, orange soda)

MFA, multiple food allergies.

Table 25.2 Modes of exposure to hidden/unexpected food allergens

Mode of exposure	Examples
Hidden ingredient in manufactured product	Undeclared ingredient, contaminant, ambiguous label, non-standard terminology
Non-food item	Pet food, shampoo, ointment
Medications	Egg, soy, and milk (often in clinically irrelevant concentrations) in a variety of medications (carriers)
Cross-contact	Shared equipment in restaurant/bakery causes contamination
Non-food allergen found in food	Dust mite contamination of grains
Unexpected exposure route	Skin contact from residual food on table/chair, inhalation of fumes during cooking, exchange of saliva (kissing, shared straws, etc.)

label and their ability to decipher the statements on the label. Errors on both fronts can occur. Sometimes mistakes are apparent from simple misunderstandings: egg substitutes may catch the eye of an egg-allergic consumer who may assume the product is egg-free and not realize that egg is clearly labeled as an ingredient. In other cases, the consumer simply cannot trust the label since ingredient labels may not accurately reflect the presence of allergens. In January 2001, the US Food and Drug Administration (FDA) reported an investigation of 85 selected food companies in Minnesota and Wisconsin [4]. The investigation was, in part, in response to a significant increase in the number of recalls of products for undeclared allergens. The firms investigated were small, medium, and large bakeries; candy manufacturers; and ice cream manufacturers and they were reviewed for their approach to food allergens. Assays were conducted to determine the presence of peanut and egg in finished products. They found that 25% of products contained undeclared allergenic ingredients, often from cross-contamination, and 47% of the firms did not check their products to ensure that the labels were accurate. The medical literature contains reports of clinical reactions to foods with allergen contamination not declared on the ingredient label for several allergens including egg, milk, and peanut [2,5–8]. The potential for minor ingredients to cause severe reactions has been recognized for decades [3,9].

Governmental oversight of manufactured products varies worldwide [10–12]. In the United States, regulations pertaining to the declaration of food ingredients and the impact on the declaration of allergens are evolving. Until January 2006, allergens may have been referred to with scientific names such as "casein" or with ambiguous terms such as "natural flavor." Several studies have described allergic reactions and confusion ascribed to these labeling practices [13,14]. The recognized deficiencies in manufacturing and labeling in the United States came under scrutiny by a variety of professional, public, governmental, and lay organizations with a variety of suggestions for improvements, resulting in new labeling laws. Labeling laws changed in the United States as the Food Allergen Labeling and Consumer Protection Act of 2004 came into effect in January 2006. The law requires that the eight major allergens or allergenic food groups – milk, egg, fish, shellfish, tree nuts, wheat, peanut, and soy – must be declared on ingredient labels using plain English words. The law requires that the specific type of allergen, in regard to grouped allergens such as nuts, fish, or shellfish, be named. The law still allows terms such as "natural flavor" or "whey" on labels, but plain English must additionally disclose a major allergen. While the law includes the listed eight major allergens/allergenic food groups, additional allergens, for example garlic, sesame, poppy, etc., may not be disclosed clearly. For example, the word "spice" may be used for these allergens. Of note, some countries include sesame as a major allergen that must be disclosed. The US law applies to all types of packaged foods except for meat, egg, and poultry products, and raw agricultural foods such as fruits and vegetables in their natural state. The plain English words used to identify the foods may be placed within the ingredient list or as a separate statement "contains." In regard to soy, terms such as soybean, soy, and soya are considered interchangeable.

The FALCPA legislation has not defined a safe "threshold" of included allergen and several food ingredients may now be included on labels that did not previously disclose them. Processing aids such as soy lecithin, a fatty derivative of soy oil which may contain minute quantities of soy protein, may now be disclosed. The law acknowledges that certain forms of highly processed oils may not contain any appreciable protein, for example, soy oil. The law which is likely to be revised by petition and updates is available from the Center for Food Safety and Applied Nutrition, a branch of the FDA (www.cfsan.fda.gov). Studies on consumer interpretation of labels and actions based on the wording used on labels indicate that the law should result in reduced allergic reactions, but will also likely result in avoidance of foods that were safely consumed before labeling was required for potential trace protein contamination [15]. In some cases where ambiguous terms remain, a manufacturer may need to be called by a consumer to clarify ingredients.

Provisionary cautions used on labels, such as "may contain," are not regulated by the FALCPA legislation. These statements have been used by companies when a particular allergen is not an ingredient of the food, but that allergen may contact or become a part of the food despite good manufacturing processes. Labeling for the possibility of allergen contact is voluntary, and various terms are used at the discretion of the manufacturer such as "processed on shared equipment with…," "manufactured in a facility that processes…," and many others. The risk is impossible to determine for the consumer. In practical terms, food-allergic individuals, specifically teenagers and young adults, are increasingly ignoring these precautionary warnings; in a study of 174 adolescent subjects, 42% were willing to eat foods labeled "may contain" an allergen [16]. The degree of risk may vary by the product/manufacturer and the degree and frequency of reactions among persons with allergies who are not heeding these warnings is unknown.

Cross-contact

Cross-contact (cross-contamination) is an issue that is relevant in and out of commercial manufacturing. Small quantities of allergens can trigger reactions, including amounts that may be carried over in various ways from an "unsafe" food to one that is purportedly free of the allergen. Simple examples of this problem abound. In the home setting, a knife used to spread peanut butter could next contact and contaminate jelly. In restaurants, shared grills, pans, food processors, and other equipment used without thorough cleaning between preparations may be a source of cross-contact. Bakeries pose similar problems as shared bowls, mixing equipment, and pans may allow for cross-contact. In ice cream shops, dipping scoops from one flavor to the next can cross-contaminate otherwise safe flavors. In the school setting, cross-contact has been identified as a possible source of inadvertent exposures to peanut and tree nut through shared utensils and cross-contact of foods [17]. A problematic issue of cross-contact, combined with false assumptions by consumers is demonstrated by "pareve" labeled products [2]. Pareve is a religious term meaning non-dairy and does not ensure absence of milk proteins. These products are often sought out by unknowing milk-allergic consumers and consequently reactions are described to products with this label due to cross-contamination by cow's milk.

Restaurant meals also pose challenges for those with food allergies. The author and colleagues evaluated allergic reactions in peanut- and tree-nut-allergic subjects that were associated with restaurants and food from establishments such as bakeries and ice cream shops [18]. Of 5149 voluntary registrants in the US National Peanut and Tree Nut Allergy Registry, 13.7% indicated that they had experienced a reaction in these types of establishments. A review of 156 episodes among 129 randomly selected registrants revealed that 39% of reactions were due to peanut or tree nut hidden in the food and not overtly identifiable to the patron (e.g. in sauces, dressing, egg rolls). In 22% of cases, cross-contact was involved primarily due to the use of shared cooking/serving supplies. There were particular problems regarding cross-contact in desserts, Asian cooking, and buffets.

The lessons learned from the study of reactions in restaurants and food establishments highlight several important issues concerning allergen exposure in these settings and others. Ideally, procedures would be in place to manage food-allergic patrons. Personnel would receive training about food allergy, the potential for trace protein contamination to trigger reactions, a variety of methods to avoid cross-contamination and how to activate emergency assistance in the event of a reaction. A clear line of communication among the patron, server, and those preparing the foods must be established and maintained. Menu items should include a description of the ingredients in the food. In addition, the restaurant personnel would be advised about the potential for cross-contamination (shared fryers/blenders/utensils/mixers/pans/grills, contamination by garnishing bars, hands, and gloves) and methods to avoid this problem (use freshly cleaned, separate equipment, change gloves). For prevention of reactions due to cross-contact to be efficacious in any setting, education of the allergic individual about these issues is paramount.

Unexpected sources of food proteins in non-food items and in medications

Allergenic food proteins may be components of a variety of items not meant for ingestion by humans. Pet foods may contain a variety of classically allergenic food proteins such as milk, peanut, soy, and seafood. Inadvertent ingestion by young children must be considered when these foods are left on the floor for household pets with curious allergic youngsters in the vicinity. A number of hair-care products and topical skin-care products contain food proteins (e.g. almond, soy). Reactions to these products applied topically are usually not severe.

Patients with food allergies and their physicians must always consider that a drug (or vaccine) reaction may be induced by a food ingredient in the drug. Well-known examples of this phenomenon include egg protein [19,20] in influenza and yellow fever vaccines and gelatin [21] in a variety of other vaccines. The measles–mumps–rubella (MMR) vaccine is no longer considered to contain appreciable egg protein. It may be administered to egg-allergic persons without increased risk, as indicated in the Red Book 2006 Report of the Committee on Infectious Diseases of the American Academy of Pediatrics. A study on influenza vaccine in children with egg allergy evaluated the risk using a vaccine with a known amount of egg protein [20] and suggested a split, two-dose (one-tenth then nine-tenths) regimen for safety. Since the amount of egg in the vaccine may vary from lot to lot, and may be unknown, the two-dose regimen may

not be universally applicable. Allergists may perform skin testing with the vaccine to better define risks. The Red Book 2006 Report of the committee on Infectious Diseases of the American Academy of Pediatrics suggests a regimen of gradual dosing in persons who are deemed to require influenza or yellow fever vaccination despite their anaphylactic egg allergy. Of note, the nasal influenza vaccine contains a higher amount of egg protein than the injection and should not be used in persons with egg allergy. Vaccines that may include gelatin include some of the diphtheria, tetanus, and pertussis vaccines; influenza vaccine; Japanese encephalitis; mumps; measles, mumps and rubella; typhoid; varicella (chicken pox) and yellow fever vaccines.

Many other food-related ingredients used in medications have not been well studied in terms of their allergic potential. Pharmaceutical-grade lactose is used in many medications and the clinical relevance of possible residual milk protein has not been well established. One report identified milk protein in the lactose used in several dry-powdered inhalers used for asthma [22]. Egg or soy lecithin and soy oil are found in a variety of medications, but the clinical relevance to most individuals with these allergies remains unexplored.

Non-food allergens in foods

There are case reports of non-food allergen contamination of foods resulting in allergic reactions. For example, dust mites may contaminate flour mixtures and cause severe reactions when ingested by dust-mite-allergic patients [23,24]. This appears to be a particular problem in tropical climates. The use of latex gloves by food handlers has resulted in unexpected reactions when these foods are ingested by latex-allergic individuals [25,26]. Indeed, latex allergens are detectable on food products following handling with powdered latex gloves [27]. Insofar as parasites are not intentionally consumed, it is worthwhile to note that the nematode *Anisakis simplex* that infests fish can induce allergic reactions. This appears to be a problem particularly in Spain and other countries with high fish consumption and is associated with undercooking [28].

Non-standard exposure routes to food allergens

There appear to be exceptional cases where topical exposure to foods result in systemic reactions [29]. More commonly, however, topical exposure leads primarily to isolated, local skin reactions. In such cases, residual food proteins on tables and chairs may induce rashes. Although not truly hidden or unexpected, school craft projects using peanut butter (peanut butter covered pine cone birdfeeders) are commonly responsible for reactions despite school's awareness about avoiding peanut as an ingestant [17].

Airborne exposure to food allergens is not unexpected in a variety of industrial food-processing settings (e.g. baker's asthma) but is a potential hidden source outside of these settings. There are several published case reports of acute allergic reactions to airborne food particles such as string bean [27], lentil [28], meats [30], and seafood [31] usually during cooking (rapidly boiling milk, frying eggs, steaming soups, sizzling fried seafood, etc). Reactions have been verified in challenge settings [32]. There are also a few reports concerning peanut reactions to inhalation of peanut dust during commercial airline flights [33–35]. In airliners, the hypothesis is that the powdery material from roasted peanuts becomes airborne [36] and can induce reactions in that setting of a closed space when many bags are being opened simultaneously. These reactions are generally isolated to the upper and sometimes lower respiratory tract.

Another source of unintended and unexpected oral exposure is through saliva from an individual who ingested an allergen, for example, through contact during kissing or sharing cups, straws, or utensils. Kissing, in particular passionate kissing, is a common route of exposure. Of 379 allergy patients in the United States with peanut/tree nut/ legume or seed allergy, 5.3% reported reactions from kissing [37]. Of 839 food-allergy patients in Denmark (self-reported) who recalled possible kissing, 16% reported a reaction [38]. These two reports also support the notion that the food was usually, but not always, recently ingested and that brushing teeth may not be sufficient for removing the allergen. A study was undertaken to determine the time course of peanut protein (a marker protein Ara h 1) in saliva after a meal of peanut butter and possible methods for cleaning [39]. Detection of Ara h 1 was performed by a monoclonal-based ELISA (detection limit, 15–20 ng/ml). Most (87%) subjects with detectable peanut after a meal had undetectable levels by 1 hour with no interventions. None had detectable levels several hours later following a peanut-free lunch. This result indicates (95% confidence) that 90% would have undetectable Ara h 1 in saliva under these circumstances. Piloted cleaning procedures only led to undetectable levels in 1 in 5 subjects, but the methods with a waiting period reduced salivary Ara h 1 to undetectable in 8 of 10 (wait-brush) and 8 of 9 (wait, gum) subjects. The studies were performed with peanut butter and results may vary with other allergens or forms of peanut. There is one case report [40] of a mild reaction to peanut despite a 2-hour wait, brushing teeth, and chewing gum. Food-allergic reactions from blood transfusion or semen are theoretically possible but highly unlikely.

Cross-reacting food allergens

When an allergic response is established toward a particular protein, presentation of a homologous form of that protein in another substance also may trigger an allergic response (cross-reaction). Hence, true allergic reactions to multiple foods may follow initial sensitization caused by one food. The initial sensitization may occur by the oral or inhaled route. In fact, as discussed in Chapter 7, the appropriate immunological response to ingested proteins is tolerance, and for most individuals food allergies do not occur despite other atopic

respiratory illnesses. However, one way that immune tolerance to foods may be bypassed is by initial sensitization that occurs to homologous proteins that contact the respiratory tree (e.g. pollen-allergy syndrome). In this way, IgE antibody toward the respiratory allergen can also induce disease when the homologous protein is ingested. As will be discussed below, the scenario of respiratory sensitization resulting in food allergy may apply to pollens, latex, and insect emanations that are airborne allergens with homologous proteins in foods. In addition to sensitization by the airborne route, typical sensitization to a particular food through the gastrointestinal tract can result in reactions to, usually related, foods containing homologous proteins. Reactions in this setting are typically more severe because they involve proteins that are capable of sensitization by ingestion and these are proteins that are typically more stable to digestion and able to enter the systemic circulation [41]. In some cases, more distantly related foods or environmental allergens contain common (conserved) homologous (pan)allergens. To complicate matters further, however, there may be homologous, allergenically important sequences (epitopes) shared even among more distantly related foods that may trigger reactions in some individuals (e.g. seed storage proteins in peanut, sesame, and tree nuts) [42].

Plant-derived proteins responsible for allergy include various families of pathogenesis-related proteins, protease and α-amylase inhibitors, peroxidases, profilins, seed storage proteins, thiol proteases, and lectins [43,44] while homologous animal proteins include muscle proteins, enzymes, and various serum proteins. Remarkably, typical food allergens derive from just these few, out of thousands, of protein families. Over 70% identity in primary sequence is generally needed for cross-reactivity [45]. The biochemical attributes of these proteins will not be discussed here, but the focus will rather be on the clinical relevance of potential cross-reactivity.

To elicit a clinical response, it is presumed that the causal food protein must maintain the ability to present the epitope in question in an immunologically relevant form. That is, evidence that there is IgE binding to a potentially cross-reactive food protein (sensitization demonstrated by prick skin test or RAST) is not evidence of clinically relevant allergy to the food. In fact, it is quite common to find food-specific IgE antibody by prick skin tests or RASTs to foods related to the one causing the index reaction. For example, using RASTs, Barnett et al. [46] screened sera from 40 peanut-allergic patients against 10 other legumes and demonstrated IgE binding to multiple legumes for 38% of patients. Similarly, Bernhisel-Broadbent and colleagues [47] studied 62 children with allergy to at least one legume and found that 79% had serological evidence of IgE binding to more than one, and 37% bound all six legumes. The scenario is similar for tree nuts [48–50]. In our studies of tree-nut-allergic children [48], 92% of 111 patients with peanut and/or tree nut allergy had IgE antibody to more than one tree nut. In all of these cases, however, it is much more common to find that the food to which there is cross-sensitization is actually tolerated when ingested [51]. Factors that determine the clinical appearance of allergy in the face of sensitization are complex and relate to the host (immune response, target organ hyperreactivity) and the allergen (liability, digestibility) [41]. Presumably, these factors also bear upon the clinical relevance of potentially cross-reactive foods. The information to follow may be of particular value in deciding on the best approach to diagnose potential allergy to cross-reactive foods (the utility of *in vivo* and *in vitro* tests).

Cross-reactions among specific foods/food families

Legumes
Despite the high rate of cross-sensitization to legumes (beans), clinical cross-reactions are uncommon. Peanut and soy represent two of the most highly allergenic legumes that are dietary staples in North America, and yet the rate of clinical cross-reactivity is low. However, Bock and Atkins [52] studied 32 children with peanut allergy confirmed by DBPCFCs and found that 10 (31%) had a positive skin test to soy, but only one (3% of those with peanut allergy) had a clinical reaction to soy. In considering a wider variety of legumes, only 3 (1.8%) of 165 children with atopic dermatitis evaluated with DBPCFCs reacted to more than one legume despite 19% reacting to at least one [53]. Bernhisel-Broadbent and Sampson [47] specifically addressed the issue of legume cross-reactivity by performing open or DBPCFCs in 69 highly atopic children with at least one positive skin test to a legume. Oral challenges to the 5 legumes (peanut, soybean, pea, lima bean, green bean) resulted in 43 reactions in 41 patients (59%). Only 2 of 41 with any one positive challenge reacted to more than one legume (5%).

There are limited data to suggest that particular legumes are more likely than others to trigger reactions and also that the types of beans consumed in various cultures (e.g. lupine used whole or as flour in breads) also impact the rate of cross-reactions [54–57]. For example, 11 of 24 (44%) French children with peanut allergy [56] had positive skin tests to lupine, and of 8 subjects who underwent DBPCFCs (6 children) or labial challenges (2 children) to lupine, 7 reacted. As a probable reflection of cultural and geographical influences on the diet, allergy to lentil is more common than to peanut in Spain [58]. Furthermore, of 22 Spanish children with lentil allergy evaluated for reactions to other legumes [59], 6 had a history of reacting to chick pea, 2 to pea, and 1 to green bean. These findings raise suspicion for multiple legume allergy in those reacting to lentil, lupine, and chick pea, but more studies in a variety of geographic settings utilizing blinded challenges to confirm reactivity are needed to quantify the risks.

In regard to a clinical approach, it is clear that multiple legume allergy is relatively uncommon, but it is common to observe positive skin tests to multiple legumes in an atopic patient with reaction to one. Thus, it is not appropriate to assume that a particular patient has multiple legume allergy; rather, a more definitive evaluation should be undertaken to ensure tolerated beans are available as personal preferences would indicate. Furthermore, tests for specific IgE antibody in this scenario may be helpful primarily when they are negative, because positive tests are common despite clinical tolerance. It must be appreciated that an individual with more than one legume allergy is at higher risk for even more legume reactions and that lentil, lupine, and chick pea may be slightly more likely to be involved in this scenario than others (pea, string bean).

Tree nuts
Clinical reactions to tree nuts can be severe [60], potentially fatal, and can occur from a first apparent exposure to a nut in patients allergic to other nuts [61]. Due to the frequency of severe reactions, there are no comprehensive studies on clinical cross-reactivity among tree nuts. Bock and Atkins [52] performed challenges to one or more nuts in 14 children and at least 2 reacted to multiple nuts (as many as 5 types). Ewan [60] reported allergy to multiple tree nuts in over a third of 34 patients evaluated for tree nut allergy. Similarly, our group noted that in 54 children with a tree nut allergy, reactions to more than one nut occurred in 37% [48]. Some nut allergens may be homologous and cause reactions (e.g. in pistachio/cashew [62]) while others may be homologous but rarely elicit clinical cross-reactivity (e.g. proteins in coconut and walnut [63]).

Legume/tree nuts/seeds
Co-sensitization to allergenic foods such as peanut, tree nuts, and seeds (sesame, poppy, mustard) is common. In a study of 731 subjects in the United Kingdom, 59% sensitized to peanut were also sensitized to hazelnut and/or Brazil nut [49]. Although clinically significant cross-reacting proteins have not yet been described, it is known that some amino acid sequences (epitopes) are highly homologous among some of the seed storage proteins that constitute the major allergens in these foods [42]. Co-allergy to peanut and tree nut has been reported between 23% and 50% in referral populations of atopic patients [48,60,64,65]. This observation raises the question: Is this high rate of co-reactivity due to homologous proteins or to expected allergies to intrinsically allergenic foods among highly atopic patients? The tools are available to answer this important question and the methodical searches are underway. Until more data are available, the clinician must consider the age of the patient, history, and sensitization in considering categorical elimination of these allergenic foods [66]. Reactions to seeds such as sesame, mustard, and poppy are being increasingly

reported [50,67–69], and cross-reactivity with foods (hazel, kiwi, other seeds) and pollens is potentially important.

The full clinical implications of possible cross-reactivity among peanuts, tree nuts, and seeds are not yet established. From a practical perspective, considering the potential severity of the allergy and issues with accurate identification of particular nuts in prepared foods, caution would seem prudent and total elimination of the nut family (perhaps with the exception of previously tolerated nuts eaten in isolation) is often suggested [48,70]. These recommendations are potentially over-restrictive. There is no consensus as to whether seeds should be considered as highly likely to elicit reactions among individuals with peanut/tree nut allergy, but based on the studies thus far, some caution is warranted.

Fish

In a prevalence study in the United States [71], reactions to multiple fish among those with any fish allergy was 67%. Among those with fish allergy ($n = 58$), 19 reported a reaction to only one type, 5 to 2 types, 13 to 3–9 types and the remainder were uncertain. In serological studies of 10 subjects with codfish allergy, sensitization to salmon was strong while sensitization to halibut, flounder, tuna, and mackerel were lower [72]. To best evaluate clinical cross-reactivity, it would be necessary to perform oral food challenges to multiple types of fish, shellfish, or mollusks in persons allergic to at least one type. The clinical studies concerning fish allergy mirror those of tree nut allergy in that clinical reactions to multiple fish is a common phenomenon, high cross-sensitization rates are even more common, and the allergic reactions tend to be severe [73–75]. A few studies have utilized DBPCFCs challenges to evaluate fish allergy. In 10 US children evaluated with DBPCFCs to 4–6 species of fish, and in whom reactions were confirmed to at least 1 species, 3 reacted to more than one type [73]. Hansen and colleagues [76] evaluated 8 adults with codfish allergy proven by DBPCFCs. Sensitization to plaice, herring, and mackerel was nearly 100% and among patients exposed to each (6, 5, and 6 patients, respectively), all had a history of clinical reactions. In a study of 6 adults from Denmark with a positive DBPCFC to at least one of 3 fish (catfish, codfish, snapper) and challenged to at least 2 types, 4 reacted to more than one species [74]. Several studies that did not utilize DBPCFCs provide additional information that is in agreement with these formal studies. In 61 children with a history of fish allergy exposed to 2–8 species, 34 (56%) reacted to all and 27 (44%) tolerated some types [75]. In a study of 20 codfish-allergic Italian children [77], a high frequency of positive skin tests (from 5% to 100% for each of 9 species tested) was documented. For those who ingested the fish to which antibody was detected, the clinical reaction rate per fish based on history was 25–100% depending on the species. Some fish were more problematic than others in these cod-allergic children. Eel, bass, sole, and tuna most frequently provoked reactions and salmon, sardine, and dogfish were least likely to induce symptoms. Regional exposure patterns are relevant. Pascual and colleagues [78] from Spain evaluated the relevance of cross-reactivity among 6 regionally important species in 79 children with fish allergy where codfish is not a common food. While all subjects had positive skin tests to multiple species, only 31 of 79 (39%) had clinical reactions, and hake and whiff had the highest while albacore had the lowest reaction rates. In contrast to the studies that indicate a high likelihood of multiple fish allergy, several reports demonstrate that isolated allergy to a single species of fish occurs (e.g. tropical sole [79], swordfish [80]). This apparently occurs because of immune responses toward species-specific allergens since there is relative absence of IgE antibody to the common fish allergens (Gad c 1). Formal studies of fish hypersensitivity have also indicated that fish proteins may be denatured when heated (canned) or lyophilized, and this must be appreciated when considering a history of specific fish that appear to be tolerated in some forms, for example reactive to salmon but not reactive to canned salmon [81].

In summary, a fish-allergic patient is at high risk for reactions to other fish, but may tolerate some fish species, and may therefore deserve further evaluation with supervised oral challenges if desirous of ingesting other fish. The facts that fish allergy can be severe and that cooking/canning and other processing can alter allergenicity must be considered during these evaluations [81].

Shellfish

The clinical impression is that reactions to multiple crustaceans are fairly common, but there are few clinical studies addressing this issue. In a prevalence study in the United States [71], reaction to multiple Crustacea for those with allergy to any was 38%, and for mollusks was 49%; only 14% with crustacean allergy reported a mollusk allergy. In that study, estimation of the rate of allergies to multiple types of seafood was complicated by the fact that not all participants were exposed to all types of seafood and, after a reaction, avoidance of multiple types of seafood was often undertaken. Among those with allergy to shrimp, lobster, and/or crab who indicated specific knowledge of an allergy among these ($n = 232$), 62% indicated allergy to one, 20% to 2, and 18% to all 3 types. Among scallops, clams, oysters, and mussels ($n = 67$), 51% reacted to one, 19% to 2, 8% to 3 and 22% to all 4 types. Forty-one persons with shellfish allergy (14%) reported an allergy to both one or more Crustaceae and one or more mollusks/bivalves.

The major shared allergenic protein is invertebrate tropomyosin found in crustaceans (shrimp, crab, lobster) [82–84] and mollusks (oyster, scallop, and squid) [85]. Not surprisingly, the rate of cross-sensitization is high. In 16 atopic, shrimp-allergic patients, >80% had positive PSTs to crab, crayfish, and lobster [86]. Unfortunately, formal clinical studies to determine the rate of clinical reactivity are lacking. In a study of 11 patients with immediate reactions to shrimp ingestion, the reaction rate to lobster, crab, and crayfish was 50–100% per species [87]. On the other hand, there are individuals who react not only to shrimp alone, but to specific species of shrimp [88].

Also poorly defined is the risk of mollusk allergy for Crustaceae or mollusk-allergic individuals. Lehrer and McCants [89] reported a study of six oyster-sensitive, seven oyster and Crustacea, and 12 Crustacea-sensitive patients in whom serologies were evaluated. Most of the reactions to oyster were isolated to the gastrointestinal tract and not associated with oyster-specific IgE antibody. However, among 19 patients with sensitivity to Crustacea, 47% had positive RASTs to oyster, indicating potential cross-reactivity. In another study evaluating 9 patients with shrimp anaphylaxis, binding to tropomyosin of 13 crustaceans and mollusks was universal [85]. These studies only evaluated serologies, so the rate of clinical reactivity is unclear but apparently not great.

Invertebrate tropomyosin is also found in airborne insect allergens found in cockroach and dust mite [85,90,91], which raises the possibility of sensitization by the respiratory route. There is a case report of a seafood restaurant worker who developed IgE to tropomyosin and occupational asthma to both scallop (mollusk) and shrimp (crustacean) [92]. In a report of wheezing induced by snail consumption in 28 patients, RAST inhibition studies indicated that house dust mite sensitization was the likely initial sensitizing event [91]. There are several reports linking allergen immunotherapy with *D. pteronyssinus* to development of severe reactions to mollusks and crustaceans. Five of six patients from the Canary Islands with anaphylaxis to limpet, a mollusk, had received immunotherapy with dust mite [93]. In a prospective study, two of 17 patients receiving dust mite immunotherapy developed cross-reactive IgE antibodies to tropomyosin and oral symptoms to shrimp [94].

Overall, Crustaceae species represent an increased risk of cross-reactivity with a potential for severe reactions and a potentially high rate of clinical symptoms. However, there are individuals who tolerate most types, so individualization, done cautiously, may be warranted. Allergy to mollusks is less well established and appears less common. Allergy to, and immunotherapy with, dust mite may be an additional risk factor, but determination of the precise risks requires further investigation.

Cereal grains

Wheat, rye, barley, and oat share homologous proteins with grass pollens and with each other [95,96] and this may account for the high rate of co-sensitization among these foods [95]. Among children with at least one grain allergy undergoing DBPCFCs to multiple grains, 80% were tolerant of all other grains. Caution is warranted, but clinical reactivity to multiple grains appears uncommon and individualization warranted for these common foods.

Avian and mammalian food products

For avian foods such as chicken, sensitization has been described to α-livetin found in feathers, egg, and meat [97]. Reactions to chicken meat is often based on reactivity to this protein (22–32%) [97,98]. Chicken meat allergy is uncommon [99], but when it occurs in the absence of egg allergy, the risk of reaction to multiple species of avian meats (turkey, pheasant, quail) may be increased. This observation is probably because a meat-specific protein, rather than within species meat–egg specific protein, is causally related to reactions [100,101]. Cross-reactive proteins among various avian eggs are also common [102], but the clinical implications have not been systematically studied. Conversely, allergy to one egg type may not guarantee reactions to others; reactions to duck and goose egg, in the absence of hen's egg allergy has been described [103].

Some patients with allergy to mammalian milks also react to mammalian meats [104]. This observation may be due to homologous proteins or, more likely, proteins that are identical and are found in meat and milk from the same animal. A study employing oral challenges showed that 10% of 62 cow's milk-allergic (CMA) children reacted to beef [105]. Heating and other cooking processes can reduce the allergenicity of beef [106], so well-cooked beef is less likely to cause a problem for those with CMA. Reactions to multiple mammalian milks are more common than milk–meat reactions. *In vitro* studies showed extensive cross-reactivity among sheep, cow, ewe, buffalo, and goat milks [107], but not to camel's milk [108]. Oral challenge studies showed goat's milk to be unsafe for patients with CMA since 92% of 26 CMA patients reacted to goat's milk [109]. Mares' milk appears comparatively safe as only 4% of 25 children with CMA reacted to it [110].

For practical purposes, it is important to note that most milk-allergic patients will tolerate beef and that cooking the meat well may improve tolerability, but that some highly milk-allergic individuals do experience reactions. Overall, individualization is usually warranted. It may be less important to try to identify a mammalian milk for those with CMA since cross-reactivity is very high and suitable alternatives (soy milk, rice milk) are available. Cross-sensitization is more common within than between avian and mammalian meats, but clinical correlation with sensitization is generally under 50%, so individualization is also warranted [111].

Fruit, pollens, and latex
Oral allergy syndrome
Oral allergy syndrome (pollen–food allergy syndrome) is described elsewhere (Chapter 11) and the focus here will be on cross-reactions within families of fruits. Several studies have selected patients based on particular fruit allergies, rather

than pollen allergies, and evaluated for reactions to related fruits. Rodriguez and colleagues [112] evaluated 34 adults in Madrid with reported allergy to Rosaceae foods (peach, apple, apricot, almond, plum, pear, and strawberry). Eighty-two percent had positive PSTs and/or RASTs to at least one of the foods with a median of five positive foods per patient. Clinical reactivity determined by DBPCFCs was less than 10% for those positive to pear and up to 90% for peach (overall, 35% with a positive skin test reacted to a given food). Multiple fruit allergy was common in the 22 who reacted to at least one fruit (46%). Peach was the dominant allergenic fruit; 46% reactive to peach reacted to another Rosaceae fruit. Pastorello and colleagues [113] studied patients selected for a history of reactions to peach confirmed through open oral food challenges; among the 19 patients evaluated, 63% reacted to at least one other fruit among cherry, apricot, and plum. Of 19 patients with melon allergy confirmed by DBPCFC (of 54 patients suspected), 94% reacted to at least one of the following related fruits: watermelon, avocado, kiwi, chestnut, banana, peach [114].

Severity of reactions to these foods is an important issue. Pollen-related fruit allergy is usually mild (oral allergy syndrome) and yet in one study, 8.7% experienced associated systemic symptoms outside of the gastrointestinal tract [115], 3% at some time experienced systemic symptoms without oral symptoms, and 1.7% experienced anaphylactic shock. It is becoming clear why some patients are more likely to experience severe reactions. There is evidence that when fruit allergy develops in the absence of pollen allergy, reactions are directed not only to Bet v 1 or profilins, but also to lipid transfer proteins (LTP). Reactions involving fruits with homologous LTPs are more likely to be severe [116,117]. Fernandez-Rivas and colleagues [118] compared patients with Rosaceae fruit allergy with and without pollenosis and found that systemic reactions occurred in 82% without pollenosis compared to 45% with pollinosis. Anaphylactic shock was also more common in the former (36% versus 9%, respectively). A similar theme was noted for hazelnut, where patients without pollinosis experienced severe reactions and had IgE binding to hazelnut proteins that were heat-stable [119]. Asero [120] found that individuals with positive skin tests to commercial Rosaceae food extracts were more likely to experience systemic reactions than those only positive to fresh extracts, (64% versus 6%, $p < 0.001$). This observation is presumably explained by the likelihood that more stable allergens are present in the commercial extract compared to fresh fruit proteins, which include labile proteins that are more likely to induce only symptoms of oral allergy. Crespo *et al.* [121] evaluated 65 adults diagnosed with clinical allergy to one or more fruits for allergy to other related foods. Thirty-four of those tested (52%) were found to be clinically allergic to more than one fruit. Food challenges with potential cross-reactive foods uncovered 18 further reactions in 14 (22%) out of 65. Only 8% (18/223) of positive results for allergy

tests to potential cross-reactive foods investigated were clinically relevant. Therefore, elimination of related fruits without oral challenge testing, that is based on skin test or RAST results, could have resulted in unnecessary restriction of 205 foods in the 65 people studied. However, it was worrisome that 18 food reactions in one-fifth (14/65) of patients could have been missed if oral challenges/evaluations were not pursued. The clinical lesson is that once a patient experiences more than oral symptoms to a fruit, a careful search by history and/or challenge may be warranted to prove the safety of related fruits. Furthermore, positive skin tests to commercial extracts and a lack of pollen allergy may indicate a higher risk of significant reactions.

Latex–food syndrome

Commonly reported latex cross-reactive foods include banana, avocado, kiwi, chestnut, potato, and papaya, and numerous latex allergens cross-react with food and pollen proteins [122,123]. In a study of 136 latex-allergic patients evaluated by RAST to 12 foods reported to be involved in latex–food reactions, 69% were positive to at least one food and 49% were positive to more than one [124]. Challenges were not performed, but only one-third of the 42% of patients who reported reactions to the particular fruit had a positive RAST. In another study of 47 latex-allergic patients, 100 of 376 food skin tests were positive but only 27 (7.2%) were associated with clinical reactions [125]. In evaluating the converse situation of fruit-allergic patients (excluded if there was a well-known risk factor for latex allergy) for sensitization to latex, 86% of 57 patients had serum latex-specific IgE antibody, and 11% experienced clinical reactions to latex [126].

Evaluation of natural rubber latex–food cross-reactivity is complicated by cross-reacting pollens, foods, and co-allergy to various substances with potential allergenic relationships. There may be clinical value in differentiating individuals with isolated food, pollen, or latex sensitization [127]. Levy and colleagues [128] evaluated adults with latex allergy with ($n = 24$) and without ($n = 20$) pollenosis and a group without latex allergy and with pollenosis ($n = 25$) for allergies to 12 foods (by convincing history) classically associated with latex and pollen allergy. In those with isolated latex allergy, reactions were reported to banana (4), avocado (4), kiwi (2), melon and peach (1 each) while those with pollinosis were more likely to react to Rosaceae foods and celery. In the pollen-allergic groups, positive skin tests to the foods were found in 45%, but for isolated latex allergy, only 24% were positive. The numbers of reactions among those with positive tests were generally less than 25%, except for reactions to banana, avocado, and kiwi, which approached 50% in those with isolated latex allergy. Overall, caution is warranted and individualization is necessary, but for patients with allergy to latex, banana, avocado, or kiwi, it may be prudent to consider potential reactions to the related foods.

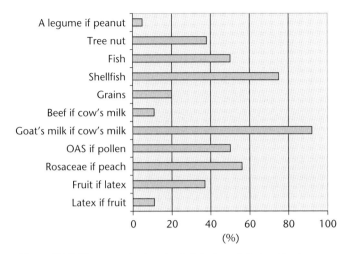

Figure 25.1 The approximate rate of clinical reactivity to at least one other related food. The probability of reacting to related foods varies, depending on numerous factors (data reviewed in Sicherer [51]). OAS, oral allergy syndrome/pollen–food syndrome.

Summary and management

As outlined in preceding sections, there is a high likelihood of sensitization to foods that bear homologous allergens, but clinical reactivity correlates poorly. It is therefore necessary to consider a variety of issues when evaluating a patient for the possibility of multiple food hypersensitivities on the basis of possible cross-reactions. Among these are *a priori* reasoning about likelihood of reactions (Fig. 25.1), severity of reactions, social and nutritional importance of the food, and the (poor) predictive value of tests for IgE antibody in this setting. However, for most foods and for most patients, multiple food allergies are relatively uncommon and the extra effort to prove which foods are or are not tolerated is worthwhile.

References

1 Steinman HA. "Hidden" allergens in foods. *J Allergy Clin Immunol* 1996;98:241–50.

2 Gern J, Yang E, Evrard H, Sampson H. Allergic reactions to milk-contaminated "non-dairy" products. *N Engl J Med* 1991; 324:976–9.

3 Lockey Sr SD. Reactions to hidden agents in foods, beverages and drugs. *Ann Allergy* 1971;29:461–6.

4 Vierk K, Falci K, Wolyniak C, Klontz KC. Recalls of foods containing undeclared allergens reported to the US Food and Drug Administration, fiscal year 1999. *J Allergy Clin Immunol* 2002; 109:1022–6.

5 Jones RT, Squillace DL, Yunginger JW. Anaphylaxis in a milk-allergic child after ingestion of milk-contaminated kosher-pareve-labeled "dairy-free" dessert [see comments]. *Ann Allergy* 1992;68:223–7.

6 Enrique E, Cistero-Bahima A, Alonso R, San Miguel MM. Egg protein: a hidden allergen in candies. *Ann Allergy Asthma Immunol* 2000;84:636.

7 Cantani A. Hidden presence of cow's milk proteins in foods. *J Investig Allergol Clin Immunol* 1999;9:141–5.

8 McKenna C, Klontz KC. Systemic allergic reaction following ingestion of undeclared peanut flour in a peanut-sensitive woman. *Ann Allergy Asthma Immunol* 1997;79:234–6.

9 Cowen DE. Hidden allergens – vehicles and excipients. *Ann Allergy* 1967;25:161–4.

10 Leitch I, Blair IS, McDowell DA. The role of environmental health officers in the protection of allergic consumers. *Int J Environ Health Res* 2001;11:51–61.

11 Hogendijk S, Eigenmann PA, Hauser C. The problem of hidden food allergens: two cases of anaphylaxis to peanut proteins concealed in a pizza sauce. *Schweiz Med Wochenschr* 1998;128:1134–7.

12 Taylor SL, Hefle SL. Food allergen labeling in the USA and Europe. *Curr Opin Allergy Clin Immunol* 2006;6:186–90.

13 Joshi P, Mofidi S, Sicherer SH. Interpretation of commercial food ingredient labels by parents of food-allergic children. *J Allergy Clin Immunol* 2002;109:1019–21.

14 Altschul AS, Scherrer DL, Munoz-Furlong A, Sicherer SH. Manufacturing and labeling issues for commercial products: relevance to food allergy. *J Allergy Clin Immunol* 2001;108:468.

15 Simons E, Weiss CC, Furlong TJ, Sicherer SH. Impact of ingredient labeling practices on food allergic consumers. *Ann Allergy Asthma Immunol* 2005;95:426–8.

16 Sampson MA, Muñoz-Furlong A, Sicherer SH. Risk-taking and coping strategies of adolescents and young adults with food allergy. *J Allergy Clin Immunol* 2006;117:1440–5.

17 Sicherer SH, Furlong TJ, DeSimone J, Sampson HA. The US Peanut and Tree Nut Allergy Registry: characteristics of reactions in schools and day care. *J Pediatr* 2001;138:560–5.

18 Furlong TJ, DeSimone J, Sicherer SH. Peanut and tree nut allergic reactions in restaurants and other food establishments. *J Allergy Clin Immunol* 2001;108:867–70.

19 Kelso JM. Raw egg allergy – a potential issue in vaccine allergy. *J Allergy Clin Immunol* 2000;106:990.

20 James JM, Zeiger RS, Lester MR, *et al.* Safe administration of influenza vaccine to patients with egg allergy. *J Pediatr* 1998;133:624–8.

21 Sakaguchi M, Miyazawa H, Inouye S. Specific IgE and IgG to gelatin in children with systemic cutaneous reactions to Japanese encephalitis vaccines. *Allergy* 2001;56:536–9.

22 Nowak-Wegrzyn A, Shapiro GG, Beyer K, *et al.* Contamination of dry powder inhalers for asthma with milk proteins containing lactose. *J Allergy Clin Immunol* 2004;113:558–60.

23 Erben AM, Rodriguez JL, McCullough J, Ownby DR. Anaphylaxis after ingestion of beignets contaminated with *Dermatophagoides farinae*. *J Allergy Clin Immunol* 1993;92:846–9.

24 Sanchez-Borges M, Capriles-Hulett A, Fernandez-Caldas E, *et al.* Mite-contaminated foods as a cause of anaphylaxis. *J Allergy Clin Immunol* 1997;99:738–43.

25 Franklin W, Pandolfo J. Latex as a food allergen. *N Engl J Med* 1999;341:1858.

26 Schwartz HJ. Latex: a potential hidden "food" allergen in fast food restaurants. *J Allergy Clin Immunol* 1995;95:139–40.

27 Beezhold DH, Reschke JE, Allen JH, *et al*. Latex protein: a hidden "food" allergen? *Allergy Asthma Proc* 2000;21:301–6.

28 Daschner A, Alonso-Gómez A, Cabañas R, *et al*. Gastroallergic anisakiasis: borderline between food allergy and parasitic disease-clinical and allergologic evaluation of 20 patients with confirmed acute parasitism by *Anisakis simplex*. *J Allergy Clin Immunol* 2000;105:176–81.

29 Tan BM, Sher MR, Good RA, Bahna SL. Severe food allergies by skin contact. *Ann Allergy Asthma Immunol* 2001; 86:583–6.

30 Polasani R, Melgar L, Reisman R, Ballow M. Hot dog vapor-induced status asthmaticus. *Ann Allergy Asthma Immunol* 1997; 78:35–6.

31 Taylor AV, Swanson MC, Jones RT, *et al*. Detection and quantitation of raw fish aeroallergens from an open-air fish market. *J Allergy Clin Immunol* 2000;105:166–9.

32 Roberts G, Golder N, Lack G. Bronchial challenges with aerosolized food in asthmatic, food-allergic children. *Allergy* 2002; 57:713–17.

33 Sicherer SH, Furlong TJ, DeSimone J, Sampson HA. Self-reported allergic reactions to peanut on commercial airliners. *J Allergy Clin Immunol* 1999;103:186–9.

34 Dawe RS, Ferguson J. Allergy to peanut. *Lancet* 1996;348: 1522–3.

35 Carlston J. Injection immunotherapy trial in inhalant food allergy. *Ann Allergy* 1988;61:80–2.

36 Jones RT, Stark D, Sussman G, Yunginger JW. Recovery of peanut allergens from ventilation filters of commercial airliners (abstract). *J Allergy Clin Immunol* 1996;97:423.

37 Hallett R, Haapanen LA, Teuber SS. Food allergies and kissing. *N Engl J Med* 2002;346:1833–4.

38 Eriksson NE, Moller C, Werner S, *et al*. The hazards of kissing when you are food allergic. A survey on the occurrence of kiss-induced allergic reactions among 1139 patients with self-reported food hypersensitivity. *J Investig Allergol Clin Immunol* 2003;13:149–54.

39 Maloney JM, Chapman MD, Sicherer SH. Peanut allergen exposure through saliva: assessment and interventions to reduce exposure. *J Allergy Clin Immunol* 2006;118:719–24.

40 Wuthrich B, Dascher M, Borelli S. Kiss-induced allergy to peanut. *Allergy* 2001;56:913.

41 Sicherer SH. Determinants of systemic manifestations of food allergy. *J Allergy Clin Immunol* 2000;106:S251–7.

42 Beyer K, Bardina L, Grishina G, Sampson HA. Identification of four major sesame seed allergens by 2D-proteonomics and Edman sequencing-seed storage proteins as common food allergens. *J Allergy Clin Immunol* 2002;109:S288.

43 Breiteneder H, Ebner C. Molecular and biochemical classification of plant-derived food allergens. *J Allergy Clin Immunol* 2000;106:27–36.

44 Breiteneder H, Radauer C. A classification of plant food allergens. *J Allergy Clin Immunol* 2004;113:821–30.

45 Aalberse RC. Structural biology of allergens. *J Allergy Clin Immunol* 2000;106:228–38.

46 Barnett D, Bonham B, Howden ME. Allergenic cross-reactions among legume foods – an *in vitro* study. *J Allergy Clin Immunol* 1987;79:433–8.

47 Bernhisel-Broadbent J, Sampson HA. Cross-allergenicity in the legume botanical family in children with food hypersensitivity. *J Allergy Clin Immunol* 1989;83:435–40.

48 Sicherer SH, Burks AW, Sampson HA. Clinical features of acute allergic reactions to peanut and tree nuts in children. *Pediatrics* 1998;102:e6.

49 Pumphrey RS, Wilson PB, Faragher EB, Edwards SR. Specific immunoglobulin E to peanut, hazelnut and Brazil nut in 731 patients: similar patterns found at all ages. *Clin Exp Allergy* 1999;29:1256–9.

50 Vocks E, Borga A, Szliska C, *et al*. Common allergenic structures in hazelnut, rye grain, sesame seeds, kiwi, and poppy seeds. *Allergy* 1993;48:168–72.

51 Sicherer SH. Clinical implications of cross-reactive food allergens. *J Allergy Clin Immunol* 2001;108:881–90.

52 Bock SA, Atkins FM. The natural history of peanut allergy. *J Allergy Clin Immunol* 1989;83:900–4.

53 Burks AW, James JM, Hiegel A, *et al*. Atopic dermatitis and food hypersensitivity reactions. *J Pediatr* 1998;132:132–6.

54 Matheu V, de Barrio M, Sierra Z, *et al*. Lupine-induced anaphylaxis. *Ann Allergy Asthma Immunol* 1999;83:406–8.

55 Hefle SL, Lemanske RFJ, Bush RK. Adverse reaction to lupine-fortified pasta. *J Allergy Clin Immunol* 1994;94:167–72.

56 Moneret-Vautrin DA, Guerin L, Kanny G, *et al*. Cross-allergenicity of peanut and lupine: the risk of lupine allergy in patients allergic to peanuts. *J Allergy Clin Immunol* 1999;104: 883–8.

57 Radcliffe M, Scadding G, Brown HM. Lupin flour anaphylaxis. *Lancet* 2005;365:1360.

58 Crespo JF, Pascual C, Burks AW, *et al*. Frequency of food allergy in a pediatric population from Spain. *Pediatr Allergy Immunol* 1995;6:39–43.

59 Pascual CY, Fernandez-Crespo J, Sanchez-Pastor S, *et al*. Allergy to lentils in Mediterranean pediatric patients. *J Allergy Clin Immunol* 1999;103:154–8.

60 Ewan PW. Clinical study of peanut and nut allergy in 62 consecutive patients: new features and associations. *BMJ* 1996; 312:1074–8.

61 Bock SA, Munoz-Furlong A, Sampson HA. Fatalities due to anaphylactic reactions to foods. *J Allergy Clin Immunol* 2001; 107:191–3.

62 Garcia F, Moneo I, Fernandez B, *et al*. Allergy to Anacardiaceae: description of cashew and pistachio nut allergens. *J Investig Allergol Clin Immunol* 2000;10:173–7.

63 Teuber SS, Peterson WR. Systemic allergic reaction to coconut (*Cocos nucifera*) in 2 subjects with hypersensitivity to tree nut and demonstration of cross-reactivity to legumin-like seed storage proteins: new coconut and walnut food allergens. *J Allergy Clin Immunol* 1999;103:1180–5.

64 Hourihane JO'B, Kilburn SA, Dean P, Warner JO. Clinical characteristics of peanut allergy. *Clin Exp Allergy* 1997;27:634–9.

65 Sicherer SH, Furlong TJ, Muñoz-Furlong A, *et al*. A voluntary registry for peanut and tree nut allergy: characteristics of the first 5,149 registrants. *J Allergy Clin Immunol* 2001;108:138–42.

66 Committee on Nutrition. American Academy of Pediatrics. Hypoallergenic infant formulas. *Pediatrics* 2000;106:346–9.

67 Asero R, Mistrello G, Roncarolo D, *et al*. A case of sesame seed-induced anaphylaxis. *Allergy* 1999;54:526–7.

68 Rance F, Dutau G, Abbal M. Mustard allergy in children. *Allergy* 2000;55:496–500.

69 Derby CJ, Gowland MH, Hourihane JO. Sesame allergy in Britain: a questionnaire survey of members of the Anaphylaxis Campaign. *Pediatr Allergy Immunol* 2005;16:171–5.

70 Hourihane JO, Dean TP, Warner JO. Peanut allergy in relation to heredity, maternal diet, and other atopic diseases: results of a questionnaire survey, skin prick testing, and food challenges. *BMJ* 1996;313:518–21.

71 Sicherer SH, Muñoz-Furlong A, Sampson HA. Prevalence of seafood allergy in the United States determined by a random telephone survey. *J Allergy Clin Immunol* 2004;114:159–65.

72 Van Do T, Elsayed S, Florvaag E, *et al*. Allergy to fish parvalbumins: studies on the cross-reactivity of allergens from 9 commonly consumed fish. *J Allergy Clin Immunol* 2005;116:1314–20.

73 Bernhisel-Broadbent J, Scanlon SM, Sampson HA. Fish hypersensitivity. I. *In vitro* and oral challenge results in fish-allergic patients. *J Allergy Clin Immunol* 1992;89:730–7.

74 Helbling A, Haydel R, McCants ML, *et al*. Fish allergy: Is cross-reactivity among fish species relevant? Double-blind placebo-controlled food challenge studies of fish allergic adults. *Ann Allergy Asthma Immunol* 1999;83:517–23.

75 Aas K. Studies of hypersensitivity to fish. A clinical study. *Int Arch Allergy Clin Immun* 1966;29:346–63.

76 Hansen TK, Bindslev JC, Skov PS, Poulsen LK. Codfish allergy in adults: IgE cross-reactivity among fish species. *Ann Allergy Asthma Immunol* 1997;78:187–94.

77 de Martino M, Novembre E, Galli L, *et al*. Allergy to different fish species in cod-allergic children: *in vivo* and *in vitro* studies. *J Allergy Clin Immunol* 1990;86:909–14.

78 Pascual C, Martin EM, Crespo JF. Fish allergy: evaluation of the importance of cross-reactivity. *J Pediatr* 1992;121:S29–34.

79 Asero R, Mistrello G, Roncarolo D, *et al*. True monosensitivity to a tropical sole. *Allergy* 1999;54:1228–9.

80 Kelso JM, Jones RT, Yunginger JW. Monospecific allergy to swordfish. *Ann Allergy Asthma Immunol* 1996;77:227–8.

81 Bernhisel-Broadbent J, Strause D, Sampson HA. Fish hypersensitivity. II. Clinical relevance of altered fish allergenicity caused by various preparation methods. *J Allergy Clin Immunol* 1992;90:622–9.

82 Daul CB, Slattery M, Reese G, Lehrer SB. Identification of the major brown shrimp (*Penaeus aztecus*) allergen as the muscle protein tropomyosin. *Int Arch Allergy Immunol* 1994;105:49–55.

83 Leung PS, Chen YC, Gershwin ME, *et al*. Identification and molecular characterization of *Charybdis feriatus* tropomy-osin, the major crab allergen. *J Allergy Clin Immunol* 1998;102:847–52.

84 Leung PS, Chen YC, Mykles DL, *et al*. Molecular identification of the lobster muscle protein tropomyosin as a seafood allergen. *Mol Mar Biol Biotechnol* 1998;7:12–20.

85 Leung PS, Chow WK, Duffey S, *et al*. IgE reactivity against a cross-reactive allergen in Crustacea and Mollusca: evidence for tropomyosin as the common allergen. *J Allergy Clin Immunol* 1996;98:954–61.

86 Daul CB, Morgan JE, Waring NP, *et al*. Immunologic evaluation of shrimp-allergic individuals. *J Allergy Clin Immunol* 1987;80:716–22.

87 Waring NP, Daul CB, deShazo RD, *et al*. Hypersensitivity reactions to ingested Crustacea: clinical evaluation and diagnostic studies in shrimp-sensitive individuals. *J Allergy Clin Immunol* 1985;76:440–5.

88 Morgan JE, O'Neil CE, Daul CB, Lehrer SB. Species-specific shrimp allergens: RAST and RAST-inhibition studies. *J Allergy Clin Immunol* 1989;83:1112–17.

89 Lehrer SB, McCants ML. Reactivity of IgE antibodies with Crustacea and oyster allergens: evidence for common antigenic structures. *J Allergy Clin Immunol* 1987;80:133–9.

90 Santos AB, Chapman MD, Aalberse RC, *et al*. Cockroach allergens and asthma in Brazil: identification of tropomyosin as a major allergen with potential cross-reactivity with mite and shrimp allergens. *J Allergy Clin Immunol* 1999;104:329–37.

91 van Ree R, Antonicelli L, Akkerdaas JH, *et al*. Asthma after consumption of snails in house-dust-mite-allergic patients: a case of IgE cross-reactivity. *Allergy* 1996;51:387–93.

92 Goetz DW, Whisman BA. Occupational asthma in a seafood restaurant worker: cross-reactivity of shrimp and scallops. *Ann Allergy Asthma Immunol* 2000;85:461–6.

93 Carrillo T, de Rodriguez C, Blanco C, *et al*. Anaphylaxis due to limpet ingestion. *Ann Allergy* 1994;73:504–8.

94 van RR, Antonicelli L, Akkerdaas JH, *et al*. Possible induction of food allergy during mite immunotherapy. *Allergy* 1996;51:108–13.

95 Jones SM, Magnolfi CF, Cooke SK, Sampson HA. Immunologic cross-reactivity among cereal grains and grasses in children with food hypersensitivity. *J Allergy Clin Immunol* 1995;96:341–51.

96 Donovan GR, Baldo BA. Crossreactivity of IgE antibodies from sera of subjects allergic to both ryegrass pollen and wheat endosperm proteins: evidence for common allergenic determinants. *Clin Exp Allergy* 1990;20:501–9.

97 Bausela BA, Garcia AM, Martin EM, *et al*. Peculiarities of egg allergy in children with bird protein sensitization. *Ann Allergy Asthma Immunol* 1997;78:213–16.

98 Szepfalusi Z, Ebner C, Pandjaitan R, *et al*. Egg yolk a-livetin (chicken serum albumin) is a cross-reactive allergen in the bird-egg syndrome. *J Allergy Clin Immunol* 1994;93:932–42.

99 Bock SA, Sampson HA, Atkins FM, *et al*. Double-blind, placebo-controlled food challenge (DBPCFC) as an office procedure: a manual. *J Allergy Clin Immunol* 1988;82:986–97.

100 Kelso JM, Cockrell GE, Helm RM, Burks AW. Common allergens in avian meats. *J Allergy Clin Immunol* 1999;104:202–4.

101 Cahen YD, Fritsch R, Wuthrich B. Food allergy with monovalent sensitivity to poultry meat. *Clin Exp Allergy* 1998;28:1026–30.

102 Langland T. A clinical and immunological study of allergy to hen's egg white. VI. Occurrence of proteins cross-reacting with allergens in hen's egg white as studied in egg white from turkey, duck, goose, seagull, and in hen egg yolk, and hen and chicken sera and flesh. *Allergy* 1983;38:399–412.

103 Anibarro B, Seoane FJ, Vila C, Lombardero M. Allergy to eggs from duck and goose without sensitization to hen egg proteins. *J Allergy Clin Immunol* 2000;105:834–6.

104 Martelli A, De Chiara A, Corvo M, et al. Beef allergy in children with cow's milk allergy; cow's milk allergy in children with beef allergy. *Ann Allergy Asthma Immunol* 2002;89:38–43.

105 Werfel SJ, Cooke SK, Sampson HA. Clinical reactivity to beef in children allergic to cow's milk. *J Allergy Clin Immunol* 1997;99:293–300.

106 Fiocchi A, Restani P, Riva E, et al. Heat treatment modifies the allergenicity of beef and bovine serum albumin. *Allergy* 1998;53:798–802.

107 Spuergin P, Walter M, Schiltz E, et al. Allergenicity of alpha-caseins from cow, sheep, and goat. *Allergy* 1997;52:293–8.

108 Restani P, Gaiaschi A, Plebani A, et al. Cross-reactivity between milk proteins from different animal species. *Clin Exp Allergy* 1999;29:997–1004.

109 Bellioni-Businco B, Paganelli R, Lucenti P, et al. Allergenicity of goat's milk in children with cow's milk allergy. *J Allergy Clin Immunol* 1999;103:1191–4.

110 Businco L, Giampietro PG, Lucenti P, et al. Allergenicity of mare's milk in children with cow's milk allergy. *J Allergy Clin Immunol* 2000;105:1031–4.

111 Ayuso R, Lehrer SB, Tanaka L, et al. IgE antibody response to vertebrate meat proteins including tropomyosin. *Ann Allergy Asthma Immunol* 1999;83:399–405.

112 Rodriguez J, Crespo JF, Lopez-Rubio A, et al. Clinical cross-reactivity among foods of the Rosaceae family. *J Allergy Clin Immunol* 2000;106:183–9.

113 Pastorello E, Ortolani C, Farioli L, et al. Allergenic cross-reactivity among peach, apricot, plum, and cherry in patients with oral allergy syndrome: an *in vivo* and *in vitro* study. *J Allergy Clin Immunol* 1994;94:699–707.

114 Rodriguez J, Crespo JF, Burks W, et al. Randomized, double-blind, crossover challenge study in 53 subjects reporting adverse reactions to melon (*Cucumis melo*). *J Allergy Clin Immunol* 2000;106:968–72.

115 Ortolani C, Pastorello EA, Farioli L, et al. IgE-mediated allergy from vegetable allergens. *Ann Allergy* 1993;71:470–6.

116 Pastorello EA, Farioli L, Pravettoni V, et al. The major allergen of peach (*Prunus persica*) is a lipid transfer protein. *J Allergy Clin Immunol* 1999;103:520–6.

117 Cuesta-Herranz J, Lazaro M, Martinez A, et al. Pollen allergy in peach-allergic patients: sensitization and cross-reactivity to taxonomically unrelated pollens. *J Allergy Clin Immunol* 1999;104:688–94.

118 Fernandez-Rivas M, van Ree R, Cuevas M. Allergy to Rosaceae fruits without related pollinosis. *J Allergy Clin Immunol* 1997;100:728–33.

119 Schocker F, Luttkopf D, Muller U, et al. IgE binding to unique hazelnut allergens: identification of non pollen-related and heat-stable hazelnut allergens eliciting severe allergic reactions. *Eur J Nutr* 2000;39:172–80.

120 Asero R. Detection and clinical characterization of patients with oral allergy syndrome caused by stable allergens in Rosaceae and nuts. *Ann Allergy Asthma Immunol* 1999;83:377–83.

121 Crespo JF, Rodriguez J, James JM, et al. Reactivity to potential cross-reactive foods in fruit-allergic patients: implications for prescribing food avoidance. *Allergy* 2002;57:946–9.

122 Nel A, Gujuluva C. Latex antigens: identification and use in clinical and experimental studies, including crossreactivity with food and pollen allergens. *Ann Allergy Asthma Immunol* 1998;81:388–96.

123 Blanco C, Carrillo T, Castillo R, et al. Latex allergy: clinical features and cross-reactivity with fruits. *Ann Allergy* 1994;73:309–14.

124 Brehler R, Theissen U, Mohr C, Luger T. "Latex–fruit syndrome": frequency of cross-reacting IgE antibodies. *Allergy* 1997;52:404–10.

125 Beezhold DH, Sussman GL, Liss GM, Chang NS. Latex allergy can induce clinical reactions to specific foods. *Clin Exp Allergy* 1996;26:416–22.

126 Garcia Ortiz JC, Moyano JC, Alvarez M, Bellido J. Latex allergy in fruit-allergic patients. *Allergy* 1998;53:532–6.

127 Reche M, Pascual CY, Vicente J, et al. Tomato allergy in children and young adults: cross-reactivity with latex and potato. *Allergy* 2001;56:1197–201.

128 Levy DA, Mounedji N, Noirot C, Leynadier F. Allergic sensitization and clinical reactions to latex, food and pollen in adult patients. *Clin Exp Allergy* 2000;30:270–5.

CHAPTER 26

Controversial Practices and Unproven Methods in Allergy

Jennifer A. Namazy and Ronald A. Simon

KEY CONCEPTS

- There have been an increasing number of patients who are using complementary therapies for chronic conditions.
- Unproven methods are increasingly being used for the diagnosis and treatment of allergic diseases.
- Unproven methods are procedures or therapies that are not supported by scientific evidence and have no basis in the pathophysiology of allergic disease.
- Inappropriate methods are procedures and therapies that are legitimate but are used inappropriately.
- It is important for the practicing allergist to become familiar with both accepted and unproven practices.

Introduction

The process of diagnosing and treating allergic disease is complex and at times elusive. It requires a thorough history and physical examination and, in certain situations, complementary laboratory tests. Most of the tests which are performed today have undergone rigorous scientific evaluation for proof of effectiveness and safety. They must also have established physiological significance when used to diagnose a particular disease. Nevertheless, there are a growing number of unconventional, unproven, and inappropriate procedures used by some in order to diagnose allergic disease. Some of these "tests" are legitimate but are misused in their application to the diagnosis of allergy. Other "tests" have no basis in the pathophysiology of allergic disease. It is important for those practicing allergy and immunology to become familiar with all diagnostic procedures. Some may be unsuitable for allergy diagnosis for several reasons. For example, a procedure may be based on an unproven theory. Others are legitimate tests used inappropriately. Some procedures do not have the ability to diagnose any disease. It thus becomes apparent that standardization and a controlled evaluation of procedures before their use are imperative for proper patient care. The following information should be useful because there have been an increasing number of patients who are using complementary therapies for chronic

conditions. One study found that complementary therapies were usually used alongside conventional treatment [1]. Patients felt empowered to take control over their condition rather than feel dependent on medication [1]. These patients may present at the beginning of their search with a multitude of questions regarding a proposed specific diagnostic procedure or they may present having been involved is a questionable, perhaps expensive procedure, resulting in a questionable diagnoses.

Definitions

Standard practice is that which is performed by the majority of physicians in the community. It encompasses those procedures and treatments which have been scientifically proven to be effective and safe. Before describing and critiquing the following procedures and therapies it is important to first attempt to categorize each one. Thus first certain approaches can be considered to be "unproven," and are also at times referred to as "complementary" or "alternative." These types of tests or treatments are those that are not based on any clear rationale based on acceptable allergy pathophysiology, and their effectiveness is not supported by scientific evidence. Although they may appear well-constructed they do not seem capable of either diagnosing or treating an allergic disease. Some of these procedures have been loosely adapted from proven methods that are currently available for the diagnosis and treatment of allergic disease. Often one of the reasons why these tests have not been examined scientifically is that their methodology

Food Allergy: Adverse Reactions to Foods and Food Additives, 4th edition.
Edited by Dean D. Metcalfe, Hugh A. Sampson, and Ronald A. Simon.
© 2008 Blackwell Publishing, ISBN: 978-1-4501-5129-0.

is vague and is often difficult to reproduce. Other procedures are categorized as being "inappropriate." This means that the test itself is a validated test used to diagnose certain conditions; however, in these cases the procedure is being inappropriately applied.

"Controversial" tests

Skin endpoint titration

During the 1940s, Rinkel developed the method of endpoint skin testing [2]. He found that this method was a useful guide in determining a patient's sensitivity and the information found could be used in determining a safe and effective dose for immunotherapy. Variations of this method have been used for both the diagnosis and treatment of inhalant and food allergies.

Method

The procedure involves intradermal testing with 5-fold serial dilutions of extract. A 7-mm whealing response is considered reactive. The endpoint is defined as the weakest dilution that produces a positive skin reaction and initiates a progressive increase in the diameter of the wheals with each stronger dilution tested [3]. The optimal starting dose is usually 0.01–0.02 ml of extract. The optimal therapeutic dose, defined as a dose at which symptoms are controlled on immunotherapy, is reached after the endpoint dilution is given weekly in increasing increments. Rinkel anticipated a relief of patient symptoms at a dose of 0.5 ml of the endpoint dilution.

Conclusion

There have been several trials over the years that have looked at the efficacy of the Rinkel method. Van Metre *et al.* published several studies which supported the Rinkel method as valid in quantifying skin sensitivity to ragweed pollen and found the method comparable with *in vitro* leukocyte histamine release and radioallergosorbent assay testing (RAST) [4]. While variations of this method of skin testing are being practiced today without any risks, using the results to determine optimal dosing of immunotherapy is questionable. In the opinion of many, most of the time this "dose" is an underestimation resulting in ineffective treatment.

Unproven tests

Applied kinesiology

Kinesiology refers to the science of motion techniques. It is a belief by some that certain diseases, including allergic reactions, may cause a weakening of skeletal musculature. Some believe that by using applied kinesiology one may diagnose allergic disease. This is commonly applied to the diagnosis of food allergy.

Method

Allergens to be tested are placed in stoppered glass bottles. In some cases a glass vial containing a specific allergen is placed on or near the body of the patient, or in other cases, the patient is asked to hold the vial. During allergen "exposure," muscle strength is tested. A positive test is said to be indicated by observed weakening in muscle strength. There are variations to the standard test which include "surrogate" testing in which a relative of the patient undergoes testing for the patient.

Conclusion

In 1988, Garrow [5] published a study of blinded and open challenges of allergen using applied kinesiology and looking at the reproducibility and efficacy of the test. The study reported no significant difference between frequencies of positive reactions to placebo versus allergen. Therefore, at this time, there appears to be no proof of the efficacy or reproducibility of the method of kinesiology in diagnosing food allergy.

Provocative testing and neutralization

Elicitation of a limited reaction by delivering allergen via the transdermal, subcutaneous, intradermal, or bronchial route are a part of an allergy practice. These procedures provide a wealth of information in the diagnosis of several allergic diseases. Such tests include: prick and intradermal skin test, intranasal, subconjunctival, oral tests and methacholine challenge. These approaches differ from provocative testing and neutralization in that they have undergone repeated scientific validation in studies with both patients and normal controls.

The provocative–neutralization method was introduced by Lee in 1961 for the diagnosis of food allergy [6]. The provocation is performed by intradermal, subcutaneous, or sublingual routes. It is currently used to diagnose and treat allergic disease and sensitivities to a wide variety of substances. The items tested are not necessarily those suspected by the history. They can include such chemicals as: formaldehyde, phenol, ethanol, and hormones such as progesterone [7].

Method

The patient is given an intradermal/subcutaneous dose of allergen extract using 5-fold serial dilutions (Rinkel method). The patient is observed for 10 minutes and any symptoms are recorded. If the patient remains symptom free then increasing doses of extract are given until symptoms do occur. Once these symptoms occur, the patient is immediately given injections of weaker dilutions of the same extract until symptoms are resolved. This amount of extract is considered the "neutralizing dose" and is then used for future treatment [8].

The technique appears vague and imprecise. There is no generally established validated protocol for performing the provocative testing and neutralization. In addition, there is no consensus on establishing what a positive test is. Symptoms may be quite extensive and non-specific and may include: headache, nasal symptoms, chest symptoms, ear reactions, gastrointestinal reactions, skin eruptions or itching, or general reactions such as fatigue, chills, muscle pain, or drowsiness [9]. There has been no general agreement on the role of wheal diameter in reporting a positive test. Some interpret an increase in wheal size as a further indication of a positive test.

Sublingual provocation testing and neutralization has been advocated by some in the diagnosis and treatment of food allergy. It was first described by Hansel in 1953 [10] as a diagnostic and therapeutic technique. The method consists of placing allergenic extract underneath the tongue and waiting 10 minutes for the appearance of symptoms. If symptoms occur then the patient is given a more dilute solution of the same extract. The neutralizing dose is used as treatment prior to or after eating meals containing the offending food if the food cannot be avoided.

Given the fact that a single item needs to be tested one at a time and requires waiting 10 minutes between each dilution, it comes as no surprise that a single complete provocative–neutralization might take an entire day. Testing multiple items may take many days. Therefore, this test is time consuming and can be costly.

Conclusion

There have been approximately 15 studies published looking primarily at the efficacy of provocative testing and neutralization. Eight of these studies were double-blinded. Only one study contained a control group. The majority of the studies were not able to demonstrate any benefit from neutralizing solution compared with placebo. Crawford *et al.* [11] performed a double-blinded study in 61 subjects with a history of reactions to five common foods. The authors were unable to demonstrate reproducibility of results from sublingual food testing. Kallin and Collier [12] in a double-blind study compared neutralizing effects of sublingual or subcutaneous food extracts versus saline placebo. The authors found that in 70% of patients, treatment with saline placebo was "relieving." Draper [13] in a study of 121 patients with inhalant allergy, found that only 38% of positive provocation tests correlated with a positive food challenge test. One of the most well-structured double-blind studies was that by Jewett *et al.* [14]. This study of 18 patients with symptoms previously provoked by intracutaneous testing were tested with food extracts or placebo. The rate of positive responses was similar between placebo and food extracts.

In conclusion, overall these studies fail to confirm the efficacy of provocative testing and neutralization in the diagnosis and treatment of allergic disease.

Neutralization therapy

Neutralization of allergic symptoms is an extension of provocation–neutralization testing described earlier. This type of treatment, also called "relieving therapy," consists of self-administered doses of allergen extract at a concentration which "neutralizes" symptoms provoked during the prior provocation testing [7]. This treatment may be used by some to relieve present symptoms and to prevent anticipated symptoms and for continuous maintenance doses twice weekly. These doses can be given either by injection or sublingual. The patient can change and discontinue or restart treatment as they deem necessary.

Theory

A number of theories have been brought forth to try and explain neutralization of symptoms. A common belief among some practitioners is that this type of therapy induces immunological tolerance. Controlled, double-blind, multicenter studies have reported that sublingual, provocative food testing did not discriminate between placebo controls and food extracts used in neutralization therapy [9]. In addition, there appear to be no long- or short-term studies looking at the efficacy of this therapy.

Conclusion

As a result, since there is no known mechanism for neutralization of symptoms and no clear scientific evidence demonstrating its effectiveness, this form of therapy is not generally recommended in the treatment of allergic conditions such as food allergy.

Cytotoxic leukocyte testing

Also known as "Bryan's" test, this form of allergy testing was adapted by Bryan in the 1960s. Initially designed to help aid physicians in diagnosing allergy, the theory behind the test is that the addition of specific allergen *in vitro* to whole blood or to serum leukocyte suspension will reduce the white blood cell count or result in the death of leukocytes. It has been claimed by some to be useful for the diagnosis of both food and inhalant allergy [15]. The newer ALCAT test currently available functions in a similar way in that it measures volumetric shifts in white blood cells upon incubation with antigens. The blood cells are passed after an incubation period through a narrow channel and are measured by an electronic instrument. The sizes are displayed as either cell diameters or as cell volumes. The company claims that their test will identify exactly which foods or chemicals are responsible for triggering a variety of symptoms including: joint pain, headaches, asthma, obesity, ADD/hyperreactivity, chronic fatigue among others.

Method

The technique involves collecting the buffy coat from a drop of patient's blood and placing it on a microscope slide coated with dried extract of food or other allergen/substance and then observed microscopically for alteration in the appearance of white blood cells [16]. Once a fair number of white cells have been located, they are rated for degree of destruction. A single sample of blood can be tested to a panel of foods and other substances.

Conclusion

There is no theoretical basis for the cytotoxic test, since there is no evidence for a general cytotoxic mechanism in allergic disease. The test itself is not standardized and has never been shown in controlled trials to be effective in the diagnosis of food or inhalant allergy. Franklin and Lowell [17] reported that there was no significant difference in white blood cell counts in blood exposed to ragweed extract versus saline in ragweed-sensitive individuals. Lieberman et al. [18] could not demonstrate clinical correlation with test results in study patients and found inconsistent results when patients were tested more than once. Benson and Arkins [19] found the test was associated with a high degree of false positives. In regards to ALCAT, one abstract, from the company homepage, assessed the degree of correlation between ALCAT and the results of oral double-blinded food challenges found an almost 84% correlation between the two tests. However, this small study had some significant limitations and no recent larger studies are available [20].

Electrodiagnosis (Vega testing)

Electrodiagnosis is also known as electroacupuncture according to Voll (EAV), electrodermal screening (EDS), bioelectric functions diagnosis (BFD), or bioenergy regulatory technique (BER) [21]. Some practitioners believe that the presence of specific allergy can lead to a change in the electrical potential of the skin. These changes are then said to be detected by Vega machines or bioresonance devices.

Method

In this procedure a sample of food extract is placed in a container in contact with an aluminum plate. This is then placed between the skin of the patient and a galvanometer. Electrical activity of the skin is measured at certain "allergy points." For example, there are certain points on the lower extremities which are said to correspond to food allergy and points on the upper extremities which are said to correspond to inhalant allergies [15]. These results are entered into a computer which prints a list of allergies for the patient. Children are assessed by testing the parent first, and repeated with the parent holding the child's hand.

Conclusion

This type of procedure appeals to those patients who are reluctant to undergo any involved and potentially uncomfortable diagnostic procedures such as skin testing. Also, the use of computers, galvanometers, and "print outs" appear "state of the art" to some patients. Semizzi et al. [22] assessed the accuracy of electrodermal testing in 72 allergic patients compared with healthy controls. They found no significant difference in skin electrical response between the two groups.

Radionics
Method
Radionics is based on the concept that all life forms are submerged in the electromagnetic energy field of the earth. And that a disease will be reflected by changes or "imbalances: in an individual's electromagnetic field said to lie outside the normal electromagnetic spectrum. Practitioners claim to treat disease by restoring normal energy balance. Sometimes the operator is with the patient, and sometimes the operator "connects" with the patient at a distance using an object such as a lock of hair, blood sample, or photograph.

Conclusion
This technique has not been subject to formal study, and there is no published evidence that it is effective for the assessment or treatment of any disorder [23].

Iridology
Method
This is based on the concept that each part of the body is represented by a corresponding part of the iris. A person's state of health is determined by the color, texture, and location of pigment flecks in the eye. Imbalances are treated with dietary supplements or herbal medicines.

Conclusion
Studies have shown that iridologists are unable to distinguish patients with disease from those who are healthy [23,24].

Body chemical analysis
Some practitioners claim that detection of any amount of inorganic or organic chemical in body fluid may indicate a toxic exposure and may explain the presence of disease. They postulate that certain substances may be toxic to the immune system leading to a state of sensitivity to the environment [2]. Some of these substances include: vitamins, drugs, chlorinated hydrocarbons, volatile organic chemicals, pesticides, and metals.

Method
Specific tests include gas chromatographic mass spectrophotometry analysis of body fluids and tissue, quantitation of chemicals in serum and other body fluids and breath analysis [3].

Conclusion
These procedures are highly sensitive and are able to identify chemicals in virtually every individual, even those who

do not report symptoms. This is why a strong clinical correlation is important in conjunction with this type of testing. In certain situations and in certain individuals, it may be appropriate to evaluate for chemical poisoning in order to properly diagnose a disorder. It is important to note that many of the laboratories performing these tests are deficient with respect to quality assurance so, for example, contamination of samples remains a major source of error [3].

Inappropriate tests

IgG antibodies

Immunoglobulin E (IgE) antibody in response to allergens causes the release of mast cell mediators which are important in the immediate-type symptoms of anaphylaxis or atopic disease. Sensitivities to certain allergens can be diagnosed by detecting IgE in the serum by RAST. Many laboratories can test in a similar fashion for the presence of immunoglobulin G (IgG) to certain foods. There are those practitioners who measure circulating IgG antibody reactive with food antigens in diagnosing food allergy. The patient then may receive therapy in the form of elimination and rotation diets. It is this construct, that while IgG may not be important in the immediate-type reactions to certain foods, it may be important in delayed-type reactions such as depression, apathy, fatigue, myalgias, and gastrointestinal complaints [25]. Diagnosis of delayed-type reactions is challenging and while conventional IgE RAST alone cannot diagnose these types of reactions there are no published double-blind, placebo-controlled studies that demonstrate that such symptoms are related to particular foods as identified using such tests.

IgG antibodies are not known to have a role in the pathogenesis of atopic disease and food allergy. Certain levels of IgG to food antigens as well as other environmental antigens may be found normally and their presence, as of yet, has not been shown to be associated with atopic disease. Therefore, measurement of antigen-specific IgG has not been recommended as a form of diagnosing food allergy in the clinical setting.

Lymphocyte subset counts

Quantitative counting of leukocytes bearing one or more surface markers known as cluster of differentiation (CD) markers is helpful in the diagnosis of some forms of lymphocyte cellular immunodeficiencies. For example, measuring CD4 lymphocytes is part of the standard procedure for diagnosis and management in human immunodeficiency virus [2]. Lymphocyte subset counts may be labile and nonspecific. Levels may not be elevated in traditional allergic diseases but may be elevated in those with viral illnesses, for example. Use of these tests to diagnose forms of allergy or other presumed immunological disorders is generally considered inappropriate and can lead to inappropriate treatment of a patient.

Pulse test

Coca in 1953 reported that tachycardia occurring 5–90 minutes after exposure to a food or inhaled material is a reliable indicator of food allergy [26].

Method

The test dose can be given by any route including injection. A change of 10 bpm is thought to be diagnostic by some, but the procedure has never been standardized. This test has no relationship to the diagnosis of allergic disease.

Unproven therapy

Neutralization therapy

This topic is discussed earlier in the section entitled "Provocation–Neutralization."

Rotation diets
Theory

This particular type of diet recommends that a certain food not be eaten more than once every four to five days [3]. Part of the rationale is that if the patient is allergic to most or all foods, by eating them frequently, he or she runs the risk of becoming increasingly sensitized to that food and possibly other foods.

Conclusion

If a patient does have clinical sensitivity to a particular food then he or she will develop symptoms after contact with that food irrespective of rotation schedule. However, if a patient demonstrates "subclinical sensitivity" to a certain food, that is, no symptoms but evidence of specific IgE by testing, then each exposure to that food will increase sensitivity and likelihood of a future reaction. There is thus no scientific data supporting the efficacy of this type of diet.

Buteyko breathing technique
Theory

This technique is promoted as a drug-free asthma therapy. It is based on the concept that carbon dioxide is a natural bronchodilator. Slowing the rate of breathing by this logic would then raise carbon dioxide levels, resulting in symptomatic improvement. One recently visited website made a "12-month unconditional guarantee" that by following these exercises you could "outgrow your asthma."

Conclusion

Controlled studies have demonstrated symptomatic improvement and reduction in medication use in some patients, but no changes in carbon dioxide levels or measurements of lung function [27]. There is no evidence that there is any impact on the inflammatory components of asthma.

Advanced allergy elimination
Theory
This treatment is based on the concept that "allergen" is perceived by the brain as a threat to the body's well being. Exposure to allergen disrupts the flow of nervous energies from the brain to the body via "meridians," resulting in symptoms [23]. Acupressure is applied to both sides of the spinal column while the patient is in direct contact to purported allergen.

Conclusion
This approach lacks scientific rationale or published evidence of efficacy.

Orthomolecular therapy
Theory
This refers to the use of supplements and/or vitamins administered in large quantities either parenterally or orally to treat numerous medical and psychiatric conditions [3]. Practitioners of this therapy will commonly measure levels of vitamins in the serum or urine to determine the amount needed for correction. This type of therapy has been used in a wide variety of diseases. For example, antioxidant supplements such as vitamin E, C and glutathione have been used to treat allergic disease based on the theory that allergic inflammation generates free radicals which can cause oxidative damage to tissues [28].

Conclusion
There have been no controlled studies looking at this type of therapy and is not a recommended treatment of any disease at this time. Large doses of certain vitamins can accumulate in the body and lead to toxic effects.

Mercury amalgam removal
Theory
Silver–mercury amalgam has been used in dental fillings for over 100 years. There have been many claims from physicians and dentists that certain patients may develop sensitivity to this material. Subsequently, it has been blamed for the development of a wide array of symptoms [3]. These claims have led to the removal of these types of fillings.

Conclusion
There is no sound clinical evidence for the claims that mercury amalgam is responsible for the development of a multiplicity of somatic complaints.

Urine autoinjections
In 1930 Oriel and Barber reportedly found protein-like substances in the urine of allergic individuals during acute exacerbations of allergic disease [29]. Urine obtained from sensitive individuals applied intradermally to those individuals with the same sensitivities resulted in a positive skin test. This was not the case for the same urine applied intradermally in a non-atopic individual [25]. These practitioners felt that these "urine proteins" can be isolated by chemical extraction and given to the patient as a form of therapy in a series of intradermal/subcutaneous injections.

In 1947, the procedure was reintroduced by Plesch [30]. He describes a system of collecting fresh urine from a patient and after sterilization, injecting set amounts intramuscularly. Various reactions would occur within hours of injection and include: fever, diarrhea, hypotension, shortness of breath, and vomiting. He found that by performing these injections in patients with various syndromes such as jaundice, allergic disease, gastrointestinal symptoms, and dermatological symptoms there was a decrease in symptoms. There are however, no controlled studies to support neither the efficacy nor the safety of the procedure. In fact, in rabbits, urine autoinjection may lead to the formation of autoantibodies to glomerular basement membrane (GBM) and result in nephritis. Although this has not been demonstrated directly in humans, it is possible that receiving these urine autoinjections could induce immune complex disease. It has been established that in humans, anti-GBM antibodies can lead to the development of Goodpasture's syndrome. Therefore, at this time, the American Academy of Allergy and Immunology has taken the position that this procedure is unproven, without scientific basis, and potentially dangerous [15].

Inappropriate therapy

Clinical ecology
Clinical ecology is based generally on two concepts. One is that a large number of chemicals and foods can be responsible for illness in the absence of abnormal laboratory tests and physical findings; and the other is that the immune system is functionally depressed as a result of exposure to certain chemicals in the environment [31]. This is not to be confused with toxic illnesses which produce a number of symptoms and abnormal laboratory tests in response to a particular toxin. Those who practice clinical ecology believe that patients with chemical hypersensitivity syndrome, also known as environmental hypersensitivity disorder, or 20th century disease, or induced immune dysregulation syndrome have symptoms which are a result of low-level, long-term exposure to environmental chemicals. The doses which cause these syndromes are far below those established in the general population to cause harmful effects [32]. The agents are sometimes referred to as "incitants" or "offenders," and they include foods, food additives, and synthetic and natural chemicals such as: pesticides, detergents, perfumes, vehicle exhaust, and natural gas. Symptoms are often generalized, frequently affecting more than one organ system including the cardiac, gastrointestinal, respiratory, genitourinary, and neurological systems.

Theory

Clinical ecologists [33] have theorized that environmental illness is a result of the development of sensitivity to novel synthetic chemicals. Others believe that these chemicals act as haptens inducing IgG formation and immune complex formation [34]. Environmental illness has also been thought to be the result of a non-specific autoimmune process. What still needs to be established is a possible mechanism for this disease process; however, there are several concepts that clinical ecologists use to account for patient symptoms. "Total body load" and "Chemical overload" draw an analogy between the immune system and a container. The immune system is said to have a limited capacity for handling antigens. Once a patient develops symptoms in response to an environmental antigen this then indicates that the immune system has been exceeded. "Masking" is a concept in which a patient, who is sensitive to a certain food, may eliminate symptoms by eating the food on a regular basis. "Spreading phenomenon" refers to sensitivity to one antigen leading to the development of sensitivity to multiple other antigens [3].

Diagnosis

A detailed history within provocation–neutralization testing remains the mainstay of diagnosing environmental illness by clinical ecologists. Occasionally blood tests looking at immunoglobulin, complement, or specific chemical levels are used to aid in diagnosis.

Treatment

Consists mainly of avoidance measures, elimination diets, neutralization therapy, and in some cases as in *Candida* hypersensitivity syndrome, drug therapy.

Anti-*Candida* **drugs for** *Candida* **hypersensitivity syndrome**
Theory

Candida albicans is yeast which maintains a role as part of the body's normal flora. There are those who believe that it is this particular organism that is the cause of a condition termed "yeast hypersensitivity syndrome" or "*Candida* hypersensitivity syndrome." Proponents of this hypothesis believe that the syndrome is caused by an overgrowth of *Candida albicans* in the gastrointestinal tract leading to local inflammation as well as a more generalized toxic response. This response is thought to be secondary to a hypersensitivity reaction to a toxin which the organism secretes. As a result, symptoms range from recurrent or persistent candidal infections to chronic gastrointestinal symptoms such as bloating, diarrhea, constipation, and heartburn. Central nervous system symptoms have also been reported including depression, chronic fatigue, and memory problem [3].

Methods

There is no established method of diagnosing this syndrome. Diagnosis is most commonly made by history alone and not with specific laboratory measures. There have been reports of practitioners performing allergy testing in order to document sensitivity to *candida*.

Treatment

Patients are first warned to avoid broad-spectrum antibiotics and systemic steroids since these medications may potentiate *candida*. They are given minute doses of oral nystatin until symptoms have resolved. If symptoms persist, treatment can be changed to another anti-candidal drug such as ketoconazole or amphotericin B. In addition to anti-candidal drugs, patients are also started on yeast-free, sugar-free diets. It is thought by some that by eating simple sugars there is an increase in growth of *candida* in the gut [35] Candida allergy shots are also included in the treatment regimen of some patients.

Conclusion

Books and lay press articles have been published; support groups have been formed, all in the hopes of establishing a connection between yeast and disease. However, a scientific basis for this syndrome has never been established. The reports that do circulate are largely anecdotal. In 1990, Dismukes *et al.* [36] published the first randomized, double-blind, crossover study looking specifically at the effect of treatment with oral and vaginal nystatin compared with placebo in 42 pre-menopausal women presumed to have *Candida* hypersensitivity syndrome. Results from their work showed that while nystatin therapy did reduce vaginal symptoms, the efficacy of treatment for systemic symptoms including depression and chronic fatigue was not established. There was no significant reduction in systemic symptoms compared with placebo. Therefore, the study could not establish a therapeutic benefit of nystatin therapy in a patient with *Candida* hypersensitivity syndrome.

Elimination diets
Theory

The elimination of multiple foods has been recommended by some practitioners when multiple food allergies have been discovered on skin testing. This type or diet is also recommended by others who believe that through elimination diets one may "boost" the immune system [3].

Methods

Once the patient is diagnosed with sensitivity to multiple foods, either by unconventional testing or perhaps history, they are placed on highly restrictive diets in order to prevent further symptoms. Most of the time patients are given supplements of vitamin, minerals, or amino acids [21].

Conclusion

There is no evidence that by eliminating multiple foods one may improve the functioning of the immune system.

In fact, placing patients on such restrictive diets may lead to harmful effects of malnutrition.

Multiple chemical sensitivity syndrome

Theory
Multiple chemical sensitivity (MCS) syndrome or idiopathic environmental intolerances (IEI), as suggested by the WHO/IPCS workshop in 1996, has been used to describe a constellation of symptoms which overlap with those of environmental illness but overall remains a distinct entity. This disorder is characterized by a wide variety of symptoms including somatic, cognitive, and affective symptoms, caused by low-level exposure to environmental chemicals [37]. Symptoms commonly involve almost every major organ system and are thought to result from sensitivity to certain chemicals. Chronic fatigue, depression, headache, and dizziness are commonly reported symptoms. Little is known about the pathophysiology of this condition, but its proponents claim that through certain mechanisms such as disruption of immunological/allergy processes, alterations in nervous system function, changes in biochemical pathways, or changes in neurobehavioral function chemicals cause tissue damage [38]. This may be accomplished through processes such as free radical generation, immune complex formation, or hapten formation.

Methods
Patients with this condition often manifest certain psychological features such as anxiety, depression, somatization, conversion, and phobia [3]. This makes it especially challenging in establishing a diagnosis of MCS. The diagnosis of MCS is, however, made if symptoms cannot be explained by abnormal tests but are associated with a documented environmental exposure. The lack of objective findings of disease such as: physical exam and laboratory tests cast doubt on the validity of MCS as a clinical disease.

Critique
The concept of multiple chemical sensitivities in the absence of any objective data remains its advocates' greatest challenge. At the present time, there is no scientific evidence that MCS should be regarded as a true clinical entity, but rather it appears to be based on an association of a wide range of symptoms to a particular or varied number of varied environmental chemicals.

Clinical ecology is inadequately supported in the literature. Both diagnostics and treatments have not been proven to be of any consistent efficacy or benefit. Part of the difficulty in evaluating clinical ecology and environmental disorders is that it is virtually impossible to establish a cause and effect relationship. There is such a varied number of possible "triggers" of symptoms.

Conclusion
Many of the subspecialty groups including the American Academy of Allergy Asthma and Immunology and the American College of Physicians have issued position papers looking at several of the above-mentioned procedures and therapies. It was the goal of this chapter to provide definitions of controversial, unproven, and inappropriate procedures and treatments and provide examples of each so that it might provide insight into remote practices of allergy. There appears no reproducible scientific basis for any of the treatments, conditions, or procedures discussed. By examining each theory and method, we can become more aware of the importance of scientific evidence and standardization of procedures in our daily practice. The history, physical exam, selective skin tests, and appropriate laboratory tests remain the standard of care in first evaluating the allergy patient. However, as we have seen this may not always be the case. Patients may be asked to undergo rigorous, expensive, invalidated and even painful testing. They may be given diagnoses and treatments, which may lead to both physical and mental deterioration. We have also seen that many "validated" tests can be misused to diagnose allergic disease. Many supporters of these procedures have misinformed the public by implying that they have been clinically proven. Therefore, it becomes the responsibility of physicians to educate patients regarding such practices of allergy. It also becomes our responsibility to design proper clinical trials to definitively establish the merit or failure of these tests.

References

1 Shaw A, Thompson EA, Sharp D. Complementary therapy used by patients and parents of children with asthma and the implications for NHS care: a qualitative study. *BMC Health Serv Res* 2006;6:76.

2 Barton M, Oleske J, LaBraico J. Controversial techniques in allergy treatment. *J Natl Med Assoc* 1983;75:831–4.

3 Van Metre Jr TE. Critique of controversial and unproven procedures for diagnosis and therapy of allergic disorders. *Pediatr Clin North Am* 1983;30:807–17.

4 Van Metre Jr TE, Adkinson Jr NF, Lichtenstein LM, *et al.* A controlled study of the effectiveness of the Rinkel method of immunotherapy for ragweed pollen hay fever. *J Allergy Clin Immunol* 1980;65:288–97.

5 Garrow JS. Kinesiology and food allergy. *BMJ* 1988;296:1573.

6 Lee CH. A new test for diagnosis and treatment of food allergens. *Buchanan Co Med Bull* 1961;25:9–12.

7 AAAI Training Program Directors' Committee. A training program directors' committee report: topics related to controversial practices that should be taught in allergy and immunology training program. *J Allergy Clin Immunol* 1994;93:955–66.

8 Middleton Jr E, Ellis EF, Yunginer JW, *et al.* (eds.) *Allergy Principles and Practice*, 5th edn. St. Louis, MO: Mosby, 1998.

9 Spector SL. Controversial and unproven techniques. Position statement from the ACCP section on allergy and clinical immunology. *Chest* 1984;86:132–3.

10 Hansel FK. *Allergy and Immunology in Otolaryngology*. Rochester, MN: American Academy of Ophthalmology and Otolaryngology, 1968:134–5.

11 Crawford LV, Lieberman P, Harfi HA, *et al*. A double-blind study of subcutaneous food testing sponsored by the Food Committee of the American Academy of Allergy. *J Allergy Clin Immunol* 1976;57:236.

12 Kailin EW, Collier R. "Relieving" therapy for antigen exposure. *JAMA* 1971;217:78–82.

13 Draper LW. Food testing in allergy: intradermal, provocative, or deliberate feeding. *Arch Otolaryngol* 1972;95:169–74.

14 Jewett DL, Greenberg MR. Placebo responses in intradermal provocation testing with food extracts (abstract). *J Allergy Clin Immunol* 1985;75:205.

15 American Academy of Allergy. Position statements – controversial techniques. *J Allergy Clin Immunol* 1981;67:333–8.

16 Terr AI. Controversial and unproven diagnostic tests for allergic and immunologic diseases. *Clin Allergy Immunol* 2000;15:307–20.

17 Franklin W, Lowell FC. Failure of ragweed pollen extract to destroy white cells from ragweed-sensitive patients. *J Allergy* 1949;20:375.

18 Lieberman P, Crawford L, Bjelland J, *et al*. Controlled study of the cytotoxic food test. *JAMA* 1974;231:728.

19 Benson TE, Arkins JA. Cytotoxic testing for food allergy: evaluations of reproducibility in correlation. *J Allergy Clin Immunol* 1976;58:471–6.

20 Fell PJ, Brostoff J, Pasula MJ. High correlation of the ALCAT test results with double blind challenge in food sensitivity (abstract). *45th Annual Congree of the American College of Allergy and Immunology*, Los Angeles, CA, 1988.

21 Wuthrich B. Unproven techniques in allergy diagnosis. *J Invest Allergol Clin Immunol* 2005;15(2):86–90.

22 Semizzi M, Senna G, Crivellaro M, *et al*. A double-blind, placebo-controlled study on the diagnostic accuracy of an electrodermal test in allergic subjects. *Clin Exp Allergy* 2002;32(6):928–32.

23 ASCIA Position Statement: Unorthodox techniques for the diagnosis and treatment of allergy, asthma, and immune disorders, *ASCIA 2004*.

24 Niggemann B, Gruber C. Unproven diagnostic procedures in IgE-mediated allergic diseases. *Allergy* 2004;59:806–8.

25 Goldberg BJ, Kaplan MS. Controversial concepts and techniques in the diagnosis and management of food allergies. *Immunol Allergy Clin North Am* 1991;11:863–84.

26 Coca AF. *Familial Nonreaginic Food Allergy*, 3rd edn. Springfield, IL: Charles C. Thomas, 1953.

27 McHugh P, Aitcheson F, Duncan B, Houghton F. Buteyko breathing technique for asthma: an effective intervention. *NZ J Med* 2003;16:U710.

28 Levine SA, Reinhardt JH. Biochemical-pathology initiated by free radicals, oxidant chemicals, and therapeutic drugs in the etiology of chemical hypersensitivity disease. *Orthomol Psychiat* 1983;12:166.

29 Oriel GH, Barber HW. Proteases in urine, excreted in anaphylactic and allergic conditions. *Lancet* 1930;2:1304.

30 Plesch J. Urine therapy. *Med Press* 1947;218:128.

31 Terr AI. Clinical ecology. *Ann Intern Med* 1989;111:168–77.

32 Sparks PJ, Daniell W, Black DW, *et al*. Multiple chemical sensitivity syndrome: a clinical perspective. I. Case definition, theories of pathogenesis, and research needs. *J Occup Med* 1994;36:718.

33 Randolph TG. The specific adaptation syndrome. *J Lab Clin Invest* 1956;48:934.

34 Rea WJ, Bell IR, Suits CW, *et al*. Food and chemical susceptibility after environmental chemical overexposure: case histories. *Ann Allergy* 1978;41:101–9.

35 Bennett JE. Searching for the yeast connection. *N Engl J Med* 2002;323:1766–7.

36 Dismukes WE, Wade JS, Lee JY, *et al*. A randomized, double-blind trial of nystatin therapy for the candidiasis hypersensitivity syndrome. *N Engl J Med* 1990; 323:1717–22.

37 Labarge XS, McCaffrey RJ. Multiple chemical sensitivity: a review of the theoretical and research literature. *Neuropsychol Rev* 2000;10:183–211.

38 Winder C. Mechanisms of multiple chemical sensitivity. *Toxicol Lett* 2002;128:85–97.

PART 4

Adverse Reactions to Food Additives

CHAPTER 27

Asthma and Food Additives

Robert K. Bush and Michelle M. Montalbano

KEY CONCEPTS

- Food additives are an uncommon cause of asthma exacerbations.
- Sulfiting agents can provoke acute and occasionally severe episodes of bronchoconstriction.
- Monosodium glutamate is unlikely to provoke bronchoconstriction.
- Tartrazine has not been definitely shown to cause airflow obstruction.
- A definite diagnosis of food-additive-induced asthma requires properly performed challenges.

Introduction

Food additives are substances added to food products for a wide variety of functions, including coloring, flavoring, nutrient, and antimicrobial purposes. Because additives are typically minor ingredients in food, the intake of additives is usually small. An estimated 23–67% of asthmatics perceive that food additives exacerbate their asthma. However, the prevalence rate of food-additive-induced asthma exacerbations obtained by double-blind, placebo-controlled trials is less than 5%. Because the current therapy for food-additive-induced asthma is avoidance or elimination of inciting agents, a correct diagnosis is imperative to avoid unnecessary dietary restriction. Sulfites, monosodium glutamate (MSG), and tartrazine will be discussed in detail in this chapter.

Evaluating asthma studies

A variety of data are available implicating sulfites, MSG, and tartrazine in asthma exacerbations, but many of the studies are of poor design.

Well-designed studies in asthmatic subjects require stable lung function at baseline. When the subjects have wide variability in peak expiratory flow rate (PEFR) or forced expiratory volume in 1 second (FEV1) at baseline, variability seen during the challenge may be related to the substance or a reflection of poor asthma control. If asthma medications are discontinued, the timing in relation to the challenge must be carefully evaluated. For example, anti-asthmatic and

Food Allergy: Adverse Reactions to Foods and Food Additives, 4th edition.
Edited by Dean D. Metcalfe, Hugh A. Sampson, and Ronald A. Simon.
© 2008 Blackwell Publishing. ISBN: 978-1-4501-5129-0.

anti-allergic medications that can inhibit a response must be withheld before a challenge. β_2-agonists are typically withheld the day of the challenge, and cromolyn sodium or antihistamines are withheld 24 hours prior to the challenge. Asthma controller medications such as theophylline and inhaled or oral corticosteroids may be continued, since they do not interfere with the response.

If rescue medications are given within 3 hours of a challenge, lung function declines 6 hours after challenge, the decline is more likely due to a waning of medication effect rather than bronchoconstriction from the challenge substance. Consistent timing of challenges is important to exclude confounding due to the physiologic diurnal variability in PEFR. To eliminate observer bias, challenges should be double-blinded and placebo-controlled.

The method of administration of challenge substance may influence results. For example, some asthmatics respond to oral capsule challenges, while others respond only to challenge with solutions (e.g. sulfites). The route of administration chosen in diagnostic challenges should be tailored to the patient's history.

The reliability of the pulmonary function measure used is another key aspect. The flow–volume loop obtained with spirometry is precise and reproducible, while PEFR is more variable. Criteria used to define positive challenges should be considered.

Duration of subject evaluation following a challenge is also important. For MSG, subjects are evaluated for as few as 2 or as many as 14 hours following challenge. Determining when reactions are most likely to occur and still be linked to the challenge substance will help determine the length of time subjects should be observed.

For sulfites, MSG, and tartrazine, various data are presented and evaluated using the criteria outlined above.

Sulfites

Sulfiting agents have been used in foods for many years. Although sulfites are often added to foods, they occur naturally in certain foods such as mushrooms and Parmesan cheese.

Adding sulfites to foods serves many purposes, for example, inhibition of enzymatic and non-enzymatic browning, antimicrobial actions, bleaching, and as a dough conditioner. Sulfites are also used in pharmaceutical agents, including medications for the treatment of allergic diseases and asthma.

Common forms of sulfites used as food or drug additives include sulfur dioxide (SO_2), inorganic sulfite salts, sodium or potassium metabisulfite ($Na_2S_2O_5$ or $K_2S_2O_5$), sodium or potassium bisulfite ($NaHSO_3$ or $KHSO_3$), and sodium or potassium sulfite ($Na_2S_2O_3$ or $K_2S_2O_3$). Sulfites can react with a variety of food constituents. Dissociable forms of sulfite can serve as reservoirs of "free" sulfites. Irreversibly bound sulfites are removed permanently from the pool of sulfites that may exist in foods.

The form of sulfite present in foods is affected by pH. For example, a low-pH favors H_2SO_3, intermediate pH (4.0) favors HSO_3^-, and high-pH favors SO_3^{2-}. In solution, especially at an acid pH (saliva, gastric juice) and in the presence of heat (stomach), sulfites are readily transformed into bisulfite and sulfurous acid. These substances may then be volatilized to SO_2, which has been implicated in causing bronchoconstriction.

The estimated prevalence of sulfite sensitivity in adult asthmatics is approximately 5%, with a higher prevalence in moderate to severe persistent asthmatics. Two hundred and three patients initially underwent a single-blind challenge with sulfite-containing capsules. If the single-blind challenge were positive (20% or greater decrease in FEV1 from baseline), a double-blind challenge followed. In the single-blind challenge, 16 of 83 moderate to severe persistent asthmatics had a positive response, while only 5 of 120 less severe asthmatics had a positive response. When these results were confirmed with double-blind challenges, three of seven more severe asthmatics and one of five less severe asthmatics had a positive response. The estimated prevalence of sulfite sensitivity in non-steroid-dependent asthmatics based on the double-blind challenge results was 0.8%. In the more severe asthmatics, the prevalence was higher (8.4%). The estimated prevalence of sulfite sensitivity in the asthmatic population as a whole is less than 3.9% and those with moderate to severe persistent asthma are at most risk.

The largest group of sulfite-sensitive asthmatics are individuals who respond to ingestion of acidic sulfite solutions. Among these patients, some react to acidic sulfite solution challenge and others do not, a phenomenon perhaps explained by variable inhalation of SO_2.

The mechanism by which sulfites induce asthma symptoms has not yet been fully elucidated. Various hypotheses have been proposed to explain the bronchoconstriction by SO_2: a cholinergic reflex mechanism, an IgE-mediated mechanism, or deficiency of sulfite oxidase. The cholinergic reflex mechanism suggests that inhaled SO_2, such might occur when swallowing an acidic sulfited beverage, acts on irritant receptors in the lung. This hypothesis is supported by the fact that the response in sulfite-sensitive individuals can be blocked by the administration of anticholinergic drugs, such as inhaled atropine or doxepin, an antihistamine with anticholinergic properties.

Another proposed mechanism is an IgE-mediated mechanism. This mechanism has not yet been proven, but is supported by the presence of positive skin prick tests to sulfites and by anaphylaxis in certain individuals.

Sulfite oxidase deficiency has also been proposed as an explanation. Sulfite oxidase metabolizes sulfite (SO_3) to inactive sulfate (SO_4), and a decrease in sulfite oxidase activity has been seen in skin fibroblasts of sulfite-sensitive asthmatics compared with controls [1].

Although sulfite-induced asthma is typically triggered by the ingestion of a sulfited food, beverage, or drug, inhalation of SO_2 can also be a trigger. Several factors determine the likelihood of an adverse reaction: the nature of the food, the level and form of residual sulfite in the food, and the sensitivity of the patient. Sulfite-sensitive asthmatics are most likely to respond to "free" sulfites. However, the degree of sensitivity these patients have to the various forms of sulfites in foods has yet to be elucidated.

The levels of sulfiting agents in foods are usually expressed as SO_2 equivalents because sulfite salts can release SO_2 under some assay conditions. In the United States, total daily *per capita* intake of sulfites in foods is approximately 6-mg SO_2. The threshold response to challenges with sulfites in sensitive asthmatics is typically between 12- and 30-mg SO_2 equivalents (20 to 50-mg potassium metabisulfite).

The levels of sulfites in foods vary (see Chapter 29) and are typically expressed as parts per million (ppm). One part per million equals one microgram per gram. The highest levels (up to 1000 ppm) are contained in dried fruits and lemon, lime, grape, and sauerkraut juices. Food processing and preparation may decrease sulfite levels. Therefore, the amounts of sulfite used initially to treat foods will not necessarily reflect residue levels after processing, storage, and preparation. Food processing also differs in various countries, so caution must be used in interpreting reports from other countries that implicate sulfites in eliciting asthma symptoms.

Inhaling as little as 1 ppm SO_2 has been demonstrated to cause bronchoconstriction in asthmatics. In doses of 1–50 ppm, 99% of inhaled SO_2 is absorbed by the upper airway. The resulting bronchospasm may be initiated by stimulation of superficial afferent nerve endings in the larynx or tracheobronchial tree and then mediated by parasympathetic pathways in the bronchi.

Although the precise mechanism has yet to be elucidated, the bronchoconstriction caused by exposure to sulfites in sensitive asthmatics can be severe and potentially life threatening. Therefore, accurate diagnosis is imperative. But because history does not always correlate with a positive challenge, history alone is insufficient for the diagnosis of sulfite-induced asthma. Skin prick tests and serologic tests are also not reliable in the diagnosis of sulfite-induced asthma. The diagnostic tool with the highest reproducibility is a double-blind, placebo-controlled challenge. However, there is no standardized procedure for challenging with sulfiting agents (see Tables 29.1 and 29.2 for suggested protocols for sulfite challenges). Patients may be challenged with capsules, neutral solutions, or acidic solutions of metabisulfite. A capsule challenge may be preferred, as most exposures are to sulfites in bound form in foods rather than to sulfites in free form, such as in lettuce. Variable thresholds for bronchospastic responses have been seen, from 5 to 200 mg of encapsulated metabisulfite. A challenge with sulfites in solution is optimal for patients who have reacted to beverages such as sulfited wines. In patients with a history of response to particular foods, food challenges are used diagnostically. Challenges, therefore, can be tailored to a patient's history of reaction.

Challenges should be conducted very carefully, with availability of equipment necessary to treat severe bronchospastic or anaphylactic reactions. Because certain drugs can inhibit the response to sulfites, anti-asthmatic and anti-allergic medications, such as β_2-agonists, cromolyn, and antihistamines, should be withheld before challenges. β_2-agonists are typically withheld the day of the challenge, while cromolyn and antihistamines are withheld at least 24 hours prior to the challenge. Theophylline and corticosteroids (inhaled and oral) can be continued, for these drugs do not interfere with sulfite-induced reactions.

Typically, if a single-blind challenge is positive, the results should be confirmed with a double-blind challenge. Randomization of administration of active and placebo challenges should be done, possibly with a third challenge day, to avoid an order effect of challenge. An order effect of challenge has been seen in patients who receive placebo on the first day and do not react but do react on subsequent challenge days regardless of whether they receive placebo or active challenge.

Given the diagnosis of sulfite-induced asthma with an appropriately performed challenge study and the establishment of a threshold dose of sulfite that provokes asthma, treatment is strict avoidance of sulfite-treated foods and drugs, especially those containing greater than 100-ppm SO_2 equivalents. In the United States federal regulations requires foods and alcoholic beverages containing greater than 10-ppm total SO_2, be labeled. Unlabeled sulfited foods still exist in restaurants, although the use of sulfites in fresh foods such as fruits and vegetables in salad bars has been banned. Residue levels of sulfites in shrimp, which are used to prevent enzymatic browning (black spot formation), are still permitted. Imported table grapes are treated with sulfites to inhibit mold growth, but they must be detained at their port of entry until sulfite residues are no longer detected. Potatoes can be sulfited, so patients with sulfite-sensitive asthma should avoid all potatoes in restaurants, except those baked with intact skins. Sulfite-sensitive asthmatics should avoid sulfite-containing pharmaceutical agents such as certain bronchodilator solutions, subcutaneous lidocaine, and intravenous corticosteroids. Pharmaceutical corporations have eliminated the use of sulfites in many products used for the treatment of asthmatics, although epinephrine contains sulfites as antioxidants because there is no alternative agent. The positive effects of the epinephrine overwhelmingly negate any negative effects of sulfites. Epinephrine therefore should *never* be withheld from sulfite-sensitive asthmatics when indicated.

Complete avoidance of sulfites is difficult, and reactions can be severe. Management of reactions includes administration of β_2-agonist medications or nebulized atropine and self-administered epinephrine for severe episodes of sulfite-induced asthma.

Monosodium glutamate

Just as sulfites have been linked to asthma exacerbations in some asthmatics, MSG has also been implicated. Unlike sulfites, however, there is little data to confirm that MSG causes bronchospasm.

MSG is a sodium salt of the non-essential amino acid, L-glutamic acid. MSG occurs naturally in a wide variety of foods. MSG exists in free form and bound to proteins and is used as a flavor enhancer in processed foods. In the United States, the average daily intake of MSG is 0.2–0.5 g. As much as 4–6 g might be ingested in a highly seasoned restaurant meal.

Because MSG is perceived as a food chemical likely to cause bronchoconstriction, it is a frequently avoided food item. However, the role of MSG in exacerbating asthma has not been firmly established. Levels of MSG precipitating adverse events are much higher than the usual dietary exposure (2.5–3 g versus 0.2–0.5 g daily exposure) and occur in the absence of food.

Thirty-two asthmatic patients with a history of MSG-induced asthmatic reactions were evaluated via single-blind, placebo-controlled oral challenge with MSG. PEFR were followed hourly for 14 hours after oral challenge. Thirteen exhibited significant declines in PEFR. Patients were given placebo on day 1 of the study and then challenged with MSG on days 2 and 3, augmenting the lack of daily controller medications, which were stopped just prior to commencement of the study. Some patients were allowed to have rescue medication within 3 hours of initial challenge, therefore declines in PEFR 6 hours or more after challenge were most likely due to waning effects of β_2-agonist rather than to bronchoconstrictive effects of MSG. The results of this study were not reproduced; a non-blinded challenge was repeated in only one patient.

Oral challenges with 1.5 g of MSG in 12 asthmatic patients found no changes in FEV1 that was statistically different from placebo. The number of patients evaluated was small, and subjects were only evaluated for 2 hours after challenge, rather than 12 hours or more as in other studies. This study does suggest that in the usual quantities found in food, MSG is unlikely to induce bronchoconstriction.

Another study evaluated 12 asthmatics, all of whom had a history of asthma exacerbation with MSG ingestion. This was a double-blind, placebo-controlled study to evaluate for MSG-induced bronchial hyperresponsiveness. Methacholine challenge was performed before and after oral challenge with MSG. The results of this study were completely negative. This study involved a small number of subjects, and patients were directly monitored for only 4 hours after challenge. Nevertheless, MSG-induced asthma was not demonstrated in this group of adult asthmatics with prior history of asthma symptoms precipitated by MSG.

A single-blind, placebo-controlled study evaluated 100 asthmatic patients, 30 of whom reported prior asthma exacerbations with MSG exposure. Subjects were given 2.5 g of MSG, and FEV1 was measured at hourly intervals for 12 hours. No significant drop in FEV1 occurred, and no patients developed asthma symptoms.

In contrast to the general perception that MSG-induced asthma exists, well-designed studies with oral challenges of MSG clearly have not demonstrated changes in FEV1 or symptoms of asthma. Currently, there is limited evidence that patients with asthma are more at risk for adverse effects from MSG than the general population [2].

When patients are concerned that a reaction may be occurring to MSG, an oral challenge can be performed (Table 27.1). Maintenance asthma medications should be continued. An initial single-blind, placebo-controlled challenge should be done. FEV1 should be monitored hourly after each of five doses of placebo. If the FEV1 changes by more than 10%, the patient has failed the placebo challenge. If the FEV1 is stable (change of less than 10%), a second placebo challenge should be performed and FEV1 monitored hourly for up to 12 hours.

If patients "pass" the placebo challenge day with less than 10% variability in FEV1, a single-blind challenge with MSG should be performed. MSG is given in five 500 mg capsules, totaling 2.5 g. FEV1 is monitored hourly for a total of 12 hours. Five placebo capsules should be given at the 6-hour point to maintain a sequence similar to the placebo challenge day. A positive response is defined as a drop in FEV1

Table 27.1 Protocol for MSG Oral Challenge

Single-blind challenge
Continue maintenance asthma medications
Perform on initial single-blind placebo challenge
- Administer five placebo capsules of 500-mg sucrose each
- Monitor FEV1 hourly
- Failure of placebo challenge is a change in FEV1 > 10%
- If FEV1 remains stable, perform a second placebo challenge, monitoring FEV1 hourly
- Total duration of placebo day: 12 hours

If patients pass the placebo challenge day, perform single-blind challenge with MSG
- Give five capsules MSG totaling 2.5 g
- Monitor FEV1 hourly for total of 12 hours
- Six hours after MSG administered, administer five placebo capsules to maintain a sequence similar to the placebo challenge day
- Positive response is FEV1 drop > 20% (perform double-blind challenge to confirm)

Double-blind challenge
- Continue maintenance asthma medications
- Repeat 12-hour placebo challenge on 1 day
- Request repeat MSG challenge as above on another day
- Challenge day (placebo or active) should be in random order.

of greater than 20%. If patients have a positive response to a single-blind challenge, a double-blind challenge should be performed.

Tartrazine

Synthetic colorants are often added to foods. One such example is the azo dye, tartrazine, also known as FD&C Yellow #5. As with MSG, many of the reported studies have design flaws. No well-designed study has corroborated claims that tartrazine provokes asthma exacerbations, for example, lack of baseline asthma stability, withholding of asthma medications, or proper controls.

In 194 aspirin-sensitive patients evaluated for tartrazine sensitivity by oral challenge, no cross-sensitivity between aspirin and tartrazine was demonstrated. The authors conclude that reports of tartrazine-induced bronchospasm represent spontaneous asthma coincidentally associated with ingestion of tartrazine, rather than bronchospasm caused by tartrazine. None of the subjects had positive reactions when double-blind, placebo-controlled challenges were performed [3].

If a patient is concerned about reactions to tartrazine, an oral challenge can be performed (Table 27.2). An initial challenge should involve hourly FEV1 monitoring throughout the challenge. Placebo should be administered first. If FEV1 remains stable after 3 hours, 25-mg tartrazine can be given. If after another 3 hours, FEV1 is still stable, 50-mg tartrazine can be administered. A "conditionally positive"

Table 27.2 Protocol for tartrazine oral challenge

Initial challenge

Administer placebo first

Monitor FEV1 hourly

If FEV1 stable after 3 hours, administer 25-mg tartrazine

If FEV1 stable after 3 hours, administer 50-mg tartrazine

A "conditionally positive" test consists of FEV1 drop of 25% or more
after the 25- or 50-mg dose tartrazine

Double-blind challenge

Begin with a full day of placebo challenge using three doses of placebo
administered 3 hours apart

Monitor FEV1 hourly

On the following day, follow protocol for initial challenge using
suspected provoking dose of tartrazine and two placebos

---

test consists of an FEV1 drop of 25% or more after the 25- or 50-mg dose of tartrazine.

When the initial challenge is positive, a double-blind challenge should be done, using the suspected provoking dose of tartrazine and two placebos. This double-blind challenge should be preceded by a full day of challenge using three doses of placebo administered 3 hours apart. FEV1 should be monitored hourly throughout the placebo challenge and active challenge.

Conclusions

Despite that a multitude of food additives exist, only a few are commonly implicated in asthma: sulfites, MSG, and tartrazine. Of these three, only sulfites have been found to incite bronchoconstriction in some asthmatics, who should avoid sulfite exposure. In contrast, due to the lack of evidence in well-designed studies linking MSG and tartrazine to asthma exacerbation, asthmatic patients need not avoid exposure to MSG or tartrazine if a double-blind, placebo-controlled challenge is negative.

References

1 Simon RA. Update on sulfite sensitivity. *Allergy* 1998;53:78–9.

2 Geha RS, Beiser A, Ren C, *et al.* Review of alleged reaction to monosodium glutamate and outcome of a multicenter double-blind placebo-controlled study. *J Nutr* 2000;130:1058S–62.

3 Stevenson DD, Simon RA, Lumry WR, Mathison DA. Pulmonary reactions to tartrazine. *Pediatr Allergy Immunol* 1992;3:222–7.

CHAPTER 28

Urticaria, Angioedema, and Anaphylaxis Provoked by Food and Drug Additives

John V. Bosso and Ronald A. Simon

KEY CONCEPTS

- Only a small fraction of the thousands of agents added to our foods have been associated with cutaneous and/or anaphylactic hypersensitivity responses.

- Early (pre-1990) literature overestimated the prevalence of such reactions due to poorly controlled studies.

- Additive-induced urticaria, angioedema, and anaphylaxis is relatively rare.

- Hypersensitivity responses to "natural" additives appear to be primarily IgE based, while the basis of most reactions to synthetic additives is unclear.

- Chronic idiopathic urticaria/angioedema is rarely associated with food-additive hypersensitivity.

- Recommendations for food-additive challenge protocols for patients with urticaria, angioedema, and/or anaphylaxis are reviewed in the text.

Many agents are added to foods that we consume [1], the number ranges from 2000 to 20,000. These substances include preservatives, stabilizers, conditioners, thickeners, colorings, flavorings, sweeteners, and antioxidants. Despite the multitude of additives known, only a surprisingly small number have been associated with hypersensitivity reactions.

Urticaria, angioedema, and anaphylaxis from food additives should be suspected when adverse reactions after food or beverage consumption occur; some, but not all the time, suggesting that the reaction occurs only when an additive is present.

A number of investigators have suggested that urticaria, angioedema, and anaphylaxis related to the ingestion of food additives are relatively common. This apparent misconception is based on several poorly controlled studies, mostly reported before 1990. Emerging evidence appears to contradict this notion, suggesting that the incidence of such reactions is relatively low.

Table 28.1 lists the food and drug additives that may be associated with adverse reactions. In this chapter, these additives are discussed in detail as they relate to urticaria and angioedema, as well as to anaphylaxis or anaphylactoid reactions.

General considerations and description of some additives

A brief overview of selected additives follows [2]. For additional information, the reader is referred to Chapters 27, 29–34 in this book.

Food dyes

Dyes approved under the Food, Drug and Cosmetic (FD & C) Act are coal tar derivatives, the best known of which is tartrazine (FD & C Yellow No. 5). In addition to tartrazine, the group of azo dyes include ponceau (FD & C Red No. 4) and sunset yellow (FD & C Yellow No. 6). Amaranth (FD & C Red No. 2) was banned from use in the United States in 1975 because of claims related to carcinogenicity. Non-azo dyes include brilliant blue (FD & C Blue No. 1), erythrosine (FD & C Red No. 3), and indigotine (FD & C Blue No. 2).

Sulfites

Sulfites and the burning of sulfur-containing coal have been used for centuries to preserve food. In addition, sulfiting agents (including sulfur dioxide and sodium or potassium sulfite, bisulfite, and metabisulfite) are used by the fermentation industry to sanitize containers and to inhibit the growth of undesirable microorganisms. Sulfites act as potent antioxidants, which explains their widespread use in foods as preventatives against oxidative discoloration (browning)

Food Allergy: Adverse Reactions to Foods and Food Additives, 4th edition.
Edited by Dean D. Metcalfe, Hugh A. Sampson, and Ronald A. Simon.
© 2008 Blackwell Publishing. ISBN: 978-1-4501-5129-0.

Table 28.1 Additives associated with adverse reactions

Synthetic additives
FD & C dyes
 Azo dyes
  Tartrazine (FD & C Yellow No. 5)
  Sunset yellow (FD & C Yellow No. 6)
  Ponceau (FD & C Red No. 4)
  Amaranth (FD & C Red No. 2)
 Non-azo dyes
  Brilliant blue (FD & C Blue No. 1)
  Erythrosine (FD & C Red No. 3)
  Indigotine (FD & C Blue No. 2)
Parabens
 p-hydroxybenzoic acid
 Methyl-, ethyl-, butyl-, and propyl-paraben
Sodium benzoate
Butylated hydroxyanisole (BHA)
Butylated hydroxytoluene (BHT)
Nitrates/nitrites
Monosodium glutamate (MSG)
Sulfites
 Sulfur dioxide
 Sodium sulfite
 Sodium/potassium bisulfite
 Sodium/potassium metabisulfite
Aspartame
Isosulfan blue (medical diagnostic agent)

Natural additives (Plant/animal sources)
Annatto
Carmine
Saffron
Mannitol

and as fresheners. Many packaged foods, including fresh and frozen cellophane-wrapped fruits and vegetables, processed grain foods (crackers and cookies), and citrus-flavored beverages, may contain sulfites.

The highest levels, however, occur in potatoes (any peeled variety), dried fruits (apricots and white raisins), and possibly shrimp and other seafood, which may be sprayed with sulfiting agents after unloading on the dock. Sulfites are listed as ingredients in prepared and packaged foods or drink that contain at least 10 ppm SO_2 equivalents. In 1986, the US Food and Drug Administration (FDA) banned the use of sulfites on foods marketed as "fresh."

Parabens

Parabens are aliphatic esters of *p*-hydroxybenzoic acid. They include methyl-, ethyl-, propyl-, and butyl-parabens. Sodium benzoate is a closely related substance, usually reported to cross-react with these compounds. These agents are widely used as preservatives in both foods and drugs, and are well recognized as causes of severe contact dermatitis.

Monosodium glutamate

Glutamic acid is a non-essential dicarboxylic amino acid that constitutes 20% of dietary protein. Glutamate occurs naturally in some foods in significant amounts: 100 g of Camembert cheese, for example, contains as much as 1 g of monosodium glutamate (MSG). The greatest exposure to MSG, however, occurs through its role as a flavor enhancer. Manufacturers and restaurateurs add MSG to a wide variety of foods. About 85 years ago a Japanese chemist established that MSG produced the flavor-enhancing properties of seaweed, a traditional component of Japanese cooking. Large amounts of MSG are sometimes added to Chinese, Japanese, and other Southeast Asian cooking. As much as 6 g of MSG may be ingested in a highly seasoned oriental meal, and a single bowl of wonton soup may contain 2.5 g of MSG. MSG may also be found in manufactured meat and chicken products.

MSG has been reported to provoke, within minutes to hours of eating, a syndrome characterized by headache, a burning sensation along the back of the neck, chest tightness, nausea, and sweating. Recently, a trend toward reducing MSG use in Asian cooking has emerged, likely in response to consumer dissatisfaction related to the occurrence of the syndrome.

Aspartame

Aspartame is a dipeptide composed of aspartic acid and the methyl ester of phenylalanine. This popular low-calorie artificial sweetener is 180 times sweeter than sucrose.

Butylated hydroxyanisole and butylated hydroxytoluene

Butylated hydroxyanisole (BHA) and butylated hydroxytoluene (BHT) are antioxidants used in cereal and other grain products.

Nitrates/nitrites

Nitrates and nitrites are widely used preservatives. Their popularity stems from both flavoring and coloring attributes. These agents are found mostly in processed meats such as frankfurters and salami [3].

Isosulfan blue

Isosulfan blue (ISB; Lymphazurin 1%, US Surgical Corporation) is an isomer of the triphenylmethane dye patent blue. It is a contrast agent for the delineation of lymphatic vessels. Following subcutaneous administration, this dye binds to interstitial proteins in lymphatic vessels, imparting a bright blue appearance that makes the lymphatics more readily discernable from surrounding tissue. ISB is indicated as an adjunct to lymphangiography, assessing lymph node response to therapeutic modalities and for visualization of the lymphatic system draining the region of injection [4].

Annatto

Annatto dye is an orange-yellow food coloring extracted from the seeds of the tree *Bixa orelana*, a large fast-growing shrub cultivated in the tropics. It is frequently used in cereals, beverages, cheese, and snack foods.

Carmine

Carmine (or cochineal extract) is a biologically derived red colorant derived from the dried bodies of female cochineal insects (*Nopalea coccinelliferna*). It is commonly used in cosmetics, textiles, and foods. It is responsible for giving the liqueur Campari its characteristic color. It is often designated E 120 .

Saffron

Saffron color, a dark yellow-orange, derives from the crocus plant. The saffron spice consists of the dried stigmas and style of the crocus bulb, while the saffron colorant, crocin, also comes from the dried stigmas and style. It is used to color soups, bouillabaisse, sauces, rice dishes (paella, "risotto Milanese"), cakes, cheese, and liqueurs [5].

Mannitol

Mannitol is a sugar alcohol widely distributed in plants. It is a white, crystalline sweetener added to processed foods for the purpose of thickening, stabilizing, and sweetening. It is also widely used as a drug excipient. In addition, it is widely used as a therapeutic agent for glaucoma, increased intracranial pressure, drug intoxication, and oliguric renal failure [6].

Mechanisms of additive-induced urticaria, angioedema, and anaphylaxis

As of now, the mechanisms underlying additive-induced urticaria, angioedema, and anaphylaxis remain largely unknown. It seems reasonable to postulate, however, that multiple mechanisms are responsible for these adverse reactions, given the heterogeneity of chemical structures found among these additives (Fig. 28.1). Natural food colorants (e.g. annatto and carmine) are derived from proteins with molecular weights consistent with common food allergens.

Immediate (IgE-mediated) hypersensitivity

Naturally derived food colorings, such as annatto and carmine, contain proteins recognized in sodium dodecyl sulphate-polyacrylamide gel electrophoresis (SDS-PAGE), appearing as gel bands that appear in the 10–100 kDa range. Therefore, these colorants can be expected to potentially elicit IgE-mediated responses in some atopic individuals. Synthetic

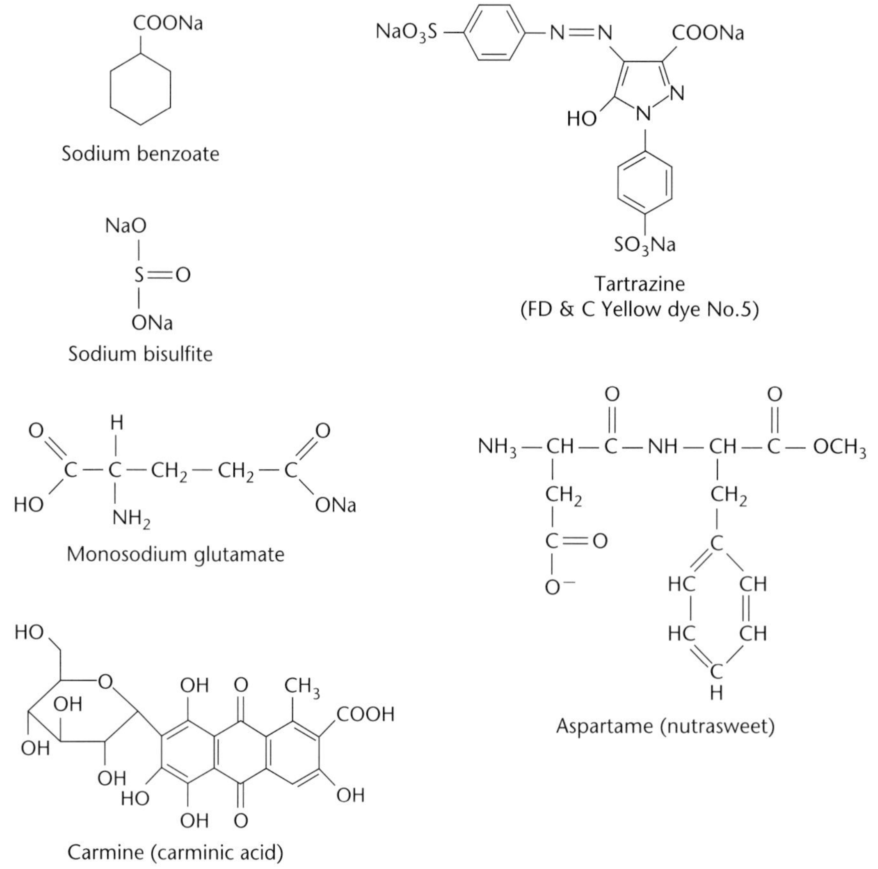

Figure 28.1 Chemical structure of common food additives.

additives would appear to have to act as haptens to create a response mediated by IgE. Only a few reports have suggested IgE-mediated reactions to synthetic additives, notably to sulfites and parabens. Instead, the overwhelming majority of these reactions are not of the immediate hypersensitivity type. In fact, many cases of additive-provoked urticaria are said to occur as late as 24 hour after challenge, arguing against an IgE-mediated mechanism.

Evidence for an IgE-mediated mechanism as the cause for identified anaphylactic episodes associated with carmine-colored foods derives from studies that have demonstrated associated positive skin prick test (SPTs), a positive Prausnitz–Küstner (PK) test, a positive basophile histamine release assay, positive IgE RAST (radioallergosorbent test) studies, and positive SDS-PAGE with IgE immunoblot [7–11]. Chung et al. [12] identified (in minced cochineal insect extracts) several protein SDS-PAGE bands of 23–88 kDa. The sera from three patients with episodic urticaria/angioedema/anaphylaxis occurring 3–5 hours after ingestion of foods containing carmine recognized these bands on immunoblot. This reactivity was inhibited by carmine. Patient reactivity to specific bands varied. Commercial carmine appears to retain proteinaceous material from the source insects. These insect-derived proteins, possibly complexed with carminic acid, are responsible for IgE-mediated carmine allergy.

Nish et al. [13] reported on a case of annatto dye-induced anaphylaxis. SPTs to annatto were strongly positive with negative control results. SDS-PAGE demonstrated two bands in the range of 50 kDa. Immunoblotting showed patient IgE specific for one of these bands and controls showed no binding. Residual or contaminating seed protein was the likely responsible antigen in this rare cast. Revan et al. [14] reported their experience with annatto at the University of Michigan allergy clinic. They found 9 (12%) of 77 atopic patients were SPT positive to liquid undiluted annatto. However, only 2 of these 9 subjects had symptomatic annatto allergy: 1 patient with a 4+ SPT had a history of annatto-induced anaphylaxis, and another with a 3+ SPT had angioedema. Only one SPT-positive reactor was challenged (2+) and was negative. The negative predictive value (NPV) of SPT in this cohort was 100%; however, the positive predictive value (PPV) was low (22%). Perhaps the undiluted extract was too potent to differentiate between true reactors and an irritant response. Double-blind, placebo-controlled (DBPC) challenges are needed to confirm these results.

In 1976, Prenner and Stevens reported an anaphylactic reaction occurring after the ingestion of food sprayed with sodium bisulfite [15]. Minutes after eating a restaurant lunch, this 50-year-old male experienced generalized urticaria, pruritus, swelling of the tongue, difficulty swallowing, and tightness in the chest. He responded promptly to treatment with subcutaneous epinephrine. Subsequently, the patient's SPT and an intradermal test gave positive results (with negative controls). The authors were able to demonstrate

PK transfer to a non-atopic subject. Yang and associates [16] also described one patient with a history of sulfite-provoked anaphylaxis. A borderline result was obtained via intradermal skin test, followed by a positive response to a single-blind oral provocation challenge with 5 mg of potassium metabisulfite. This patient's cutaneous reactivity was also passively transferred via the PK reaction. However, this group was unable to elicit positive responses from challenges in nine patients with histories of hives related to eating restaurant food. In addition, Sokol and Hydick [17] reported a case of sulfite-induced anaphylaxis that provided evidence for specific IgE-mediated mechanism. Despite these isolated reports, IgE-mediated immediate hypersensitivity reactions to sulfites (possibly via a hapten mechanism) appear to occur only rarely.

Studies measuring serum levels of neutrophil chemotactic factor of anaphylaxis (NCF-A) did not find an increase in this mast cell (MC) mediator post-challenge in subjects with negative metabisulfite skin tests, suggesting that MC degranulation is not associated with non-IgE-mediated sulfite reactions [18]. Cromolyn pre-treatment did not ablate an urticarial reaction in an individual sensitive to potassium metabisulfite [19]. In the overwhelming majority of cases, the mechanisms behind sulfite-provoked urticaria, angioedema, and anaphylaxis (or anaphylactoid reactions) remain unknown.

At least three cases of apparent IgE-mediated, paraben-induced urticaria and angioedema have been reported [20,21]. All of these cases concerned reactions to benzoates used as pharmaceutical preservatives. The three patients had positive skin test responses to parabens, but negative results when exposed to the drugs themselves minus the paraben preservatives. These subjects, however, could tolerate oral benzoates in their diets without reactions. Macy et al. [22] recently reported a series of 287 patients who underwent immediate hypersensitivity skin test to methylparaben-preserved local anesthetics. Only three patients had positive skin tests. These three individuals underwent skin testing as well as provocative dose testing to 0.1% methylparaben, in addition to local anesthetic without preservative. All three reacted definitely to the methylparaben, suggesting that methylparaben is a potential cause for local immediate hypersensitivity reactions previously attributed to the local anesthetics themselves.

Delayed (type IV) hypersensitivity

Another suggested mechanism focuses on delayed hypersensitivity. Studies in this area have been few in number and often of questionable design. Warrington and co-workers [23] measured the release of a T-lymphocyte-derived leukocyte-migration inhibition factor in response to incubation with tartrazine, sodium benzoate, and aspirin (acetylsalicylic acid) in vitro using peripheral blood mononuclear cells from patients with chronic urticaria, with or without associated additive or aspirin sensitivity. Significant production of the inhibitory factor occurred in response to tartrazine and sodium benzoate in individuals with chronic additive-induced urticaria. The groups of patients studied (four patients per group) reportedly exhibited sensitivity to tartrazine, sodium benzoate, and aspirin as determined either by response to elimination diet alone or by challenge-proved sensitivity. In this study, the potential for false-positive reactions on the basis of response to diet alone presented a problem. Essentially no details of the challenge procedures were given.

Valverde and associates [24] studied *in vitro* lymphocyte stimulation in 258 patients with chronic urticaria, angioedema, or both, using a series of food extracts and additives that included tartrazine, benzoic acid, and aspirin. They found positive stimulation (using the lymphocyte transformation test) to additives in 18% of subjects. After the patients were placed on a diet that excluded the offending additives, 62% had total remission of symptoms and 22% had partial remission. The investigators concluded that this response to diet lent credence to the lymphocyte transformation test as an *in vitro* diagnostic test for chronic urticaria and angioedema related to food additives. However, no provocation challenges were performed in this study. No definitive conclusions regarding the presence or absence of a delayed-type hypersensitivity mechanism in additive-provoked urticaria can be made from the studies described above. It does seem reasonable to conclude that a reaction with an onset between 30 minutes and 6 hours after exposure to the material in question (most reactions began within the first 6 hours) is not typical of a type IV mechanism.

Cyclooxygenase, aspirin, and tartrazine

The possibility of tartrazine sensitivity remains controversial. Many claims of cross-reactivity between aspirin and tartrazine have been made; estimates of its incidence based on earlier studies ranged from 21% to 100% [25–29]. In a DBPC study (with objective reaction criteria and withholding of antihistamines for 72 hours prior to challenge), only 1 (4.2%) of 24 patients experienced urticaria after challenge with 50 mg of tartrazine [30]. When challenged with 975 mg of aspirin, this patient did not react, suggesting that cross-reactivity between aspirin and tartrazine may not occur. An earlier DBPC crossover challenge with 0.22 mg of tartrazine found sensitivity in 3 (8%) of 38 patients with chronic urticaria and 2 (20%) of 10 patients with aspirin intolerance [28]. This dose of tartrazine is similar to that used to color medication tablets, but remains far less than that typically encountered in the diet. The report did not mention, however, whether antihistamines were withheld during the challenges. No convincing evidence has been found to prove that tartrazine inhibits the enzyme cyclooxygenase (in the arachidonic acid cascade), an often-suggested mechanism for aspirin sensitivity.

Neurologically mediated hypersensitivity

Considerable evidence exists that MSG has both neuroexcitatory and neurotoxic effects in animals [31] and humans [32]. Neurologically mediated urticarias have been described [33]. Several factors, including heat, exercise, and stress, may induce cholinergic urticaria. This mechanism represents only a theoretical basis for MSG-induced urticaria, possibly via release of cutaneous neuropeptides.

Anticoagulation

In 1986, Zimmerman and Czarnetzki [34] sought to disprove claims by earlier investigators that changes in bleeding time play an important role in diagnosing anaphylactoid reactions to aspirin, other non-steroidal anti-inflammatory drugs (NSAIDs), and food additives. They measured bleeding time, prothrombin time, and partial thromboplastin times in 10 patients with histories of anaphylactoid reactions to these drugs and various food additives. Challenges were not placebo-controlled, nor were they blinded. Nevertheless, the investigators found no correlation between patient's reactions and the aforementioned coagulation parameters.

Conclusion

Thus, aside from several case reports describing IgE-mediated reactions to sulfites and parabens, the majority of synthetic additive-induced urticaria, angioedema, and anaphylactic reactions involve mechanisms that have not been elucidated. This stands in contrast to the natural food additives carmine and annatto, which show definite IgE binding to residual source protein antigens.

Food additive challenge studies in patients with urticaria/angioedema

Patient selection

Selection of patients for study of urticaria/angioedema has included three types of subjects: (1) all available patients with chronic urticaria (or only those with chronic idiopathic urticaria); (2) patients with histories suggestive of food additive-provoked urticaria; or (3) patients who have responded to a diet free of commonly implicated additives. The percentage of positive reactors will depend on the group selected. This variability adds more confusion to the already difficult task of comparing results from differing studies.

Activity of urticaria at the time of study

The relative degree of activity or inactivity of urticaria or angioedema at the time of challenge appears to affect the ability to obtain cutaneous responses to food additives. Challenges performed on patients with active urticaria are more likely to yield false-positive results. Challenges performed on patients whose urticaria is in remission, on the other hand, are more likely to yield false-negative results. In a study by Mathison and colleagues [35], only 1 of 15 patients whose urticaria was in remission experienced a reaction to aspirin, whereas 7 of 10 patients with active urticaria reacted to aspirin. These challenges were performed using objective reaction criteria, and the reactions observed were then compared with base-line observations.

Medications

Several studies made no reference to whether medications – particularly antihistamines – were continued or withheld during challenge. The following caveats must be considered when interpreting such challenge studies: (1) Discontinuation of antihistamines immediately before or within 24 hours of challenge often facilitates more false-positive results. (2) Continuation of antihistamines during challenges may block milder additive-induced cutaneous responses and, there-fore, give more false-negative results. (3) Subjects become increasingly likely to experience breakthrough urticaria as the interval from the last antihistamine dose to the "posi-tive challenge" increases. Such results would be even more confusing if placebo-controlled challenges preceded additive challenges.

Reaction criteria

Often no period of baseline observation is made by the investigators for comparison with reaction data. Most chal-lenge studies performed have employed a loosely defined and rather subjective means to define urticarial responses. The reaction criteria might simply consist of "clear signs of urticaria developing within 24 hours." The studies by Stevenson et al. [30] and Mathison et al. [35], in contrast, utilized an objective system of scoring urticarial responses.

Placebo controls

The use of placebo-controlled studies in additive challenge protocols is desirable because studies without these controls are difficult to interpret when assessing positive urticarial challenge responses. Nevertheless, a number of reported additive challenge studies do not employ placebo controls. Even in many placebo-controlled studies, the placebo is always the first challenge, followed by aspirin, and finally by an additive. Thus, a spontaneous flare of urticaria would be least likely to coincide with the first placebo challenge. We also question the validity of having only a single pla-cebo in challenge studies that test large numbers of additives. A need exists for multiple placebos and randomization of placebo usage in the order of challenges.

Blinding

Among the most important features of any protocol for food additive challenge is a double-blind challenge, because urticaria may be exacerbated by emotional stress. In addition, it is necessary to eliminate observer bias given the subjective nature of positive responses. Open challenges are useful tools for ruling out additive-associated reactions. Positive challenge responses, in contrast, need double-blinded confirmation before they can be accepted as "true positives."

Multiple additive challenges in patients with chronic urticaria

Examples of studies with less stringent design criteria

One of the earliest additive challenge studies in patients with chronic urticaria was reported by Doeglas [36]. Seven (30.4%) subjects reacted to tartrazine and "four or five" (17.4% or 22.7%) reacted to sodium benzoate. Placebo-controlled challenges were not performed. Thune and Granholt [37] reported that 20 (21%) of 96 patients reacted to tartrazine, 13 (15%) of 86 reacted to sunset yellow, 5 (71%) of 7 reacted to parabens, and 6 (13%) of 47 reacted to BHA and BHT. Furthermore, in the group of patients with chronic idiopathic urticaria, 62 (62%) of the 100 patients challenged reacted to at least 1 of the 22 different agents used. The challenges were not placebo-controlled, however, so any conclusions about the incidence of reactions to a particular agent derived from this study would be difficult to support.

In a study of 330 patients with recurrent urticaria, Juhlin [38] performed single-blind challenges using multiple addi-tives and a single placebo, which always preceded the addi-tive challenge. He found that one or more positive reactions occurred in 102 (31%) of patients tested. Reaction criteria were relatively subjective in this study. In fact, 109 (33%) of patients had reactions judged to be "uncertain" because, as the author stated, "Judging whether a reaction is positive or negative is not always easy." Furthermore, if patients reacted to the lactose placebo, retesting involved a wheat starch placebo. Questionable reactors were retested. If the repeat test gave a positive result, the first test was assumed to be posi-tive as well; the same logic applied for negative retesting.

Supramaniam and Warner [39] described 24 of 43 chil-dren as reacting to one or more additives used in their double-blind challenge study. No baseline observation period was established, however, and only one placebo was inter-spersed among the nine additives used for challenge. Furthermore, no mention was made about whether anti-histamines were withheld prior to or during challenges.

In 1985, Genton and co-workers [40] performed single-blind additive challenges on 17 patients with chronic urticaria or angioedema. The patients were placed on a 14-day elim-ination diet (free of food additives) before challenge and medications were discontinued at the beginning of the diet. Of the 17 patients in the study, 15 reacted to at least one of the six additives used for challenge.

Examples of studies with more stringent design criteria

In 1988, Ortolani and associates [41] reported 396 patients with recurrent chronic urticaria and angioedema; this report was a follow-up to a study performed in 1984 [42]. DBPC oral food provocations were performed on patients that had experienced significant remissions while following an elimination diet. The diet was maintained, but medications were discontinued during challenges. The report did not describe the timing of discontinuation of medications. On the basis of history alone, 179 patients were considered for an elimination diet for suspected food or food additive intolerance; only 135 patients ultimately participated in the study. Eight (9.2%) of 87 patients who had significantly improved on the diet after 2 weeks gave positive responses to food challenges. Of the 79 patients with negative responses to food challenges, 72 underwent DBPC, oral food additive provocations. Twelve (17%) of these patients experienced positive responses to challenges with one or more additives. Many of these patients reacted to two or three additives. Five (31%) of the 16 patients with positive responses to aspirin challenges gave positive responses to additive challenges; four of these subjects tested positive to sodium salicylate.

The similarity in chemical structure observed between aspirin and sodium salicylate supports the possibility of cross-reactivity between these agents. They differ in that sodium salicylate is a "non-acetylated" salicylate. The doses used (>400 mg) in the sodium salicylate challenge, however, far exceed the levels encountered in most conventional diets. Furthermore, although it is important in assessing food sensitivity, a patient's history is usually a poor indicator of a possible additive hypersensitivity, because patients are usually unaware of all additives that they consume daily.

Hannuksela and Lahti [43] challenged 44 chronic urticaria patients with several food additives, including sodium metabisulfite, BHA or BHT, β-carotene, and benzoic acid in a prospective, DBPC study. Only 1 (2.2%) of the 44 patients had a positive response to challenge, reacting positively to benzoic acid. Another patient also reacted to the placebo challenge. All medications were discontinued 72 hours before the first challenge and during the study. Patients were not placed on an additive-free diet prior to the challenge. The challenge dose of metabisulfite was low, only 9 mg. Similarly, Kellet and associates noted that approximately 10% of 44 chronic idiopathic urticaria patients reacted to benzoates, tartrazine, or both, but 10% of the subjects reacted to placebo challenges [44].

Elimination diet studies

An alternative strategy for investigating additive-induced urticaria involves the elimination of all additives from the diet and the observation of its effects on hives. Unfortunately, there are no reported blinded or placebo-controlled studies of this nature. In uncontrolled studies, Ros and co-workers [45] reported an additive-free diet to be "completely helpful" in 24% of patients with chronic urticaria; 57% of patients were deemed "much improved," and 19% were "slightly better" or experienced no change in their urticaria. Rudzki and associates [46] reported that 50 (32%) of 158 patients

responded to a diet that eliminated salicylates, benzoates, and azo dyes. These studies did not address the question of which, if any, additives constituted the cause of the problem.

Gibson and Clancy [47] found that 54 (71%) of 76 patients who underwent a 2-week, additive-free diet "responded." They then challenged the responders with individual additives. Although the challenges were controlled, the patients always received the placebo first. No mention was made of whether the challenges were blinded. A diet that eliminated the offending additive was then continued for 6–18 months, followed by repeat challenge. All three patients who initially responded positively to tartrazine challenge had negative results upon re-challenge, as did one of the four patients with initially positive responses to benzoate challenges. Thus, despite this approach, the incidence of additive sensitivity in urticaria remains unknown.

Reports of single additive challenge studies

Sulfites

The reports by Prenner and Stevens [15] and Yang et al. [16] discussed earlier presented single cases of sulfite-provoked anaphylaxis and gave skin test and PK-transfer evidence to suggest that an IgE-mediated mechanism played a role in these reactions. In addition, Yang et al. [16] performed a single-blind oral challenge. Their patient responded positively to a challenge with 5 mg of potassium metabisulfite.

In 1980, Clayton and Busse [48] described a non-atopic female who developed generalized urticaria that progressed to life-threatening anaphylaxis within 15 minutes of drinking wine. Her symptoms were not reproduced by ingestion of other alcoholic beverages. This case may have involved sulfite-provoked urticaria and anaphylaxis.

Habenicht and co-workers [49] described two patients who experienced several episodes of urticaria and angioedema after consuming restaurant meals. Only one of these individuals underwent a single-blind oral challenge with potassium metabisulfite. Generalized urticarial lesions developed in this patient within 15 minutes of receiving a 25-mg challenge dose. No placebo challenge was performed. Avoidance of potential sulfite sources apparently resolved this patient's recurrent symptoms.

Schwartz reported two patients with restaurant-related symptoms who underwent oral challenges with metabisulfite [50]. Both subjects had symptoms temporally related to ingestion of salads: weakness, a feeling of dissociation from the body, dizziness, borderline hypotension, and bradycardia. These signs and symptoms are more consistent with vasovagal reactions than with anaphylaxis. One report has described a patient who received less than 2 ml of procaine (Novocaine) with epinephrine administered subcutaneously by her dentist [51]. Within several minutes, she developed flushing, a sense of warmth, and pruritus, followed by scattered urticaria, dyspnea, and anxiety. Skin tests of various local anesthetics and sulfite proved negative. Thirty minutes after receiving a single-blind, oral dose of 10 mg of sodium bisulfite, she developed "a sense of fullness in her head, nasal congestion, and a pruritic erythematous blotchy eruption." No respiratory symptoms developed and the investigators did not observe any pulmonary function test abnormalities. This patient was able to tolerate local anesthetics without epinephrine. Importantly, this patient did not describe a history of food-related symptoms. Furthermore, the usual dose of aqueous epinephrine (adrenalin) contains only 0.3 mg of sulfite and local anesthetics contain only as much as 2 mg/ml of sulfite. Thus, the usual doses, even in the most sensitive persons, would not provoke reactions. The mechanism of this patient's reaction cannot be definitively linked to sulfite and likely was a vasomotor response to the effects of epinephrine.

A DBPC challenge that reproduced urticaria after challenge with 25 mg of potassium metabisulfite was reported by Belchi-Hernandez et al. [19]. Skin tests were negative in this subject.

Two reports have demonstrated the inability to provoke reactions to sulfites in patients with idiopathic anaphylaxis, some of whom had histories of restaurant-associated symptoms [52,53]. In a study describing food-related skin testing in 102 patients with idiopathic anaphylaxis, only one patient was found to have metabisulfite sensitivity [54]. In addition, the authors performed sulfite-ingestion challenges in 25 patients with chronic idiopathic urticaria and angioedema without a reaction (unpublished observations). At present, sulfite-induced urticaria, angioedema, or anaphylaxis appears to be a rare phenomenon.

Acute urticaria associated with leukocytoclastic vasculitis and eosinophilia was induced by a single placebo-controlled challenge with 50-mg sodium bisulfite in a subject suffering from recurrent urticaria and angioedema of unclear etiology. Blinded challenges were performed during a symptom-free period, followed by biopsy confirmation of the leukocytoclasis. Conscious avoidance of sulfites reduced the frequency of subsequent reactions dramatically [55].

Tartrazine/azo dyes

Murdoch et al. [56] found at least 2 (8.3%) of 24 patients who developed hives after ingesting a panel of four azo dyes, including tartrazine. As previously indicated, Stevenson et al. [30] found that only 1 (4.2%) of 24 aspirin-sensitive subjects undergoing double-blind challenge with 50-mg tartrazine developed urticaria. It appears, therefore, that tartrazine and other azo dyes rarely induce urticaria. The tartrazine-sensitive individual identified in Stevenson's study did not react to a blinded challenge with doses of aspirin of as much as 975 mg, suggesting a lack of cross-reactivity between tartrazine and aspirin.

Aspartame

Two cases of aspartame-provoked urticaria and angioedema have been reported. In these individuals, hives emerged only after aspartame's 1983 approval as a sweetener in carbonated beverages. Both patients reported the onset of urticaria within 1 hour of ingesting aspartame-sweetened soft drinks. DBPC challenges induced urticaria with doses of aspartame (25–75 mg) that fell below the amount contained in typical 12-oz cans (100–150 mg) [57].

In a multi-center, randomized, placebo-controlled crossover study, Geha et al. [58] challenged 21 subjects with histories of a temporal (minutes to hours) association between aspartame ingestion and urticaria/angioedema. These subjects were identified after an extensive recruiting process spanning 4 years. Only four urticarial reactions were observed: two following aspartame consumption and two following placebo ingestion. Doses ranged as high as 600 mg of aspartame.

Butylated hydroxyanisole and butylated hydroxytoluene

In a DBPC study, Goodman et al. [59] challenged two patients with chronic idiopathic urticaria who experienced remissions following dye- and preservative-elimination diets. Both patients noted significant exacerbations of their urticaria after challenge with BHA and BHT. Subsequent avoidance of foods containing these antioxidants resulted in marked abatement of the frequency, severity, and duration of urticaria episodes. Long-term follow-up revealed urticarial flares after dietary indiscretion, but an otherwise quiescent disease.

Monosodium glutamate

Squire described a 50-year-old man with recurrent angioedema of the face and extremities that was related to a history involving ingestion of soup-containing MSG [60]. A single-blind, placebo-controlled challenge with the soup base resulted in "a sensation of imminent swelling" within a few hours, with visible angioedema emerging 24 hours after the challenge. In a graded challenge with only MSG, angioedema occurred 16 hours after challenge with a dose of 250 mg. Avoidance of MSG led to an extended remission. Details of the challenge were not reported, nor did the author mention whether medications were withheld during challenges.

Nitrates/nitrites

Hawkins and Katelaris [61] reported a single case of recurrent anaphylaxis occurring after eating take-out food. DBPC capsule challenge with 25 mg each of sodium nitrates and sodium nitrite resulted in an acute anaphylactic reaction, with hypotension within 15 minutes of the active challenge.

Sodium benzoate

Nettis et al. [62] performed DBPC challenges on 47 patients suspected to have acute urticaria/angioedema induced by sodium-benzoate-containing foods. Only one subject (2%) had a reaction after the ingestion of 75 mg of sodium benzoate without an adverse reaction to placebo, suggesting that even when confronted with suspected historical data on potential reactions to sodium benzoate, true sensitivity rates are quite low.

Food additive sensitivity in chronic idiopathic urticaria/angioedema

Malamin and Kalimo [9] performed prick and scratch skin tests on 91 individuals with chronic idiopathic urticaria/angioedema (CIUA), utilizing a panel of 18 food additives and preservatives. A positive response was defined as a wheal greater than or equal to the size of the histamine control. Sixty-four (26%) subjects had at least one positive skin test as compared with 25 (10%) of 247 non-urticaria control subjects. Ten of the 24 CIUA patients with positive skin tests underwent oral provocation with the additives that gave the positive skin test results. Details of the challenge procedure were not provided. Only one patient reacted, experiencing an urticarial reaction to benzoic acid. The activity level of the patient's prechallenge urticaria was not noted.

At Scripps Clinic and Research Foundation, patients with CIUA are undergoing single-blinded challenges with a panel of additives. Amounts of each additive are listed in Table 28.2. Positive reactors are confirmed with DBPC challenges. To date, no true positive reactors have been identified among more than 100 patients [63 and unpublished data]. From these data, we can conclude with a 95% confidence limit that sensitivity to any of the 11 food and drug additives in patients with CIUA is less than 1%.

Volonakis and colleagues [64] performed an extensive analysis of etiologic factors in 226 children with chronic urticaria. Elimination of food additives and DBPC challenges performed with a panel of four additives (tartrazine, sodium benzoate, nitrates, and sorbic acid) plus aspirin resulted in an overall incidence of 6 (2.6%) of the 226 cases attributable to these additives. Half of these patients (3 of 226, or 1.3%) reacted to aspirin (a known exacerbator of chronic urticaria), and the remaining 3 subjects (1.3%) reacted to tartrazine. No benzoate, nitrate, or sorbic acid reactions occurred among these subjects.

Table 28.2 Suggested maximum doses for additives used in challenge protocols

Yellow dyes No.5 and No.6: 50 mg
Sulfites: 100 mg
MSG: 2.5 g
Aspartame: 150 mg
Parabens/benzoates: 100 mg
BHA/BHT: 250 mg
Nitrates/nitrites: 50 mg

Di Lorenzo and colleagues [65] studied a large series of 838 patients with recurrent chronic idiopathic urticaria for sensitivity to a panel of common food additives. After undergoing historical screenings, all patients had negative food allergen SPTs. After a 4-week food-additive-free diet (FAFD), patients were then screened with a DBPC mixed additive challenge, consisting of tartrazine, erythrosin, sodium benzoate, p-hydroxybenzoate, sodium metabisulfite, and MSG. Positive reactors underwent DBPC single challenges with individual additives with 1-week intervals between challenges. An additional control used included patients with negative DBPC mixed challenges. The incidence of patients having positive histories, clinical response to FAFD, positive DBPC mixed, and DBPC single challenges was only 16 of the 838 patients studied (1.9%; 95% CI 1–3%). Twenty-four total reactions occurred in these 16 patients, due to some individuals reacting to multiple agents.

Food and drug additive skin test and case report studies

Carmine

Several cases of carmine-induced urticaria, angioedema, and anaphylaxis have been described [7,10–12]. These have followed the initial case reports of carmine-induced anaphylaxis by Kagi et al. [66] and Beaudouin et al. [67]. The food products reported implicated in the past include campari-orange liquer, Yoplait brand custard style strawberry–banana yogurt, imitation crab meat, Good Humor SnoFruit Popsicle, and ruby red grapefruit juice. SPTs were positive with undiluted carmine in the history positive patients and negative in control subjects. Contact urticaria associated with carmine-colored cosmetics has also been reported [12]. Specific challenges have not been performed with carmine in any of the above reports, with the exception of Baldwin et al. [10], whose patient showed negative oral challenges to each of the other components of the Good Humor SnoFruit Popsicle. As noted above, these collaborators at the University of Michigan have demonstrated that an IgE-mediated mechanism is responsible for these reactions.

Annatto

Case reports of anaphylactic reactions to annatto dye have been documented. Revan et al. [14] describe one patient with anaphylaxis (4+ SPT with undiluted extract) and one with angioedema (3+ SPT with undiluted extract) after ingesting annatto-containing foods. Neither patient was challenged.

Saffron

Saffron-induced near-fatal anaphylaxis was reported by Wuthrich [5]. The subject, a 21-year-old atopic farmer, developed violent abdominal cramps, laryngeal edema, and generalized urticaria a few minutes after a meal of saffron rice and mushrooms. This progressed to pulse-less collapse which responded to advanced cardiac life support. SPTs to ingredients of the meal were negative except for a strong reaction to saffron. RAST testing to two saffron preparations were both positive. SDS-PAGE and immunoblotting showed five IgE-binding bands with molecular weights between 40 and 90 kDa.

Mannitol

One report of mannitol-induced anaphylaxis has been well described by Hegde and Venkatesh. An individual who demonstrated anaphylactic reactions to mannitol found in pomegranate and cultivated mushroom also experienced severe allergic reactions to mannitol as an excipient in the chewable pharmaceutical cisapride. The authors utilized SPTs, serum mannitol-specific IgE by enzyme-linked immuno-sorbent assay (ELISA), and multiple chemical purification techniques for mannitol separation to demonstrate an immediate hypersensitivity mechanism to mannitol as the explanation for the reactions [6].

Parabens/benzoate

One local anesthetic analysis noted above strongly suggested that methylparaben is a cause of local immediate hypersensitivity reactions previously attributed to the local anesthetics themselves [22]. One isolated case report of sodium-benzoate-induced anaphylaxis was reported by Michils [8].

Isosulfan blue

Askenazi et al. [68] reported three cases of anaphylactic shock to ISB dye used as a lymphatic contrast agent. All three patients reacted within 30 minutes of subcutaneous injection of ISB and all three have positive ISB skin tests. All of the 10 control subjects had negative skin tests to ISB. Two patients had elevated tryptase levels, indicating MC degranulation. All three patients were re-exposed to latex and the other perioperative concomitant medications after their reactions to ISB and demonstrated tolerance to them. Previous retrospective analyses demonstrate an acute allergic reaction rate of 1.1–2.0% [69,70].

Nitrates

Asero [71] reported a case of chronic generalized pruritis without skin eruption that disappeared on an additive-free diet. DBPC challenge with multiple additives resulted in symptom reproducibility within 60 minutes of the 10-mg sodium nitrate challenge. The patient did not react to seven other additives and multiple placebos.

Recommendations for food additive challenge protocols in patients with urticaria, angioedema, and/or anaphylaxis

A review of the literature on food and drug additive challenges in patients with urticaria suggests that more rigorously conducted studies are needed. With the use of more objective criteria and stringent design, more meaningful conclusions may be drawn regarding the true incidence of food additive-induced urticaria, angioedema, and anaphylaxis. Our recommendations for future additive challenge protocols in patients with chronic or acute urticaria/angioedema are presented in the following sections.

Patient selection

In view of the ubiquitous and frequent dietary exposure to food and drug additives, the study population should be selected from patients with chronic "idiopathic" urticaria or angioedema, unless the study is intended to examine another defined subgroup of patients with acute or intermittent urticaria, angioedema, and/or anaphylaxis (e.g. patients with a convincingly positive acute history or patients responsive to an elimination diet). The diagnosis of chronic idiopathic urticaria or angioedema should be made in subjects with recurrent urticaria of at least 6 weeks duration without identifiable cause. In addition, appropriate challenges should be conducted to ascertain any physical urticarias. After a negative workup, a patient's urticaria may then be considered idiopathic [72].

Activity of urticaria

Chronic urticaria should preferably be in an active phase (e.g. some lesions should have appeared within 1 month prior to challenge), as additives may not only provoke urticaria de novo, but also exacerbate ongoing urticaria, as is true with aspirin [35]. For patients with an intermittent and/or acute anaphylactic history associated with an additive, challenges should not be conducted for at least 2 weeks time after the acute reaction.

Medications

Antihistamines should be withheld for 3–5 days prior to the challenges, if possible. For patients with intractable chronic symptoms, antihistamines should be tapered to the minimal effective dose. Although corticosteroids are not first-line treatment for chronic urticaria/angioedema, when necessary their use should also be tapered to the minimal effective dose.

Food-additive-free diet

Patients should be placed on a diet free of all additives included in the challenge protocol at least 1 week prior to challenge.

Reaction criteria

Reaction criteria should be as objective as possible. The "rule of nines" used for assessing thermal burns provides a useful method for estimating skin surface area. On each of the 11 divided areas of the body, the investigator assigns a score of 0–4, then derives a total scored (0–44 points). A positive urticarial response may be defined as either an absolute increase in the total score of 9 points or an increase of more than 300% from the baseline score determined immediately before challenge. A positive angioedema response may be defined as a relative increase in size of more than 50% in the body part affected.

Baseline observation

Prior to any challenges, skin scores should be recorded at the same intervals during a baseline period of observation as during challenges. The appropriate length of the baseline observation period depends on factors such as the activity of the patient's urticaria, the interval of time between discontinuation of antihistamines and the challenges, and the length of the challenge protocol.

In general, 1 day of pure observation with skin scoring should be followed by 1 day of single-blind placebo challenge with skin scoring, except perhaps in patients who are completely free of hives at challenge (in this instance, 1 day of placebo challenge should be sufficient). Skin scores on those 2 days should not vary by more than 3 points or 30% (whichever is greater) before proceeding to additive and further placebo challenges.

Placebo controls

Placebo challenge should be conducted in a randomized fashion. Ideally, at least an equal number of placebo and active challenges should be undertaken. Screening open challenges may be performed without placebo. Here, a negative result does not require further confirmation, but positive reactors must undergo a placebo-controlled protocol, preferably double-blinded (DBPC).

Blinding

Confirmatory challenges should preferably be conducted in a double-blind manner. Coded opaque capsules will serve for this purpose. The code should not be broken until the completion of all challenges. Screening challenges may be performed open or single-blinded. Any "positive challenges" should be confirmed with a double-blind protocol.

Additive doses

The additive doses used in challenge protocols should reflect natural exposure to each agent. Suggested limits for some common additives are listed in Table 28.2. Starting doses should be individualized on the basis of the patient's history, but usually consist of 1/100 of the maximum dose. Challenges must be performed with informed consent and in a setting where severe reactions may be appropriately treated.

Conclusion

Only a small number of well-designed clinical studies have been conducted in the area of additive-provoked urticaria, angioedema, and anaphylaxis. The true incidence of such

reactions remains unknown, although it appears to be relatively rare, despite claims in earlier (pre-1990) additive literature.

Most natural additives (carmine, annatto, and saffron) contain source proteins capable of inducting direct IgE-mediated immediate hypersensitivity reactions. Perhaps the route of sensitization for a subset of the carmine-sensitive patients derives from exposure to topically applied carmine-containing cosmetics, as contact urticaria to this natural additive has been described.

The case for similar immediate hypersensitivity mechanisms is less compelling when the synthetic additive group is analyzed. A relatively small number of case reports describing IgE-mediated reactions to sulfites and parabens exist, compared with the overall number of positive challenges reported.

It is now well accepted that many cases of CIUA have an autoimmune basis, as demonstrated by the presence of autoantibodies directed against the IgE receptor and/or IgE itself [72]. CIUA is frequently associated with other autoimmune syndromes, most notably thyroid autoimmunity [72]. Most studies attempting to link causation and/or exacerbation of this condition by food or drug additives have been poorly designed. Emerging evidence appears to refute the earlier notion that these additives are frequently associated with chronic urticaria. Guidelines for conducting additive challenges in CIUA as well as in episodic urticaria/angioedema patients are reviewed in the text.

Although rare, IgE-mediated paraben reactions can confound the diagnostic evaluation of local anesthetic allergy, given the use of this preservative in multi-dose vials of these medications.

Finally, given the anticipated widespread usage of ISB as a lymphangiography contrast agent, the incidence of reported hypersensitivity reactions to this agent may escalate in the future.

Further well-designed trials addressing additive-provoked urticaria, angioedema, and anaphylaxis are needed before more complete practice parameters can evolve.

References

1 Collins WC. Intolerance to additives. *Ann Allergy* 1983;51:315–16.

2 Marmion DM. *Handbook of US Colorants: Foods, Drugs, Cosmetics and Medical Devices*, 3rd edn. New York: Wiley, 1991.

3 Simon RA. Adverse reactions to food additives. *N Engl Reg Allergy Proc* 1986;7:533–42.

4 Lymphazurin 1% [package insert]. Norwalk, CT: United States Surgical Corporation 2007.

5 Wuthrich B, Schmid-Grendelmeyer P, Lundberg M. Anaphylaxis to saffron. *Allergy* 1997;52:476–7.

6 Hegde VL, Venkatesh YP. Anaphylaxis to excipient mannitol: evidence for an immunoglobulin E-mediated mechanism. *Clin Exp Allergy* 2004;34:1602–9.

7 Acero S, Taber AI, Lizaso MT, *et al*. Occupational asthma due to carmine in a spices handler. European Association of Allergy and Clinical Immunology, Abstract No. 689, 1997.

8 Michils A, Vandermoten G, Duchateau J, *et al*. Anaphylaxis with sodium benzoate. *Lancet* 1991;337:1424–5.

9 Malamin G, Kalimo K. The results of skin testing with food additives and the effect of elimination diet in chronic and recurrent urticaria and recurrent angioedema. *Clin Exp Allergy* 1989;19:539–43.

10 Baldwin JL, Chou AH, Solomon WR. Popsicle-induced anaphylaxis due to carmine allergy. *Ann Allergy Asthma Immunol* 1997;79:415–19.

11 Wuthrich B, Kagi MK, Stucker W. Anaphylactic reactions to ingested carmine (E120). *Allergy* 1997;52:1133–7.

12 Chung K, Baker JR, Baldwin JL, Chou A. Identification of carmine allergens among three carmine allergy patients. *Allergy* 1997;56:73–7.

13 Nish WA, Whisman BA, Goetz DW, Ramirez DA. Anaphylaxis to annatto dye: a case report. *Ann Allergy* 1991;66:129–31.

14 Revan VB, Gold B, Baldwin JL. Annatto experience with skin testing at a University Allergy Clinic. Presented at American College Allergy, Asthma, and Immunology Annual Meeting, Abstract P-70, November 2001.

15 Prenner BM, Stevens JJ. Anaphylaxis after ingestion of sodium bisulfite. *Ann Allergy* 1976;37:180–2.

16 Yang W, Purchase E, Rivington RN. Positive skin tests and Prausnitz–Küstner reactions in metabisulfite-sensitive subjects. *J Allergy Clin Immunol* 1986;78:443–9.

17 Sokol WN, Hydick IB. Nasal congestion, urticaria and angioedema caused by an IgE mediated reaction to sodium metabisulfite. *Ann Allergy* 1990;65:233–8.

18 Sprenger JD, Altman LC, Marshall SG, *et al*. Studies of neutrophil chemotactic factor of anaphylaxis in metabisulfite sensitivity. *Ann Allergy* 1989;62:117–21.

19 Belchi-Hernandez J, Florido-Lopez JF, *et al*. Sulfite induced urticaria. *Ann Allergy* 1993;71:230–2.

20 Nagel JE, Fuscaldo JT, Fireman P. Paraben allergy. *JAMA* 1977;237:1594–5.

21 Aldrete JA, Johnson DA. Allergy to local anesthetics. *JAMA* 1969;207:356–7.

22 Macy E, Schatz M, Zeiger RS. Methylparaben immediate hypersensitivity is a rare cause of false positive local anesthetic provocative dose testing. *J Allergy Clin Immunol* 2002;109:S149.

23 Warrington RJ, Sauder PJ, McPhillips S. Cell-mediated immune responses to artificial food additives in chronic urticaria. *Clin Allergy* 1986;16:527–33.

24 Valverde E, Vich JM, Garcia-Calderone JV, Garcia-Calderone PA. *In vitro* stimulation of lymphocytes in patients with chronic urticaria induced by additives and food. *Clin Allergy* 1980;10:691–8.

25 Juhlin L, Michaelsson G, Zetterstrom O. Urticaria and asthma induced by food and drug additives in patients with aspirin sensitivity. *J Allergy Clin Immunol* 1972;50:92–8.

26 Michaelsson G, Juhlin L. Urticaria induced by preservatives and dye additives in food and drugs. *Br J Dermatol* 1973;88:525–32.

27 Ros A, Juhlin L, Michaelsson G. A follow-up study of patients with recurrent urticaria and hypersensitivity to aspirin, benzoates and azo dyes. *Br J Dermatol* 1976;95:19–24.

28 Settipane GA, Pudupakkam RK. Aspirin tolerance. III. Subtypes, familial occurrence and cross-reactivity with tartrazine. *J Allergy Clin Immunol* 1975;56:215–21.

29 Settipane GA, Chafee FH, Postman M, Levine MI. Significance of tartrazine sensitivity in chronic urticaria of unknown etiology. *J Allergy Clin Immunol* 1976;57:541–6.

30 Stevenson DD, Simon RA, Lumry WR, Mathison DA. Adverse reactions to tartrazine. *J Allergy Clin Immunol* 1986;78:182–91.

31 Blake JL, Lawrence N, Bennet J, *et al*. Late endocrine effects of administering monosodium glutamate to neonatal rats. *Neuroendocrinology* 1978;26:220–3.

32 Allen DH, Van Nunen S, Loblay R, *et al*. Adverse reactions to foods. *Med J Aust* 1984;141:S37–42.

33 Casale TB, Sampson HA, Hanifin J. Guide to physical urticarias. *J Allergy Clin Immunol* 1988;82:758–63.

34 Zimmerman RE, Czarnetzki BM. Changes in the coagulation system during pseudo allergic anaphylactoid reactions to drugs and food additives. *Int Arch Allergy Appl Immunol* 1986;81:375–7.

35 Mathison DA, Lumry WR, Stevenson DD, Curd JG. Aspirin in chronic urticaria and/or angioedema. Studies of sensitivity and desensitization (abstract). *J Allergy Clin Immunol* 1982;69:135.

36 Doeglas HM. Reactions to aspirin and food additives in patients with chronic urticaria, including the physical urticarias. *Br J Dermatol* 1975;93:135–44.

37 Thune P, Granholt A. Provocation tests with anti-phlogistica and food additives in recurrent urticaria. *Dermatologica* 1975; 151:136–67.

38 Juhlin L. Recurrent urticaria: clinical investigation of 330 patients. *Br J Dermatol* 1981;104:369–81.

39 Supramaniam G, Warner JO. Artificial food additive intolerance in patients with angio-oedema and urticaria. *Lancet* 1986;2:907–10.

40 Genton C, Frei PC, Pecoud A. Value of oral provocation tests to aspirin and food additives in the routine investigation of asthma and chronic urticaria. *J Allergy Clin Immunol* 1985;76:40–5.

41 Ortolani C, Pasterello E, Fontana A, *et al*. Chemicals and drugs as triggers of food-associated disorder. *Ann Allergy* 1988;60:358–66.

42 Ortolani C, Pasterello E, Luraghi MI, *et al*. Diagnosis of intolerance to food additives. *Ann Allergy* 1984;53:587–91.

43 Hannuksela M, Lahti A. Peroral challenge tests with food additives in urticaria and atopic dermatitis. *Int J Dermatol* 1986;25:178–80.

44 Kellet JK, August PJ, Beck MH. Double-blinded challenge tests with food additives in chronic urticaria. *Br J Dermatol* 1984;111:32.

45 Ros AM, Juhlin L, Michaelsson G. A follow-up study of patients with recurrent urticaria and hypersensitivity to aspirin, benzoates and azo dyes. *Br J Dermatol* 1976;95:19–24.

46 Rudzki E, Czubalski K, Grzywa Z. Detection of urticaria with food additive intolerance by means of diet. *Dermatologica* 1980;161:57–62.

47 Gibson A, Clancy R. Management of chronic idiopathic urticaria by the identification and exclusion of dietary factors. *Clin Allergy* 1980;10:699–704.

48 Clayton DE, Busse W. Anaphylaxis to wine. *Clin Allergy* 1980;10:341–3.

49 Habenicht HA, Preuss L, Lovell RG. Sensitivity to ingested metabisulfites: cause of bronchospasm and urticaria. *Immunol Allergy Pract* 1983;5:243–5.

50 Schwartz HJ. Sensitivity to ingested metabisulfite, variations in clinical presentation. *J Allergy Clin Immunol* 1985;75:487–9.

51 Schwartz HJ, Sher TH. Bisulfite sensitivity manifesting as allergy to local dental anaesthesia. *J Allergy Clin Immunol* 1985;75:525–7.

52 Sonin L, Patterson R. Metabisulfite challenge in patients with idiopathic anaphylaxis. *J Allergy Clin Immunol* 1985;75:67–9.

53 Meggs WJ, Atkins FM, Wright IH. Sulfite challenges in patients with systematic mastocytosis or unexplained anaphylaxis. *J Allergy Clin Immunol* 1985;75:144.

54 Stricker WE, Anorve-Lopez E, Reed CE. Food skin testing in patients with idiopathic anaphylaxis. *J Allergy Clin Immunol* 1986;77:516–19.

55 Wuthrich B, Kägi MK, Hafner I. Disulfite-induced acute intermittent urticaria with vasculitis [Letter]. *Dermatology* 1993;186:274.

56 Murdoch RD, Pollock I, Young E, et al. Food additive induced urticaria: studies of mediator release during provocation tests. *J R Coll Phys Lond* 1987;21:262.

57 Kulczycki A. Aspartame-induced urticaria. *Ann Intern Med* 1986;104:207–8.

58 Geha R, Buckley CE, Greenberger P, et al. Aspartame is no more likely than placebo to cause urticaria/angioedema. Results of a multicenter randomized, double-blind, placebo-controlled, crossover study. *J Allergy Clin Immunol* 1993;92:513–20.

59 Goodman DL, McDonnell JT, Nelson HS, et al. Chronic urticaria exacerbated by the antioxidant food preservative, butylated hydroxyanisole (BHA) and butylated hydroxyl toluene (BHT). *J Allergy Clin Immunol* 1990;86:570–5.

60 Squire EN. Angio-oedema and monosodium glutamate (MSG). *Lancet* 1987;1:998.

61 Hawkins CA, Katelaris CH. Nitrate anaphylaxis. *Ann Allergy Asthma Immunol* 2000;85:74–6.

62 Nettis E, Colonardi MC, Ferrannini A, Tursi A. Sodium benzoate-induced repeated episodes of acute urticaria/angioedema: randomized controlled trial. *Br J Dermatol* 2004;151:898–902.

63 Simon RA, Bosso JV, Daffern PD, Ward B. Prevalence of sensitivity to food/drug additives in patients with chronic idiopathic urticaria/angioedema (CIUA). *J Allergy Clin Immunol* 1998;101:S154–5.

64 Volonakis M, Katsarou-Katsari A, Stratigos I. Etiologic factors on childhood chronic urticaria. *Ann Allergy* 1992;69:61–5.

65 Di Lorenzo G, Pacor ML, Mansueto P, et al. Food-additive-induced urticaria: a survey of 838 patients with recurrent chronic idiopathic urticaria. *Int Arch Allergy Immunol* 2005;138:235–42.

66 Kagi MK, Wuthrich B, Johansson SGO. Campari-orange anaphylaxis due to carmine allergy. *Lancet* 1994;344:60–1.

67 Beaudouin E, Kanny G, Lambert H, et al. Food anaphylaxis following ingestion of carmine. *Ann Allergy* 1995;74:427–30.

68 Askenazi N, Sheets M, Gewurz A. Three cases of anaphylaxis to isosulfan blue. *J Allergy Clin Immunol* 2002;109:S150–1.

69 Cimmino VM, Braun AC, Szocik JF, et al. Allergic reactions to isosulfan blue during sentinel lymph node biopsy – a common event. *Surgery* 2001;130:439–42.

70 Albo D, Wayne JD, Hunt KK, et al. Anaphylactic reactions to isosulfan blue dye during sentinel lymph node biopsy for breast cancer. *Am J Surg* 2001;182:393–8.

71 Asero R. Chronic generalized pruritis caused by nitrate intolerance. *J Allergy Clin Immunol* 1999;104:1110–11.

72 Kaplan AP. Clinical practice. Chronic urticaria and angioedema. *N Engl J Med* 2002;346:175–9.

29

CHAPTER 29

Sulfites

Steve L. Taylor, Robert K. Bush, and Julie A. Nordlee

KEY CONCEPTS

- Sulfites are frequently used food and drug additives.
- Ingestion of sulfite residues has been documented to trigger asthmatic reactions in sensitive individuals.
- Sulfite-induced asthma occurs in less than 5% of asthmatic individuals and those with severe, persistent asthma are at greatest risk.
- The diagnosis of sulfite-induced asthma is best made by blinded oral challenge with assessment of lung function.
- Labeling regulations in the United States alert sulfite-sensitive individuals to the presence of sulfites in foods which must then be avoided.

Introduction

Sulfites or sulfiting agents include sulfur dioxide (SO_2), sulfurous acid (H_2SO_3), and any of several inorganic sulfite salts that may liberate SO_2 under their conditions of use. The inorganic sulfite salts include sodium and potassium metabisulfite ($Na_2S_2O_5$, $K_2S_2O_5$), sodium and potassium bisulfite ($NaHSO_3$, $KHSO_3$), and sodium and potassium sulfite (Na_2SO_3, K_2SO_3). Sulfites have a long history of use as food ingredients, although potassium sulfite and sulfurous acid are not permitted for use in foods in the United States [1]. Sulfites occur naturally in many foods, especially fermented foods such as wines [1]. In addition, sulfites have long been used as ingredients in pharmaceuticals [2,3].

Over the past 25 years, questions have arisen about the safety of the continued use of sulfites in foods and drugs. These concerns were first voiced following the independent observations in 1981 by David Allen in Australia and Donald Stevenson and Ronald Simon in the United States of the role of sulfites in triggering asthmatic reactions in some sensitive individuals [4–6]. While it is now apparent that sulfite sensitivity affects only a small subgroup of the asthmatic population [6,7], concerns remain because sulfite-induced asthma can be severe – even life threatening – in some sensitive individuals.

As a consequence of the concerns related to sulfite-induced asthma, the use of sulfites in foods and drugs has changed considerably over the years. Sulfites have been replaced in some products; and the search for effective alternatives continues; in addition, levels of sulfites used have been reduced in other products. Federal regulations have further restricted the use of sulfites in certain food products in the United States. Nevertheless, the sulfite-sensitive individual must stay alert to avoid inadvertent exposure to sulfites.

Clinical manifestations of sulfite sensitivity

A host of adverse reactions have been attributed to sulfiting agents, including asthma, diarrhea, abdominal pain and cramping, nausea and vomiting, urticaria, pruritus, localized angioedema, difficulty in swallowing, faintness, headache, chest pain, loss of consciousness, "change in body temperature," "change in heart rate," and non-specific rashes. With the notable exception of the role of sulfites in asthma, diagnostic challenges were not undertaken to confirm the causative role for sulfites in the reported adverse reactions. For normal individuals, exposure to sulfiting agents appears to pose little risk. Toxicity studies in normal volunteers showed that ingestion of 400 mg of sulfite daily for 25 days had no adverse effect [8].

Non-asthmatic responses on oral exposure to sulfites

Various authors have suggested adverse reactions involving several organ systems, but for the most part these effects have not been substantiated by double-blind, placebo-controlled (DBPC) provocation studies. Schmidt et al. [9] posited that sulfiting agents may have caused the appearance of a cardiac

Food Allergy: Adverse Reactions to Foods and Food Additives, 4th edition.
Edited by Dean D. Metcalfe, Hugh A. Sampson, and Ronald A. Simon.
© 2008 Blackwell Publishing, ISBN: 978-1-4501-5129-0.

arrhythmia in a patient given intravenous dexamethasone. This relationship was never confirmed by appropriate challenge. Hallaby and Maddocks [10] attributed central nervous system toxicity to the absorption of sodium bisulfite from peritoneal dialysis solutions. Wang *et al.* [11] described eight patients who developed chronic neurological defects after receiving an epidural anesthetic agent that contained sodium bisulfite as a preservative. Using an animal model, they demonstrated that the sulfiting agent produced a similar defect. Whether the clinical manifestation in humans was directly attributable to the sodium bisulfite is unknown. In a preliminary report, Flaherty *et al.* [12] presented a patient who appeared to have hepatotoxicity as manifested by changes in liver function tests following challenge with potassium metabisulfite. Meggs *et al.* [13] failed to demonstrate any role for sulfites among eight individuals with systemic mastocytosis. Schwartz [14] described two non-asthmatic subjects who developed abdominal distress and hypotension associated with oral challenge with potassium metabisulfite. Placebo-controlled challenges proved negative, however.

Cutaneous adverse reactions suggestive of hypersensitivity responses have been observed in a few individuals. cutaneous exposure to sulfites can on rare occasions, apparently elicit contact sensitivity reactions [15]. Epstein [15] described a patient who developed contact sensitivity, as confirmed by appropriate patch testing, through exposure to sulfiting agents used in a restaurant. The ingestion of sulfites has been reported to elicit urticaria in a very few cases as confirmed by DBPC challenges [16], single-blind challenges [17,18], or open challenges [19]; in other cases, an urticarial response was not confirmed by oral challenge [20]. Angioedema attributable to the ingestion of sulfiting agents was reported in two of these patients, but only urticaria was confirmed by open challenge with potassium metabisulfite [19]. Wuthrich [17] conducted single-blind, placebo-controlled challenges with sodium bisulfite in 245 patients with suspected sulfite sensitivity. Fifty-seven of the challenges were positive including 17 patients with urticaria/angioedema, 7 patients with rhinitis, and 5 patients with local anesthetic reactions. Wuthrich *et al.* [18] reported a case of acute intermittent urticaria with an associated vasculitis due to sulfites, based on a placebo-controlled, single-blind challenge. Huang and Frazier [21] presented an individual who developed palmar and plantar pruritus, generalized urticaria, laryngeal edema, and severe abdominal pain with fulminant diarrhea after ingesting sulfiting agents. In a controlled challenge with a local anesthetic containing 0.9μg of sodium metabisulfite, the patient experienced palmar pruritus but no generalized urticaria. The toxicological mechanism involved in these cutaneous reactions has not been elucidated.

Anaphylaxis-like events have been described in several individuals, although appropriate confirmatory testing was only performed in some instances. Prenner and Stevens [22] described a non-asthmatic individual who developed urticaria, pruritus, and angioedema after eating sulfited foods in a restaurant. A single-blind challenge with no placebo controls was conducted with sodium metabisulfite. Some of the symptoms (nausea, coughing, erythema of the patient's skin) were reproduced by this challenge. Clayton and Busse [23] reported a patient who developed anaphylaxis after ingesting wine. An open challenge with wine reproduced the patient's symptoms of urticaria, angioedema, and hypotension. While this patient represents a possible case of sulfite sensitivity, specific testing with sulfites was not conducted, nor was any association with sulfiting agents in wine recognized at that time.

Sokol and Hydick [24] identified a single case of sulfite-induced anaphylaxis presenting with urticaria, angioedema, nasal congestion, and nasal polyp swelling that was later confirmed by multiple, single-blind, placebo-controlled oral challenge trials. The patient, who had a history of similar food-related reactions, also produced a positive skin test to sulfite, and histamine could be released from her basophils following incubation with sulfites. Yang *et al.* [25] described three patients with systemic anaphylactic symptoms (rhinorrhea with asthma in one; urticaria with asthma in the second; asthma only in the third) confirmed by sulfite challenge. These three patients had positive skin tests to sulfites and two of the three had positive Prausnitz–Küstner (PK) tests. One individual subsequently died, allegedly after ingestion of sulfited food.

Sulfites have also been implicated as possible causative factors in persistent rhinitis [26]. The role of sulfites was evaluated in a group of 226 patients with persistent rhinitis using DBPC challenges after 1 month on an additive-free diet. Challenges with up to 20mg of sodium metabisulfite elicited both objective (sneezing and rhinorrhea) and subject (nasal blockage and itching) symptoms in 6 of 20 individuals who reported improvement in rhinitis on the additive-free diet [26]. A reduction of greater than or equal to 20% in nasal peak inspiratory flow rate was also observed in these six subjects [26].

Studies have been undertaken to determine whether sulfiting agent sensitivity frequently causes idiopathic anaphylaxis or chronic idiopathic urticaria (CIU) [13,27–29]. Sonin and Patterson [27] conducted sodium metabisulfite challenges on 12 individuals with idiopathic anaphylaxis, nine of whom reported episodes associated with restaurant meals. None of the patients responded to the challenge. One additional patient with CIU and restaurant-associated symptoms was also challenged; this individual also failed to react to the challenge. Meggs *et al.* [13] studied 25 patients with idiopathic anaphylaxis. Two of the individuals reacted on single-blind challenge; after repeating the sulfite and placebo challenge, one of these patients was subsequently found not to be sulfite sensitive. Another individual appeared to react on repeated challenge and not to placebo. However, institution of a sulfite-free diet had no effect on this patient's subsequent episodes. In a preliminary report on 65 adults with CIU, none reacted to sulfites when appropriately challenged [28]. Using a rigorous blinded, placebo-controlled trial and objective criteria for positive reactions, Simon [29] was unable to demonstrate a positive reaction to encapsulated metabisulfite (200 mg maximum dose) in 75 patients with chronic urticaria and/or anaphylaxis with a history suggestive of sulfite sensitivity.

Thus, although many adverse reactions have been ascribed to sulfiting agents, the risk appears to be rather low for the non-asthmatic subject. Properly performed DBPC challenges are necessary to confirm whether sulfite sensitivity was responsible for suspected adverse reactions.

Adverse reactions to sulfites on inhalation or intravenous exposures

In addition, systemic adverse reactions have been attributed to intravenous and inhalation administration of sulfiting agents contained in pharmaceutical products. While receiving bronchodilator therapy with isoetharine, an asthmatic subject developed acute respiratory failure that required mechanical ventilation [30]. The patient subsequently experienced erythematous flushing with urticaria upon intravenous administration of metaclopramide that contained a sulfiting agent. In placebo-controlled oral provocation with sodium metabisulfite, this patient developed flushing without urticaria, as well as a significant decrease in pulmonary function. Jamieson et al. [31] performed inhalation challenge in a patient with presumed sulfite sensitivity. This individual experienced intense pruritus, tingling of the mouth, nausea, chest tightness, and a feeling of impending doom. No placebo challenge was undertaken, however.

Asthmatic responses on oral exposure to sulfites

Although sulfiting agents play a very limited and somewhat controversial role in the causation of non-asthmatic adverse reactions, their role in the causation of bronchospasm and severe asthma is better established. Kochen [32] was among the first to suggest that ingestion of sulfited food can cause bronchospasm. He described a child with mild asthma who repeatedly experienced coughing, shortness of breath, and wheezing when exposed to dehydrated fruits treated with sulfur dioxide that were packaged in hermetically sealed plastic bags. No direct challenge studies were conducted to confirm this observation. Single-dose, open challenges without placebo control performed in a group of asthmatics by Freedman [33,34] suggested that sulfiting agents could trigger asthma. Eight of 14 subjects with a history of wheezing following consumption of sulfited orange drinks were shown to experience changes in pulmonary function upon administration of an acidic solution containing 100 ppm (100 mg/l) of sodium metabisulfite.

The role of sulfite sensitivity in asthma became more widely recognized after reports of Stevenson and Simon [5] and Baker et al. [4]. The initial studies of Stevenson and Simon [5] demonstrated that placebo-controlled oral challenges with potassium metabisulfite could produce significant changes in pulmonary function in certain asthmatics. Their first subjects had severe persistent asthma. In addition to their asthmatic response, these individuals experienced flushing, tingling, and faintness following sulfite challenges. Baker et al. [4] showed that oral ingestion and intravenous administration of sulfites could cause significant bronchoconstriction to the point of respiratory arrest in two individuals with severe, persistent asthma. Exposure to sulfiting agents may occur through ingestion and other routes. Sulfur dioxide generated from sulfited foods and drugs may be inhaled. Werth [35] described an asthmatic individual who developed wheezing, flushing, and diaphoresis upon inhaling the vapors released from a bag of dried apricots. The patient did not respond to ingested metabisulfite in capsule form, but reacted to inhalation of nebulized metabisulfite in distilled water. Reports have described several patients who suffered paradoxical responses to the inhalation of bronchodilator solutions. Koepke et al. [36,37] demonstrated that sodium bisulfite used as a preservative in bronchodilator solutions was capable of producing bronchoconstriction. Other studies from this group [38] confirmed that the concentration of metabisulfite contained in bronchodilator solutions could potentially generate 0.8–1.2 ppm of sulfur dioxide. Four of 10 subjects who tested negative to a capsule challenge with metabisulfite reacted upon inhalation, whereas 10 non-asthmatic controls did not respond.

In addition to sulfiting agents administered intravenously, orally, or via inhalation, patients may respond to the topical application of sulfiting agents. Schwartz and Sher [39] reported an individual who experienced a 25% decrease in forced expiratory volume in one second (FEV1) after application of one drop of a 0.75-mg/ml potassium metabisulfite solution to the eye. This patient had previously experienced episodes of bronchoconstriction from the use of eye drops containing sulfite preservatives for the treatment of glaucoma.

Asthmatic subjects may develop bronchoconstriction in response to a wide variety of stimuli. Interestingly, a patient has been described [40] who failed to respond to typical triggers of bronchoconstriction, including inhalation of methacholine and cold air hyperventilation, but who nevertheless experienced increased airway resistance and decreased specific airway conductance following oral challenge with potassium metabisulfite. The significance of this response remains unknown, as no changes in other parameters of pulmonary function, including FEV1, were observed.

The potential for fatal reactions from sulfite exposure has been confirmed [25,41]. In many instances, individuals who supposedly died from an adverse reaction to sulfite had not undergone appropriate diagnostic challenges. Nonetheless,

76 Nordlee JA, Naidu SG, Taylor SL. False positive and false negative reactions encountered in the use of sulfite test strips for the detection of sulfite-treated foods. *J Allergy Clin Immunol* 1988;81:537–41.

77 Wedzicha B. *Chemistry of Sulfur Dioxide in Foods.* Barking, England: Elsevier Applied Science Publishers, 1984.

78 Otwell WS, Iyengar R, McEvily AJ. Inhibition of shrimp melanosis by 4-hexylresorcinol. *J Aquatic Food Prod Technol* 1992;1:53–65.

79 Monsalve-Gonzalez A, Barbosa-Canovas GV, Cavalieri RP, *et al.* Control of browning during storage of apple slices preserved by combined methods: 4-hexylresorcinol as anti-browning agent. *J Food Sci* 1993;58:797–800.

80 McWeeny DJ, Knowles ME, Hearne JF. The chemistry of non-enzymatic browing in foods and its control by sulfites. *J Sci Food Agric* 1974;25:735–46.

81 Roberts AC, McWeeny DJ. The uses of sulfur dioxide in the food industry – a review. *J Food Technol* 1972;7:221–38.

82 Nelson KE. Effects of in-package sulfur dioxide generators, package liners, and temperature on decay and desiccation of table grapes. *Am J Enol Vitic* 1983;34:10–16.

83 Wade P. Action of sodium metabisulfite on the properties of hard sweet biscuit dough. *J Sci Food Agric* 1972;23:333–6.

84 Simon RA. Sulfite sensitivity. *Ann Allergy* 1987;59:100–5.

85 Martin LB, Nordlee JA, Taylor SL. Sulfite residues in restaurant salads. *J Food Prot* 1986;49:126–9.

86 Taylor SL, Bush RK, Busse WW. The sulfite story. *Assoc Food Drug Off Quart Bull* 1985;49:185–93.

87 Halpern GM, Gershwin E, Ough C, *et al.* The effect of white wine upon pulmonary function of asthmatic subjects. *Ann Allergy* 1985;55:686–90.

88 Howland WA, Simon RA. Restaurant-provoked asthma: sulfite sensitivity? (abstract). *J Allergy Clin Immunol* 1985;75:145.

89 Helrich K (ed.). *Official Methods of Analysis of the Association of Official Analytical Chemists,* 15th edn. Arlington, VA: Association of Official Analytical Chemists, 1990:1157–8.

90 Timbo B, Koehler KM, Wolyniak C, *et al.* Sulfites – a Food and Drug Administration review of recalls and reported adverse events. *J Food Prot* 2004;67:1806–11.

CHAPTER 30

Monosodium Glutamate

Katharine M. Woessner

KEY CONCEPTS

- Glutamate is recognized by distinct taste receptors on the tongue as "umami" (savory) along with sweet, sour, salty, and bitter.

- Monosodium glutamate (MSG) is rapidly and efficiently metabolized by the intestinal mucosa and liver in both adults and infants. Despite high maternal intake of MSG, levels remain low in fetal circulation. Therefore, no limitation for MSG ingestion in pregnant women and infants is recommended.

- MSG has been anecdotally associated with a diverse array of conditions including migraine headache, which have not been validated in carefully controlled challenge studies. Low-MSG diets should not be empirically recommended for migraine sufferers, as there is no science to back up such a recommendation.

- MSG symptom complex (formally the Chinese restaurant syndrome) may occur with high-dose MSG ($\geq 3\,g$) in the absence of food in some people and is a self-limited condition.

- MSG is generally recognized as safe by the Food and Drug Administration. Numerous studies have failed to show that MSG causes any serious acute or chronic medical problems in the general population.

A 1968 letter to the editors of the *New England Journal of Medicine* by Dr. Robert Kwok describing what he termed the Chinese restaurant syndrome (CRS) with "numbness at the back of the neck ... radiating to both arms and the back, general weakness and palpitation" which he experienced only when dining in Chinese restaurants, initiated the public controversy surrounding monosodium glutamate (MSG) which continues to this day [1]. Although Dr. Kwok hypothesized that his symptom complex was due to the alcohol in Chinese cooking wine, sodium content, or the flavoring ingredient MSG, attention became focused on MSG. Since the 1960s, the role of MSG has been questioned in not only what has become known as the MSG symptom complex, but also a number of other potential adverse reactions. In addition to the MSG symptom complex, MSG ingestion has been anecdotally associated with asthma, urticaria, and angioedema, headache, shudder attacks in children, psychiatric disorders, and convulsions. In the three decades since the publication of Dr. Kwok's letter, extensive research has failed to demonstrate a clear and consistent relationship between MSG ingestion and the development

of these or any adverse reactions in humans. Despite this, strong suspicion regarding MSG persists in the public arena.

The fifth taste: L-glutamate

Humans can detect four primary tastes: sweet, salty, bitter, and sour. There is also a fifth taste called umami. Umami describes the palatability or deliciousness of a food, and has been called a "brothy mouth-watering sensation" [2]. Glutamic acid is a non-essential amino acid that constitutes approximately 20% of dietary proteins. When added to foods in the form of a sodium, potassium, or calcium salt, glutamate enhances the palatability of foods. Ikeda first documented the unique taste- and flavor-enhancing qualities of MSG in 1908 after isolating it from the seaweed *Laminaria japonica*, which has been used for centuries in Japanese cooking as a flavor enhancer [3]. Its characteristic taste, umami, is imparted through its stereochemical structure, monosodium L-glutamate; the D-isomer has no characteristic taste. MSG became widely available in the United States during the 1940s.

MSG is commercially synthesized by taking protein, usually derived from wheat or soy, through an acid wash to isolate amino acids. A neutralizing agent, sodium hydroxide, is then added to form the sodium salt of each amino acid.

Food Allergy: Adverse Reactions to Foods and Food Additives, 4th edition.
Edited by Dean D. Metcalfe, Hugh A. Sampson, and Ronald A. Simon.
© 2008 Blackwell Publishing. ISBN: 978-1-4501-5129-0.

Table 30.1 Food labeling of MSG

Free glutamate	Bound glutamate
MSG	HVP
Monopotassium glutamate	HPP
Monoammonium glutamate	HSP
Glutamic acid	Natural flavorings
Glutamic acid hydrochloride	Flavor(s) or flavoring
Glutamate	Seasoning
	Kombu extract
	Autolyzed yeast extract

Typically, MSG constitutes 10–30% of the mixture. When other amino acids are present it is referred to as hydrolyzed vegetable protein (HVP). MSG is also produced by fermentation of beetroot pulp or sugarcane. It is then purified to 98% purity. Table 30.1 lists the Food and Drug Administration (FDA) approved names of MSG. Since 1986, the FDA has permitted glutamate to be indirectly identified on food labels as HVP (hydrolyzed vegetable protein), HPP (hydrolyzed plant protein), or HSP (hydrolyzed soy protein) [4]. The glutamate salts are used widely in the food manufacturing and restaurant industries and flavor a wide spectrum of foods including crackers, potato chips, canned and dry soups, canned seafood, meats, frozen dinners, salad dressings, Chinese, and other Asian foods. When MSG is added to food, the FDA requires "MSG" to be listed on the label. Other salts of glutamic acid – such as monopotassium glutamate and monoammonium glutamate – also have to be declared on labels and cannot be lumped together under "spices," "natural flavoring," or other general terms. The salts quickly dissociate in aqueous solution releasing free glutamate.

Normal dietary intake of MSG in the United States is approximately 1 g/day in its free form. An additional 0.55 g/day comes from added MSG. Some foods contain naturally occurring high levels of free glutamate such as tomatoes (0.34% MSG), Parmesan cheese (1.5% MSG), and soy sauce (1.3% MSG) [5]. In the body, the turnover rate for MSG is 5–10 g/hour [5]. Glutamate is metabolized in a number of ways, including oxidative deamination, transamination, decarboxylation, and amidation. MSG is readily transaminated to α-ketoglutarate, which is converted to energy by the Krebs cycle [6]. Studies on humans indicate that MSG ingested with meals results only in a very small increase in plasma glutamate concentration when compared with the levels achieved when it is consumed while dissolved in water or consommé [7]. The presence of carbohydrates appears to greatly reduce the levels of free glutamate in plasma after meals, even those containing very high levels of MSG. Even when MSG is administered in large quantities (>30 mg/kg body weight) without food, serum levels are only slightly elevated due to the very efficient metabolism of glutamate in the intestines and liver [8]. Elevated plasma levels due to doses exceeding 5 g of MSG return to basal levels in less than 2 hours [8].

Fetal and neonatal exposure to glutamate is likely to be small. Though glutamate can cross the placenta, fetal plasma concentrations do not increase significantly even with maternal ingestion of 100 mg/kg of MSG [9]. Studies by Stegink *et al.* in pregnant rhesus monkeys showed that it was not until the maternal plasma level of MSG exceeded 2000 μmol/l that there was a slight increase in fetal MSG levels [10]. This data suggests that transfer of glutamate from the mother to the fetus is unlikely even with very high maternal oral intake. Infants, including premature babies, can metabolize greater than 100-mg MSG/kg body weight administered in infant formulas [11]. Free glutamate is found in breast milk in conjunction with other free amino acids and is among the most prevalent amino acids along with glutamine and taurine [12]. The free glutamate in breast milk is speculated to have a protective role in assuring intestinal growth and supplying functional substrates to the nervous tissue [13].

Monosodium glutamate and neurotoxicity

By the late 1960s, concerns were raised regarding the possible neurotoxicity of MSG. Olney reported MSG-induced toxicity in the nervous system of rodents when glutamate was given in large amounts by non-dietary routes to neonatal mice [14]. The resulting focal necrosis of the arcuate nucleus of the hypothalamus led to functional alteration of the reproductive capability and body weight regulation in mice. The proposed mechanism for neuronal damage is passage across the blood–brain barrier by glutamate whereby glutamate, as an excitatory transmitter, leads to continuous excitation of the glutaminergic receptors, depleting ATP and leading to cell death. This appears to be a phenomenon to which neonatal mice are particularly susceptible. There have been at least 21 studies looking for effects of MSG-induced neurotoxicity in primates and only two were positive and came from the same laboratory [15,16]. The threshold blood levels associated with neuronal damage in the mouse are 100–130 μmol/dl in neonates rising to 380 μmol/dl in weanlings and greater than 630 μmol/dl in adult mice [17]. In humans, such levels have not been recorded even after very high bolus doses of MSG. It has been noted by the Joint Food and Agriculture Organization (FAO) of the United Nations and the World Health Organization (WHO) Expert Committee on Food Additives (JECFA) that the oral ED$_{50}$ for production of hypothalamic lesions in the neonatal mouse is ~500-mg MSG/kg body weight by gavage. In humans, the largest palatable dose of MSG is ~60 mg/kg body weight with higher doses causing nausea, making voluntary ingestion of higher doses very unlikely [17].

Neuroendocrine effects of high-dose glutamate administration have been demonstrated in rodents including a reduction in hypothalamic growth hormone releasing hormone (GHRH) release and pituitary growth hormone (GH) secretion as well as an increase in serum leutenizing hormone (LH) levels [5,18,19]. Such effects have not been shown in humans and the implications of these findings remain unknown. Acute toxicity of glutamate has been determined with a LD_{50} value of 16–20 g/kg body weight [20]. There is no evidence to date of MSG-associated carcinogenicity or teratogenicity [21–26].

MSG is classified by the FDA as generally recognized as safe (GRAS). The amount of MSG that can be added to foods is limited only by its palatability. The Joint FAO/WHO JECFA has evaluated MSG and has determined that no numerical limitation is necessary for its use in food [27]. In addition, there was no evidence to support recommendations limiting intake of MSG in pregnant women or infants. However, they did contend that food additives, in general, should not be added to infant foods to be consumed before 12 weeks of age [27]. Around the time of the discovery of MSG-induced neurotoxicity in mice, large amounts of MSG were routinely added to infant formulas in the United States. After these data became available, however, manufacturers of infant formula voluntarily removed MSG from their products.

MSG symptom complex

The controversy surrounding MSG as a food additive first came to light after Dr. Kwok published a letter to the editors in the *New England Journal of Medicine* in 1968 detailing a set of symptoms he experienced when eating at Chinese restaurants [1]. He described the experience of numbness at the back of the neck, general weakness, and palpitations. This set of symptoms became known as the CRS. More recently, it has been renamed as the MSG symptom complex. As defined by Settipane, a restaurant syndrome is an adverse reaction to foods occurring within 20 minutes of ingestion, frequently while patients are still dining in restaurants [28]. After Dr. Kwok's letter in 1968, a series of anecdotes implicated MSG as the agent responsible for the CRS. In 1968, Schaumburg reported on his own experiences which included tightening of facial muscles, lacrimation, periorbital fasiculations, numbness of the neck and hands, palpitations, and syncope occurring within 20 minutes of eating Chinese food on separate occasions, with symptoms resolving in 45 minutes. He reported having as many as eight experiences per day without sequelae [29]. Over the ensuing 30 years, numerous human challenge studies have been conducted in an attempt to determine the association of MSG with the clinical entity of the MSG symptoms complex.

In general, challenge studies with MSG pose great difficulty because of the distinct taste properties of MSG that makes adequate blinding hard to achieve. Interpretation of some reported challenge studies has been hampered by the lack of a food vehicle. As pointed out earlier, the metabolism of MSG is greatly enhanced by the presence of metabolizable carbohydrates, which characterizes most dietary encounters with MSG. Extrapolation of food-free challenges to "in-use" situations may not be valid [30].

In one of the first challenge studies with MSG, Schaumburg *et al.* found an oral dose–response curve to MSG and concluded that all of the subjects they tested would eventually experience the sensory phenomena if they ingested enough MSG [31]. Double-blind studies by Kenney [32] and Kenney and Tidball [33] identified individuals who experienced symptoms specific to MSG on a relatively regular basis but only when the MSG was given in amounts or concentrations far greater than that normally encountered in a regular diet. Double-blind studies from Italy and the United Kingdom found no difference between the sensation experienced after MSG or placebo [34,35].

Geha *et al.* [36,37] undertook an ambitious multi-center double-blind placebo-controlled (DBPC) challenge study with a crossover design to evaluate reactions allegedly due to MSG in 130 self-identified MSG-sensitive subjects. Their efforts included meeting the criteria set forth by the August 1995 Federation of American Societies for Experimental Biology (FASEB) report on MSG which recommended that in order to confirm the MSG symptom complex, three DBPC challenges administered on separate occasions must reproduce the symptoms with ingestion of MSG and produce no response with placebo [38]. In three of their four protocols (A–D), MSG was administered without food. A positive response was defined as the presence of at least two of ten symptoms reported to occur after ingestion of MSG-containing foods. They had 110 subjects who underwent four consecutive 5-g MSG placebo-controlled challenges. Only 2 of the 110 subjects or 1.8%, who had previously self-identified themselves to be MSG reactors, responded to 5 g of MSG in the four challenges. The data from their study suggests that large doses of MSG given without food may elicit more symptoms than placebo in individuals who believe that they react adversely to MSG. However, neither persistent nor serious effects from MSG ingestion were observed and the frequency of responses was very low [36,37]. The responses were not observed when MSG was given with food. Their data again confirms the rarity of the MSG symptom complex even among individuals who believe themselves to be MSG sensitive.

Determining the prevalence of MSG sensitivity in the general population has been difficult. Estimating adverse reactions to a particular food ingredient through questionnaires is potentially fraught with subjectivity and bias. This has complicated the estimation of incidence of the MSG symptom complex in the general population. Reif-Lehrer reported that 25% of a population surveyed by questionnaire felt they had experienced MSG-related symptoms [39]. This survey included several leading, close-ended questions, which likely evoked many false-positive responses. In a 1977 questionnaire survey, Kerr *et al.* showed that in the Harvard University Medical School community, no one reported experiencing the triad of symptoms in the CRS and that 3–7% of subjects could be classified as having experienced "possible CRS" [40]. In a 1979 study, Kerr *et al.* used a National Consumer Panel to select a representative group to improve the accuracy of extrapolation to the US population at large, and found the prevalence of the MSG symptom complex to be 2% [41]. As the clinical studies have shown, the incidence of MSG symptom complex appears to be quite low.

The pathophysiology of the MSG symptom complex remains elusive. It is clearly not the result of an IgE-mediated process. Many theories have been put forth to explain the condition. Ghadimi *et al.* proposed that the symptoms of the MSG symptom complex are linked to an increase in acetylcholine; this group was able to show an attenuation of symptoms in subjects pretreated with atropine [42]. Gajalakshmi *et al.* lent further support to this theory when they demonstrated MSG's ability to produce spasmogenic effects on isolated guinea pig ileum; these effects were also blocked with by atropine [43]. Glutamic acid is a precursor to acetylcholine, which may account for these findings. Folkers *et al.* suggested that vitamin B6 deficiency may play a role in the development of the MSG symptom complex [44,45]. While Kenney has suggested that the clinical symptoms result from esophageal dysfunction or reflux esophagitis [33]. More recently, Scher and Scher have proposed that nitric oxide production may be the mediator in the pathogenesis of the MSG symptom complex [46]. Nguyen-Duong in 2001 demonstrated that glutamate-induced vasorelaxation of porcine coronary arteries was potentiated by glycine and proposed that this vasodilatory action might be responsible for the flushing and palpitations associated with the complex [47]. Despite these assorted hypotheses and 30 years of research, the causative mechanism remains unknown.

Asthma

In the early 1980s, several reports suggested that MSG could provoke bronchospasm in asthmatics. In 1981, Allen and Baker reported their experience with two young women who had developed life-threatening asthma after ingestion of MSG in meals from Chinese restaurants [48]. The asthma developed 12–14 hours after ingestion of the MSG-containing meals. Allen and Baker performed single-blind, oral challenge studies on both patients and found that 2.5-g MSG capsules resulted in asthma 11–12 hours after ingestion. Subsequently in 1987, Allen *et al.* performed in-hospital, single-blind, placebo-controlled MSG challenges in 32 asthmatic subjects; 14 were suspected MSG reactors by history and 18 were unstable asthmatics with bronchospasm due to aspirin, benzoic acid, tartrazine,

or sulfites [49]. As described by Stevenson in 2000, several problems were associated with this study: theophylline was discontinued 1 day prior to placebo challenges, some patients received inhaled bronchodilator therapy within 3 hours prior to their first challenge, bronchospasm was measured by effort-dependent peak expiratory flow rates (PEFR) rather than flow-volume loops, and baseline PEFR exhibited large variations consistent with unstable asthma [50]. Although Allen *et al.* concluded that 14 patients developed asthma exacerbations 1–12 hours after ingesting MSG, these limiting factors rendered the results difficult to interpret [49]. What was interpreted by the study authors, as MSG-provoked asthma may merely have been peak flow variability indicative of underlying active asthma.

Five additional studies attempted to clarify the issue of whether MSG induces bronchospasm in asthmatics using double-blind challenges. Schwartzstein *et al.* found no exacerbation of asthma from MSG in 12 asthmatics challenged with 25-mg MSG/kg body weight [51]. This study involved mild asthmatics with no history of MSG or Chinese restaurant meal-induced symptoms. In addition, the doses of MSG were lower than those used by Allen and Baker's 1987 study. In a second study, Moneret-Vautrin published a report of delayed bronchospasm occurring in 2 of 30 asthmatics challenged with MSG [52]. Evidence of bronchoconstriction was defined by a 15% decline in peak flow rate determinations. If the same criteria for bronchospasticity found in the Allen and Baker paper (20% decline from baseline or the lowest value recorded during placebo single-blind challenge) were applied to Moneret-Vautrin's subjects, the two patients would not fit the definition of a positive response, as the decline was less than 20%.

A third study by Germano *et al.* reported that 1 of 30 asthmatics, during single-blind screening oral challenges with MSG (up to 6 g), experienced a significant reduction in FEV1 values [53]. However, when the one preliminary reactor was re-challenged with the same dose (6-g MSG), under double-blind, placebo-controlled conditions, the response to MSG challenge was negative. This study was criticized for having only 2 of their 30 asthmatics with a positive history of asthma exacerbations after a Chinese restaurant meal. The report also exists in abstract form. A 1998 double-blind, placebo-controlled study by Woods *et al.* [54] challenged 12 asthmatics who reported that MSG caused them to have asthma attacks. They incorporated elaborate controls in their study, including strict dietary avoidance of MSG, home spirometry (PEFR measurements) before and after the challenges, as well as a double-blind, placebo-controlled protocol. The patients were challenged with 1 and 5 g of MSG. The study was completely negative, with none of the subjects reacting at either dose. One minor criticism of this paper is the small number of subjects.

Although it had been previously suggested by Allen *et al.* that those asthmatics with bronchoconstriction due to food additives or aspirin were more likely to experience MSG-related bronchospasm, a study by Woessner *et al.* [55] in 1999 demonstrated this not to be the case. In this study, two groups were tested: 30 asthmatics who believed MSG ingestion exacerbated their asthma, and 70 subjects with proven aspirin exacerbated respiratory disease (AERD), a population identified by Allen and Baker as being at high risk for MSG-provoked bronchospasm [49]. Asthma maintenance medications including inhaled and systemic corticosteroids and theophylline were continued, though inhaled β-agonists were not. Patients were enrolled in an in-patient DBPC challenge if their FEV1 values were at least 70% predicted off on inhaled bronchodilators. The first day consisted of a single-blind placebo day to assess pulmonary baseline. If FEV1 values varied by 10% or less on placebo day, the patients were challenged with 2.5-g MSG after a low-MSG breakfast. Adverse symptoms and FEV1 values were recorded during the following 24 hours. Patients whose FEV1 values decreased by at least 20% next underwent two additional MSG challenges in a blinded, placebo-controlled manner. On initial MSG challenge, only 1 of the 30 patients experienced a decline in FEV1 of 20% although she remained asymptomatic. She did not have any drop in her FEV1 on the two subsequent DBPC MSG challenges. None of the 70 AERD patients had a positive MSG challenge.

There does not appear to be any strong evidence that MSG can provoke bronchospasm in asthmatics. Because of the limited number of studies performed to date, further research is needed before any firm claims can be made that MSG provokes bronchospasm.

Urticaria and angioedema

Very few case reports of MSG-induced angioedema or urticaria have appeared in the literature. A report by Squire [56] in the Lancet described a 50-year-old man with recurrent angioedema of the face and extremities that was temporally related to the ingestion of a soup mix high in MSG. A single-blind, placebo-controlled challenge with the soup base resulted in angioedema 24 hours after the ingestion. In a graded challenge using only MSG, angioedema was provoked 16 hours after challenge. Avoidance of MSG-containing foods reportedly caused remission of the angioedema episodes.

Though not extensively evaluated, there have been several studies evaluating the role of MSG in urticaria. Genton *et al.* [57] in 1985 studied 19 subjects with chronic idiopathic urticaria (CIU) for sensitivity to 28 food additives, including MSG. In a single-blind protocol, 4 of the 19 subjects reacted, defined by an increase in urticaria within 18 hours following challenge. In 1986, Supramaniam and Warner [58] evaluated 36 children with asthma or urticaria. There were three reactors in this placebo-controlled study in which one placebo, eight additives, and aspirin were administered at 4-hour increments. Whether the reactions were pulmonary

or dermatologic was not specified. A 1998 study in Spain by Botey *et al.* [59] detailed the work-up of five children with angioedema or urticaria who presented for evaluation of possible drug allergy. Particular attention was paid to the dietary history regarding additives including MSG. Following a 2-day diet without known additives, these patients were administered 50-mg MSG orally in a single-blinded fashion: if there was no reaction in 1 hour, an additional 100 mg was given. Three of the five children had recurrence of urticaria at 1, 2, and 12 hours following ingestion; one developed pruritic erythema of the skin at 1 hour; and the fifth developed abdominal pain and diarrhea following ingestion of 50-mg MSG.

Reports in the literature of possible MSG-induced urticaria or angioedema do not clarify whether MSG was the inciting agent. Evaluation of MSG-induced urticaria or angioedema must be approached in a double-blind, placebo-controlled protocol to obtain a clearer picture of the role of MSG in urticaria and angioedema. Simon [60] addressed these concerns in a 2000 report of food additive challenges in 65 patients with chronic urticaria. The subjects initially underwent single-blinded 2.5-g MSG challenges. A baseline urticaria skin score (reminiscent of a burn score) was obtained. This scoring system is based on the "rule of nines" in which the body is divided into areas of 9%. Each of these body areas is then scored on a scale from 0 to 4 (0 = no urticaria; 1 = urticaria involving up to 25% of that surface area; 2 = up to 50% of that area; 3 = urticaria involving up to 75%; and 4 = diffuse urticaria in that area). A score of 9 or a 30% increase in the score from baseline urticaria was considered a positive challenge. Two subjects had positive single-blind challenges. Neither had a positive DBPC MSG challenge. Therefore, as is the case for MSG provoking the MSG symptom complex and bronchspasm, the role in development of urticaria and angioedema is likely to be quite rare.

Headache

Though many people believe they have adverse reactions to foods and food additives, few people have confirmed sensitivity on objective examination. It is not surprising, therefore, that MSG has been associated with a myriad of physical and psychiatric complaints. Of all the adverse symptoms thought to be attributable to MSG ingestion, headache was the symptom most often reported to the FDA's Adverse Reaction Monitoring System between 1980 and 1995 [61]. In 1969, Schaumburg *et al.* [31] performed one of the first formal studies of the symptoms potentially associated with MSG ingestion. Their study suggested that the three main symptoms consisted of a burning sensation, facial pressure or tightness, and chest pain. Headache occurred in a minority of the subjects. Ratner *et al.* [62] in 1984 described four patients with MSG-related headaches. They were evaluated with double-blind testing consisting of sublingually administered soy sauce with and without 1.5–2.0 g added MSG. These patients developed recurrent headaches within 15 minutes to 2 hours of sublingual administration of MSG soy sauce but not to "placebo" soy sauce, and reportedly had relief with of symptoms with MSG avoidance. No attempt was made to disguise the taste of the two soy sauce formulations. Furthermore, it could be argued that they truly did not have a negative control due to the high glutamate content naturally occurring in soy sauce. Scopp in 1991 described two chronic headache patients who decreased the frequency of their headaches through MSG avoidance. No objective testing was performed [63]. Yang *et al.* [64] undertook placebo-controlled 5-g MSG challenge in self-identified MSG-sensitive subjects. A positive response was two or more index symptoms. The rates of reaction to MSG or placebo were not statistically different in this group of 61 self-identified MSG-sensitive subjects. If the subjects had a positive challenge they were brought back for blinded placebo-controlled graded MSG challenges. Again, there was a high rate of response to placebo but they did have some patients who developed statistically significant associations of symptoms with MSG such as headache, flushing, muscle tightness, numbness/tingling, and generalized weakness.

Theories regarding the etiology of MSG-induced headache are scarce. Merritt *et al.* in 1990 found that high concentrations of glutamate caused concentration-dependent contractions of excised rabbit aorta [65]. These authors suggested that a similar vascular response might account for MSG-induced headache. However, there is little data that suggests that MSG can cross the intact blood–brain barrier. Despite a widespread belief that MSG can trigger migraine headaches, there is a striking paucity of literature to support this claim. As a result, low-MSG diets should not be empirically recommended for the chronic headache patients since they are not based on clear scientific fact and are only likely to be an unnecessary burden for these patients.

Monosodium glutamate and the Food and Drug Administration

Because of continuing reports of adverse reactions to MSG, the FDA contracted with FASEB in 1992 to perform a scientific safety review of the effects of glutamates in foods. The FASEB report was submitted in 1995. The MSG symptoms complex was defined as an acute, temporary, and self-limiting complex including the following: (1) a burning sensation at the back of neck, forearms, and chest; (2) facial pressure or tightness; (3) chest pain; (4) headache; (5) nausea; (6) upper body tingling and weakness; (7) palpitation; (8) numbness at the back of the neck, arms, and back; (9) bronchospasm (in asthmatics only); and (10) drowsiness. The report concluded that, although there was no scientifically verifiable evidence of adverse effects in most individuals exposed to high levels

of MSG, there is sufficient documentation to indicate that there is a subgroup of presumably healthy individuals that responds, generally within 1 hour of exposure with manifestations of the MSG symptom complex when exposed to an oral dose of MSG of 3 g in the absence of food [66]. This report pointed out that the key data relate to single-dose challenges in capsules or solutions and are limited in their ability to predict adverse reactions resulting from the use of MSG in food. It is well known that carbohydrates greatly modulate the uptake of MSG making extrapolation to real-world experience very difficult. The Hattan memorandum also indicates that the FDA did not consider the evidence regarding the sensitivity of asthmatics to MSG to be compelling and questioned its inclusion in the MSG symptom complex [66].

The FASEB report concludes that there is no evidence to support a role for dietary MSG or other forms of free glutamate in causing or exacerbating serious, long-term medical problems resulting from degenerative nerve cell damage [67]. It was accepted that neurotoxicologic effects of MSG are limited to animals given very large doses by parenteral, pharmacologic, or other non-dietary conditions.

Conclusion

Overall, the available data on MSG reflect that it is safe for use as a food additive in the population at large. MSG toxicologic data has not demonstrated serious nervous system effects in humans. Furthermore, metabolic studies performed in infants and adults have shown ready and rapid utilization of excess glutamate with failure of serum glutamate levels to rise even when very large amounts of MSG were ingested with carbohydrate. The carefully done DBPC studies indicate that MSG ingestion is likely to be without adverse effect even in people suspecting themselves to be MSG reactors [36,37,55]. MSG has not been clearly documented to cause bronchospasm, urticaria or angioedema, or migraine headache. It is possible that large doses in excess of 3 g of MSG ingested on an empty stomach without concommitant food administration may elicit the MSG symptom complex. This syndrome is likely to be infrequent and transient, resolving without treatment. In conclusion, there is no clear evidence in the current scientific literature documenting MSG as cause of any serious acute or chronic medical problem in the general population.

References

1 Kwok R. Chinese restaurant syndrome. *N Engl J Med* 1968;178:796.

2 Yamaguchi S. *Fundamental Properties of Umami in Human Taste Sensation.* New York: Marcel Dekker, 1987.

3 Ikeda K. On the taste of the salt of glutamic acid (new seasonings). *J Tokyo Chem Soc* 1909:820–36.

4 Schultz W. Food labeling; declaration of free glutamate in food. *Federal Register*, 21 CFR Past 101 [Docket No 96N–0244]. 1996;61:48102–10.

5 Filer Jr LJ, Stegink LD. A report of the proceedings of an MSG workshop held August 1991. *Crit Rev Food Sci Nutr* 1994;34:159–74.

6 Meisler A. Biochemistry of glutamate, glutamine and glutathione. In: Filer LJ, Garattini S, Kare MR, Reynolds WA, Wurtman RJ (eds.) *Glutamic Acid: Advances in Biochemistry and Physiology*. New York: Raven Press, 1979;69–84.

7 Stegink LD, Bell E, Daabees TT, *et al.* Factors influencing utilization of glycine, glutamate and aspartate in clinical products. In: Blackburn GL, Grant JP, Young VR (eds.) *Amino Acids: Metabolism and Medical Applications*. MA: John Wrist, 1983:123–41.

8 Filer LJ, Stegink LD (eds.). A report of the proceedings of a MSG workshop held August 1991. *Clin Rev Food Sci Nutr* 1991;34:159–74.

9 Stegink LD, Baker, GL. Monosodium glutamate: effect of plasma and breast milk levels in lactating women. *Proc Soc Exp Biol Med* 1972;140:836–41.

10 Stegink LD, Pitkin, RM, Reynolds, WA, *et al.* Placental transfer of glutamate and its metabolites in the primate. *Am J Obstet Gynecol* 1975;122:70–8.

11 Tung TC, Tung TS. Serum free amino acid levels after oral glutamate intake in infant and adult humans. *Nutr Rep Int* 1980;22:431–43.

12 Agostoni C, Carratu B, Boniglia C, *et al.* Free amino acid content in standard infant formulas: comparison with human milk. *J Am Coll Nutr* 2000;19:434–8.

13 Agostoni C, Jochum F, Meinardus P, *et al.* Total glutamine content in preterm and term human breast milk. *Acta Paediatr* 2006;95:985–90.

14 Olney JW. Brain lesions, obesity, and other disturbances in mice treated with monosodium glutamate. *Science* 1969; 164:719–21.

15 Olney JW, Sharpe, LG. Brain lesions in an infant rhesus monkey treated with monosodium glutamate. *Science* 1969;166:386–8.

16 Olney JW, Sharpe, LG, Fergin, LD. Glutamate-induced brain damage in infant primates. *J Neuropathol Exp Neurol* 1972;31:464–88.

17 Walker R, Lupien JR. The safety evaluation of monosodium glutamate. *J Nutr* 2000;130:1049S–52S.

18 Wakabayashi I, Hatano, H, Minami, S, *et al.* Effects of neonatal monosodium glutamate on plasma growth hormone (GH) response to GH-releasing factor in adult male and female rats. *Brain Res* 1986;372:361–6.

19 Olney JW, Cicero TJ, Meyer ER, *et al.* Acute glutamate-induced elevations in serum testosterone and leutenizing hormone. *Brain Res* 1976;112:420–4.

20 Morikyi HIM. Acute toxicity of monosodium L-glutamate in mice and rats. *Pharmacometrics* 1979;5:433–6.

21 Ebert AG. Adverse effects of monosodium glutamate. *J Asthma* 1983;20:159–64.

22 Shibata MA, Tanaka H, Kawabe M, *et al.* Lack of carcinogenicity of monosodium L-glutamate in Fischer 344 rats. *Food Chem Toxicol* 1995;33:383–91.

23 Ebert AG. The dietary administration of monosodium glutamate or glutamic acid to c-57 black mice for two years. *Toxicol Lett* 1979b;3:65–70.

24 Ebert AG. The dietary administration of L-monosodium glutamate, DL-monosodium glutamate and L-gluatmic acid to rats. *Toxicol Lett* 1979a;3:71–8.

25 Ishidate Jr MST, Yoshikawa K, Hayashi M, *et al.* Primary mutagenicity screening of food additives currently used in Japan. *Food Chem Toxicol* 1984;22:623–36.

26 Owen G, Cherry CP, Prentice DE, Worden, AN. The feeding of diets containing up to 10% MSG to beagle dogs for two years. *Toxicol Lett* 1978;1:217–19.

27 WHO. L-Glutamic acid and its ammonium, calcium, and monosodium and potassium salts. *Toxicological Evaluation of Certain Food Additives 31st Meeting of the Joint FAO/WHO Expert Committee on Food Additives*. New York: Cambridge University Press, 1988:97–161.

28 Settipane GA. The restaurant syndromes. *N Engl Reg Allergy Proc* 1987;8:39–46.

29 Schaumburg HH, Byck R. Sin cib-syn: accent on glutamate. *N Engl J Med* 1968;279:105.

30 Tarasoff L, Kelly MF. Monosodium L-glutamate: a double-blind study and review. *Food Chem Toxicol* 1993;31:1019–35.

31 Schaumburg HH, Byck R, Gerstl R, *et al.* Monosodium L-glutamate: its pharmacology and role in the Chinese restaurant syndrome. *Science* 1969;163:826–8.

32 Kenney RA. Placebo controlled studies of human reaction to oral monosodium L-glutamate. In: Filer LJ, Garattini S, Kare MR, Reynolds WA, Wurtman RJ (eds.) *Glutamic Acid: Advances in Biochemistry and Physiology*. New York: Raven Press, 1979:363–73.

33 Kenney RA, Tidball CS. Human susceptibility to oral monosodium L-glutamate. *Am J Clin Nutr* 1972;25:140–6.

34 Morselli PL, Garattini, S. Monosodium glutamate and the Chinese restaurant syndrome. *Science* 1979;227:611–12.

35 Zanda G, Franciosi P, Tognoni G, *et al.* A double blind study on the effects of monosodium glutamate in man. *Biomedicine* 1973;10;19:202–4.

36 Geha RS, Beiser A, Ren C, *et al.* Multicenter, double-blind, placebo-controlled, multiple-challenge evaluation of reported reactions to monosodium glutamate. *J Allergy Clin Immunol* 2000;106:973–80.

37 Geha RS, Beiser A, Ren C, *et al.* Review of alleged reaction to monosodium glutamate and outcome of a multicenter double-blind placebo-controlled study. *J Nutr* 2000;130:1058S–62S.

38 Raiten DJ, Talbo, JM, Fisher KD. *Analysis of Adverse Reactions to Monosodium Glutamate (MSG)*. American Institute of Nutrition, Bethesda MD 1995.

39 Reif-Lehrer L. A questionnaire study of the prevalence Chinese restaurant syndrome. *Fed Am Soc Exp Biol* 1977;36:1617–23.

40 Kerr GR, Wu-Lee M, El-Lozy M, *et al.* Objectivity of food-symptomatology surveys. Questionnaire on the "Chinese restaurant syndrome". *J Am Diet Assoc* 1977;71:263–8.

41 Kerr GR, Wu-Lee M, El-Lozy M, *et al.* Food symptomatology questionnaires: risks of demand-bias questions and population-based surveys. In: Filer LJ, Garattini S, Kare MR, Reynolds WA,

challenges with tartrazine. Whether or not asthma medications were withheld during the challenges was not stated.

Stenius and Lemola conducted oral challenge studies using small doses of tartrazine (0.1–10 mg). Following ingestion of tartrazine, 25/114 (22%) unselected asthmatics dropped their peak flow measurements by 20% from baseline values. In the same study, a separate population of 25 aspirin-sensitive asthmatics underwent tartrazine challenges and 12 (50%) reacted with a >20% decline in peak flow values.

It is generally agreed that peak flow measurements are less reproducible than timed flow/volume measurements [21,22]. Most investigators use flow/volume spirometry and obtain FEV1 values during repetitive measurements of lung function. This subject was reviewed in detail by Stevenson [23]. During placebo challenges, in patients with irritable airways, FEV1 values have been documented to decline by as much as 43%. Therefore, it is incumbent upon the investigator to treat the underlying asthma, demonstrate that the FEV1 values do not vary by more than 10% during placebo challenges even before beginning single- or double-blind challenge studies. Most investigators use a 20% or more decline in FEV1 as evidence of bronchospasm during challenge studies, assuming that the baseline challenge with placebo was stable [23]. Despite everything stated above, in a 1977 report by Freedman, a 14% decline in FEV1 was used as an endpoint for "an asthmatic reaction to tartrazine" and was provided as proof that a tartrazine-induced bronchospastic reaction had occurred [24].

Spector and co-workers conducted one of the largest studies investigating the prevalence of tartrazine-associated bronchospasm [25]. In their studies, bronchodilators were withheld for 6–12 hours before beginning double-blind oral challenges with one challenge substance (or placebo) each day during inpatient hospitalizations. A 20% decline in FEV1 values, when compared to the placebo day, was considered to be evidence of a bronchospastic reaction. Tartrazine provoking doses ranged from 1 to 50 mg. The results of their study are summarized as follows. There were 277 asthmatic patients in their study. All were challenged with aspirin and 44/277 (16%) experienced respiratory reactions. Of the remaining 233 aspirin-tolerant patients, none experienced a 20% decline in FEV1 values on the days they ingested tartrazine. By contrast, when the 44 aspirin-sensitive asthmatics were challenged with tartrazine, 11 (25%) experienced a 20% decline in FEV1 values. Unfortunately, of the 11 tartrazine reactors, "5 did not undergo placebo challenges" (i.e. did not have a placebo challenge baseline day with proven airway stability before challenges with tartrazine). Thus the authors, stopped anti-asthmatic medications in a group of aspirin-sensitive asthmatics, whose asthma was severe enough to be admitted to National Jewish Hospital, failed to consistently perform baseline placebo challenges and then noted a 20% decline in FEV1 values during challenges with tartrazine. Were these changes in lung function due to

discontinuing anti-asthmatic medications, inherent hyper-irritability of the airways or did these patients have tartrazine- and aspirin-induced asthma?

The most revealing study in this area of controversy was performed by Weber and associates [26]. Using standard single-blind oral aspirin challenges, they identified 13 of 44 asthmatic patients as having aspirin-sensitive asthma. After challenges with tartrazine, in doses ranging from 2.5 to 25 mg and withholding morning bronchodilators, 7/44 (16%) of the patients experienced a 20% decline in FEV1 values. Tartrazine challenges were repeated in the same 7 patients 1 week later and this time they received their morning bronchodilator medications. During these follow-up challenges, using the same "provoking dose" of tartrazine, FEV1 values remained steady throughout the testing period and therefore none could be categorized as having tartrazine-induced asthma. These patients were also challenged with six other azo dyes and did not experience any reactions. If one took the position that morning bronchodilator treatment prevented the tartrazine reactions, one is faced with the task of explaining why 13/44 (30%) of these patients experienced a 20% or more decline in their FEV1 values during oral challenges with aspirin while taking the same bronchodilators. In a study by Vedanthan and associates, 49 aspirin-tolerant children and 5 aspirin-sensitive asthmatic children underwent oral challenges with tartrazine [27]. Standard asthma medications, including cromolyn, theophylline, and corticosteroids, were continued during the challenges. None of the subjects reacted to tartrazine. The 5 aspirin-sensitive asthmatics, during aspirin challenges, experienced a >20% decline in FEV1 values. Therefore, the endpoint of a 20% decline in FEV1 values, as evidence of induced bronchospasm, was sensitive enough to detect changes in bronchial airways during aspirin challenges. If tartrazine was comparable to aspirin and could actually provoke bronchospasm, might we have expected this to occur in some of the 5 aspirin-sensitive asthmatic children?

In a study of adult asthmatics by Tarlo and Broder bronchodilators were continued. One of 26 aspirin-tolerant asthmatics experienced a "wheezing reaction" and a >20% decline in FEV1 values during a double-blind challenge with tartrazine [28]. The first point of this chapter is the disassociation between aspirin sensitivity and tartrazine-induced asthma. Secondly, the authors stated that elimination of tartrazine from the diet in this patient did not have any effect on the course of her asthma. This chapter is instructive, since the original premise of detecting tartrazine-induced asthma was to then advise the patient to avoid tartrazine and improve their asthma. Although, one patient provides only an anecdotal report, proponents of the theory that "dietary tartrazine causes asthma" did not gain support from this patient's clinical course [17,20,25].

In the largest series of aspirin-sensitive asthmatics undergoing single-blind, tartrazine challenges, Stevenson and associates were unable to detect tartrazine-induced asthma in any of 150 aspirin-sensitive asthmatics [13]. The protocol for this study was as follows. All patients were admitted to an inpatient General Clinical Research Center. Regular asthma controller medications were continued (inhaled corticosteroids, theophylline, long-acting bronchodilators, and in a minority of patients systemic corticosteroids). All patients underwent single-blind, placebo-controlled oral challenges. If the baseline placebo challenges were stable (<10% change in FEV1 values over 3 hours), tartrazine 25 mg in a green capsule was given. If FEV1 did not decline by 20% from baseline at 3 hours, 50 mg of tartrazine was given and FEV1 values were obtained every hour for an additional 3 hours. If FEV1 values dropped by 20% during one of the tartrazine challenges, patients were re-scheduled for a repeat double-blind tartrazine challenge at a later date. However, if the single-blind tartrazine challenge was negative (<15% change in FEV1), the patient was classified as not having tartrazine-induced asthma. After tartrazine challenges were completed, all 150 patients underwent single-blind oral aspirin challenges on the next day while taking the same four controller medications. Asthmatic reactions (>20% decline in FEV1) occurred in all 150 patients. Only those patients with a positive oral aspirin challenge were classified as having aspirin-sensitive asthma and were included in this study.

Of the 150 patients, 6 experienced a 20% or more drop in FEV1 values, compared to placebo challenges during the single-blind screening challenges with tartrazine (either coinciding with the 25- or 50-mg tartrazine doses). These six patients were re-challenged with the same provoking dose of tartrazine in a double-blind, placebo-controlled oral challenge protocol at a later date. None reacted to tartrazine during these double-blind challenges. At the time of re-challenge, none of the patients were participating in aspirin-desensitization treatment and all were taking the same or less asthma controller medications as they were during the first tartrazine challenges. These studies were extended when another 44 aspirin-sensitive asthmatic patients underwent oral single-blind tartrazine challenges at the same institution [29]. Again, none of the patients reacted to 25 and 50 mg of tartrazine.

A 1986 study from Poland identified tartrazine sensitivity during oral challenges in 16/51 (31.4%) of aspirin-sensitive asthmatic patients [30]. The authors reported that 5 of the 18 aspirin-sensitive asthmatics also experienced reactions (dyspnea) to tartrazine and when these same 5 were desensitized to aspirin they could then take tartrazine without adverse effects. Obviously, there was something radically different about the results of this study and the study by Stevenson *et al.* [13]. If the study from Poland was accurate, with a tartrazine cross-challenge rate of 31.4% [30], Stevenson *et al.* [13,29] should have identified 61/194 (31.4%) tartrazine-sensitive patients in order to equal the percentage identified by this Polish study.

In a large multi-institutional study in Europe, including patients from Poland, 156 known aspirin-sensitive asthmatic patients underwent screening single-blind oral challenges with tartrazine [31]. Of the 156 participants, 4 (2.6%) reacted to 25 mg of tartrazine with a 25% decline in FEV1 values during single-blind challenges. At another time, these four patients were re-challenged with the same dose of tartrazine. Again, the four patients experienced a 25% decline in FEV1 values during double-blind tartrazine challenges. A full day of placebo challenges may have been performed for each patient before starting tartrazine single-blind challenges but was not reported in their paper. However, comparative placebo challenges were conducted as part of the double-blind, placebo-controlled follow-up challenges. The authors of this study are well-known investigators with extensive experience in conducting oral challenges. The extremely low prevalence of positive single- and double-blind challenge studies with tartrazine (2.6%) in the 1988 European study contrasts sharply with the 31.4% prevalence in the 1986 study from Poland. Assuming that Polish patients were equally represented in the 1988 study, within 2 years, the prevalence of tartrazine sensitivity appeared to drop by 29%. Such a decline seems unlikely.

On the basis of scientific facts, what conclusions can be drawn from the literature on this subject? First, many of the early studies reporting large numbers of asthmatics with tartrazine reactions were actually measuring spontaneous asthma in patients whose anti-asthmatic medications were inadequate or had been discontinued before the challenges. Most of the high prevalence rates of positive respiratory reactions to tartrazine are simply not credible. Even the very large study by Spector *et al.* [25] where 11/44 (25%) aspirin-sensitive asthmatics were said to have tartrazine-induced asthma had serious methodological flaws in the performance of the challenges.

Second, there are probably a few patients with reactions to tartrazine, which include urticaria [13] and or bronchospasm [28,31]. Whether or not these reactions are IgE mediated is unknown. However, such a mechanistic explanation is more attractive than the idea that tartrazine participates in COX-1 inhibiting cross-reactions. In fact, it has been shown that tartrazine does not inhibit cyclooxygenase *in vitro* [32]. Since inhibition of COX-1 is the mechanism by which NSAIDs and aspirin cross-react, the Gerber data [32] eliminate any possibility that tartrazine and aspirin are cross-reactors. COX-1 inhibiting NSAIDs, on a dose-dependent basis, cross-react in aspirin-sensitive asthmatics 100% of the time and the weak inhibitors of COX-1, acetaminophen and salsalate, cross-react 34% and 20% when given in usually therapeutic doses, respectively [33–37]. Since all the NSAIDs that cross-react with aspirin inhibit COX-1 and tartrazine does not inhibit COX-1, there is no rational reason to suspect cross-reactivity between aspirin and tartrazine.

Except for the Samter study in 1968 [20], Spector study in 1979 [25], and the 1986 Polish study [30], the link

[17]. BHT, however, increased the incidence of liver tumors in male C3H mice [18]. The same study showed increased colon cancer in BALB/c mice following one chemical carcinogen, dimethylhydrazine, but not another, methylnitrosourea. BHA, on the other hand, appeared to protect against the acute liver toxicity of a colon-specific carcinogen, methylazoxymethanol acetate [19]. However, high-dose BHA was shown several years ago to produce cancers of the forestomach in rats [5]. Since man does not have a forestomach, and doses about 10,000 times higher than likely human consumption were used, it was felt by the FAO/WHO Joint Expert Committee on review of the data that the benefits of BHA outweighed the potential risks [5]. The Netherlands Cohort Study found no significant association with stomach cancer risk with usual intake levels of BHA and BHT [8].

BHT may have anti-atherogenic effects. Using a cholesterol-fed rabbit model, Xiu and colleagues showed BHT prevented decreased blood flow and vessel diameter in the microcirculation [20]. The same group more recently demonstrated that this effect is mediated through induction of increased triglyceride levels [21].

Using human lymphocytes, Klein and Bruser demonstrated BHT cytotoxicity with concentrations >100 μg/ml [22]. At 50 μg/ml, BHT inhibited the mixed lymphocyte reaction, but not phytohemagglutinin (PHA) stimulation. A synergistic effect of PHA suppression was seen with co-incubation with either cortisol or prednisolone.

In mice studies, BHA inhibited several microsomal enzymes, but long-term administration also induced specific P450 cytochrome enzymes [23]. In humans, BHA 0.5 mg/kg for 10 days had no appreciable effects on biotransformation capacity [24]. Antipyrine and paracetamol (acetaminophen) metabolism were unaffected. Urinary excretion of BHA metabolites was significantly increased on days 3 and 7 compared to day 1, suggesting either an inhibition of BHA metabolizing enzymes or bioaccumulation of BHA and/or its metabolites in the body.

Asthma/rhinitis

Despite a wealth of animal toxicology literature on these antioxidants, there are only scattered reports of adverse reactions to BHA and BHT in humans. In 1973, Fisherman and Cohen reported on seven patients with asthma, vasomotor rhinitis with or without nasal polyps, or the combination, who were suspected of intolerance to BHA and BHT [25]. There were no clinical details given as to why BHA and BHT were suspected. These patients were identified following open challenge with capsule ingestion of 125–250 mg of BHA/BHT and reproduction of symptoms of worsening vasomotor rhinitis, headache, flushing, asthma, conjunctival suffusion, dull retrosternal pain radiating to the back, diaphoresis, or somnolence. No objective measures were noted. BHA/BHT intolerance was additionally documented by a doubling of a Duke earlobe bleeding time (termed the sequential vascular response by the authors) in all cases. No rationale for the reported effect on the bleeding time was given, other than a supposed similarity to aspirin intolerance. In a follow-up paper the same year, dealing with aspirin cross-reactivity, these authors had apparently found 21 patients with intolerance to BHA/BHT via the bleeding time, of which 17 had clinical symptoms on challenge, with no clinical details given [26].

The following year, in an unsuccessful attempt to duplicate Fisherman and Cohen's initial findings, Cloninger and Novey performed a similar study using oral ingestion of 300–850 mg BHA in five asthmatics and two rhinitics [27]. They reported that the baseline earlobe bleeding time was not reproducible. None of the patients had clinical exacerbations, changes in peak flows, or more than a 50% change in the bleeding times; there was a non-dose-related effect of drowsiness noted in four of seven patients. These authors questioned the validity of clinical BHA intolerance as well as the validity and reproducibility of the sequential vascular response. Goodman and colleagues, as discussed further below, in a case of well-documented BHA/BHT-induced chronic urticaria, could not demonstrate a positive effect of either BHA 250 mg or placebo on the earlobe bleeding time in either the patient or two controls [28].

Weber and colleagues, in a study where single-blind challenges were validated by subsequent double-blind challenges, found no asthmatic responses of >25% drop in forced expiratory volume in 1 second (FEV1) in 43 moderately severe perennial asthmatics undergoing single-blind capsule challenges with sequential doses of 125 and 250 mg of BHA and BHT [29]. Aspirin sensitivity was documented in 44% of the patients, and reactivity to p-hydroxybenzoic acid, sodium benzoate, non-azo or azo dyes in 2–5%. The author is aware of one unpublished case of a drop of pulmonary function following double-blind challenge with BHT 250 mg in a patient with food anaphylaxis and oral allergy syndrome, but this was not validated with additional blinded challenges. Therefore, at the present time, there are no published reports of BHA or BHT challenges resulting in well-documented, reproducible asthmatic responses.

Urticaria

In 1975, Thune and Granholt reported 100 patients with recurrent urticaria evaluated with provocative food additive challenges [30]. Sixty-two patients had positive challenges, with two-thirds reacting to multiple substances. Positivity rates for individual dyes, preservatives, or anti-inflammatory drugs ranged from 10% to 30%. Most reactions occurred within 1–2 hours, with a number occurring between 12 and >20 hours. Six of 47 (12.7%) tested to BHA reacted, and 6 of 43 (13.9%) reacted to BHT; it is unclear whether these were the same six patients. Test doses were given in two to three increments, with the total dose of BHA and BHT being 17 mg. The provocative challenges were not blinded, nor did the authors state criteria for a positive challenge.

In 1977, Fisherman and Cohen reported the results of provocative oral or intradermal challenges of a large number of suspected agents on the bleeding time (sequential vascular response) in the assessment of 215 patients with chronic urticaria [31]. Medications were withdrawn 12 hours prior to challenge, with the exception of hydroxyzine, which was held for 72 hours. Intolerance was found in 19 patients with challenges of 250–500 mg of BHA and BHT. Slight details of four reactors challenged with 250 mg each of BHA and BHT were included in a table: in addition to doubling of the earlobe bleeding time, two developed nasal congestion, and three had urticaria, although it is not clear whether this was increased over baseline. These authors felt they made a determination of "single or partial etiologies" in 203 of the 215 patients (94.4%), an astounding success rate in a clinical entity known for its resistance to defined etiology. Obviously, the same criticism of the lack of conceivable mechanism and the non-reproducibility of the test in other hands holds for these authors' urticaria evaluations as well as the asthma challenges.

Juhlin mentioned in a review on urticaria in 1977 the results of provocative challenges with a mix of BHA and BHT in 130 urticaria patients [32]. Incremental doses of 1, 10, and 50 mg each of BHA and BHT resulted in nine positive and five probably positive challenges (6.9–10.8%). Details as to the nature of the patients' symptoms, criteria for positive response, or the blinding of the challenges were not given. Four years later, Juhlin published the results of an evaluation of 330 patients with recurrent urticaria [33]. He used a 15-day single-blind challenge battery of dyes, preservatives, and placebo. Antihistamines were withheld from 4 to 5 days before the commencement of the challenge sequence. Testing was accomplished when patients had "no or slight symptoms." Tests were judged positive if "clear signs of urticaria or angioedema" occurred within 24 hours. Slightly less than half of the 330 patients (156) received a BHA/BHT challenge with cumulative doses of 1, 10, 50, and 50 mg given (total dose 111 mg). Fifteen percent had positive reactions, and 12% had equivocal reactions. Lactose placebo was given in two doses on days 1, 3, 9, and 12, although modifications in the order did occur. Active substances were given in single to six divided doses at hourly intervals. Most patients did not undergo the entire challenge schedule; one third did not receive a placebo challenge.

In 1986, Hannuksela and Lahti published their results of an extensive double-blind challenge study [34]. They evaluated 44 patients with chronic urticaria of >2 months duration, 91 atopic dermatitis patients, and 123 patients with resolved contact dermatitis. They used wheat starch as their placebo rather than lactose since Juhlin had reported positive responses to lactose placebo. Patients were challenged to

sodium metabisulfite 9 mg, benzoic acid 200 mg, BHA and BHT mixture of 50 mg each, and β-carotene and β-apo-carotenal mixture 200 mg each. Positive reactions were repeated 4 days later to validate the response: challenges were rated as positive if the patient responded both times, and as equivocal if the repeat was negative. Of the 44 urticaria patients none had reproducible positive reactions to BHA/BHT, two responded to the first challenge but not the second. The same response occurred with the atopic dermatitis patients; two had equivocal reactions to BHA/BHT. None of the contact dermatitis patients reacted to the antioxidants. One urticaria patient had reproducible responses to the wheat placebo, and another to benzoic acid, and one had an equivocal response to metabisulfite. One atopic dermatitis patient had positive reactions to carotenal/carotene, and another had an equivocal reaction to metabisulfite. One contact dermatitis patient had an equivocal reaction to the wheat placebo (second challenge not done). The authors contrasted their results to those of Juhlin, and cited challenge differences to explain their lack of responses. They also wondered whether a prolonged refractory period following the initial positive challenges could account for the negative follow-up trials, since they had waited only 4 days. In general, however, the authors felt that ordinary amounts of food additives do not provoke urticaria or influence atopic dermatitis [34].

In 1990, Goodman and colleagues reported the first double-blind, placebo-controlled multiple challenge protocol documenting the link of BHA and BHT with chronic urticaria [28]. The demonstration of symptom aggravation did not rest on single challenges: two patients with chronic urticaria and angioedema of 3–4 years duration underwent oral challenges with several agents performed 2–3 times for verification. The patients had demonstrated improvement on restricted diets, but had lost 20–30 pounds in the process. Both patients were admitted, placed on an elemental diet formula, and observed for 5–7 days to establish baseline activity. The patients ranked pruritus severity, and skin lesions were ranked from 0 to 4+ based on degree of body distribution. Only challenges inducing lesions within 12 hours of ingestion and involving an entire extremity or body area, or generalized, were considered positive. Those occurring 12–24 hours were considered equivocal. A mixture of 125 mg each of BHA and BHT was given, with 250 mg of each given 2–4 hours later if no major reaction had occurred. One patient was additionally challenged to BHA 250 mg alone. Placebo capsules were either dextrose or lactose. The patients were also challenged to sodium benzoate, p-hydroxybenzoic acid, tartrazine, and other azo dyes. Both patients reacted within 1–6 hours to BHA and BHT at all times, and did not react to the other additives or placebo on numerous trials. There were no delayed reactions.

Oatmeal one patient had been routinely ingesting for breakfast contained BHA and BHT. Both patients were placed on diets specifically avoiding BHA and BHT, resulting in

There has been some interest in linking the prevalence of hyperactivity in children to food-additive intolerance. The initial reports linked hyperactivity to artificial food flavors and colors [53]. Recently, a large study of 3-year old children from the Isle of Wight, UK attempted to address the possible link between food additives and hyperactivity in children in a population-based study [54]. The study was designed to test the hypothesis that food additives have a pharmacological effect on behavior that is irrespective of other characteristics of the child, specifically hyperactivity at baseline and atopy. Bateman *et al.* attempted to enroll all children resident on the Isle of Wight with birth dates in a specified date range who were registered with a general practitioner. Phase 1 of the trial involved screening with a behavioral questionnaire and was followed by skin prick testing for atopy (phase 2). A total of 397 children were selected to enter the challenge stage of the trial, phase 3. Based on results of the behavior questionnaire and skin prick testing, the children were divided into four groups: hyperactive/atopic, non-hyperactive/atopic, hyperactive/non-atopic, and non-hyperactive/non-atopic. After assessment, each group was subjected to a diet eliminating artificial colorings and benzoate preservatives for 1 week. In the subsequent 3 weeks the subjects underwent a double-blind crossover study where they received periods of dietary challenge with a drink containing artificial colorings and sodium benzoate or a placebo mixture. Behavior was then assessed by a tester blind to the subjects' dietary status and by parent's ratings. The study found significant reductions in hyperactive behavior during the additive-free diet phase by parental report. There were also significantly greater increases in hyperactive behavior during the additive versus placebo period based on parental reports. There was no correlation with presence or absence of hyperactivity neither at baseline nor by the presence of atopy. The authors concluded that there is a general adverse effect of artificial food coloring and benzoate preservatives on the behavior of 3-year old children. However, there are aspects of the study that make it difficult to interpret. There were a significant number of dietary mistakes reported where children consumed products that contained preservatives and/or artificial colorings. Also, research psychologists using validated tests were unable to associate the subjects' hyperactivity with consumption of the additive drink versus placebo. Further study of the relationship between childhood hyperactivity and food additives needs to be carried out before any firm conclusions can be made.

Summary and conclusions

Benzoates and parabens are used extensively as chemical preservatives in foods and beverages in the United States and throughout much of the developed world. These compounds have essentially no toxicity at approved concentrations and considering their widespread consumption, are extremely well tolerated. Benzoates and parabens have been investigated frequently in association with chronic urticaria–angioedema. Many studies with less stringent design criteria have implicated these agents, particularly the benzoates, as relatively frequent exacerbating factors. On the other hand, more rigorously designed protocols suggest that these chemicals are unusual provoking or exacerbating agents among urticaria patients.

Asthmatic reactions have also been reported and investigated in association with food additives including benzoates and parabens. Well-designed trials have not provided a conclusive link between persistent asthma and benzoates or parabens.

The association of atopic dermatitis with food additives has received relatively limited attention in the medical literature. No well-designed study has implicated benzoates or parabens individually as pathogenic factors. Studies by Worm *et al.* using multiple food additives including benzoates provide evidence that at least some of these substances may be provoking factors in a minority of patients and a potential mechanism may be increased production of leukotrienes.

Rarely, anaphylactic-type reactions have been reported with ingested benzoates but definitive evidence of systemic anaphylaxis is lacking. Oral parabens have not been reported as potential causes of anaphylaxis. However, parabens have been implicated in systemic reactions related to their use in pharmaceutical agents, particularly local anesthetic preparations. Other miscellaneous reports have appeared suggesting benzoates as occasional inciting agents in cutaneous vasculitis.

Reports of hyperactivity in children induced by food additives have been present in the literature for several decades, but further study is needed to confirm this association.

References

1 US FDA. *Everything Added to Food in the US*. Boca Raton, FL: CK Smoley, 1993:149.

2 Williams AE. Benzoic acid. In: Kirk-Othmer (ed.) *Encyclopedia of Chemical Technology*. New York: Wiley-Interscience, 1978:778–92.

3 Lueck E. *Antimicrobial Food Additives*. New York: Springer-Verlag, 1980.

4 Juhlin L. Intolerance to food additives. In: Marzulli FM, Maibach HI (eds.) *Advances in Modern Toxicology, Vol. 4. Dermatotoxicology and Pharmacology*. New York: John Wiley, 1977:455–63.

5 Elder RL. Final report on the safety assessment of methylparaben, ethylparaben propylparaben and butylparaben. *J Am Coll Toxicol* 1984;3:147–209.

6 Soni MG, Burdock GA, Taylor SL, Greenberg NA. Safety assessment of propyl paraben: a review of the published literature. *Food Chem Toxicol* 2001;39:513–32.

7 Aalto TR, Foirman MC, Rigler NE. *p*-hydroxybenzoic acid esters as preservatives. I. Uses, antibacterial and antifungal studies, properties and determination. *J Am Pharm Assoc* 1953;42:449–57.

8   Moir CJ, Eyles MJ. Inhibition, injury, and inactivation of four psychotrophic foodborne bacteria by the preservatives methyl *p*-hydroxybenzoate and potassium sorbate. *J Food Protection* 1992; 55:360–6.

9   Lumry WR, Mathison DA, Stevenson DD, Curd JC. Aspirin in chronic urticaria and/or angioedema: studies of sensitivity and desensitization. *J Allergy Clin Immunol* 1982;69:135.

10 Doeglas HMG. Reactions to aspirin and food additives in patients with chronic urticaria, including the physical urticarias. *Br J Dermatol* 1975;93:135–44.

11 Thune P, Granholt A. Provocation tests with antiphlogistic and food additives in recurrent urticaria. *Dermatologica* 1975; 151:360–7.

12 Juhlin L. Recurrent urticaria: clinical investigation of 330 patients. *Br J Dermatol* 1981;104:369–81.

13 Michaelsson G, Juhlin L. Urticaria induced by preservatives and dye additives in food and drugs. *Br J Dermatol* 1973;88:525–32.

14 Ros AM, Juhlin L, Michaelsson G. A follow-up study of patients with recurrent urticaria and hypersensitivity to aspirin, benzoates and azo dyes. *Br J Dermatol* 1976;95:19–24.

15 Supramaniam G, Warner JO. Artificial food additive intolerance in patients with angio-oedema and urticaria. *Lancet* 1986;2:907–9.

16 Genton C, Frei PC, Pecond A. Value of oral provocation tests to aspirin and food additives in the routine investigation of asthma and chronic urticaria. *J Allergy Clin Immunol* 1985;76:40–5.

17 Ortolani C, Pastorello E, Luraghi MT, *et al.* Diagnosis of intolerance to food additives. *Ann Allergy* 1984;53:587–91.

18 Hannuksela M, Lahti A. Peroral challenge tests with food additives in urticaria and atopic dermatitis. *Int J Dermatol* 1986;25:178–80.

19 Kellett JK, August PJ, Beck MH. Double-blind challenge tests with food additives in chronic urticaria. *Br J Dermatol* 1984;111:32.

20 Simon RA. Additive-induced urticaria: experience with mono-sodium glutamate. *J Nutr* 2000;130:1063S–6S.

21 Nettis E, Colanardi MC, Ferrannini A, Tursi A. Sodium benzoate-induced repeated episodes of acute urticaria/angio-oedema: randomized controlled trial. *Br J Dermatol* 2004;151:898–902.

22 Rudzki E, Czubalski K, Grzywa Z. Detection of urticaria with food additive intolerance by means of diet. *Dermatologica* 1980;1 61:57–62.

23 Gibson A, Clancy R. Management of chronic idiopathic urticaria by the identification and exclusion of dietary factors. *Clin Allergy* 1980;10:699–704.

24 Ehlers I, Niggemann B, Binder C, Zuberbier T. Role of nonallergic hypersensitivity reactions in children with chronic urticaria. *Allergy* 1998;53:1074–7.

25 Malanin G, Kalimo K. The results of skin testing with food additives and the effect of an elimination diet in chronic and recurrent urticaria and recurrent angioedema. *Clin Exp Allergy* 1989;19:539–43.

26 Weber RW, Hoffman M, Raine DA, Nelson HS. Incidence of bronchoconstriction due to aspirin, azo dyes, non-azo dyes, and preservatives in a population of perennial asthmatics. *J Allergy Clin Immunol* 1979;64:32–7.

27 Tarlo SM, Broder I. Tartrazine and benzoate challenge and dietary avoidance in chronic asthma. *Clin Allergy* 1982;12:303–12.

28 Osterhalle O, Taudoroff E, Hashr J. Intolerance to aspirin, food-colouring agents and food preservatives in childhood asthma. *Ogeskr Laeger* 1979;141:1908–10.

29 Garcia HJ, Alvarez MMN, Selles FJS, Aleman JAP. Reacciones adversas a conservatanes alimentarios. *Allergol Immunopathol (Madr)* 1986;14:55–63.

30 Juhlin L, Michaelsson G, Zetterstrom O. Urticaria and asthma induced by food and drug additives in patients with aspirin sensitivity. *J Allergy Clin Immunol* 1972;50:92–8.

31 Rosenhall L, Zetterstrom O. Asthma provoked by analgesics, cold colorants and food preservatives. *Lakartidningen* 1973;70: 1417–19.

32 Hodge L, Yan KY, Loblay RL. Assessment of food chemical intolerance in adult asthmatic subjects. *Thorax* 1996;51:805–9.

33 Kinsey RE, Wright DO. Reaction following ingestion of sodium benzoate in a patient with severe liver damage. *J Lab Clin Med* 1944;29:188–96.

34 Michels A, Vandermoten G, Duchateau J, *et al.* Anaphylaxis with sodium benzoate. *Lancet* 1991;337:1424–5.

35 Nagel JE, Fuscaldo JT, Fireman P. Paraben allergy. *JAMA* 1977; 237:1594–5.

36 Carr TW. Severe allergic reaction to an intraurethral ligno-caine preparation containing parabens preservatives. *Br J Urol* 1990;66:98.

37 Veien NK, Hattel T, Laurberg G. Oral challenge with parabens in paraben-sensitive patients. *Contact Dermatitis* 1996;34:433.

38 Munoz FJ. Perioral contact urticaria from sodium benzoate in a toothpaste. *Contact Dermatitis* 1996;35:51.

39 Van Bever HP, Docx M, Stevens WJ. Food and food additives in severe atopic dermatitis. *Allergy* 1989;44:588–94.

40 Worm M, Ehlers I, Sterry W, Zuberbier T. Clinical relevance of food additives in adult patients with atopic dermatitis. *Clin Exp Allergy* 2000;30:407–14.

41 Worm M, Vieth W, Ehlers I, *et al.* Increased leukotriene production by food additives in patients with atopic dermatitis and proven food intolerance. *Clin Exp Allergy* 2001;31:265–73.

42 Fauler J, Neumann CH, Tsikas D, *et al.* Enhanced synthesis of cysteinyl leukotrienes in atopic dermatitis. *Br J Dermatol* 1993; 128:627–30.

43 Pacor ML, Di Lorenzo G, Martinelli N, *et al.* Monosodium benzoate hypersensitivity in subjects with persistent rhinitis. *Allergy* 2004;59:192–7.

44 Vogt T. Sodium benzoate-induced acute leukocytoclastic vasculitis with unusual clinical appearance. *Arch Dermatol* 1999;135:726–7.

45 Wuthrich B. Adverse reactions to food additives. *Ann Allergy* 1993;71:379–84.

46 Lunardi C, Bambara LM, Biasi D, *et al.* Elimination diet in the treatment of selected patients with hypersensitivity vasculitis. *Clin Exp Rheumatol* 1992;10:131–5.

47 Lamey PJ, Lewis MA. Oral medicine in practice: orofacial allergic reactions. *Br Dent J* 1990;168:59–63.

48 Patton DW, Ferguson MM, Forsyth A, James J. Oro-facial granulomatosis: a possible allergic basis. *Br J Oral Maxillofac Surg* 1985;23:235–42.

49 Sweatman MC, Tasker R, Warner JO, *et al.* Oro-facial granulomatosis. Response to elemental diet and provocation by food additives. *Clin Allergy* 1986;16:331–8.

50 Pachor ML, Ubani G, Cortina P, *et al.* Is the Melkersson–Rosenthal syndrome related to the exposure to food additives? *Oral Surg Oral Med Oral Pathol* 1996;67:393–5.

51 McKenna KE, Walsh MY, Burrows D. The Melkersson–Rosenthal syndrome and food additive hypersensitivity. *Br J Dermatol* 1994; 131:921–2.

52 Morales C, Penarrocha M, Bagan JV, *et al.* Immunological study of Melkersson–Rosenthal syndrome: lack of response to food additive challenge. *Clin Exp Allergy* 1995;25:260–4.

53 Feingold BF. Hyperkinesis and learning disabilities linked to artificial food flavors and colors. *Am J Nurs* 1975;75:797–803.

54 Bateman B, Warner JO, Hutchinson E, Dean T, *et al.* The effects of a double blind, placebo controlled, artificial food colourings and benzoate preservative challenge on hyperactivity in a general population sample of preschool children. *Arch Dis Child* 2004;89:506–11.

34

CHAPTER 34

Food Colorings and Flavors

Matthew Greenhawt and James L. Baldwin

KEY CONCEPTS

- Food flavorings and colorings are often derived from potential allergens.
- The overall prevalence of reactions attributable to food colorings and flavorings is thought to be low.
- Carmine/cochineal extract, annatto and spices are the most commonly implicated agents in this group.
- Current labeling regulations for these agents make identification of potential allergens a difficult task.
- The Food and Drug Administration has proposed a change in labeling requirements for carmine/cochineal extract.

Food colorings and flavors are essential parts of the experience of eating that have existed for centuries. Though their inclusion is often an afterthought in our consumption, ultimately, the colorings and flavorings are at the core of what we enjoy about eating our favorite foods. In many processed foods, coloring and flavoring are inseparable from the food's identity in the eyes of the consumer and the corporate production of the food itself.

The use of both synthetic and biogenic sources for color and flavor is a common practice. Most of these pose no risk of adverse events. However, there is a growing body of medical literature regarding adverse reactions involving food colorings and flavors derived from both synthetic and non-synthetic sources.

This chapter will discuss non-synthetic food colorings and flavorings that have been implicated in adverse food reactions. We will review known mechanisms of reaction, treatment strategy, and legislation involved in changing the way that colors and flavors are used in foods. Synthetic color additives are discussed elsewhere in this book.

Food colorings

Background history

According to the United States Food and Drug Administration (FDA), food colorants are any dye, pigment, or substance that imparts color when applied to food. Both synthetic and biogenic sources are used for this purpose [1]. Coloring influences one's acceptance of food, but also aids food

manufacturing in several ways. Coloring is essential to correcting loss of a product's true color from exposure to light, air, temperature, moisture, or the elements involved in storage. It can be useful in correcting natural variations in color between products, to make them appear more uniform in quality to the consumer, or to enhance and augment an appearance of a natural occurring color. Coloring is also a useful marketing tactic to give otherwise colorless substances identity, or to make them appear more festive. Coloring can also be essential to protect vitamins and flavors that can be damaged from direct sunlight [2–4].

There is a lengthy relationship between food coloring and adverse reactions attributed to such coloring. One of the first recorded case reports was from 1848, involving 21 individuals at a public dinner poisoned by copper arsenite, which was used to color a dessert green [4]. By 1900, it was estimated that there were 80 synthetic color additives available for use in foods, but there were no regulations pertaining to the quality and use for these dyes. The Food and Drug Act of 1906 created the first seven dyes "certified" for use in foods, and established a voluntary certification program for quality and purity. Initial control of this process was under the United States Department of Agriculture (USDA). However, in 1938, authority and responsibility for this process was transferred to the FDA [1–3,5]. Three separate categories were additionally created to delineate food manufacturing processes from other use of colors: FD&C (Food, Drug, and Cosmetic), D&C (Drug and Cosmetic), and External D&C (External Drug and Cosmetic) [1–3,5].

There was a paucity of further legislation until the Food Additive Amendment of 1958, which declared that food additives safely in use before 1958 were exempted from obtaining FDA approval. However, in 1960, the Color Additive

Food Allergy: Adverse Reactions to Foods and Food Additives, 4th edition.
Edited by Dean D. Metcalfe, Hugh A. Sampson, and Ronald A. Simon.
© 2008 Blackwell Publishing, ISBN: 978-1-4501-5129-0.

Amendments to the FDA act of 1906 created a "provisional" listing for all known colors in use for foodstuff [1–3,5,6]. This act required that all previously certified dyes and colors used in food undergo further testing to establish safety before they were re-certified. Manufacturers were given a provisional time allotment in which they could continue using the particular color on the market, while submitting the required data regarding safety to the FDA. Other types of additives were exempted from this act. This act also set limits to usable amounts of color in products, deemed good manufacturing practices [1–3,5].

Specifically, one section of the 1960 amendment, known as the Delaney Clause, placed a strict prohibition on the use of any amount of a substance shown to be carcinogenic in humans or laboratory animals [1–3,5,6]. This clause was applied to additives as well, though they were exempt from the rest of the amendment. The market effect of the 1960 Color Additive Amendments was the reduction of a list of 200 provisionally approved colors to a final list of 90 that were deemed safe for human consumption, after meeting newly applied regulations [1–3,5,6]. Colors that did not meet the new standards were removed from the market. Interestingly, the Delaney Clause had a vague definition of safety beyond establishing lack of carcinogenesis, and established no absolute standard for safety beyond "convincing evidence that establishes with reasonable certainty that no harm will result from the intended use of the color additive" [3,6].

The amendment also designated two distinct classes of colorants: certified and non-certified [1–3,5–7]. Colors exempt from certification were given this designation if certification was deemed unnecessary in the interest of public health to examine the color batch physical properties, including: purity, moisture, residual salts, unreacted intermediates, color

Table 34.1 Colors exempt from FDA certification (Adapted from www.cfsan.fda.gov, updated September 2006.)

Color additives approved for use in Human Food Part 73, Subpart A: Color additives exempt from batch certification:

21 CFR section	Straight color	EEC#	Year approved	Uses and restrictions
73.30	Annatto extract	E160b	1963	Foods generally
73.40	Dehydrated beets (beet powder)	E162	1967	Foods generally
73.75	Canthaxanthin	E161g	1969	Foods generally, NTE 30 mg/lb of solid or semi-solid food or per pint of liquid food; May also be used in broiler chicken feed
73.85	Caramel	E150a–d	1963	Foods generally
73.90	-Apo-8'-carotenal	E160e	1963	Foods generally, NTE: 15 mg/lb solid, 15 mg/pt liquid
73.95	-Carotene	E160a	1964	Foods generally
73.100	Cochineal extract	E120	1969	Foods generally
	Carmine		1967	
73.140	Toasted partially defatted cooked cottonseed flour	–	1964	Foods generally
73.160	Ferrous gluconate	–	1967	Ripe olives
73.165	Ferrous lactate	–	1996	Ripe olives
73.169	Grape color extract	E163?	1981	Non-beverage food
73.170	Grape skin extract (enocianina)	E163?	1966	Still and carbonated drinks and ades; beverage bases; alcoholic beverages (restrict. 27 CFR Parts 4 & 5)
73.200	Synthetic iron oxide	E172	1994	Sausage casings NTE 0.1% (by wt)
73.250	Fruit juice	–	1966	Foods generally
			1995	Dried color additive
73.260	Vegetable juice	–	1966	Foods generally
			1995	Dried color additive, water infusion
73.300	Carrot oil	–	1967	Foods generally
73.340	Paprika	E160c	1966	Foods generally
73.345	Paprika oleoresin	E160c	1966	Foods generally
73.450	Riboflavin	E101	1967	Foods generally
73.500	Saffron	E164	1966	Foods generally
73.575	Titanium dioxide	E171	1966	Foods generally; NTE 1% (by wt)
73.600	Turmeric	E100	1966	Foods generally
73.615	Turmeric oleoresin	E100	1966	Foods generally

NTE: Not to exceed.

impurities, other specified impurities, and presence of heavy metals [5]. Generally, this exemption was applied to a particular color that was from a biogenic source, with a history of use prior to the amendment, and without complaints of toxicity or allergic reactions to the FDA or its manufacturer [1–3, 5–7]. Colors exempt from FD&C certification are still subject to the standards of the Delaney Clause of the Color Additive Amendment [6]. In reality, there are virtually no restrictions applied to use of either non-certified colors in food manufacturing. One notable exception is for colors to be used in meat and poultry, which requires additional authorization from the USDA Food Safety Inspection Service (FSIS) above the FDA approval (Table 34.1 and Fig. 34.1) [5].

Color additives in the United States are regulated by the FDA Title 21 of the Code of Federal Regulations (CFR) part 73, subpart A (colors not subject to batch certification) and part 74, subpart A (colors subject to batch certification) [8]. As part of this legislation, all certified colors carry an FD&C or D&C color label and have undergone rigorous testing to establish their safety and batch purity, in contrast to their non-certified counterparts, as explained in the previous section. In 1990, the National Labeling and Education Act (NLEA) required that certified color additives must be declared on package labeling as individual ingredients as of July 1, 1991, regardless of their quantity in the item [9]. Biogenic colors were exempt from this requirement and

therefore may be referred to on labels as "artificial color," "artificial color added," or "color added" [8]. The use of the term "natural color" is not allowed as it could imply that the coloring might be derived from the food item itself, when in fact it is referring to an additive. As will be discussed in detail in the section on carmine, the unique labeling requirements for non-certified colors has become a controversial issue, as there are increasing numbers of case reports of biogenic color induced hypersensitivity [10]. Since certified colors (azo and non-azo dyes) are discussed in detail elsewhere in this book, henceforth, we will be referring to colors exempt from certification only.

An important distinction of how colors are used in foods and drugs is between dyes and lakes. A color dye is a water-soluble form of color (liquid, powder, or granule), and a lake is a water-insoluble form. Lakes are more stable than dyes and are better for use with fat or oil. Most pharmaceuticals use lakes in their coatings. A major technical advantage of certified colors is that they often require less chemical to produce an intense color, allow for more uniform distribution of color, and do not influence the flavor [1,2].

Biogenic colors are believed to contain low molecular weight non-protein chemicals, most likely acting as haptens when they elicit reactions. Reactions to this class of colorants can be both immunologic and non-immunologic. There is growing concern that biologic source contamination

Name	Hue	Common uses
Annatto	Orange	Dairy products, popcorn oil, butter mixes, baked goods, icings, snacks, ice cream, salad dressing, yogurts
Beta-carotene	Orange	Margarine, non-dairy creamers
Beet powder	Purple	Ice cream, cake icings, mixes, yogurt, gelatin desserts, fruit chews, frozen products, chewable tablets
Caramel color	Brown to red	Dairy foods, drinks, colas, iced tea, cocoa, beer, coffee, icings, cereals, popcorn, gravies, sauces, candies
Carrot oil	Orange	
Carmine	Wine red	Cake icings, hard candy, bakery products, yogurt, ice cream, gelatin desserts, fruit syrups, pet foods, jams/preserves
Fruit juice	Many colors	Beverages, jellies, candy, gelatin desserts, dry mixes, dark chocolate
Paprika	Red-orange	Sausage, cheese sauces, gravies, condiments, salad dressings, baked goods, snacks, icings, cereals
Riboflavin	Yellow-orange	
Saffron	Yellow-orange	
Turmeric	Yellow	Baked products, dairy products, ice cream, yogurts, cakes, cookies, popcorn, candy, cake icings, cereals, sauces, gelatins
Vegetable juice	Many colors	

Figure 34.1 Pictorial of the non-certified color additives. (Adapted and modified from www.red40.com.)

in the colorant is the source of IgE-mediated reactions attributed to them [7,10]. Annato and carmine/cochineal extract have both been linked to such reactions in the literature [7]. Because these colors are non-certified, it is difficult to ascertain the purity of a particular lot of these dyes. Thus, there could be varying levels of biogenic protein contamination due to technical discrepancies in different batches. There have been a few reports of SDS-PAGE analysis of carmine and cochineal insect protein fractions to determine their allergenicity, but there has been nothing conclusively nor consistently proven in this analysis [11–15]. At present time, despite several lobbying efforts by consumer groups, there has been no change made to the reporting of biogenic colors on food labels, though a specific petition to declare carmine on food labels is under consideration [16]. This petition and the subsequent FDA recommendation will be discussed in detail in the section covering carmine.

Biogenic colorants involved in hypersensitivity reactions

Only a few biogenic substances have been linked to allergic type reactions. These include carmine (cochineal extract), annatto, turmeric, saffron, beta-carotenoid, and grape anthocyanins. However, the majority of the literature pertains to carmine, with a small amount pertaining to annatto.

Carmine

Carmine is a red color derived from the female insect *Coccus cacti* or *Dactylopius cocus costa* [3,7,10,17–19]. This insect is commonly found in Peru, Central America, and the Canary Islands, where it grows as a parasite on the prickly pear cactus *Noplae coccinelliferna*. Its origins in Europe date back to the 1500s, when Hernando Cortez discovered its use by the Aztecs and brought the cochineal insects back to Spain [20]. The color is produced from the aqueous–alcohol extract of the dried, gravid, female insect, resulting in cochineal extract. Cochineal extract contains approximately 10% carminic acid, a hydroxyanthraquinone, and the rest is the residual insect body. Cochineal extract is acidic, and the color variation from deep red to orange is dependent on the pH. Carmine is produced from the aluminum or calcium aluminum lake on an aluminum hydroxide substrate of carminic acid. Since the lake is minimally soluble in water, strong acids or bases can be used to make the color more soluble. Commercial preparations of carmine are estimated to contain approximately 20–50% carminic acid, but it is usually diluted to 2–4% for sale. Commercial cochineal extract contains 1.8% carminic acid. Carmine is relatively expensive to produce. It is estimated that it requires 70,000 dried insects to make 1 lb of dye (Figs 34.2 and 34.3) [3,7,18].

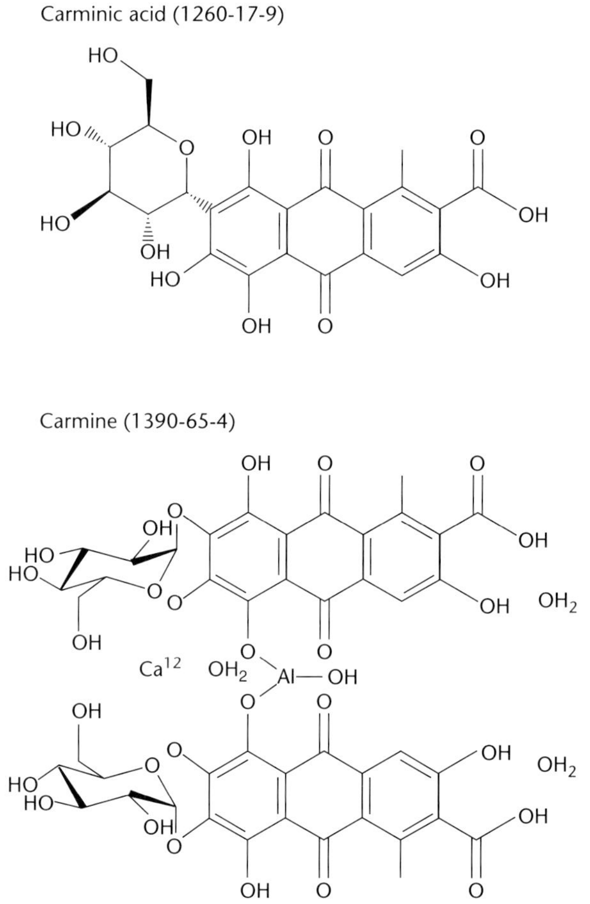

Carmine was given approval by the FDA for use in food in 1967, and cochineal extract in 1968 [21,22]. As part of this approval, it was determined that carmine or cochineal extract had no carcinogenic or teratogenic properties in

Carminic acid (1260-17-9)

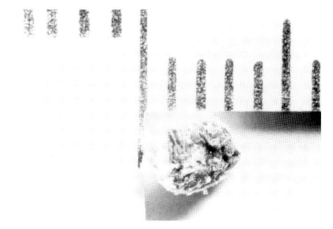

Figure 34.2 Chemical structures of carminic acid and carmine.

Figure 34.3 Photo of dried cochineal insect.

studies on rats. Carmine, as a biogenic color, is not certified, and therefore is exempt from specific declaration on food labels. It is generally labeled as "color added," "artificial color" or "artificial color added," "colored with carmine," "cochineal extract," or "carmine color." In Europe it is designated as E120 by the European Union, and may be labeled as "Natural Red No. 4" or CI 75470 (color index).

Table 34.2 Commercial uses of carmine/cochineal extract

Water-insoluble carmine colors	Water-soluble carmine colors	Water-soluble cochineal
Cosmetics	Yogurt	Beverages
Pharmaceuticals	Ice cream	Yogurt
Dairy products	Fruit-based drinks	Ice cream
Baked goods	Beverages	Fruit fillings
Condiments	Fruit fillings	Puddings
	Puddings	Confections
	Bakery mixes	
	Confections	
	Cosmetics	
	Pharmaceuticals	

Carmine is also used in cosmetics, where it had been required to be declared as an ingredient since 1977, but in order of its relative weight per volume of cosmetic (Table 34.2) [3,7,8,10,23].

Most foods colored with carmine contain very low levels that would limit exposure when consumed [7]. However, there are several case reports of hypersensitivity reactions attributed to carmine ranging from anaphylaxis to occupational asthma (see Table 34.3). Though these reports are uncommon, the actual incidence of these reactions is unknown under the current labeling regulations. This is because suspicion for a substance not listed by name on a label is generally non-existent. Hence, it is important for an allergist to be aware that this is a potential allergen.

Since levels of carmine in food are low, our group (Baldwin *et al.*) and others have hypothesized another likely route of sensitization (e.g. respiratory or dermatologic). Most of the reported cases involve workers with occupational exposure, or females with a prior history of use of carmine containing cosmetics [12]. Carmine was approved for use in cosmetics as a non-certified color in 1977, and is the only biogenic color allowed to be used around the eyes [23]. It is plausible that persons using makeup containing carmine can become sensitized through a cutaneous route. Upon re-exposure to carmine in food, an IgE-mediated reaction can occur. Similarly, occupational inhalation could cause sensitization in textile or dye workers exposed to high levels of carmine powder in the environment and cause an IgE-mediated reaction upon ingestion of carmine containing food or beverage. Carminic acid is a low-molecular weight molecule and may act as a hapten during sensitization. Protein remnants from the cochineal insects are likely candidate antigens as well. Most authors believe that there is chemical modification of the protein contaminants in the processing of the extracted carminic acid from the insect. Once sensitization occurs, low levels of exposure could result in hypersensitivity. However, no mechanism of sensitization has definitively been proven to date [7,10–12,19].

As of 2005, there were 35 reported patient-cases of hypersensitivity to carmine; 11 of these have been reported to the FDA under the MedWatch program, and the rest reported in the medical literature. There are no known reports of fatalities related to carmine [10,12]. The range of symptoms reported includes occupational asthma, extrinsic allergic aveolitis, chelitis, and food allergy manifesting as anaphylaxis, angioedema, bronchospasm and urticaria. There have been no consistent reports pertaining to time from exposure to symptoms, nor dose required to elicit symptoms [10,12]. The first case was reported in 1961, involving chelitis from a lip-salve that contained carmine [24]. In 1997, our group successfully showed there was a definitive IgE-mediated reaction in a 27-year-old-woman with anaphylaxis to a red-colored ice-pop containing carmine by the use of a Prausnitz–Küstner test [19]. Other groups have shown the reactions were IgE mediated through prick skin tests (PSTs)[11–15,19, 25–32], leukocyte histamine release test [29], radioallergosorbent testing (RAST) [12,27,28,30–32], and immunoblotting for specific IgE [11–15].

Reactions have been reported with two common predominating phenotypes, food hypersensitivity and occupational respiratory disease. In the occupational respiratory disease phenotype, these cases involve predominately males with no atopic background. In the food hypersensitivity phenotype, all case reports have involved females, half of whom were atopic. Two of these females also showed occupational disease features, and many have described prior episodes of itching and burning with application of makeup, suspicious for contact reactions [12]. There have been four distinct reports via the FDA MedWatch program of contact dermatitis, comprising a small third phenotype of reaction [10].

Immunoblot analysis of persons with occupational respiratory disease and food hypersensitivity phenotypes have shown mixed results. Typically, authors have used both carmine and pulverized cochineal insect extract, subjected to SDS-PAGE and column chromatography fractionation to determine protein bands. Subsequent immunoblotting with patient sera has determined IgE-recognized protein bands [10]. However, investigators who have performed these experiments have not found consistent recognition of any particular protein band in either carmine, pulverized cochineal insect, or carminic acid [11–15]. Our group found that commercial carmine could inhibit recognition of pulverized cochineal insect bands, strong evidence that there is insect protein contaminant in the commercial dye [25]. A recent immunoblot study confirmed this finding and inferred that these proteins undergo chemical modification in the commercial processing of carmine [12]. Groups have identified proteins 17, 28, 38, 50, 88, and 40–97 kDa in size. However, there is no universally recognized specific protein band found in carmine or cochineal extract, and there is considerable overlap when examining the reported data [11–15]. Considering that carmine is non-certified and exempt from

418

Table 34.5 Reported allergic reactions to spices

Spice	Family	Allergy	Specific IgE	Bet v 1 homolog	Profilin homolog	Other protein	Reference
Allspice	Myrtaceae	Contact dermatitis	None	None	None		[37,107]
Anice	Apiaceae	Rhinoconjunctivitis, anaphylaxis	12, 20, 33, 34, 35, 37, 39, 40, 42, 48, 50–70kDa	Pim a 1	Pim a 2		[59, 108–115]
Basil	Lamiaceae	Contact dermatitis	PST, CAP-RAST	None	None		[115–119]
Bay leaf	Lauraceae	Contact dermatitis, perioral dermatitis, asthma	PST, RAST	None	None		[120–123]
Caraway seed	Apiaceae	Rhinoconjunctivitis, GI	20, 33, 34, 37, 39, 42, 48kDa	None	None		[59]
Cardamom	Zingiberaceae	Dermatitis	PST	None	None		[124,125]
Cayenne	Solanaceae	Atopic dermatitis, bronchospasm	PST, RAST	None	None		[123,126–130]
Celery	Apiaceae	Anapylaxis, OAS	30–70kDa, including 55/58kDa (Api g 5)	Api g 1	Api g 4		[131–135]
Chervil	Apiaceae		None	None	None		None
Chili	Solanaceae	Atopic dermatitis, bronchospasm	None	None	None		[123,126–130]
Chives	Alliaceae	Contact dermatitis		None	None		[136]
Cinnamon	Canellaceae	Bronchospasm, rhinoconjunctivitis, contact dermatitis, stomatitis, Type IV hypersensitivity	None	None	None		[37,59,85,107,117,121, 124,125,128,137–155]
Cloves	Myrtaceae	Contact dermatitis	None	None	None		[37,85,137,151,153, 154]
Coriander	Apiaceae	Bronchospasm, anaphylaxis, contact dermatitis	12, 20, 21, 33, 34, 35, 37, 39, 40, 42, 34, 35, 37, 39, 40, 42, 48, ~70kDa	Cor s 1	Cor s 2		[59,85,108,117, 126–128,155–160]
Cumin	Apiaceae	Anaphylaxis, contact dermatitis	20, 33, 34, 37, 39, 42, 48, ~70kDa	Cum c 1	Cum c 2		[59,108,109,155,161]
Dill	Apiaceae	Anaphylaxis, contact urticaria	12, 21, 35, 40kDa	None	None		[59,111,162–165]
Fennel	Apiaceae	Rhinoconjunctivitis, bronchospasm, atopic dermatitis	20, 33, 34, 37, 39, 42, 48, 50–70, 65, 75kDa	Foe v 1	Foe v 2		[59,108,110,130,155, 166–173]
Garlic	Alliaceae	Contact dermatitis, bronchospasm, rhinitis, anaphylaxis	10, 12, 20, 31–60, 40, 42, 54, 56kDa (alliin lyase)	None	None		[166,174–200]
Ginger	Zingiberaceae	Contact dermatitis, bronchospasm, contact dermatitis	14, 23, 34kDa	None	None		[111,117,128,155,158, 201,202]
Jalapeno	Solanaceae	Same as chili	None	None	None		[123,126–130]
Lovage	Apiaceae		None	None	None		None
Mace	Myristicaceae	Bronchospasm, contact dermatitis	See nutmeg	None	None		[85,117,120,123,125, 128,155,157,158,201, 203–205]
Marjoram	Lamiaceae	Atopic dermatitis, perioral dermatitis	PST, RAST				[119,121,206,207]

Mustard		Anaphylaxis, Type IV hypersensitivity, contact urticaria	None	None	None	14 kDa (Bra j 1, Sin a 1) seed storage proteins	[89,127,158,208–212, 311]
Allspice	Myrtaceae						
Nutmeg	Myristicaceae	Bronchospasm, contact dermatitis	PST, RAST, histamine release assay	None	None	None	[85,117,120,123,125, 128,155,157,158,201, 203–205]
Onion	Alliaceae	Anaphylaxis, bronchospasm, contact dermatitis, rhinoconjunctivitis	12, 43 kDa	None	None	15 kDa lipid transferase	[182,193,213–222]
Oregano	Lamiaceae	Systemic reactions	PST, RAST	None	None		[117,119,123,207]
Paprika	Solanaceae	Contact urticaria, rhinoconjunctivitis	10, 17, 23 (Cap a 1w = osmotin-like), 24, 28, 29, 30, 32, 36, 40, 46, 69 kDa	None	Cap a 2		[63,64,85,105,106, 120,127,128,158,202, 223–231]
Parsley	Apiaceae	Angioedema, urticaria	None	Pet c 1	Pet c 2		[167,193,232–235]
Pepper	Piperaceae	Bronchospasm, contact dermatitis	11.8, 13.6, 14, 25, 28 (glucagon-like peptide), 30, 35, 40, 60 kDa	None	None		[63,85,120,124,126, 128,155,157,224,227, 229–231,236–239]
Pink peppercorns	Anacardiaceae	Atopic dermatitis (canine)	None	None	None		[240]
Peppermint	Lamiaceae	Contact allergy, anaphylactoid reactions, stomatitis	PST	None	None		[119,151,241–247]
Poppy seed	Papaveraceae	Anaphylaxis, exercise-induced anaphylaxis	5, 20, 25, 30, 34, 40, 45 kDa	None	None		[248–256]
Rosemary	Lamiaceae	Bronchospasm, contact dermatitis	PST, RAST	None	None		[123,257,258]
Saffron	Iridaceae	Anaphylaxis, bronchospasm, rhinoconjunctivitis	21 kDa (Cro s 1)	None	None		[51,52,93,201]
Sage	Lamiaceae	Bronchospasm, contact dermatitis	PST	None	None		[117,119,259–261]
Savory	Lamiaceae	Bronchospasm	PST	None	None		[123]
Sesame seed	Pedaliaceae	Anaphylaxis, bronchospasm, rhinitis, urticaria	10, 12, 14, 15–20, 15 (Ses i 5, oleosin),17 (Ses i 4, oleosin), 25, 29, 32, 34, 45, (Ses i 3, vicilin-type globulin), 45, 52, 30–67, 78 kDa, Ses i 4, Ses i 5	None	None	7 (Ses i 2 2S), 9 kDa (Ses i 1 2S) seed storage proteins	[250,262–286]
Star anise	Illiaceae	Contact dermatitis	None	None	None		[287,288]
Tarragon	Asteraceae	Subglottic edema	28–46, 60 kDa in related mugwort (Artemisia vulgaris)	None	None		[285,289]
Thyme	Lamiaceae	Bronchospasm, atopic dermatitis, systemic reactions	PST, RAST	None	None		[119,123,206,290]
Turmeric	Zingiberaceae	Bronchospasm, contact dermatitis	None	None	None		[93,117,291–294]
Vanilla	Orchidaceae	Atopic dermatitis, contact dermatitis	None	None	None		[152–154,295–298,312]

Adapted and modified from Ref. [85].

Table 35.1 Physiologic responses elicited by histamine

Responses mediated by H1 receptors
    Smooth muscle contraction
    Increased vascular permeability
    Mucous gland secretion
Responses mediated by H2 receptors
    Gastric acid secretion
    Inhibition of basophile histamine release
    Inhibition of lymphokine release
Responses mediated by H1 and H2 receptors
    Vasodilation
    Hypotension
    Flush
    Headache
    Tachycardia

appear to be roughly dose dependent. Ingestion of 25–50 mg of histamine may precipitate headache, whereas 100–150 mg may induce flushing [6]. These values are only rough estimates, however, and scombroid toxicity has been described with ingestion of as little as 2.5 mg of histamine [7].

Metabolism

The duration of histamine's effect depends on its metabolism. In normal physiology, conversion of histamine to its major inactive metabolites by either histamine methyltransferase or diamine oxidase (DAO) generally occurs rapidly [8,9]. Figure 35.1 shows the two routes of histamine metabolism. Prolonged binding of histamine from normal dietary sources to H1 and H2 receptors is uncommon, and symptoms rarely occur with such incidental ingestions. When large ingestions of histamine occur (e.g. scombroid poisoning), however, the metabolic capacity is temporarily exceeded and a multitude of histamine-mediated effects are observed. Experimental administration of large oral quantities of histamine yields similar clinical responses [10].

Although methylation appears to be the primary route for metabolism of histamine administered by both the oral and intravenous routes, DAO is important as well. DAO is present in the intestinal mucosa in almost all mammalian species examined [11]. Ingestion of a histamine-containing meal along with ingestion of drugs that inhibit DAO can produce histamine-induced symptoms. Isoniazid is a potent DAO inhibitor and, when combined with a histamine-containing meal, has resulted in severe histamine-induced symptoms [12,13,21]. *In vitro* experiments have shown a number of drugs (e.g. chloraquine, pentamidine, clavulanic acid, dobutamine, pancuronium, imipenem, and others) to be potent human intestinal mucosal DAO inhibitors. The *in vivo* clinical relevance of these findings remains uncertain [14].

Histamine-containing foods

Certain foods are generally accepted as having higher histamine content than others [15,16]. Three cheeses (Parmesan, Blue, and Roquefort), two vegetables (spinach and eggplant), two red wines (Chianti and Burgundy), yeast extract, and scombroid fish have histamine content adequate to raise postprandial 24-hour urinary histamine levels [15]. For this reason, dietary histamine restrictions are recommended for patients undergoing 24-hour urinary histamine determinations.

The histamine content in red wines is commonly cited as one of the possible causes of wine intolerance. The symptoms most often reported by susceptible individuals include flushing of the face, headache, nasal congestion, and/or respiratory distress. A French study, however, found no significant difference in the occurrence of adverse reactions in wine-intolerant individuals who underwent two double-blind provocation tests, one with a wine poor in histamine (0.4 mg/l) and one with a wine rich in histamine (13.8 mg/l) [17]. The histamine-rich wine also contained higher levels of other biogenic amines including tyramine, ethylamine, putrescine, and phenylethylamine [17]. This suggests that the histamine content of wine may not be directly linked to adverse reactions to wines. It is also interesting to note that fermented cheeses contain amounts of histamine that are much greater than those found in wines, yet signs typical of intolerance to histamine have rarely been reported after ingestion of cheeses [18].

Several symptoms generally attributed to monosodium glutamate (MSG) resemble those associated with histamine toxicity. Using a radio enzymatic assay technique, the histamine content of several common Asian dishes, condiments, and basic ingredients was measured. Although the amount of histamine in individual food portions was determined to fall below the level generally thought necessary to induce symptoms, consumption of multiple portions could result in ingestion of enough histamine to produce symptoms [18].

Scombroid poisoning

Histamine poisoning from ingestion of foods with high histamine content is well documented. The prototype for this kind of histamine toxicity is scombroid poisoning. Marine bacteria such as *Morganella morganii*, *Klebsiella pneumoniae*, and *Photobacterium phosphoreum* generate histamine from histadine through a chemical reaction involving histadine decarboxylase. In a recent publication this gene was cloned from *P. phosphoreum* and sequenced [19]. Improperly refrigerated scombroid fish (e.g. tuna, mackerel, skipjack, and bonito) and non-scombroid fish (e.g. mahimahi, bluefish, amberjack, herring, sardines, marlin, and anchovies) develop an enriched histamine content through this bacterial action. Laboratory confirmation of scombroid is established by sampling the muscle of the suspected meal and finding a histamine level over 50 ppm [20]. Since the last edition of this text two additional reports of outbreaks of scombroid poisoning have been reported. Ninety-four cases occurred at a kindergarten as a result of spoiled sailfish and the other as a result of saury fish paste in six patients on a TB ward who were

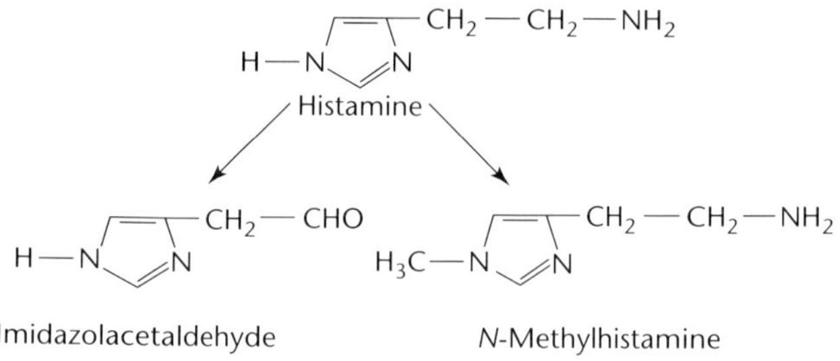

Figure 35.1 Histamine metabolism.

concomitantly taking isoniazid [21,22]. The US Food and Drug Administration (FDA) recognizes the issue of scromboid poisoning as a continuing problem and has conducted a study to base recommendations regarding fish handling to prevent histamine formation. Mahimahi, skipjack, and yellowfin tuna were tested for the formation of histamine after storage. At 26°C, over 12 hours of incubation was required before a histamine concentration of 50 ppm was reached, however at 35°C 50 ppm of histamine was formed by 9 hours [23].

Ingestion of such fish causes a clinical picture bearing strong resemblance to anaphylaxis. Symptoms generally begin within an hour of ingestion and include flushing, sweating, nausea, vomiting, abdominal cramps, diarrhea, headache, palpitations, urticaria, dizziness, a metallic, sharp, or peppery taste, and, in severe cases, hypotension and bronchospasm [7,24]. Outbreaks of scombroid poisoning continue to appear in the literature. The US FDA has established a hazard concentration for histamine poisoning of greater than 450 μg per 100 g of tuna [24]. Levels from 2.5 to 250 mg of histamine per 100 g of fish have been reported in most cases of scombroid poisoning. Treatment is supportive and includes H1 and H2 receptor blockade. Improper warming between the time that the fish is caught and when it is prepared can lead to histamine production sufficient to cause poisoning. Scombroid poisoning can be prevented only by proper handling and refrigeration of fish [23,25,26].

Histamine-releasing foods
Some foods without significant histamine content may contain substances capable of triggering degranulation of tissue mast cells (MCs), with resultant histamine release. Substances thought to be responsible for this histamine-releasing activity include enzymes in foods, such as trypsin, and other agents from both animal and vegetable sources, such as peptone. Foods with this unproven intrinsic histamine-releasing capacity include egg whites, crustaceans, chocolate, strawberries, ethanol, tomatoes, and citrus fruits [27].

Monoamines

Synthesis
Naturally occurring amino acids are converted into vasoactive monoamines by a number of microorganisms that possess amino acid decarboxylases necessary for this conversion. For example, tyrosine is the precursor for both dopamine and tyramine, phenylalanine is the precursor for phenylethylamine, and tryptophan is the precursor for serotonin. Amine production by these microorganisms varies depending on a variety of different conditions, including pH, temperature, and sodium chloride content [27].

Metabolism
The vasoactive monoamines are metabolized by the enzyme monoamine oxidase (MAO), which includes two subtypes: MAO-A and MAO-B. The genes for both MAO-A and MAO-B have been mapped to the short arm of the X chromosome (Xp11.23) [28], and appear to be derived from a duplication of a common ancestral gene [29]. MAO is found in a variety of tissues, where it is localized to the outer membrane of mitochondria. It catalyzes the oxidative deamination of a variety of neurotransmitters as well as the monoamines of dietary significance. Dopamine and tyramine can be metabolized by both MAO-A and MAO-B. The polar amines (serotonin, epinephrine, and norepinephrine) are metabolized primarily by MAO-A, whereas the non-polar amine phenylethylamine metabolizes primarily by MAO-B [30].

Patients with rare deletions in their MAO-A gene have increased levels of serotonin, epinephrine, and norepinephrine detectable in their urine, whereas MAO-B deficient subjects have increased urinary phenylethylamine levels [31]. Although no studies have examined pharmacologic food reactions in these individuals, it is interesting to note that the MAO-A deficient individuals clinically have problems with impaired impulse control, including a propensity toward stress-induced aggression. MAO-B deficient individuals do not seem to have clinically apparent disturbances in their behavior [31]. Although the reasons for these clinical differences are not known, it may be that raised serotonin levels in MAO-A deficient individuals have a disruptive effect on the developing brain [31].

Specific monoamines
Tyramine
Many fermented foods contain tyramine derived from the bacterial decarboxylation of tyrosine. Foods with particularly high levels of tyramine include Camembert and Cheddar cheeses, yeast extract, wine (especially Chianti), pickled herring, fermented bean curd, fermented soybean, soy sauces, miso soup, and chicken liver. Smaller but still detectable amounts are present in avocados, bananas, figs, red plums, eggplant, and tomato [32–34].

Although tyramine exerts an indirect sympathomimetic effect by releasing endogenous norepinephrine [35], dietary tyramine usually does not cause detectable clinical effects. However, it is suggested to be responsible for adverse clinical

Food Allergy Action plan

Students's Name:_____ **D.O.B:**_____ **Teacher:**_____

ALLERGY TO:_____

Asthmatic   Yes* ☐   No ☐   *Higher risk for severe reaction

Place Child's Picture Here

◆ STEP 1: TREATMENT ◆

Symptoms:		Give Checked Medication**: **(To be determined by physician authorizing treatment)	
■	If a food allergen has been ingested, but *no symptoms*:	☐ Epinephrine	☐ Antihistamine
■ Mouth	Itching, tingling, or swelling of lips, tongue, mouth	☐ Epinephrine	☐ Antihistamine
■ Skin	Hives, itchy rash, swelling of the face or extremities	☐ Epinephrine	☐ Antihistamine
■ Gut	Nausea, abdominal cramps, vomiting, diarrhea	☐ Epinephrine	☐ Antihistamine
■ Throat†	Tightening of throat, hoarseness, hacking cough	☐ Epinephrine	☐ Antihistamine
■ Lung†	Shortness of breath, repetitive coughing, wheezing	☐ Epinephrine	☐ Antihistamine
■ Heart†	Weak or thready pulse, low blood pressure, fainting, pale, blueness	☐ Epinephrine	☐ Antihistamine
■ Other†	_____	☐ Epinephrine	☐ Antihistamine
■	If reaction is progressing (several of the above areas affected), give:	☐ Epinephrine	☐ Antihistamine

†Potentially life-threatening. The severity of symptoms can quickly change.

DOSAGE

Epinephrine: inject intramuscularly (circle one) EpiPen® EpiPen® Jr., Twinject® 0.3 mg Twinject® 0.15 mg
(see reverse side for instructions)

Antihistamine: give _____
medication/dose/route

Other: give _____
medication/dose/route

IMPORTANT: Asthma inhalers and/or antihistamines cannot be depended on to replace epinephrine in anaphylaxis.

◆ STEP 2: EMERGENCY CALLS ◆

1. Call 911 (or Rescue Squad:_____). State that an allergic reaction has been treated, and additional epinephrine may be needed.

2. Dr. _____   Phone Number: _____

3. Parent _____   Phone Number(s) _____

4. Emergency contacts:
   Name/Relationship   Phone Number(s)

a. _____   1. _____   2. _____

b. _____   1. _____   2. _____

EVEN IF PARENT/GUARDIAN CANNOT BE REACHED, DO NOT HESITATE TO MEDICATE OR TAKE CHILD TO MEDICAL FACILITY!

Parent/Guardian's Signature _____   Date _____

Doctor's Signature _____   Date _____
(Required)

Figure 36.1 Food Allergy Action Plan.

TRAINED STAFF MEMBERS

1. _____   Room _____

2. _____   Room _____

3. _____   Room _____

EpiPen® and EpiPen® Jr. Directions

- Pull off gray activation cap.

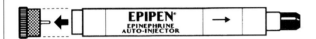

- Hold black tip near outer thigh (always apply to thigh).

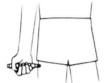

- Swing and jab firmly into outer thigh until Auto-Injector mechanism functions. Hold in place and count to 10. Remove the EpiPen® unit and massage the injection area for 10 seconds.

Twinject® 0.3 mg and Twinject® 0.15 mg Directions

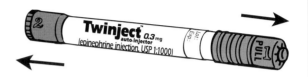

- Remove caps labeled "1" and "2."

- Place rounded tip against outer thigh, press down hard until needle penetrates. Hold for 10 seconds, then remove.

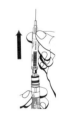

SECOND DOSE ADMINISTRATION:
If symptoms don't improve after 10 minutes, administer second dose:

- Unscrew rounded tip. Pull syringe from barrel by holding blue collar at needle base.

- Slide yellow collar off plunger.

- Put needle into thigh through skin, push plunger down all the way, and remove.

Once EpiPen® or Twinject® is used, call the Rescue Squad. Take the used unit with you to the Emergency Room. Plan to stay for observation at the Emergency Room for at least 4 hours.

For children with multiple food allergies, consider providing separate Action Plans for different foods.

**Medication checklist adapted from the Authorization of Emergency Treatment form developed by the Mount Sinai School of Medicine. Used with permission.

The Food Allergy & Anaphylaxis Network

June 2007

Figure 36.1 (*Continued*)

Eating away from home

When food is consumed that is not personally prepared and served in one's home, the risk of encountering a hidden allergen increases. As an example, a peanut-sensitive teenager made her own jam sandwich while on a camping trip [35]. She was not aware that the knife had been used earlier to spread peanut butter and had been wiped but not washed. She died minutes after eating the sandwich. Another individual suffered a reaction after eating ice cream that should not have contained nuts. It was later discovered that the wait staff mistakenly put the wrong flavor ice cream on the child's ice cream cone.

Food-allergic patients must be on heightened alert when dining away from home. Common ingredients can appear in unexpected places, for example eggs in meat loaf or peanut butter in meat sauce. Convincing the wait staff that food allergies are real, and that it is critical that they give accurate information about ingredients, are just some of the obstacles patients must be prepared to address.

From the restaurateur's perspective, high staff turnover and part-time staff make training or standardization of food allergy policies difficult to implement. When dining in a restaurant, patients should address food allergy queries to the restaurant manager. The manager is often more seasoned and less distracted than harried wait staff, increasing the chances that the patient will receive accurate information [36].

Furlong et al. reported that reactions in restaurants were caused by a number of factors: the food-allergic individual not telling the wait staff about the food allergy; cross-contact between foods (primarily from shared ice cream equipment, from cooking surfaces, and serving utensils); and establishment error (e.g. switching ingredients and not notifying the wait staff). Half of the reactions were caused by allergens in unexpected places, for example, in sauces, dressings, or in egg rolls. Desserts accounted for 43% of the reactions, followed by entrées (35%), appetizers (13%), and others (9%) [16].

There are some simple strategies for avoiding a reaction in a restaurant setting. Individuals who are allergic to peanuts or tree nuts should not eat in Chinese, Thai, Indian, or other Asian-type restaurants. These ingredients are commonly used in many dishes and cross-contact between foods during meal preparation and cooking is likely. Peanut-allergic individuals have reported reactions after eating Mexican food. These restaurants are now using peanut butter in some dishes, an example is enchilada sauce.

Patients who are allergic to fish or shellfish should avoid eating at seafood restaurants. The oil, grill, and other cooking areas are likely to contain small amounts of fish or shellfish protein that could come into contact with the fish-free meal. Some individuals are so sensitive to a food that simply breathing the aerosolized protein in steam can cause a severe or even fatal reaction. A shrimp-sensitive woman is said to have suffered fatal anaphylaxis within minutes after a waiter in a restaurant walked past her carrying a sizzling shrimp dish [8].

Buffet-style service offers another potentially high risk for cross-contact. The food is often placed in serving dishes that are close to each other, and small amounts of one food may fall into another serving dish; diners often dip one spoon into several dishes. Finally, dishes and their ingredients are rarely identified. One woman learned after she had a reaction that the food she ate contained walnuts.

While eating in a fast-serve or fast-food restaurant, it is not prudent to assume that what is safe in one restaurant will necessarily be safe in another. Although food preparation at chain restaurants is usually standardized, regional differences may exist in products served or ingredients used [37]. Franchise owners may not follow corporate policy regarding separation of various foods during cooking and preparation.

When eating in restaurants, individuals with food allergies will minimize the chance for an allergic reaction if they identify themselves to the wait staff and manager, ask questions about ingredients used, cooking methods, that is whether the grill is greased with butter, the use of "secret ingredients," and ask for advice on selecting menu items. Patients should order simply prepared foods with as few ingredients as possible, for example, a baked potato without the toppings.

A peanut-sensitive teenager died after eating an egg roll at an oriental restaurant [38]. He apparently had asked the waiter if any of the food was cooked in peanut oil, and was assured that the restaurant did not use any peanut oil. He may not have inquired about the use of peanut butter, which the restaurant used in its egg rolls. As a rule, if the patient has any doubt about whether his or her questions and concerns are being taken seriously, the individual should eat elsewhere.

To discreetly and consistently convey information to the restaurant staff, some teens and young adults prefer to use a "chef card" (Fig. 36.2). These personalized cards usually include the list of synonyms for the allergen, a caution about food preparation, and the symptoms of a reaction (to convey the seriousness of the food allergy). Some use a brightly colored laminated card; others have business cards printed with this information.

When it comes to menu selection, avoidance of high-risk foods on a menu, such as sauces and desserts, foods prepared in a pastry covering, combination foods (such as stews), and fried foods, may help patients avoid an allergic reaction.

Surprise use of allergens include almonds in dressings for chicken entrees, sauces used on fresh fruit and in baked goods. Eggs used to create foam for milk toppings on

Sample Chef Card

To the Chef:

WARNING! I am allergic to peanuts. In order to avoid a life-threatening reaction, I must avoid the following ingredients:

Artificial nuts

Beer nuts

Cold pressed, expelled, or extruded peanut oil

Ground nuts

Mandelonas

Mixed nuts

Monkey nuts

Nut pieces

Peanut

Peanut butter

Peanut flour

Please ensure any utensils and equipment used to prepare my meal, as well as prep surfaces, are thoroughly cleaned prior to use. Thanks for your cooperation.

Figure 36.2 Sample chef card.

specialty coffee drinks, as a binder in meatballs or meatloaf and as a glaze on baked goods. Peanut butter used to thicken chili, Mexican salsa, spaghetti sauce, hot chocolate, and brown gravy [15]. It also has been used as the "glue" to hold egg rolls and Rice Krispie treats together, to add crunch and texture to piecrusts and cheesecakes, and to add flavor to brownies.

Nuts and other toppings are often accidentally dropped into containers of ice cream. Furthermore, the scoopers for the various flavors are often placed in a common tub of water, which may contain protein from all of the different flavors.

It is a common industry policy for restaurants to cook several types of foods in the same deep-fat fryer. This can pose a risk to the allergic individual who has no way of knowing what other foods were fried in that cooking oil. In one case, an individual with a fish allergy reacted to French fries that had been cooked in the same oil as the fish.

In spite of their precautions, however, mistakes can occur in the kitchen during meal preparation, as well. Several reactions have occurred after the kitchen staff simply removed the allergen rather than making a new dish. To avoid this risk, if a food-allergic individual is served an allergen-containing dish at a restaurant (a cheeseburger instead of a plain burger), the individual should keep the original dish at their table to ensure that a new dish is prepared.

Dining away from home

Selection of low-risk restaurants is key for minimizing the chances of an allergic reaction

Avoiding desserts, sauces, fried foods, and foods in covered pastry will help minimize the chance of an accidental ingestion of an allergen

Teens can use a "chef card" to identify themselves to the wait staff in restaurants

If an order is incorrect, the allergic individual should keep it until a new dish is served

Buffets offer a tremendous risk for cross-contact with allergens and are best avoided

Special occasions

Preparation, planning ahead, and minimizing risks are the key ingredients for success during special occasions such as birthday parties, family gatherings, vacations, and air travel.

Before attending a birthday party or visiting a relative's house, the hostess should be alerted of the food allergy. Some families prefer to bring their own "safe" food for their peace of mind. For vacations, many rent condominiums or cottages with kitchens so they can prepare the child's meals themselves. Those that choose this option often bring food with them or ship staples such as bread and cereals to their vacation destination. For sleep away camps the options may include providing the child's food or reviewing the menu to determine what foods the child can eat. Careful attention should be given to camp activities that will require the children to be in remote areas to be sure emergency-medical services are available if needed.

Regarding air travel, the best policy is to avoid eating any food served by the airline, as ingredient lists are not usually available and the meals are prepared in large warehouses with many opportunities for mistakes or cross-contact to occur. Some families of children with peanut allergy request peanut-free flights. No airline can guarantee a peanut-free flight. There may be peanut ingredients in meals; other passengers may carry peanuts on the plane with them. Some airlines will serve a non-peanut snack upon request; others make no such accommodations. Families would do well to check with the airline when booking their flights, confirm the arrangements before the trip, and keep in mind that airlines change their policy without warning. As a precaution, all families should keep their child's medications stored in a carry-on bag, and be prepared to treat a reaction should one occur.

According to the Transportation Security Administration (TSA), passengers are permitted to bring self-injectable epinephrine on board, provided that the medication features a professionally printed label identifying the medication or the manufacturer's name. FAAN recommends that patients carry additional documentation such as a doctor's note and the prescription label from the pharmacy. A sample doctor's note is available on the FAAN web site.

When traveling outside the United States, other problems may arise. In some parts of Europe, for example, product labels do not have to list all ingredients and emergency services differ from country to country. FAAN's booklet *Travel Guide: Tips for Traveling with Food Allergy* includes information and advice for managing meals while traveling [39].

Treatment of a food-allergic reaction

Since ingestion of food allergens can occur even with stringent avoidance measures, a treatment protocol must be prescribed that is immediately available in case of inadvertent ingestion of the offending allergen. The booklet "*Just One Little Bite Can Hurt*" and "*It Only Takes One Bite*" video (FAAN) are references that can be recommended to patients to raise their own awareness, and that of their families, friends, and teachers, to the potential severity of food allergy [20].

Treatment of a mild reaction

Recently an NIAID-FAAN multi-specialty working group published criteria for diagnosing anaphylaxis (Table 36.3) [40]. In addition, a grading system for the severity of anaphylaxis

has also been recommended (Table 36.4). The working group sought to distinguish allergic reactions from anaphylactic reactions. A mild allergic reaction is considered to be urticaria/angioedema only with no other systemic symptoms appearing in a patient who is not at high risk for serious anaphylaxis, that is, has never had a previous severe reaction and/or does not have asthma. Alternatively, it might consist of mouth itching only, in a subject who has the oral allergy syndrome [41] and no risk factors. Risk factors for serious reactions to foods include asthma [42], peanut or nut allergy [4,43,44], previous history of severe reaction to any food [4], extreme atopy (with elevated IgE and multiple positive skin tests, atopic dermatitis, food allergy, and asthma) [4,45,46], and use of β-blocking medications [45] (Table 36.5).

For an individual who presents with a mild reaction to a food and has none of the risk factors listed above, treatment may be limited to an antihistamine, preferably liquid diphenhydramine or cetirizine. It should be clearly understood that antihistamines possess no anti-anaphylactic activity and are never a substitute for epinephrine. Whether such a subject who has experienced a mild allergic reaction to a food should routinely carry epinephrine remains the subject of some debate [4,45–47]. However, all patients with IgE-mediated food allergy should be warned about the possibility

Table 36.3 Diagnostic criteria for anaphylaxis

Anaphylaxis is highly likely when any one of the following three criteria is fulfilled:

1 Acute onset of an illness (minutes to several hours) with involvement of the skin, mucosal tissue, or both (e.g. generalized hives, pruritus, or flushing, swollen lips–tongue–uvula)
  And at least one of the following:
  (a) Respiratory compromise (e.g. dyspnea, wheeze-bronchospasm, stridor, reduced peak expiratory flow, hypoxemia)
  (b) Reduced blood pressure or associated symptoms of end-organ dysfunction (e.g. hypotonia (collapse), syncope, incontinence)

2 Two or more of the following that occur rapidly after exposure *to a likely allergen for that patient* (minutes to several hours):
  (a) Involvement of the skin-mucosal tissue (e.g. generalized hives, itch-flush, swollen lips-tongue-uvula)
  (b) Respiratory compromise (e.g. dyspnea, wheeze-bronchospasm, stridor, reduced peak expiratory flow, hypoxemia)
  (c) Reduced blood pressure or associated symptoms of end-organ dysfunction (e.g. hypotonia (collapse), syncope, incontinence)
  (d) Persistent gastrointestinal symptoms (e.g. crampy abdominal pain, vomiting)

3 Reduced blood pressure after exposure *to known allergen for that patient* (minutes to several hours):
  (a) *Infants and children*: low systolic blood pressure (age specific) or greater than 30% decrease in systolic blood pressure*
  (b) *Adults*: systolic blood pressure less than 90 mmHg or greater than 30% decrease from that patient's baseline

(Reproduced from Sampson HA *et al.* [40], with permission from Elsevier.)
*Low systolic blood pressure for children: 1 month to 1 year < 70 mmHg; 1–10 years < (70 mmHg + (2 × age)); 11–17 years < 90 mmHg

Table 36.4 Grading severity of anaphylaxis

Grade	Defined by
1 *Mild* (skin and subcutaneous tissues, gastrointestinal, and/or mild respiratory)	Flushing, urticaria, periorbital erythema, or angioedema; mild dyspnea, wheezing, and upper respiratory symptoms; mild abdominal pain and/or emesis
2 *Moderate* (mild symptoms + features suggesting moderate respiratory, cardiovascular, or gastrointestinal symptoms)	Marked dysphagia, hoarseness, and/or stridor; shortness of breath, wheezing and retractions; crampy abdominal pain, recurrent vomiting, and/or diarrhea; and/or mild dizziness
3 *Severe* (hypoxia, hypotension, or neurological compromise)	Cyanosis or $SpO_2 \leqslant 92\%$ at any stage, hypotension, confusion, collapse, loss of consciousness; or incontinence

Table 36.5 Risk factors for a severe allergic reaction to food

Asthma
Extreme atopy
History of anaphylactic reaction to any food
β-blocker treatment
Peanut or tree nut as the allergen
Adolescent or young adult
Lack of readily available epinephrine

of developing a more severe anaphylactic reaction. In addition, parents of young children with food allergy should be advised to contact their physician if their child develops wheezing from any cause, for example viral infection, because evidence of airway hyperreactivity moves the child into a higher-risk group. In some cases, parents of children with mild reactions may prefer to keep epinephrine available for use, but reserve actual administration to occasions on which more severe symptoms develop. All individuals should be instructed in the signs and symptoms of anaphylaxis (Table 36.6) and warned to use epinephrine immediately and seek emergency care if significant symptoms develop (see Chapter 13). A written Food Allergy Action Plan clearly describing what symptoms to look for and what to do if a reaction occurs should be provided to these patients and their caregivers.

Treatment of moderate to severe reactions

Any individual who has a history of an IgE-mediated reaction to a food, especially if it was more severe than urticaria only, mouth itching only, mild tightness in the throat, and/or who has any of the risk factors listed above should be considered at risk for a more serious subsequent reaction. Some of the most severe reactions may not, in fact, have urticaria associated with the symptom complex [4,45,46,48–52]. The treatment of choice in such cases is epinephrine administered by intramuscular injection [52,53]. The point at which to administer epinephrine remains controversial. Traditionally, administration was delayed until the onset of serious symptoms, but evidence suggests that it may be a poor policy to wait for severe symptoms to develop in high-risk subjects [4,7,50]. *In any patient with a history of a severe reaction, epinephrine should be administered as soon as it is realized that the allergenic food has been ingested.*

Table 36.6 Clinical features of anaphylaxis

Cutaneous	Urticaria, angioedema, pruritus, flushing, morbilliform rash
Respiratory	Upper airway – rhinorrhea, congestion, sneezing, **stridor**, **hoarseness**, **"lump in throat"*** **lower airway – cough**, **wheeze**, **dyspnea**, **chest tightness**, **cyanosis**
Cardiovascular	Tachycardia, arrhythmia, **syncope**, **hypotension**, **shock**
Gastrointestinal	Pruritus or edema of the lips/tongue/palate, metallic taste in the mouth, nausea, vomiting, abdominal cramps, diarrhea
Genitourinary	Uterine cramping, uterine bleeding
Neurological	Anxiety, headache, seizure, **syncope**, **loss of consciousness**
Ocular	Pruritus, conjunctival injection, lacrimation

*Patients presenting with any of the symptoms depicted in bold should be given epinephrine immediately.

Epinephrine is currently available in pre-measured doses for patient use from only one source. The EpiPen® (Dey; Napa, CA) and Twinject® (Verus Pharmaceuticals; San Diego, CA) are single and double unit-dose devices, respectively, for use in adults and children weighing 28 kg or more [54,55]. They deliver 0.3 mg of epinephrine as 0.3 ml of 1:1000 solution in an automatic syringe preloaded for intramuscular injection. The EpiPen® Jr. (Dey, Napa, CA) and Twinject® Jr. (Verus Pharmaceuticals; San Diego, CA) are intended for smaller children; it delivers 0.15 mg of epinephrine in 0.3 ml of 1:2000 dilution of epinephrine. In children weighing less than 10–15 kg, one may either administer the EpiPen® Jr. For children less than 10 kg, a needle, syringe, and vials of epinephrine may be prescribed, but the reliability of dosing administered by parents is highly variable [56]. The usual dose of epinephrine is 0.01 mg/kg body weight up to a maximum of 0.3 ml, but larger doses may be well tolerated. Epinephrine kits ideally should be stored between 59°F and 86°F.

Inhaled epinephrine delivered by metered-dose devices has been compared with injected epinephrine [57,58]. Theoretically, this treatment could allow more rapid deposition of epinephrine at the site of laryngeal edema. Doses of 10–20 puffs of metered-dose inhaler-delivered epinephrine comparable to those provided with the injection of 0.3 ml of 1:1000 epinephrine, although the duration of effect may be somewhat shorter. While anecdotal reports of successful use of this treatment are known [46], but a study by Simons has shown that children are not able to inhale adequate amounts of epinephrine by this method [59].

A rapidly absorbed antihistamine (H1 antagonist) should be prescribed for all patients with IgE-mediated food allergy. Liquid diphenhydramine, 1 mg/kg up to 75 mg, or cetirazine, 0.25 mg up to 10 mg, are rapidly absorbed and may ameliorate some symptoms of anaphylaxis. However, antihistamines should never be considered as a substitute for epinephrine in the treatment of anaphylaxis.

Corticosteroids provide no immediate effect, but are usually recommended for use early in the treatment of moderate to severe anaphylaxis, in the hope that they will prevent or ameliorate a prolonged or biphasic reaction [50,60]. Furthermore, they restore the responsiveness of β-receptors to their agonists. Patients who have severe anaphylaxis or who have received corticosteroid therapy during the previous 6 months should receive pharmacological doses of corticosteroids [50].

Individuals who have food allergy and asthma appear to be at higher risk for severe allergic reactions than those without asthma and food allergy [4,52]. Bronchodilators may be used during a reaction. However, these or other asthma medications should never be used as a substitute for epinephrine.

Treatment of extremely severe reactions

Life-threatening anaphylaxis from food ingestion typically involves severe compromise of the upper and lower respiratory

Table 36.7 Management of anaphylaxis

Assessment
 Check airway; secure if necessary
 Assess level of consciousness
 Obtain vital signs
 Estimate body weight

Initial therapy
 Epinephrine

Further treatment based on evaluation of clinical condition
 General
  H1 antihistamine
  Corticosteroids
  Oxygen
  Elevate legs and lie flat if tolerated
 Respiratory symptoms
  Nebulized β-agonist
  Aminophylline
  Nebulized epinephrine
 Cardiovascular symptoms
  Intravenous fluids (colloid or crystalloid)
 H2 antihistamine
 Inotropic agent
 Vasopressors
 Glucagon
 Assisted ventilation

tract, although cardiovascular reactions, including dysrhythmias and shock can develop [61,62] (see Chapter 13 for further discussion). The treatment approach should be tailored to the condition of the patient (Table 36.7). If any question arises about the adequacy of cardiopulmonary function, the caregiver should administer supplemental oxygen, secure an intravenous line, and begin cardiac monitoring.

In the hypotensive patient, the combination of H1 and H2 antihistamines in addition to intravenous fluids may represent an additional treatment strategy. Studies suggest that this combination could protect against the decrease in diastolic blood pressure linked to histamine [63,64]. For example, 1-mg/kg diphenhydramine and 4-mg/kg cimetidine could be infused slowly [65]. The effectiveness of this therapy as a prophylactic agent in preventing histamine-induced hypotension is generally accepted [66]; however, its use in the treatment of acute anaphylaxis remains more controversial [67,68].

Respiratory symptoms

Food allergy may provoke severe asthmatic attacks, which result in death or require mechanical ventilation [42,45]. In addition to intramuscular epinephrine, the treatment approach to severe bronchospasm resembles that for any asthma attack, with the understanding that recurrent or prolonged severe obstruction may occur, necessitating the need for observation to continue for at least 4 hours after a satisfactory response to treatment [4,52]. A β-agonist such as albuterol, nebulized with oxygen, provides the basis of treatment. If upper airway edema appears, nebulized racemic epinephrine may be administered. In the face of severe bronchospasm, intravenous aminophylline may be used, although albuterol, aminophylline, and hypoxia carry some risk of additive cardiac toxicity [69]. Intubation and assisted ventilation may be necessary [50,61,70]. Edema of the upper airway, a less common effect, may also occur [50,71]. Intubation or cricothyroidotomy may be necessary.

Advice to patients for treating a reaction

All patients with food allergy should be instructed in avoidance of the incriminated food. However, in spite of best efforts to avoid the food allergen, reactions are likely to occur from "hidden" ingredients. Vander Leek reported that 60% of 83 peanut-allergic children had a total of 115 documented adverse reactions caused by accidental exposure to peanuts during follow up [3,30].

Patients need to be taught the early warning symptoms of a reaction to a food. Even if they have previously had only mild reactions, they should be educated about all possible symptoms that may develop in more severe allergic reactions. Each food-allergic subject must maintain constant scrutiny of his/her diet. All food-allergic individuals should receive information concerning emergency medical identification systems such as MedicAlert® (www.medicalert.org).

Some debate has arisen about which patients should receive a prescription for epinephrine, although all agree that subjects at risk for a severe food-allergic reaction should carry epinephrine [4,50]. The medical record should include documentation of patient instruction in the identification and treatment of an allergic reaction. The patient needs to be given written instructions for when and how to use the prescribed epinephrine auto-injector, urged to carry epinephrine at all times, and to use it early in the course of a reaction, as lack of epinephrine administration can prove catastrophic [4,5,72]. *Up to a third of food-allergic patients experiencing moderate to severe reactions may develop biphasic reactions.* Therefore, all patients must seek professional medical care after using epinephrine, even if symptoms appear to have resolved [50,70]. They must remain under observation for 4–6 hours, as a precaution. Patients should be warned that, while an H1 antihistamine may ease symptoms of itching and urticaria, this medication is not a substitute for epinephrine. Likewise, asthma medications should not be used in place of epinephrine.

In the United States, many states do not allow Emergency Medical Technical (EMT), Basic EMTs, who represent 72% of all emergency medical service personnel, to carry and administer epinephrine. The EMT Basics are usually the first to arrive in response to a 911 call. Patients should be advised to call their rescue squad ahead of time, warn them of their need for epinephrine in case of a medical emergency, and set up an acceptable safety net. In some cases, if they tell the 911-dispatcher that they need epinephrine, an Advanced Life Support (ALS) vehicle and paramedics will be sent. All ALS vehicles in the United States are staffed by paramedics who can carry and administer epinephrine.

Prevention of food allergy

In addition to allergen avoidance, prevention of food allergy may include preventing sensitization to allergens by means of early allergen avoidance, as discussed further in Chapter 38, administering drugs to allow ingestion of the food culprit, and altering established food sensitivity through immunological modification.

Prevention of sensitization

Since 1936, when Grulee and Sanford reported that infants who were breast-fed developed less eczema than those who received cow's milk, the idea of manipulating the infant's diet to decrease the development of allergic disease has drawn great attention [73]. This topic has been extensively reviewed [74–76]. The picture that emerges does not present a strong argument for the success of this approach [76].

Studies performed primarily in Sweden have shown that neither avoidance nor ingestion of large amounts of cow's milk or egg during the third trimester of pregnancy affect the development of atopic disease from birth to 5 years of age [77–79]. Many studies have found that dietary intervention after delivery may result in a lower incidence of food allergy and atopic dermatitis by age 12–24 months [77,80–85]. Such dietary intervention has included modalities such as strict breast-feeding combined with avoidance of highly allergenic foods by the lactating mother, or the use of protein hydrolysate formula instead of breast-feeding and diet regulation. Zeiger *et al.* published an outcome study on 165 children aged 7 years who were at high risk to develop atopic disease [86]. These children had been followed since birth in a prospective randomized-controlled study of food allergen avoidance. In the prophylaxis group, the mother had avoided cow's milk, egg, and peanut in the last trimester of pregnancy and throughout lactation, and the infant had avoided cow's milk until age 1, eggs until age 2, and fish until age 3 years. The control infants followed standard infant feeding practices. Although a significant reduction in food allergy and atopic dermatitis was noted in the prophylaxis group by age 1 year, this effect had faded by age 2 years and disappeared by age 4 years [80,87]. By age 7 years, no difference was found in the development of food allergy or any other atopic disease in either group [86]. Even in carefully designed studies, it appears that dietary manipulation might lessen the frequency of food allergy during infancy – a time when it may be quite troublesome – but it does not seem to affect the eventual outcome of food allergy, and has not resulted in any decrease in the frequency of respiratory allergic diseases [84,86,88]. Prophylactic feeding with soy formula has not been found to be effective in preventing the development of food allergy [89].

The American Academy of Pediatrics policy statement titled, "Hypoallergenic Infant Formulas" recommends, "Infants at high risk for developing allergy, identified by a strong (biparental, parent, and sibling) family history of allergy may benefit from exclusive breast-feeding or hypoallergenic formula or possibly a partial hydrolysate formula." For these infants, solid foods should not be introduced until 6 months of age. Dairy products should not be introduced until age 1; eggs at age 2; and peanuts, tree nuts, and fish at age 3 years [90]. However, new guidelines will be released soon that are similar to what has been recommended in Europe [84], which do not promote allergen exclusion diets.

Drug treatment

Although the major emphasis in preventing food allergy involves avoidance with instructions for treatment if accidental ingestion occurs, it is not always possible to avoid a food entity completely. It would be desirable to have a drug that could be taken either before deliberate ingestion of a food or on a regular basis to decrease reaction to an accidentally or episodically ingested food, but no such drug is available at the present time. As discussed further in Chapter 42, Traditional Chinese Herbal Medicines may provide a means of treating patients prophylactically in certain "high-risk" situations.

Allergen immunotherapy

Allergen immunotherapy remains a time-honored treatment for allergy. In view of the severe and persistent nature of peanut allergy, it was hoped that a trial of immunotherapy could alter the natural course of this condition. Oppenheimer *et al.* reported the results of a double-blind, placebo-controlled study in three subjects with anaphylactic sensitivity to peanuts that underwent rush desensitization with peanut allergen [91]. A follow-up study of this group 1 month after rush immunotherapy revealed a 10- to 100-fold reduction in prick skin test sensitivity and a 2- to 20-fold increase in antigen dose on double-blind, placebo-controlled challenge [92]. Both rush and maintenance immunotherapies were associated with a significant frequency of generalized reactions; 23% during the build-up phase and 37% during maintenance. It was concluded that traditional immunotherapy was not feasible for the treatment of food allergy. Recently there has been renewed interest in oral immunotherapy [93–95] and sublingual immunotherapy [96], and although promising, more placebo-controlled trials are necessary to determine the efficacy of these forms of therapy. In addition, a number of novel immunotherapeutic strategies, including anti-IgE therapy [97], use of recombinant "engineered" proteins [98], etc. are being investigated, as discussed in Chapter 42.

Summary

The diagnosis of food allergy impacts the patient, family, and other caregivers. Education regarding label reading, identification of symptoms, and a written emergency action plan should be given to all patients with food allergies. Access to newsletters such as *Food Allergy News* (published by FAAN; Fairfax, VA), warning jewelry (MedicAlert, Turlock, CA), and careful planning are all essential in managing food allergy and allowing the patient to receive the education and emotional support necessary for managing food allergies. At present, efforts to prevent sensitization to foods or to allow the deliberate ingestion of food allergens with drug pre-treatment remain at the experimental stage, as does the use of allergen immunotherapy to desensitize the food-allergic patient.

References

1 Hefle SL, Nordlee JA, Taylor SL. Allergenic foods. *Crit Rev Food Sci Nutr* 1996;36:S69–89.

2 James JM, Burks AW. Food-associated gastrointestinal disease. *Curr Opin Pediatr* 1996;8:471–5.

3 Vander Leek TK, Liu AH, Stefanski K, *et al.* The natural history of peanut allergy in young children and its association with serum peanut-specific IgE. *J Pediatr* 2000;137:749–55.

4 Sampson HA, Mendelson L, Rosen JP. Fatal and near-fatal anaphylactic reactions to food in children and adolescents. *N Engl J Med* 1992;327:380–4.

5 Bock SA, Munoz-Furlong A, Sampson HA. Fatalities due to anaphylactic reactions to foods. *J Allergy Clin Immunol* 2001;107:191–3.

6 Rhim GS, McMorris MS. School readiness for children with food allergies. *Ann Allergy Asthma Immunol* 2001;86:172–6.

7 Yunginger JW, Sweeney KG, Sturner WQ, *et al.* Fatal food-induced anaphylaxis. *JAMA* 1988;260:1450–2.

8 Meff E. Hatfield woman's allergy reaction rare, but deadly. *Reporter Thursday*, A4, 12-15-1994.

9 Dominguez C, Ojeda I, Crespo JF, *et al.* Allergic reactions following skin contact with fish. *Allergy Asthma Proc* 1996;17:83–7.

10 Joshi P, Mofidi S, Sicherer SH. Interpretation of commercial food ingredient labels by parents of food-allergic children. *J Allergy Clin Immunol* 2002;109:1019–21.

11 Regenstein JM, Regenstein CE. Kosher foods and allergies. *Food Allergy News* 1994;1(7).

12 Gern JE, Yang E, Evrard HM, Sampson HA. Allergic reactions to milk-contaminated "nondairy" products. *N Engl J Med* 1991;324:976–9.

13 Shank FR. Notice to manufacturers: label declaration of allergenic substances in foods, 6-10-1996. US Food and Drug Administration Center for Food Safety and Applied Nutrition.

14 Hefle SL, Furlong TJ, Niemann L, *et al.* Consumer attitudes and risks associated with packaged foods having advisory labeling regarding the presence of peanuts. *J Allergy Clin Immunol* 2007;120:171–6.

15 Taylor SL, Munoz-Furlong A. *Understanding Food Labels*. Fairfax, VA: Food Allergy & Anaphylaxis Network, 1994.

16 Furlong TJ, DeSimone J, Sicherer SH. Peanut and tree nut allergic reactions in restaurants and other food establishments. *J Allergy Clin Immunol* 2001;108:867–70.

17 Koerner CB. Diet dilemas. *Food Allergy News* 1993;2(6).

18 Taylor SL. Choose your ice cream flavor wisely. *Food Allergy News* 1995;4(7).

19 FARRP. Notes from FARRP Meeting, 2006.

20 Food Allergy & Anaphylaxis Network. *It Only Takes One Bite.* 1993. Fairfax, VA: Food Allergy & Anaphylaxis Network.

21 Sicherer SH, Noone SA, Munoz-Furlong A. The impact of childhood food allergy on quality of life. *Ann Allergy Asthma Immunol* 2001;87:461–4.

22 Marklund B, Ahlstedt S, Nordstrom G. Health-related quality of life in food hypersensitive schoolchildren and their families: parents' perceptions. *Health Qual Life Outcome* 2006;4:48.

23 Bollinger ME, Dahlquist LM, Mudd K, *et al.* The impact of food allergy on the daily activities of children and their families. *Ann Allergy Asthma Immunol* 2006;96:415–21.

24 FAAN Member, 2006.

25 Sampson MA, Munoz-Furlong A, Sicherer SH. Risk-taking and coping strategies of adolescents and young adults with food allergy. *J Allergy Clin Immunol* 2006;117:1440–5.

26 Nowak-Wegrzyn A, Conover-Walker MK, Wood RA. Food-allergic reactions in schools and preschools. *Arch Pediatr Adolesc Med* 2001;155:790–5.

27 Weiss C, Munoz-Furlong A, Furlong TJ, Arbit J. Impact of food allergies on school nursing practice. *J Sch Nurs* 2004;20:268–78.

28 Simonte SJ, Ma S, Mofidi S, Sicherer SH. Relevance of casual contact with peanut butter in children with peanut allergy. *J Allergy Clin Immunol* 2003;112:180–2.

29 Perry TT, Conover-Walker MK, Pomes A, *et al.* Distribution of peanut allergen in the environment. *J Allergy Clin Immunol* 2004;113:973–6.

30 Sicherer SH, Furlong TJ, DeSimone J, Sampson HA. The US Peanut and Tree Nut Allergy Registry: characteristics of reactions in schools and day care. *J Pediatr* 2001;138:560–5.

31 McIntyre CL, Sheetz AH, Carroll CR, Young MC. Administration of epinephrine for life-threatening allergic reactions in school settings. *Pediatrics* 2005;116:1134–40.

32 National Association of School Nurses. *Position Statement: Individual Health Care Plans*, 2003.

33 The Food Allergy & Anaphylaxis Network. *Schools: What's New?* November 2007. http://www.foodallergy.org/advocacy/advocacy-schools.html.

34 United States Department of Education OfCR. The Civil Rights of Students with Hidden Disabilities under Section 504 of the Rehabilitation Act of 1973, 1973.

35 Duncanson J, Freed DA. Allergy to nuts kills teen on school trip. *Toronto Star*, A1, A11, 7-19-1994.

36 Food Allergy & Anaphylaxis Network. *Restaurant Program*. 2006. Fairfax, VA, Food Allergy & Anaphylaxis Network.

37 Munoz-Furlong A. Dining tips and strategies. *Food Allergy News* 1993;1(7).

38 Hoffman SGC. Fatal allergy suspected; student reacts after egg roll. *Cincinnati Enquirer*, C1, C4, 3-7-1995.

39 Munoz-Furlong A. *Travel Guide*. Fairfax, VA: Food Allergy & Anaphylaxis Network, 1994.

40 Sampson HA, Munoz-Furlong A, Campbell RL, *et al*. Second symposium on the definition and management of anaphylaxis: summary report. *J Allergy Clin Immunol* 2006;117(2):391–7.

41 Pastorello EA, Ortolani C, Farioli L, *et al*. Allergenic cross-reactivity among peach, apricot, plum, and cherry in patients with oral allergy syndrome: an *in vivo* and *in vitro* study. *J Allergy Clin Immunol* 1994;944:699–707.

42 Settipane GA. Anaphylactic deaths in asthmatic patients. *Allergy Proc* 1989;10:271–4.

43 Yunginger JW, Squillace DL, Jones RT, Helm RM. Fatal anaphylactic reactions induced by peanuts. *Allergy Proc* 1989;10:249–53.

44 Sampson HA. Peanut anaphylaxis. *J Allergy Clin Immunol* 1990;86:1–3.

45 Patel L, Radivan FS, David TJ. Management of anaphylactic reactions to food. *Arch Dis Child* 1994;71:370–5.

46 Hourihane JO, Warner JO. Management of anaphylactic reactions to food. *Arch Dis Child* 1995;72:274.

47 Sicherer SH, Simons FE. Quandaries in prescribing an emergency action plan and self-injectable epinephrine for first-aid management of anaphylaxis in the community. *J Allergy Clin Immunol* 2005;115:575–83.

48 Webb LM, Lieberman P. Anaphylaxis: a review of 601 cases. *Ann Allergy Asthma Immunol* 2006;97:39–43.

49 Lieberman P, Camargo Jr CA, Bohlke K, *et al*. Epidemiology of anaphylaxis: findings of the American College of Allergy, Asthma and Immunology Epidemiology of Anaphylaxis Working Group. *Ann Allergy Asthma Immunol* 2006;97:596–602.

50 Sampson HA, Munoz-Furlong A, Bock SA, *et al*. Symposium on the definition and management of anaphylaxis: summary report. *J Allergy Clin Immunol* 2005;115:584–91.

51 Brown SG, Mullins RJ, Gold MS. Anaphylaxis: diagnosis and management. *Med J Aust* 2006;185:283–9.

52 Simons FE, Frew AJ, Ansotegui IJ, *et al*. Risk assessment in anaphylaxis: current and future approaches. *J Allergy Clin Immunol* 2007;120:S2–24.

53 Sampson HA, Munoz-Furlong A, Campbell RL, *et al*. Second symposium on the definition and management of anaphylaxis: summary report – *Second National Institute of Allergy and Infectious Disease/Food Allergy and Anaphylaxis Network Symposium*. *J Allergy Clin Immunol* 2006;117:391–7.

54 Simons FE, Gu X, Silver NA, Simons KJ. EpiPen Jr versus EpiPen in young children weighing 15 to 30 kg at risk for anaphylaxis. *J Allergy Clin Immunol* 2002;109:171–5.

55 Saryan JA, O'Loughlin JM. Anaphylaxis in children. *Pediatr Ann* 1992;21:590–8.

56 Simons FE, Chan ES, Gu X, Simons KJ. Epinephrine for the out-of-hospital (first-aid) treatment of anaphylaxis in infants: Is the ampule/syringe/needle method practical? *J Allergy Clin Immunol* 2001;108:1040–4.

57 Warren JB, Doble N, Dalton N, Ewan PW. Systemic absorption of inhaled epinephrine. *Clin Pharmacol Ther* 1986;40:673–8.

58 Heilborn H, Hjemdahl P, Daleskog M, Adamsson U. Comparison of subcutaneous injection and high-dose inhalation of epinephrine – implications for self-treatment to prevent anaphylaxis. *J Allergy Clin Immunol* 1986;78:1174–9.

59 Simons FE, Gu X, Johnston LM, Simons KJ. Can epinephrine inhalations be substituted for epinephrine injection in children at risk for systemic anaphylaxis? *Pediatrics* 2000;106:1040–4.

60 Stark BJ, Sullivan TJ. Biphasic and protracted anaphylaxis. *J Allergy Clin Immunol* 1986;78:76–83.

61 Smith PL, Kagey-Sobotka A, Bleecker ER, *et al*. Physiologic manifestations of human anaphylaxis. *J Clin Invest* 1980;66:1072–80.

62 Delage C, Irey NS. Anaphylactic deaths: a clinicopathologic study of 43 cases. *J Forensic Sci* 1972;17:525–40.

63 Kaliner M, Sigler R, Summers R, Shelhamer JH. Effects of infused histamine: analysis of the effects of H-1 and H-2 histamine receptor antagonists on cardiovascular and pulmonary responses. *J Allergy Clin Immunol* 1981;68:365–71.

64 Kaliner M, Shelhamer JH, Ottesen EA. Effects of infused histamine: correlation of plasma histamine levels and symptoms. *J Allergy Clin Immunol* 1982;69:283–9.

65 Bochner BS, Lichtenstein LM. Anaphylaxis. *N Engl J Med* 1991;324:1785–90.

66 Ring J, Behrendt H. H1- and H2-antagonists in allergic and pseudoallergic diseases. *Clin Exp Allergy* 1990;20:43–9.

67 Kelly JS, Prielipp RC. Is cimetidine indicated in the treatment of acute anaphylactic shock? *Anesth Analg* 1990;71:104–5.

68 Brown SG. Cardiovascular aspects of anaphylaxis: implications for treatment and diagnosis. *Curr Opin Allergy Clin Immunol* 2005;5:359–64.

69 Perkin RM, Anas NG. Mechanisms and management of anaphylactic shock not responding to traditional therapy. *Ann Allergy* 1985;54:202–8.

70 The diagnosis and management of anaphylaxis: an updated practice parameter1. *J Allergy Clin Immunol* 2005;115: S483–523.

71 Lieberman P. Anaphylaxis. *Med Clin North Am* 2006;90:77–95, viii.

72 Bock SA, Munoz-Furlong A, Sampson HA. Further fatalities caused by anaphylactic reactions to food, 2001–2006. *J Allergy Clin Immunol* 2007;119:1016–8.

73 Grulee C, Sanford H. The influence of breast feeding and artificial feeding in infantile eczema. *J Pediatr* 1936;9:223–5.

74 Kramer MS, Kakuma R. Maternal dietary antigen avoidance during pregnancy or lactation, or both, for preventing or treating atopic disease in the child. *Cochrane Database Syst Rev* 2006;3: CD000133.

75 Zeiger R. Breast-feeding and dietary avoidance. In: de Weck A, Sampson H (Eds.) *Intestinal Immunology and Food Allergy.* New York: Raven Press, 1995:203–22.

76 Muraro A, Dreborg S, Halken S, *et al.* Dietary prevention of allergic diseases in infants and small children. Part II. Evaluation of methods in allergy prevention studies and sensitization markers. Definitions and diagnostic criteria of allergic diseases. *Pediatr Allergy Immunol* 2004;15:196–205.

77 Lilja G, Dannaeus A, Falth-Magnusson K, *et al.* Immune response of the atopic woman and foetus: effects of high- and low-dose food allergen intake during late pregnancy. *Clin Allergy* 1988;18:131–42.

78 Lilja G, Dannaeus A, Foucard T, *et al.* Effects of maternal diet during late pregnancy and lactation on the development of atopic diseases in infants up to 18 months of age – *in-vivo* results. *Clin Exp Allergy* 1989;19:473–9.

79 Falth-Magnusson K, Kjellman NI. Allergy prevention by maternal elimination diet during late pregnancy – a 5-year follow-up of a randomized study. *J Allergy Clin Immunol* 1992;89:709–13.

80 Zeiger RS, Heller S, Mellon MH, *et al.* Effect of combined maternal and infant food-allergen avoidance on development of atopy in early infancy: a randomized study. *J Allergy Clin Immunol* 1989;84:72–89.

81 Halken S, Host A, Hansen LG, Osterballe O. Preventive effect of feeding high-risk infants a casein hydrolysate formula or an ultra-filtrated whey hydrolysate formula. A prospective, randomized, comparative clinical study. *Pediatr Allergy Immunol* 1993;4:173–81.

82 Businco L, Dreborg S, Einarsson R, *et al.* Hydrolysed cow's milk formulae. Allergenicity and use in treatment and prevention. An ESPACI position paper. European Society of Pediatric Allergy and Clinical Immunology. *Pediatr Allergy Immunol* 1993;4:101–11.

83 Arshad SH, Matthews S, Gant C, Hide DW. Effect of allergen avoidance on development of allergic disorders in infancy. *Lancet* 1992;339:1493–7.

84 Muraro A, Dreborg S, Halken S, *et al.* Dietary prevention of allergic diseases in infants and small children. Part III. Critical review of published peer-reviewed observational and interventional studies and final recommendations. *Pediatr Allergy Immunol* 2004;15:291–307.

85 von Berg A, Koletzko S, Filipiak-Pittroff B, *et al.* Certain hydrolyzed formulas reduce the incidence of atopic dermatitis but not that of asthma: three-year results of the German Infant Nutritional Intervention Study. *J Allergy Clin Immunol* 2007;119:718–25.

86 Zeiger RS, Heller S. The development and prediction of atopy in high-risk children: follow-up at age seven years in a prospective randomized study of combined maternal and infant food allergen avoidance. *J Allergy Clin Immunol* 1995;95:1179–90.

87 Zeiger RS, Heller S, Mellon MH, *et al.* Genetic and environmental factors affecting the development of atopy through age 4 in children of atopic parents: a prospective randomized study of food allergen avoidance. *Pediatr Allergy Immunol* 1992;3:110–27.

88 Sigurs N, Hattevig G, Kjellman B. Maternal avoidance of eggs, cow's milk, and fish during lactation: effect on allergic manifestations, skin-prick tests, and specific IgE antibodies in children at age 4 years. *Pediatrics* 1992;89:735–9.

89 Osborn DA, Sinn J. Soy formula for prevention of allergy and food intolerance in infants. *Cochrane Database Syst Rev* 2006;4:CD003741.

90 American Academy of Pediatrics. Committee on Nutrition. Hypoallergenic infant formulas. *Pediatrics* 2000;106:346–9.

91 Oppenheimer JJ, Nelson HS, Bock SA, *et al.* Treatment of peanut allergy with rush immunotherapy. *J Allergy Clin Immunol* 1992;90:256–62.

92 Nelson HS, Lahr J, Rule R, *et al.* Treatment of anaphylactic sensitivity to peanuts by immunotherapy with injections of aqueous peanut extract. *J Allergy Clin Immunol* 1997;99:744–51.

93 Patriarca G, Nucera E, Roncallo C, *et al.* Oral desensitizing treatment in food allergy: clinical and immunological results. *Aliment Pharmacol Ther* 2003;17:459–65.

94 Meglio P, Bartone E, Plantamura M, *et al.* A protocol for oral desensitization in children with IgE-mediated cow's milk allergy. *Allergy* 2004;59:980–7.

95 Morisset M, Moneret-Vautrin DA, Guenard L, *et al.* Oral desensitization in children with milk and egg allergies obtains recovery in a significant proportion of cases. A randomized study in 60 children with cow's milk allergy and 90 children with egg allergy. *Allergy Immunol (Paris)* 2007;39:12–9.

96 Enrique E, Pineda F, Malek T, *et al.* Sublingual immunotherapy for hazelnut food allergy: a randomized, double-blind, placebo-controlled study with a standardized hazelnut extract. *J Allergy Clin Immunol* 2005;116:1073–9.

97 Leung DY, Sampson HA, Yunginger JW, *et al.* Effect of anti-IgE therapy in patients with peanut allergy. *N Engl J Med* 2003;348:986–93.

98 Li XM, Srivastava K, Grishin A, *et al.* Persistent protective effect of heat-killed *Escherichia coli* producing "engineered," recombinant peanut proteins in a murine model of peanut allergy. *J Allergy Clin Immunol* 2003;112:159–67.

CHAPTER 37

The Natural History of Food Allergy

Robert A. Wood

KEY CONCEPTS

- The natural history of food allergy is generally positive.
- Natural history varies widely from one food to another.
- Peanut, tree nuts, fish, and shellfish allergies tend to be most persistent.
- Natural history varies widely for individual foods from one individual to another.
- Regular follow-up is important to monitor food-allergic patients over time.

Introduction

The natural history of food allergy refers to both the acquisition of allergic sensitivities and their natural course over time. Food allergy most often begins in the first 1–2 years of life with the process of sensitization, by which the immune system responds to specific food proteins, most often with the development of allergen-specific immunoglobulin E (IgE). Over time, most food allergy is lost, although allergy to some foods is more often long-lived. For example, while most milk and egg allergy is outgrown, most peanut and tree nut allergies are not. This chapter will review the development of food allergy and the natural history of food sensitivities over time.

When considering the natural history of food allergy, it is critical that the criteria used to define food allergy be carefully considered. Some studies report solely on rates of sensitization while others focus on clinical reactivity to specific foods. The definition of clinical reactivity is also not consistent between studies, with some relying solely on parental reports of food reactions, while others utilize food challenges and other more objective evidence of true food allergy. These details are important in that a history of an adverse food reaction, or even evidence of sensitization, does not necessarily mean that a patient will exhibit a clinical reaction upon exposure to that food. The specific criteria used to diagnose food allergy may therefore have a significant impact on the results of these studies, especially those used to measure the prevalence of food allergy.

Studies on the development of food allergy

Most food allergy is acquired in the first 1–2 years of life. The prevalence of food allergy peaks at 5–8% at 1 year of age and then falls progressively until late childhood, after which the prevalence remains stable at about 3.5% [1]. In this section studies on the development of food allergy will be reviewed.

Bock prospectively followed 480 children, recruited from a single pediatric practice, for the development of food allergy from birth through the age of 3 years [2]. Foods that were suspected of causing adverse reactions were eliminated from the diet and then reintroduced in either open or blinded challenges at regular intervals. Limited allergy testing was performed, so it was not possible to characterize the proportion of reactions that were IgE mediated. Overall, 28% of the children were reported to have an adverse food reaction and the reactions were confirmed by challenge in 8%. Eighty percent of these reactions occurred in the first year of life and the majority of the foods could be successfully reintroduced into the diet within 1 year of the onset of the allergy.

Another prevalence study was conducted in Finland in a cohort of 866 children who were followed for the occurrence of food allergy at ages 1, 2, 3, and 6 years [3]. The diagnosis of food allergy was based on a history of either rash or vomiting and all suspected reactions were confirmed by elimination and home re-challenge. Allergy testing was not otherwise conducted. Based on these criteria, the prevalence of adverse food reactions was 19% at age 1, 22% at age 2, 27% at age 3, and 8% at age 6 years. In order of prevalence, the foods most commonly implicated at all ages were citrus fruits, tomato, egg, strawberry, and fish.

Food Allergy: Adverse Reactions to Foods and Food Additives, 4th edition.
Edited by Dean D. Metcalfe, Hugh A. Sampson, and Ronald A. Simon.
© 2008 Blackwell Publishing, ISBN: 978-1-4501-5129-0.

An even larger cohort study was recently conducted in Norway [4–6]. For the first part of the study, a population-based cohort of 3623 children was followed from birth until the age of 2 years [3], during which parents completed questionnaires regarding adverse food reactions at 6-month intervals. The cumulative incidence of adverse food reactions was 35% by age 2 years, with milk being the single food item most commonly incriminated at 11.6%. The duration of the reactions was overall short, with approximately two-thirds of the reactions resolving within 6 months of their onset.

In the second phase of the study, those children who had persistent complaints of milk or egg allergy underwent a more detailed evaluation at the age of 2–2.5 years [5–6], including skin testing and open and double-blind oral challenges. The point prevalence of cow's milk and egg allergy or intolerance at the age of 2.5 years were estimated to be 1.1% and 1.6%, respectively. Most milk reactions were not IgE mediated and only 33% of parental reports of adverse milk reactions were confirmed, while most egg reactions were IgE mediated and 56% of parental reports were confirmed.

Host and Halken sought to determine the prevalence of milk allergy by prospectively following 1749 Danish children from birth through age 3 years [7]. The children were carefully evaluated by history, milk elimination, oral challenge, and skin tests or radioallergosorbent tests (RAST). Milk allergy was suspected in 117 children (6.7%) and confirmed in 39 (2.2%). Of those, 21 had IgE-mediated allergy and the remaining 18 were classified as non-IgE mediated. All milk allergy developed in the first year of life and most of the allergic children were able to tolerate milk by age 3 years (56% by age 1, 77% by age 2, and 87% by age 3 years). All children with non-IgE-mediated allergy were tolerant by age 3, compared to 75% with IgE-mediated allergy. Also of note, of those with IgE-mediated allergy, 35% had other food allergies by age 3 and 25% had other food allergies by age 10 years [8]. Those children were also more likely to develop inhalant allergies over time.

Tariq and colleagues followed a cohort of children for the development of peanut and tree nut sensitization through the age of 4 years [9]. All children born on the Isle of Wight in a 1-year period were recruited and evaluated at ages 1, 2, and 4 years. Fifteen (1.2%) of the 1218 children were sensitized to peanut or tree nuts. Thirteen were sensitive to peanut and six had had allergic reactions to peanut (0.5% of the population), while one child each had had a reaction to hazelnuts and cashews.

One final study of importance followed the development of sensitization to common food allergens in a large cohort of children, without clinical confirmation of food sensitivity. Two hundred and sixteen children from a birth cohort of 4082 children in the Multicenter Allergy Study conducted in Germany were assessed for allergy by RAST at 1, 2, 3, 5, and 6 years of age [10]. The overall annual incidence rates for food sensitization decreased from a peak of 10% at age

1 to 3% at age 6 years. Sensitization to egg and milk were most common at all ages, followed by wheat and soy. This study also found that there was a high rate of aeroallergen sensitization in children who began with food sensitivities, especially to egg [11–12]. Remarkably, if a child had both a positive family history of allergy and an egg-specific IgE level above 2 kU$_A$/l at the age of 12 months, there was a 78% positive predictive value and a 99% specificity for the development of inhalant allergen sensitivity by the age of 3 years [11].

Several points are worth emphasizing from these studies. First, suspected food allergy is extraordinarily common in early childhood, with at least one-fourth of all parents reporting one or more adverse food reactions. Second, adverse food reactions can be confirmed in 5–10% of young children with a peak prevalence at around 1 year of age. Third, most food allergy is lost over time. And finally, children who begin with one food allergy, especially if it is IgE mediated, have a very high chance of developing additional food allergies, as well as inhalant allergies. It is therefore critical that children with food allergy be identified as early as possible, both to initiate an appropriate diet for their existing allergies and to consider preventative measures that may help to reduce their chance of developing additional food allergies, as well as asthma and allergic rhinitis.

Studies on the loss of food allergy

Most food allergy is indeed lost over time. The process of outgrowing food allergies, by which a patient becomes completely tolerant to a food that had previously caused a reaction, varies a great deal for different foods and among individual patients. In the study by Bock described above [2], almost all of the adverse food reactions had been lost by the age of 3 years. Among these, there were 11 children with confirmed milk allergy and 14 children with probable milk allergy, all of whom were able to tolerate milk by the age of 3 years. The median duration of adverse reactions to milk was in fact only 9 months. In a second study by Bock, nine children who had had severe reactions to milk, egg, and/or soy at 2–15 months of age were followed for 3–9 years [13]. Over time, three of the nine children were able to fully tolerate the offending food, four could tolerate small amounts, and two continued to have reactions with small exposures.

Dannaeus and Inganas followed 82 children between the ages of 6 months and 14 years with a variety of food allergies for a period of 2–5 years [14]. Of the 12 children who were allergic to milk, 4 developed complete tolerance, 7 had reduced sensitivity, and only 1 remained unchanged by the completion of their follow-up. Fifty-five children had egg allergy, of whom 20 developed complete tolerance, 24 had reduced sensitivity, and 11 remained unchanged. The results were very different for fish and peanut/tree nut allergy, with only 5 of 32 patients with fish allergy and 0 of 35 patients with peanut or tree nut allergy developing tolerance.

Sampson and Scanlon followed a group of 75 patients between the ages of 3 and 18 years with atopic dermatitis and food allergy that had been diagnosed by skin testing, RASTs, and double-blind, placebo-controlled food challenges (DBPCFCs) [15]. Patients were re-challenged yearly to each of the foods that had previously elicited a positive challenge and after 1 year, 19 of the 75 had lost all food allergy, including 15 of 45 patients allergic to one food and 4 of 21 allergic to two foods. A total of 38 of 121 specific food sensitivities had been lost after 1 year. After 2 years, an additional 4 of 44 patients lost their food allergy, while none of the 20 patients re-challenged after 3 years had a negative challenge. The results for specific foods after 1–2 years of follow-up are represented in Table 37.1, showing that egg allergy had been lost in 24%, milk in 19%, soy in 50%, wheat in 33%, and peanut in 20%. In a similar study by Sampson, follow-up data was provided on 40 of 113 patients with food allergy and atopic dermatitis

1–2 years after their original diagnosis [16]. In that study, egg allergy had been outgrown in 14 of 20 patients (30%), compared to 4 of 7 with milk allergy (57%), 1 of 4 with wheat allergy (25%), and 2 of 3 with soy allergy (67%).

Shek *et al.* monitored food-specific IgE levels in 88 patients with egg allergy and 49 patients with cow's milk allergy (CMA) who also underwent repeated double-blind, placebo controlled [17]. Twenty-eight of the 66 egg-allergic and 16 of the 33 milk-allergic patients lost their allergy over time. For egg, the decrease in serum IgE (sIgE) levels was significantly related to the probability of developing clinical tolerance, with the duration between challenges having an influence. For milk, there was also a significant relationship between the decrease in sIgE levels and the probability of developing tolerance to milk but no significant contribution with regard to time. Stratification into two age groups, those below 4 years of age and those above 4 years of age at the time of first challenge, had an effect, with the younger age group being more likely to develop clinical tolerance in relation to the rate of decrease in sIgE. The median food sIgE level at diagnosis was significantly less for the group developing tolerance to egg, and a similar trend was seen for milk allergy ($p=0.06$).

Milk allergy

The natural history of milk allergy has been most extensively studied [18–27]. However, as summarized in Table 37.2, the results of these studies do not provide a completely clear and consistent picture.

Dannaeus and Johansson followed 47 infants with milk allergy for 6 months to 4 years [19]. In children with immediate-type, IgE-mediated reactions, 29% developed complete tolerance to milk over the course of the study,

Table 37.1 The persistence or loss of specific food sensitivities over 1–2 years in children with atopic dermatitis

Allergen	Total	Challenge	
		Positive	Negative
Egg	59	45 (76%)	14 (24%)
Milk	21	17 (81%)	4 (19%)
Soy	10	5 (50%)	5 (50%)
Wheat	6	4 (67%)	2 (33%)
Peanut	10	8 (80%)	2 (20%)
Other	15	5 (33%)	10 (66%)

Reproduced from Dannaeus A and Inganas M [14], with permission from Blackwell Publishing.

Table 37.2 Studies on the natural history of milk allergy

Author (reference)	N	Age at diagnosis	Duration of follow-up	Percent tolerant at completion of study	
				IgE-mediated (or immediate-type) reactions	Non-IgE-mediated (or delayed-type) reactions
Dannaeus [14]	47	14 days to 20 months	6 months to 4 years (mean 28 months)	29%	74%
Host [6]	39	0–12 months	Up to age 3 years	76%	100%
Hill [19]	47	3–66 months	6–39 months (mean 16 months)	40%	38%
Bishop [21]	100	1–98 months (median 16 months)	5 years	67%	86%*
Hill [22]	98	4–100 months (median 24 months)	6–73 months (mean 24 months)	22%	59%
James [26]	29	3–14 years (median 3 years)	3 years	38%	NA
Saarinen [23]	116	Mean 7 months	Up to 8.6 years	85%	100%
Skripak [24]	807	1–209 months (median 13 months)	4–285 months (median 55 months)	19% at age 4, 42% at age 8, 79% at age 16	NA

*Combines immediate and late reactors.

compared to 74% of those with delayed-type, non-IgE-mediated reactions. The trend for non-IgE-mediated milk allergy to be outgrown more quickly than IgE-mediated allergy has been demonstrated in most studies, including the study by Host and Halken [7], in which the vast majority of all children were milk tolerant by age 3 years.

A series of studies on milk allergy have been published by Hill and colleagues [20–23]. In their first natural history study [20], 47 children from 3 to 66 months of age with challenge-confirmed milk allergy were followed for a median of 16 months (range 6–39 months). Overall, 38% of the children were able to tolerate milk by the completion of the study. When the children were divided into groups based on having immediate, intermediate, or late milk reactions, tolerance occurred in 40%, 42%, and 25%, respectively. Milk-specific IgE, IgA, IgM, and IgG levels were measured and no specific immunologic changes were clearly associated with the development of milk tolerance.

In the second study from this group, a cohort of 100 children with challenge-confirmed milk allergy were followed for 5 years [22]. Overall, milk tolerance had occurred in 28% of patients by age 2, 56% by age 4, and 78% by age 6 years. When the children were again divided into groups based on having immediate, intermediate, or late reactions, tolerance had occurred by the completion of the study in 67%, 87%, and 83%, respectively. Adverse reactions to other foods were also common in this cohort, occurring to egg in 58%, soy in 47%, and peanut in 34%. Most children also developed one or more other atopic diseases, such that at the completion of the study 40% had asthma, 43% had allergic rhinitis, and 21% had eczema.

A final study from this group followed 98 children with milk allergy for a median of 2 years (range 6–72 months) [23]. In this study, the children were divided into two groups: 69 had IgE antibodies to milk with immediate-type reactions and 29 had delayed-type reactions. Over the period of follow-up, 15 of 69 (22%) with IgE-mediated disease developed tolerance, compared to 17 of the 29 (59%) with non-IgE-mediated reactions. For those children with IgE-mediated milk sensitivity, the development of tolerance was associated with lower milk-specific IgE levels at the time of diagnosis and at study completion, as well a significant reduction in their milk skin test reactivity. However, it is also important to note that 8 of the 15 who developed tolerance still had strongly positive skin tests at that time.

In the largest prospective study to date, Saarinen et al. followed 118 children diagnosed with milk allergy from a birth cohort study of over 6000 children [24]. Eighty-six (73%) had IgE-mediated milk and of those, 51% had become tolerant by age 2 years and 85% were tolerant at age 8.6 years. All children with IgE-negative CMA were tolerant by age 5.0 years. By age 8.6 years, children with IgE-positive CMA more frequently had asthma, rhinoconjunctivitis, atopic eczema, and sensitization to any allergen than control subjects. They concluded that IgE-mediated milk allergy often persists to school age and is a risk factor for other atopy, while non-IgE-mediated milk allergy is a benign infantile condition.

In the largest overall study to date, our group retrospectively collected data on 807 patients with IgE-mediated milk allergy [25]. Patients were considered to have become tolerant if they passed a challenge, or experienced no reactions in the past 12 months and had a cow's milk IgE level $<3\,kU_A/l$. Using that definition, the rates of resolution were 19% at age 4, 42% by age 8, 64% by age 12, and 79% by age 16 years. Patients with persistent allergy had higher cow's milk IgE levels at all ages up to age 16 years. The highest cow's milk IgE for each patient, defined as "peak" CM-IgE, was found to be highly predictive of outcome. Of note, some patients developed tolerance during adolescence, indicating that follow-up and re-evaluation of CMA patients is an important component of their care.

Three additional studies have focused specifically on the immunologic changes associated with the development of milk tolerance. From a group of 80 milk-allergic children, James and Sampson reported on a subset of 29 who were followed for a minimum of 3 years [27]. Evaluations included annual DBPCFCs, skin tests, and measurement of casein-specific and β-lactoglobulin-specific IgE, IgG, IgG1, and IgG4 antibody concentrations. All children had specific IgE to milk as well as positive skin tests and 80% had atopic dermatitis. The median age at the time of study entry was 3 years with a range from 1 month to 11 years. Of the 29 children, 11 (38%) developed tolerance at a median age of 7 years. In those who became tolerant to milk, specific IgE and IgE/IgG ratios to both milk proteins were lower initially and decreased significantly over time.

Two even more detailed studies on antibody responses to milk proteins and the development of milk tolerance were reported by Chatchatee et al. [28,29]. In the first study, IgE- and IgG-binding epitopes on α_{s1}-casein were identified using the sera of 24 milk-allergic children, and the patterns of epitope recognition were analyzed to determine if they might help predict the natural history of milk allergy. When comparing epitope recognition of patients with persistent milk allergy to younger children likely to outgrow their allergy, they found that two IgE-binding regions were recognized by all of the older children with persistent milk allergy but none of the younger children. In the second study, a similar analysis was performed of IgE- and IgG-binding epitopes on β- and κ-casein in milk-allergic patients. Three IgE-binding regions on β-casein and six on κ-casein were recognized by the majority of patients in the older age group but none of the younger patients. In addition to a more clear definition of the antibody responses to specific milk proteins/epitopes, these studies suggest that it may eventually be possible to develop clinical tests, in essence epitope-specific IgE levels that may help to identify children at risk for more persistent milk allergy.

A summary of studies on the natural history of milk allergy is presented in Table 37.2. As one examines this information, a somewhat confusing picture emerges. For example, in the study by Host and Halken [7], which in many ways is the best study on milk allergy yet performed, 76% of those with IgE-mediated milk allergy and 100% of those with non-IgE-mediated milk allergy were milk tolerant by the age of 3 years. These numbers are far higher than those presented in the other studies. The only numbers that approach those are from the study by Bishop et al. [21], although it took until age 6 for 78% of those children to become milk tolerant. The differences in these studies are almost certainly a result of selection biases. The study by Host and Halken was a population-based study that would therefore include all degrees of milk sensitivity, whereas the other studies included children who were under the care of an allergy specialist, indicating that they may have had a more severe form of milk allergy. For the primary care physician, it is therefore likely that the more optimistic numbers will be correct, while the allergist might expect a slower rate of loss of milk allergy in their patients over time, as well as a higher percentage of patients with persistent milk allergy.

Egg allergy

Only two studies have specifically focused on the natural history of egg allergy. Ford and Taylor followed 25 children from 7 months to 9 years of age (median 17 months) with challenge-confirmed egg allergy for 2–2.5 years [30]. Egg allergy resolved in 11 of 25 (44%) and persisted in the other 14. Skin tests were negative or diminished in size in those who lost their egg reactivity compared to those with ongoing reactivity. This is similar to the 36% of children in the Dannaeus study [14] who became egg tolerant, although they also reported that an additional 44% had become less sensitive over time. The largest and most recent prospective study of the natural history of egg allergy is from a Spanish cohort of 58 children, in which 50% of egg-allergic children developed tolerance by age 4–4.5 years [31]. These data would agree with the clinical observation that a slight majority of egg allergy is outgrown by the school-age years.

Peanut allergy

Until recently, the dogma had been that peanut allergy is rarely, if ever, outgrown and studies had in fact suggested that that was the case. For example, Bock followed 32 children, 1–14 years of age, with challenge-confirmed peanut allergy over a period of 2–14 years and found that 24 had had accidental peanut exposures/reactions and no patients appeared to outgrow their allergy [32].

Evidence that a subset of children with peanut allergy may indeed lose their sensitivity was first reported by Hourihane et al. [33]. They evaluated 230 children with a diagnosis of peanut allergy and performed oral challenges in 120. A total of 22 children between the ages of 2 and 9 years had a negative challenge, equaling 18% of those challenged or 9.8% of the total group. They found that a negative challenge was associated with a smaller skin test size and fewer allergies to other foods compared to those with persistent peanut allergy.

Spergel et al. retrospectively reviewed 293 patients with a diagnosis of peanut allergy [34]. All families were offered a peanut challenge to confirm their diagnosis and a total of 33 children between the ages of 18 months and 8 years with a convincing history of peanut allergy and a positive skin test were actually challenged. Of those, 14 passed their challenge and were felt to have resolved their peanut allergy. None of the 5 patients with a history of peanut anaphylaxis developed tolerance, compared to 9 of 17 with a history of urticaria and 4 of 10 with a history of atopic dermatitis. In addition, those developing tolerance had significantly smaller skin test responses than the 19 with a positive challenge.

Skolnick et al. performed a detailed evaluation of 223 children with a diagnosis of peanut allergy [35], including an oral peanut challenge in those who had not had a reaction in the past year and who had a peanut-specific IgE (PN-IgE) $<20\,kU_A/l$. As shown in Table 37.3, 97 children were not challenged because they were considered to still be peanut allergic based on either a history of a recent reaction or a PN-IgE level $>20\,kU_A/l$ [36], and an additional 41 children were eligible to be challenged but declined. Of the 85 children who were challenged, 48 (21.5% of the total group) passed the challenge and were felt to have outgrown their peanut allergy. The PN-IgE level as measured by UniCap® (Phadia; Uppsala, Sweden) was the best predictor of a negative challenge, with 61% of those with a PN-IgE level $<5\,KU_A/l$ and 67% with a level $<2\,KU_A/l$ passing their challenge. The presence of other atopic diseases and the severity of initial peanut reactions did not predict the probability of losing peanut allergy, and even one patient who had had severe anaphylaxis with his initial reaction outgrew his allergy.

A final study on the natural history of peanut allergy was reported by VanderLeek et al. [37]. Eighty-five children with peanut allergy were studied, including 55 who were followed for at least 5 years. Among those patients, 58% who had been followed for 5 years and 75% who had been followed for at least 10 years had had at least one reaction due to an accidental exposure. In addition, the majority of these reactions were more severe than initial reactions and 52% included potentially life-threatening symptoms. Severe reactions were associated with higher PN-IgE levels compared to those with purely cutaneous reactions. The only positive note from this study was that four children did outgrow their peanut allergy.

Peanut allergy is therefore likely to be lifelong for most but not all patients. Given the fact that a substantial minority of patients do appear to lose their sensitivity over time, it is appropriate to re-evaluate children with peanut allergy on

Table 37.3 Characteristics of patients with persistent and resolved peanut allergy

	Passed challenge (N = 48)	Failed challenge (N = 37)	Unable to be challenged (N = 97)	Refused challenge (N = 41)	Total (N = 223)
Age at diagnosis					
Range	8 months to 12 years	6 months to 4 years	2 months to 10 years	8 months to 15 years	2 months to 15 years
Median (year)	1.5	1.5	1.5	2	1.5
Current age (year)					
Range	4 to 17.5	4 to 13	4 to 20	4 to 16.5	4 to 20
Median	6	6.5	7	7	6.5
PN-IgE at diagnosis*					
Range	<0.35 to 52.9	1.8 to 24.4	4.5 to >100	0.64 to >100	<0.35 to >100
Median	2.2	2.91	>100	6.27	19.8
Current PN-IgE*					
Range	<0.35 to 20.4	<0.35 to 18.2	16.8 to >100	<0.35 to 16.9	<0.35 to >100
Median	0.69	2.06	>100	4.98	10.7

PN-IgE refers to peanut-specific IgE level in kU_A/l. A level <0.35 is considered negative and any level over 100 is reported as >100.
Reproduced from Ford RPK and Taylor B [30], with permission from the BMJ Publishing Group.

a regular basis. Those patients who have not had reactions in the past 1–2 years and who have a low PN-IgE level should be considered for an oral challenge in a supervised setting. If a patient is still peanut allergic by late childhood or adolescence, it is very unlikely that they will subsequently lose their allergy and regular retesting may no longer be warranted.

One additional issue in the natural history of peanut allergy relates to the potential for the recurrence of the allergy in some patients with resolved peanut allergy.

Busse et al. first reported such recurrences and estimated a recurrence rate of 14% after 3 of their 21 patients had recurrences [38]. Each of these patients reported consuming peanut intermittently in small amounts after passing a food challenge to peanut, and then reacquired their allergy 1–2 years later. Next, Fleischer et al. surveyed 64 patients who had outgrown their peanut allergy to see whether patients ate peanut products since passing their challenge, what types of peanut-containing foods they ate, and how frequently they ate them, and whether there were any allergic reactions to peanuts [39]. They found that although 97% had eaten peanut since passing their challenge, ongoing aversion to peanut is common, with 70% of patients eating peanut infrequently and in small amounts. Two of the 64 patients had suspicious allergic reactions to peanut.

Because of concerns that more patients might have had recurrences and did not know it because of their ongoing peanut avoidance, Fleischer et al. invited all patients from their center who had outgrown peanut allergy to undergo re-evaluation, including questionnaires, skin tests, peanut-specific IgE levels, and DBPCFCs [40]. Of 68 patients, 47 continued to tolerate peanut, of which 34 ingested concentrated peanut products at least once per month and 13 ate peanut infrequently or in limited amounts but passed a DBPCFC. The status of 18 patients was indeterminate

because they ate peanut infrequently or in limited amounts and declined to have a DBPCFC. The overall recurrence rate was 7.9 (95% CI 1.7–21.4%). They concluded that children who outgrow peanut allergy are at risk for recurrence, and this risk is significantly higher for patients who continue to largely avoid peanut after resolution of their allergy. Based on these findings, they recommended that patients eat peanut frequently and carry epinephrine indefinitely until they have demonstrated ongoing peanut tolerance.

Tree nuts allergy

The study by Dannaeus [14] did include 26 patients with tree nut allergy, none of whom lost their sensitivity in a 2–5 year follow-up. Our group evaluated 278 patients with tree nut allergy, defined as a history of reaction on ingestion and evidence of tree nut-specific IgE or positive tree nut-specific IgE level but no history of ingestion [41]. If all current tree nut-specific IgE levels were <10 kU_A/l, DBPCFCs were offered. One hundred and one of the 278 (36%) had a history of acute reactions, 12 (12%) of whom had reactions to multiple tree nuts and 73 (63%) of whom had a history of moderate-to-severe reactions. Nine of 20 patients who had previously reacted to a tree nuts passed challenges, so that 9 (8.9%; 95% CI, 4–16%) of 101 patients with a history of prior tree nut reactions outgrew their allergy. Fourteen of 19 who had never ingested tree nuts but had detectable tree nut-specific IgE levels passed challenges. One hundred and sixty-one did not meet the challenge criteria, and 78 met the criteria but declined challenges. Fifty-eight percent with tree nut-specific IgE levels of 5 kU_A/l or less and 63% with tree nut IgE levels of 2 kU_A/l or less passed challenges. We concluded that approximately 9% of patients outgrow tree nut allergy, including some who had prior severe reactions.

Other foods

Far less has been published about the natural history of other food allergies. Among the other most common food allergens, it is clinically recognized that soy and wheat allergy are typically outgrown in the pre-school-age years, but no large studies have focused on the natural course of these food allergies. In the studies by Sampson of children with food allergy and atopic dermatitis (1516), soy allergy was outgrown in 50% and 67% of children over a 1–2 year follow-up, compared to 25% and 33% for wheat. The few children in the studies of Bock [2] and Host [7] who had soy and wheat allergy had lost these allergies by the age of 3 years. Hill *et al.* did report on 18 infants with intolerance to both soy and extensively hydrolyzed infant formulas through the age of 3 years [42]. However, while they report that two children were tolerant of soy by age 3 years, the true frequency of soy tolerance could not be determined since soy had still not been reintroduced to 13 children at the completion of the study.

As was noted above in a number of studies, adverse reactions to fruits, vegetables, and other cereal grains are typically very short-lived [2–3,14]. While some children do have severe, IgE-mediated allergies to these foods that may persist over time, for most children they can be successfully reintroduced into the diet within a period of 6–12 months. Many of these may in fact represent intolerances or irritant reactions than true allergy as well.

On the contrary, although actual studies are limited, it has been appreciated that allergies to fish, shellfish, and seeds are usually not outgrown. The study by Dannaeus [14] did include 32 children with fish allergy, of whom 5 became tolerant. One additional study followed 11 patients with shrimp allergy over a 2-year period and found that there were no significant changes in allergen-specific antibody levels over that period of time [43].

Food allergy in adults

Most study on the natural course of food allergy has logically involved children. The most common food sensitivities in adults include peanut, tree nuts, fish, and shellfish, all of which are most often lifelong. In fact, it is their persistent nature that makes them the most common food allergies in adults, in that most of these allergies are actually acquired in childhood and persist into adulthood.

One study, however, did focus on the natural history of food allergies in adults [44]. Twenty-three adults with allergies to a variety of foods underwent baseline DBPCFCs, in which clear reactions in 10 patients to a total of 13 food were identified. They were then placed on strict dietary avoidance of the offending food for 1–2 years and re-challenged. Five (38%) of the 13 previously offending foods were well tolerated, including milk in two patients

and wheat, egg, and tomato in one patient each. The two patients with nut allergy continued to react, as did two patients with milk allergy and one patient each with allergies to potato, garlic, and rice.

Follow-up of the food-allergic child

It is imperative that food-allergic children undergo regular follow-up. This is necessary to monitor growth, signs, and symptoms of ongoing food allergy, adherence to the recommended avoidance diet, and objective measures of food allergy. Any reactions that have occurred need to be reviewed with particular attention to how the reaction might have been prevented and whether the treatment provided was appropriate.

All children with food allergy should also be re-evaluated at regular intervals to determine if the allergy has been outgrown. This typically should be done annually, although for some food allergies a shorter or longer interval might be appropriate. For example, an infant with adverse reactions to fruits or vegetables might deserve re-evaluation after 3–6 months whereas an older child who clearly has persistent peanut or tree nut allergy may no longer need repeat testing, although regular follow-up is still important to review avoidance procedures and treatment protocols.

The re-evaluation process may include skin testing, measurement of specific IgE levels, and/or oral food challenges, depending on the specific clinical scenario. It is very important to note, however, that a positive skin test or IgE level does not necessarily mean that the food allergy has not been outgrown, since these tests can remain positive even when the patient is no longer clinically sensitive. Quantitative IgE levels (e.g. UniCAP® or CAP System FEIA®) have increasingly become the test of choice to monitor food allergies over time and to help guide decisions about the timing of oral food challenges. In the end, a food challenge will usually be necessary to prove that an allergy has been outgrown. These must be performed with caution because severe reactions may at times occur even when the testing suggested that the food allergy had most likely been outgrown.

Until an allergy has been outgrown, it is recommended that a strict avoidance diet be maintained. However, while the clinical impression has been that strict avoidance increases the chance of outgrowing a food allergy and may even hasten the process, there is very little data to support this notion [27,44]. In addition, it is clear that some children rapidly outgrow their food allergies without strict avoidance while others who fail to lose their allergies even with the most stringent diet. Since strict avoidance is so difficult, it would be ideal if we could somehow identify, such as with epitope mapping, those children who might be equally likely to outgrow their food allergies with or without a strict diet. However, until we have further information on this issue, it is still likely that the majority of children with food allergy will benefit from very strict avoidance, at least to avoid symptoms and hopefully to promote the outgrowing process.

Conclusions

An understanding of the natural history and prevention of food hypersensitivity is extremely important to the management of food-allergic patients. Although the various studies on these topics are not completely consistent, there are trends in the data that provide several clear messages. First, food allergy is very common. Second, the vast majority of food allergy has its onset in the first 1–2 years of life. Third, most food allergy is outgrown, although there are notable exceptions to this generally positive outcome. Fourth, food allergy is often the first of the atopic diseases, with most children going on to develop respiratory allergies over time. Finally, at least some food allergy can be prevented by avoiding major food antigens in infancy and early childhood.

It is also important to stress the importance of making early, accurate diagnoses of childhood food allergy. Only this will allow for the initiation of the key elements necessary for the care of the food-allergic patient, including education about avoidance diets and the development of emergency care plans for the treatment of allergic reactions. Avoidance diets are complex and require detailed education, without which the child will be at risk for accidental reactions and possibly even more persistent food allergy. In addition, measures that might help to prevent the development of additional food allergies, as well as inhalant allergies, should be initiated at the time of the initial diagnosis.

References

1 Sicherer SH, Sampson HA. Food allergy. *J Allergy Clin Immunol* 2006;117:S470–5.

2 Bock SA. Prospective appraisal of complaints of adverse reactions to foods in children during the first 3 years of life. *Pediatrics* 1987;79:683–8.

3 Kajosaari M. Food allergy in Finnish children aged 1 to 6 years. *Acta Paediatr Can* 1982;71:815–19.

4 Eggesbo M, Halvorsen R, Tambs K, Botten G. Prevalence of parentally perceived adverse reactions to food in young children. *Pediatr Allergy Immunol* 1999;10:122–32.

5 Eggesbo M, Botten G, Halvorsen R, Magnus P. The prevalence of CMA/CMPI in young children: the validity of parentally perceived reactions in a population-based study. *Allergy* 2001;56:393–402.

6 Eggesbo M, Botten G, Halvorsen R, Magnus P. The prevalence of allergy to egg: a population-based study in young children. *Allergy* 2001;56:403–11.

7 Host A, Halken S. A prospective study of cow milk allergy in Danish infants during the first 3 years of life. Clinical course in relation to clinical and immunological type of hypersensitivity reaction. *Allergy* 1990;45:587–96.

8 Host A, Halken S, Jacobsen HP, *et al.* The natural course of cow's milk protein allergy/intolerance (abstract). *J Allergy Clin Immunol* 1997;99:S490.

9 Tariq SM, Stevens M, Matthews S, *et al.* Cohort study of peanut and tree nut sensitization by the age of 4 years. *BMJ* 1996; 313:514–17.

10 Kulig M, Bergmann R, Klettke U, *et al.* Natural course of sensitization to food and inhalant allergens during the first 6 years of life. *J Allergy Clin Immunol* 1999;103:1173–9.

11 Nickel R, Kulig M, Forster J, *et al.* Sensitization to hen's egg at the age of 12 months is predictive for allergic sensitization to common indoor and outdoor allergens at the age of 3 years. *J Allergy Clin Immunol* 1997;99:613–17.

12 Kulig M, Bergmann R, Niggermann B, *et al.* Prediction of sensitization to inhalant allergens in childhood: evaluating family history, atopic dermatitis and sensitization to food allergens. *Clin Exp Allergy* 1998;28:1397–403.

13 Bock SA. Natural history of severe reactions to foods in young children. *J Pediatr* 1985;107:676–80.

14 Dannaeus A, Inganas M. A follow-up study of children with food allergy. Clinical course in relation to serum IgE- and IgG-antibody levels to milk, egg, and fish. *Clin Allergy* 1981;11:533–9.

15 Sampson HA, Scanlon SM. Natural history of food hypersensitivity in children with atopic dermatitis. *J Pediatr* 1989;115:23–7.

16 Sampson HA, McCaskill CC. Food hypersensitivity and atopic dermatitis: evaluation of 113 patients. *J Pediatr* 1985;107:669–75.

17 Shek LP, Soderstrom L, Ahlstedt S, *et al.* Determination of food specific IgE levels over time can predict the development of tolerance in cow's milk and hen's egg allergy. *J Allergy Clin Immunol* 2004;114:387–91.

18 Businco L, Benincori N, Cantani A, *et al.* Chronic diarrhea due to cow's milk allergy. A 4- to 10-year follow-up study. *Ann Allergy* 1985;55:844–7.

19 Dannaeus A, Johansson SGO. A follow-up of infants with adverse reactions to cow's milk. *Acta Paediatr Scand* 1979;68:377–82.

20 Hill DJ, Firer MA, Ball G, Hosking CS. Recovery from milk allergy in early childhood: antibody studies. *J Pediatr* 1989;114:761–6.

21 Hill DJ, Firer MA, Shelton MJ, Hosking CS. Manifestations of milk allergy in infancy: clinical and immunologic findings. *J Pediatr* 1986;109:270–6.

22 Bishop JM, Hill DJ, Hosking CS. Natural history of cow milk allergy: clinical outcome. *J Pediatr* 1990;116:862–7.

23 Hill DJ, Firer MA, Ball G, Hosking CS. Natural history of cows' milk allergy in children: immunological outcome over 2 years. *Clin Exp Allergy* 1993;23:124–31.

24 Saarinen KM, Pelkonen AS, Makela MJ, Savilahti E. Clinical course and prognosis of cow's milk allergy are dependent on milk-specific IgE status. *J Allergy Clin Immunol* 2005;116: 869–75.

25 Skripak J, Matsui EC, Mudd K, Wood RA. The natural history of milk allergy. *J Allergy Clin Immunol* (In Press).

26 Host A, Jacobsen HP, Halken S, Holmenlund D. The natural history of cow's milk protein allergy/intolerance. *Eur J Clin Nutr* 1995;49:S13–18.

27 James JM, Sampson HA. Immunologic changes associated with the development of tolerance in children with cow milk allergy. *J Pediatr* 1992;121:371–7.

28 Chatchatee P, Jarvinen K-M, Bardina L, *et al*. Identification of IgE- and IgG-binding epitopes on α_{s1}-casein: differences in patients with persistent and transient cow's milk allergy. *J Allergy Clin Immunol* 2001;107:379–83.

29 Chatchatee P, Jarvinen K-M, Bardina L, *et al*. Identification of IgE- and IgG-binding epitopes on β- and κ-casein in cow's milk allergic patients. *Clin Exp Allergy* 2001;31:1256–62.

30 Ford RPK, Taylor B. Natural history of egg hypersensitivity. *Arch Dis Child* 1982;57:649–52.

31 Boyano-Martínez T, García-Ara C, Díaz-Pena JM, Martín-Esteban M. Prediction of tolerance on the basis of quantification of egg white-specific IgE antibodies in children with egg allergy. *J Allergy Clin Immunol* 2002;110:304–9.

32 Bock SA, Atkins FM. The natural history of peanut allergy. *J Allergy Clin Immunol* 1989;83:900–4.

33 Hourihane JO, Roberts SA, Warner JO. Resolution of peanut allergy: case-control study. *BMJ* 1998;316:1271–5.

34 Spergel JM, Beausoleil JL, Pawlowski NA. Resolution of childhood peanut allergy. *Ann Allergy Asthma Immunol* 2000;85:473–6.

35 Skolnick HS, Conover-Walker MK, Barnes-Koerner C, *et al*. The natural history of peanut allergy. *J Allergy Clin Immunol* 2001;107:367–74.

36 Sampson HA, Ho DG. Relationship between food specific IgE concentrations and the risk of positive food challenges in children and adolescent. *J Allergy Clin Immunol* 1997;100:444–51.

37 Vander Leek TK, Liu AH, Stefanski K, *et al*. The natural history of peanut allergy in young children and its association with serum peanut-specific IgE. *J Pediatr* 2000;137:749–55.

38 Busse PJ, Nowak-Wegrzyn AH, Noone SA, *et al*. Recurrent peanut allergy. *N Engl J Med* 2002;347:1535–6.

39 Fleischer DM, Conover-Walker MK, Christie L, *et al*. The natural progression of peanut allergy: resolution and the risk of recurrence. *J Allergy Clin Immunol* 2003;112:183–9.

40 Fleischer DM, Conover-Walker MK, Matsui EC, Wood RA. Peanut allergy: recurrence and its management. *J Allergy Clin Immunol* 2005;116:1087–93.

41 Fleischer DM, Conover-Walker MK, Matsui EC, Wood RA. The natural history of tree nut allergy. *J Allergy Clin Immunol* 2005;116:1087–93.

42 Hill DJ, Heine RG, Cameron DJ, *et al*. The natural history of intolerance to soy and extensively hydrolyzed formula in infants with multiple food protein intolerance. *J Pediatr* 1999;135:118–21.

43 Daul CB, Morgan JE, Lehrer SB. The natural history of shrimp-specific immunity. *J Allergy Clin Immunol* 1990;86:88–93.

44 Pastorello EA, Stocchi L, Pravettoni V, *et al*. Role of elimination diet in adults with food allergy. *J Allergy Clin Immunol* 1989;84:475–83.

38 CHAPTER 38
Prevention of Food Allergy

Gideon Lack and George Du Toit

KEY CONCEPTS

- Despite a trend toward delayed weaning, food allergies have increased in the past decades.

- Exclusive breast-feeding for the first 3 months of life may have a protective effect on allergy outcomes, but not specifically food allergies.

- There is no consistent evidence to support exclusive breast-feeding beyond 3 months of age as means to prevent food allergy or atopic disease.

- Hydrolyzed formulas in high-risk infants reduce symptoms of eczema.

- There is a need for randomized-controlled studies to test novel prevention strategies such as oral tolerance induction.

Introduction

The prevalence of IgE-mediated food allergy appears to have increased over the last few decades with approximately 3–6% of children in the developed world affected [1]. The increase in food allergy is best described for peanut allergy [2–4]. For example, in the United Kingdom three sequential studies (cohorts born 1989–2000) demonstrate an increase in the prevalence of peanut allergy from 0.6% to 1.8% over the last 10 years [3]. Food allergy is now considered a public health concern as the condition is associated with significant morbidity and occasional mortality. Although genetic factors are clearly important in the development of food allergy, the increase in food allergy has occurred over a short period of time and is therefore unlikely to be due to germ-line genetic changes alone. It seems plausible therefore that one or more environmental exposures may, through epigenetic changes, result in the interruption of the "default immunological state" of tolerance to foods. Strategies are therefore required for the prevention of food allergy: primary prevention strategies seek to prevent the onset of IgE sensitization, secondary prevention seeks to interrupt the development of food allergy in IgE-sensitized children, and tertiary prevention seeks to reduce the expression of "end-organ" allergic disease in children with established food allergy.

This chapter does not seek to replicate the many reviews in this field. Rather it aims to highlight the important

conclusions derived from these reviews and focuses on novel strategies that help advance contemporaneous thinking in this field.

Methodological challenges

In this section we examine the methodological aspects which complicate the interpretation of the many studies performed in the field of allergy prevention (summarized in Table 38.1).

Numerous studies have assessed different strategies for the prevention of food allergy. Despite this extensive body of work, findings have generally proved ineffective. The fact that no single intervention, or combination of interventions is able to repeatedly demonstrate a strong protective effect against food allergy, reflects either on the interventions themselves or alternatively, the study methods used to measure them.

A major limitation of many food allergy prevention studies lies in the study design, with few nutritional studies being randomized due to the necessary ethical restrictions which surround randomization of infants to anything but breast milk.

A second major limitation of studies in this field is the phenotypic description of food allergy, particularly for young children. Few studies make use of food challenge procedures. Whilst the determination of tolerance is adequately determined by an open food challenge, the gold standard for the determination of food allergy is the double–blind, placebo-controlled food challenge (DBPCFC). Such challenges are laborious and may be difficult to perform, particularly in young children who may be unwilling to eat unfamiliar

Food Allergy: Adverse Reactions to Foods and Food Additives, 4th edition.
Edited by Dean D. Metcalfe, Hugh A. Sampson, and Ronald A. Simon.
© 2008 Blackwell Publishing, ISBN: 978-1-4501-5129-0.

Table 38.1 Methodological issues known to complicate the interpretation of studies aimed at the prevention of food allergy

Issue	Problem	Recommended approach
Study design	The majority of studies in this field are observational studies.	RDBPC trials reduce unmeasured and unknown sources of bias.
Reverse causality	Early signs of suspected allergic disease (such as eczema) will result in altered feeding patterns.	If possible, trials should adopt RDBPC methodologies for food challenging.
Randomization	There are necessary ethical restraints which limit randomization to dietary interventions. This is especially so for studies involving infant milks.	Breast-feeding should always be encouraged. Studies which wish to assess the effect of complementary feeds should randomize within the breast-fed group.
Blinding of dietary interventions	Blinding of specific dietary interventions may not be possible due to safety concerns or practical limitations.	It may not always be possible to have a placebo arm to infant nutritional studies.
Determination of food allergy	Few studies make use of the oral food challenges (OFC) for the diagnosis of food allergy. The diagnosis of food allergy is therefore often inadequate both at study entry and exit. Too many studies rely exclusively on the presence of specific IgE (as determined by skin prick testing and/or specific IgE).	Aim to perform oral challenges in all participants. For children who do not undergo OFCs, *a priori* diagnostic algorithms are required which will then reach a diagnosis through the combination of history, examination, skin prick testing, and specific IgE determination.
Surrogate markers	Eczema, rhinitis, and asthma are often used as surrogate markers of food allergy.	As above
Natural history of food allergy	Tolerance is anticipated for many, but not all, childhood food allergies.	Account for natural remission rate of a disease before assessing for a study effect.
Nomenclature	There is insufficient consensus within the allergy community with respect to the terminology of common allergic conditions.	Consensus with respect to the allergy nomenclature, of common allergic disorders will greatly facilitate research in this field.
Allergy diagnosis	There is little consensus within the allergy community with respect to the ideal diagnostic criteria to be sued for common allergic conditions, particularly in early childhood. For example, many studies refer to generic terms such as "allergy" or "atopy." Definitions for each of these conditions are open to great variability.	Consensus with respect to the diagnosis of common allergic disorders is desperately required between specialist allergy organizations.
Determination of diet	The determination of food consumption is usually by retrospective Food Frequency Questionnaire (FFQ). FFQs are prone to many forms of bias.	Use should be made of prospective food diaries which have been validated for context, language, and consistency.
Dietary variables and measurement thereof	Few dietary analyses consider all variables; these include age of introduction, quantity ingested (individual and cumulative), frequency of exposure, variability of allergens, allergen processing, and concomitant breast-feeding at time of commencing complementary feeds.	Well-designed validated tools are required in order to accurately record all dietary variables.
Definitions: weaning	Use of the term "weaning" is not consistent and is usually limited to the introduction of solid foods only.	Adopt the term "complementary feeding" which incorporates any nutrient-containing food or liquid other than breast milk given to young children during the period of complementary feeding.
High-risk markers	Many studies are aimed at high-risk atopic populations. However, such populations are difficult to define.	Studies should include entire study populations (i.e. both low and high risk). At-risk populations should be defined *a priori*. Better high-risk markers are required.
Separation of specific effects when interventions are combined	Multiple interventions are often studied at different time points. For example, probiotic administration may be to mother (during pregnancy and/or breast-feeding) and/or newborn infant. This makes it difficult to determine the specific effect of each intervention at each time point.	Preliminary proof-of-concept studies need to separate the effects of each intervention.
Introduction of complementary feeds is associated with multiple variables	The early cessation of breast-feeding and introduction of complementary feeds have been associated with cultural, socio-economic factors as well as specific factors such as maternal age, formula feeding, and maternal smoking.	Regression analysis should control for as many relevant confounders as possible, especially in observational studies. This highlights the need for randomized-controlled trials.
Monitoring adherence	Monitoring of adherence to interventions, particularly dietary interventions is difficult.	Better tools for monitoring dietary adherence are required.

food/s. In addition, entry-level oral challenges cannot be performed in those children assigned to the avoidance arm of intervention studies. The true phenotype of infants at time of enrollment or exit from studies is therefore seldom certain. This limitation is particularly problematic for the diagnosis of cow's milk allergy (CMA) which is a common and frequently studied childhood allergy associated with both immediate onset IgE-mediated and delayed onset non-IgE-mediated reactions.

The most frequently used surrogate marker for the determination of food allergy is the outcome of IgE sensitization (determined by skin prick test results and/or specific IgE determination). Although IgE-mediated food allergy requires the state of "sensitization," the majority of children who are sensitized to foods are not food allergic.

Eczema is also a commonly used surrogate for food allergy. Whereas eczema has been shown to be a risk factor for the development of food allergy, not all food allergic children have eczema [5,6]. Hence, although eczema is strongly associated with food allergy, the two are not synonymous, as evidenced by studies which demonstrate an improvement in eczema but not food allergy. In addition, most studies which report an effect on eczema do not assess the severity of the eczema. Mild eczema has been shown to run a transient course when compared with moderate–severe eczema [7]. It may therefore be that studies which claim to prevent eczema are actually treating eczema (i.e. tertiary prevention) in children who entered the study with food allergy. Alternatively, study effects may be limited to the transient disease of mild eczema. Similar limitations apply to the diagnosis of asthma and rhino-conjunctivitis.

Additional limitations of the surrogate markers used for the diagnosis of food allergy include inconsistencies in nomenclature and difficulties in accurately diagnosing these conditions in infants and young children. For example, different terms are used to describe the "eczematous" condition. This results not only in disease misclassification, but may describe different immunological conditions. Indeed, the role of atopic sensitization in childhood eczema remains obscure as it is neither a prerequisite nor a uniform cause of the disease.

Nutritional studies are prone to selection bias and reverse causality. Such bias may arise when atopic families – if aware of public health recommendations – are increasingly motivated to alter dietary practices, either in their own diet or in the diet of their infants. The effects of reverse causality are highlighted in various studies and for different allergic outcomes. For example, in the Avon Longitudinal Study of Parents and Children (ALSPAC), a history of an allergic reaction to peanut was associated with prolonged breast-feeding [5]. However, when adjusted for infantile eczema by regression analysis, there was no effect of breast-feeding on the development of peanut allergy.

Childhood food allergies are dynamic with the general trend being for resolution of many but not all during the first decade of life. This is also true for mild eczema and selects asthma phenotypes. Study planning needs to take these natural histories into account prior to assessing for long-term study outcomes.

Observational studies (as most studies in this field are) are vulnerable to bias from both unmeasured, and unknown, sources. In an ideal world, study hypothesis would therefore only be assessed by randomized double–blind, placebo-controlled (RDBPC) studies. The inclusion of a placebo in nutritional studies is not always practical, or safe. Randomized-controlled studies in infants testing the early or delayed introduction of a food or foods cannot practically incorporate a placebo in the control group.

Above all, study interventions should be safe for both mother and child. Safety concerns have nonetheless arisen in select studies. For example, dietary interventions have been noted to compromise fetal and maternal well-being [8] and studies using probiotics have shown increased rates of sensitization and allergic outcomes in separate studies [9,10].

Prevention studies are often aimed at high-risk families. The high-risk population is however difficult to define. For example, approximately 10% of children without an allergic first degree relative develop allergic disease, compared to 20–30% with single allergic heredity (parent or sibling) and 40–50% with double-allergic heredity [11]. In addition, the definition of the term "atopy" is inconsistent.

Many interventions are introduced to both mother and child. This complicates the understanding of specific study effects as it is unclear whether the immunological effects were achieved pre- or postnatally or whether effects should be attributed to a single or multiple factors.

The determination of dietary intake is usually performed by Food Frequency Questionnaires (FFQs). FFQs are known to be subject to substantial forms of bias. FFQs do not always assess all relevant dietary variables such as age of introduction, recurrence of exposure, quantity (single and cumulative) of exposure, variability of allergens consumed, and allergen processing. In addition, it is often difficult to disguise those questions which relate to the specific food/s of interest. Prospective food diaries are cumbersome as they demand detailed information and effort by parents.

It is difficult to measure food allergen exposures which occur via routes other than the oral route (e.g. through an abraded skin barrier). For example, the nursing mother who ingests peanut butter is also likely to transfer this allergen to the infant through kiss and touch-contact [12,13]. In addition, it is often the nursing mother who determines consumption patterns within the household, which further increases (or decreases) the opportunity for environmental food allergen exposure to foods which the mother likes (or dislikes). A different problem arises if the intervention is one of avoidance as the elimination of one or more foods from the diet is likely to impact the diet. Such changes may be anticipated and therefore measured, or unknown and missed.

Onset of sensitization and food allergy

It remains unclear as to when prevention strategies should be implemented. It is therefore important to determine whether sensitization occurs *in utero*. Prerequisites for the development of food allergy (particularly in genetically susceptible individuals) are thought to include allergen exposure, uptake, recognition, and processing. The fact that *in utero* sensitization to foods is possible is suggested by the early clinical presentation of IgE-mediated food allergies. This is usually apparent within the first year of life. Non-IgE-mediated food-induced immunological reactions such as cow's milk–protein (CMP)-induced colitis usually present in the first year of life.

There is some data that food and aero-allergens can be transmitted via the placenta [14]. However, the analysis of specific IgE to foods in cord blood in two large birth cohort studies was unable to demonstrate measurable food specific IgE in cord blood, even in those children who subsequently developed clinical or immunological food sensitization [5,15].

Summary

Although possible on theoretical grounds, there is no firm evidence to support the hypothesis that sensitization and allergy to foods commences *in utero*.

Maternal diet (during pregnancy and/or breast-feeding) and the prevention of food allergy

In this section we examine the effect of maternal diet during pregnancy and/or lactation on the development of food allergy.

There are three studies which assess the effects (with respect to allergy prevention) of maternal dietary avoidance of one or more common food allergens during pregnancy [16–18]. In a Cochrane review, Kramer *et al.* [19] assessed the evidence for allergy prevention through prescribing an antigen avoidance diet during lactation. They include four trials involving 334 women. Their findings suggested a protective effect of maternal antigen avoidance on the incidence of atopic eczema during the child's first 12–18 months of life. There was no effect on asthma or rhinitis. They however also noted the methodological shortcomings in all three trials and argued for caution in applying these results. Most importantly, one trial reported that a restricted diet (egg and CMP) during pregnancy was associated with both maternal and fetal nutritional compromise.

Given the uncertainty of these findings, and potential safety concerns, specialist allergy organizations do not recommend the avoidance of either egg or milk during pregnancy [20–25]. However, there are recommendations for the avoidance of peanut in high-risk scenarios by both the American Association of Pediatrics (AAP) [26] and the UK Government

Department of Health (DoH) [27]. This recommendation was not evidence based and came about as a response to the public health concern of peanut allergy. There are no studies which assess effects of modifying maternal diet during lactation only. There are however studies which modify the maternal diet during pregnancy or both pregnancy and lactation; these have not shown a protective role against infant food allergy through maternal dietary avoidance of cow's milk, egg, and fish during either pregnancy and/or breast-feeding. In addition, the ALSPAC study showed no effect of maternal peanut consumption in pregnancy or lactation on the development of immunological or clinical reaction to peanuts on follow-up at 4–6 years of age [5].

Breast milk contains low concentrations of dietary proteins which are present in maternal serum. Indeed, β-lactoglobulin is found in the breast milk of 95% of mothers consuming cow's milk during lactation. Whether at-risk infants are protected by the many beneficial immunological properties of breast milk or put at risk by this low-dose allergen exposure is an ongoing debate. There are studies which modify the maternal diet during both pregnancy and lactation. Neither the study by Hattevig *et al.* [7] nor the study by Herman *et al.* [28] demonstrate a protective role against infant food allergy through maternal dietary avoidance of cow's milk, egg, and fish during either pregnancy or both pregnancy and lactation. The study by Herman *et al.* did however note effects for eczema.

Summary

Manipulation of the maternal diet during pregnancy and/or breast-feeding has not consistently been shown to exert protective effects on the development of allergy; however preventative effects are noted for eczema. Such strategies carry the risk of nutritional compromise for both mother and child.

Complementary infant feeding and the prevention of food allergy

In this section we examine the effect of complementary feeding on the development of food allergy.

The World Health Organization (WHO) now recommend that the term "weaning" be replaced by the term "complementary feeding" which incorporates any nutrient-containing food or liquid other than breast milk. Most studies in this field consider weaning to be the introduction of solid foods only. However, the biophysical properties of allergens are complex and there is no reason to believe that the allergenic potential of liquid feeds is different from that of solid or semi-solid feeds. For example, both cow's milk and hen's egg allergy are common childhood allergies despite being ingested as liquid and solid, respectively. An infant who is breast-fed whilst receiving cow's milk formula (CMF) supplementation is no more or less weaned than a breast-fed infant who is fed rice cereal mixed with expressed breast milk. It is therefore arbitrary to restrict the usage of the term "weaning" to solids.

Breast milk provides a rich and favorable source of immune-regulating substances and possesses numerous other qualities which have the capability of directly influencing allergic disease expression. For example, breast milk regulates food antigen absorption and processing which may delay or prevent the development of food allergy. Breast milk has also been shown to decrease lower respiratory tract infections (LRTIs) in the first year of life and LRTIs are known risk factors for the development of asthma. That worldwide breast-feeding is initiated in only 60–80% of newborns and exclusive breast-feeding rates remain below WHO targets.

There are numerous health care specialist allergy organizations which offer advice with respect to infant feeding in at-risk infants [20–24]. Whilst there is consensus that breast milk remains unchallenged as the milk of choice for all infants, advice with respect to the duration of exclusive breast-feeding and the avoidance of common food allergens differ between organizations.

Studies which support a protective effect of breast-feeding over CMFs date back to the 1930s when Grulee and Sanford demonstrated a protective effect of breast-feeding on the development of eczema in the first 12–48 months of life in a large ($n \approx 20,000$) observational study [29]. Not all of the observational studies which followed supported these early findings. In a 2007 review by the Paediatric Section of EAACI, Muraro et al. [30] suggested an overall protective effect (for at-risk children) of exclusive breast-feeding during the first 3 months of life on atopic eczema and asthma, but not childhood allergic rhinitis.

While exclusive breast-feeding for 3 months may protect against the development of allergy taken in the context of the numerous studies done in this field, the consensus however is that prolonged exclusive breast-feeding beyond 3 months of age has not been shown to consistently protect against the development of food allergy, or atopy. Kramer et al. [31] performed a WHO commissioned systematic review of the available evidence concerning the effects of exclusive breast-feeding for 6 months versus exclusive breast-feeding for 3–4 months followed by mixed breast-feeding (complementary liquid or solid foods with continued breast-feeding) to 6 months, on eczema, asthma, and other atopic outcomes. This extensive review covers 20 independent observational studies. They were unable to establish evidence for a significant reduction in the risk of atopic eczema, asthma, or other atopic outcomes amongst those infants who were exclusively breast-fed for 6 months compared with those exclusively breast-fed for 3–4 months followed by mixed feeding.

It is therefore surprising that the WHO [32] recommendations use the justification of reduction in atopy to support exclusive breast-feeding for the first 6 months of the infant's life. While there are other beneficial health effects

of prolonged exclusive breast-feeding, prevention of allergy does not provide a justification.

Kramer et al. [33] in a recent large (n = 13 889) cluster randomised trial indicate that the experimental intervention to promote breastfeeding did not reduce the risk of asthma, hay fever, or eczema at age 6.5 years despite large increases in the duration of exclusivity of breast feeding; nor did the intervention succeed in reducing the prevalence of positive skin prick tests. Indeed, there was a suggestion that atopic sensitisation by skins tests to inhalent allergens was increased in the intervention group.

There are only two randomized studies looking at the introduction of CMP formula against exclusive breast-feeding on the development of food allergy and atopy. Lucas et al. [34] in a large (n = 777) randomized interventional study of premature infants, compared the effects of human breast milk, standard preterm formula, and nutrient-enriched preterm formula. Interestingly, at 18 months after term there was no overall difference in the incidence of food-allergic reactions between dietary groups, although a subgroup effect was noted for the group of infants with a family history of atopy. Similarly, in a large (n = 1693) randomized intervention study of term infants, De Jong et al. [35] found that early (first 3 days of life) high-dose exposure to CMP (as frequently occurs in nurseries) was not associated with an increase in allergic disease or symptoms. In addition, no increase in sensitization or allergy to CMP was found between the groups up to 5 years of age.

There are indeed some observational studies which demonstrate an increased risk in the development of allergic disorders in breast-fed infants. In a large (n = 1037 children) observational study, Sears et al. [36] followed up children until 21 years of age. They found that breast-feeding (for at least 4 weeks) did not protect against childhood atopy and asthma. Indeed, significantly more breast-fed children were atopic to common aero-allergens at the age of 13 than non-breast-fed children. Breast-feeding also increased the likelihood of asthma at age 9 and 21 years. Findings were similar when breast-feeding was considered over longer periods (8–12 weeks). Exclusive breast-feeding did not offer any protection against atopy and there was even a suggestion that the risk of atopy was increased. Likewise, in the large Multicenter Allergy Study (MAS) observational birth cohort (n = 1314 infants born in 1990), Bergman et al. [37] found that each month of breast-feeding elevated the risk of developing atopic eczema in the first 7 years by approximately 3%. It was noted, however, that breast-feeding persisted for longer if at least one parent had eczema, the mother was older, did not smoke in pregnancy, or the family had a high social status. Reverse causality could not be ruled out in this study.

The WHO recommendations that exclusive breast-feeding be continued until 6 months of age is a change to their previous recommendations and different from the 1999 joint

European Allergy Statement which recommended exclusive breast-feeding for between 4 and 6 months. Interestingly, there has, since 1975, been a significant trend in developed countries toward the later introduction of solid foods. For example, in the United Kingdom, the proportion of infants given solids by 8 weeks of age has decreased, 49% in 1975, 24% in 1980 and 1985, and 19% in 1990 [38]. It is interesting that this decrease to a third of what it was has coincided with a 3-fold increase in allergy in children [39]. Reasons for differences in weaning are complex and early weaning has been associated with cultural, socio-economic, as well as specific factors such as maternal age, formula feeding, and maternal smoking. All of these factors need to be controlled for in study analyses.

A review of the evidence for the relationship between the early (defined as less than 4 months of age) introduction of solid foods to infants and the development of allergic disease was recently performed by Tarini et al. [40]. Thirteen studies met their criteria for review, of which only one was a controlled study. Studies were not limited to at-risk study populations. They concluded that there was insufficient evidence to suggest that, on its own, the early introduction of solids to infants was associated with an increased risk of asthma, food allergy, or allergic rhinitis. They noted the consistent association between the persistence of eczema and the introduction of solid foods before 4 months of age that is supported by long-term follow-up studies and the dose-dependent nature of the association.

Fergusson et al.'s [41] article is the only study to report an increased risk of persistent eczema with the early introduction of solids. They reported a 2.9 times greater risk of chronic or recurrent eczema amongst children fed four or more solids before 4 months of age compared with those not fed solids before 4 months of age. This difference was still apparent at 10 years of age. When they assessed the effect of exposure to individual foods such as cow's milk, egg, cereals, vegetables, meat products, or fruits they found no increased risk of developing atopic dermatitis (AD). Zutavern et al. [42] more recently conducted a large multicenter study which controlled for the effects of reverse causality whilst assessing for the effect of early life diet on allergy outcomes. They found no evidence of a protective effect of late introduction of solids on the development of pre-school wheezing, transient wheezing, atopy, or eczema. There was no evidence for a protective effect of the delayed introduction of solids beyond 4 months of age on the development of sensitization to foods. On the contrary, there was a statistically significant increased risk of eczema in relation to late introduction of egg and milk. The late introduction of egg was also associated with a non-significant increased risk of pre-school wheezing.

Although exclusive breast-feeding does not have proven effects in the prevention of allergy, there have been numerous studies examining the protective effects of different types of formulas especially CMP-hydrolysates as a substitute for breast milk where the mother is unable to or chooses not to breast-feed. There are several studies and a meta-analysis of the evidence for the role of infant formula in the prevention of allergic disease in high-risk infants who are unable to breast-feed. Cochrane review by Osborn et al. [43] found no evidence to support feeding with a hydrolyzed formula for the prevention of allergy compared to exclusive breast-feeding. For high-risk infants who are unable to be completely breast-fed, they found limited evidence that prolonged feeding with a hydrolyzed formula compared to a CMF-reduced infant and childhood allergy and infant CMA. The general consensus among the reviews is that the use of hydrolyzed milk formula in at-risk infants offers at least some protection against allergic disease, and in particular eczema. These findings are reflected in the recommendations of specialist allergy organizations [20–24].

One recent study in this field is the German Infant Nutritional Interventional (GINI) study [42,43]. This is a large (n = 2252) randomized multicenter study in which von Berg et al. allocate high-risk infants to one of four milks; CMF, partially hydrolyzed whey formula (pHW-F), extensively hydrolyzed whey formula (eHW-F), or extensively hydrolyzed casein formula (eHC-F). A significant reduction in the incidence of AD was achieved at 1 and 3 years of age with the eHC-F and the pHW-F. The greater reduction in eczema at 1 year of age in high-risk children with a pHW-F and eHC-F rather than with an eHW-F is difficult to explain. In this study, hydrolyzed formula did not protect against wheezing. The clinical benefits demonstrated by the GINI study are convincing. However it remains unclear whether dietary modification has truly prevented allergic disease. The GINI study [44,45] was not able to clearly define the endpoint of food allergy by DBPCFC as many parents declined. The reduction in eczema could therefore either be due to the primary prevention of eczema through dietary modification or alternatively reflect the beneficial effect of removing CMP from the diet of infants with concomitant eczema and milk allergy.

Soy formulas have long been used as CMF alternatives. In a recent Cochrane review, Osborn et al. [46] found three studies which met their inclusion criteria. They concluded that, on current evidence, the use of soy formulas could not be recommended for the prevention of allergy or food intolerance in at-risk infants. No study demonstrated an increase in soy allergy. There is also no evidence to support the use of "other" mammalian milks for the prevention of food allergy.

Summary

There is some evidence of a protective effect against the development of allergy in high-risk infants when exclusively breast-feeding for the first 3 months of life. There is no convincing effect noted beyond 3 months of life in both high-risk infants and normal infants. Some studies suggest that prolonged exclusive breast-feeding may increase the risk of allergies, although reverse causality may be an explanation. The use of CM-hydrolysates in high-risk infants shows amelioration of eczema – but not food allergy – at 1 and 3 years of age (in the GINI study). There is no evidence that hydrolyzed formulas prevent against the development of other allergies. There is no evidence to support the use of soy formula or "other" mammalian milk formula for the prevention of allergy.

Combined maternal and infant dietary measures and the prevention of food allergy

It seems intuitive that of all dietary interventions aimed at the prevention of food allergy the combined approach should offer the greatest hope as it covers many routes of allergen exposure at immunologically vulnerable time points.

In a Cochrane review, Kramer et al. [19] assessed the evidence for the prevention of allergic disease through maternal dietary antigen avoidance during pregnancy or lactation, or both. Their analysis found that the prescription of an antigen avoidance diet to high-risk woman during pregnancy was unlikely to substantially reduce her child's risk of atopic disease.

There are two randomized studies which adopted a multi-intervention approach. Zeiger et al. [47] in a study of 165 mother/infant pairs randomized participants to either a prophylactic group (*maternal avoidance of cow's milk, egg, and peanut during the last trimester of pregnancy and lactation, and infants diet free of cow's milk until age 1 year and using a hydrolysate formula as supplement, egg until age 2 years, and peanut and fish until age 3 years*) or a control group (*following standard feeding practice*). Findings demonstrate a significant reduction in cow's milk sensitization and eczema before the age of 2 years but no significant reduction in food allergy, AD, allergic rhinitis, asthma, any atopic disease, lung function, food or aeroallergen sensitization or serum IgE level at 7 years of age. No difference in skin prick testing or specific IgE testing was shown for the other food allergens tested, including peanut, which was the most common skin test-positive food allergen at 7 years of age. This indicates that the beneficial effect of the dietary interventions was mainly in reducing CMA.

Arshad et al. [48] in a study of 120 infants randomized participants to either a prophylactic group (*breast-fed with mother on a low allergen diet or given an extensively hydrolyzed formula and house dust mite reduction*) or a control group (*who followed standard UK DoH advice*). Findings demonstrate a reduction in allergic disease (asthma, atopy, rhinitis, and eczema) at least for the first 8 years of life in the prophylactic group. Repeated measurement analysis, adjusted for all relevant confounding variables, confirmed a preventive effect on asthma, AD, rhinitis, and atopy. The protective effects were primarily observed in the subgroup of children with persistent disease (symptoms at all visits) and in those with evidence of allergic

sensitization. Study powering did not allow for the assessment of food allergy at 8 years of age, but earlier transient effects were noted.

Summary

There are randomized trials which adopt a multi-intervention approach (dietary modification of both maternal diet – during pregnancy and/or lactation – and infant diet) that have demonstrated a reduction in allergic disease. Whilst findings in one study were transient and no longer observed at 7 years of age, in a second study, the effects in allergy reduction were still observed at 8 years of age. The effects with respect to a reduction in food allergy appear to predominantly apply to CMA. Caution is required prior to the recommendation of such interventions due to the potential for nutritional compromise in both mother and child.

Routes of sensitization, cross-sensitization, and oral tolerance induction

Until recently, preventive strategies have focused on oral exposure to foods. However, the oral route of exposure is not the only route as exposure to food allergens may occur through aerosolized allergen exposure (e.g. fish and milk cooking vapors) or via the skin (as detailed above). The ALSPAC study [5] followed a large cohort of children (*n* = 13,971) from birth; the results of this study showed a positive associaion between peanut allergy and eczema, and an even greater association with an oozing or crusting skin rash. They also found an increased use of skin preparations using peanut oil in children with peanut allergy (this was limited to cutaneous rather than oral exposure). The observations support the occupational health findings in adults that sensitization may occur through contact with the skin, particularly through abraded skin.

There is a significant body of evidence in animal models that a single oral dose of antigen is sufficient to induce oral tolerance [49–51]. This phenomenon has been demonstrated for different antigens and in different experimental models. The data is consistent; uniformly showing that a single dose of oral protein administration effectively causes immunological tolerance and prevents the expression of related clinical disease.

Poole et al. [52] in a large prospective cohort study in Colorado (*n* = 1612) found an association between age at initial exposure to cereal grains and the development of wheat allergy. Their date suggested that delaying introduction of cereal grains until after 6 months was not protective against development of wheat allergy, but that it may in fact increase the child's risk of wheat allergy. This study excluded children with celiac disease (positive tissue transglutaminase autoantibodies) and controlled for family history of allergy, prior food allergy, breast-feeding duration, and whether the child was breast-fed when first exposed to cereals.

There are no interventional studies that examine the potential role of oral tolerance induction to foods in childhood. There is one adult human study that showed that feeding key-hole limpet hemocyanin (KLH) resulted in immunological tolerance to KLH antigen [53]. Ecological data suggests that African, Asian, and Middle Eastern countries [54] where peanuts are consumed throughout pregnancy and early childhood have low rates of peanut allergy compared to Western industrialized societies such as the United Kingdom and United States where peanut allergy is high despite peanut avoidance during pregnancy and infancy. However, differential predisposition to atopy due to both genetic and environmental factors could however explain these differences.

The high prevalence of peanut allergy in the United Kingdom occurs despite DoH recommendations which advocate avoidance of peanut during pregnancy, breast-feeding, and the first 3 years of life in high-risk children. Recent data suggests that the average age for peanut introduction in the United Kingdom is at 33 months as opposed to 12 months in 1985. The US National Institute of Health and Immune Tolerance Network (NIH/ITN) sponsored interventional study (LEAP Study) is currently underway and seeks to randomize infants less than 11 months of age with risk factors for the development of peanut allergy (moderate–severe eczema and/or egg allergy) to either peanut consumption or avoidance. A final assessment for peanut allergy will be made by oral food challenge at 5 years of age.

There are observational studies to other foods that lend weight to the hypothesis of tolerance induction through early oral exposure. A large observational cohort of children, by Poole et al. [52] demonstrated that delaying the initial exposure to cereal grains until after 6 months may increase the risk of developing IgE-mediated wheat allergy. In a population-based observational study, Saarinen et al. [55], fish and citrus allergy was determined at 3 years of age by oral food challenge. They then found no difference in the cumulative incidence of fish and citrus allergy at 3 years of age between children with fish introduced early or late (after 1 year of age).

Summary

Recent observational and animal studies raise the question of whether sensitization to food antigens may occur via the cutaneous route. There is a body of literature in animal models which demonstrates the effect of tolerance induction following early high-dose food allergen consumption. Human trials are awaited.

Unpasteurized milk and the use of probiotics and prebiotics

It is hypothesized that the increase in allergic disease may be due to a relative lack of microbial stimulation of the infantile gut immune system. This is in keeping with other observations which provide support for the "hygiene hypothesis" whereby dietary, or other immune-modulating factors associated with the anthroposophic lifestyle, lead to lower rates of allergic disease [56].

Observations from rural environments suggest an inverse association between consumption of farm-produced dairy products and the prevalence of allergic disease. Waser et al. [57] conducted a cross-sectional multicenter study, which demonstrated that the consumption of farm milk might offer protection against asthma and allergy. These associations were independent of farm-related co-exposures and other farm-produced products, but were not independently related to any allergy-related health outcome. Similarly, Perkins et al. [53] conducted a two-stage cross-sectional study which demonstrated that unpasteurized milk might be a modifiable influence on allergic sensitization in children. The effect was seen in all children, independent of farming status.

Other strategies have sought to alter the commensal gut flora either directly through the administration of living micro-organisms (probiotics) or indirectly through the provision of non-digestible growth-enhancing substrates (prebiotics). There are many variables between studies performed in this field; these include probiotic strain and viability, dose, and duration. In addition, not all studies treat both mother (during pregnancy and/or breast-feeding) and child. Hence, clinical trial results from one probiotic strain in one population cannot be automatically generalized to other strains or to different populations. There is also great variability with respect to patient groups recruited in trials to date. Boyle et al. [58] published a review in 2005 of the evidence for the use of probiotics in the management of allergic disease. They found evidence for the use of probiotics in the treatment of eczema, but the level of evidence regarding the role of probiotics for the prevention of eczema was "weak."

More recently, Kukkonene et al. [59] in a large randomized trial (n = 925) assessed the combined role of prebiotics (galacto-oligosaccharides) and probiotics (four bacterial strains) in the prevention of allergic disease in a high-risk population. They randomized pregnant women to probiotic or placebo for 2–3 weeks before delivery; their infants received the same intervention or a placebo for 6 months. Results indicate that the prebiotic–probiotic combination treatment, when compared with placebo, showed no effect on the cumulative incidence of allergic disease at 2 years of age. However, the prebiotic–probiotic combination treatment did reduce eczema and atopic eczema (in both IgE- and non-IgE-sensitized children). Taylor et al. [10] randomized high-risk newborns (n = 231) to either receive Lactobacillus acidophilus or placebo daily for the first 6 months of life. They were unable to demonstrate a significant difference in eczema between the groups at 6 and 12 months of age, and found that the proportion of children with positive skin prick tests and eczema was significantly higher in the probiotic group.

Whether probiotic-induced microbiota changes – and associated clinical effects – persist after administration ceases remains unclear. For example, in a study by Kalliomaki et al. [9,60] initial findings at 4 years of age suggested a reduction in eczema, rhinitis, and asthma, however at 7 years of age, the overall risk for developing eczema remained lower in the LGG probiotic group whilst allergic rhinitis and asthma were more common. Interestingly, both the Kukkonene et al. and Kalliomaki et al. studies find the preventive effect on eczema not to be associated with IgE changes [9,59].

Boyle et al. [61] recently highlighted the known and theoretical safety concerns of probiotics; these include infection, deleterious metabolic activities, immune deviation, excessive immune stimulation, and microbial resistance.

It has been shown that infant formulas which are fortified with prebiotics can bias the microbiota to more closely resemble that of breast milk (the so-called "bifidogenic" effect). The clinical relevance of these prebiotic-induced changes remains unclear. Cochrane reviews into the use of pre- and probiotics in the prevention of allergy are currently underway.

Summary

Observational studies suggest that the consumption of unpasteurized milk may reduce the prevalence of allergic sensitization and disease. There are safety concerns regarding unpasteurized milk and this cannot therefore be recommended for the prevention of food allergy. Although some studies do show that the use of probiotics (and in one study a mixture of both pro- and prebiotics) reduces eczema, these effects are not consistent in all studies and are not associated with a reduction in atopy. Currently neither prebiotics nor probiotics can be recommended as a strategy to prevent food allergies or other allergic disease, and safety concerns need to be considered.

Nutritional supplements

There are ecological observations which note that the geographical distribution of allergy prevalence is linked with regional dietary practices [62]. In recent years, there has been a focus on the role of vitamins, antioxidants, fruits, and vegetables, as well as fatty acid intake on the prevention or treatment of allergies.

(a) *Fatty acids*: Dietary lipids, especially n-3 and n-6 long-chain polyunsaturated fatty acids (LCPUFAs) regulate immune function, and may modify the adherence of microbes in the mucosa thereby contributing to host–microbe interactions. There are studies in this field which demonstrate a positive effect with respect to the prevention of allergies, however outcomes are inconsistent. Peat et al. [63] randomized 616 high-risk pregnant mothers (at 36 weeks gestation) to either an intervention group (omega-3-fatty acid supplementation and house dust mite reduction measures) or placebo. They demonstrate a reduction in the outcomes for dust mite sensitization and cough (in atopic children only)

for infants in the intervention group. No significant differences in wheeze were found with either intervention. There was however limited perinatal intervention in this study. Kull et al. [64] in a large prospective birth cohort assessed for the effect of fish (a rich source of omega-3 fatty acids) consumption on allergy outcomes in a large prospective birth cohort. After controlling for confounding factors (parental allergy and early onset eczema or wheeze), regular fish consumption during the first year of life was associated with a reduced risk for allergic sensitization to foods by age 4 years. It is unclear whether such an effect could be explained by oral tolerance induction to food proteins or whether omega-3 fatty acids could have a generic anti-allergic effect. Negative study findings include those by Almqvist et al. [65] who conducted a large (n = 516) randomized, placebo-controlled trial in high-risk children and found that dietary fatty acids (in the first 5 years of life) did not reduce the risk of asthma or allergic disease at 5 years of age. Despite these conflicting findings, many infant formulas are supplemented with LCPUFAs such as *arachadonic acid* and *docosahexaenoic acid*.

(b) *Vitamins*: Dietary vitamins have potent immune-modulating effects. It has been possible to study the effect of vitamin supplementation in young children with respect to allergy outcomes, as many countries advocate routine vitamin supplementation during early childhood. Separate studies in Finland [66] and the United States [67] observed an increased association between vitamin D supplementation in infancy and atopic disease. However, study outcomes were restricted to rhinitis in adulthood in the first study, and select subgroups in the second study; asthma in black children and food allergies (as defined by a medical professional) in the exclusively formula-fed population.

Kull et al. [68] in a large (n = 4089) prospective birth cohort investigated the association between the supplementation of vitamins A and D (administered in either a water- or peanut-oil-based vehicle) during the first year of life and the outcome of allergic disease up to 4 years of age. Children supplemented with vitamins A and D in the water-soluble vehicle during the first year of life had an almost 2-fold increased risk of asthma, food hypersensitivity (determined by parental questionnaire), and sensitization (to common food and airborne allergens) at age 4 years, when compared with those receiving vitamins in peanut oil. There are various possible explanations for these findings. Vitamin A and/or D may protect against the risk of developing allergy; the study findings would then hinge on better absorption of vitamins A and D from the oil-based vehicle than from a water-based vehicle. Alternatively, vitamin A and/or D may actually increase the risk of the development of allergic disease; the absorption of vitamin A and/or D would then need to be superior when the vitamins were administered in the water-based vehicle. Systemic uptake was unfortunately not measured in this study. It is not known how the rates of allergy in the two study groups compare with children who had not received vitamin supplementation at all (less than 2% of children in this cohort did not receive vitamin supplementation). It may also be that vitamin A and/or D has no effect on allergy outcomes and the effects observed are due to the use of peanut oil itself. However, the fatty acids in peanut oil are strongly biased toward the pro-inflammatory omega-6 fatty acids in a ratio of omega-6:omega-3 fatty acids of 34:1. Were this effect to be significant, a higher rate of allergy would have been expected in the group of children who received the oil-based supplement. It is therefore difficult to interpret these findings.

(c) *Antioxidants and trace elements*: Antioxidants are free radical scavengers shown to decrease inflammatory processes. There are no interventional studies which assess the effect of antioxidant supplementation on the prevention of food allergy; however, ecological observations suggest that the higher intake of fresh fruits and vegetables in certain European countries is associated with a decreased prevalence of food allergy [62]. In addition, preliminary findings from the ALSPAC cohort suggest that low cord blood selenium and iron may be associated with a higher subsequent risk of persistent wheeze and eczema [69].

Summary

Randomized-controlled studies provide conflicting results with respect to LCPUFA supplementation for the prevention of allergy. Studies which show a positive effect do so for different allergic disease outcomes. Observational studies which examine the effect of vitamins A and D supplementation during the first year of life suggests an increased rate of sensitization and allergy at 4 years of age, but only when administered in a water-soluble vehicle. It remains unclear as to why vitamins A and D supplementation in different vehicles should exert different clinical effects.

Ecological observations, and preliminary studies, suggest that the higher intake of foods rich in antioxidants may confer protection against allergy outcomes. Although the role of nutritional supplements for the prevention of allergy is interesting, further randomized interventional studies are required.

Conclusions

The natural history of food allergy suggests "plasticity" within the developing immune system as many common food allergies (such as egg and milk allergy) are outgrown. Indeed, the switch from a state of allergy to tolerance may even occur during the first few years of life. Turcanu *et al.* [70] demonstrated that the resolution of peanut allergy was accompanied by a reversal of the Th2- to Th1-skewed, allergen-specific, immune response. These findings are encouraging as it raises the possibility that immune responses are susceptible to prevention strategies.

The conventional wisdom is that early exposure to allergenic food proteins during pregnancy, lactation, or infancy leads to food allergies, and that prevention strategies should aim to eliminate allergenic food proteins during these periods of "immunological vulnerability," especially in high-risk subgroups. There is some evidence to support the use of dietary interventions in high-risk pregnant and/or lactating women, especially for the outcome of atopic eczema. Such interventions may however compromise maternal and fetal nutrition. Exclusive breast-feeding for at least the first 3 months of life offers some protection against allergic disease in high-risk infants. The protective effect of exclusive breast-feeding beyond 4 months of age remains uncertain. For high-risk infants who are not exclusively breast-fed, or where supplementation of breast-feeding is required, the use of hydrolyzed formula may offer some protection against the development of eczema. The findings of dietary interventions such as LCPUFAs, antioxidants, pre- and probiotics, and vitamin supplementation are unconvincing, inconsistent, or not adequately tested. There are safety concerns surrounding some of the interventions trialled to date.

Future studies will need to overcome the methodological challenges detailed in this chapter, many of which are unique to this field of research. Better markers are required to identify high-risk populations, as not all children who develop food allergy are born to atopic families. With current advances in the field of gene–environment interactions, it may also be that future studies need to focus their interventions at specifically defined groups of children, whose genotyping identifies them at being at-risk of (or protected from) specific environmental exposures.

Finally, in order for the field of food allergy prevention to significantly advance, strategies will need to be put to the test using rigorous study design methodologies.

References

1 Sicherer SH, Sampson HA. 9. Food allergy. *J Allergy Clin Immunol* 2006;117:S470–5.

2 Grundy J, Matthews S, Bateman B, *et al.* Rising prevalence of allergy to peanut in children: data from 2 sequential cohorts. *J Allergy Clin Immunol* 2002;110:784–9.

3 Hourihane JO, *et al.* The impact of government advice to pregnant mothers regarding peanut avoidance on the prevalence of peanut allergy in United Kingdom children at school entry. *J Allergy Clin Immunol* 2007;119:1197–1202.

4 Sicherer SH, Munoz-Furlong A, Sampson HA. Prevalence of peanut and tree nut allergy in the United States determined by means of a random digit dial telephone survey: a 5-year follow-up study. *J Allergy Clin Immunol* 2003;112:1203–7.

5 Lack G, Fox D, Northstone K, Golding J. Factors associated with the development of peanut allergy in childhood. *N Engl J Med* 2003;348:977–85.

6 Hill DJ, Hosking CS. Food allergy and atopic dermatitis in infancy: an epidemiologic study. *Pediatr Allergy Immunol* 2004;15:421–7.

7 Hattevig G, *et al.* The effect of maternal avoidance of eggs, cow's milk, and fish during lactation on the development of IgE, IgG, and IgA antibodies in infants. *J Allergy Clin Immunol* 1990;85:108–15.

8 Zeiger RS. Food allergen avoidance in the prevention of food allergy in infants and children. *Pediatrics* 2003;111:1662–71.

9 Kalliomaki M, Salminen S, Poussa T, Isolauri E. Probiotics during the first 7 years of life: a cumulative risk reduction of eczema in a randomized, placebo-controlled trial. *J Allergy Clin Immunol* 2007;119:1019–21.

10 Taylor AL, Dunstan JA, Prescott SL. Probiotic supplementation for the first 6 months of life fails to reduce the risk of atopic dermatitis and increases the risk of allergen sensitization in high-risk children: a randomized controlled trial. *J Allergy Clin Immunol* 2007;119:184–91.

11 Sigurs N, *et al.* Appearance of atopic disease in relation to serum IgE antibodies in children followed up from birth for 4 to 15 years. *J Allergy Clin Immunol* 1994;94:757–63.

12 Maloney JM, Chapman MD, Sicherer SH. Peanut allergen exposure through saliva: assessment and interventions to reduce exposure. *J Allergy Clin Immunol* 2006;118:719–24.

13 Nolan RC, de Leon MP, Rolland JM, *et al.* What's in a kiss: peanut allergen transmission as a sensitizer? *J Allergy Clin Immunol* 2007;119:755.

14 Vance GH, *et al.* Exposure of the fetus and infant to hens' egg ovalbumin via the placenta and breast milk in relation to maternal intake of dietary egg. *Clin Exp Allergy* 2005;35:1318–26.

15 Arshad SH, Kurukulaaratchy RJ, Fenn M, Matthews S. Early life risk factors for current wheeze, asthma, and bronchial hyperresponsiveness at 10 years of age. *Chest* 2005;127:502–8.

16 Falth-Magnusson K, Kjellman NI. Allergy prevention by maternal elimination diet during late pregnancy – a 5-year follow-up of a randomized study. *J Allergy Clin Immunol* 1992;89:709–13.

17 Falth-Magnusson K, Kjellman NI. Development of atopic disease in babies whose mothers were receiving exclusion diet during pregnancy – a randomized study. *J Allergy Clin Immunol* 1987;80:868–75.

18 Lilja G, *et al.* Effects of maternal diet during late pregnancy and lactation on the development of atopic diseases in infants up to 18 months of age – *in-vivo* results. *Clin Exp Allergy* 1989;19:473–9.

19 Kramer MS, Kakuma R. Maternal dietary antigen avoidance during pregnancy or lactation, or both, for preventing or treating atopic disease in the child. *Cochrane Database Syst Rev* 2006;3: CD000133.

20 Fifty-Fourth World Health Assembly. Provisional Agenda Item 13.1.1. *Global Strategy for Infant and Young Child Feeding: The Optimal Duration of Exclusive Breastfeeding.* Geneva: World Health Organization, 2001.

21 Department of Health. *1. Peanut Allergy.* Committee on the Toxicity of Chemicals in Food, Consumer Products and the Environment, 1998:35–7.

22 Fiocchi A, Assa'ad A, Bahna S. Food allergy and the introduction of solid foods to infants: a consensus document. Adverse Reactions to Foods Committee, American College of Allergy, Asthma and Immunology. *Ann Allergy Asthma Immunol* 2006; 97:10–20.

23 Gartner LM, *et al.* Breastfeeding and the use of human milk. *Pediatrics* 2005;115:496–506.

24 Prescott SL, Tang ML. The Australasian Society of Clinical Immunology and Allergy Position Statement: summary of allergy prevention in children. *Med J Aust* 2005;182:464–7.

25 Host A, *et al.* Dietary products used in infants for treatment and prevention of food allergy. Joint Statement of the European Society for Paediatric Allergology and Clinical Immunology (ESPACI) Committee on Hypoallergenic Formulas and the European Society for Paediatric Gastroenterology, Hepatology and Nutrition (ESPGHAN) Committee on Nutrition. *Arch Dis Child* 1999;81:80–4.

26 Gartner LM, *et al.* Breastfeeding and the use of human milk. *Pediatrics* 2005;115:496–506.

27 *Weaning and the Weaning Diet*, 2007. COMA working group on the weaning diet. Department of Health, London, 1-1-1994.

28 Herrmann ME, *et al.* Prospective study of the atopy preventive effect of maternal avoidance of milk and eggs during pregnancy and lactation. *Eur J Pediatr* 1996;155:770–4.

29 Grulee CG. The influence of breast and artificial feeding on infantile eczema. *J Pediatr* 1930;9:223–5.

30 Muraro A, *et al.* Dietary prevention of allergic diseases in infants and small children. Part III. Critical review of published peer-reviewed observational and interventional studies and final recommendations. *Pediatr Allergy Immunol* 2004;15:291–307.

31 Kramer MS, Kakuma R. The optimal duration of exclusive breastfeeding: a systematic review. *Adv Exp Med Biol* 2004;554:63–77.

32 WHO Report. The optimal duration of exclusive breast feeding. Report of an expert consultation, Geneva, Switzerland. Pg2. 2001.

33 Kramer MS, *et al.* Effect of prolonged and exclusive breast feeding on risk of allergy and asthma: cluster randomised trial. *BMJ* 11 Sept 2007.

34 Lucas A, Brooke OG, Morley R, *et al.* Early diet of preterm infants and development of allergic or atopic disease: randomized prospective study. *BMJ* 1990;300:837–40.

35 de Jong MH, Scharp-Van Der Linden VT, Aalberse R, *et al.* The effect of brief neonatal exposure to cows' milk on atopic symptoms up to age 5. *Arch Dis Child* 2002;86:365–9.

36 Sears MR, *et al.* Long-term relation between breastfeeding and development of atopy and asthma in children and young adults: a longitudinal study. *Lancet* 2002;360:901–7.

37 Bergmann RL, *et al.* Breastfeeding duration is a risk factor for atopic eczema. *Clin Exp Allergy* 2002;32:205–9.

38 COMA working group on the weaning diet. Weaning and the weaning diet. Report of the Working Group on the Weaning Diet of the Committee on Medical Aspects of Food Policy. Page 13 of DH Report on Health and Social Subjects 45 Weaning and The Weaning Diet, 1994. London.

39 Asher MI, *et al.* Worldwide time trends in the prevalence of symptoms of asthma, allergic rhinoconjunctivitis, and eczema in childhood: ISAAC Phases One and Three repeat multicountry cross-sectional surveys. *Lancet* 2006;368:733–43.

40 Tarini BA, Carroll AE, Sox CM, Christakis DA. Systematic review of the relationship between early introduction of solid foods to infants and the development of allergic disease. *Arch Pediatr Adolesc Med* 2006;160:502–7.

41 Fergusson DM, Horwood LJ, Shannon FT. Early solid feeding and recurrent childhood eczema: a 10-year longitudinal study. *Pediatrics* 1990;86:541–6.

42 Zutavern A, *et al.* The introduction of solids in relation to asthma and eczema. *Arch Dis Child* 2004;89:303–8.

43 Osborn DA, Sinn J. Formulas containing hydrolysed protein for prevention of allergy and food intolerance in infants. *Cochrane Database Syst Rev* 2003:CD003664.

44 von Berg A, *et al.* The effect of hydrolyzed cow's milk formula for allergy prevention in the first year of life: the German Infant Nutritional Intervention Study, a randomized double-blind trial. *J Allergy Clin Immunol* 2003;111:533–40.

45 von Berg A, *et al.* Certain hydrolyzed formulas reduce the incidence of atopic dermatitis but not that of asthma: three-year results of the German Infant Nutritional Intervention Study. *J Allergy Clin Immunol* 2007;119:718–25.

46 Osborn DA, Sinn J. Soy formula for prevention of allergy and food intolerance in infants. *Cochrane Database Syst Rev* 2006: CD003741.

47 Zeiger RS, Heller S. The development and prediction of atopy in high-risk children: follow-up at age seven years in a prospective randomized study of combined maternal and infant food allergen avoidance. *J Allergy Clin Immunol* 1995;95:1179–90.

48 Arshad SH, Bateman B, Sadeghnejad A, *et al.* Prevention of allergic disease during childhood by allergen avoidance: the Isle of Wight prevention study. *J Allergy Clin Immunol* 2007; 119:307–13.

49 Strid J, Thomson M, Hourihane J, *et al.* A novel model of sensitization and oral tolerance to peanut protein. *Immunology* 2004;113:293–303.

50 Strid J, Hourihane J, Kimber I, *et al.* Disruption of the stratum corneum allows potent epicutaneous immunization with protein antigens resulting in a dominant systemic Th2 response. *Eur J Immunol* 2004;34:2100–9.

51 Strid J, Hourihane J, Kimber I, *et al.* Epicutaneous exposure to peanut protein prevents oral tolerance and enhances allergic sensitization. *Clin Exp Allergy* 2005;35:757–66.

52 Poole JA, *et al.* Timing of initial exposure to cereal grains and the risk of wheat allergy. *Pediatrics* 2006;117:2175–82.

53 Perkin MR, Strachan DP. Which aspects of the farming lifestyle explain the inverse association with childhood allergy? *J Allergy Clin Immunol* 2006;117:1374–81.

54 Levy Y, Broides A, Segal N, Danon YL. Peanut and tree nut allergy in children: role of peanut snacks in Israel? *Allergy* 2003;58:1206–7.

55 Saarinen UM, Kajosaari M. Does dietary elimination in infancy prevent or only postpone a food allergy? A study of fish and citrus allergy in 375 children. *Lancet* 1980;1:166–7.

56 Strachan DP. Family size, infection and atopy: the first decade of the "hygiene hypothesis". *Thorax* 2000;55:S2–10.

57 Waser M, *et al.* Inverse association of farm milk consumption with asthma and allergy in rural and suburban populations across Europe. *Clin Exp Allergy* 2007;37:661–70.

58 Boyle RJ, Tang ML. The role of probiotics in the management of allergic disease. *Clin Exp Allergy* 2006;36:568–76.

59 Kukkonen K, *et al.* Probiotics and prebiotic galacto-oligosaccharides in the prevention of allergic diseases: a randomized, double-blind, placebo-controlled trial. *J Allergy Clin Immunol* 2007;119:192–8.

60 Kalliomaki M, Salminen S, Poussa T, *et al.* Probiotics and prevention of atopic disease: 4-year follow-up of a randomized placebo-controlled trial. *Lancet* 2003;361:1869–71.

61 Boyle RJ, Robins-Browne RM, Tang ML. Probiotic use in clinical practice: What are the risks? *Am J Clin Nutr* 2006;83:1256–64.

62 Heinrich J, Holscher B, Bolte G, Winkler G. Allergic sensitization and diet: ecological analysis in selected European cities. *Eur Respir J* 2001;17:395–402.

63 Peat JK, *et al.* Three-year outcomes of dietary fatty acid modification and house dust mite reduction in the Childhood Asthma Prevention Study. *J Allergy Clin Immunol* 2004;114:807–13.

64 Kull I, Bergstrom A, Lilja G, *et al.* Fish consumption during the first year of life and development of allergic diseases during childhood. *Allergy* 2006;61:1009–15.

65 Almqvist C, *et al.* Omega-3 and omega-6 fatty acid exposure from early life does not affect atopy and asthma at age 5 years. *J Allergy Clin Immunol* 2007;119:1438–44.

66 Hypponen E, Laara E, Reunanen A, *et al.* Intake of vitamin D and risk of type 1 diabetes: a birth-cohort study. *Lancet* 2001; 358:1500–3.

67 Milner JD, Stein DM, McCarter R, Moon RY. Early infant multivitamin supplementation is associated with increased risk for food allergy and asthma. *Pediatrics* 2004;114:27–32.

68 Kull I, *et al.* Early-life supplementation of vitamins A and D, in water-soluble form or in peanut oil, and allergic diseases during childhood. *J Allergy Clin Immunol* 2006;118:1299–1304.

69 Shaheen SO, *et al.* Umbilical cord trace elements and minerals and risk of early childhood wheezing and eczema. *Eur Respir J* 2004;24:292–7.

70 Turcanu V, Maleki SJ, Lack G. Characterization of lymphocyte responses to peanuts in normal children, peanut-allergic children, and allergic children who acquired tolerance to peanuts. *J Clin Invest* 2003;111:1065–72.

CHAPTER 39
Diets and Nutrition

Marion Groetch

KEY TERMS

- Food Allergy Labeling and Consumer Protection Act of 2004 (FALCPA) – FALCPA mandates the labeling of all food ingredients derived from commonly allergenic foods.

- Dietary reference intakes (DRI) – A new set of reference values of nutrient intakes that not only prevent nutritional deficiencies, but also reduce the risk of chronic disease.

- Essential fatty acids (EFAs) – EFAs are fatty acids that must be provided through the diet.

- Indispensable amino acids (IAAs) – IAAs are amino acids that cannot be biosynthesized, therefore must be provided through the diet.

- Waterlow classification – Waterlow classification defines acute and chronic states of malnutrition.

KEY CONCEPTS

- Allergen avoidance is currently the only treatment option available for the prevention of food-allergic reactions.

- The ability to accurately identify food allergens on product labels is fundamental to the success of allergen avoidance.

- Hidden allergens may be present in foods due to unintentional contamination during manufacturing or food preparation.

- Comprehensive nutrition education should include how to avoid the allergen and how to safely and appropriately substitute for eliminated foods and the nutrients in those foods.

- Children with food allergies may be at greater risk of inadequate growth and suboptimal nutrition and therefore require more stringent monitoring of growth and nutritional status.

Introduction

At this time there are no available prophylactic agents that have been consistently shown to prevent IgE-mediated reactions to food [1]. Although hopeful treatment options are being explored, immunotherapy to food proteins is experimental and should not be relied upon for the treatment of food allergies. Currently, strict dietary avoidance is the only therapeutic option available for the prevention of food-allergic reactions. The increasing prevalence of atopic disease presents a growing need for health care professionals who can effectively manage the dietary needs of those with food hypersensitivity.

As food elimination diets pose a challenge to providing a nutritionally balanced diet, it is essential that they are prescribed only when needed for the treatment of a properly diagnosed food allergy or for diagnostic purposes on a short-term basis. The physician prescribing the diet should understand the great burden placed on patients and their families with the introduction of an allergen-restricted diet. The social, psychological, and nutritional impact of such a dietary prescription must be measured against the necessity or potential benefit of treatment. The time required for meal planning and food preparation may be greatly increased. Eating out in restaurants or at friends' homes may become difficult or impossible, which may impact the socialization of the individual. Anxiety issues may arise about food and eating situations in general. In children, the acquisition of feeding skills may be delayed when food elimination diets present challenges to finding safe and appropriate textures required in developing oral motor feeding skills. Finally, food elimination diets may impact nutrient intake, and great care must be taken to ensure that the restricted diet continues to provide adequate nutrition. Comprehensive education should include not only how to avoid specific allergens, but also how to safely and appropriately substitute for eliminated foods and the nutrients inherent in those foods.

Food Allergy: Adverse Reactions to Foods and Food Additives, 4th edition.
Edited by Dean D. Metcalfe, Hugh A. Sampson, and Ronald A. Simon.
© 2008 Blackwell Publishing, ISBN: 978-1-4501-5129-0.

Food elimination diets: general overview

It may seem an easy task to eliminate a single allergen from the diet. However, the elimination of a single allergen, such as milk protein, makes it necessary to avoid many common foods including not only milk, butter, cheese, yogurt, and ice cream, but also numerous manufactured products such as many breads, cookies, cakes, crackers, cereals, processed meats, and cold cuts that may also contain milk protein as an ingredient [2]. In order for the diet to be successful, the patient must be able to comply with the dietary restrictions. The more diverse and appealing the diet, the less likely the patient will be tempted to risk an unsafe food. The diet must therefore be planned to provide the greatest possible variety in products, reflect the taste preferences of the individual, and minimize the social consequences, while remaining safe and nutritionally adequate. This is a tall order and important for any age group, but perhaps especially important in the teenage population where risky behavior is generally more common and the strain of social restriction may seem most daunting. A recent study of 174 adolescents and young adults reported that 54% of the participants indicated intentional ingestion of a potentially unsafe food and 42% reported a willingness to eat a food labeled "may contain (allergen)" [3]. Therefore, providing instruction for a diet that is safe, but also reflects the individual's tastes as well as social and nutritional needs is crucial.

Label reading

Fundamental to the success of any elimination diet is the ability to accurately identify food allergens on product labels. A study in 2002 by Joshi *et al.* reported that many food-allergic individuals or their caretakers were unable to correctly identify ingredients derived from major allergens on a variety of food labels, with milk and soy presenting the greatest challenges to families of children with food allergies [4]. Of 60 participants (parents of milk-allergic children), only 4 (7%) could correctly identify milk on all 14 labels that indicated the presence of milk protein. This study strongly highlighted the need for improved labeling that consumers with food allergies could more easily interpret [4]. In recognition of this need, new food labeling legislation came into effect in the European Union (EU) in November 2005 and in the United States in January 2006 to help make ingredient identification on manufactured foods easier [5,6].

In European countries, the EU directive 2003/89/EC, requires that 12 common food allergens be clearly identified on the ingredient label of all packaged foods manufactured after November 25, 2004. The 12 ingredients required to be listed on the package label in the European Union are the following:
- Milk
- Egg
- Peanut

- Tree nuts
- Fish
- Crustacean shell fish
- Soybean
- Gluten (wheat, rye, barley, oat, spelt, kamut, and their hybrid strains)
- Celery
- Mustard
- Sesame
- Sulfur dioxide and sulfites at concentrations of more than 10 mg/kg or 10 mg/l expressed as SO_2.

The EU directive applies to all prepackaged food but does not apply to foods sold loose or foods pre-packed for direct sale such as freshly made bread or cakes sold in supermarkets in which they have been packaged for hygienic purposes, foods sold in restaurants, or fancy confectionery products [6,7].

Previously in the European Union, the "25% rule" exempted the labeling of individual ingredients making up a compound ingredient in any food in which the compound comprised less than 25% of the finished product (e.g. a pudding filling in a cake). This obviously allowed for significant levels of allergens to be present in food products without any identification on the ingredient label. The EU directive has changed the "25% rule" to the "5% rule", but only for compounds whose compositions are defined by EU law, such as in foods like jam [7]. Fortunately, the "5% rule" does not override the allergen labeling requirements. Therefore all intentional sources of the 12 common allergens, regardless of whether or not the ingredient is part of a compound ingredient, must be identified on the ingredient label [6].

Currently, the EU Safety Authority has granted exemption for fermentation substrates and their bacterial cultures and enzymes, but no other permanent exemptions have been made. Temporary exemptions have been granted for several ingredients including highly refined soybean oil, wheat starch hydrolysate, and fish gelatin [7]. Manufacturers are granted a limited period of time to provide scientific data to support the lack of allergenic hazard of these ingredients for permanent exemption status.

In the United States, The Food Allergen Labeling and Consumer Protection Act of 2004, or FALCPA, mandates that food products must clearly list on the package label, in plain English language, ingredients derived from commonly allergenic foods. Conventional food products, including those imported for sale in the United States, dietary supplements, infant formulas and medical foods are all affected by FALCPA; raw agricultural commodities are not [5].

Allergic reactions may occur to a vast range of food ingredients; however, eight foods are responsible for 90% of all food allergic reactions. The ingredients subject to FALCPA, identified as the major food allergens, are those derived from these eight major food allergens:
- Milk
- Egg

- Soybean
- Wheat
- Peanut
- Tree nut
- Fish
- Crustacean shellfish

Additionally, manufacturers must list the specific tree nut (almond, Brazil nut, cashew, hazelnut, pecan, pistachio, walnut, etc.), fish (salmon, tuna, cod, etc.), or crustacean shellfish (crab, lobster, shrimp, etc.) used as an ingredient. Mollusks (clam, muscles, oyster, scallops, etc.) are not considered major food allergens under FALCPA [5].

Prior to January 2006, ingredients could be listed by their scientific or usual name, such as casein or whey, without any reference to the source of the ingredient, making identification of allergens difficult for the consumer. The plain language stipulation now requires the presence of a major food allergen to be listed on the product label in one of the following ways:

1 In the ingredient list for example: milk, egg, or soy.

2 Parenthetically following the food protein derivative for example: casein (milk).

3 Immediately below the ingredient list in a "contains" statement for example: *contains wheat* [7].

Only one of these methods is required and therefore consumers should be cautioned to avoid looking only for "contains" statements. However, if a "contains" statement is used and one or more major allergens are present in a product, they must all be listed in the "contains" statement even if one or more of the allergens were listed elsewhere on the label. For example, if casein, egg white, and almond are listed in the ingredient list, a "contains" statement would be necessary as casein was not identified as milk. The "contains" statement must however list all of the ingredients derived from major allergens; therefore, the following statement must be included on the label: *"contains milk, egg, and almond"* [9].

Additionally, a major food allergen may no longer be omitted from the product label if it is only an incidental ingredient such as in a spice, flavoring, coloring, or additive, or used merely as a processing aid in a product [5]. Consumers should be aware that these regulations apply only to ingredients derived from the eight foods that are considered the major allergens. An individual with sensitivity to an ingredient not covered under FALCPA, such as mustard, garlic, or sesame, would still need to call the manufacturer to ascertain if mustard, garlic, sesame, or sesame oil was included as an ingredient in a spice or natural flavoring of a product.

While it is likely that thresholds exist below which the vast majority of allergic individuals would not react, there is no consensus established on thresholds for most allergens at this time [7,10]. In addition, variability in individual threshold doses occurs as some people are clearly more sensitive than others to the same food allergen. This makes it difficult to determine if an ingredient with a very low risk of allergenicity should be included on a product label. So while an ingredient may be derived from an allergenic source, it may contain insignificant amounts of the allergenic protein. One example would be lecithin, which may be derived from soy, but is generally tolerated by most individuals with soy allergy due to the low levels of allergenic protein and the minute amount of ingredient use in any given product. Another example is kosher gelatin, derived from fish, which has a very low relative allergenicity [7,10].

FALCPA does provide for notification and petition processes that could lead to the exclusion of labeling requirements for some ingredients. Any person may petition the Secretary of Health and Human Services, under 21 USC 343 (w) [7], for exemption of a food ingredient from the allergen labeling requirement. The petition process for exemption of an ingredient requires that the petitioner "provide scientific evidence (including the analytical method used to produce the evidence) that demonstrates that such a food ingredient, as derived by the method specified in the petition, does not cause an allergic response that poses a risk to human health." US Food and Drug Administration (FDA) has 90 days to object to a notification. If an objection is not made, the food ingredient is exempt from FALCPAs labeling requirements for major food allergens. Currently FALCPA allows for highly refined vegetable oils derived from major food allergens to be exempt from the labeling requirement since highly refined oils have almost complete removal of allergenic protein and have not been shown to pose a risk to human health [5,7,11]. A petition for exemption of an ingredient from the labeling requirements of FALCPA may be sent to:

Food Labeling and Standards Staff (HFS-820)

Food and Drug Administration

5100 Paint Branch Parkway, Rm 4D-045

College Park, MD 20740

A consumer's ability to accurately identify intentional ingredients derived from a major food allergen will be improved by FALCPA and by the EU directive, but these laws do not yet address the issue of unintentional ingredients. Products may unintentionally come in contact with a potential allergen during customary methods of growing and harvesting crops, or from the use of shared storage, transportation, or production equipment, which may lead to significant levels of allergens in the product without any identification on the label [7,9]. In a study of 659 total food products classified for recall in the United States during fiscal year 1999, 36% of those products were recalled because they were contaminated with one or more undeclared allergens. The primary factors in this study contributing to the presence of undeclared allergens were ingredient-statement omissions and errors (51%), manufacturing equipment cross-contact (40%); and errors by ingredient suppliers or manufacturing firm employees (5%) [12].

Some manufacturers are beginning to address the issue of unintentional ingredients with advisory labeling such as "may contain (allergen)" or "produced in a facility that also produces (allergen)". These statements are appearing on more and more food product labels making the addition of many manufactured foods in the diet of individuals with food allergies quite difficult. FALCPA does not speak to the use of advisory labeling, but it does require FDA to submit a report to Congress to assess the use of advisory labeling as well as consumer preferences about advisory labeling. Previously, FDA advised that labeling such as "may contain (allergen)" should not be used as a substitute for adherence to current good manufacturing practices and it must be truthful and not misleading [9]. The consumer needs also be aware that while many manufacturers are adding advisory statements regarding the risk of cross-contact, these statements are voluntary in the United States and European Union. The absence of a "may contain" statement does not mean that there is no risk of cross-contact with the product. Consumers are still, in many cases, required to call manufacturers to ascertain the risk of cross-contact as well as to ascertain allergenicity of ingredients identified on the label or in "may contain" statements before including the food product in the diet. This puts the burden of responsibility on the consumer, and health care professionals must be prepared to offer extensive education to patients with food allergies, so safe food selections can be made. Health care professionals must continue to counsel their patients to avoid products that may contain their specific allergen [13].

Although label ambiguities continue to exist, the new food labeling laws in the European Union and the United States have begun a process directed at providing information greatly needed by those with food allergies to make safer food selections.

Food preparation safety

Individuals with food allergies must be diligent about risk assessment of all food purchased and consumed. Cross-contamination occurs outside of the manufacturing industry. It may occur in the home during food preparation as well as while eating out. Meals for the family member with allergies should be prepared first, covered, and then the other foods for the home prepared. The food preparation should be done in a clean environment with clean utensils and cooking equipment. Those with food allergies are especially at risk while dining out since restaurants are not required to list ingredients and the servers are generally ignorant about the ingredients in a dish. Cross-contact is common such as when the same grill is used to make a cheese burger that was used for a plain hamburger, or the French fries might have been cooked in the same fryer as the coconut shrimp. The same tongs may be used to assemble the green salad as is used to assemble the salad with walnuts. Consumers should be taught to speak directly to the chef or food service manager to inquire about ingredients and cross-contact risk. They should feel confident that the staff understands the severity of their food allergy as well as how to prepare a safe meal and be willing to leave the restaurant if they do not feel confident that a safe meal can be prepared [13].

Resources

The Food Allergy and Anaphylaxis Network or FAAN (www.foodallergy.org or 1 (800) 929-4040), is a non-profit organization whose mission is to raise public awareness, to provide advocacy and education, and to advance research on behalf of those affected by food allergies and anaphylaxis. Their medical advisory board ensures accuracy of information provided. FAAN is a valuable resource for patients with food allergies and their families providing a wealth of information and resources including conferences, newsletters, recipes, cookbooks, and videos as well as a limited number of a free school food allergy programs for elementary, intermediate, and high schools. The program is a comprehensive, multimedia program for schools to learn how to safely and effectively manage their students with food allergies.

Nutrition

The nutrient needs of each individual must be determined and a plan devised to meet those needs within the context of the allergen-restricted diet. In general, there is no good source of evidence describing altered nutritional needs in individuals with food allergies compared to their non-allergic peers. An exception would be the patient with atopic dermatitis who may have increased energy and protein needs due to loses through the compromised skin barrier and energy required for repair [2]. Other altered nutritional states such as increased protein needs for individuals whose food allergies contribute to protein losing enteropathy may be more apparent. There also remains some question as to the protein utilization of amino acid formulas potentially necessitating an increase in protein intake for individuals whose sole protein source is from an amino acid formula [14]. In general, however, the food-allergic individual is at greater nutritional risk primarily due to the restrictions in the diet.

Dietary reference intakes

In 1997, The Food and Nutrition Board of the National Academy of Science began a revision of the recommended dietary allowances (RDAs) that resulted in a new set of nutrient references called the *dietary reference intakes* or the DRIs. The DRIs have been established to provide reference values of nutrient intakes that not only prevent nutritional deficiencies, but also reduce the risk of chronic diseases such as osteoporosis, cancer, and cardiovascular disease.

DRIs have been established for vitamins, minerals, energy, and macronutrients such as dietary fat, fatty acids, protein, amino acids, carbohydrates, sugars, and dietary fiber. The DRIs contain four distinct reference values, plus a value used exclusively for energy, which are defined below [15].

Recommended dietary allowance

The RDA is the average daily dietary nutrient intake level sufficient to meet the nutrient requirement of nearly all healthy individuals (97–98%) in a particular life stage and gender group [16].

Adequate intake

The adequate intake (AI) is the recommended average daily intake level based on observed or experimentally determined approximations or estimates of nutrient intake by a group (or groups) of apparently healthy people that are assumed to be adequate. The AI is used when an RDA cannot be determined and when sufficient scientific evidence is not available to derive an estimated average requirement. The AI is set at a level thought to meet or exceed the needs of virtually all members of a life stage and gender group. Therefore in assessing individuals, if intake usually meets or exceeds the AI, a conclusion can be made that dietary intake is adequate. On the other hand, if intake regularly falls below the AI, prevalence of inadequacy cannot be determined as AI is set to meet or exceed the needs of most people [15,16].

Tolerable upper intake level

The tolerable upper intake level (UL) is the highest average daily nutrient intake level that is likely to pose no risk of adverse health effects to almost all individuals in the general population. As intake increases above the UL, the potential risk of adverse effects increases [16].

Estimate average requirement

The estimate average requirement (EAR) is the average daily nutrient intake level estimated to meet the requirement of half the healthy individuals in a particular life stage and gender group. The EAR exceeds the requirements of half the group and falls below the requirements of the other half as the EAR is actually the median requirement rather than the average [15,16].

Estimated energy requirement (EER), defined below, is a reference value used specifically for energy needs.

Energy

The EER is the average dietary energy intake that is predicted to maintain energy balance in a healthy adult for a defined age, gender, weight, height, and level of physical activity consistent with good health. In children and pregnant or lactating women, the EER includes the needs associated with the deposition of tissues or the secretion of milk at rates consistent with good health. There is no established RDA for energy because energy intakes exceeding the EER would be expected to result in excessive weight gain. EER can be calculated using the equations provided in the DRI reports and can be found at www.nap.edu.

In individuals with food allergy, dietary boredom and severely restrictive diets may contribute to inadequate energy intake. Additionally, certain food-allergic disorders, such as allergic eosinophilic esophagitis or gastroenteritis, may negatively affect appetite or contribute to early satiety, hence impacting adequate energy intake [17].

Energy is provided in the diet through three major classes of substrates or macronutrients, which are proteins, carbohydrates, and fats. Alcohol, another source of energy in the diet, will not be addressed here.

Protein

Many commonly allergenic foods are also excellent sources of protein: milk, egg, soy, fish, peanut, and tree nuts. Diets must be carefully planned to meet protein needs when high-quality protein sources are eliminated from the diet. The Food and Nutrition Board has set Acceptable Macronutrient Distribution Ranges (AMDR) for protein (and all macronutrients), which have been provided in Table 39.1. An AMDR is defined as "a range of intakes for a particular energy source that is associated with a reduced risk of chronic disease while providing AI of essential nutrients" [16]. Dietary protein needs may also be estimated using the DRI, which can be found in Table 39.2. The RDAs are based on nitrogen balance; the level at which the amount of dietary protein ingested will maintain a neutral or slightly positive nitrogen balance. The RDAs for infants, children, and pregnant and lactating women are determined to account for accretion of tissue. In assessing adequacy of protein in the diet, quality and quantity of dietary protein need to be considered as well as total energy intake [16].

Dietary protein recommendations are based on the assumption that energy intake is adequate. Amino acids liberated from dietary protein are either oxidized for energy, incorporated into protein in the body, or used for the formation of other nitrogen-containing compounds. There is an interrelation between energy needs and protein needs. If energy intake is insufficient, free amino acids will be oxidized for energy, allowing for less available amino acids for anabolic and synthetic pathways [18].

The quality of dietary protein will also impact nitrogen balance. Proteins are composed of amino acids and those amino acids that cannot be biosynthesized by enzymatic pathways are termed indispensable. These indispensable amino acids

Table 39.1 Acceptable macronutrient distribution range*

Age	Carbohydrate	Protein	Fat	EFA n-3	EFA n-6
Infant					
0–6 months	45–65				
7–12 months	45–65				
Children					
1–3 year	45–65	5–20	30–40	5–10	0.6–1.2
4–8 year	45–65	10–30	25–35	5–10	0.6–1.2
9–18 year	45–65	10–30	20–35	5–10	0.6–1.2
Adults	45–65	10–35	20–35	5–10	0.6–1.2

*Acceptable macronutrient distribution range (AMDR) is the range of intake for a particular energy source, expressed as a percentage of total caloric intake that is associated with reduced risk of chronic disease while providing intakes of essential nutrients.

For infants, an AMDR for protein and fats has not been established due to insufficient data regarding adverse effects of excess intakes.

Protein, dietary fat, and EFAs are vital in the diets of infants and a RDA/AI has been established for these nutrients.

Source: Dietary reference intakes for energy, carbohydrate, fiber, fat, fatty acids, cholesterol, protein, and amino acids (2002/2005). The entire report is available at www.nap.edu

Table 39.2 Dietary reference intakes for dietary protein

Age/life stage (group)	RDA (g/kg body weight/day)
Infants	
0–6 months	1.52*
7–12 months	1.2
Children	
1–3 years	1.05
4–13 years	0.95
14–18 years	0.85
Adults	
>18 years	0.80
Pregnancy	1.1
Lactation	1.3

*Adequate intake

Source: Dietary reference intakes for energy, carbohydrate, fiber, fat, fatty acids, cholesterol, protein, and amino acids (2002/2005). The entire report is available at www.nap.edu

(IAAs) must be provided through the diet. An estimated 65–70% of protein needs should be of high biological value, meaning animal products. While animal products contain a full complement of all IAAs, most other protein sources do not. Animal products are not necessary to provide optimal protein, but alternative sources from plants, legumes, grains, nuts, seeds, and vegetables do not contain a full complement of IAAs and therefore greater dietary planning will be required. Of additional concern to the food-allergic individual is the use of amino acid formulas, which may increase nitrogen losses as compared to intact protein formulas [14].

Greater protein intake may be required to counter nitrogen losses in individuals whose main protein source is from amino acid formulas [2,14]. Recommended dietary intakes for individual amino acids have been revised and can be accessed in the DRI reports at www.nap.edu [16].

Fat

Dietary fats provide energy and serve as a carrier for the absorption of fat-soluble vitamins. Adequate fat in the diet is also necessary to provide the fatty acids that are considered essential for human health. While too much fat can negatively impact health, a certain amount of fat is essential. The type of fat as well as the total amount of fat consumed will determine if fat intake is appropriate and healthful.

Table 39.1 provides the AMDR of dietary fat as a percentage of total energy intakes. An AMDR for infants has not been established but the AI for total fat for infants 0–6 months of age is 31 g/day and for infants 7–12 months of age is 30 g/day and can be found in Table 39.3 [16]. Intakes below 20% of total caloric intake increase risk of hypocaloric, vitamin E deficient and essential fatty acid (EFA) deficient diets while intakes greater than 35% (except in children under 3 years of age) are not recommended as they will likely increase intake of saturated fat and excess calories.

Dietary fats are largely present in the triacylglycerol (triglyceride) form, which consists of three fatty acids and a glycerol molecule. Fatty acids can be either saturated, polyunsaturated, monounsaturated, or present as trans-fatty acids. Although some trans-fatty acids occur naturally, they are predominantly present in our food supply through hydrogenated oils in margarines, cookies, cakes, crackers, and other snack foods. Saturated fatty acids are found in full fat dairy products, fatty meats, and tropical oils such as coconut and palm kernel oil. Since there is no required role for dietary saturated and trans-fatty acids, individuals should consume predominantly polyunsaturated and monounsaturated fat sources.

Unsaturated fatty acids can have either one (monounsaturated or MUFA) or more (polyunsaturated or PUFA) double bonds on the carbon chain. PUFAs are further categorized on the basis of the location of the first double bond. Human cells can introduce double bonds in all positions on the fatty acid chain except the omega-3 (n-3) and the omega-6 (n-6) positions, hence the n-3 α-linolenic acid (ALA) and the n-6 linoleic acid (LA) are considered essential and must be provided through the diet [18]. EFA are metabolized to their long chain metabolites, arachidonic acid and dihomo-γ-linolenic acid from LA, and eicosapentaenoic acid and docohexaenoic acid from ALA. These long chain metabolites form precursors to respective prostaglandins, thromboxanes, and leukotrienes that regulate a large number of vital functions in the body, including blood pressure, blood clotting, blood lipid levels, the immune response, and the inflammation response to injury and infection [18,19].

Table 39.3 Dietary reference intakes for dietary fat and EFAs in infants

Age	Omega-3 EFA AI (g/day)	Omega-6 EFA AI (g/day)	Total fat AI (g/day)
Infant			
0–6 months	0.5	4.4	31
7–12 months	0.5	4.6	30

Source: Dietary reference intakes for energy, carbohydrate, fiber, fat, fatty acids, cholesterol, protein, and amino acids (2002/2005). The entire report is available at www.nap.edu

EFA deficiency is rare and the challenge to all people including those with food allergies is finding a healthy balance between the two EFAs. There has been an increased interest in n-3 fatty acids as several lines of research have suggested that a high ratio of n-6 to n-3 fatty acids may contribute to a number of chronic diseases [19,20]. LA or n-6 fatty acid is generally provided abundantly in the diet and found in a wide variety of vegetable oils including safflower, sunflower, soy, and corn oils. ALA is less abundantly found and the sources tend to be from more commonly allergenic foods. Dietary sources that provide 10% or more of the RDA/AI for ALA or n-3 fatty acids are fish, fish oils, canola or rapeseed oil, soybean oil, flaxseed, walnuts, and wheat germ [18].

The FNB has set AMDR for dietary fat and EFAs for individuals 1 year of age and older, which can be found in Table 39.1. There is no determined AMDR for dietary fat or EFAs for infants up to 12 months of age, but the AI is set to meet the requirement for neural development and growth and can be found in Table 39.3 [16]. AIs for the EFAs, which vary by age group and sex, as well as during pregnancy and lactation, can be accessed in the DRI reports at www.nap.edu [16].

Dietary fat is an important source of energy, supports the transport of fat-soluble vitamins, and provides the two fatty acids that are essential in the human diet. Maintaining a healthy balance of dietary fats including n-3 to n-6 fatty acids may pose a challenge to those with food allergies as the primary sources or n-3 fatty acids are from commonly allergenic foods. For the individual with food allergies, and especially in the pediatric population, adequate fat intake may be compromised due to dietary restrictions. The addition of vegetable oils to the allergen-restricted diet may be required to meet fat and EFA needs [2]. The amount and type of oil required will need to be individualized based on current dietary intake and degree and type of dietary restrictions.

Carbohydrates

Carbohydrates make up the remaining energy sources and are an important supply of numerous micronutrients. The AMDR for carbohydrate is between 45% and 65% of total caloric intake [16]. The RDA is based on carbohydrates role as the primary source of energy for the brain and is set at

130g/day for children and adults 1 year of age or older. AI established for infants 0–6 months and for infants 7–12 months is 60 and 95 grams or carbohydrates daily, respectively [16]. Grains, fruits, and vegetables provide dietary carbohydrates. Foods with added sugars also contribute carbohydrates and additional energy, but are of little further nutritional benefit and should be limited to no more than 25% of total energy intake [16]. Adequate carbohydrate intake prevents ketosis and excessive intake of dietary fats while contributing to AI of dietary fiber. Individuals with grain allergies may have an especially difficult time ingesting sufficient carbohydrates.

Micronutrients

Variety in the diet contributes to adequacy of all nutrients provided. When a food group is eliminated, many nutrients provided by that food group must now be provided by other dietary sources. A recent study by Salman *et al.* reviewed nutrient intakes of children with food allergies and noted that several nutrients including calcium, vitamin D, vitamin E, iron, and zinc were found to be insufficiently provided, less than 67% of the RDAs for those nutrients [21]. While it is important to ensure an appropriate intake of all essential nutrients, certain nutrients will be at greater risk of insufficiency depending on the food allergen. The specific nutrients lost must be adequately replaced by other foods in the diet. When dietary modifications are inadequate to meet vitamin, mineral, and trace element needs, appropriate supplementation may be considered. Health care professionals should be aware that many dietary supplements pose a risk of contamination with food allergens (even those labeled allergen free) [2] and they should be chosen carefully with consideration for safe ingredients as well as risk assessment of potential cross-contact during manufacturing. Appropriate dietary substitutions should always be the first, and will likely be the safest option for those with food allergies.

Pediatric nutrition

A special focus on the nutritional status of children with food allergies is warranted as food allergy and multiple food allergies are more prevalent in the pediatric population. The prevalence of food allergy in infants and young children is 6% with the major allergens being milk, soy, egg, wheat, and peanut [8,22]. Christie *et al.* reported that children with two or more food allergies were shorter, based on height-for-age percentiles than those with only one food allergy. Furthermore, children with cow's milk allergy or multiple food allergies consumed dietary calcium less than age- and gender-specific recommendations compared with children without cow's milk allergy and/or one food allergy [22]. Since children with food allergies are at greater risk of inadequate growth and suboptimal nutrition, pediatricians may need to screen these patients more carefully, and refer them for nutritional counseling at the first signs of growth faltering, rather than take a "wait and see" position. Interventions aimed at meeting the distinct nutritional needs of children are imperative as poor nutrition may adversely affect growth and development, and dietary counseling may significantly improve nutritional intake.

Growth in the pediatric population is a sensitive indicator of the provision of adequate energy and protein. Individual micronutrient deficiencies may not be reflected in growth alone, certainly not in the short term, and therefore the measurement and assessment of growth is only one aspect of the nutrition assessment. In addition to growth, physical assessment, biochemical indices, clinical diagnoses, dietary intake including the frequency, amount and type of feeding, allergies and intolerances, aversions and food preferences, and the use of supplements and medications must all be taken into consideration [23].

Pediatricians generally track a patient's growth from birth and therefore have the best information regarding the child's growth patterns. A child's current weight gives an incomplete picture. Current weight needs to be compared to reference standards as well as to typical growth patterns for that child. Plotting a child's weight history on the appropriate National Center for Health Statistics (NCHS) growth chart provides a way to compare growth of that child with that of the healthy reference population (www.cdc.gov/growthchart) [24]. It also allows for a child's individual growth over a period of time to be assessed. Weight is the most sensitive measure of adequate energy and is affected earlier and to a greater extent than stature by dietary inadequacies.

Stature can be delayed due to dietary protein inadequacy or chronic energy deficits. Children less than 2 years of age should have their length measured in the supine position while those 3 years of age or older may have their height measured standing. Children between 2 and 3 years of age may be measured by either technique although they should be plotted on the appropriate corresponding NCHS chart. A supine length is actually greater than a standing height; therefore, if a child is measured standing but plotted on a length growth chart, he will appear to be shorter. A recent randomized-controlled intervention trial of 878 children in 55 pediatric facilities reported accurate growth measurements in only 30% of children [25]. Since children grow 5 cm/year on average between the ages of 2 years and the onset of puberty, with measurements generally taken annually at well visits, accuracy is of the essence. Body mass index (BMI), defined as weight in kilograms divided by the square of height in meters, may be used after 2 years of age and is helpful as it takes into consideration weight for height [24]. The Centers for Disease Control and Prevention (CDC) defined underweight in children as a BMI of less than the 5th percentile. Children are considered to be at risk of overweight when their BMI is greater than the 85th percentile and overweight when their BMI is greater than the 95th percentile.

Significant changes in growth velocity are not expected as normal development typically follows predictable increases in both height and weight. When malnutrition is suspected due to changes in growth velocity, the degree of malnutrition may be assessed using Waterlow classification [26,27]. Waterlow classification, found in Table 39.4, is based on height for age and weight for height and defines acute and chronic nutritional states. Acute malnutrition (wasting) refers to adequate height but inadequate weight for height. Chronic malnutrition (stunting) refers to inadequate height for age. Children may be both chronically and acutely malnourished. Waterlow classification utilizes anthropometric measurements that are made as described above and percentages which are determined using the NCHS growth charts. The following equations can be used to determine acute and chronic nutritional status as defined by Waterlow classification [23]:

$$\textit{Acute nutritional status} = \frac{\text{Actual weight}}{\substack{\text{50th percentile} \\ \text{weight for height}}} \times 100$$

$$\textit{Chronic nutritional status} = \frac{\text{Actual height}}{\substack{\text{50th percentile} \\ \text{height for age}}} \times 100$$

The 50th percentile weight for height may be calculated by finding first the height age, which is the age at which the patient's length or height would be reflected at the 50th percentile on the appropriate NCHS growth chart. The 50th percentile weight for height therefore is the weight at the 50th percentile for the patient's height age or the ideal body weight for height age. To illustrate, take the example of a 4-year-old male with a height of 96 cm and a weight of 12 kg. His height would be reflected at the 50th percentile on the NCHS growth chart for a 3.25-year-old boy and therefore he would have a height age of 3.25 years. His weight for the 50th percentile for height would be 15 kg. Using the above equations for acute and chronic nutritional status, he would have an acute nutritional status of 80% and a chronic nutritional status of 94%; therefore, he is moderately wasted and mildly stunted. When determining caloric and protein need for catch-up growth, ideal body weight for height age should be used.

Table 39.4 Waterlow's classification to define acute and chronic nutritional status

Nutritional status	Acute	Chronic
Stage 0 (normal)	>90%	>95%
Stage 1 (mild)	81–90%	90–95%
Stage 2 (moderate)	70–80%	85–89%
Stage 3 (severe)	<70%	<85%

Table 39.6 Primary functions and significant dietary sources of vitamins

Vitamin	Chief functions in the body	Significant sources
Vitamin A	Visual adaptation to light and dark; growth of skin and mucous membrane	Retinol (animal foods): liver, egg yolk, fortified milk, cheese, cream, butter, and fortified margarine; carotene (plant foods): spinach and other dark leafy greens, broccoli, deep orange fruits (apricots and cantaloupe), and vegetables (squash, carrots, sweet potato, and pumpkin)
Vitamin D	Absorption of calcium and phosphorus; calcification of bones	Self-synthesis from sunlight; fortified milk, fortified margarine, eggs, liver, and fish oils
Vitamin E	Antioxidant, stabilization of cell membranes, protection of PUFAs and vitamin A	Polyunsaturated plant oils, green and leafy vegetables, wheat germ, whole grain products, nuts, and seeds
Vitamin K	Normal blood clotting	Bacterial synthesis in the digestive tract; green leafy vegetables, milk and dairy products, meats, eggs, and cereals
Thiamin (B1)	Coenzyme in carbohydrate metabolism; normal function of the heart, nerves, and muscle	Pork, beef, liver, whole or enriched grains, legumes, and nuts
Riboflavin (B2)	Coenzyme in protein and energy metabolism	Milk, yogurt, cottage cheese, meat, leafy green vegetables, whole or enriched grains, and cereals
Niacin (B3)	Coenzyme in energy production, health of skin, normal activity of stomach, intestines, and nervous system	Meat, peanuts, legumes, and whole or enriched grains
Pyridoxine (B6)	Coenzyme in amino acid metabolism; helps convert tryptophan to niacin; heme formation	Grains, seeds, liver, meats, milk, eggs, and vegetables
Cyanocobalamin (B12)	Coenzyme in synthesis of heme in hemoglobin; normal blood cell formation	Animal products (meat, fish, poultry, shellfish, milk, cheese, and eggs)
Folic acid	Part of DNA; growth and development of red blood cells	Liver, leafy green vegetables, legumes, seeds, and yeast
Pantothenic acid	Part of coenzyme A, which is used in energy metabolism; formation of fat, cholesterol, and heme; activation of amino acids	Meats, cereals, legumes, milk, fruits, and vegetables
Biotin	Part of coenzyme A, which is used in energy metabolism; involved in lipid synthesis, amino acid metabolism, and glycogen synthesis	Liver, egg yolk, soy flour, cereals, tomatoes, and yeast
Vitamin C	Collagen synthesis (strengthens blood vessel walls, forms scar tissue, matrix for bone growth); antioxidant; thyroxine synthesis; strengthens resistance to infection; helps with absorption of iron	Citrus fruits, tomato, cabbage, dark leafy green vegetables, broccoli, chard, turnip greens, potatoes, peppers, cantaloupe, strawberries, melons, papayas, and mango

Reproduced from Mofidi, S. [2], with permission from the American Academy of Pediatrics.

Wheat allergy

The wheat-allergic patient must avoid all wheat-containing products resulting in the elimination of many processed and manufactured products. Wheat is a component of most commercial bread, cereal, pasta, crackers, cookies, and cakes. Those with wheat allergy should be aware that wheat starch is commonly used as a minor ingredient in other commercial food products such as condiments and marinades, cold cuts, soups, soy sauce, some low or non-fat products, hard candies, licorice, and jelly beans.

Nutritionally, wheat contributes necessary carbohydrates, the major source of energy in the diet, as well as many micronutrients such as thiamin, niacin, riboflavin, iron, and folate. Whole grain wheat products also contribute fiber to the diet. Four servings of wheat-based products such as whole grain and enriched cereals or breads generally provide greater than 50% of the RDA/AI for carbohydrate, iron, thiamin, riboflavin, and niacin for individuals 1 year of age and older as well as a significant source of vitamin B6 and magnesium. Elimination of wheat products from the diet has great nutritional impact. Table 39.5 lists the major nutrients provided by wheat in the diet. Alternative sources of these nutrients may be found in Tables 39.6 and 39.7.

Many alternative flours are available to patients with wheat allergy, including rice, corn, oat, barley, buckwheat, rye, amaranth, millet, and quinoa. Cereal grain proteins may be cross-reactive and therefore those with wheat allergy

Table 39.7 Primary functions and food sources of minerals and trace elements

Mineral	Primary functions in the body	Significant sources
Calcium	Bone and teeth formation; involved in normal muscle contraction and relaxation, nerve functioning, blood clotting, and blood pressure	Milk and milk products; small fish (with bones); greens; legumes; calcium-fortified tofu; calcium-fortified juices; calcium-fortified rice, soy, or potato milks
Chloride	Part of hydrochloric acid found in the stomach, necessary for proper digestion	Salt, soy sauce; moderate quantities in whole, unprocessed foods, large amounts in processed foods
Chromium	Cofactor for insulin	Molasses, nuts, whole grains, and seafood
Copper	Cofactor for enzymes; necessary for iron metabolism; cross-linking of elastin	Liver, shellfish, whole-grain cereals, legumes, and nuts
Fluoride	Structural component in calcium hydroxyapatite of bones and teeth	Seafood, meat, fluoridated water
Iodide	A component of the thyroid hormone, thyroxin, which helps to regulate growth, development, and metabolic rate	Iodized salt and seafood
Iron	Structural component of hemoglobin (which carries oxygen in the blood) and myoglobin (which makes oxygen available for muscle contraction) and other enzymes; necessary for the utilization of energy	Red meats, fish, poultry, shellfish, legumes, dried fruits
Magnesium	One of the factors involved in bone mineralization; maintain electrical potential in nerves and muscle membranes; involved in building of proteins, enzyme action, normal muscular contraction, transmission of nerve impulses, and maintenance of teeth	Widely distributed in most foods with nuts, fruits, vegetables, and cereals as best sources
Manganese	Cofactor for enzymes	Whole grains, leafy green vegetables, and wheat germ
Molybdenum	Xanthine oxidase, aldehyde oxidase	Legumes, whole grains, and wheat
Phosphorus	Bone and teeth formation; regulation of acid–base balance; present in cell's genetic material as phospholipids, in energy transfer, and in buffering systems	Milk, poultry, fish, meat, and carbonated beverages
Potassium	Regulation of osmotic pressure and acid–base balance; activation of a number of intracellular enzymes; nerve and muscle contraction	All whole foods; meats, milk, fruits, vegetables, grains, and legumes
Selenium	Part of glutathione peroxidase (an enzyme that breaks down reactive chemicals that harm cells); works with vitamin E	Seafood, organ meats, muscle meats, grains, and vegetables depending on soil conditions
Sodium	Regulation of pH, osmotic pressure, and water balance; conductivity or excitability of nerves and muscles; active transport of glucose and amino acids	Salt, soy sauce, seafood, dairy products, and processed foods
Zinc	Part of the hormone insulin and many enzymes; taste perception; wound healing; metabolism of nucleic acids	Red meat; seafood, especially oysters; and bean

Reproduced from Mofidi, S. [2], with permission from the American Academy of Pediatrics.

may test positive on prick skin testing to other grains as well. It has been reported that 20% of individuals with grain allergy may be clinically reactive to another grain; therefore, use of these products should be individualized and based on tolerance as determined by the patient's allergist [34]. If a patient has tolerance to alternative grains, these flours may improve the nutritional quality, variety, and convenience of the wheat-restricted diet; not only are these flours commercially available, but there are now many wheat- and gluten-free products made from these flours. As many of these flours may not be fortified, those with wheat allergies may choose to substitute fortified infant cereal for a portion of the alternative flour used in baked products for added nutrients such as iron, thiamin, riboflavin, niacin, and zinc [2].

Soybean allergy

Soybean allergy is relatively common in early childhood. Soy protein is present in our food supply in a variety of forms and can be found in a surprising array of products including baked goods, cereals, crackers, canned tuna and soups, reduced-fat peanut butter, pre-basted meat products, cold cuts, and hotdogs. Soy protein may be found in many vegetarian-based products and is often the base for hydrolyzed vegetable or hydrolyzed plant protein. Studies show that the vast majority of soy-allergic individuals can tolerate soy oil and soy lecithin [10]. This is an important piece of knowledge, since soy oil and soy lecithin are pervasive in processed foods and avoidance of these two soy-derived ingredients eliminates an extensive list of processed or manufactured foods that might otherwise be tolerated. Highly refined soy oil is exempt from allergen labeling, but soy lecithin is not, and therefore products that contain soy lecithin with a "contains soy" statement may in fact be safe for consumption by many soy-allergic consumers. Patients should never assume that a product is safe, however, and should first call the manufacturer to determine if any other soy protein ingredients are contained in a product.

While soy itself contains a number of vital nutrients including protein, thiamin, riboflavin, pyridoxine, folate, calcium, phosphorus, magnesium, iron and zinc, it generally is not a major component of the diet, and therefore the nutrients lost due to soy elimination may easily be replaced. The result of eliminating many manufactured foods with soy as an ingredient, however, will impact the variety of manufactured products available for consumption. Table 39.5 lists the major nutrients provided by soy in the diet. Alternative sources of these nutrients may be found in Tables 39.6 and 39.7.

Peanut allergy

Recent studies have indicated that the prevalence of peanut allergy has doubled among children less than 5 years of age in the last decade [8,35]. Peanut allergy is common, affecting approximately 0.6% of the general population in the United States with both children and adults affected [8]. While food-protein-induced anaphylaxis can be caused by any food allergen, the most common cause of fatal anaphylaxis is peanut ingestion.

Peanuts have become popular ingredients in our food; however, it is easier to avoid foods that contain peanut than it is to avoid, say milk or wheat, in the typical Western diet. Furthermore, avoidance of peanuts and tree nuts in the diet does not pose any specific nutritional risk although peanuts are a good source of protein, fat, vitamin E, niacin, magnesium, manganese, and chromium. Peanuts are a common ingredient in cereal, crackers, cookies, candy, and frozen desserts. Peanut butter or peanut flour can be found in unexpected places such as in chili, stew, and pasta sauce where it may be added as a thickener. Peanut butter is sometimes used as an ingredient in egg rolls to seal the roll before frying. Peanut flours may also be used in protein bars and other high protein products. Individuals with peanut allergy need to take additional precautions when eating in restaurants. Certain ethnic cuisines such as Chinese, Thai, etc. are considered high risk as peanut and tree nuts are pervasive ingredients in these cuisines and often cooking utensils and woks are merely wiped clean before preparing the next dish, potentially leaving enough residual protein to cause a reaction. Ice cream parlors are also considered high risk for those with nut allergies due to the likelihood of cross-contact. Ice cream scoopers are used for all flavors of ice cream including those flavors which contain nuts. Using a clean scooper does not alleviate the risk as a previous scooper may already have contaminated

the ice cream. Highly processed peanut oil has been shown to be safe for those with peanut allergy, although cold pressed, expressed, or expelled oils may contain sufficient protein to cause an allergic reaction [11]. Individuals with peanut allergy may choose to avoid peanut oil as information on how the oil was processed may not always be available and the variety of alternative vegetable oils is vast.

Exposure to peanut allergen, through saliva via kissing, shared utensils or young children sharing and mouthing the same toys, can cause local- and systemic-allergic reactions. A recently published study by Maloney *et al.* evaluated the time course to clear the presence of peanut allergen in saliva after the ingestion of two tablespoons of peanut butter. While peanut protein in the saliva varied considerably after ingestion, peanut protein was undetectable in all participants after waiting several hours and ingesting a peanut-free meal. Interestingly, brushing the teeth, rinsing the mouth, and chewing gum were ineffective at accelerating the elimination of peanut protein from the saliva. This study suggests that waiting several hours after ingestion of a peanut-containing meal and then eating a peanut-free meal is the safest way to eliminate peanut allergen from the saliva [36].

It was once believed that a peanut allergy was always a lifelong allergy, but it is now known that approximately 20% of young children with peanut allergy may eventually develop clinical tolerance [35]. Children with a peanut allergy are at greater risk for tree nut allergies. In fact, about 35% of those allergic to peanut will react to at least one tree nut although these two foods are botanically different, peanut being a legume rather than a nut. Clinical reactivity is generally specific and clinical cross-reactivity between more than one member of a botanical species is not common [8]. Cross-reactivity between peanuts and legumes is rare with only 5% of those with a peanut hypersensitivity reacting to another legume [34]. Certain types of legumes, however, appear to be more cross-reactive. Lupine, a legume used predominantly in Europe, often as a flour mixed with wheat flour in baked goods, appears to have a higher risk of cross-reactivity to peanut. Lupine is also beginning to appear in high protein and low carbohydrate versions of products (such as pasta) in the United States. Moneraet-Vautrin *et al.* reported that 44% of those allergic to peanut have a positive prick skin test response to lupine. Of those with a positive prick skin test, seven of eight of those who were challenged were clinically reactive to lupine flour [37].

Tree nut allergy

Tree nuts (almond, Brazil nut, cashew, chestnut, filbert/hazelnut, macadamia, pecan, pine nut, pistachio, and walnut) are added to numerous products, similar to those products containing peanut. Tree nut oils may be added to lotions and soaps, so these labels must also be carefully read. Artificial nuts can be made from peanuts that are flavored with a tree nut flavor such as walnut or pecan, and therefore are not safe for those with a tree nut allergy. Additionally, marinades and some brands of barbeque sauce are now adding tree nut oils and flavoring to their products.

Clinical reactions to tree nuts can be severe and cross-reactivity among the nuts is relatively high with 37% of patients with an allergy to one tree nut having IgE binding and clinical reactivity to another tree nut [34]. Patients are often advised to avoid all tree nuts if one is proven to be allergic to one tree nut due to the high risk of cross-reactivity, the potential for severe reactions, and the risk of cross-contact in handling. However, if a specific tree nut had previously been eaten and tolerated, the patient may be advised to proceed with caution but to always contact the manufacturer to ascertain the safety of the tree nut from a cross-contact perspective [34].

Coconut and the following tree nuts also require disclosure on food labeling by US law: Beech nut, Ginkgo, shea nut, Butter nut, Hickory, Chinquapin, Lyctree nut, and Pili nut. Coconut allergy in patients with tree nut allergy is rare and coconut is generally not restricted in the diets of those with tree nut allergies. However, while rare, reactions to coconut have occurred and are most likely due to clinical cross-reactive proteins with walnut protein [38]. Including coconut in the diet of those allergic to tree nuts is likely safe, but should be individualized by the patient's allergist. The risk of allergic reaction to these other less common tree nuts has not been extensively studied. Nutmeg is not a nut and is safe to include in the diet of those with tree nut allergies.

Fish allergy

Fish is an excellent source of dietary protein and in some cultures, the primary source. Fish and more specifically the individual fish species must be listed on the food ingredient label and may no longer be "hidden" in a product. Those with fish allergies should be aware that fish is a common ingredient in Worcestershire sauce, Surimi, and other imitation shellfish. The major allergens responsible for cross-reactivity among species of fish are parvalbumins. IgE binding to multiple fish species in patients with fish allergy is often the case and while clinical cross-reactivity occurs, isolated allergy to a single species of fish also occurs [34]. It has been estimated that approximately 50% of individuals with fish allergy are at risk of reacting to at least one other fish species [34]. A patient with a confirmed fish allergy should be advised to avoid all other fish species until the patient is further evaluated by an allergist and a fish species is proven safe to eat by oral food challenge. Patients should always proceed with caution as cross-contact of fish species in seafood stores and restaurants is common.

Shellfish allergy

Allergic reactions to shellfish are the most common form of food allergy in adults, affecting 2% of the population. Shellfish represent a high risk for cross-reactivity, with a potential for severe reactions. Those who are allergic to a specific species of shellfish have a 75% risk of reacting to another species of shellfish [34]. Crustacean shellfish (shrimp, lobster, crab and crawfish) are considered major allergens in the United States and European Union, and therefore must be listed on the product label even if a minor ingredient such as a flavoring. Mollusks (clams, mussels, oysters, scallops and squid) are not considered major allergens under new food labeling laws. Although shellfish are not commonly used as a hidden ingredient in a product, those with an allergy to clam, for instance, may need to call the manufacturer to determine if clam was used in seafood flavoring. Those with shellfish allergy should avoid seafood restaurants because cross-contact is likely even if a non-shellfish dish is ordered. Also, some sensitive individuals may react to aerosolized shellfish protein through cooking vapors. There have been reported cases of fatal reactions caused by inhalation of shrimp protein from cooking fumes [13].

Sesame seed allergy

While sesame seed is not considered a major allergen in the United States, it is in the European Union and allergic reactions to sesame seed protein appear to be growing in prevalence in many countries, including the United States. Allergic reactions to sesame have been reported to be severe with respiratory symptoms and anaphylactic shock not uncommon. Sesame oil is a crude oil and not highly refined, and therefore may contain significant amounts of sesame protein. In a recent study by Morisset *et al.*, five of six patients with sesame allergy were positive on double-blind, placebo-controlled food challenge to sesame oil and two of these patients experienced anaphylactic reactions. Of note, these subjects reacted to only a few milligrams of sesame protein in the sesame oil, but when challenged to sesame protein in crushed sesame seeds, the threshold for reaction was 100 mg – 7 g of sesame protein. The authors contend that the considerable increase in allergenicity of the sesame protein in sesame oil may be due to the interaction between sesame allergens and the lipid matrix [39].

Food ingredients that contain sesame seed protein are sesame seeds, Tahini (sesame seed paste), sesame oil, and sesame flour. Products to be aware of that may contain sesame seed protein are breads, bread crumbs and breading, hummus, halvah, falafel, high protein energy bars and snacks, vegetarian burgers and cold cuts, salad dressings and marinades, some herbal drinks, and certain brands of cereals (e.g. kashi brand cereals) which routinely use sesame flour as part of their grain mixture. Cross-contact with sesame may occur in manufacturing and most especially in bakeries and bagel shops as well as pizza parlors.

Summary

Dietary management of food allergy requires extensive education regarding the elimination of the allergenic food as well as how to replace the nutrients usually provided by the food or foods to be eliminated. Worldwide, the use of manufactured foods presents a risk due to unintentional contamination. Even with the advent of new food allergen labeling laws, the use of packaged products continues to pose a threat to those with food allergies. Patients should be advised to include predominantly fresh whole foods such as safe meats, fruits and vegetables, and individual ingredients, and to limit as much as possible the use of packaged convenience foods. When packaged foods are used, understanding the food ingredient label and calling the manufacturer for further information to ascertain the safety of the product is imperative.

At their initial visit to the allergist, patients diagnosed with food allergy must absorb an overwhelming amount of new information. They must understand their emergency action plans, how to use their emergency medications and maintenance medications for chronic atopic disease, as well as the concept of dietary avoidance. Dietary issues may not be discussed extensively at the initial assessment and questions may arise after the patient has gone home and no longer has access to accurate information. Ideally, a patient with food allergies should be referred for dietary counseling upon diagnosis. In the pediatric population, growth should be closely monitored and pediatricians have a specific responsibility in assessing growth and referring patients to a registered dietitian for evaluation if dietary inadequacies are suspected. Success in dietary management depends on the practitioner's ability to educate the patient on dietary avoidance as well as how to substitute safe and appropriate foods to meet nutritional needs.

References

1 Nowak-Wegrzyn A. Immunotherapy for food allergy. *Inflamm Allergy Drug Targets* 2006;5:23–34.

2 Mofidi S. Nutritional management of pediatric food hypersensitivity. *Pediatrics* 2003;111:1645–53.

3 Sampson MA, Munoz-Furlong A, Sicherer SH. Risk-taking and coping strategies of adolescents and young adults with food allergy. *J Allergy Clin Immunol* 2006;117:1440–5.

4 Joshi P, Mofidi S, Sicherer SH. Interpretation of commercial food ingredient labels by parents of food-allergic children. *J Allergy Clin Immunol* 2002;109:1019–21.

5 *Food Allergen Labeling Consumer Protection Act of 2004.* Available from: http://www.cfsan.fda.gov.

6 MacDonald A. Better European food labelling laws to help people with food intolerances. *Matern Child Nutr* 2005;1:223–4.

7 Taylor SL, Hefle SL. Food allergen labeling in the USA and Europe. *Curr Opin Allergy Clin Immunol* 2006;6:186–90.

8 Sampson HA. Update on food allergy. *J Allergy Clin Immunol* 2004;113:805–19; quiz 820.

9 *Questions and Answers Regarding Food Allergens including the Food Allergen Labeling Consumer Protection Act of 2004*, 3rd edn.

10 Taylor SL, Hefle SL, Bindslev-Jensen C, *et al.* Factors affecting the determination of threshold doses for allergenic foods: How much is too much? *J Allergy Clin Immunol* 2002;109:24–30.

11 Crevel RWR, Kerkhoff MAT, Konig MMG. Allergenicity of refined vegetable oils. *Food Chem Toxicol* 2000;38:385–93.

12 Vierk K, Falci K, Wolyniak C, Klontz KC. Recalls of foods containing undeclared allergens reported to the US Food and Drug Administration, fiscal year 1999. *J Allergy Clin Immunol* 2002;109:1022–6.

13 Munoz-Furlong A. Daily coping strategies for patients and their families. *Pediatrics* 2003;111:1654–61.

14 Jones B, Lees R, Andrews J, Frost P. Comparison of an elemental and polymeric enteral diet in patients with normal gastointestinal function. *Gut* 1983;24:78–84.

15 Barr SI, Murphy SP, Poos MI. Interpreting and using the dietary references intakes in dietary assessment of individuals and groups. *J Am Diet Assoc* 2002;102:780–8.

16 Trumbo P, Schlicker S, Yates AA, Poos M. Food and Nutrition Board of the Institute of Medicine, The National Academies. Dietary reference intakes for energy, carbohydrate, fiber, fat, fatty acids, cholesterol, protein and amino acids. *J Am Diet Assoc* 2002;102:1621–30.

17 Pentiuk SP, Miller CK, Kaul A. Eosinophilic esophagitis in infants and toddlers. *Dysphagia* 2007 Jan;22(1):44–8.

18 Shils M, Shike M, Ross A, *et al.* Modern nutrition in Health and Disease. 10th edn. Lippincott Williams & Wilkins, Philadelphia, Baltimore, New York, 2006.

19 Effects of Omega-3 Fatty Acids on Lipids and Glycemic Control in Type II Diabetes and the Metabolic Syndrome and on Inflammatory Bowel Disease, Rheumatoid Arthritis, Renal Disease, Systemic Lupus Erythmatosus, and Osteoporosis. Evidence Report/Technology Assessment No. 89 (Prepared by Southern California/RAND Evidence-Based Practise Center, under Contract No. 290-02-0003). AHRQ Publication No. 04-E012-2. Rockville, MD: Agency for Healthcare Research and Quality, 2004.

20 James MJ, Gibson RA, Cleland LG. Dietary polyunsaturated fatty acids and inflammatory mediator production. *Am J Clin Nutr* 2000;71:S343–8.

21 Salman S, Christie L, Burks AW. Dietary intakes of children with food allergies: comparison of the Food Guide Pyramid and the Recommended Dietary Allowances, 10th edn. *J Allergy Clin Immunol* 2002;109:S214.

22 Christie L, Hine RJ, Parker JG, Burks W. Food allergies in children affect nutrient intake and growth. *J Am Diet Assoc* 2002;102:1648–51.

23 *Pediatric Manual of Clinical Dietetics.* Parkman Williams C (ed.). The American Dietetic Association, Chicago, 1998:19–34.

24 Kuszmarski RJ, Ogden CL, Guo SS, *et al.* Growth charts for the United States: methods and development. *Vital Health Stat* 2002;290:1–190.

25 Lipman TH, Hench KD, Benyi T, *et al.* A multicentre randomised controlled trial of an intervention to improve the accuracy of linear growth measurement. *Arch Dis Child* 2004;89:342–6.

26 Waterlow JC. Note on the assessment and classification of protein-energy malnutrition in children. *Lancet* 1973;2:87–9.

27 Waterlow JC. Classification and definition of protein-calorie malnutrition. *BMJ* 1972;3:566–9.

28 Shirley Walberg Ekvall. Nutrition assessment and early intervention. In: Ekvall S (ed.) *Pediatric Nutrition in Chronic Diseases and Developmental Disorders.* Oxford University Press, New York, Oxford, 1998.

29 Scherer SH. Food allergy. *Lancet* 2002;360:701–10.

30 Committee on Nutrition. American Academy of Pediatrics: hypoallergenic infant formulas. *Pediatrics* 2000;106:346–9.

31 Moneret-Vautrin DA, Morisset M, Cordebar V, *et al.* Probiotics may be unsafe in infants allergic to cow's milk. *Allergy* 2006;61:507–8.

32 Kalliomaki M, Salminen S, Arvilommi H, *et al.* Probiotics in primary prevention of atopic disease: a randomised placebo-controlled trial. *Lancet* 2001;357:1076–9.

33 Han DK, Kim MK, Yoo JE, *et al.* Food sensitization in infants and young children with atopic dermatitis. *Yonsei Med J* 2004;45:803–9.

34 Sicherer SH. Clinical implications of cross-reactive food allergens. *J Allergy Clin Immunol* 2001;108:881–90.

35 Sicherer SH. Clinical update on peanut allergy. *Ann Allergy Asthma Immunol* 2002;88:350–61; quiz 361–2, 394.

36 Maloney JM, Chapman MD, Sicherer SH. Peanut allergen exposure through saliva: assessment and interventions to reduce exposure. *J Allergy Clin Immunol* 2006;118:719–24.

37 Moneret-Vautrin DA, Guerin L, Kanny G, *et al.* Cross-allergenicity of peanut and lupine: the risk of lupine allergy in patients allergic to peanuts. *J Allergy Clin Immunol* 1999;104:883–8.

38 Teuber SS, Peterson WR. Systemic allergic reaction to coconut (Cocos nucifera) in 2 subjects with hypersensitivity to tree nut and demonstration of cross-reactivity to legumin-like seed storage proteins: new coconut and walnut food allergens. *J Allergy Clin Immunol* 1999;103:1180–5.

39 Morisset M, Moneret-Vautrin DA, Kanny G, *et al.* Thresholds of clinical reactivity to milk, egg, peanut and sesame in immunoglobulin E-dependent allergies: evaluation by double-blind or single-blind placebo-controlled oral challenges. *Clin Exp Allergy* 2003;33:1046–51.

CHAPTER 40

Food Toxicology

Steve L. Taylor

KEY CONCEPTS

- Food intoxications are caused by chemicals in foods including both synthetic and naturally occurring substances.

- The central axiom of toxicology is that all chemicals are toxic, it is the dose that makes the poison.

- Certain naturally occurring constituents (e.g. the toxins in poisonous mushrooms) and contaminants (e.g. the algal toxins causing paralytic shellfish poisoning and ciguatera poisoning) can be particularly hazardous to consumers causing serious and acute symptoms if ingested.

- Food additives do not typically elicit toxic reactions in consumers if used in accordance with governmental regulations and ingested in doses consistent with those practices.

- Lactose intolerance results from a deficiency of β-galactosidase in the small intestine so that ingestion of milk sugar or lactose elicits acute gastrointestinal complaints including flatulence, abdominal pain, and frothy diarrhea.

Food toxicology could be defined as the science that establishes the basis for judgments about the safety of foodborne chemicals. The central axiom of toxicology as set forth by Paracelsus in the 1500s states: "Everything is poison. Only the dose makes a thing not a poison." Thus, all chemicals in foods, whether natural or synthetic, inherent, adventitious, or added, are potentially toxic. The vast majority of foodborne chemicals are not hazardous because the amounts of each foodborne chemical in the typical diet are not sufficient to cause injury. The degree of risk posed by exposure to any specific foodborne chemicals is determined by the dose, duration, and frequency of exposure (and especially in the case of allergies, the degree of sensitivity of the individual). The age-old wisdom about the benefits of eating moderate amounts of a varied diet protects most consumers from any harm. Foodborne chemicals that are considered to be toxicants are those chemicals where the dose, duration, and frequency of exposure can, in at least some circumstances, be sufficient to elicit adverse reactions. Unusual diets can sometimes result in intoxications from chemicals that would normally be considered safe and desirable. For example, polar explorers experienced toxic responses to excessive intake of vitamin A as the result of consuming large amounts of polar bear liver.

Food Allergy: Adverse Reactions to Foods and Food Additives, 4th edition.
Edited by Dean D. Metcalfe, Hugh A. Sampson, and Ronald A. Simon.
© 2008 Blackwell Publishing, ISBN: 978-1-4501-5129-0.

Acute adverse reactions to foods can occur through many mechanisms including infections (viral, bacterial, parasitic), various intoxications, and allergies and intolerances. Food allergies are the major focus of this book. Other medical conditions including some food intoxications can cause symptoms resembling food allergies. These other conditions must be considered and eliminated in diagnosing food allergy.

Toxic reactions to food encompass all food-associated illnesses that are caused by chemicals in food, although foodborne chemicals vary greatly in toxicity. All consumers are susceptible to most food intoxications, although differences will exist primarily related to the dose of exposure and body weight (infants versus adults). Food allergy can be viewed as a category of food intoxication that affects only certain individuals in the population. Other categories of food intoxications, such as metabolic food disorders, also affect only certain individuals in the population. This chapter will focus on some of the more common types of acute foodborne intoxications including the most common metabolic food disorders. Some of the selected examples have certain manifestations in common with food allergies and intolerances and are thus of some importance in the differential diagnosis of food allergies.

Intoxications caused by synthetic chemicals in foods

Most of the synthetic chemicals in foods including food additives, agricultural chemical residues, and chemicals migrating from packaging materials have been rigorously tested for toxicity. These synthetic chemicals are typically safe under normal circumstances of exposure, although adverse reactions can occur from misuse, either intentional or accidental. In most situations, the concentrations of chemicals in these categories are well below any levels that might be associated with adverse reactions. The focus here will be on a few intentional food additives, agricultural chemical residues, packaging migrants, and other man-made chemicals that can occur in foods at concentrations sufficient to cause concern.

Food additives

These examples were chosen because some of the manifestations are similar to symptoms that can occur during IgE-mediated allergic reactions.

Niacin

Excessive consumption of niacin (nicotinic acid), which is part of the B vitamin complex, can cause an acute onset of flushing, pruritus, rash, and burning or warmth in the skin especially on the face and upper trunk [1]. Gastrointestinal (GI) discomfort is noted by some patients. Outbreaks have sporadically occurred from the excessive enrichment of grain products as the result of inaccurate or inadequate labeling of food ingredient containers. Such episodes are rare because the amount of niacin required to elicit such symptoms is at least 50 times the recommended dietary allowance [2]. The symptoms of niacin intoxication are self-limited and without sequelae.

Sorbitol and other polyhydric alcohols

Sugar alcohols, such as sorbitol, are widely used sweeteners in dietetic food products. They are especially common in candy and chewing gum because they are non-cariogenic. Diarrhea can result from the excessive consumption of sugar alcohols [3]. Sorbitol and the other sugar alcohols are not as easily absorbed as sugar. Because of their slow absorption, these sweeteners can cause an osmotic-type diarrhea if excessive amounts are ingested. For adults, outbreaks occur from ingesting more than 20g of these sweeteners per day [3]. Infants are susceptible to lower doses. The illness is self-limited.

Toxic oil poisoning

In 1981 and 1982, an epidemic occurred in Spain linked to the ingestion of unlabeled, illegally marketed cooking oils [4]. A total of 19,828 cases and 315 deaths were recorded in this epidemic [5]. The illicit cooking oil contained oils from both plant and animal sources but some of the oils were denatured and intended for industrial rather than food uses. The causative toxin in the oils remains unknown, although fatty acid anilides resulting from the denaturation process are suspected to be at least partially responsible [5].

The clinical manifestations of this illness involved multiple organ systems [5]. In the first few days after ingestion of the oil, patients experienced fever, chills, headache, tachycardia, cough, chest pain, and pruritus. Physical examinations revealed various skin exanthema, splenomegaly, and generalized adenopathy. Pulmonary infiltrates were noted in 84% of patients probably as the result of increased capillary permeability. The intermediate phase of the illness tended to begin in the second week and persist through the eighth week post-ingestion. GI symptoms, primarily abdominal pain, nausea, and diarrhea, predominated. Clinical examination revealed marked eosinophilia in 42% of patients, high IgE levels, thrombocytopenia, abnormal coagulation patterns, and evidence of hepatic dysfunction with abnormal enzymes. Some patients became jaundiced, and many had hepatomegaly. The late phase of the illness developed in 23% of cases and began after 2 months of illness. This phase was characterized initially by neuromuscular and joint involvement. Later, patients developed vasculitis and a scleroderma-like syndrome. Patients complained of intense muscular pain, edema, and progressive muscular weakness. Muscular atrophy was apparent in some patients. Neurological involvement included depressed deep tendon reflexes, anesthesia, and dysesthesia. Respiratory problems developed due to neuromuscular weakness and progressed to pulmonary hypertension and thromboembolic phenomena. The sclerodermalike symptoms included Raynaud's phenomenon, sicca syndrome, dysphagia, and contractures due to thickening collagen in the skin. Vascular lesions were noted in all organs apparently resulting from endothelial proliferation and thrombosis. All patients in the late group had antinuclear antibody and many had antibodies against smooth muscle and skeletal muscle [6]. The pathological and clinical features are consistent with an autoimmune mechanism for this illness. Since the precise causative agent and its mechanism have not been delineated, a recurrence is not impossible [5]. Also, the toxin, if present in small amounts in other foods, may be producing or aggravating other clinical conditions [5].

Agricultural chemicals

A wide diversity of chemicals are used in modern agricultural practices. Residues of these chemicals can occur in raw and processed foods, although federal regulatory agencies evaluate the use and safety of such chemicals. The major categories of agricultural chemicals would include insecticides, herbicides, fungicides, fertilizers, and veterinary drugs including antibiotics.

Insecticides

Insecticides are added to foods to control the extent of insect contamination. The major categories of insecticides include organochlorine compounds (DDT, chlordane, and others, many of which are now banned), organophosphate compounds (e.g. parathion and malathion), carbamate compounds (e.g. carbaryl and aldicarb), botanical compounds (e.g. nicotine and pyrethrum), and inorganic compounds (e.g. arsenicals).

The exceedingly low residue levels of insecticides found in most foods are not particularly hazardous especially on an acute basis. Large doses of insecticides can be toxic to humans. For example, the organophosphates and carbamates are cholinesterase inhibitors and act as neurotoxins by blocking synaptic nerve transmission. Several reasons exist for the low degree of hazard posed by insecticide residues in foods: (i) the level of exposure is very low, (ii) some insecticides are not very toxic to humans, (iii) some insecticides decompose rapidly in the environment, and (iv) many different insecticides are used, which limits exposure to any one particular insecticide.

No food poisoning incidents have ever been attributed to the proper use of insecticides on foods. However, problems have occasionally arisen from the inappropriate use of certain insecticides [7]. An outbreak of aldicarb intoxication from watermelons occurred on the West Coast of the United States in 1985 [8]. Aldicarb use on watermelons is not allowed in the United States because excessive levels of aldicarb become concentrated in the edible portion of the melon. In this episode, several farmers used aldicarb illegally resulting in consumer illnesses and the recall and destruction of thousands of watermelons. A total of 1373 illness reports were received in this outbreak with 78% classified as probable or possible aldicarb poisoning cases [8]. This episode is thus the largest known outbreak of pesticide poisoning in North America [8]. Aldicarb has also been involved in several food poisoning outbreaks associated with ingestion of hydroponically grown cucumbers [9]. The symptoms of aldicarb intoxication include nausea, vomiting, diarrhea, and mild neurological manifestations such as dizziness, headache, blurred vision, and loss of balance [8,9]. Many other episodes of pesticide intoxications have resulted from the misuse of pesticides including contamination of foods during storage and transport, the use of pesticides in food preparation due to their mistaken identity as common food ingredients such as sugar and salt, and their misuse in agricultural practice as in the examples noted above [7].

Herbicides

Herbicides are applied to control the growth of weeds. Among the more important herbicides are chlorophenoxy compounds (e.g. 2,4-D), dinitrophenols (e.g. dinitroorthocresol), bipyridyl compounds (e.g. paraquat), substituted ureas (e.g. monuron), carbamates (e.g. propham), and triazines (e.g. simazine). Generally, herbicide residues in foods are not a hazard to consumers. No food poisoning incidents have resulted from the proper use of herbicides on food crops. The lack of hazard from herbicide residues is associated with the low level of exposure, their low degree of toxicity to humans and selective toxicity toward plants, and the use of many different herbicides which limits exposure to any particular herbicide.

Since most herbicides are selectively toxic to plants, they pose little hazard to humans in the amounts normally used for weed control. The bipyridyl compounds are an exception. These non-selective herbicides are rather toxic to humans and tend to exert their toxic effects on the lung [10]. However, no food poisoning incidents have ever been attributed to inappropriate use of the bipyridyl compounds.

Fungicides

Fungicides are used to prevent the growth of molds on food crops. Important fungicides include captan, folpet, dithiocarbamates, pentachlorophenol, and the mercurials. The hazards from foodborne fungicides are miniscule because exposure is quite low, most fungicides do not accumulate in the environment, and fungicides are typically not very toxic.

Exceptions are the mercurial compounds and hexachlorobenzene. The mercurials are often used to treat seed grains to prevent mold growth during storage. These seed grains are usually colored pink and are clearly intended for planting rather than consumption. However, on several occasions, consumers have eaten these treated seed grains and developed mercury poisoning [7]. Although some severe episodes have resulted in deaths, mild cases of mercury intoxication can be manifested in GI symptoms such as abdominal cramps, nausea, vomiting, and diarrhea, and dermal symptoms such as acrodynia and itching [7]. Hexachlorobenzene caused one of the most massive outbreaks of pesticide poisoning in recorded history affecting over 3000 individuals in Turkey from 1955 through 1959 [11]. Hexachlorobenzene-treated seed grain was consumed rather than planted resulting in severe symptoms including prophyria cutanea tarda, ulcerated skin lesions, alopecia, porphyrinuria, hepatomegaly, thyroid enlargement, and a 10% mortality rate [11].

Fertilizers

The commonly used fertilizers are combinations of nitrogen and phosphorus compounds. Nitrogen fertilizers are oxidized to nitrate and nitrite in the soil. Both nitrate and nitrite are hazardous to humans if ingested in large amounts. Infants are particularly susceptible to nitrate and nitrite intoxication. Some plants, such as spinach, can accumulate nitrate to hazardous levels if allowed to grow on overly fertilized fields. Because nitrite is more toxic than nitrate, the situation can be worsened if nitrate-reducing bacteria are allowed to proliferate on these foods.

Acute nitrite intoxications have occurred. In low doses, the symptoms include flushing of the face and extremities, GI discomfort, and headache; in larger doses, cyanosis, methemoglobinemia, nausea, vomiting, abdominal pain, collapse, and death can occur. The lethal dose of nitrite is estimated at about 1g in adults. Illnesses have occurred from ingestion of over-fertilized spinach in which bacterial action on the nitrate-rich, unprocessed spinach allows conversion to nitrite before ingestion. Illnesses have also resulted from the improper storage of carrot juice that allowed the proliferation of nitrate-reducing bacteria resulting in the accumulation of hazardous levels of nitrite [12].

Veterinary drugs and antibiotics

Food-producing animals can be treated with a variety of veterinary drugs especially antibiotics. Residues in foods are typically quite low. Acute food poisoning incidents have not occurred as a result of properly used veterinary drugs and antibiotics. Penicillin is probably one of the major concerns because of the potential for allergic reactions to penicillin residues. However, the likelihood of allergic reactions to the very low levels of penicillin residues found in foods is quite remote [13].

Chemicals migrating from packaging materials and containers

Chemicals migrating from packaging materials into foods and beverages are not a significant source of chemical exposure. A variety of chemicals, including plastics monomers, plasticizers, stabilizers, printing inks, and others, do migrate at extremely low levels into foods. These chemicals do not often create any known hazards for consumers. Lead, copper, and tin are perhaps the main concerns associated with packaging materials. The storage of acidic foods in inappropriate containers can result in the leaching of toxic heavy metals, such as zinc. Contact of acidic beverages with copper can also release potentially hazardous levels of copper into the beverage.

Lead

Lead (Pb) exposure from foods has always been a comparatively moderate contributor to overall environmental lead exposure. The migration of Pb from Pb-soldered cans was previously a source of some concern. However, Pb-soldered cans have been successfully phased out of use in the United States. The main issue with Pb contamination remains the occasional use of Pb-based glazes on pottery or paint on glassware that may come in contact with acidic foods or beverages. Pb is a well-known toxicant that can affect the nervous system, the kidney, and the bone.

Tin

Tin plate is commonly used in the construction of metal cans for foods. The inner surfaces of these cans are lined with a lacquer material when cans are used for acidic foods or beverages. Acute tin intoxication has occurred from the inappropriate placement of tomato juice or fruit cocktail in unlined cans. Since tin is poorly absorbed, the primary symptoms are bloating, nausea, abdominal cramps, vomiting, diarrhea, and headache occurring 30 minutes to 2 hours after consumption of the acidic product.

Copper

Copper poisoning, characterized primarily by nausea and vomiting, most commonly occurs from faulty check valves in soft drink vending machines. The check valves prevent contact between the acidic, carbonated beverage, and the copper tubing that delivers the water or ice in the machine. Several outbreaks of copper poisoning have resulted from such occurrences. Copper poisoning results in acute gastroenteritis.

Zinc

Zinc intoxication typically results from the unwise storage of acidic foods or beverages in galvanized containers. Zinc is a potent emetic. The symptoms of zinc intoxication include irritation of the mouth, throat, and abdomen; nausea and vomiting; dizziness; and collapse.

Industrial chemicals

Industrial and/or environmental pollutants often migrate into foods in small amounts. On rare occasions, hazardous levels of such chemicals enter the food supply often with devastating consequences.

Polychlorinated biphenyls and polybrominated biphenyls

The contamination of foods with polychlorinated biphenyls (PCBs) and polybrominated biphenyls (PBBs) has occurred on several occasions. PCBs and PBBs are quite persistent in the environment and are considered to be toxic pollutants from industrial practices. PBBs are commonly used as fire retardants, while PCBs are frequently used in transformer fluid. PCBs and PBBs are not worrisome acute toxicants in foods. However, since they are lipid-soluble, the chronic effects of exposure to these contaminants in foods are of concern. The most infamous incident involved the accidental contamination of dairy feed in Michigan with PBBs. This incident resulted in the destruction of many cows and their milk. Leaking transformers have contributed to the contamination of feeds with PCBs which led to the destruction of chickens, eggs, and egg-containing food products.

Mercury

Minamata disease, due to mercury (Hg) intoxication, is the classic example of the contamination of foods by industrial pollutants [14]. An industrial firm located on the shores of Minamata Bay in Japan dumped Hg-containing wastes into the bay where bacteria converted the inorganic Hg into highly toxic methylmercury. Fish in the bay became contaminated with the methylmercury. Over 1200 cases of Hg intoxication occurred among consumers of Minamata Bay fish [14]. The symptoms included tremors and other neurotoxic effects and kidney failure.

Intoxications caused by naturally occurring chemicals in foods

The naturally occurring chemicals in foods are less frequently tested for their potential toxic effects than synthetic chemicals. While the vast majority of naturally occurring chemicals in foods are safe under the normal circumstances of exposure, some potentially hazardous situations do exist. Those naturally occurring chemicals with significant pharmacological activity including the vasoactive amines, methylxanthines, ethanol, and myristicin are covered elsewhere. However, naturally occurring chemicals in foods can elicit a wide variety of adverse reactions including both acute and chronic intoxication. Naturally occurring toxicants could be defined as those naturally occurring chemicals in foods that might be hazardous under typical circumstances of exposure. Naturally occurring chemicals in foods are more likely to be hazardous under typical circumstances of exposure than are synthetic chemicals. Although chronic illnesses, such as cancer, are undeniably important, this chapter will focus exclusively on acute intoxications caused by natural, foodborne toxicants.

Naturally occurring contaminants

Naturally occurring contaminants can be produced in foods as the result of contamination by bacteria, molds, algae, and insects. The chemicals produced from these biological sources can remain in foods even after the living organism has been removed or destroyed. Naturally occurring contaminants are not always present in foods and can be avoided, if contamination is prevented. Such contaminants represent the most important and potentially hazardous chemicals of natural origin existing in foods. The bacterial and insect toxins will not be discussed in detail. The bacterial toxins cause very familiar diseases including staphylococcal food poisoning and botulism. The insect toxins have not been studied to any extent, and their impact on human health is uncertain.

The toxicants produced by algal species that bioaccumulate in seafoods are among the most common causes of foodborne illness of chemical etiology. These algal toxicants are involved with several of the seafood poisonings including ciguatera poisoning and paralytic shellfish poisoning. Mycotoxins produced by foodborne molds are a source of considerable toxicological concern and occur at low levels rather frequently in certain stored foods. Several of the mycotoxins will be discussed in some detail because they are confirmed to be involved in acute foodborne illness. A bigger concern with the mycotoxins is their potential involvement with chronic toxicity. The chronic toxicity of mycotoxins will not be described here because it is unlikely to be relevant to the investigation of allergic reactions.

Ciguatera poisoning

Ciguatera poisoning results from the ingestion of fish that have fed on toxic dinoflagellate algae. Ciguatera poisoning is the most common cause of acute foodborne disease of chemical etiology reported to the Centers for Disease Control. This foodborne illness is common throughout the Caribbean, South Pacific, and Indian Ocean areas, but is now encountered around the world due to the improved distribution of fish [15,16]. In the United States, the illness occurs most frequently in Florida, Hawaii, and the Virgin Islands. The fish most commonly implicated in cases of ciguatera poisoning are large tropical and semi-tropical reef fishes such as grouper, barracuda, sea bass, Spanish mackerel, snappers, and sea perches, although as many as 400 different fish species have been implicated in this illness. Curiously, although most cases involve tropical or semi-tropical fishes, at least one outbreak has involved farm-raised salmon [17].

With the tropical and semi-tropical reef fishes, the fish acquire the toxic agent(s) by feeding on smaller fishes that acquire the toxin from the poisonous planktonic algae [16]. Several species of dinoflagellate algae appear able to produce toxins of the type associated with ciguatera poisoning; *Gambierdiscus toxicus* is one of the most prominent [16]. Several toxins may be involved in ciguatera poisoning [16,18]. The major toxins, known as ciguatoxins, are lipid-soluble, heat-stable, polyether compounds with an approximate molecular weight of 1110 Da [16,18]. Ciguatoxin has ionophoric properties, which selectively opens voltage-sensitive sodium channels of the neuromuscular junction. Maitotoxin also appears to be responsible to a lesser extent for ciguatera poisoning [16,18]. Maitotoxin is a water-soluble compound of molecular weight of 3424 Da which activates both voltage-sensitive and receptor-operated calcium channels in the plasma membranes of cells. The toxins accumulate in the liver and viscera of the fish, but enough can enter the muscle tissues to result in ciguatera poisoning among humans ingesting these fish [16]. Larger fish pose a greater risk than smaller fish. The toxins are heat-stable and are unaffecting by processing or cooking practices.

The symptoms of ciguatera poisoning tend to be somewhat variable perhaps confirming the role of several different dinoflagellate algae and several different toxins in this syndrome [15,16]. GI and neurological manifestations are the predominant symptoms associated with ciguatera poisoning, although in some cases, the GI symptoms predominate, while in other cases, the neurological symptoms predominate. The GI symptoms include nausea, vomiting, diarrhea, and abdominal cramps. The neurological symptoms include dysesthesia, paresthesia especially in the perioral region and extremities, pruritus, vertigo, muscle weakness, malaise, headache, and myalgia. A peculiar reversal of hot and cold sensations occurs in about 65% of all patients [18]. In severe cases, the neurological manifestations can progress to delirium, pruritus, dyspnea, prostration, brachycardia, and coma [18]. Many patients recover within a few days or weeks, although treatment is difficult and deaths from cardiovascular collapse have been encountered in about 0.1% of cases [19].

Paralytic shellfish poisoning

Paralytic shellfish poisoning results from the ingestion of molluscan shellfish, such as clams, mussels, cockles, and scallops, that have become poisonous by feeding on toxic dinoflagellate algae [15,20]. Paralytic shellfish poisoning occurs worldwide but is commonly encountered along the Pacific and North Atlantic coasts of North America, the coastal areas of Japan, and the coasts of Chile and Argentina [16]. Several species of toxic dinoflagellate algae have been implicated in paralytic shellfish poisoning; *Alexandrium catanella* (formerly *Gonyaulax catanella*) and *A. tamarensis* are two of the most common ones. "Blooms" of the toxic dinoflagellates are sporadic, so most shellfish will be hazardous only during the times of the blooms. While most shellfish species clear the toxins from their system within a few weeks after the end of the dinoflagellate bloom, a few species, such as the Alaskan butter clam, seem to retain the toxin for long periods [21]. The toxins involved in paralytic shellfish poisoning are known as saxitoxins [22]. Saxitoxins are neurotoxins that bind to and block the sodium channels in nerve membranes [16]. The saxitoxins are heat-stable so processing and cooking have no effect on the toxicity of the shellfish.

Through the blocking of nerve transmission, the saxitoxins are very potent neurotoxins. The symptoms of paralytic shellfish poisoning include a tingling sensation and numbness of the lips, tongue, and fingertips followed by numbness in the legs, arms, and neck, ataxia, giddiness, staggering, drowsiness, incoherent speech progressing to aphasia, rash, fever, and respiratory and muscular paralysis [15,16]. Death from respiratory failure occurs frequently, usually within 2–12 hours depending on the dose ingested. No antidotes are known, although prognosis is good if the victim survives the first 24 hours of the illness.

Amnesic shellfish poisoning

Amnesic shellfish poisoning was first recognized following an outbreak in Canada in late 1987 [23]. Amnesic shellfish poisoning was associated with the ingestion of mussels from Prince Edward Island which resulted in over 100 cases and at least four deaths [23,24]. The source of the toxin was a planktonic algae, *Nitzschia pungens*, which was blooming in an isolated area of Prince Edward Island at the time of the outbreak [25]. The toxin involved was identified as domoic acid, a neuroexcitatory amino acid [24]. Amnesic shellfish poisoning is characterized by GI symptoms and unusual neurological abnormalities [24]. The GI symptoms, which occurred within the first 24 hours, were vomiting, abdominal cramps, and diarrhea. The neurological symptoms, which had onset within 48 hours, were severe incapacitating headaches, confusion, loss of short-term memory, and, in a few cases, seizures and coma. Severely affected patients

who did not die experienced prolonged neurologic sequelae including memory deficits and motor or sensorimotor neuronopathy or axonopathy [24].

Diarrhetic shellfish poisoning

Diarrhetic shellfish poisoning is primarily associated with the ingestion of clams that have become toxic through the ingestion of toxic dinoflagellate algae of the genus *Dinophysis* and *Prorocentrum* [16]. No confirmed outbreaks have occurred in North America but outbreaks have occurred primarily in Japan and Europe [19]. The toxins responsible for diarrhetic shellfish poisoning are polyether compounds: okadaic acid and its derivatives, the dinophysistoxins [16]. The symptoms include diarrhea, nausea, vomiting, and abdominal cramps [19].

Pufferfish poisoning

Pufferfish poisoning occurs primarily in Japan and China, the only parts of the world where pufferfish are frequently consumed. While about 30 species of pufferfish are found worldwide, most species are not toxic. The most hazardous pufferfish belong to the genus *Fugu*, which are considered in Japan and China to be delicacies. The toxin in pufferfish is a potent neurotoxin called tetrodotoxin [26]. For many years, the toxin was thought to be produced by the fish, but evidence now exists that marine bacteria may be the original source of the toxin [27]. Tetrodotoxin is heat-stable and, like saxitoxin, acts by blocking the sodium channels in nerve cell membranes. The symptoms of tetrodotoxin poisoning usually begin with a tingling sensation of the fingers, toes, lips, and tongue, followed by nausea, vomiting, diarrhea, and epigastric pain [26]. Twitching, tremors, ataxia, paralysis, and death often ensue [26]. The fatality rate is about 60% in untreated cases. Most of the tetrodotoxin accumulates in the liver, viscera, and roe of the pufferfish. Careful cleaning of the fish, before ingestion of the edible muscle, is required to safeguard against tetrodotoxin intoxication.

Mycotoxins

Mycotoxins are produced by a wide variety of molds which can grow and produce toxins on a wide variety of foods [28]. Most of the known mycotoxins have been recognized because of their toxicity to domestic animals fed moldy feed grains. However, a few mycotoxins are noteworthy because they are known hazards for humans.

Ergotism

Ergotism was the first recognized mycotoxin-associated illness. The responsible mold is *Claviceps purpurea*, which can infect the grains of rye, wheat, barley, and oats. The last recorded outbreak of ergotism occurred in Europe in 1951. Ergotism is caused by a group of toxins known as the ergot alkaloids. Ergotism is manifested in two forms: gangrenous ergotism and convulsive ergotism. Gangrenous ergotism, also known as Saint Anthony's fire, is characterized by a burning sensation in the feet and hands followed by progressive restriction of blood flow to the hands and feet resulting ultimately in gangrene and loss of limbs. Convulsive ergotism is characterized by hallucinations leading to convulsive seizures and sometimes death. Modern agricultural practices and grain milling procedures have virtually eliminated ergotism as a concern.

Alimentary toxic aleukia

Alimentary toxic aleukia (ALA) was observed in Russia during World War II and was associated with the consumption of over-wintered millet that contained trichothecene mycotoxins. Trichothecenes are a group of mycotoxins produced by molds of the genus *Fusarium*. ALA occurs in four stages. In the first stage, affected individuals experience burning sensations in the mouth, throat, and esophagus followed 1–3 days later by diarrhea, nausea, and vomiting. The GI symptoms cease after about 9 days. The second stage of ALA begins during the second week and lasts through the second month. This stage involves bone marrow destruction, leukemia, agranulocytosis, anemia, and loss of platelets. Small hemorrhages begin to appear at the end of this stage. The third stage of ALA lasts for 5–20 days and involves total loss of bone marrow with necrotic angina, sepsis, total agranulocytosis, moderate fever, larger hemorrhages on the skin, and the appearance of necrotic skin lesions. Bronchial pneumonia usually develops along with abscesses and hemorrhages in the lungs. The fourth stage of ALA is death, which occurred in about 80% of cases within 3 months of the onset of symptoms. Due to the circumstances at the time of this outbreak, the identification of the exact species of *Fusarium* and the trichothecenes responsible for ALA were not accomplished. The level of contamination of the millet with trichothecenes was not determined.

Fusarium molds are very common on grain crops worldwide. Trichothecene mycotoxins continue to occur at low levels in many cereal foods. However, no acute illnesses in humans including ALA have been attributed to trichothecene intoxication since the original outbreak. The effects of ingestion of low levels of toxic trichothecenes on humans remain uncertain.

Naturally occurring constituents

Many fungi, some plants, and a few animals contain hazardous levels of various naturally occurring toxicants. Such fungi, plants, and animals should not be eaten, but are accidentally or intentionally consumed on occasion resulting in foodborne illness. Furthermore, many plants and animals contain levels of naturally occurring toxicants that are probably not hazardous to humans ingesting typical amounts of these foods. The ingestion of abnormally large quantities of such foods and their naturally occurring toxicants is potentially hazardous. Some naturally occurring toxicants are inactivated or removed during processing or preparation of foods prior to consumption. The failure to adhere to such processing and preparation practices can result in foodborne illness.

Poisonous animals

Very few animal species are poisonous, although several species of poisonous fish and other marine animals are known to exist. Pufferfish is the best-known example, although the toxin in pufferfish may actually emanate from bacteria [27].

Animal tissues and products also contain very few naturally occurring toxicants that could cause adverse reactions if ingested in abnormally large quantities. Fat-soluble vitamins, most notably vitamin A, serve as an example. Cases of vitamin A intoxication have occurred in polar explorers ingesting polar bear liver and in infants resulting from feeding diets rich in vitamin A (e.g. chicken livers and fortified milk) and carotenoids (e.g. pureed carrots), while also administering daily vitamin supplements [29].

Poisonous plants

Many poisonous plants exist in nature [30]. Classic examples would include water hemlock and nightshade which were used in centuries past to poison one's enemies. While consumers purchasing foods from commercial sources can usually avoid the ingestion of poisonous plants, intoxications occur among individuals who have harvested their own foods in the wild. For example, an elderly couple succumbed after mistaking foxglove for comfrey while harvesting herbs for tea; foxglove contains digitalis. In another example, a team member in a desert survival course died after eating a salad prepared in part from a *Datura* species, jimsonweed. Jimsonweed contains tropane alkaloids including atropine. While atropine is a useful pharmaceutical agent, its ingestion from natural sources in uncontrolled doses can be fatal. Atropine has potent anticholinergic properties, and individuals ingesting jimsonweed and other plants containing tropane alkaloids suffer neurotoxic effects. Many more such examples could be provided.

More rarely, intoxications from poisonous plants occur with products purchased from commercial sources. In one well-investigated outbreak, a commercial herbal tea was contaminated with *Senecio longilobis*, a well-known poisonous plant [31]. The herbal tea, called gordolobo yerba, was sold to the Mexican-American population in Arizona, and promoted as a cure for colic, viral infections, and nasal congestion in infants. Several infants died from the ingestion of this contaminated herbal tea. *Senecio* and many other plants contain a group of chemicals known as pyrrolizidine alkaloids. The pyrrolizidine alkaloids can cause both acute and chronic symptoms. Chronic low doses produce liver cancer and cirrhosis. The acute symptoms associated with the contaminated herbal tea included ascites, hepatomegaly, veno-occlusive liver disease, abdominal pain, nausea, vomiting, headache, and diarrhea [31]. Death resulted from liver failure.

Occasionally, intoxications from poisonous plants occur from the intentional addition of such materials to foods. The intentional addition of marijuana to bakery items is the most common example.

Many plant-derived foods contain naturally occurring toxicants at doses that are not hazardous, at least on an acute basis, unless large quantities of the food are eaten. Examples would include solanine and chaconine in potatoes, oxalates in spinach and rhubarb, furan compounds in mold-damaged sweet potatoes, and cyanogenic glycosides in lima beans, cassava, and many fruit pits [32].

The cyanogenic glycosides, for example, can release cyanide from enzymatic action occurring during the storage and processing of the foods, or on contact with stomach acid. Commercial varieties of lima beans contain minimal amounts of these cyanogenic glycosides having a hydrogen cyanide (HCN) yield of 10 mg per 100 g of lima beans (wet weight). The lethal oral dose of cyanide for humans is 0.5 mg/kg, so a 70-kg adult would need to ingest 35 mg of cyanide, an amount that would require the ingestion of at least 350 g of lima beans. Such levels of consumption are quite unlikely, and human illnesses from cyanide intoxication from lima bean ingestion have not been reported. Wild varieties of lima beans contain much higher levels of the cyanogenic glycosides (up to 300 mg HCN/100 g) and would likely be hazardous to consume. Cyanide intoxications have occurred in Africa and South America due to the consumption of cassava which is sometimes ingested in large quantities due to a lack of other foods [32]. Cyanide intoxication has also occurred from the ingestion of fruit pits, especially by the grinding of pits with the fruit in food processors during the preparation of jams and wines. The symptoms of cyanide intoxication include a rapid onset of peripheral numbness and dizziness, mental confusion, stupor, cyanosis, twitching, convulsions, coma, and death.

Many toxic constituents of plants are inactivated or removed during processing and preparation. For example, raw soybeans contain trypsin inhibitors, lectins, amylase inhibitors, saponins, and various antivitamins. Fortunately, these toxicants are inactivated during the heating and fermentation processes used with soybeans. Failure to remove or inactivate these toxicants can result in foodborne illness. For example, raw kidney beans contain lectins which are typically inactivated during cooking. In the United Kingdom, immigrants who did not appreciate the importance of thorough cooking of kidney beans have ingested undercooked kidney beans leading to the onset of nausea, vomiting, abdominal pain, and bloody diarrhea from the lectins.

Poisonous mushrooms

Many species of mushrooms are poisonous. The harvesting of mushrooms in the wild can be a hazardous practice. Intoxications occur each year in the United States from the ingestion of poisonous mushrooms. Poisonous mushrooms contain a variety of naturally occurring toxicants which can be classified into Groups I–VI [33].

The Group I toxins are the most hazardous and include amatoxin and phallotoxin. Amatoxin is produced by *Amanita phalloides*, the death cap mushroom. Amatoxin poisoning occurs in three stages. The first stage involves abdominal pain, nausea, vomiting, diarrhea, and hyperglycemia beginning 6–24 hours after ingestion of the mushrooms. A short period of remission then occurs. The third and often fatal stage involves severe liver and kidney dysfunction, hypoglycemia, convulsions, coma, and death. Death resulting from hypoglycemic shock occurs 4–7 days after the onset of symptoms.

The Group II toxins are hydrazines; gyromitrin is the best-known example. Gyromitrin is produced by *Gyromitra esculenta* or false morel mushrooms. The symptoms elicited by ingestion of these mushrooms include a bloated feeling, nausea, vomiting, watery or bloody diarrhea, abdominal pain, muscle cramps, faintness, and ataxia occurring with a 6–12 hour onset time.

The Group III toxins are characterized by muscarine and affect the autonomic nervous system. Muscarine is found in fly agaric (*Amanita muscarina*) sometimes in association with the Group I toxins. Symptoms include perspiration, salivation, lacrimation with blurred vision, abdominal cramps, watery diarrhea, constriction of the pupils, hypotension, and a slowed pulse occurring rapidly following the ingestion of the poisonous mushrooms.

The Group IV toxins cause symptoms only when ingested with alcoholic beverages. Coprine, a Group IV toxin produced by *Coprinus atramentarius*, is the best example. Symptoms include flushing of the neck and face, distension of the veins in the neck, swelling and tingling of the hands, metallic taste, tachycardia, and hypotension progressing to nausea and vomiting. Symptoms begin within 30 minutes of ingestion of the mushrooms and can last for up to 5 days.

The Group V and VI toxins act primarily on the central nervous system causing hallucinations. The Group V toxins include ibotenic acid and muscimol and cause dizziness, drowsiness followed by hyperkinetic activity, confusion, delerium, incoordination, staggering, muscular spasms, partial amnesia, a coma-like sleep, and hallucinations beginning 30 minutes to 2 hours after ingestion. Fly agaric is a good source of the Group V toxins.

The Group VI toxins include psilocybin and psilocin. The symptoms of the Group VI toxins include pleasant or aggressive mood, anxiety, unmotivated laughter and hilarity, compulsive movements, muscle weakness, drowsiness, hallucinations, and sleep. The Group VI toxins are found in Mexican mushrooms, *Psilocybe mexicana*. Symptoms usually begin 30–60 minutes after ingestion of the mushrooms, and recovery is often spontaneous in 5–10 hours. When the dose of the Group VI toxins is high, prolonged and severe sequelae, even death, can occur.

Metabolic food disorders

Like food allergies, metabolic food disorders affect only certain individuals in the population. These individuals display increased sensitivity to certain chemicals in foods because they lack an enzyme necessary to metabolize that particular chemical or because they have a genetic abnormality that makes them especially susceptible to the toxic effects of a particular foodborne chemical. The best examples of metabolic food disorders are lactose intolerance and favism.

Lactose intolerance

Lactose intolerance is associated with an inherited deficiency in the amount of the enzyme, ß-galactosidase, in the small intestine [34]. ß-galactosidase is needed for the hydrolysis of the milk disaccharide, lactose, into its constituent monosaccharides, glucose and galactose. While glucose and galactose can be absorbed and used for metabolic energy, lactose cannot be absorbed without prior hydrolysis. If the activity of ß-galactosidase is insufficient, the lactose from milk or dairy products will be incompletely hydrolyzed. Undigested lactose will pass into the colon where the large numbers of bacteria will convert it to CO_2, H_2, and H_2O. The symptoms associated with lactose intolerance are abdominal cramps, flatulence, and frothy diarrhea.

Almost all individuals are born with sufficient levels of ß-galactosidase activity. However, with increasing age, the levels of enzyme activity diminish. At some point, the levels of ß-galactosidase activity may be insufficient to handle the load of lactose ingested in the diet. Symptoms of lactose intolerance can begin to appear in the early teen years and often worsen with advancing age. Many lactose-intolerant individuals can tolerate some lactose in their diets, often as much as the amount found in an 8-oz glass of milk [35]. The degree of tolerance may lessen with advancing age.

Lactose intolerance is an inherited trait. It affects only about 6–12% of all Caucasians, but ultimately affects 60–90% of some ethnic groups including black Americans, Native Americans, Hispanics, Asians, Jews, and Arabs [34].

Lactose intolerance is treated with dairy product avoidance diets, although some dairy products can usually be ingested without harm. Lactose-intolerant individuals can often safely consume yogurt if the yogurt contains live bacterial cultures with ß-galactosidase [34]. Lactose-hydrolyzed milk is also available in many markets.

Favism

Favism is caused by the ingestion of fava beans or the inhalation of pollen from the *Vicia faba* plant by individuals with a deficiency of the enzyme, glucose-6-phosphate dehydrogenase (G6PDH), in their erythrocytes [36]. Erythrocyte G6PDH deficiency is the most common enzyme deficiency in the world, affecting perhaps 100 million individuals.Erythrocyte G6PDH deficiency is most prevalent among Kurds, Iraqis, Iranians, Sardinians, Cypriot Greeks,

American blacks, and some African populations. This deficiency is virtually unknown in northern Europeans, North American Indians, and Eskimos. G6PDH is a critical enzyme which is essential for the maintenance of adequate levels of the reduced form of glutathione (GSH) and nicotinamide dinucleotide phosphate (NADPH) in erythrocytes. GSH and NADPH protect the erythrocyte membrane from oxidation. Fava beans contain two potent, naturally occurring oxidants, vicine and convicine. These oxidants can damage the erythrocyte membranes in G6PDH-deficient individuals, but not normal persons. Exposure to fava beans in sensitive individuals results in acute hemolytic anemia. The typical symptoms are pallor, fatigue, dyspnea, nausea, abdominal and/or back pain, fever, and chills. In a few severe cases, hemoglobinuria, jaundice, and renal failure may occur. Favism is not a common malady in the United States because fava beans are rarely ingested here. Favism occurs primarily in the Mediterranean area, the Middle East, China, and Bulgaria where the genetic trait is fairly prevalent and fava beans are more frequently consumed.

References

1 Press E, Yeager L. Food "poisoning" due to sodium nicotinate – report of an outbreak and a review of the literature. *Am J Public Health* 1962;52:1720–8.

2 Burkhalter J, Shore M, Wollstadt L, et al. Illness associated with high levels of niacin in cornmeal – Illinois. *CDC MMWR* 1981;30:11–12.

3 Taylor SL, Byron B. Probable case of sorbitol-induced diarrhea. *J Food Prot* 1984;47:249.

4 Kilbourne EM, Rigau-Perez JG, Heath Jr CW, et al. Clinical epidemiology of toxic oil syndrome: manifestations of a new illness. *N Engl J Med* 1983;309:1408–14.

5 Condemi JJ. Unusual presentations. In: Frieri M, Kettelhut B (eds.) *Food Hypersensitivity and Adverse Reactions – a Practical Guide to Diagnosis and Management*. New York: Marcel Dekker, 1999: 331–46.

6 Rodriguez M, Nogura AE, Del Villaras S, et al. Toxic synovitis from denatured rapeseed oil. *Arthritis Rheum* 1982;25: 1477–80.

7 Ferrer A, Cabral R. Toxic epidemics caused by alimentary exposure to pesticides. *Food Addit Contam* 1991;8:755–76.

8 Goldman LR, Beller M, Jackson RL. Aldicarb food poisonings in California, 1985–1988; toxicity estimates for humans. *Arch Environ Health* 1990;45:141–7.

9 Goes EA, Savage EP, Gibbons G, et al. Suspected foodborne carbamate pesticide intoxication associated with ingestion of hydroponic cucumbers. *Am J Epidemiol* 1980;111:254–60.

10 Taylor SL, Nordlee JA, Kapels LM. Foodborne toxicants affecting the lung. *Pediatr Allergy Immunol* 1991;3:180–7.

11 Schmid R. Cutaneous porphyria in Turkey. *N Engl J Med* 1960; 268:397–8.

12 Keating JP, Lell ME, Straus AW, *et al*. Infantile methemoglob-inemia caused by carrot juice. *N Engl J Med* 1973;288:825–6.

13 Dewdney JM, Edwards RG. Penicillin hypersensitivity – Is milk a significant hazard? A review. *J Royal Soc Med* 1984;77:866–77.

14 Kurland LT, Faro SN, Siedler H. Minamata disease. *World Neurol* 1960;1:370–95.

15 Isbister GK, Kiernan MC. Neurotoxic marine poisoning. *Lancet Neurol* 2005;4:219–28.

16 Whittle K, Gallacher S. Marine toxins. *Br Med Bull* 2000; 56:236–53.

17 DiNubile MJ, Hokama Y. The ciguatera poisoning syndrome from farm-raised salmon. *Ann Intern Med* 1995;122:113–14.

18 Russell FE, Egen NB. Ciguatoxic fishes, ciguatoxin (CTX) and ciguatera poisoning. *J Toxicol Toxin Revs* 1991;10:37–62.

19 Mines D, Stahmer S, Shephard SM. Poisonings – food, fish, shellfish. *Emerg Clin North Am* 1997;13:157–77.

20 Lipp EK, Rose JB. The role of seafood in foodborne disease in the United States of America. *Rev Sci Tech* 1997;16:620–33.

21 Gessner BD, Middaugh JP. Paralytic shellfish poisoning in Alaska: a 20-year retrospective analysis. *Am J Epidemiol* 1995; 141:766–70.

22 Okada K, Niwa M. Marine toxins implicated in food poisoning. *J Toxicol Toxin Revs* 1998;17:373–84.

23 Perl TM, Bedard L, Kosatsky T, *et al*. An outbreak of toxic encephalopathy caused by eating mussels contaminated with domoic acid. *N Engl J Med* 1990;322:1775–80.

24 Todd ECD. Domoic acid and amnesic shellfish poisoning – a review. *J Food Prot* 1993;56:69–83.

25 Bates SS, Bird CJ, DeFreitas ASW, *et al*. Pennate diatom *Nitzchia pungens* as the primary source of domoic acid, a toxin in shell-fish from eastern Prince Edward Island, Canada. *Can J Fish Aquatic Sci* 1989;46:1203–15.

26 Noguchi T, Ebesu JSM. Puffer poisoning: epidemiology and treatment. *J Toxicol Toxin Rev* 2001;20:1–10.

27 Miyazawa K, Noguchi T. Distribution and origin of tetrodo-toxin. *J Toxicol Toxin Rev* 2001;20:11–33.

28 Van Genderen H. Adverse effects of naturally occurring nonnu-tritive substances. In: deVries J (ed.) *Food Safety and Toxicology*. Boca Raton, FL: CRC Press, 1997:147–62.

29 Food and Nutrition Board, Institute of Medicine. *Dietary Reference Intakes – A Risk Assessment Model for Establishing Upper Intake Levels for Nutrients*. Washington, DC: National Academy Press, 1998.

30 Smith RA. Poisonous plants. In: Hui YH, Gorham JR, Murrell KD, Cliver DO (eds.) *Foodborne Disease Handbook. Vol. 3. Diseases Caused by Hazardous Substances*. New York: Marcel Dekker, 1994:187–226.

31 Huxtable RJ. Herbal teas and toxins: novel aspects of pyrrolizi-dine poisoning in the United States. *Perspect Biol Med* 1980; 24:1–14.

32 Beier RC, Nigg HN. Toxicology of naturally occurring chemicals in foods. In: Hui YH, Gorham JR, Murrell KD, Cliver DO (eds.) *Foodborne Disease Handbook. Vol. 3. Diseases Caused by Hazardous Substances*. New York: Marcel Dekker, 1994:1–186.

33 Spoerke Jr DG. Mushrooms: epidemiology and medical man-agement. In: Hui YH, Gorham JR, Murrell KD, Cliver DO (eds.) *Foodborne Disease Handbook. Vol. 3. Diseases Caused by Hazardous Substances*. New York: Marcel Dekker, 1994:433–62.

34 Stear GIJ, Horsburgh K, Steinman HA. Lactose intolerance – a review. *Curr Allergy Clin Immunol* 2005;18:114–19.

35 Lisker R, Aguilas L. Double blind study of milk lactose intoler-ance. *Gastroenterology* 1978;74:1283–5.

36 Marquardt RR, Wang N, Arbid MS. Pyrimidine glycosides. In: D'Mello JPF (ed.) *Handbook of Plant and Fungal Toxicants*. Boca Raton, FL: CRC Press, 1997:139–55.

CHAPTER 41

Seafood Toxins

Soheil Chegini and Dean D. Metcalfe

KEY CONCEPTS

- Seafood poisoning is uncommon in non-endemic regions, but may be responsible for adverse reactions to seafood.

- Marine toxins produce syndromes with primarily acute gastrointestinal and neurological manifestations that frequently masquerade as allergic reactions.

- Seafood poisoning may result in similar symptoms in several individuals who shared the seafood and display an "endemic" nature.

- The absence of prior history of allergy to seafood and its subsequent tolerance point away from an allergic etiology and suggest poisoning.

- Knowledge of specific seafood toxic syndromes is necessary to consider them in the differential diagnosis and obtain the appropriate history and collect specimens to confirm the diagnosis and institute the correct treatment.

Introduction

Fish and shellfish are nutritious foods that constitute desirable components of a healthy diet. However, seafood, including fish, shrimp, lobster, crabs, crayfish, mussels, and clams, are listed among the most frequent causes of food allergy [1–3]. The differential diagnosis of seafood allergy is extensive. It includes true hypersensitivity reactions to non-seafood components, such as peanut or tree nuts, foods that may cross-react with seafood allergens or food contaminants, such as antibiotic residues contained in seafood, adverse reactions to food additives, such as sulfites, monosodium glutamate (MSG), and tartrazine, as well as seafood-associated poisoning (Table 41.1). Seafood poisoning primarily results in acute gastrointestinal and neurological manifestations that frequently masquerade as allergic reactions on presentation to emergency departments and urgent care clinics and are often misdiagnosed [4–8]. Bacteria and bacterial toxins may cause gastrointestinal and systemic symptoms that can also be confused with food allergy. In the United States, seafood poisoning, principally scombroid and ciguatera fish poisoning (Table 41.2), was responsible for about 4% of all reported food-borne disease outbreaks reported by the Centers for Disease

Table 41.1 Differential diagnosis of seafood-associated poisoning

A. Common seafood poisons
   1. Fish poisoning
      a. Ciguatera
      b. Scombroid
      c. Tetrodon poisoning
   2. Shellfish poisoning
      a. Paralytic
      b. Neurotoxic
      c. Amnesic
      d. Diarrhetic

B. Less common seafood poisoning
   1. Fish
      a. Clupeotoxin
      b. Elasmobranch
   2. Mollusks
      a. Red whelks

C. Infections and bacterial intoxications
   1. Bacterial toxins
      a. *Clostridium botulinum*
      b. *Staphylococcus aureus*
   2. Bacterial infections
      a. *Vibrio cholerae*
      b. *Vibrio parahemolyticus*
      c. *Vibrio vulnificus*
   3. Viral infections
      a. Norwalk and Norwalk-like enteric viruses

Food Allergy: Adverse Reactions to Foods and Food Additives, 4th edition.
Edited by Dean D. Metcalfe, Hugh A. Sampson, and Ronald A. Simon.
© 2008 Blackwell Publishing, ISBN: 978-1-4501-5129-0.

Table 41.2 Epidemiology of seafood poisoning in the United States from 1978 through 2004*

Year	Scombroid Outbreaks	Cases	Ciguatera Outbreaks	Cases	PSP Outbreaks	Cases	NSP Outbreaks	Cases	AFP Outbreaks	Cases	PFP Outbreaks	Cases
1978	7	30	19	56	4	10	0	0	0	0	0	0
1979	14	134	21	91	1	3	0	0	0	0	0	0
1980	28	151	15	52	5	116	0	0	0	0	0	0
1981	9	93	30	219	0	0	0	0	0	0	0	0
1982	18	58	8	37	1	5	0	0	0	0	0	0
1983	13	271	13	43	0	0	0	0	0	0	0	0
1984	12	53	18	78	0	0	0	0	0	0	0	0
1985	14	56	26	104	2	3	0	0	0	0	0	0
1986	20	60	18	70	0	0	0	0	0	0	0	0
1987	22	98	11	35	0	0	0	0	0	0	0	0
1988	16	65	4	8	1	6	0	0	0	0	0	0
1989	17	80	19	66	0	0	0	0	0	0	0	0
1990	11	194	11	44	2	24	0	0	0	0	0	0
1991	17	40	7	50	2	35	0	0	1	29	0	0
1992	15	135	1	8	0	0	0	0	0	0	0	0
1993	5	21	13	44	0	0	0	0	0	0	0	0
1994	21	83	11	54	3	29	0	0	0	0	0	0
1995	16	91	10	27	1	7	0	0	0	0	0	0
1996	19	55	9	32	0	0	1	3	0	1	1	3
1997	22	92	18	65	2	4	0	0	0	0	0	0
1998	27	124	16	73	1	6	0	0	0	0	0	0
1999	19	59	11	41	0	0	0	0	0	0	0	0
2000	19	73	12	46	3	9	0	0	0	0	0	0
2001	27	126	23	79	0	0	0	0	0	0	0	0
2002	21	59	20	68	1	21	0	0	0	0	0	0
2003	33	187	16	55	1	2	0	0	0	0	0	0
2004	18	48	10	31	2	4	0	0	0	0	0	0
1978–2004	480	2536	390	1576	32	284	1	3	1	30	1	3

*Number of outbreaks and cases (in parenthesis) reported to the Center for Disease Control and Prevention (CDC) (data from [9–11]).

Control from 1988 through 2002 [9,10] (Table 41.3). This was significantly smaller than 17.8% reported for the period 1978–1987 [11]. In Australia from 1995 to 2000, ciguatera and scombroid poisoning were responsible for 11% and 3% of all foodborne outbreaks, respectively [12]. Wordwide ciguatera is the most frequently reported poisoning associated with seafood [13].

National surveillance data on seafood-related poisoning in the United States is based on outbreaks of acute foodborne disease reported by state health departments to the CDC. From 1978 through 2004 there were 480 outbreaks with 2536 cases of scombroid poisoning and 390 outbreaks and 1576 cases of ciguatera poisoning. Thirty-two outbreaks of paralytic shellfish poisoning (PSP) involving 284 people were reported that included two large California outbreaks in 1980. There was one case each of puffer fish poisoning, neurotoxic shellfish poisoning (NSP), and amnesic shellfish poisoning (ASP) during this period [9,10,14,15]. However, these figures are likely to underrepresent the true

incidence of seafood poisoning, since some cases remain undiagnosed and many are not reported to health authorities. For instance, even in the endemic area of Queensland, Australia, it is estimated that only about 20% of ciguatera cases are reported to the local database [16].

Based on the presence or absence of the toxin at the time of capture, fish poisoning can be classified into two categories. In ciguatera and puffer fish poisoning the toxin is present in the live fish, whereas in scombroid it is produced only after the capture in the fish flesh by contaminating bacteria that spoil improperly refrigerated fish. Puffer fish poisoning is associated with a high rate of mortality, as opposed to scombroid and ciguatera that are self-limiting illnesses and resolve spontaneously in the vast majority of cases.

The bulk of shellfish-associated illness is infectious in nature, which can be either bacterial or viral, with the Norwalk virus likely to account for most cases of gastroenteritis. Ingestion of contaminated shellfish results in a wide variety of symptoms, depending on the toxins present, their

Table 41.3 Number of outbreaks and cases associated with seafood toxins and their relative contribution to the foodborne diseases (1988–2002)

Year	Outbreaks of seafood poisoning	Cases of seafood poisoning	Percentage of outbreaks of seafood poisoning	Percentage of cases of seafood poisoning	Total outbreaks of foodborne illness	Total cases of foodborne illness
1988	21	79	4.66	0.502	451	15,732
1989	36	146	7.13	0.92	505	15,867
1990	24	262	4.5	0.136	533	19,231
1991	27	149	5.08	0.99	531	15,052
1992	16	143	3.89	1.29	411	11,083
1993	18	65	3.5	0.46	514	14,080
1994	35	166	5.07	0.997	690	16,995
1995	27	125	4.19	0.927	645	13,497
1996	30	93	4.98	0.603	602	15,421
1997	42	161	5.21	0.856	806	18,802
1998	44	203	3.35	0.76	1314	26,719
1999	30	100	2.23	0.532	1344	18,802
2000	34	128	2.4	0.491	1417	26,043
2001	50	205	4.04	0.819	1238	25,035
2002	42	148	3.15	0.593	1332	24,971
1988–2002	476	2173	3.86	0.734	12,333	277,330

Calculated from [9,10].

concentrations in the shellfish, and the amount of contaminated shellfish consumed. Five different types of shellfish poisoning have been identified including paralytic, neurotoxic, diarrhetic, amnesic, and azaspiracid (AZA) poisonings. PSP may be severe and life threatening, but other shellfish poisonings are usually transient, self-limited, and rarely fatal. Except for scombroid, there is no antidote for seafood poisoning and treatment is primarily supportive.

Toxins responsible for the clinical manifestations are generally produced by microscopic marine algae in the warmer summer months, which are then concentrated in filter-feeding bivalve mollusks, such as clams and mussels. These toxins are retained and concentrated over time. Of the estimated 4000 species of marine algae worldwide, <2% produce toxins [17]. Only about 30 dinoflagellates and a few diatom species are known to cause human illness, and fewer still are potentially lethal [18]. Generally marine toxins do not alter the appearance, taste, or smell of seafood, and are not inactivated by heat or gastric acid. Anthropogenic eutrophication has been incriminated in the higher frequency of harmful algal blooms and increased production of biointoxins by marine dinoflagellates [19]. However, the incidence of shellfish poisoning has been declining, most likely because of careful monitoring, beach closures, and improved public awareness. It is recommended that the public should avoid collecting shellfish from areas where red tides are known to occur and refrain from consumption of suspect shellfish that should be submitted to health authorities for investigation [20].

Seafood poisoning is largely a regional problem and cases are usually concentrated in endemic areas. However, poisonings associated with imported seafood are an exception, since they occur sporadically and do not follow geographic patterns. At present well over half the seafood supply in the United States is imported; and as reef fish are increasingly exported from the tropical areas, seafood poisoning has become a more widespread problem. Most current health risks associated with seafood contamination originate in the environment and should be dealt with by control of harvest or at the point of capture by application of principles of hazard analysis and critical control point (HACCP). Some seafood poisonings, although not a problem in the United States, could become one, as international tourism increases and seafood from different regions of the world becomes available. Thus, knowledge about some of these clinical syndromes is helpful.

Some marine toxins are allelopathic and function in nature to inhibit the growth of other microalgae as an adaptive mechanism. Animals may have evolved to acquire toxicity by sequestration of toxic compounds in their food source, which provides protection from predators that have learned to avoid them. Recently, two new classes of marine toxins that can cause human disease were discovered: azaspiracid and spirolides. The sources of these toxins have also been identified in phytoplanktons that have widespread presence in Atlantic waters. The occurrence of these toxin classes in seafood presents new challenges to the seafood industry and the regulatory agencies. Aquaculture is gaining an ever-increasing importance in production of seafood, which introduces new challenges to health care and the practicing physician. Use of algicides, antibiotics, and antiparasitic medications that leave detectable residues in farm-raised seafood is a potential human health hazard. Genetic engineering and neo-antigens incorporated into seafood or introduced into other food from a marine origin can present an alternative source of antigen that could potentially lead to allergic sensitization.

In this chapter, special emphasis is placed on important aspects of the clinical picture, the marine species most commonly involved, and their general geographic distribution; information that we hope will be helpful in recognizing these reactions, making the correct diagnosis, and differentiating them from seafood allergy. Current knowledge on mechanisms of toxicity and methods of detection and quantification of various seafood toxins are reviewed and general treatment and preventive measures are discussed.

Common intoxications associated with fish

Scombroid (histamine poisoning)

A constellation of gastrointestinal, neurological, cardiovascular, and cutaneous symptoms such as nausea, vomiting, diarrhea, abdominal cramping, throbbing headache, palpitations, flushing, tingling, burning, itching, hypotension, urticaria, and angioedema characterize scombroid. In severe cases and in persons with asthma, bronchospasm may develop. The most frequent symptoms are tingling and burning sensations around the mouth, gastrointestinal complaints, and a skin rash. Patients sometimes describe a peppery or bitter taste to the fish, but often the fish tastes completely normal. In general the onset of symptoms is rapid, usually within 10–30 minutes of ingesting fish. Physical signs may include a diffuse blanching erythema, tachycardia, wheezing, and hypotension or hypertension. Immediate reactions may be indistinguishable from anaphylaxis and scombroid is often misdiagnosed as an allergic reaction [4–8]. Scombroid intoxication results from ingestion of fish containing high levels of free histamine. Since histamine is resistant to heat, cooking the fish and even high temperatures used in canning process will not prevent scombroid poisoning [21]. Because the symptoms are usually self-limited and resolve in the vast majority of cases within 4–10 hours without any sequelae, there is often no need for specific treatment. However, H1 and H2 antihistamines ameliorate the symptoms in severe cases [22]. The mildness and transient nature of scombroid contribute to underreporting of the disease.

Initially, the disease was associated with consumption of scombroid fish. Scombroid means like mackerel (*Scomber*); fish belonging to the Scombroidea family that are found in temperate and tropical waters including tuna, mackerel, bonito, and saury. More recently, other non-scombroid species have been identified as causing the intoxication, including mahi-mahi, bluefish, jack, mackerel, amberjack, herring, sardine, and anchovy. Some of these species constitute highly commercialized marine products and have been among the most valuable resources of the canning industry [23]. In the United States between 1978 and 1999, scombroid poisoning owing to mahi-mahi, tuna, and bluefish accounted for the majority of the cases reported to CDC [9–11].

The histamine is not present when the fish are caught, but is later produced during spoilage by decarboxylation of free histidine, which is naturally present at high levels in species of fish implicated in scombroid [24]. The production of histamine is due to the action of histidine decarboxylase, an enzyme produced by bacteria growing on the fish. The enteric bacteria *Morganella morganii*, *Klebsiella pneumonias*, and *Hafnia alvei* are most frequently implicated. These organisms are not considered as natural flora of living fish and contamination probably occurs during catching and handling [25]. This reaction occurs optimally between 20°C and 30°C and is prevented by refrigeration or chemical decontamination. Experimental studies have shown that histamine formation is negligible in fish stored at 0°C [26].

Even though histamine levels may not be correlated with any obvious signs of decomposition, histamine content may be used as an index of spoilage in certain fish. Fresh fish normally contain histamine levels of <10 ppm or 1 mg/100 g of fish flesh. Laboratory confirmation of scombroid is based on demonstrating elevated histamine levels >50 ppm in the muscle tissue of incriminated fish using an enzyme-linked immunosorbent assay (ELISA) [27,28].

Although histamine was first suggested as the causative toxin over 50 years ago, it was not until 1991 that urinary excretion of histamine, in quantities far exceeding those required to produce toxicity, was documented *in vivo* in humans in association with the clinical syndrome [29]. Subsequently, elevated plasma histamine levels were demonstrated in scombroid [30]. Various hypotheses have been put forward to explain why histamine consumed in spoiled fish is more toxic than pure histamine taken orally; one postulates a role for other heat-stable substances produced in fish by putrefactive bacteria that inhibit the metabolism of histamine by intestinal flora and permit absorption of a more substantial portion of the ingested histamine. A second hypothesis suggests that urocanic acid, another imidazole compound derived from histidine in spoiling fish, may induce mast cell degranulation, and endogenous histamine release may augment the exogenous histamine consumed in spoiled fish [31]. There is still controversy about the exact mechanism and none has proved totally satisfactory.

Scombroid is preventable by proper handling and prompt refrigeration of fish at the time of capture and during subsequent storage, processing, and distribution until it is preserved or cooked. Fish should be chilled rapidly to temperatures below 10°C within 4 hours after capture and stored at 0–4°C to keep bacterial numbers and histamine levels low. Despite the huge expansion in trade in recent years, great progress has been made in ensuring the quality and safety of fish products. This is largely the result of the introduction of international standards of food hygiene and the application of HACCP principles [31].

Ciguatera

Ciguatera fish poisoning is a clinical syndrome that presents after consumption of ciguatoxic fish with characteristic gastrointestinal, neurological, and, occasionally, cardiovascular symptoms [32]. The onset of the symptoms ranges between 30 minutes and 12 hours after ingestion of contaminated fish, depending on the severity of intoxication. Nausea, vomiting, watery diarrhea, and abdominal pain usually develop within 3–6 hours and typically last 12–24 hours. Neurological symptoms develop over 24 hours and tend to be the most distinctive and enduring. They include paresthesias that initially involve the lips, tongue, and throat, which later may extend to the extremities, hypoesthesia, dysesthesias, pruritus, generalized weakness, and anxiety. Cold allodynia (burning dysesthesia or sensation of heat upon touching cold water or objects) is almost pathognomonic for ciguatera and is often incorrectly referred to as "temperature reversal" [16,30]. Paresthesias do not follow dermatome patterns [33,34]. Neurological symptoms are often aggravated by alcohol consumption, stress, and physical activity [35]. Other less common symptoms include diaphoresis, chills, dizziness, headache, blurred vision, prostration, myalgias, dry mouth, taste disturbances or a metallic taste, and pain or a loose sensation in the teeth. Weakness may last for 1–7 days. Mean duration of acute illness is typically 8.5 days, although it is not unusual for neurological symptoms such as paresthesias or cold allodynia to periodically reoccur for a month or longer. Diminished or increased reflexes and dilated pupils may also be noted which usually resolve in 2–3 days. Cardiovascular symptoms are found in 10–15% of cases, most commonly in individuals previously exposed to the toxin but, when present, bradycardia or hypotension may require urgent management [36]. In cases of severe intoxication, seizures, coma, and respiratory paralysis may occur and which, in the absence of adequate life support, may be fatal [33,35]. Ciguatera fish poisoning is usually a self-limiting disease, but symptoms may be extremely debilitating, resulting in extended periods of disability.

Current estimates place the annual number of ciguatera cases at 50,000 worldwide [37]. This poisoning spans the globe and generally is observed in warm waters between latitudes within 35° of the equator [38]. It is the most common type of fish poisoning in the Caribbean [39]. In the United States during the period from 1978 through 2004, 390 outbreaks of ciguatera involving 1576 persons were reported to CDC. No ciguatera-related deaths were reported [9,10,15]. In Hawaii the average annual incidence of ciguatera was 8.7/100,000 population based on 150 outbreaks involving

462 individuals that were reported to the State Department of Health during a 5-year interval from January 1984 through December 1988 [41]. These figures however are substantially higher than the CDC statistics which accounted only for 75 outbreaks and 295 cases in the US during that period. Of the 297 outbreaks between 1983 and 2004, 236 were reported from Hawaii and 40 from Florida [10,40]. Reported outbreaks in other states have been related, in most cases, to travel to the endemic areas, or from eating fish caught in endemic ciguatera areas; and there is concern that many cases are not recognized by mainland US physicians [40,42]. Despite its exceedingly low incidence outside endemic areas, as the domestic fish industry expands its sources of supply, the diagnosis of this "tropical" disease must also be considered in areas where coral reef fish are not native.

Ciguatoxins (CTX), the toxins responsible for ciguatera, are produced by *Gambierdiscus toxicus*, a marine dinoflagellate that belongs to the family of benthic macroalgae. They usually grow attached to dead coral and are ingested by small herbivores off the reef [32]. They are lipid-soluble polyether toxins, which when ingested by certain subtropical and tropical finfish can accumulate in their tissues. Biotransformation of CTX in fish increases their polarity and thus their toxicity. The toxins and their metabolites are concentrated when carnivorous reef fish (e.g. barracuda, grouper, and amberjacks) prey on smaller herbivorous fish. Thus, the toxic effect is amplified in large predatory fish that become the most toxic to humans at the end of the food chain [36]. Factors influencing the concentration of CTX that accumulate in fish include the rate of dietary intake, the efficiency of assimilation, the degree and nature of any toxin biotransformation, the rate of depuration, and the rate of growth of fish [43]. More than 400 species of fish can be vectors of CTX, but generally only a relatively small number of species of reef fish belonging to the family Carrangidae are regularly incriminated in ciguatera. The fish most commonly implicated include amberjack, snapper, grouper, barracuda, and goatfish. The toxin may be most concentrated in the head, liver, intestines, testes, ovaries, and roe. CTX activate voltage-dependent sodium channels, causing cell membrane excitability and instability [44]. *In vitro* studies suggest that CTX causes a nerve conduction block after initial neural stimulation [45].

Maitotoxins (MTX) are water-soluble polyether phytotoxins also produced by *G. toxicus*, which are distinct from CTX. MTX induce severe pathological changes involving the stomach, heart, and lymphoid tissues of experimental mice and rats when injected intraperitoneally [46]. They also display hemolytic and ichthyotoxic activities. MTX-induced hemolysis is dependent on calmodulin and phospholipase A2 activity. Toxicity to fish is dependent on pH and Ca^{2+} concentration [47]. MTX are potent activators of a voltage-independent, non-selective cationic channel that results in elevation of the intracellular Ca^{2+} concentration, which is ultimately responsible for toxicity [48]. MTX have low oral potency and poor ability to accumulate in fish flesh, consequently they are unlikely to play a significant role in causing human illness. To date, no compelling evidence exists to support a role for water-soluble toxins, including MTX, in ciguatera [16].

Ciguatera often affects only a discrete region of a reef, with flare-ups of ciguatera being both temporally and spatially unpredictable [41]. While low levels of *G. toxicus* are found throughout tropical and subtropical waters, the presence of bloom numbers is unpredictable and patchy. Only certain genetic strains produce CTX, and environmental triggers for increasing toxin production are unknown [49]. However, there is concern as to whether disruptions in the reef ecosystem may shift the balance toward a higher rate of toxin-producing *G. toxicus* and an increased incidence of ciguatera poisoning [50].

CTX are heat stable, so are not inactivated by either cooking or freezing. They are not affected by gastric acid and are harmless to the fish itself. Since they are odorless, colorless, and tasteless, ciguateric fish look, taste, and smell normal, and detection of toxins in fish remains a problem. A radioimmunoassay (RIA) and subsequently a stick-enzyme immunoassay and a solid-phase immunobead assay have been developed to detect even negligible amounts of toxins in suspect fish flesh [51–53]. The stick-enzyme immunoassay has been improved and has become a simple, rapid, sensitive, and specific test for CTX [54]. A kit (Cigua-Check, Oceanit Test Systems, Inc) using this detection method is available for use by sports fisherman that could screen fish for CTX. However, its cost and lack of awareness remain an obstacle to its utilization. Because there is no approved assay for CTX in human tissues, the diagnosis is based on a history of recent consumption of potentially ciguateric fish, clinical findings, and by the detection of toxin in samples of fish. Thus, any uneaten portions of fish should be saved in a freezer and submitted to state or local public health officials when suspected cases are reported to assist with the investigation and control of a possible outbreak [55].

There is no immunity and no known antidote for CTX poisoning. Treatment is primarily supportive and for relief of symptoms; however, intravenous mannitol may be effective early in the course of illness in reducing the associated neurological and muscular symptoms [56–58]. The initially promising results with mannitol were not confirmed in a more recent randomized, placebo-controlled trial; thus it cannot be endorsed as a general therapeutic recommendation [59]. To prevent ciguatera, persons living in or traveling to areas where ciguatera toxin is endemic should follow these general precautions [55]:

1 Avoid consuming large, predatory reef fish, especially barracuda and amberjack.
2 Avoid eating the head, viscera, or roe of any reef fish.
3 Avoid eating fish caught at sites with known ciguatera toxins.

Puffer fish (tetrodon) poisoning

Symptoms begin with paresthesias 10–45 minutes after ingestion, initially usually a stinging of the lips, tongue, and inner surface of the mouth. Common symptoms that follow include headache, lightheadedness, dizziness, vomiting, diaphoresis, pallor, weakness, malaise, and feelings of doom [59]. Some patients may experience a floating sensation, salivation, muscle twitching, and pleuritic chest pain. Depending on the amount of tetrodotoxin (TTX) ingested, the patient may experience ataxia, dysphagia, aphonia, and convulsions. Severe poisoning is indicated by hypotension, bradycardia, depressed corneal reflexes, and fixed dilated pupils. An ascending paralysis may develop and death can occur within 6–24 hours secondary to respiratory muscle paralysis [11]. Petechial hemorrhage, blistering and desquamation, and hematemesis have also been reported. Prognosis is good if the patient survives the first 24 hours [59].

Diagnosis is based on clinical symptoms and a history of recent consumption of suspect fish. Treatment is supportive, including active airway management and ventilatory and circulatory support as needed. To minimize the amount of toxin absorbed, gastric lavage and activated charcoal may be beneficial soon after the ingestion. There is no specific antitoxin for human use; however 4-aminopyridine has been reported to effectively reverse neuromuscular blockade and cardiorespiratory depression in a guinea pig model of TTX poisoning [60].

Puffer fish poisoning is rare in the United States and since 1951 only 10 cases have been reported, including three fatalities [61,62]. It is far more common in Japan where 20–100 fatal cases occur each year [11]. The mortality rate is high and approaches 60% [36].

Puffer fish poisoning results from ingestion of the flesh of certain species of fish belonging to the order Tetraodontidae that includes ocean sunfishes, porcupine fishes, and fugu, which are among the most poisonous of all marine life [63,64]. These fish get their name because they characteristically inflate to several times normal size by swallowing air or water when feel threatened. The liver, gonads, intestines, and skin of these fish contain TTX; but the flesh is edible if cleaned and prepared properly, and considered a delicacy by some persons in Japan, who may pay the equivalent of 400 US dollars for one meal. Rigid public health standards including training and certification of fugu chefs have decreased the incidence of puffer fish poisoning; but it has not eliminated the risk associated with consumption of fugu, which remains a common cause of fatal food poisoning in Japan. All puffer species in US waters, including *Sphoeroides maculates, Sphoeroides annulatus,* and *Arothron hispidus,* have been implicated in fatalities and it would seem prudent to consider them potentially toxic. Note the Food and Drug Administration (FDA) has permitted fugu to be imported and served in Japanese restaurants by certified fugu chefs on special occasions. A cooperative agreement with the Japanese Ministry of Health and Welfare ensures that fugu is properly processed and certified safe for consumption by the government of Japan before export [62].

TTX is a heat-stable alkaloid that blocks sodium conductance and neuronal transmission in skeletal muscle. TTX is also present in several other marine and terrestrial species such as blue-ringed octopus, some newts and toads [65,66]. TTX concentration in puffer fish fluctuates drastically with the reproductive cycle, reaching a peak around the spawning season; and is considerably higher in the female than the male [59]. TTX is not present in cultured puffer fish, nor is it found in all puffer fish of the same species caught in the wild. These observations and the marked individual, regional, and seasonal variability in TTX concentration suggest that all TTX-bearing animals do not themselves produce the toxin, but harbor TTX-producing microorganisms within their bodies. This hypothesis was confirmed when the natural source of TTX was identified in marine *Vibrio* species that are part of puffer fish microflora, and it was proven the fish itself merely accumulated the toxin in its tissue [67–69]. Several other TTX-producing bacteria have since been isolated from various marine organisms including *Alteromonas, Bacillus,* and *Pseudomonas* species [70]. The consumption of as little as 10 g of the toxic tissue may be fatal and 1–4 mg of TTX constitutes a lethal dose for humans [11].

Common intoxications associated with shellfish

Paralytic shellfish poisoning

PSP, which is caused by saxitoxins (STX), is the best known of the shellfish poisonings and causes the most severe symptoms. It is a serious illness in which neurological symptoms predominate. The first and most consistent symptoms are numbness, tingling, and/or burning of the lips, tongue, and throat that begin within 30 minutes of ingestion. Paresthesia spreads to the face and neck and often to the fingertips and toes. This precedes muscular weakness that affects the upper and lower limbs and in more severe cases is followed by dysphonia, dysphagia, and ataxia. Paralysis may follow within 2–12 hours, and may persist for as long as 72 hours. The sensation of floating in air, dizziness, weakness, drowsiness, headache, salivation, intense thirst, and throat tightness are commonly described. Diaphoresis, nausea, vomiting, diarrhea, tachycardia, and temporary blindness may also occur. Reflexes may be normal or absent, and most patients remain calm and conscious throughout. Death can result from paralysis of the respiratory muscles within 2–24 hours, depending on the dose. Prognosis is good for individuals surviving past 12 hours. The duration of the illness may be from a few hours to a few days, but occasionally muscular weakness can persist for weeks following recovery [20].

Diagnosis is based on characteristic symptoms and on a history of recent ingestion of shellfish. There is no specific laboratory diagnostic test for a patient with PSP. However, examination of water samples for toxic algae and laboratory tests on the suspect food can provide supportive evidence.

Treatment is symptomatic. Gastric emptying has been advocated by some authors as an early treatment and activated charcoal has generally been recommended to help block further absorption of the toxins. Airway management and ventilatory support is the mainstay of treatment and can be life saving. However, larger doses of poison may result in death despite this treatment. Fluid therapy facilitates renal excretion of the toxin and intravenous administration of sodium bicarbonate may be beneficial to correct possible acidosis. Since the half-life of elimination of the toxin from the body is about 90 minutes, 9 hours should be adequate in most cases for physiological reduction of toxin concentration to relatively harmless levels. There is no immunity to PSP and the second attack may be more severe than the first. No effective antidote is available, but experimental results with 4-aminopyridine are promising in a guinea pig model of PSP [60].

In the United States, PSP is a problem primarily in the New England states on the East Coast and in Alaska, California, and Washington on the West Coast. Most disease incidents involve mussels and clams gathered and eaten by recreational collectors, often from closed areas, reflecting the effectiveness of current testing and control measures for commercially produced shellfish. The CDC listed 32 outbreaks involving 284 people with four fatal cases during 1978–2004 suggesting a mortality rate of <2% [9–11,14,15]. The case-fatality rate has been quoted at about 8.5% [71], but at present it is probably <1% in developed countries [72]. Although PSP is an extremely dangerous disease that can cause death, there is reason to believe that mild cases due to consumption of marginally toxic clams by recreational diggers are never reported to health authorities or are misdiagnosed.

The first case of PSP was described in 1793 as poisoning by mussels in explorers of coastline of British Columbia, Canada [73]. The dinoflagellate, *Alexandrium catenella* (then called *Gonyaulax catenella*), was identified as the actual cause about 1927 [74]. Bivalve mollusks, such as mussels, clams, and oysters, assimilate and temporarily store STX, a complex of neurotoxins produced by dinoflagellates; and thus they function as vectors for the toxin. The primary sources of STX include three morphologically distinct genera of saltwater dinoflagellates: *Alexandrium* spp. (previously *Gonyaulax*), *Pyrodinium* spp., and *Gymnodinium* spp. [75]; and four species of freshwater blue-green algae: *Aphanizomenon flos-aquae, Anabaena circinalis, Lyngbya wollei,* and *Cylindrospermopsis raciborskii* [20]. The STX are a family of water-soluble alkaloids that consist of various sulfonated and hydroxylated derivatives that contain the basic structure of a tetrahydropurine skeleton and two guanidinium groups. They are among the most potent neurotoxins known. More than 20 STX analogs have been described. The positively charged guanidinium group of the toxins binds specifically to a negatively charged site of the sodium (Na^+) channel on the extracellular side of plasma membrane of nerve and muscle cells, thus blocking the flow of Na$^+$ through the channel. As Na$^+$ entry through the nerve cell membrane is essential for impulse transmission, blockage interferes with signal transmission and results in paralysis [75]. Most shellfish contain a mixture of several STX, depending on the species of algae, geographic area, and type of marine animal involved. Biotransformation of the toxin results in generation of more toxic forms. The higher the net charge, the greater is the toxicity. The potency of STX is expressed in mouse units per milligram (MU/mg). One MU is the amount of toxin required to kill a mouse weighing 20 g in 15 minutes after intraperitoneal injection and is equivalent to 0.18 μg STX. Toxicity of the STX is generally expressed in terms of saxitoxin equivalents (STX eq) per 100 g of shellfish meat. There is great variation in individual susceptibility and children are thought to be more susceptible. As little as 120–180 μg of STX can induce moderate symptoms in adults, and fatalities have been associated with levels of 0.3–12 mg [20]. Although normal steaming or boiling will not inactivate the toxins, exposure of toxic shellfish to high temperatures (e.g. in the sterilization step of the canning process) substantially reduces STX concentrations. However, the effectiveness of canning as a means of reducing STX levels below the statutory limit depends on the initial toxicity and must be used with caution [76].

The mouse bioassay has been the classical method for analysis of STX. It is a standardized procedure in which mice are injected with toxin extracts, and their responses are compared with known amounts of toxin. It is rather insensitive with a detection limit of only 40 μg STX eq/100 g shellfish meat [77]. High-performance liquid chromatography (HPLC) is quite rapid and has been considered as a possible replacement for the mouse bioassay. HPLC detection limits are generally an order of magnitude lower than that of the mouse bioassay [78]. A direct enzyme immunoassay (EIA) has been available for determination of STX in shellfish that correlates closely with mouse bioassay [79]. A lateral flow immunochromatographic (LFI) assay has been developed and is termed the MIST Alert dipstick test for PSP. It can detect toxic shellfish (i.e. STX >80 μg/100 g) with 100% sensitivity and detects 95% for samples in the range 32–80 μg/100 g. It has a false-positive rate of 15% at <32 μg/100 g, which is below detection limit of the mouse bioassay [80]. MIST Alert has also been evaluated for the rapid identification of PSP toxins in the water column and benthos. PSP toxins are detected at 100 cells per sample with no false-negative responses. It appears to be an effective tool for broad scale monitoring of algal toxins in coastal waters and has the potential to replace existing surveillance techniques [81]. In addition, the tests for the detection of STX in shellfish tissue have shown a sensitivity of 100% above 80 μg STX eq/100 g, which is the current FDA tolerance level. MIST Alert detected reliably STX above 40 μg STX eq/100 g and identified the majority of extracts above 32 μg STX eq/100 g, which is the mouse bioassay detection limit with a false-positive rate of 6% below 20 μg STX eq/100 g [82,83]. STX is a potent inhibitor of

the membrane depolarizing effects of the sodium channel activator veratridine. Based on this property, a membrane potential assay using mouse brain synaptoneurosomes has been developed. PSP toxins contained in shellfish extracts can be detected by inhibition of veratridine-induced depolarization using the fluorescent probe rhodamine 6G. This technique has yet to be validated in field tests to determine its sensitivity and specificity [84].

In the United States, the toxigenic dinoflagellates causing PSP are *A. catenella* and *A. tamarense*; the first being most dominant on the West Coast responsible for PSP outbreaks in the Pacific and the second on the East Coast associated with New England outbreaks [85]. When the dinoflagellates proliferate or "bloom," they often give the water a red or reddish-brown discoloration, giving rise to a "red tide." Outbreaks of PSP tend to cluster from shortly before, up to several weeks after, the appearance of red tide [86]. It should be noted that some *Alexandrium* species do not produce toxins and not all red tides are caused by toxic algae [87]. Conversely, shellfish may also become toxic in the absence of red tide [33]. Anthropogenic eutrophication has been incriminated to result in a higher frequency of red tides or harmful algal blooms and increased production of biointoxins by marine dinoflagellates [19,88].

STX persist in shellfish for varying periods, depending on the shellfish and the tissue involved [85]. Mussels become highly toxic within a few hours to a few days of the onset of a red tide, but lose their toxin rapidly. Clams and oysters generally do not become as toxic as mussels. They require more time to accumulate high levels of toxins and longer to cleanse themselves. The Alaska butter clam, once contaminated, may never be safe for consumption as it retains paralytic shellfish toxins for years [74]. Sea scallops can take up large amounts of STX, even in the absence of algal blooms, but generally do not pose a threat because their adductor muscle, the only part of the scallop that is usually consumed, does not accumulate toxins. Gastropods can also accumulate significant amounts of STX, and in Spain levels as high as 44 ppm have been recorded in meat of abalone. Even though paralytic shellfish toxins have been reported in the viscera of rock lobsters and crabs, STX do not appear to accumulate in significant amounts in muscle tissue. Similarly, they can accumulate up to 50 ppm in intestine, liver, and gills of Atlantic mackerel, but not to any extent in muscle. Therefore, crustaceans and finfish do not appear to present a threat of PSP unless consumed whole or unless livers are consumed [20].

The rate of accumulation and loss of toxin differ between marine species. Thus, even though mussels, once they are in non-contaminated waters, can lose their toxicity within weeks, it can take the Alaskan butter clam as long as 2 years or more to lose toxicity after the initial accumulation of toxin from a red tide. Shellfish containing STX cannot be detoxified by depuration, and the toxins can persist within shellfish at dangerous levels for weeks or months after the algae are no longer present in the growing waters. Seafood containing STX looks and tastes normal and cooking or steaming only partially destroys the toxins [71]. The most effective way of protecting consumers is to establish and maintain comprehensive monitoring programs for toxic algal blooms and toxins in shellfish in all growing areas. When toxic algal species are present in significant numbers, seafood products must be tested for toxicity and withheld from marketing if necessary. The FDA and European "alert level" for STX is 0.8 ppm (80 µg/100 g) in shellfish meat [89,90]. Commercial shellfish harvesting in United States and European Union must be suspended if higher concentrations are detected in routine monitoring programs. Toxin levels can exceed 10 mg/100 g mussels [89]. As illness has been reported to occur in adults at a total oral dose of only 120 µg and death at 300 µg, this maximum permitted level is not particularly conservative. The best way to prevent PSP is to adhere to the public health agency guidelines on harvesting, processing, and consumption of shellfish. To further minimize the risk of PSP, the public should avoid collecting shellfish from areas of known red tides and refrain from consuming suspect shellfish. In addition, since the toxins are water soluble, they can dissolve and concentrate in the cooking broth, which should be discarded after cooking or steaming [20].

Neurotoxic shellfish poisoning

NSP is characterized by both gastrointestinal and neurological symptoms. The illness resembles a mild case of ciguatera or PSP, but with neuroexcitation rather than flaccid paralysis. The onset is rapid and symptoms occur within 3 hours following the ingestion of contaminated shellfish. Symptoms include numbness of the lips, tongue, and throat; and paresthesias, initially circumoral, which then spread to other parts of the body, "temperature reversal," myalgias, vertigo, headache, nausea, vomiting, diarrhea, and abdominal pain. Less commonly, victims may experience a feeling of inebriation, burning pain in the rectum, dysphagia, ataxia, tremor, decreased reflexes, mydriasis, and bradycardia. The intoxication is usually self-limited and resolves spontaneously within a few hours. Treatment is supportive and generally all patients recover within a few days with no after effects. No fatalities have been reported. There are no known antidotes for the toxin [91]. From 1978 through 2004 the CDC reported only a single small outbreak involving three members of a family that consumed toxic small clams harvested from Sarasota Bay, Florida, in June 1996 [10]. The diagnosis was confirmed by detection of the causative toxins, brevetoxins (BTX), in the urine of the patients and in extracts of shellfish collected from the same location by RIA and by receptor-binding assay (RBA) [92]. A competitive ELISA has been developed that detects BTX in body fluids such as urine and serum, seawater, and shellfish extract, with a detection limit of 2.5 µg/100 g shellfish meat. It appears to be a useful tool for monitoring shellfish and seawater, and for diagnostic investigations [93].

Unlike other shellfish toxins, BTX can aerosolize by surf and wave action along the beach during red tides. Irritant toxin aerosols produce a syndrome characterized by conjunctival irritation, sneezing, and rhinorrhea that resembles an allergic response. Shortness of breath, non-productive cough, and wheezing due to bronchospasm are also triggered in individuals with underlying asthma or chronic obstructive pulmonary disease. The syndrome is self-limited and treatment of the bronchospastic episodes due exposure to aerosolized toxins is symptomatic. *In vitro* data indicate that BTX produce contraction of human lower airway smooth muscle via stimulation of cholinergic nerve fibers through activation of sodium channels [94]. In 1987 during a red tide off the coast of North Carolina, 48 individuals were reported that experienced upper and/or lower respiratory symptoms [95].

Karenia brevis (formerly *Gymnodinium breve*) is the dinoflagellate that synthesizes BTX, a group of related, heat-stable toxins responsible for clinical manifestations of NSP. BTX are lipid-soluble polyether toxins of unique structure and pharmacological function. They are active *in vivo* in the nanomolar to picomolar concentration range. Their excitatory effect is mediated by the enhancement of cellular Na^+ influx through the voltage-sensitive sodium channel [96]. Filter-feeding bivalve mollusks, such as oysters, clams, and mussels, that consume *K. brevis* concentrate the toxins in various organs and become toxic to humans but remain unaffected. NSP in the United States is generally associated with the consumption of shellfish harvested along the coast of the Gulf of Mexico from Florida to Texas, and, sporadically, along the southern Atlantic coast. This is identical with the geographic distribution of *K. Brevis* blooms or "red tides." These red tides occur in many areas within the Gulf of Mexico and may result in massive fish kills. The earliest record of fish kills, later attributed to a *K. brevis* bloom, was in 1844 off the West Coast of Florida, where they still occur most frequently, but may be carried north in the Gulf Stream, affecting the coastline of adjacent states. Red tides occur throughout the world and there was a significant outbreak of NSP in New Zealand involving 186 cases, as well as reported outbreaks in the coastal waters of Japan [89,97].

K. Brevis blooms are initiated on the continental shelf or at the shelf edge, over 40 miles offshore, rather than near the shore where they produce the most deleterious effects. Bloom initiation is characteristically associated with intrusion of deeper, offshore waters onto the shelf. Once dense blooms move inshore, they cannot be sustained without maintaining a minimum nutrient level. Thus human inputs of nutrients could be responsible for extending the duration and impacts of red tides when blooms enter the nearshore waters [98]. These blooms on the Southwest Florida shelf served as a source for cells inoculating the Florida East Coast and North Carolina in 1987–1988 [99]. Concern has been raised that human activity may increase the frequency of harmful algal blooms and disseminate *K. Brevis* and other toxic phytoplanktons to non-indigenous waters and result in globalization [100,101].

K. brevis is well adapted and is able to out-compete or otherwise exclude other phytoplankton species. Low concentrations (<1000 cells/l) of the organism occur in off-shore waters throughout the year and can be detected microscopically. Typically in late summer and fall when nutrients are abundant, and physical, chemical, and biological conditions are favorable, *K. brevis* grows rapidly, gradually building high densities that in 2–8 weeks reach bloom concentrations (1–25×10^5 cells/l).

During severe blooms, fish die rapidly from the neurotoxic effects and do not survive to accumulate high toxin concentrations in their tissues. However, fish exposed to sub-lethal concentrations may accumulate these toxins. Such bioaccumulation in fish eaten by marine mammals, such as dolphins and manatees, results in their demise due to BTX exposure and may also affect human health.

Chlorophyll in *K. brevis* results in discoloration of surface water at 10–100 mg/m^3 and is a good surrogate for biomass. It can be detected by satellite color sensors at densities three orders of magnitude less than when water discoloration is visible to human eye, at about 10^6 cells/l. However, it cannot detect deep patches or distinguish *K. brevis* from other algae, which limit the utility of this technology as an early warning system for a ban on shellfish harvest and beach closure. Local authorities may close shellfish harvesting to industries and the public. The basis for closure is the occurrence of more than 5000 *K. brevis* cells per liter of seawater, and reopening of harvest is dependent on demonstrated absence of BTX in shellfish meat [102,103]. The FDA has established a guidance level for BTX at 0.8 ppm (80 μg/100 g) BTX-2 equivalent (20 mouse units/100 g) in shellfish meat, and shellfish harvesting is banned if higher concentrations are detected in monitored areas [89]. The small number of cases of NSP testifies to the effectiveness of the surveillance and closure systems operated by the states.

Amnesic shellfish poisoning

ASP presents initially with vomiting, diarrhea, and abdominal cramps within 24 hours post-ingestion of contaminated shellfish. In some cases, varying degrees of neurological dysfunction follow within 48 hours, including confusion, loss of memory, and disorientation. Other neurological symptoms are headache, hyporeflexia, hemiparesis, ophthalmoplegia, and abnormalities of arousal ranging from agitation to coma, seizures, and myoclonus, especially affecting the face. The acute symptoms are milder compared with PSP. Loss of short-term memory is unique among the marine poisonings, hence the name ASP [104]. It is the most persistent symptom and can be permanent.

The syndrome was first described in a series of outbreaks in individuals that had eaten mussels cultivated in the river estuaries of Prince Edward Island in Canada from November through December 1987 [105]. In this cohort, the frequency of acute symptoms were vomiting (76%), abdominal cramps (50%), diarrhea (4%), severe headache (43%), and loss of short-term memory (25%). Gastrointestinal symptoms were present in all but 7 of the 107 cases. Onset of symptoms after mussel ingestion ranged from 15 minutes to 38 hours, with a median of 5.5 hours. Nineteen patients (18%) were hospitalized, of whom 12 required intensive care because of seizures, coma, profuse respiratory secretions, or unstable blood pressure. Severity of the disease and permanent neurological sequelae, especially cognitive dysfunction, are associated with age over 60 years, male sex and with pre-existing illnesses, as well as the amount of mussels consumed. Three elderly patients died directly and one died indirectly from the intoxication. Neuropathological studies in these four fatal cases showed neuronal necrosis in the hippocampus and amygdala [106]. The clinical records of 14 more severely affected patients that displayed neurological manifestations were reviewed. All 14 patients reported confusion and disorientation within 1.5–48 hours after ingestion and exhibited a variety of neurological abnormalities including coma [9], mutism [11], seizures [8], purposeless chewing and grimacing [6], and uncontrolled crying, or aggressiveness [6]. In neuropsychological testing performed in those 14 patients several months after the acute episode, 12 had severe anterograde-memory deficits, with relative preservation of other cognitive functions. Eleven from the 14 individuals had clinical and electromyographic evidence of pure motor or sensory motor neuronopathy or axonopathy. The maximal neurological deficits were seen 4 hours post-ingestion in the least affected patients and 72 hours in those most affected, with maximal improvement 24 hours to 12 weeks post-ingestion. Acute coma was associated with the slowest recovery. Seizures ceased by 4 months but were frequent up to 8 weeks [107]. Relative preservation of intellect and higher cortical function appears to distinguish ASP from Alzheimer's disease, and the absence of confabulation with well-preserved frontal lobe function differentiates it from Korsakoff's syndrome.

In mussels left uneaten by the patients, as well as mussels harvested later from the same estuaries, the toxic agent was isolated and identified as domoic acid (DA). Its concentration ranged from 31 to 128 mg/100 g of mussel meat that suggested an estimated ingestion of 60–290 mg of DA per patient [104].

Diagnosis is based on a recent history of shellfish ingestion and is made on clinical grounds. It is confirmed by demonstration of DA in shellfish samples. At this point, the treatment of ASP is symptomatic and supportive. Seizures respond well to parenteral benzodiazepins and phenobarbital. There is no antidote and immunity does not develop.

The source of DA in the Prince Edward Island outbreak was subsequently identified as the phytoplanktonic diatom *Psendo-nitzschia multiseries*, formerly known as *Nitzschia pungens* [107]. ASP is the only shellfish poisoning caused by diatoms. Ten isomers of DA (isodomoic acids) have been identified in marine samples, but are minor constituents in ASP relative to DA [108]. DA is a potent neurotoxin that accumulates in mussels and clams that feed on toxic planktons during a bloom. On the Pacific Coast, DA is produced by *P. multiseries* and two other species *P. australis* and *P. pseudo-delicatissima* that bloom in late summer and fall. DA is water soluble and heat stable, similar in structure and function to another excitatory neurotoxin known as kainic acid (KA), which is found in the Japanese seaweed, *Digenea simplex*. DA and KA both appear to produce neurotoxic effects by activating the glutamate receptors [109]. These receptors are ligand-gated, voltage-dependent Ca^{2+} channels that are activated by glutamic acid, mediating a fast excitatory synaptic transmission in the mammalian central nervous system (CNS). Persistent activation of KA receptors results in elevated levels of intracellular calcium (Ca^{2+}) that causes neurotoxicity with subsequent lesions in areas of the brain where glutaminergic pathways are heavily concentrated [110]. The observations that the glutamate receptors are present within the cardiac conducting system, intramural ganglia, and cardiac nerve fibers could explain some of the clinical manifestations such as the arrhythmia described with DA intoxication in humans. Hence individuals with pre-morbid cardiac conditions may be at higher risk of the toxic effects of these excitatory compounds [111]. In animals, DA is 3 times as potent as KA and 30–100 more potent than glutamic acid [112].

DA poisoning first became a noticeable problem in the West Coast of the United States in September 1991 when it was reported that brown pelicans had died after eating anchovies in Monterey Bay off the coast of California. It was subsequently found that the death of these pelicans was due to the bloom of *P. multiseries* that produced high levels of DA [113]. Since this time and until December 2004, 29 cases of ASP have been reported to the CDC, all of which occurred in November 1991 and were caused by razor clams harvested in Washington [10]. No fatalities have occurred in the United States; however, mortality rate was 3.7% in the 1987 Canadian outbreak.

Traditionally a mouse bioassay has been used for detection of DA, which is the same assay as for PSP, however the relative potency of DA appears to be less than STX. There are several newer methods used to detect DA in seawater and shellfish such as HPLC, immunoassay, and an RBA. Also, two indirect competitive EIA for measurement of DA in shellfish and seawater have been developed. One utilizes polyclonal ovine antibodies and the other uses monoclonal murine antibodies. They have a working range of 0.15–15 μg/l and 0.15–10 μg/l, respectively, and a quantification limit of <4 μg/100 g of shellfish flesh [114,115]. The RBA measures the competitive displacement of radiolabeled KA bound to a cloned glutamate receptor (GluR6) by DA in a sample. A comparison of the latter two methods showed that the RBA has a larger working range whereas EIA is more sensitive. The detection limit and working range are 3.1 and 5–100 μg/l for the RBA and 0.01 and 0.15–15 μg/l for the EIA, respectively. RBA and EIA yield statistically equivalent results for detection of DA in seawater [116]. An LFI assay, the MIST Alert dipstick test for ASP, is a newer assay and has a detection limit of approximately 8–12 μg/g DA in shellfish extracts, which is about half the regulatory limit a sensitivity approaching 100% [80].

In Canada, to prevent future outbreaks of ASP, sacks of mussels are now labeled with respect to time and place of harvesting; in addition both water column and shellfish are monitored for the presence of *Psendo-nitzschia* and DA, respectively. Since an estimated concentration of 20 mg/100 g wet weight DA has affected some consumers, applying a safety factor of 1/10, Canadian surveillance authorities have set 2 mg/100 g (20 ppm) as the threshold level above which shellfish commercial operations are suspended.

On the Pacific Coast, DA poisoning has been a serious problem affecting razor clams and Dungeness crabs in Washington; and oysters, bay and razor clams, and mussels in Oregon. Authorities in Washington, Oregon, and California now randomly analyze samples of commercially harvested or cultivated shellfish for DA. The FDA and the European Union have adopted the level of 20 ppm (2 mg/100 g) for DA and when higher levels are detected in seafood closure of beds is enforced [89,90]. The viscera of Dungeness crabs are an exception, where 30 ppm is permitted [89,117]. States in the northeastern United States also monitor shellfish for DA, which is present at low levels that do not necessitate quarantine.

Diarrhetic shellfish poisoning

Diarrhetic shellfish poisoning (DSP) is the mildest and most benign of the toxic shellfish poisonings. Clinical features are generally limited to the gastrointestinal tract and include diarrhea (92%), nausea (80%), vomiting (79%), abdominal pain and cramps (53%). Chills, fever, or headache may also be present in up to 10% of cases [118]. The symptoms usually manifest in a period ranging from 30 minutes to 6 hours after ingestion of contaminated shellfish and persist on average for 36 hours. No known fatalities have occurred, and total recovery is expected within 3 days. Due to the transient nature of the illness and its spontaneous resolution, often patients do not seek medical attention, however the duration could be shortened with charcoal, which reduces the bioavailability of the toxins and its repeated administration interrupts their enterohepatic recirculation. Treatment, if required, is limited to alleviation of symptoms.

DSP is associated with the consumption of mussels, scallops, clams, and oysters contaminated with biotoxins produced by toxic marine dinoflagellates during their blooms in the summer. *Dinophysis* and *Prorocentrum* species have been identified as the source of DSP toxins that are heat stable and not denatured by normal cooking. Although to date there has been no documented DSP outbreak in the United States, toxin-producing *Dinophysis* species are present in US waters and in 1990 caused an outbreak in eastern Canada. The disease occurs worldwide in temperate waters. It is common in Japan, where over 200 cases are reported annually and has become a public health problem in Europe. Sporadic outbreaks have also been documented in Southeast Asia, Chile, Australia, New Zealand, and eastern Canada [89].

At least 10 different toxins have been isolated from dinoflagellates and shellfish in association with DSP. The major toxins are high molecular weight polyethers including okadaic acid (OA), dinophysistoxins (DTX), and several of their metabolites, as well as pectenotoxins (PTX) and yessotoxin (YTX) [119]. OA is most commonly encountered in Europe where *Dinophysis acuminata* is the usual agent, whereas in Japan mixtures of OA, DTX, and PTX are detected usually involving *D. fortii* [120]. OA is a highly selective inhibitor of protein phosphatases that causes dramatic increases in phosphorylation of numerous proteins and can act as a potent tumor promoter. It induces diarrhea by increasing paracellular permeability of intestinal epithelial lining without inducing cytotoxicity [121]. DTX are structurally related to OA and cause in laboratory experiments highly similar intestinal lesions that appear within 5 minutes of dosing and resolve completely within 2 days [122]. PTX, although non-diarrheagenic, are potently cytotoxic and have been found to be tumor promoters in animals [123]. YTX is only a weak cytotoxin, and is not orally lethal to mice. It does not cause accumulation of intestinal fluid or inhibit protein phosphatase and has no diarrheagenic or hemolytic effects suggesting that it should not be classed as a DSP toxin [124]. The DSP toxins, particularly, OA and some DTX, are potent microalgal inhibitors. They are probably an evolutionary adaptive mechanism and are produced by toxic dinoflagellates to create a survival advantage against other competing microalgae [125].

A mouse bioassay is the standard method for DSP surveillance; however, it is non-specific and lacks sensitivity. HPLC is an alternative technique and has a low detection limit of 26 μg/100 g of shellfish for both OA and DTX, but is cumbersome and requires calibration [126]. Most of the recent developments in rapid screening methods for OA detection are based either on the use of specific antibodies or on its ability to inhibit protein phosphatase coupled with use of fluorescence substrates. The fluorimetric assay achieves a detection limit of 1 μg/100 g OA in mussel tissue, which is well below 20 μg/100 g that has been established by FDA as toxicity threshold level [89,127]. The European Union has adopted a level of 160 μg of OA eq/kg (16 μg/100 g) for the total amount of OA, DTX, and PTX, whereas the alert level for YTX is 1 mg/kg [90]. Commercially available EIA kits detect OA and some of its metabolites but not all DSP toxins. Thus EIA kits underestimate total toxin present in crude toxic shellfish [128,129]. Both the HPLC and protein phosphatase

inhibition (PPI) assays correlate with each other and with the standard mouse bioassay. Although EIA does not accurately and consistently detect low DSP toxin concentrations, it offers advantages of rapidity and ease of use [126].

At present, for the US consumer, the risk of DSP is limited to imported products and should be controllable by import regulations that permit import of shellfish only from countries that test it for the presence of toxins. Nevertheless, because *Dinophysis* does occur in US coastal waters, regulatory agencies in the United States should be alert for the possibility of an outbreak [130].

Less common seafood poisonings

Clupeotoxism

Clupeotoxism is a potentially fatal form of human intoxication due to ingestion of clupeidae (herring-like fish). It is a rare poisoning, occurring in the tropics only during the warm summer months. Like ciguatera, it occurs sporadically and over an extensive area of the tropical Pacific and Indian Ocean coasts. A few cases have been reported from Madagascar related to eating sardines, including one fatality in 1994. Symptoms include nausea, vomiting, diarrhea, abdominal pain, headache, dry mouth, sweats, chills, lightheadedness, and paresthesia; and in one report one of the two patients with clupeotoxism died [131]. Physical findings may include tachycardia, hypotension, tachypnea, and cyanosis. Treatment is supportive and no specific antidote is available. The causative toxin was identified as palytoxin, one of the most potent phycotoxins known [132]. It is tasteless and odorless and not inactivated by cooking. Palytoxin has been reported to induce rhabdomyolysis after eating parrotfish. Patients presented with weakness and myalgia within 5 hours of ingestion and recovered without complications or fatalities. In one case, myocardial damage was also present as indicated by electrocardiographic changes and elevation of cardiac enzymes [133,134]. A more recent report of 11 cases, also from Japan, described typical features of rhabdomyolysis including myalgia, back pain, dark discoloration of urine, and elevated serum creatine kinase [135]. The benthic dinoflagellate *Ostreopsis siamensis* has been identified as the source of palytoxin [132]. *O. siamensis* is found in African, Caribbean, and Indo-Pacific Coastal waters and plankton feeders such as herring, pilchard, tarpon, and anchovies that ingest it can become toxic. In most cases, the fish have been captured close to shore, indicating that the toxin was obtained from benthic algae in the bottom sediments.

Palytoxin alters the function of excitable cells and acts as a hemolysin. Its hemolytic activity against sheep erythrocytes can be inhibited by polyclonal rabbit anti-palytoxin antibodies. The mechanism of toxicity of palytoxin has been elucidated, and it was shown to bind to Na$^+$/K$^+$ pump and convert it into a non-selective cation channel [136]. Consequently it results in reduction of the membrane potential and depolarization, which triggers secondary activation of voltage-dependent Ca^{2+} channels and results in neurotransmitter release by nerve terminals and contractions of striated and smooth muscle cells [137].

Elasmobranch poisoning

Elasmobranch poisoning is caused by the ingestion of contaminated meat or liver from several species of sharks, most notably the Greenland sleeper shark [138]. The disease is characterized by gastrointestinal and neurological symptoms including nausea, vomiting, diarrhea, abdominal pain, headache, and perioral paresthesia. Malaise, weakness, muscle cramps, ataxia, and visual disturbances may also develop. Severe progressive respiratory distress, hyporeflexia, and coma usually precede death. The onset of symptoms is 30 minutes to 5 hours following ingestion. The shark and its meat do not display any unusual characteristics. The toxicity is not affected by cooking. Trimethylamine has been proposed as the cause of this poisoning [138]. In November 1993, a large outbreak involving 188 people who ate the meat from a single shark was reported from Madagascar. The patients presented within 5–10 hours after ingestion with neurological symptoms. Ataxia was almost universally present and of moderate to severe intensity. Gastrointestinal symptoms, like diarrhea and vomiting, were rare. The attack rate approached 100% and the overall case mortality was close to 30%. Carchatoxin-A and -B, two novel lipid-soluble toxins were isolated from the shark's liver, which were distinct from other known marine toxins [139].

Red whelk poisoning

In red whelk poisoning symptoms develop within 30–120 minutes, which include headache, dizziness, blurred vision or diplopia, paresthesia, dry mouth, muscular twitching or cramps, ataxia, weakness, and collapse. Nausea, vomiting, and diarrhea may also be present in some patients [140]. The red whelk (*Neptunea antiqua*) is a gastropod species common in Japan and Northern European waters and is distinguished from the edible whelk (*Buccinam undatum*), by its larger size and its smooth shell that has a distinctive pale orange coloration [141]. It contains a heat-stable water-soluble toxin, tetramine that is present in the salivary gland [142]. The concentration of tetramine shows significant seasonal fluctuations [143]. Tetramine possesses curare-like effect and produces short-lived symptoms that resolve rapidly and recovery is complete within 24 hours. As a result few people are likely to seek medical attention and intoxication is rarely reported. It is notably more common in Japan [141].

Newly discovered marine biotoxins

Azaspiracid

AZA is a structurally novel phycotoxin that contains a unique spiro ring assembly found to be responsible for outbreaks of diarrhetic food poisoning associated with consumption of contaminated shellfish in Europe. The first outbreak was reported in November 1995 in the Netherlands following the consumption of mussels harvested on the west coast of Ireland and initially was mistaken for DSP; but was subsequently proven to be azaspiracid shellfish poisoning (AZP). Since then, outbreaks have been reported in other European countries, including France, Italy, Ireland, Norway, and the United Kingdom [144]. The onset is 12–24 hours after consumption of mussels and the symptoms of the illness include severe diarrhea, vomiting, nausea, abdominal cramps, headaches, and chills, which resolve in 2–5 days [145]. Scallops have been also reported to cause AZP; and in several instances toxin levels in crabs harvested in Norway have exceeded the safety levels of the European Unions [90,146,147].

There are up to 10 forms of AZA and these toxins are not affected by heat or freezing [148]. The causative organism is *Protoperidinium crassipes*, a dinoflagellate found in North Atlantic waters. While AZA was initially classified as a DSP toxin, it was subsequently re-classified into a new poisoning category known as AZA poisoning. AZA has a number of unique properties that set it apart from the "classic" DSP toxins, OA, DTX, and YTX. In animal experiments AZA administered orally, induces pronounced neurotoxic effects and causes necrosis in the lamina propria of the small intestine, liver, and lymphoid tissues in the Peyer's patches, spleen, and thymus; whereas toxic effects of OA are limited to the gastrointestinal mucosa [149].

In mice, AZA leads to progressive paralysis, and is rapidly fatal within 5–60 minutes; while OA and DTX cause convulsions and prostration and ultimately death over a longer period of time. OA, DTX, and YTX are known to be located exclusively within the hepatopancreas (HP) of the shellfish, while AZA may initially concentrate in HP but eventually distributes throughout the body and migrates also into the flesh. Since depuration occurs in the HP first, mussels contaminated with AZA may take longer to depuriate. In addition, surveillance of shellfish toxicity based on the assessment of toxin concentration in HP will underestimate AZA hazard and may allow toxic shellfish to be harvested [150]. Consequently, it has been recommended to determine toxin levels in the whole shellfish and a threshold concentration of $16 \mu g$ AZA eq/100 g as a regulatory standard in Europe has been successful in preventing AZP outbreaks since 2001 [90,147]. A liquid chromatography–multiple tandem mass spectrometry method for determination of AZA has been developed that is capable of detecting each of the 10 AZA with limit <20 pg within a few minutes and is far more sensitive than the mouse bioassay [151].

Spirolides

Spirolides are a novel family of lipophilic shellfish toxins that were recently isolated from the marine dinoflagellate, *Alexandrium ostenfeldii*. They consist of a spiro-linked tricyclic ether ring system and an unusual seven-membered spiro-linked cyclic iminium moiety; hence the name spirolide

[152]. To date no human disease has been associated with spirolides. However, based on toxicity profile they should be viewed as a potential cause of seafood poisoning. They were discovered in 1991 during routine biotoxin monitoring of shellfish in eastern Canada. Their distinct toxicological and chemical properties differentiate them from other known lipophilic shellfish toxins. Spirolides are macrocyclic imines that were initially labeled as fast-acting neurotoxin, since in mouse bioassay they rapidly resulted in neurological symptoms and death in 3–20 minutes. They appear to activate muscarinic receptors in the brain and particularly affect the brain stem. The rapid lethal action in rodents is probably due to compromise of cardiorespiratory centers in the brain stem [153]. Liquid chromatography–mass spectrometry is a highly sensitive analytical assay that can detect spirolides in concentrations as low as 2 μg/l; and is the method currently used for surveillance of biotoxins in Canada [154].

Potential allergens associated with seafood

Residues of bioactive substances from aquaculture

Aquaculture is an important source of food worldwide and now contributes up to 15% of the US seafood supply [155]. Traditionally, the environmental safety risks of seafood products have been subdivided into natural hazards such as biotoxins, and anthropogenic contaminants such as synthetic chemicals. In aquaculture, the latter hazard becomes more prominent as more synthetic products are used in the seafood industry. The use and misuse of antibiotics to control diseases in aquacultured species appears widespread. Similarly, the improper or illegal use of chemicals to control pond pests and algae can also result in human health hazards. Natural products that are not present in aquatic environments can also become health hazards when misused or abused; for instance raw chicken manure as pond fertilizer may result in the transmission of *Salmonella* from manure to the cultured product [156].

Compounds commonly used in aquaculture include chemicals that might be considered a potential threat to human health include drugs and biologics, pesticides, disinfectants, and water-treatment products. FDA oversees the use of drugs in aquaculture and has approved oxytetracycline, sulfadimethoxine/ormetoprim, formalin, and tricaine for use in various aquatic species [157]. Many more drugs are believed to be used in an off-label fashion in aquaculture. FDA Office of Seafood began a monitoring program for animal drug residues in farmed seafood in 1991 and has detected some instances of residues of chloramphenicol in shrimp and oxolinic acid in salmon [158].

Oxytetracycline is a prototype antibiotic approved by the FDA for use in fish farming to control certain diseases in salmonids and catfish [159]. The normal method of administration of oxytetracycline to fish is to mix the drug into feed. As a consequence, the concentration of the drug in feed and the composition of feed can influence the disposition of the drug itself [160]. Oxytetracycline is depleted over a period following the completion of the treatment and detectable residues are present in the fish and could be transferred to human if the fish is marketed during that period [161]. In addition, use of other antibiotics as, for example, chloramphenicol in shrimp culture, may similarly result in significant levels in the harvested product. Likewise other bioactive substances, such as antiparasitic agents and algicides, can accumulate in the aquaculture products. For instance, mebendazole and its metabolites have been shown to leave detectable residues in cultured eel [162].

Allergic reactions have been reported following the ingestion of penicillin containing milk in a few previously sensitized patients. Primary sensitization of humans to antimicrobials through the consumption of drug residues in foods has never been clearly documented and evidence suggests that the residue levels in food may be too low to cause sensitization. Drug toxicity, other than allergic reactions, appears not to result from residues of antimicrobial drugs in food [163,164]. Although the available data suggests that these cases are exceedingly rare, they illustrate the continuing need to control antibiotic residues. The human risk can be minimized by the judicious use of antibiotics and observance of washout periods [164].

Genetically engineered neo-antigens

Food biotechnology, the use of recombinant-DNA and cell-fusion techniques to confer selected characteristics on plants and animals used for food, can be used to increase agricultural productivity. The transfer of genes from microbes, plants, or animals into foods raises issues about the unintended consequences of such manipulations. Allergenicity could be one such consequence, since genes encode proteins, which potentially could be allergenic [165]. Even though several bioengineered products have been introduced into the human diet since 1990, they have not yet resulted in any confirmed reported case of food allergy.

An allergen from a food known to be allergenic can be transferred into another food by genetic engineering. This situation occurred when Brazil nut 2S albumin, which is probably one of its major allergens, was introduced into soybeans to improve their nutritional quality. Recognizing the potential problem, the company that had developed the transgenic soybeans discontinued plans to market them [166]. Thus products of food biotechnology should be subjected to a careful and complete safety assessment including the potential allergenicity of the novel proteins introduced into these foods before commercialization [167].

Polar fish produce antifreeze proteins (AFPs), which even at low concentrations decrease the freezing point of solutions and inhibit ice crystal growth. Transgenic expression of AFP in plants can prevent frost damage to crops and improve the quality of frozen fruits and vegetables. Genes encoding for fish AFPs have been successfully expressed in tobacco and tomato plants [168]; and AFP genes transferred from winter flounder to Atlantic salmon, resulted in functionally effective levels of AFP [169]. Fish AFP do not belong to known fish allergens, but they may acquire allergenic properties when expressed in a different host or consumed in larger amounts. Using the same technique, other genes can be transferred from marine species to other animals or plants that could create neo-antigens and result in allergic sensitization. On the other hand, fish can be recipients of transgenes that enhance disease resistance, increase growth rate and size, improve food conversion ratio, or benefit consumers by enhancing nutritional value or palatability. Transgenic expression of growth hormone has been achieved in commercially farmed fish, such as tilapia, catfish, trout, and salmon [170–172]. Limited data are available on the safety of biotechnology products in aquaculture; however, no post-marketing rise in incidence of seafood allergy has been clearly documented and in a published trial no adverse effects were detected in healthy subjects after the consumption of growth hormone-transgenic tilapia [173].

Poisoning due to bacterial toxins

Botulism

Foodborne botulism is acquired from ingestion of food contaminated with preformed toxin that is produced by *Clostridium botulinum*, a sporulating, anaerobic Gram-positive bacillus. It is characterized by symmetric, descending, flaccid paralysis of motor and autonomic nerves, usually beginning with the cranial nerves, which may be fatal due to respiratory failure. Onset is abrupt, usually 12–36 hours after ingestion of toxin. The first manifestations are often dry mouth, diplopia, blurred vision, blepharoptosis, and photophobia due to loss of papillary light reflex, but may be preceded by gastrointestinal symptoms, such as nausea, vomiting, abdominal pain, and diarrhea. Other common symptoms are generalized weakness, dysphagia, dysarthria, nasal voice, and constipation due to paralytic ileus. Sensory disturbances, fever, and tachycardia are typically absent. The diagnosis of botulism is based on clinical findings; history of exposure to suspect foods; and is confirmed by detection of toxin in serum, stool, or gastric contents of the patient or in leftover fish. The differential diagnosis includes the Guillain–Barre syndrome, myasthenia gravis, basilar meningitis, and stroke [174].

C. botulinum elaborates seven types of toxin. Types A, B, and E are usually involved in human poisoning. Botulism from seafood products is most frequently caused by type E toxin, which is the most predominant type in Alaska and Great Lakes area. Type E spores have been demonstrated in lakeshore mud, coastal sands, and sea bottom silt in northern latitudes that can contaminate the intestinal tract of fish. Outbreaks of botulism have been reported after eating unviscerated, salted, air-dried whitefish and mullet, known as kapchunka and faseikh, respectively [175,176]. In Alaska, cases have been linked to Alaska Native foods, such as marinated raw fish aged in plastic bags, seal meat stored in oil, and smoked salmon wrapped in seal skins [177].

The spores are highly heat resistant and may not be inactivated by boiling for several hours. However, commercial canning procedures that use moist heat at temperatures above 250°F (121°C) will kill the spores. Although the majority of reported cases of botulism have been associated with the consumption of inadequately processed home-canned food, about 10% of outbreaks have resulted from contamination of commercially canned fish. In these cases, post-processing contamination owing to faulty cans or inadequate heating during the process have been found to be responsible for the outbreaks [174,178]. Toxins, on the other hand, are readily destroyed by heat and are inactivated by boiling for 10 minutes, or by heating at 80°C for 30 minutes. They are, however, resistant to digestive enzymes and are readily absorbed into circulation from the gastrointestinal tract. The toxins are zinc metalloproteinases that cleave specific components of the synaptic membrane docking and fusion complex, which prevents the release of acetylcholine at the neuromuscular junction and autonomic synapses [179].

Treatment includes close medical supervision, supportive care, and early use of trivalent equine antitoxin (types A, B, and E) and GI decontamination. The source of an outbreak must be determined to prevent further cases. Only prompt recognition, therapy, and epidemiological investigation can reduce the death toll from botulism [180]. In Alaska, where approximately 27% of US foodborne botulism cases occur, early diagnosis and antitoxin treatment have contributed to the decline of the case-fatality rate from approximately 31% during 1950–1959 to no deaths since 1994 [181].

Staphylococcal food poisoning

Acute gastroenteritis is caused by the ingestion of food contaminated with preformed staphylococcal enterotoxin. The onset is abrupt and ranges 2–8 hours post-ingestion. Symptoms start with characteristically severe nausea and vomiting. Other symptoms may include abdominal cramps, diarrhea, and occasionally headache and fever. The attack is brief, most often lasting only 3–6 hours, and recovery is complete; but in severe cases it may lead to dehydration, prostration, and shock. Diagnosis is clinical and can be confirmed by demonstration of coagulase-positive staphylococci in the suspected food or vomitus. Treatment is symptomatic [182]. The disease is caused by the enterotoxins produced by *Staphylococcus aureus*, rather than the organism *per se*, which can multiply in a wide temperature range from 39°F to 115°F (4°C to 46°C). Fish, along with cream pastries, milk, processed meat, and mayonnaise, provide excellent media and if contaminated and allowed to remain at room temperature, these organisms can rapidly multiply and produce toxins. Currently nine enterotoxins have been identified. They are resistant to heat and are only destroyed by prolonged boiling [183].

Bacterial and viral infections

Vibrio species

Nine marine *Vibrio* species have been associated with food-borne disease in humans. *Vibrios* are not detected by standard methods of monitoring coastal waters for bacterial contamination, and standard commercial decontamination techniques do not rid shellfish of these organisms.

Vibrio cholera infection is most prevalent during the summer months. It is characterized by abrupt onset and watery diarrhea; vomiting occasionally occurs [34]. It is endemic in the coastal waters of the Indian Ocean. The largest outbreak in the United States in a century involving l8 persons was reported in 1986 in Louisiana. It was associated with undercooked crabs, which are the most important vehicle for *V. cholerae* infection in the United States; but shrimp and oysters can also transmit the disease. A persisting reservoir along the Gulf Coast may continue to cause sporadic cases [184].

Vibrio parahemolyticus is found in coastal waters throughout the world. This agent is the leading cause of acute diarrheal disease in Japan, presumably because of the frequency of ingestion of raw seafood. In the United States, it has been related to inadequately cooked seafood, usually shrimp, and was recently reported to be associated with crayfish consumption [185]. *V. parahemolyticus* damages the intestinal mucosa and the stool may be bloody. Diarrhea develops 12–48 hours after ingestion of contaminated food, and is associated with abdominal cramps. Chills and fever are observed in over half the cases. Between 1973 and 2004, 60 outbreaks of *V. parahemolyticus* infections were reported to the CDC, and involved about 1200 individuals [10,186]. Most of these outbreaks occurred during the warmer months and were attributed to seafood, particularly shellfish. Of patients with acute *V. parahemolyticus* gastroenteritis, 88% reported having eaten raw oysters during the week before their illness occurred. The median attack rate among persons who consumed the implicated seafood was 56% [186].

Although quite rare, infection of immunocompromised persons with *V. vulnificus* can be associated with high mortality (50%). It appears to be part of the normal bacterial flora of estuaries along the United States, Gulf, Atlantic, and Pacific coasts. The septicemia induced by *V. vulnificus* is associated with eating raw oysters. Of patients with primary septicemia, which accounts for approximately half of the cases, 96% consumed raw oysters and 61% died, usually in association with underlying liver disease. Oysters harvested in the Gulf of Mexico grown and water temperature exceeding 72°F (22°C) closely correlated with the infection [187].

Norwalk virus

In the United States, about 55% of reported shellfish-related incidents are registered as unknown etiology, but are believed to be due mainly to Norwalk, Norwalk-like, or human enteric virus infections, with a smaller proportion caused by *Vibrio* bacteria [188]. The first documented shellfish-associated gastroenteritis involving Norwalk virus was in Australia in 1979, with more than 2000 cases [189]. Since then, many outbreaks of Norwalk or Norwalk-like viral gastroenteritis have been reported in the United States. Incubation periods were generally 24–48 hours. The most common symptoms were nausea (100%), vomiting (83%), diarrhea (50%), and abdominal cramps; and were of brief duration and resolved within 24–48 hours [190,191]. The diagnosis is clinical, with typically unrevealing bacterial studies on stool and shellfish specimens. It can be confirmed by demonstration of seroconversion and the formation of IgM antibody to Norwalk virus. In addition, Norwalk virus was identified by RIA in clam and oyster specimens. The reported incidents have increased in the last decade.

Shellfish-borne disease occurs mostly from mollusks consumed raw or lightly heated. In a confirmed outbreak of Norwalk virus gastroenteritis, 83% of persons who ate raw oysters became ill versus only 7% of people who did not, suggesting a relative risk, 11.9% for consumption of raw oysters. The outbreak was caused by contamination of oysters in the oyster bed by stool from ill harvesters who routinely dispose their sewage overboard [192]. Steaming clams to open the shells takes about 1 minute, but to inactivate viruses it takes between 4 and 6 minutes [193]. These organisms do not multiply once released into the marine environment, but remain infectious in the presence of organic material in the water and temperatures below 50°F (10°C) [194].

Finally, marine organisms such as oysters may concentrate microorganisms including hepatitis A [195]. Contamination occurs through collection of shellfish grown in sewage-polluted waters, by contaminated waters used in irrigation and through infection of foods by food handlers.

Conclusions

This review presents the more common clinical syndromes produced by the ingestion of natural seafood toxins. For the practicing allergist, knowledge of this wide array of toxic syndromes is important for the proper differential diagnosis of seafood allergy (Table 41.4). A careful history and physical examination are essential to establish the diagnosis on clinical grounds, which can be confirmed by detection of toxins either in remnants of the seafood or in specimens collected from the patient. The history should include symptoms and their severity, time of onset with respect to ingestion of seafood, number and frequency of reactions, whether others became ill, previous history of food allergy, types of marine species ingested and where they were captured, and

Table 41.4 Summary of common toxic syndromes associated with naturally occurring toxins in seafood

Type of poisoning	Type of toxins	Source	Symptom onset	Clinical syndrome
Scombroid	Histamine	Tuna, mahi-mahi, bonita, marlin, bluefish, wahoo, mackerel, and salmon	Minutes to 4 hours	Severe headache, dizziness, nausea, vomiting, flushed skin, urticaria, and wheezing
Ciguatera	Ciguatoxins	Coral reef fish: amberjack, snappers, grouper, goat fish, barracuda, sea bass, surgeon fish, ulua, and papio	30 minutes to 4 hours	Abdominal pain, diarrhea, vomiting, paresthesias, cold-to-hot sensory reversal, weakness, and myalgias
Puffer fish poisoning	Tetradotoxin	Ocean sunfishes, porcupine fishes, and fugu	10–45 minutes	Paresthesias headache, vomiting, diaphoresis, and respiratory paralysis
Paralytic shellfish	Saxitoxins	Mussels, clams, and oysters	5–30 minutes	Vomiting, diarrhea, facial paresthesias, and respiratory paralysis
Neurotoxic shellfish	Brevetoxins	Mussels and clams	30 minutes to 3 hours	Diarrhea, vomiting, abdominal pain, myalgias, paresthesias, and ataxia
Amnesic shellfish	Domoic acid	Mussels, clams, crabs, and anchovies	15 minutes to 38 hours	Vomiting, diarrhea, headache, myoclonus, loss of short-term memory, seizures, coma, and hemiparesis
Diarrhetic shellfish	Okadaic acid, Dinophysistoxins, Pectenotoxins, Yessotoxin	Mussels, clams, and scallops	30 minutes to 6 hours	Diarrhea, nausea, vomiting, and abdominal pain

the quantity of food consumed, and the way in which it was prepared. Whether the food was eaten at a restaurant, the patient was traveling, alcohol was consumed, or medications were taken by the patient should be recorded.

Presence of similar symptoms in other individuals who shared the seafood meal and the "endemic" nature of the syndrome are paramount in alerting the physician to possible seafood poisoning. The absence of prior reactions to the same seafood and its subsequent tolerance without symptoms point away from an allergic etiology and should be considered as corroborative evidence in support of a toxic syndrome. Since histamine mediates the symptoms of both scombroid and type I hypersensitivity reactions, clinical manifestations of scombroid may be virtually indistinguishable from seafood allergy. History of a "peppery" taste and type of fish consumed, as well as suspected improper refrigeration, are helpful in reaching the proper diagnosis.

Neurological symptoms associated with an allergic reaction are the result of hypoperfusion of the CNS and correlate with the severity of cardiovascular involvement and hypotension in anaphylaxis. This may help the physician to distinguish ciguatera, PSP, NSP, and ASP, where neurological impairment is commonly present in the absence of hypotension. In ciguatera, knowledge of the type of fish and whether it is imported from or consumed in endemic areas, such as Caribbean, Hawaii, and Pacific Islands, will provide clinical information to differentiate it from seafood allergy. Likewise in puffer fish poisoning, consumption of fugu, a delicacy of Japanese cuisine; and in shellfish poisoning, the location where seafood was caught, for instance

Pacific Coast in cases of PSP and ASP, are crucial pieces of information. The seasonal association with algal blooms and presence of high levels of biotoxins or toxic algae that are reported by authorities surveying coastal waters should increase the index of suspicion for physicians practicing in endemic areas. In the majority of these toxic syndromes, the causative toxin does not alter the taste and appearance of the seafood and is not inactivated by normal cooking.

Treatment is supportive, with active early respiratory support, especially in cases where neurological involvement could lead to respiratory paralysis. Upper respiratory reactions in individuals with no history of atopy and exacerbation of chest symptoms in asthmatics are caused by aerosolized NSP toxins. These irritant reactions are usually associated with a red tide and should not be mistaken for allergic respiratory symptoms.

Viruses, bacteria, and bacterial toxins may cause gastrointestinal and systemic symptoms that can be confused with food allergy. Raw or lightly steamed shellfish and raw fish are potential sources of infection with hepatitis A and Norwalk virus and *Vibrio* sp. Botulism is a hazard associated with consumption of home-canned, vacuum-packed smoked, or unviscerated salt-dried fish. If alternative diagnoses cannot be ruled out and seafood allergy remains a likely diagnosis, skin prick test and oral food challenge are diagnostic procedures of choice that may be employed in the evaluation of the patient.

Most current health risks associated with seafood contamination originate in the environment and should be dealt with by control of harvest or at the point of capture using HACCP principles. The most effective way of protecting consumers is to establish and maintain comprehensive monitoring programs for toxic algae and toxins in shellfish in all growing areas. Developing a better understanding of factors that promote harmful algal blooms and lead to production of toxins by marine algae is crucial to control human exposure and deleterious environmental effects. Further research is needed in most areas of seafood poisoning. Easy, accurate, and cost-effective methods for detection of toxins in seafood, monitoring shellfish for viral and bacterial contamination, and surveillance of coastal waters for harmful marine algae and their toxins are needed. Knowledge gained from research on the mechanism of action of marine toxins should lead to more specific treatment modalities that would limit morbidity and mortality of seafood intoxications. The following general preventive measures could greatly reduce the incidence of poisoning outbreaks that are associated with seafood:

1 Avoid eating raw seafood.

2 Avoid eating lightly steamed and undercooked shellfish.

3 Adhere to the public health agency guidelines on harvesting, processing, and consumption of shellfish and avoid shellfish from areas of frequent red tides.

4 Promptly refrigerate the catch of sport fishermen.

5 Avoid eating large, predatory reef fish usually implicated in ciguatera poisoning, especially barracuda, amberjack, and snapper.

6 Avoid reef fish caught in ciguatera endemic areas, especially the head, viscera, and roe.

7 Promptly report the suspected outbreaks of seafood poisoning to local health departments.

8 Submit left-over seafood or uncooked portions of the fish or shellfish to local health departments for analysis to establish nature and amount of contaminating toxin.

Finally, the informed physician can be of great help in public health prevention through public education and involvement with the local and public agencies that deal with these health issues.

References

1 Metcalfe DD. Food allergens. *Clin Rev Allergy* 1985;3:331–49.

2 Leung PS, Chen YC, Chu KH. Seafood allergy: tropomyosins and beyond. *J Microbiol Immunol Infect* 1999;32:143–54.

3 Sampson HA. Food anaphylaxis. *Br Med Bull* 2000;56:925–35.

4 Ohnuma S, Higa M, Hamanaka S, *et al*. An outbreak of allergy-like food poisoning. *Intern Med* 2001;40:833–5.

5 Sanchez-Guerrero IM, Vidal JB, Escudero AI. Scombroid fish poisoning: a potentially life-threatening allergic-like reaction. *J Allergy Clin Immunol* 1997;100:433–4.

6 Wong RC, Katelaris CH. Adult onset restricted fish allergy. *Aust N Z J Med* 1999;29:829–30.

7 O'Connor MM, Forbes GM. Scombroid poisoning: not fish allergy. *Aust N Z J Med* 2000;30:520.

8 Taylor SL, Stratton JE, Nordlee JA. Histamine poisoning (scombroid fish poisoning): an allergy-like intoxication. *J Toxicol Clin Toxicol* 1989;27:225–40.

9 CDC. Surveillance for foodborne disease outbreaks, United States, 1988–1992. *MMWR* 1996;45:1–55.

10 CDC. National Center for Infectious Diseases, Division of Bacterial and Mycotic Diseases. Foodborne disease outbreak line listings 1990 through 2004 in http://www.cdc.gov/foodborneoutbreaks/outbreak_data.htm.

11 Ahmed FE (ed.). Naturally occurring fish and shellfish poisons, Chapter 4. *Seafood Safety. Institute of Medicine, National Academy of Sciences*. Washington, DC: National Academy Press, 1991:87–110.

12 Dalton CB, Gregory J, Kirk MD, *et al*. Foodborne disease outbreaks in Australia, 1995 to 2000. *Commun Dis Intell* 2004;28:211–24.

13 Isbister GK, Kiernan MC. Neurotoxic marine poisoning. *Lancet Neurol* 2005;4:219–28.

14 CDC. Foodborne disease outbreaks, 5-year summary, 1983–1987. *MMWR* 1990;39:15–57.

15 CDC. Surveillance for foodborne disease outbreaks, United States, 1993–1997. *MMWR* 2000;49:1–66.

16 Lewis RJ. Ciguatera: Australian perspectives on a global problem. *Toxicon* 2006;48:799–809.

17 Food poisoning caused by shellfish contaminated by marine algal toxins. *Commun Dis Rep CDR Wkly* 2001;11:19 http://www.hpa.org.uk/cdr/archives/2001/cdr1901.pdf.

18 Arnott GH. Toxic marine microalgae: a worldwide problem with major implications for seafood safety. *Adv Food Safety* 1998;1:24–34.

19 Viviani R. Eutrophication, marine biotoxins, human health. *Sci Total Environ* 1992;631–62.

20 Lehane L. *Paralytic Shellfish Poisoning: A Review. Canberra, Australia*: National Office of Animal and Plant Health Agriculture, Fisheries and Forestry – 2000.

21 Merson MH, Baine WB, Gangarosa EJ, Swanson RC. Scombroid fish poisoning. Outbreak traced to commercially canned tuna fish. *JAMA* 1974;228:1268–9.

22 Lange WR. Scombroid poisoning. *Am Fam Physician* 1988;37:163–8.

23 Concon JM. *Food Toxicology. Part B: Contaminants and Additives*. New York: Marcel Dekker, 1988;511–604.

24 Lukton A, Olcott HS. Content of free imidazole compounds in the muscle tissue of aquatic animals. *Food Res* 1958;23:611–18.

25 Taylor SL. Histamine food poisoning: toxicology and clinical aspects. *CRC Crit Rev Toxicol* 1986;17:91–128.

26 CDC. Scombroid fish poisoning – Illinois, South Carolina. *MMWR* 1989;38:140–2.

27 Hughes JM, Potter ME. Scombroid-fish poisoning. From pathogenesis to prevention. *N Engl J Med* 1991;324:766–8.

28 Werner SB. Food poisoning. *Public Health and Preventive Medicine*, 14th edn. Stanford, CT: Appleton and Lange, 1998.

29 Morrow JD, Margolies GR, Rowland J, Roberts LJ. Evidence that histamine is the causative toxin of scombroid fish poisoning. *N Engl J Med* 1991;324:716–20.

30 Bedry R, Gabinski C, Paty MC. Diagnosis of scombroid poisoning by measurement of plasma histamine. *N Engl J Med* 2000;342:520–1.

31 Lehane L, Olley J. Histamine fish poisoning revisited. *Int J Food Microbiol* 2000;58:1–37.

32 Bagnis R, Chameau S, Chungue E, *et al*. Origins of ciguatera fish poisoning: a new dinoflagellate *Gambierdiscus toxicus* Adachi and Fukuyo, definitely involved as a causal agent. *Toxicon* 1980;18:199–208.

33 Hughes JM, Merson MH. Fish and shellfish poisoning. *N Engl J Med* 1976;295:1117–20.

34 Eastaugh J, Shepherd S. Infectious and toxic syndromes from fish and shellfish consumption. A review. *Arch Intern Med* 1989;149:1735–40.

35 Lange WR. Ciguatera fish poisoning. *Am Fam Physician* 1994; 50:579–84.

36 Sims JK. A theoretical discourse on the pharmacology of toxic marine ingestions. *Ann Emerg Med* 1987;16:1006–15.

37 Ting JY, Brown AF. Ciguatera poisoning: a global issue with common management problems. *Eur J Emerg Med* 2001;8:295–300.

38 Lipp EK, Rose JB. The role of seafood in foodborne diseases in the United States of America. *Rev Sci Tech* 1997;16:620–40.

39 Stinn JF, De Sylva DP, Fleming LE, Hack E. Geographic Information Systems (GIS) and ciguatera fish poisoning in the tropical Western Atlantic region. Proceedings of the 1998 Geographic Information Systems in Public Health, 3rd National Conference San Diego, CA, 2000. http://www.atsdr.cdc.gov/gis/conference98/proceedings/html/stinn.html.

40 CDC. Ciguatera fish poisoning – Vermont. *MMWR* 1986;35:263–4.

41 Escobar LI, Salvador C, Martinez M, Vaca L. Maitotoxin, a cationic channel activator. *Neurobiology* 1998;6:59–74.

42 Gollop JH, Pon EW. Ciguatera: a review. *Hawaii Med J* 1992; 51:91–9.

43 Weisman, RS. Marine envenomations. Goldfrank's Toxicologic Emergencies. 7th ed. Goldfrank LR, Flomenbaum NE, Lewin NA, Howland MA, Hoffman RS, Nelson LS. (eds.) McGraw-Hill, New York, NY. 2002:1592–1597.

44 Lewis RJ, Holmes MJ. Origin and transfer of toxins involved in ciguatera. *Comp Biochem Physiol C* 1993;106:615–28.

45 Bidard JN, Vijuerben HPM, Frelin C, *et al*. Ciguatoxin is a novel type of Na$^+$ channel toxin. *J Biol Chem* 1984;359:8353–7.

46 Gillespie NC, Lewis RJ, Pearn JH, *et al*. Ciguatera in Australia: occurrence, clinical features, pathophysiology and management. *Med J Aust* 1986;145:584–90.

47 Terao K, Ito E, Sakamaki Y, *et al*. Histopathological studies of experimental marine toxin poisoning. II. The acute effects of maitotoxin on the stomach, heart and lymphoid tissues in mice and rats. *Toxicon* 1988;26:395–402.

48 Igarashi T, Aritake S, Yasumoto T. Mechanisms underlying the hemolytic and ichthyotoxic activities of maitotoxin. *Nat Toxins* 1999;7:71–9.

49 Lehane L, Lewis RJ. Ciguatera: recent advances but the risk remains. *Int J Food Microbiol* 2000;61:91–125.

50 Van Dolah FM. Marine algal toxins: origins, health effects, and their increased occurrence. *Environ Health Perspect* 2000; 108:133–41.

51 Hokama Y, Banner AH, Boyland D. A radioimmunoassay for the detection of ciguatoxin. *Toxicon* 1977;15:317–25.

52 Hokama Y. A rapid simplified enzyme immunoassay stick test for the detection of ciguatoxin and related polyethers from fish tissue. *Toxicon* 1985;23:939–46.

53 Hokama Y. Simplified solid-phase immunobead assay for detection of ciguatoxin and related polyethers. *J Clin Lab Anal* 1990;4:213–17.

54 Hokama Y, Nishimura K, Takenaka W, Ebesu JS. Simplified solid-phase membrane immunobead assay (MIA) with monoclonal anti-ciguatoxin antibody (MAb-CTX) for detection of ciguatoxin and related polyether toxins. *J Nat Toxins* 1998;7:1–21.

55 CDC. Ciguatera fish poisoning – Texas, 1997. *MMWR* 1998; 47:692–4.

56 Palafox NA, Jain LG, Pinano AZ, *et al*. Successful treatment of ciguatera fish poisoning with intravenous mannitol. *JAMA* 1988;259:2740–2.

57 Blythe DG, De Sylva DP, Fleming LE, *et al*. Clinical experience with IV mannitol in the treatment of ciguatera. *Bull Soc Path Ex* 1992;85:425–6.

58 Schnorf H, Taurarii M, Cundy T. Ciguatera fish poisoning: a double-blind randomized trial of mannitol therapy. *Neurology* 2002;58:873–80.

59 Halstead BW. *Poisonous and Venomous Marine Animals of the World*. Princeton, NJ: Darwin Press, 1988;525–644.

60 Chang FC, Bauer RM, Benton BJ, *et al*. 4-Aminopyridine antagonizes saxitoxin-and tetrodotoxin-induced cardiorespiratory depression. *Toxicon* 1996;34:671–90.

61 Benson J. *Tetradon* (blowfish) poisoning. A report of two fatalities. *J Forensic Sci* 1956;1:119–26.

62 CDC. Tetradotoxin poisoning associated with eating puffer fish transported from Japan – California, 1996. *MMWR* 1996;45:389–91.

63 Halstead BW. *Poisonous and Venomous Marine Animals of the World*, Vol. II. Washington, DC: US Government Printing Office, 1967:679–844.

64 Torda TA, Sinclair E, Ulyatt DB. Puffer fish (tetrodotoxin) poisoning: clinical record and suggested management. *Med J Aust* 1973;1:599–602.

65 Bradley SG, Klika LJ. A fatal poisoning from the Oregon roughskinned newt (*Taricha granulosa*). *JAMA* 1981;246:247.

66 Sheumack DD, Howden ME, Spence I, Quinn RJ. Maculotoxin: a neurotoxin from the venom glands of the octopus *Hapalochlaena maculosa* identified as tetrodotoxin. *Science* 1978;199:188–9.

67 Narita H, Matsubara S, Miwa N, *et al. Vibrio alginolyticus* a TTX-producing bacterium isolated from the starfish *Astropecten polyacanthus. Nippon Suisan Gakk* 1987;53:617–21.

68 Sugita H, Iwata J, Miyajima C, *et al*. Changes in microflora of a puffer fish *Fugu niphobles* with different water temperatures. *Mar Biol* 1989;101:299–304.

69 Lee MJ, Jeong DY, Kim WS, *et al*. A tetrodotoxin-producing *Vibrio* strain, LM-1, from the puffer fish *Fugu vermicularis radiatus. Appl Environ Microbiol* 2000;66:1698–701.

70 Wu Z, Xie L, Xia G, *et al*. A new tetrodotoxin-producing actino-mycete, *Nocardiopsis dassonvillei*, isolated from the ovaries of puffer fish *Fugu rubripes. Toxicon* 2005;45:851–9.

71 Halstead BW, Schantz EJ. *Paralytic Shellfish Poisoning*. Geneva, Switzerland: WHO Offset Publication, 1984;79:1–60.

72 Gessner BD, Middaugh JP. Paralytic shellfish poisoning in Alaska: a 20-year retrospective analysis. *Am J Epidemiol* 1995;141:766–70.

73 Kao CY. Paralytic shellfish poisoning, Chapter 4. In: Falconer IR (ed.) *Algal Toxins in Seafood and Drinking Water*. London and New York: Academic Press, 1993:75–86.

74 Schantz E. Seafood toxicants. *Toxicants Occurring Naturally in Foods*, 2nd edn. Washington, DC: National Academy Press, 1973:424–47.

75 Hall S, Strichartz G, Moczydlowski E, *et al*. The saxitoxins: sources, chemistry, and pharmacology, Chapter 3. In: Hall S, Strichartz G (eds.) *Marine Toxins: Origin, Structure and Molecular Pharmacology*. Washington, DC: American Chemical Society Symposium Series, 1990:29–65.

76 Leftley JW, Hannah F. Phycotoxins in seafood. In: Watson DH (ed.) *Natural Toxicants in Food*. Sheffield: Sheffield Academic, 1998:182–224.

77 Hungerford JM, Weckell MM. Analytical methods for marine toxins. In: Tu AT (ed.) *Handbook of Natural Toxins, Vol. 7, Food Poisoning*. New York: Marcel Dekker Inc, 1992:416–73.

78 van Egmond HP, Aune Y, Lassus P, *et al*. Paralytic and diarrhoeic shellfish poisons: occurrence in Europe, toxicity, analysis and regulation. *J Nat Toxins* 1993;2:41–83.

79 Usleber E, Donald M, Straka M, Martlbauer E. Comparison of enzyme immunoassay and mouse bioassay for determining par-alytic shellfish poisoning toxins in shellfish. *Food Addit Contam* 1997;14:193–8.

80 Jellett J, Laycock MV, Belland ER, *et al*. Rapid toxin tests: MIST Alert for PSP and ASP. In: Whyte JNC (ed.) Canadian Technical Report of Fisheries and Aquatic Sciences No. 2386. *Proceedings of the Seventh Canadian Workshop on Harmful Marine Algae*. Fisheries and Oceans Canada Pacific Biological Station, 2001:23–25.

81 Silv MA, Jellett JF, Laycock MV, *et al*. Phytoplankton moni-toring using a rapid field test: MIST Alert for paralytic shell-fish poisons. In: Whyte JNC (ed.) Canadian Technical Report of Fisheries and Aquatic Sciences No. 2386. *Proceedings of the Seventh Canadian Workshop on Harmful Marine Algae*. Fisheries and Oceans Canada Pacific Biological Station, 2001:28–34.

82 Mackintosh FH, Gallacher S, Shanks AM, Smith EA. Assessment of MIST Alert, a commercial qualitative assay for detection of paralytic shellfish poisoning toxins in bivalve molluscs. *J AOAC Int* 2002;85:632–41.

83 Jellett JF, Roberts RL, Laycock MV, *et al*. Detection of paralytic shellfish poisoning (PSP) toxins in shellfish tissue using MIST Alert, a new rapid test, in parallel with the regulatory AOAC mouse bioassay. *Toxicon* 2002;40:1407–25.

84 Nicholson RA, Guohua L, Buenaventura E, Graham D. A rapid and sensitive biochemical assay for PSP bioactives based on mouse brain synaptoneurosomes. In: Whyte JNC (ed.) Canadian Technical Report of Fisheries and Aquatic Sciences No. 2386. *Proceedings of the Seventh Canadian Workshop on Harmful Marine Algae*. Fisheries and Oceans Canada Pacific Biological Station, 2001:26.

85 Taylor SL. Marine toxins of microbial origin. *Food Tech* 1988;42:94–8.

86 Dale B, Yentsch CM. Red tide and paralytic shellfish poison-ing. *Oceanus* 1978;21:41–9.

87 Scholin CA, Anderson DM. Population analysis of toxic and non-toxic *Alexandrium* species using ribosomal RNA signature sequences. In: Smayda TJ, Shimizu Y (eds.) *Toxic Phytoplankton Blooms in the Sea*. Amsterdam, The Netherlands: Elsevier, 1993:95–102.

88 Lam CWY, Ho KC. Red tides in Tolo Harbor, Hong Kong. In: Okaichi T, Anderson DM, Nemoto T (eds.) *Red Tides: Biology Environmental Science and Toxicology*. New York: Elsevier, 1989:49–52.

89 FDA. Natural toxins, Chapter 6. *Fish and Fishery Products Hazards and Controls Guide*, 2nd edn. Washington, DC: Department of Health and Human Services, Public Health Service, Food and Drug Administration, Center for Food Safety and Applied Nutrition, Office of Seafood, 1998:65–72.

90 Regulation (EC) No. 853/2004 of the European Parliament and of the Council of 29 April 2004 laying down specific hygiene rules for food of animal origin. *Offic J Eur Union* L 226:22–82.

91 Sakamoto Y, Lockey RF, Krzanowski Jr JJ. Shellfish and fish poisoning related to the toxic dinoflagellates. *South Med J* 1987;80:866–72.

92 Poli MA, Musser SM, Dickey RW, *et al*. Neurotoxic shell-fish poisoning and brevetoxin metabolites: a case study from Florida. *Toxicon* 2000;38:981–93.

93 Naar J, Bourdelais A, Tomas C, *et al*. A competitive ELISA to detect brevetoxins from *Karenia brevis* (formerly *Gymnodinium breve*) in seawater, shellfish, and mammalian body fluid. *Environ Health Perspect* 2002;110:179–85.

94 Shimoda T, Krzanowski Jr J, Nelson R, *et al*. In vitro red tide toxin effects on human bronchial smooth muscle. *J Allergy Clin Immunol* 1988;81:1187–91.

95 Tester PA, Fowler PK. Brevetoxin contamination of *Mercenaria mercenaria* and *Crassostrea virginica*: a management issue. In: Graneli E, Sundstrom B, Edler L, Anderson DM (eds.) *Toxic Marine Phytoplankton*. New York: Elsevier Press, 1990:499–503.

96 Baden DG. Brevetoxins: unique polyether dinoflagellate tox-ins. *FASEB J* 1989;3:1807–17.

97 Sim J, Wilson N. Surveillance of marine biotoxins, 1993–96. *N Z Publ Health Rep* 1997;4:9–11.

98 Tester PA, Steidinger KA. *Gymnodynium breve* red tide: ini-tiation, transport, and consequences of surface circulation. *Limnol Oceanogr* 1997;42:1052–75.

99 Tester PA, Stumpf RP, Vukovich FM, *et al*. An expatriate red tide bloom: transport, distribution, and persistence, *Limnol Oceanogr* 1991;36:1053–61.

100 Hallegraeff GM. A review of harmful algal blooms and their apparent global increase. *Phycologia* 1993;32:79–99.

101 Carlton JT, Geller JB. Ecological roulette: the global transport of nonindigenous marine organisms. *Science* 1993;261:78–82.

102 FDA. Sanitation of shellfish growing areas. *National Shellfish Sanitation Program Manual of Operations Pan I. Food and Drug Administration*, Center for Food Safety and Applied Nutrition, Division of Cooperative Programs, Washington, DC: Shellfish Sanitation Branch, 1989.

103 DNR (Department of Natural Resources, Florida). *Contingency Plan for Control of Shellfish Potentially Contaminated by Marine Biotoxins*. St. Petersburg, FL: Bureau of Marine Research, 1985:1–10.

104 Todd ECD. Amnesic shellfish poisoning – a new seafood toxin syndrome. In: Graneli E, Sundstrom B, Edler L, Anderson DM (eds.) *Proceedings of the 4th International Conference on Toxic Marine Phytoplankton*. Amsterdam, The Netherlands: Elsevier, 1989:504–8.

105 Perl TM, Bedard L, Kosatsky T, *et al*. An outbreak of toxic encephalopathy caused by eating mussels contaminated with domoic acid. *N Engl J Med* 1990;322:1775–80.

106 Teitelbaum JS, Zatorre RJ, Carpenter S, *et al*. Neurologic sequelae of domoic acid intoxication due to the ingestion of contaminated mussels. *N Engl J Med* 1990;322:1781–7.

107 Subba RD, Quilliam M, Pocklington R. Domoic acid – a neurotoxic amino acid produced by the marine diatom *Nitzschia pungens* in culture. *Can J Fish Aquat Sci* 1988;45:2076–9.

108 Jeffery B, Barlow T, Moizer K, *et al*. Amnesic shellfish poison. *Food Chem Toxicol* 2004;42:545–57.

109 Debonnel G, Weiss M, de Montigny C. Neurotoxic effect of domoic acid: mediation by kainate receptor electrophysiological studies in the rat. *Can Dis Wkly Rep* 1990;16:59–68.

110 Tryphonas L, Iverson F. Neuropathology of excitatory neurotoxins: the domoic acid model. *Toxicol Pathol* 1990;18:165–9.

111 Gill S, Pulido O. Glutamate receptors in peripheral tissues: current knowledge, future research and implications for toxicology. *Toxicol Pathol* 2001;29:208–23.

112 Debonnel G, Beaushesne L, Demonigny C. Domoic acid, the alleged mussel toxin, might produce its neurotoxic effect through kainate receptor activation: an electrophysiologic study in the rat dorsal hippocampus. *Can J Physiol Pharmacol* 1989;67:29–33.

113 Walz PM, Garrison DL, Graham WM, *et al*. Domoic acid-producing diatom blooms in Monterey Bay, California: 1991–1993. *Nat Toxins* 1994;2:271–9.

114 Garthwaite I, Ross KM, Miles CO, *et al*. Polyclonal antibodies to domoic acid, and their use in immunoassays for domoic acid in sea water and shellfish. *Nat Toxins* 1998;6:93–104.

115 Kawatsu K, Hamano Y, Noguchi T. Production and characterization of a monoclonal antibody against domoic acid and its application to enzyme immunoassay. *Toxicon* 1999;37:1579–89.

116 Baugh KA, Wekell JC, Trainer VL. Detection methods for domoic acid in seawater. In: Whyte JNC (ed.) Canadian Technical Report of Fisheries and Aquatic Sciences No. 2386. *Proceedings of the Seventh Canadian Workshop on Harmful Marine Algae*. Fisheries and Oceans Canada Pacific Biological Station, 2001:86.

117 Washington State Department of Health. Establishing tolerable dungeness crab (*Cancer magister*) and razor clam (*Siliqua patula*) domoic acid contaminant levels. Office of Environmental Health Assessment, Olympia, WA, 1996.

118 Saavedra-Delgado AM, Metcalfe DD. Seafood toxins. *Clin Rev Allergy* 1993;11:241–60.

119 Goto H, Igarashi T, Yamamoto M, *et al*. Quantitative determination of marine toxins associated with diarrhetic shellfish poisoning by liquid chromatography coupled with mass spectrometry. *J Chromatogr A* 2001;907:181–9.

120 Yasumoto T, Murata M. Polyether toxins involved in seafood poisoning. In: Hall S, Stricharty G (eds.) *Marine Toxins: Origin, Structure and Molecular Pharmacology*. Washington, DC: American Chemical Society, 1990:120–32.

121 Tripuraneni J, Koutsouris A, Pestic L, *et al*. The toxin of diarrheic shellfish poisoning, okadaic acid, increases intestinal epithelial paracellular permeability. *Gastroenterology* 1997;112:100–8.

122 Ito E, Terao K. Injury and recovery process of intestine caused by okadaic acid and related compounds. *Nat Toxins* 1994;2:371–7.

123 Burgess V, Shaw G. Pectenotoxins – an issue for public health: a review of their comparative toxicology and metabolism. *Environ Int* 2001;27:275–83.

124 Quilliam MA. Phycotoxins. *J AOAC Int* 1999;82:773–81.

125 Windust AJ, Wright JLC, McLachlan JL. The effects of the diarrhetic shellfish poisoning toxins, okadaic acid and dinophysistoxin-1, on the growth of microalgae. *Mar Biol* 1996; 126:19–25.

126 Nunez PE, Scoging AC. Comparison of a protein phosphatase inhibition assay, HPLC assay and enzyme-linked immunosorbent assay with the mouse bioassay for the detection of diarrhetic shellfish poisoning toxins in European shellfish. *Int J Food Microbiol* 1997;36:39–48.

127 Quilliam MA. Phycotoxins. In: Quilliam MA, Williams KA (eds.) General Referee Reports: Committee on Natural Toxins and Food Allergens. *J AOAC Int* 2001;84:194–212.

128 Vale P, Sampayo MA. Comparison between HPLC and a commercial immunoassay kit for detection of okadaic acid and esters in Portuguese bivalves. *Toxicon* 1999;37:1565–77.

129 Morton SL, Tindall DR. Determination of okadaic acid content of dinoflagellate cells: a comparison of the HPLC-fluorescent method and two monoclonal antibody ELISA test kits. *Toxicon* 1996;34:947–54.

130 Freudenthal AR, Jijina JL. Potential hazards of *Dinophysis* to consumers and shellfisheries. *J Shellfish Res* 1988;7:695–701.

131 Champetier De Ribes G, Rasolofonirina RN, Ranaivoson G, *et al*. Intoxication by marine animal venoms in Madagascar (ichthyosarcotoxism and chelonitoxism): recent epidemiological data. *Bull Soc Pathol Exot* 1997;90:286–90.

132 Onuma Y, Satake M, Ukena T, *et al*. Identification of putative palytoxin as the cause of clupeotoxism. *Toxicon* 1999;37:55–65.

133 Okano H, Masuoka H, Kamei S, *et al*. Rhabdomyolysis and myocardial damage induced by palytoxin, a toxin of blue humphead parrotfish. *Intern Med* 1998;37:330–3.

134 Yoshimine K, Orita S, Okada S, *et al.* Two cases of parrotfish poisoning with rhabdomyolysis. *Nippon Naika Gakkai Zasshi* 2001;90:1339–41.

135 Taniyama S, Mahmud Y, Terada M, *et al.* Occurrence of a food poisoning incident by palytoxin from a serranid *Epinephelus* sp. in Japan. *J Nat Toxins* 2002;11:277–82.

136 Artigas P, Gadsby DC. Na+/K+-pump ligands modulate gating of palytoxin-induced ion channels. *Proc Natl Acad Sci USA* 2003;100:501–5.

137 Frelin C, Van Renterghem C. Palytoxin. Recent electrophysiological and pharmacological evidence for several mechanisms of action. *Gen Pharmacol* 1995;26:33–7.

138 Anthoni U, Christophersen C, Gram L, *et al.* Poisonings from flesh of the Greenland shark *Somniosus microcephalus* may be due to trimethylamine. *Toxicon* 1991;29:1205–12.

139 Boisier P, Ranaivoson G, Rasolofonirina N, *et al.* Fatal mass poisoning in Madagascar following ingestion of a shark (*Carcharhinus leucas*): clinical and epidemiological aspects and isolation of toxins. *Toxicon* 1995;33:1359–64.

140 Reid TM, Gould IM, Mackie IM, *et al.* Food poisoning due to the consumption of red whelks (*Neptunea antiqua*). *Epidemiol Infect* 1988;101:419–23.

141 Black NMI, O'Brian SJ, Blain B. Red spells danger for whelk eaters. *Commun Dis Rep* 1991;1:R125.

142 Anthoni U, Bohlin L, Larsen C, *et al.* The toxin tetramine from the "edible" whelk *Neptunea antiqua. Toxicon* 1989;27:717–23.

143 Power AJ, Keegan BF, Nolan K. The seasonality and role of the neurotoxin tetramine in the salivary glands of the red whelk *Neptunea antiqua. Toxicon* 2002;40:419–25.

144 McMahon T. Azaspiracid in Irish shellfish. *Report of the ICES/IOC Working Group on Harmful Algal Bloom Dynamics*, Dublin, Ireland: International Council for Exploration of the Sea, Copenhagen, Denmark, 2001:22.

145 CDR. Food poisoning caused by shellfish contaminated by marine algal toxins. *Commun Dis Rep CDR Wkly* 2001;11:19.

146 James KJ, Fidalgo Saez MJ, Furey A, Lehane M. Azaspiracid poisoning, the food-borne illness associated with shellfish consumption. *Food Addit Contam* 2004;21:879–92.

147 *Risk Assessment of Azaspiracids (AZAs) in Shellfish*: A Report of the Scientific Committee of the FSAI. August 2006. http://www.fsai.ie/publications/other/AZAs_risk_assess_aug06.pdf

148 Hess P, Nguyen L, Aasen J, *et al.* Tissue distribution, effects of cooking and parameters affecting the extraction of azaspiracids from mussels, *Mytilus edulis*, prior to analysis by liquid chromatography coupled to mass spectrometry. *Toxicon* 2005;46:62–71.

149 Ito E, Satake M, Ofuji K, *et al.* Multiple organ damage caused by a new toxin azaspiracid, isolated from mussels produced in Ireland. *Toxicon* 2000;38:917–30.

150 James KJ, Lehane M, Moroney C, *et al.* Azaspiracid shellfish poisoning: unusual toxin dynamics in shellfish and the increased risk of acute human intoxications. *Food Addit Contam* 2002;19:555–61.

151 Lehane M, Fidalgo Saez MJ, Magdalena AB, *et al.* Liquid chromatography – multiple tandem mass spectrometry for the determination of ten azaspiracids, including hydroxyl analogues in shellfish. *J Chromatogr A* 2004;1024:63–70.

152 Richard D, Arsenault E, Cembella A, Quilliam M. Investigations into the toxicology and pharmacology of spirolides – a novel group of putative biotoxins. *9th International Conference on Algal Blooms*, 2000. Hobart, Tasmania.

153 Pulido O, Richard D, Quilliam M, *et al.* Toxicological neuropathology from domoic acid to spirolides – the health Canada experience. In: Whyte, JNC. (ed.) Canadian Technical Report of Fisheries and Aquatic Science. *Proceedings of the Seventh Canadian Workshop on Harmful Marine Algae*, 2001:36–44.

154 Cembella AD, Lewis NI, Quilliam MA. Spirolide composition of micro-extracted pooled cells isolated from natural plankton assemblages and from cultures of the dinoflagellate *Alexandrium ostenfeldii. Nat Toxins* 1999;7:197–206.

155 Ratafia M. Aquaculture today: a worldwide status report. *Aquaculture News* 1994;3:12–13, 18–19.

156 Garrett ES, Lima dos Santos C, Jahncke ML. Special issue: public, animal, and environmental health implications of aquaculture. *Emerg Infect Dis* 1997;3:453–7.

157 Institute of Medicine, National Academy of Sciences. Food animal production practices, Chapter 2. *The Use of Drugs in Food Animals: Benefits and Risks*. Washington, DC: National Academy Press, 1999:27–68.

158 Institute of Medicine, National Academy of Sciences. Drug residues and microbial contamination in food, Chapter 5. *The Use of Drugs in Food Animals: Benefits and Risks*. Washington, DC: National Academy Press, 1999:110–41.

159 Stehly GR, Gingerich WH, Kiessling CR, Cutting JH. A bridging study for oxytetracycline in the edible fillet of rainbow trout: analysis by a liquid chromatographic method and the official microbial inhibition assay. *J AOAC Int* 1999;82:866–70.

160 Luzzana U, Serrini G, Moretti VM, *et al.* Effect of temperature and diet composition on residue depletion of oxytetracycline in cultured channel catfish. *Analyst* 1994;119:2757–59.

161 Brocklebank JR, Namdari R, Law FC. An oxytetracycline residue depletion study to assess the physiologically based pharmokinetic (PBPK) model in farmed Atlantic salmon. *Can Vet J* 1997;38:645–6.

162 Iosifidou EG, Haagsma N, Olling M, *et al.* Residue study of mebendazole and its metabolites hydroxy-mebendazole and amino-mebendazole in eel (*Anguilla anguilla*) after bath treatment. *Drug Metab Dispos* 1997;25:317–20.

163 Black WD. The use of antimicrobial drugs in agriculture. *Can J Physiol Pharmacol* 1984;62:1044–8.

164 Woodward KN. Hypersensitivity in humans and exposure to veterinary drugs. *Vet Hum Toxicol* 1991;33:168–72.

165 Nestle M. Allergies to transgenic foods – questions of policy. *N Engl J Med* 1996;334:726–8.

166 Nordlee JA, Taylor SL, Townsend JA, *et al.* Identification of a Brazil-nut allergen in transgenic soybeans. *N Engl J Med* 1996;334:688–92.

167 Taylor SL, Hefle SL. Will genetically modified foods be allergenic? *J Allergy Clin Immunol* 2001;107:765–71.

168 Hightower R, Baden C, Penzes E, *et al*. Expression of antifreeze proteins in transgenic plants. *Plant Mol Biol* 1991;17:1013–21.

169 Hew C, Poon R, Xiong F, *et al*. Liver-specific and seasonal expression of transgenic Atlantic salmon harboring the winter flounder antifreeze protein gene. *Transgenic Res* 1999;8:405–14.

170 Devlin RH, Biagi CA, Yesaki TY, *et al*. Growth of domesticated transgenic fish. *Nature* 2001;409:781–2.

171 Houdebine LM, Chourrout D. Transgenesis in fish. *Experientia* 1991;47:891–7.

172 Rahman MA, Mak R, Ayad H, *et al*. Expression of a novel piscine growth hormone gene results in growth enhancement in transgenic tilapia (*Oreochromis niloticus*). *Transgenic Res* 1998;7:357–69.

173 Guillen II, Berlanga J, Valenzuela CM, *et al*. Safety evaluation of transgenic tilapia with accelerated growth. *Mar Biotechnol* 1999;1:2–14.

174 Shapiro RL, Hatheway C, Swerdlow DL. Botulism in the United States: a clinical and epidemiologic review. *Ann Intern Med* 1998;129:221–8.

175 Telzak EE, Bell EP, Kautter DA, *et al*. An international outbreak of type E botulism due to uneviscerated fish. *J Infect Dis* 1990;161:340–2.

176 Weber JT, Hibbs Jr RG, Darwish A, *et al*. A massive outbreak of type E botulism associated with traditional salted fish in Cairo. *J Infect Dis* 1993;167:451–4.

177 Wainwright RB, Heyward WL, Middaugh JP, *et al*. Food-borne botulism in Alaska, 1947–1985: epidemiology and clinical findings. *J Infect Dis* 1988;157:1158–62.

178 Hayes Jr AH. The Food and Drug Administration's role in the canned salmon recalls of 1982. *Public Health Rep* 1983;98:412–15.

179 Chambers HF. Infectious diseases: bacterial and chlamydial – Botulism, Chapter 33. In: Trieney LM, McPhee SJ, Papadakis MA (eds.) *Current Medical Diagnosis and Treatment*. New York: McGraw-Hill, 2002:1407–8.

180 Eisenberg MS, Bender TR. Botulism in Alaska, 1947 through 1974. Early detection of cases and investigation of outbreaks as a means of reducing mortality. *JAMA* 1976;235:35–8.

181 CDC. Botulism outbreak associated with eating fermented food – Alaska, 2001. *MMWR* 2001;50:680–2.

182 Tranter HS. Foodborne staphylococcal illness. *Lancet* 1990;336:1044–6.

183 Balaban N, Rasooly A. Staphylococcal enterotoxins. *Int J Food Microbiol* 2000;61:1–10.

184 Lowry PW, Pavia AT, McFarland LM, *et al*. Cholera in Louisiana. Widening spectrum of seafood vehicles. *Arch Intern Med* 1989;149:2079–84.

185 Bean NH, Maloney EK, Potter ME, *et al*. Crayfish: a newly recognized vehicle for *Vibrio* infections. *Epidemiol Infect* 1998;121:269–73.

186 Daniels NA, MacKinnon L, Bishop R, *et al*. Vibrio parahaemolyticus infections in the United States, 1973–1998. *J Infect Dis*;181:1661–6.

187 Shapiro RL, Altekruse S, Hutwagner L, *et al*. The role of Gulf Coast oysters harvested in warmer months in *Vibrio vulnificus* infections in the United States, 1988–1996. *Vibrio* Working Group. *J Infect Dis* 1998;178:752–9.

188 Ahmed FE (ed.). Executive summary, Chapter 1. *Seafood Safety. Institute of Medicine, National Academy of Sciences*. Washington, DC: National Academy Press, 1991:1–20.

189 Murphy AM, Grohmann GS, Christopher PJ, *et al*. An Australia-wide outbreak of gastroenteritis from oysters caused by *Norwalk* virus. *Med J Aust* 1979;2:329–33.

190 Morse DL, Guzewich JJ, Hanrahan JP, *et al*. Widespread outbreaks of clam- and oyster-associated gastroenteritis. Role of *Norwalk virus*. *N Engl J Med* 1986;314:678–81.

191 Gunn RA, Janowski HT, Lieb S, *et al*. *Norwalk virus* gastroenteritis following raw oyster consumption. *Am J Epidemiol* 1982;115:348–51.

192 Kohn MA, Farley TA, Ando T, *et al*. An outbreak of *Norwalk virus* gastroenteritis associated with eating raw oysters. Implications for maintaining safe oyster beds. *JAMA* 1995;273:466–71.

193 DuPont HL. Consumption of raw shellfish – is the risk now unacceptable? *N Engl J Med* 1986;314:707–8.

194 Ahmed FE (ed.). Microbial and parasitic exposure and health effects, Chapter 3. *Seafood Safety. Institute of Medicine, National Academy of Sciences*. Washington, DC: National Academy Press, 1991:30–86.

195 Desenclos JC, Klontz KC, Wilder MH, *et al*. A multistate outbreak of hepatitis A caused by the consumption of raw oysters. *Am J Public Health* 1991;81:1268–72.

CHAPTER 42

Neurological Reactions to Foods and Food Additives

Richard W. Weber

KEY CONCEPTS

- Dietary factors have been suspected or demonstrated in several conditions with neurological manifestations, the most prominent being migraine and epilepsy.

- Dietary migraine is a bona fide entity, with both pharmacological and immunological mechanisms involved in subsets of migraineurs.

- The benefit of ketogenic diets for epilepsy management is well established, but the manner in which they operate remains uncertain.

- Food-induced anaphylaxis may present with neurological manifestations in one-quarter of cases.

- Neurological complications associated with gluten sensitivity are of unclear etiology.

The impact of foods or food additives on neurological functioning has received varying attention, ranging from case reports to placebo-controlled, double-blind challenges. Signs and symptoms range from those that are purely subjective to those that may be validated by objective findings. Syndromes such as food-induced migraine and epilepsy will be addressed in the present chapter.

Migraine headache

In 1962, the Ad Hoc Committee on the Classification of Headache defined migraine as "recurrent attacks of headache, widely varied in intensity, frequency, and duration." The attacks are commonly unilateral in onset; are usually associated with anorexia and, sometimes, with nausea and vomiting; in some are preceded by, or associated with, conspicuous sensory, motor, and mood disturbances; and are often familial [1]. Migraine may be divided into several clinical syndromes. "Classic migraine" presents with a prodromal "aura," frequently visual in nature, which precedes onset of the headache by 5–30 minutes. The visual disturbance is typically that of "scintillating scotomata," multicolored saw-toothed arcs, which may move across the visual field. "Common migraine" lacks a prodrome before the headache. "Complicated migraine" indicates the asso-

ciation of more significant neurological dysfunction such as hemiplegia; symptoms may persist beyond the duration of the headache but usually resolve.

Migraine headache is a common affliction, occurring in 5–30% of the general population, with a familial predisposition in 60–80% of cases, and affecting females 3-fold more often than males. A survey published in 1992 of 20,468 individuals revealed that 5.7% of males and 17.6% of females suffered one or more migraines per year, with the prevalence highest between 35 and 45 years of age [2]. It was projected in this study that in the US population 8.7 million females and 2.6 million males suffer from migraine with moderate to severe disability. However, another 1992 study from Minnesota estimated that the prevalence of migraine had increased in that region from 25% to 40% [3]. Estimates of pediatric migraine have increased 3-fold over the past 20 years [4].

Precipitating factors of migraine are varied, and include stress, bright lights or loud sounds, physical exertion, fasting, and foods. Menses or oral contraception use may precipitate headaches, but migraine frequently improves during pregnancy. There are no definitive laboratory tests to confirm the diagnosis. Electroencephalogram (EEG) abnormalities have been noted but are minimal and are more common in childhood migraine, with epileptiform discharges noted in 18 of 100 patients [5]. The diagnosis of migraine is based primarily on history. It is necessary to exclude other medical conditions that may mimic migraine: aneurysm, temporal arteritis, carcinoid tumor, pheochromocytoma, brain tumor,

Food Allergy: Adverse Reactions to Foods and Food Additives, 4th edition.
Edited by Dean D. Metcalfe, Hugh A. Sampson, and Ronald A. Simon.
© 2008 Blackwell Publishing. ISBN: 978-1-4501-5129-0.

arteriovenous malformation, glaucoma, mastocytosis, or carotid or vertebrobasilar vascular insufficiency.

Theories of migraine etiology

Despite its description centuries ago, there is still no firm consensus on the etiology of migraine. The frequently pulsatile nature of the headache suggests the vascular theory by which the aura was explained as an initial phase of regional intracerebral vasoconstriction followed by vasodilation with inflammation explaining the headache. This theory was supported by evidence of slowed intracerebral blood flow in patients with classic migraine, but patients with common migraine showed no similar changes. However, a report of spontaneous migraine during a positron-emission tomography study in a patient with common migraine revealed bilateral cerebral hypoperfusion spreading anteriorly from the occipital lobes to the temporal and parietal lobes [6].

The neurogenic theory suggested that the basic defect was in neuronal response to certain neurotransmitters and that vascular changes were secondary to neuronal impulses and the vasoactive properties of such neurotransmitters as substance P [7]. Serotonin metabolism abnormalities have been described in the platelets of patients with migraine, but it is unclear whether these are primary defects or epiphenomena from drug effects [7,8]. It has been difficult to reconcile these theories with the actions of agents that have been found empirically either to provoke or to relieve migraine.

Moskowitz and Macfarlane have emphasized that several levels of pathophysiological triggering and potentiating factors may consolidate neurogenic and vasogenic elements in migraine headache [9]. The hypothesis has been proposed that ionic and metabolic cortical mechanisms release nociceptive substances that stimulate trigeminovascular sensory fibers. These impulses cause pain and release vasoactive neuropeptides such as substance P and neurokinin A, inducing vasodilation and protein extravasation, causing further nociceptive substance release and sensory nerve ending sensitization. Receptors for 5-hydroxytryptamine on sensory nerve endings and vascular smooth muscle are central to this cascade. The large number of dural mast cells has also been implicated in this process [9]. The great variety of therapeutic modalities may be explained by the complexity of initiating and potentiating elements in the migraine reaction.

Diet manipulation in migraine

Diets may play a role in migraine severity by limiting precursor availability for generation of vasoactive mediators or nociceptor transmitters. Carbohydrate-rich, protein–tryptophan-low diets have been attempted to modify migraine headaches [10]. The rationale being that if platelet serotonin is a precipitator of the vasoconstrictory phase of migraine, the restricted dietary intake of serotonin and the serotonin precursor tryptophan may lower levels within platelets, and thereby alleviate migraine headaches. However, it has

also been suggested that increased brain serotonin levels may improve migraine through the anti-nociceptive system. Insulin release induced by carbohydrate-rich meals would increase tryptophan availability to the brain, with subsequent increased serotonin synthesis. Hasselmark and co-workers tried such a diet for 50 days (after a 30-day routine diet) in 10 migraineurs [10]. Three patients dropped out, leaving four with classic and three with common migraine. While three of four with classic migraine had a marked improvement in headache frequency, and none of the common migraineurs noted benefit from the diet, no differences in platelet serotonin uptake were found. The authors felt that the beneficial effect could be due either to a decrease in the ingestion of migraine-precipitating foods or increased brain serotonin levels. Drummond recently observed the effects of acute dietary tryptophan depletion on induction of motion sickness with a rotary drum [11]. He compared 37 controls with 39 migraineurs, who as a group are unusually susceptible to motion sickness. Tryptophan depletion raised dizziness, nausea, and illusion of motion in the controls to levels approaching that of the migraineurs, in whom depletion had little effect. It was postulated that migraineurs have chronically low central serotonin levels, or that serotonergic receptors may be less sensitive to serotonin in migraineurs than controls.

In a double-blind, crossover study, Harel and co-workers examined the benefit of dietary supplementation with fish oil rich in very-long-chain omega-3 polyunsaturated fatty acids in adolescent migraine [12]. The placebo treatment was olive oil, and 2-month treatments were followed by a 1-month washout, followed by 2 months of the other treatment. Headache frequency and severity were both reduced compared to baseline by both fish oil and olive oil ($p < 0.0001$ and $p < 0.01$–0.03, respectively). Reductions were in the range of 65–87% for severity, duration, and frequency for both treatments. The authors suggested both modalities were having an active effect, and the magnitude of the improvement argued against placebo effect.

Association of food allergy and migraine

Allergy to food is self-reported more commonly in migraineurs than those with non-migrainous headache or without headache [13]. Pinnas and Vanselow have pointed out that the association between allergy and migraine is more than a 100 years old [14]. In 1885, Trousseau had included periodic headache in the allergic diathesis; Tileston in 1918 likened migraine to asthma; and the following year, Pagniez considered migraine as a manifestation of anaphylaxis [14]. Several reports then attributed food allergy as the cause of migraine, but methodological issues made these less than compelling. In 1921, Brown linked attacks to such foods as milk, egg, fish, beef, pork, and chocolate [15]. In 1927, Vaughan reported that 10 of 33 migraine patients studied showed specific food triggers [16].

These were identified by skin testing followed by elimination and re-challenge with the incriminated foods. With the exception of a solitary blinded challenge, these were open challenges. Shortly thereafter, Eyermann reported that 69% of headache patients improved on an elimination diet [17]. Forty-four subjects had headaches with suspected foods, beginning within 3–6 hours after ingestion. The diet was directed by skin test results, but of those who did not respond to the diet, 53% had positive tests, suggesting over-interpretation of the skin test responses. Additionally, many of the patients did not have accepted criteria for migraine headache. Balyeat and Rinkel stated that of 202 consecutive migraine patients managed with food skin testing and elimination diets, 120 had 60% or greater improvement, with only 12% of the patients demonstrating little or no improvement [18]. In 1932, DeGowin reported results with 60 migraine patients who had positive prick or intradermal skin tests to foods [19]. Elimination diets in 42 patients brought about complete relief in 33% and partial relief in another 45%; incidence of headache on the reintroduction of foods was not reported.

These early studies suggested that food allergy, as determined by positive immediate skin tests, was a significant cause of migraine headache. However, they are flawed by being open studies and susceptible to expectation bias and placebo effect. Thereafter, mainstream of migraine opinion moved away from the causative role of allergy. Nonetheless, in 1952 Unger and Unger published a paper entitled "Migraine Is an Allergic Disease" [20]. Of interest, the preceding article in that issue was captioned "Is Migraine an Allergic Disease?" [21]. Schwartz detailed his extensive epidemiological work in Denmark, involving 241 asthmatics, 200 non-allergic controls, and their 3815 relatives spanning four generations. He found no difference in the frequency of migraine in relatives of asthmatics and normal controls, commenting that because migraine was so common, it was not unexpected to find it occurring in allergic kindreds.

Unger and Unger investigated 55 patients with skin tests, elimination diets, food diaries, and the "feeding test" to identify migraine-provoking foods [20]. All foods ingested for 24 hours before the onset of migraine were recorded. The patients were challenged with the suspected food after 2 weeks on an elimination diet. If no reaction occurred within 1 hour, a second portion was given, the patients recording all symptoms for the next 24 hours. Using this protocol, 35 of the 55 patients achieved complete relief of migraine symptoms, 9 had 75% or greater relief, and another 2 had 50–65% improvement. In nine patients, no benefit was derived. Food skin testing in this study was not helpful, identifying a provoking food only 5 times. This study was reminiscent of earlier work, in being an open study, but certain findings repeatedly appeared. A substantial number of migraineurs had marked improvement on elimination diets. Recurrence of headache coincided with reintroduction of certain foods, and the onset of the headache could be delayed 3–6 hours after ingestion of the provoking agent. Food skin tests were of varying help in defining diets.

A smattering of open studies over the next 25 years supported the value of elimination diets in migraine but offered little insight into mechanisms. Grant in 1979 reported remarkable results in 60 patients placed on a strict lamb-and-pear elimination diet [22]. Of an initial group of 126 migraineurs, 35 discontinued the diet, and data was reported on only 60. After 5 days of the diet, foods were reintroduced singly, with symptoms and pulse rate monitored up to 1.5 hours. This technique led to improvement in all the patients, and complete resolution in 51 (85%). Foods found to provoke symptoms for each patient ranged from 1 to 30, with a mean of 10. No blinded challenges were performed, and these results no doubt reflect substantial placebo effect. Likewise, the use of the pulse test has no documented validity and could lead to unnecessary elimination of numerous foods. Finally, the 31 patients who continued the diet but were not included in the data analysis presumably had less striking results.

Monro and co-workers reported 47 migraineurs managed with elimination and rotation diets [23]. Twenty-three of 36 patients completing the diet phase were able to identify provoking foods. Subsequently, the radioallergosorbent test (RAST) to a battery of foods found migraine provokers to have higher RAST titers than foods not producing headaches. In a further report, these workers presented nine migraine patients with reproducible food sensitivity documented by elimination diets with open challenges [24]. High-dose oral cromolyn blocked headache in five patients while placebo did not. The benefit of a strict milk-protein-free diet for classic migraine was reported in 1983 [25]. Of 26 patients, 18 improved on the diet, all of which had documented lactase deficiency. One additional deficient patient did not improve on the diet; the remainder was not lactose intolerant. Hughes and colleagues placed 21 migraine patients on a "semi-elemental" diet for a week and 19 had a marked reduction of headache severity during the week of observation [26]. These unblinded studies suggested that a large percentage of migraineurs would benefit from elimination of specific foods, and the more stringent the diet, the more likely success.

Double-blind, placebo-controlled (DBPC) challenges are necessary to clarify issues in an area where cause and effect are being assessed by subjective symptomatology such as headache. There have been only a small number of such studies. However, a preliminary report by Vaughan and colleagues in 1983 linked the value of food skin tests and DBPC food capsule challenges in adult migraine patients [27]. Also that year, Egger and associates studied 99 children who suffered from at least one migraine per week for a minimum of 6 months [28]. They were maintained for 3–4 weeks on

it is difficult to demonstrate appreciable numbers of reactors in controlled settings. Lai and associates performed clinical assessments and EEG on 38 patients with diet-induced migraine [48]. After a control day, the patients were challenged with a combination of red wine, chocolate, and sharp cheddar cheese: 16 developed headache, 4 with scotomata. Abnormalities in the EEG were demonstrated but generally did not separate headache responders from non-responders. All of the patients with headache showed photic driving of the EEG, while only 64% of the non-responders did so ($p < 0.01$); the significance of this finding is uncertain.

A number of people experience headache after the ingestion of hot dogs or cured meats. The incriminated vehicles are nitrites, which are added to meats as coloring agents. High concentrations of nitrites are found in hot dogs, bacon, ham luncheon meats, smoked fish, and some imported cheeses; it is not uncommon to find levels much higher than the FDA recommended levels of 200 ppm. The headache usually begins within minutes or hours after ingestion, is bitemporal or bifrontal, and is pulsatile about 50% of the time [49]. The mechanism is unclear.

Alcohol is commonly identified by migraineurs as a precipitant. Headache usually appears within 30–45 minutes after consumption, similar to the timing to achieve cutaneous vasodilation. Alcohol has little to no effect on cerebral blood flow, however; therefore, intracerebral vasodilation is not the mechanism by which alcohol causes headache. Depression of brain serotonin turnover by high levels of alcohol may play a role, considering the role of serotonin metabolism postulated in migraine [7,8,41]. Red wine is incriminated more often than other forms of alcohol. Littlewood and associates assembled 19 migraineurs who believed that red wine but not other forms of alcohol provoked headache [50]. Chilled red wine and vodka were consumed in a blinded fashion, and the incidence of headache compared. The alcohol content of the two preparations was similar; and the tyramine content of the wine was 2 mg/l and that ingested <1 mg. The wine produced significantly more headaches than the vodka. The authors felt that alcohol and tyramine were not responsible for the migraine headaches, suggesting other ingredients such as phenolic flavanoids (found in higher quantities in red than white wine) as possible triggers.

The "Chinese restaurant syndrome" induced by monosodium glutamate (MSG) is comprised of headache, facial tightness, warmth across the shoulders, and also dizziness, nausea, and abdominal cramps [41]. Approximately 30% of people ingesting Chinese food have symptoms, usually beginning about 20 minutes after ingestion. Thresholds vary from 1.5 to 12 g, but are commonly below 3 g, the amount found in a portion of wonton soup. Symptoms are presumed to be due to central nervous system (CNS) neuroexcitatory effects.

Since its introduction in 1981, the artificial sweetener aspartame has provoked numerous reports of adverse reactions. A large number included headache or were of a neurological or behavioral nature [51]. In 1987, a DBPC crossover study in 40 subjects reporting aspartame-induced headaches showed no differences in headache induction between the sweetener and placebo [52]. The following year, however, another study demonstrated differing results [53]. Twenty-five subjects began a 13-week study, however, only 11 completed the protocol. A 4-week baseline period was followed by randomized sequential 4-week periods with either aspartame 300 mg q.i.d. or placebo, with the crossover periods separated by a week washout. Headaches occurred twice as frequently on aspartame as on placebo or during the baseline period ($p < 0.02$). The differences were accounted for by a marked increase of headaches in 4 of the 11 subjects. Ironically, two patients have been reported with headache triggered by aspartame contained in their migraine medication [54]. Another commonly used sweetener, sucralose, has recently been reported to induce migraine [55].

Mediators and immunological mechanisms in migraine

Immunological studies have been generally unrewarding in migraine. Medina and Diamond reported no differences in total IgE between migraineurs and the normal population [40]. Merrett and colleagues examined IgE levels in 74 adults with dietary migraine, 45 with non-dietary migraine, 29 with cluster headache, and 60 normal controls [56]. They found no differences in specific and total IgE in the groups with the exception of a higher total IgE in the cluster headache patients, which they attributed to a higher percentage of smokers. Specific IgE for cheese, milk, and chocolate showed no difference between dietary and non-dietary migraine. Pradalier and co-workers performed duodenal biopsies for immunocyte enumeration in patients with common migraine [57]. Twenty consecutive migraineurs, 11 with food-induced migraine, and 9 without, had mid-duodenal biopsies examined for lamina propria IgE, IgG, IgA, or IgM containing plasmocytes. There were no differences between the two groups for histological appearance, total plasmocytes, or subsets. Ratner and associates have linked dietary migraine with lactase deficiency, and represented data on elevated IgM in 11 such migraine patients [58]. Martelletti and co-workers, using a C1q-binding assay, showed an increased incidence of circulating immune complexes in 21 patients with food-induced migraine (29% versus 10% in the control group) [59,60]. Activated T-cells showed an increase at 4 hours after challenge followed by a decrease at 72 hours. The authors speculated on the role of IL-2 receptors in food-induced migraine.

Three studies have examined mediator release in dietary migraine. Three patients in the Mansfield adult migraine study returned for repeat challenges and histamine plasma levels [30]. Headache was provoked only with the active challenge and was associated with increases in the histamine levels coinciding with or preceding the onset of the headache. Placebo challenge on two revealed no or little change in histamine. Steinberg and colleagues reported an extensively evaluated single case of beef-induced migraine in a young woman [61]. A 3-fold increase in histamine was noted as well as an increase of a PGF2α metabolite coinciding with the onset of the migraine after the ingestion of the beef. Increased intracerebral blood flow was demonstrated with Xenon computerized tomography and Doppler ultrasonography. Prick skin test and RAST to beef were negative.

Olson and colleagues reported serial histamine and Prostaglandin D_2 (PGD) levels during DBPC challenges in five patients with food-induced migraine [62]. Placebo challenges produced no changes; with active challenge, all five had a 3- to 38-fold increase in plasma histamine as well as increases in PGD_2 before or coinciding with the onset of symptoms. A second increase in the PGD_2 was noted 4–6 hours after ingestion. Histamine did not demonstrate this late increase. This discordance suggests the late recruitment of non-basophil inflammatory cells. Skin tests in this group were all negative.

Summary

There is a wealth of clinical data that supports the contention that dietary migraine is a bona fide entity, with both pharmacological and immunological mechanisms involved in subsets of migraineurs (Table 42.2). Certainly, these are not mutually exclusive conditions, and both may be operant in the same patient. What the exact pathophysiology of these reactions remains unclear, although reproducible release of immediate hypersensitivity mediators has been convincingly demonstrated. The variable results of immediate skin testing suggest that although some reactions may be IgE mediated, many are probably pseudoallergic, akin to radiocontrast media reactions. Why release of these mediators causes migraine in susceptible persons and not more traditional allergic manifestations is unclear.

What the exact frequency of dietary migraine is in migraineurs is not settled. Studies suggest that 15% may have reproducible triggers under controlled situations, but that twice that number may benefit from dietary restriction.

Table 42.2 Incriminated agents in dietary migraine

Presumed pharmacological action

Tyramine
Phenylethylamine
Phenolic flavanoids
Ethanol
Nitrites
Caffeine
Monosodium glutamate
Aspartame/sucralose

Immunological or uncertain action

Food proteins

While the majority of headache patients believe that there are connections between food intake and their headaches, fewer than half have this relationship addressed by their physicians, and fewer modify their dietary practices [63]. The evaluation of such patients seems indicated, and should begin with the appropriate history and physical examination and the exclusion of migraine-mimicking conditions. Once bona fide migraine has been established, and pharmacological control achieved, it is not unreasonable to pursue possible dietary triggers. Global dietary restrictions as suggested by some authors are most likely not indicated. Although history may identify a number of triggers, some patients with reproducible headaches on DBPC challenges could not separate the causative agents during a normal diet.

Food skin testing is likely to present both false positives and false negatives, and should not be relied on alone, and RAST is of little value. This leaves the prospect of food diaries and elimination diets. For patients with infrequent migraines, a diary listing foods ingested in the previous 48 hours to a headache may be useful. A diet eliminating wheat, corn, milk, and egg may be helpful for a period of 2–4 weeks. Patients benefiting from such a diet should reintroduce foods singly and for 3 consecutive days. Foods not provoking symptoms should be returned freely to the diet. Suspect foods should be eliminated and re-challenged. In patients with numerous suspected positives, it is wise to perform challenges under blinded conditions to remove expectation or anxiety as confounding factors, and to avoid unnecessary restriction of the diet. Consulting with a nutritionist is warranted for the rare patient who has multiple documented dietary triggers.

Epilepsy

Earlier in the last century, epilepsy was compared to the similarly episodic syndromes of anaphylaxis and the atopic disorders. Schwartz, in his monumental epidemiological study of asthma and atopy in 4256 probands and relatives in Denmark, also collected data on migraine (as mentioned above) and epilepsy [64]. He found very few cases of epilepsy in the kindreds, and no evidence for any genetic correlation between epilepsy and the atopic disorders. Nonetheless, there have been a number of reports linking allergy (frequently food induced) and epilepsy. In 1927, Ward and Patterson food skin tested 1000 epileptics and 100 controls, finding patient reactivity between 37% and 67%, and only 8% reactivity in the controls [65].

In 1951, Dees and Lowenbach reported on 37 children with epilepsy who were treated with anti-allergic therapy, environmental avoidance measures, and elimination diets as well as anti-convulsant therapy [66]. Of these, 22 met criteria for "allergic epilepsy:" personal and family history of allergy, blood eosinophilia, positive skin tests, and no organic disease of the CNS. The remainder had possible allergic disease, but did not meet all criteria, half had eosinophilia. Twenty of the "allergic" group and 13 of the "non-allergic" group had positive food skin tests. The predominant EEG finding was occipital arrhythmia (73% of both groups), a rhythm that the authors had found to be present in some allergic children without an overt seizure disorder. Thirteen in the allergic group were treated with allergen immunotherapy as well as the dietary and medical manipulations. Convulsions were controlled in 18/22 allergic children and 6/15 "non-allergic" children; anticonvulsant therapy could be stopped in 13 of the former and 1 of the latter group. The authors felt that in certain cases epilepsy could be on an allergic basis, and therefore could conceivably be controlled with appropriate anti-allergic therapy. They did not, however, provide any indication of how many epileptic children were surveyed to arrive at their study group; so while this is an interesting observation it is difficult to place it in proper perspective.

Egger and colleagues in their assessment of food factors in migraine had several patients who had epilepsy and or behavioral problems which also appears to respond to the oligoantigenic diet [28]. In a further communication, they investigated children who either had epilepsy alone, or in association with migraine, all of whom had difficult to control symptoms [67]. None of 18 with epilepsy alone improved on the oligoantigenic diet, while 40 of 45 with both epilepsy and migraine reported improvement of one or more symptoms. In follow-up ranging from 7 months to 3 years, 25 patients had complete control of their epilepsy. Thirty-two patients had seizure during reintroduction of incriminated foods. In double-blind challenges of 16 children, 7 reacted to the suspected food only, none to placebo only, and one to both. Pelliccia and colleagues have reported a total of four cases of cow's intolerance where partial idiopathic epilepsy was improved, both clinically and with electroencephalographic findings, with cow's milk-free diets, with recurrence and reintroduction [68,69].

There is a variant of reflex epilepsy where it is not the food ingested which is the precipitant of the seizure, but rather the act of eating itself. This entity is called "eating epilepsy," and while quite rare, appears to be more common in kindreds in Sri Lanka and the Indian subcontinent [70–72]. The seizure type is usually complex partial, does not occur with all meals, and usually happens at home. Many episodes are linked to the ingestion of rice, but since this is a staple of the diet, it is likely that this is not truly specific [70]. It has been postulated that stimulation of areas of the brain which receive sensory input during eating may lower the seizure threshold [73]. A recent report of two patients localized the seizure focus to the suprasylvanian and temporolimbic regions, respectively [74].

Diet manipulation in epilepsy

Some time ago it was observed that many epilepsy patients were free of seizures while fasting, the benefit persisting after return to a normal diet. It was suggested that this effect was due to ketonemia, and a "ketogenic" high fat, low carbohydrate diet was proposed for treatment. The diet was rigid, unpalatable, and difficult to maintain, requiring strict nutritional supervision [75,76]. It appeared useful, especially in younger age children whose seizures were not responsive to anti-epileptic medications. Kinsman and associates showed benefit from the diet in 58 epileptic children requiring multiple medications [76]. Seizure control improved in 67%, with reduced medication in 64%, greater alertness in 36%, and improved behavior in 23%. Seventy-five percent of these improved patients were able to maintain the diet at least 18 months. A medium chain triglyceride diet was found to be more ketogenic than the fat in the traditional diet, and felt to be more palatable; Sills and colleagues reported on their success with such a diet in 50 epileptic children [75]. Eight achieved complete control of seizures (4 without medication), 4 had seizures reduced by 90%, and 10 by 50–90%. Extra dosing of the medium chain triglycerides at bedtime was useful for control of nocturnal seizures. The diet appears to work in a variety of epileptic syndromes, and response is not predicted by age, syndrome, or etiology [77,78]. Variations on the diet have been attempted to make in easier and more palatable, and appear to be successful, as is the Atkins diet [79–81]. Gradual introduction of the ketogenic diet appears to be both better tolerated and effective [82]. The mechanisms remain unclear. Possibilities include alterations in acid–base balance, water and electrolyte distribution, or lipid concentrations, or direct action of ketone bodies [76,83]. Experimental models have shown increased plasma levels of polyunsaturates like linoleate and α-linoleate decrease seizure susceptibility either directly or through promoting ketosis [84].

Epilepsy and migraine

The link between migraine and epilepsy is apparent, but the nature of the relationship unclear. An editorial by Wilson addressed several overlapping issues [85]. If attacks and auras are brief, especially if the attacks are stereotyped, a diagnosis of epilepsy is preferred; if attacks with prodrome are longer, and if the impact on consciousness is primarily confusion, migraine may be more likely. Therapeutic trials of migraine prophylaxis and anti-epileptic drugs may help clarify the diagnosis. Several migraine–epilepsy syndromes have been identified: seizures with typical migraine prodrome; migraine with later development of epilepsy; alternating hemiplegic migraine. In the first case, impairment of cerebral blood flow associated with migraine may precipitate the seizure. In the next, repeated ischemic insult may lead to an epileptogenic focus. Despite such cases, the relationship between epilepsy and migraine remains obscure. Can one condition trigger the other, in a dually susceptible individual, or is epilepsy an epiphenomenon in a vascular disease? [85]. Both mechanisms may occur in different patients.

Summary

While the role of food is important in provoking attacks of migraine, less is known concerning dietary factors in epilepsy. The efficacy of ketogenic diets is well established, but the manner in which they operate remains uncertain. That bona fide anaphylactoid reactions could trigger convulsions in susceptible patients appears likely, but DBPC studies are absent, and would be helpful in validating the clinical observations to date. And certainly, studies investigating mediator release are needed.

Vertigo

In 1976, Dunn and Snyder reported their experience with 33 pediatric cases of benign paroxysmal vertigo, a syndrome of sporadic brief episodes of disequilibrium, nystagmus, and/or vomiting [86]. During infancy, this often manifested by paroxysmal torticollis. While food allergy was considered in all cases, in only four cases was it deemed likely. Three children had histories suggestive of milk allergy, and attacks were eliminated by removing milk from the diet, with vertigo reappearing with milk challenges. In another child chocolate was suspected, but could not be confirmed on challenge. The authors do not state whether these were open or blinded challenges. Therefore, at best, a 10th of the cases had evidence for a food etiology.

A food cause for adult vertigo or Meniere's syndrome has been postulated. In 1923, Duke had reported five cases of Meniere's improved on elimination diets [87]. There continue to be no well-performed double-blind studies. Older reports are limited to the non-reproducible technique of provocation–neutralization. A 2000 survey by Derebery, of 137 Meniere's patients who returned a questionnaire, revealed that 113 of these underwent allergen immunotherapy and/or elimination diet [88]. An analysis of pre- and post-treatment symptoms revealed improvement in both frequency and severity of vertigo, tinnitus, and unsteadiness ($p < 0.005$–0.001). Unfortunately, the mode of diagnosis of food allergy was by both skin testing and provocation–neutralization, and those that received diet manipulations were not segregated from those that received immunotherapy. Also, a quarter of the patients acknowledged not following the diet, 30% "sometimes," and about 45% followed the diet "almost always." So this survey, at best, suggests that there may be an association between diet and vertigo. Whether a food role can be substantiated in this area will require appropriately controlled studies.

Hemiplegia

Several case reports exist of transient neurological deficits following presumed allergic reaction to foods. Cooke reported transient third cranial nerve palsy associated with hemiparesis, followed by an episode of contralateral blindness and paresthesia in a food-allergic patient [89]. Symptoms resolved with avoidance of beef and pork, challenges were not performed. In 1951, Staffieri and colleagues reported a case of right-sided hemiplegia immediately following after a meal, and associated with angioedema, urticaria, purpura, and peripheral eosinophilia ranging from 34% to 40% [90]. A wheat elimination diet was attended by resolution of the symptoms within a few days. To rule out coincidence, a total of four wheat challenges (apparently single blinded) were performed over the ensuing 4 months, resulting initially in headache, with purpura and angioedema, and ultimately in the skin manifestations alone. Passive transfer of skin sensitizing antibodies was not successful. Such reports are fascinating, but probably reflect that anaphylactic reactions may be attended by edema almost anywhere, to include the central and peripheral nervous systems. Reinforcing this concept is a report of 55 cases of anaphylaxis in 50 children by Dibs and Baker, where neurological symptoms were manifest in 26% [91]. Symptoms included aura, irritability, lethargy, disorientation, dizziness, tremor, syncope, and seizure.

Gluten sensitivity and neurological abnormalities

As well reviewed by Wills and Unsworth, several neurological complications have been described with gluten sensitivity, including cerebellar ataxia, myoclonus, epilepsy, neuropathy, and dementia [92]. The majority of these are case reports. Interestingly, there is a dichotomy between finding such impairments in celiac disease patients, but not in patients with dermatitis herpetiformis. Two series have failed to find any increase in neurological problems in the latter manifestation of gluten sensitivity [93,94]. While previous reports have not shown a benefit of gluten dietary elimination in neurological symptoms, Cicarelli and colleagues did so in a series of 176 gluten-sensitive patients and 52 age-matched controls [95]. Increased occurrence of headache, dysthymia, cramps, and weakness in the patients compared to the controls were reduced in those patients adhering to a strict gluten-free diet. There was no impact on occurrence of paresthesia or hyporeflexia, however. A constellation of celiac disease, epilepsy, and occipital lobe calcifications has been described in Italians [96]. The neurological complications associated with gluten sensitivity remain of uncertain etiology, with direct neurotoxic effects, autoimmune injury, or resultant metabolic deficiency from malabsorption all possible mechanisms.

References

1 Ad Hoc Committee on the Classification of Headache. Classification of headache. *Arch Neurol* 1962;6:173–6.

2 Stewart WF, Lipton RB, Celentano DD, Reed ML. Prevalence of migraine headache in the United States: relation to age, income, race, and other sociodemographic factors. *JAMA* 1992;267:64–9.

3 Stang PE, Yanagihar PA, Swanson JW, *et al.* Incidence of migraine headache: a population-based study in Olmstead County, Minnesota. *Neurology* 1992;42:1657–62.

4 Millichap JG, Yee MM. The diet factor in pediatric and adolescent migraine. *Pediatr Neurol* 2003;28:9–15.

5 Millichap JG. Recurrent headaches in 100 children. Electroencephalographic abnormalities and response to phenytoin (Dilantin). *Childs Brain* 1978;4:95–105.

6 Woods RP, Iacoboni M, Mazziotta JC. Brief report: bilateral spreading cerebral hypoperfusion during spontaneous migraine headache. *N Engl J Med* 1994;331:1689–92.

7 Zeigler DK, Murrow RW. Headache. In: Joynt RJ (ed.). *Clinical Neurology*, Vol. 2, revised edn. Philadelphia, PA: JB Lippincott Co, 1988:1–49.

8 D'Andrea G, Welch KMA, Grunfeld S, *et al.* Reduced platelet turnover of serotonin in diet restricted migraine patients. *Cephalalgia* 1987;7:141s–3s.

9 Moskowitz MA, Macfarlane R. Neurovascular and molecular mechanisms in migraine headaches. *Cerebrovasc Brain Metab Rev* 1993;5:159–77.

10 Hasselmark L, Malmgren R, Hannerz J. Effect of a carbohydrate-rich diet, low in protein–tryptophan, in classic and common migraine. *Cephalalgia* 1987;7:87–92.

11 Drummond PD. Effect of tryptophan depletion on symptoms of motion sickness in migraineurs. *Neurology* 2005;65:620–2.

12 Harel Z, Gascon G, Riggs S, *et al.* Supplementation with omega-3 polyunsaturated fatty acids in the management of recurrent migraines in adolescents. *J Adolesc Health* 2002;31:154–61.

13 Schéle R, Ahlborg B, Ekbom K. Physical characteristics and allergic history in young men with migraine and other headaches. *Headache* 1978;18:80–6.

14 Pinnas JL, Vanselow NA. Relationship of allergy to headache. *Res Clin Stud Headache* 1976;4:85–95.

15 Brown TR. Role of diet in etiology and treatment of migraine and other types of headache. *JAMA* 1921;77:1396–400.

16 Vaughan WT. Allergic migraine. *JAMA* 1927;88:1383–6.

17 Eyermann CH. Allergic headache. *J Allergy* 1930;2:106–12.

18 Balyeat RM, Rinkel HJ. Further studies in allergic migraine: based on a series of two hundred and two consecutive cases. *Ann Intern Med* 1931;5:713–28.

19 DeGowin EL. Allergic migraine: a review of sixty cases. *J Allergy* 1932;3:557–66.

20 Unger AH, Unger L. Migraine is an allergic disease. *J Allergy* 1952;23:429–40.

21 Schwartz M. Is migraine an allergic disease? *J Allergy* 1952;23:426–8.

22 Grant EC. Food allergies and migraine. *Lancet* 1979;1:966–9.

23 Monro J, Carini C, Brostoff J. Food allergy in migraine: study of dietary exclusion and RAST. *Lancet* 1980;2:1–4.

24 Monro J, Carini C, Brostoff J. Migraine is a food allergic disease. *Lancet* 1984;2:719–21.

25 Ratner D, Shoshani E, Dubnov B. Milk protein-free diet for nonseasonal asthma and migraine in lactase-deficient patients. *Isr J Med Sci* 1983;19:806–9.

26 Hughes EC, Gott PS, Weinstein RC, Binggeli R. Migraine: a diagnostic test for etiology of food sensitivity by a nutritionally supported fast and confirmed by long term report. *Ann Allergy* 1985;55:28–32.

27 Vaughan TR, Mansfield LE, Haverly RW, *et al.* The value of cutaneous testing for food allergy in the diagnostic evaluation of migraine headache (abstract). *Ann Allergy* 1983;50:362.

28 Egger J, Wilson J, Carter CM, Turner MW. Is migraine food allergy? A double-blind controlled trial of oligoantigenic diet treatment. *Lancet* 1983;2:865–8.

29 Atkins FM, Ball BD, Bock A. The relationship between the ingestion of specific foods and the development of migraine headaches in children (abstract). *J Allergy Clin Immunol* 1988;81:185.

30 Mansfield LE, Vaughan TR, Waller SF, *et al.* Food allergy and adult migraine: double blind and mediator confirmation of an allergic etiology. *Ann Allergy* 1985;55:126–9.

31 Vaughan TR, Stafford WW, Miller BT, *et al.* Food and migraine headache (MIG): a controlled study (abstract). *Ann Allergy* 1986;56:522.

32 Weber RW, Vaughan TR. Food and migraine headache. *Immunol Allergy Clin North Am* 1991;11:831–41.

33 Vaughan TR. The role of food in the pathogenesis of migraine headache. *Clin Rev Allergy* 1994;12:167–80.

34 Curtis-Brown R. Protein poison theory: its application to treatment of headache and especially migraine. *BMJ* 1925;1:155–7.

35 Hanington E. Preliminary report on tyramine headache. *BMJ* 1967;2:550–1.

36 Smith I, Kellow AH, Hanington E. A clinical and biochemical correlation between tyramine and migraine headache. *Headache* 1970;10:43–51.

37 Moffett A, Swash M, Scott DF. Effect of tyramine in migraine: a double-blind study. *J Neurol Neurosurg Psychiatry* 1972;35:496–9.

38 Forsythe WI, Redmond A. Two controlled trials of tyramine in children with migraine. *Dev Med Child Neurol* 1974;16:794–9.

39 Zeigler DK, Stewart R. Failure of tyramine to induce migraine. *Neurol* 1977;27:725–6.

40 Medina JL, Diamond S. The role of diet in migraine. *Headache* 1978;18:31–4.

41 Raskin NH. Chemical headaches. *Ann Rev Med* 1981;32:63–71.

42 Peatfield RC, Hampton KK, Grant PJ. Plasma vasopressin levels in induced migraine attacks. *Cephalalgia* 1988;8:55–7.

43 Sandler M, Youdim MBH, Hanington E. A phenylethylamine oxidising defect in migraine. *Nature* 1974;250:335–7.

44 Schweitzer JW, Friedhoff AJ, Schwartz R. Chocolate, beta-phenylethylamine and migraine re-examined. *Nature* 1975;257:256.

45 Moffett AM, Swash M, Scott DF. Effect of chocolate in migraine: a double-blind study. *J. Neurol Neurosurg Psychiatry* 1974;37:445–448.

46 Wantke F, Götz M, Jarisch R. Histamine-free diet: treatment of choice for histamine-induced food intolerance and supporting treatment for chronical headaches. *Clin Exp Allergy* 1993;23:982–5.

47 Salfield SAW, Wardley BL, Houlsby WT, *et al.* Controlled study of exclusion of dietary vasoactive amines in migraine. *Arch Dis Child* 1987;62:458–60.

48 Lai C-W, Dean P, Ziegler DK, Hassanein RS. Clinical and electrophysiological responses to dietary challenge in migraineurs. *Headache* 1989;29:180–6.

49 Henderson WR, Raskin NH. "Hot-dog" headache: individual susceptibility to nitrite. *Lancet* 1972;2:1162–3.

50 Littlewood JT, Glover V, Davies PTG, *et al.* Red wine as a cause of migraine. *Lancet* 1988;1:558–9.

51 Centers for Disease Control (CDC). Evaluation of consumer complaints related to aspartame use. *MMWR* 1984;33:605–7.

52 Schiffman SS, Buckley III CE, Sampson HA, *et al.* Aspartame and susceptibility to headache. *N Engl J Med* 1987;317:1181–5.

53 Koehler SM, Glaros A. The effect of aspartame on migraine headache. *Headache* 1988;28:10–14.

54 Newman LC, Lipton RB. Migraine MLT-down: an unusual presentation of migraine in patients with aspartame-triggered headaches. *Headache* 2001;41:899–901.

55 Bigal ME, Krycmchantowski AV. Migraine triggered by sucralose – a case report. *Headache* 2006;46:515–17.

56 Merrett J, Peatfield RC, Rose FC, Merrett TG. Food related antibodies in headache patients. *J Neurol Neurosurg Psychiatry* 1983;46:738–42.

57 Pradalier A, De Saint Maur P, Lamy F, Launay JM. Immunocyte enumeration in duodenal biopsies of migraine without aura patients with or without food-induced migraine. *Cephalalgia* 1994;14:365–7.

58 Ratner D, Eshel E, Shneyour A, Teitler A. Elevated IgM in dietary migraine with lactase deficiency. *Isr J Med Sci* 1984;20:717–19.

59 Martelletti P, Sutherland J, Anastasi E, *et al.* Evidence for an immune-mediated mechanism in food-induced migraine from a study on activated T-cells, IgG_4 subclass, anti-IgG antibodies and circulating immune complexes. *Headache* 1989;29:664–70.

60 Martelletti P. T cells expressing IL-2 receptor in migraine. *Acta Neurol* 1991;13:448–56.

61 Steinberg M, Page R, Wolfson S, *et al.* Food induced late phase headache (abstract). *J Allergy Clin Immunol* 1988;81:185.

62 Olson GC, Vaughan TR, Ledoux R, *et al.* Food induced migraine: search for immunologic mechanisms (abstract). *J Allergy Clin Immunol* 1989;83:238.

63 Guarnieri P, Radnitz C, Blanchard EB. Assessment of dietary risk factors in chronic headache. *Biofeedback Self-Regul* 1990;15:15–25.

64 Schwartz M. Heredity in bronchial asthma: a clinical and genetic study of 191 asthma probands and 50 probands with baker's asthma. *Acta Allergol* 1952;5:14s–268s.

65 Ward RF, Patterson HA. Protein sensitization in epilepsy: a study of one thousand cases and one hundred normal controls. *Arch Neurol Psychiatry* 1927;17:427–43.

66 Dees SC, Lowenbach H. Allergic epilepsy. *Ann Allergy* 1951;9:446–58.

67 Egger J, Cater CM, Soothill JF, Wilson J. Oligoantigenic diet treatment of children with epilepsy and migraine. *J Pediatr* 1989;114:51–8.

68 Pelliccia A, Lucarelli S, Frediani T, *et al.* Partial cryptogenic epilepsy and food allergy/intolerance. A causal or a chance relationship? Reflections on three clinical cases. *Minerva Pediatr* 1999;51:153–7.

69 Frediani T, Pelliccia A, Aprile A, *et al.* Partial idiopathic epilepsy: recovery after allergen-free diet. *Pediatr Med Chir* 2004;26:196–7.

70 Ahuja GK, Pauranik A, Behari M, Prasad K. Eating epilepsy. *J Neurol* 1988;235:444–7.

71 Senanayake N. Familial eating epilepsy. *J Neurol* 1990;237:388–91.

72 Senanayake N. "Eating epilepsy" – a reappraisal. *Epilepsy Res* 1990;5:74–9.

73 Fiol ME, Leppik IE, Pretzel K. Eating epilepsy: EEG and clinical study. *Epilepsia* 1986;27:441–6.

74 Labate A, Colosimo E, Gambardella A, *et al.* Reflex periodic spasms induced by eating. *Brain Dev* 2006;28:170–4.

75 Sills MA, Forsythe WI, Haidukewych D, *et al.* The medium chain triglyceride diet and intractable epilepsy. *Arch Dis Child* 1986;61:1168–72.

76 Kinsman SL, Vining EPG, Quaskey SA, *et al.* Efficacy of the ketogenic diet for intractable seizure disorders: review of 58 cases. *Epilepsia* 1992;33:1132–6.

77 Mackay MT, Bicknell-Royle J, Nation J, *et al.* The ketogenic diet in refractory childhood epilepsy. *J Paediatr Child Health* 2005;41:353–7.

78 Caraballo RH, Cerosimo RO, Sakr D, *et al.* Ketogenic diet in patients with myoclonic-astatic epilepsy. *Epileptic Disord* 2006;8:151–5.

79 Kossoff EH, Krauss GL, McGrogan JR, Freeman JM. Efficacy of the Atkins diet as therapy for intractable epilepsy. *Neurology* 2003;61:1789–91.

80 Kossoff EH. More fat and fewer seizures: dietary therapies for epilepsy. *Lancet Neurol* 2004;3:415–20.

81 Pfieffer HH, Thiele EA. Low-glycemic-index treatment: a liberalized ketogenic diet for treatment of intractable epilepsy. *Neurology* 2005;65:1810–12.

82 Bergqvist AV, Schall JI, Gallagher PR, *et al.* Fasting versus gradual initiation of the ketogenic diet: a prospective, randomized clinical trial of efficacy. *Epilepsia* 2005;46:1810–19.

83 Papandreou D, Pavlou E, Kalimeri E, Mavromichalis I. The ketogenic diet in children with epilepsy. *Br J Nutr* 2006; 95:5–13.

84 Cunnane SC, Musa K, Ryan MA, *et al.* Potential role of polyunsaturates in seizure protection achieved with the ketogenic diet. *Prostaglandins Leukot Essent Fatty Acids* 2002;67:131–5.

85 Wilson J. Migraine and epilepsy. *Dev Med Child Neurol* 1992;34:645–7.

86 Dunn DW, Snyder CH. Benign paroxysmal vertigo of childhood. *Am J Dis Child* 1976;130:1099–100.

87 Duke WW. Meniere's syndrome caused by allergy. *JAMA* 1923;81:2179–81.

88 Derebery MJ. Allergic management of Meniere's disease: an outcome study. *Otolaryngol Head Neck Surg* 2000;122:174–82.

89 Cooke RA. Allergic neuropathies. In: Cooke RA (ed.) *Allergy in Theory and Practice*. Philadelphia, PA: WB Saunders Co, 1947:325–36.

90 Staffieri D, Bentolila L, Levit L. Hemiplegia and allergic symptoms following ingestion of certain foods. *Ann Allergy* 1951;10:38–9.

91 Dibs SD, Baker MD. Anaphylaxis in children: a 5-year experience. *Pediatrics* 1997;99:E7.

92 Wills AJ, Unsworth DJ. The neurology of gluten sensitivity: separating the wheat from the chaff. *Curr Opin Neurol* 2002;15:519–23.

93 Reunala T, Collin P. Diseases associated with dermatitis herpetiformis. *Br J Dermatol* 1997;136:315–18.

94 Wills AJ, Turner B, Lock RJ, *et al*. Dermatitis herpetiformis and neurological dysfunction. *J Neurol Neurosurg Psychiatry* 2002;72:259–61.

95 Cicarelli G, Della Rocca G, Amboni M, *et al*. Clinical and neurological abnormalities in adult celiac disease. *Neurol Sci* 2003;24:311–17.

96 Gobbi G, Bouquet F, Greco L, *et al*. Coeliac disease, epilepsy, and cerebral calcification. *Lancet* 1992;340:439–43.

CHAPTER 43

Experimental Approaches to the Study of Food Allergy

M. Cecilia Berin

KEY CONCEPTS

- Animal models of IgE-mediated anaphylaxis in response to oral challenge with common food allergens have been developed in rodents, pigs, and dogs.

- Experimental approaches have been used to show that perturbation of intestinal barrier function, digestive capacity, or the composition of the gut flora can influence the development of allergic sensitization.

- Cutaneous exposure to peanut can lead to allergic sensitization in the absence of exogenous adjuvants.

- Several therapeutic approaches have been developed that use microbial products in combination with immunotherapy to induce safe desensitization to food allergens.

Current experimental animal models of food allergy

Most experimental animal models of food allergy have focused on IgE-mediated, immediate hypersensitivity reactions and anaphylaxis. In recent years, models have also been developed to address the pathophysiology of eosinophilic disorders of the gastrointestinal tract. Other food-allergic disorders such as food protein-induced enterocolitis and proctocolitis have not yet been modeled. As we gain more understanding of these disorders from the *in vitro* study of patient samples, we may in future be able to establish appropriate new animal models for the study of additional non-IgE-mediated food-allergic disorders.

Models of IgE-mediated food allergy

The majority of experimental models of food allergy use rats or mice, where the major advantages are cost, availability of immunological reagents, and availability of genetic targeting strategies that allow for mechanistic studies of the pathophysiology of food allergy. Experimental animal models of IgE-mediated food allergy generally fall into two broad categories: oral sensitization or systemic sensitization to food allergens. Typically the systemic sensitization models have been used to study the gastrointestinal response to allergen re-challenge, while in contrast the oral sensitization

models are used to address mechanisms of sensitization or testing of protein allergenicity. (See Table 43.1 for an overview of IgE-mediated models of food allergy).

Oral sensitization models

One approach to model human food allergy has been to find strains of rodents that are susceptible to the development of allergy to oral administration of food allergens in the absence of adjuvant. The Brown–Norway (BN) rat is a high IgE-responder strain that has been shown to develop IgG and IgE antibodies in response to prolonged daily oral exposure to ovalbumin (OVA) [1]. When orally challenged with OVA, the BN rat develops an increase in intestinal permeability, suggestive of a local anaphylaxis response in the gastrointestinal tract. This was not accompanied by a drop in blood pressure or respiratory rate, however, suggesting a lack of systemic anaphylaxis [2]. The B10A strain of mouse was also shown to respond to prolonged oral OVA exposure with the development of OVA-specific IgE and IgG and release of histamine after systemic OVA challenge [3].

Recently Hogan and colleagues have developed an adjuvant-free model of allergic food sensitization by transgenic expression of the bean α-amylase inhibitor (αAI) in peas [4]. Mice orally administered αAI-pea homogenate develop αAI-specific IgE, and develop early- and late-phase hypersensitivity responses in skin when the allergen is cutaneously administered [5]. Allergic inflammation in lung in response to intratracheal administration was also reported with this model [4]. Transgenic expression of αAI was necessary

Food Allergy: Adverse Reactions to Foods and Food Additives, 4th edition.
Edited by Dean D. Metcalfe, Hugh A. Sampson, and Ronald A. Simon.
© 2008 Blackwell Publishing. ISBN: 978-1-4501-5129-0.

for allergenicity, and was associated with expression of a slightly modified form of αAI that had enhanced immuno-genicity. This finding highlights the usefulness of adjuvant-free systems for careful assessment of protein allergenicity, particularly in light of recent findings that many allergens appear to have intrinsic adjuvant-like activity [6–8].

Other models of oral sensitization have incorporated adjuvants such as cholera toxin (CT) to induce sensitization to orally delivered antigens. Snider et al. [9] showed that mice orally administered two feeds of hen's egg lysozyme (HEL) or OVA together with CT-generated antigen-specific IgE antibodies, and were primed for systemic anaphylaxis in response to systemic antigen challenge. In addition, immunization of mice with CT and HEL primed for HEL-specific secretory responses in the mouse intestine, as measured by Ussing chamber analysis of short-circuit current (Isc). Li et al. modified this model to establish models of oral sensitization to peanut [10] and whole milk [11] in C3H/HeJ mice with an outcome of systemic anaphylaxis to oral challenge. Variations of these models in C3H strains and Balb/c mice have been used to begin to address the immune mechanisms of allergic sensitization to common food allergens [12–16].

Systemic sensitization models

Models of systemic sensitization of rodents (most commonly OVA/alum sensitization of rats and mice) were developed to examine local responses to allergen challenge in the gastrointestinal tract [17–21]. Rats and mice systemically sensitized to OVA generate a local intestinal secretory response driven by active chloride secretion. One approach to study this secretory response is preparation of perfused intestinal loops of anesthetized rats where changes in water and ion content are measured in the perfusate [22]. Radioactive tracers have been used to address epithelial and vascular permeability in response to luminal allergen challenge [17,20,23]. Alternatively, Ussing chambers have been used to study active ion secretion in response to luminal or serosal allergen challenge [24–26], and also to measure gastrointestinal permeability changes in response to allergen challenge [25,27,28]. Systemically sensitized rats have also been used to study motility changes in response to allergen challenge [21]. These studies have shown that luminal allergen challenge results in an immediate hypersensitivity reaction in the gastrointestinal tract, characterized by mast cell degranulation, active ion secretion (and therefore water secretion), increased permeability to macromolecules, and disrupted intestinal motility. The pathophysiology of local hypersensitivity reactions in the gastrointestinal tract will be covered in greater detail later in the chapter.

Recent studies have extended the systemic sensitization model by administering multiple feeds of OVA to induce an in vivo allergic diarrhea response. Mice systemically sensitized to OVA with alum and then fed with multiple high-dose feeds of OVA (every second day) have severe acute

diarrhea in response to OVA challenge beginning after three feeds of OVA [29,30]. Studies by Brandt et al. demonstrated that the model is dependent on both mast cells and IgE [29]. Other investigators have used Freund's adjuvant to systemically sensitize mice to OVA, and repetitive feeding of OVA (×10) also induces a diarrheal response [31]. In contrast to the model using alum adjuvant, this model is localized to the large intestine, and is mediated by Th2 CD4+ T-cells that home to the large intestine and induce diarrhea in a STAT-6 dependent manner [31]. It is not clear if this model is also representative of an immediate allergic reaction in the intestinal mucosa.

Large animal models

Non-rodent models of food allergy have been developed that feature symptoms that may be more closely related to human food-allergic reactions than rodent models. Although these large animal models are unlikely to be used widely for mechanistic studies, they offer a unique opportunity to test potential therapeutics in a non-rodent model prior to human trials. Dogs, like humans, develop spontaneous allergic disease, most commonly atopic dermatitis. It was found that 32.7% of dogs with allergic skin disease seen at a veterinary dermatology practice had food hypersensitivity, indicating a similar association of atopic dermatitis and food hypersensitivity in dogs [32]. A colony of spontaneous food-allergic dogs (maltese/beagle cross) has been described by Jackson et al. at North Caroline State University [33,34]. These dogs have hypersensitivity to soy and corn, manifesting as pruritic skin disease, otitis, and colitis that resolves in response to a restricted diet and recurs upon food challenge.

Experimental food allergy in dogs has also been described. Dogs in an atopic spaniel/basenji dog colony maintained at the University of California, Davis, have been shown to develop allergy to peanut, tree nuts, soy, wheat, barley, and milk when immunized with allergen extracts in alum at birth [35,36]. The sensitized dogs were described as undergoing severe gastrointestinal and systemic symptoms after allergen challenge, and were treated with epinephrine, diphenhydramine, and intravenous fluids post-challenge. This dog model was used to show that immunotherapy of allergic dogs with peanut plus heat-killed Listeria monocytogenes (HKL) in incomplete Freund's adjuvant could improve symptom scores in peanut-allergic dogs [35].

A food allergy model using newborn pigs has also been described [37]. Piglets were sensitized by intraperitoneal injection of peanut extract plus CT as adjuvant. The majority of piglets responded to oral challenge on days 39 and 53 after sensitization with Grade 2 symptoms, described as including vomiting, lethargy/malaise, tremors, convulsions, reduced activity not activated by prodding, or major areas of edematous rashes. A minority of animals had severe respiratory distress requiring epinephrine. Gastrointestinal manifestations of food allergy included diarrhea in the majority

Table 43.1 Animal models of food allergy

Model	Sensitization	Challenge	Outcome
OVA: systemic (Various rat/mice)	OVA + alum systemic	Single, gastrointestinal	Immediate changes in GI physiology (secretion, motility, permeability); late-phase inflammation
Allergic diarrhea (1) (Balb/c mice)	OVA + alum systemic	Multiple, gastrointestinal	Acute diarrhea beginning at ~3rd feed, allergic inflammation in small intestine
Allergic diarrhea (2) (Balb/c mice)	OVA + CFA systemic	Multiple, gastrointestinal	Acute diarrhea beginning at ~10th feed, allergic inflammation in large intestine
CT adjuvant models	Allergen + CT oral	Single, gastrointestinal	Systemic anaphylaxis (susceptible strains) or "local anaphylaxis"
CT adjuvant models	Allergen + CT oral	Single, systemic	Systemic anaphylaxis
Brown–Norway rat	OVA (oral)	Systemic	Plasma histamine
Transgenic pea	αAI-pea (oral)	Respiratory or cutaneous	Allergic inflammation of lung or skin dependent on challenge site
Allergic dog	Allergens + alum subcutaneous	Graded food challenge	Vomiting, diarrhea, lethargy
Neonatal swine	Peanut + CT i.p.	Repeated food challenges	Diarrhea, respiratory distress, anaphylaxis

CFA, Complete Freund's Adjuvant.

of responders, and changes in the mucosal architecture of the small intestine including vascular engorgement, villous tip damage, and submucosal edema. Therefore, while separate rodent models are used to study anaphylaxis versus gastrointestinal manifestations of food allergy, the newborn pig model has the advantage of producing both types of immediate reactions to food allergens.

Models of eosinophilic-allergic disorders

The models outlined above are focused on IgE-mediated immediate hypersensitivity reactions to food allergens. Although gastrointestinal eosinophilia is a feature in some of these models, eosinophils do not appear to play a pathological role in the immediate hypersensitivity reactions. To address gastrointestinal eosinophilic disorders, Hogan *et al.* developed a murine model of eosinophilic gastroenteritis [38,39]. As with the IgE-mediated models of allergic diarrhea, the model was initiated by systemic sensitization of Balb/c mice with OVA in alum. To induce gastrointestinal eosinophilia, mice were administered encapsulated OVA followed by acidified water to release the OVA in the small intestine. Sensitized mice fed encapsulated OVA had an eotaxin-dependent infiltration of eosinophils in the jejunum and priming of OVA-specific IgE and IgG1 in the serum [39]. This was associated with weight loss, gastromegaly, and impaired gastric emptying. Weight loss and gastromegaly were eotaxin dependent [38]. How eosinophils induce gastrointestinal pathology, how they become activated, and interactions with other cell types such as

enteric nerves remain to be determined using this model. The reader is referred to Chapter 15 for an in-depth review of the pathophysiology of eosinophilic disorders of the gastrointestinal tract.

Pathophysiology of food allergy: progress with animal models

Mechanisms of sensitization

A working hypothesis in experimental food allergy research is that allergic sensitization to food proteins occurs via the gastrointestinal tract. It is also well accepted that the normal response to protein antigens delivered via the oral route is one of active tolerance mediated by the induction of regulatory cells (see Chapter 7 for a discussion of immunological tolerance). Therefore one area of research focus has been to determine the conditions that could skew a tolerogenic response to an allergenic response.

Gut barrier

It has been hypothesized that age of exposure to food allergens is a critical factor since infants have not yet developed a mature intestinal barrier. The barrier function is composed of many components, including tight junction formation between intestinal epithelial cells, secretion of IgA, and gastric and duodenal digestion of proteins. The role of these factors in allergic sensitization has been addressed in a number of studies. The role of gastric digestion was tested by interfering with gastric acid in mice prior to administration of fish proteins by gavage [40]. Mice treated with ranitidine or omeprazole to suppress gastric acid had a significant enhancement of allergen-specific IgE to the fed allergens compared to mice administered the fish allergens without acid suppression. In contrast, there was no development of IgE reactivity to mouse chow. These results suggest that in the absence of pre-existing tolerance, interference with normal digestion can promote sensitization.

IgA is thought to be protective against allergy by interfering with uptake of antigens from the intestinal lumen. Fecal antigen-specific IgA has been shown to be upregulated in mice with tolerance, but not sensitization to the milk protein β-lactoglobulin (BLG) [15]. The role of IgA in experimental food allergy has not yet been directly tested through the use of mice deficient in IgA or the polymeric immunoglobulin receptor.

Factors that influence epithelial permeability have also been shown to be associated with sensitization to food proteins. In rats, psychological stress is commonly modeled by cold-restraint or water-avoidance protocols, which induce a corticotropin-releasing hormone (CRH)-mediated increase in epithelial permeability in the jejunum and colon [41,42]. Stress has recently been shown to enhance sensitization to orally delivered antigens [43]. Unstressed rats that were intragastrically administered the antigen horseradish peroxidase (HRP) in adjuvants (alum and pertussis toxin) did not develop sensitization to HRP (as measured by IgE or presence of local immediate hypersensitivity reactions upon re-challenge). However, if rats were subjected to water avoidance stress prior to administration of HRP in adjuvants, there was sensitization to HRP. *In vitro* antigen challenge of intestinal segments from sensitized rats showed characteristic increases in ion secretion and epithelial permeability, responses previously shown to be mast cell and IgE dependent. It should be noted that stress also has a number of effects on the immune system that may contribute to sensitization by other mechanisms. It was recently shown that mice colonized with *Candida albicans* develop a mast-cell-dependent defect in the gut barrier against macromolecules [44]. When infected mice were administered OVA, there was a significant rise in OVA-specific immunoglobulin production (IgE, IgG) compared to uninfected mice. Like stress, infection likely has many other effects beyond perturbation of barrier function, so these studies do not directly indicate that increasing delivery of an antigen across the epithelial barrier is in itself sufficient to induce sensitization. However, combined with the data on gastric acid suppression they suggest that normal gastrointestinal barrier function is required for tolerance to food proteins.

Immune mechanisms of allergic sensitization to food proteins

A number of groups have started to examine the host immune mechanisms, rather than external factors, by which an allergenic immune response to an orally delivered protein is induced instead of the predicted response of tolerance. Signaling of T-cells through CTLA-4 rather than CD28 inhibits T-cell activation, and CTLA-4 pathways have been shown to be important in the generation of oral tolerance [45]. Blockade of CTLA-4 was tested in a murine model of peanut allergy, and was shown to significantly increase the IgE and clinical response to peanut when administered with CT, but not in the absence of CT [46]. Therefore CTLA-4 is an important suppressive factor preventing allergic sensitization, but absence of CTLA-4 signaling does not appear to convert a tolerogenic response to an allergenic response, and other factors (provided experimentally by adjuvant) are required for development of sensitization to peanut. Other groups have shown that T-cells isolated from liver [47], mesenteric lymph node, or spleen [16] can transfer the allergen-specific immunoglobulin response, indicating that allergen-specific T-cells are generated locally within the gastrointestinal tract. CT, which is used experimentally to generate an allergic response to co-administered antigens, has been shown to induce the migration and maturation of dendritic cells (DCs) to the mesenteric lymph node [48] and migration of DCs to T-cell areas in the Peyer's patch [49]. This maturation results in more robust T-cell activation, and migration is necessary for delivery of captured antigens to sites of efficient T-cell interaction. It is not yet understood how food allergens initiate the same response in the absence of experimental adjuvants such as CT, but the very interesting finding that peanut itself has intrinsic adjuvant activity [6] suggests that these additional migratory or maturation signals may be provided by the allergen or associated proteins.

Gut flora

The composition of the gut flora has been hypothesized to have a critical role in the development of allergic sensitization. One of the first indications that this could be true was the finding that the development of oral tolerance was impaired in germ-free rodents [50]. However, there are conflicting data on the role of gut flora in oral tolerance. Investigators using particulate antigens (sheep red blood cells) or haptens have described a lack of tolerance development in germ-free mice [50], while results with a soluble antigen such as OVA have been conflicting [51–53]. A confounding factor is the impact of the gut flora on the development of the mucosal immune system, such that impairment in oral tolerance may not be due to conditioning of the mucosal immune system by gut flora, but rather may be due to the underdeveloped gastrointestinal-associated lymphoid tissue. This may be of particular relevance to antigens trafficking through the Peyer's patches, as particulate antigens such as sheep red blood cells would be expected to do.

Bashir *et al.* examined the impact of TLR4 deficiency on oral sensitization to peanut in a mouse model of anaphylaxis

[54]. They found that TLR4 deficiency was associated with susceptibility to peanut sensitization and associated with enhanced peanut-specific IgE production, increased Th2 cytokine production and increased severity of peanut-induced anaphylaxis. In addition, treatment of TLR4+/+ mice with broad-spectrum antibiotics to suppress the gut flora resulted in enhanced sensitization to peanut. We also observed that TLR4 deficient mice had enhanced Th2 cytokine production and increased severity of peanut-induced anaphylaxis [55], but this was not observed in all strains of mice or to the milk allergen BLG [55] or OVA (unpublished observations). The difference in TLR4 influence on allergic responsiveness to peanut versus other allergens could potentially relate to the route of sensitization, for example peanut has been shown to traffic through the Peyer's patch [56]. Alternatively, the unique interaction between TLR4 and peanut sensitization may relate to the ability of peanut to bind DC-SIGN and have adjuvant-like activity on DCs as recently shown by Shreffler *et al.* [6].

Cutaneous sensitization

Although the natural site of exposure to food proteins in humans is through the gastrointestinal tract, several studies have also indicated that sensitization may occur through skin. The skin is a common site of symptoms in food-allergic patients, and patients often have food-related skin symptoms (urticaria or atopic dermatitis) in the absence of any gastrointestinal symptoms. One potential explanation for this common observation is that sensitization occurs cutaneously and when cells are re-exposed they will home back to the skin using skin-specific homing markers (cutaneous lymphocyte-associated antigen (CLA)) and chemokines (e.g. CCL17, CCL27) [57]. A number of studies have shown that mice can be sensitized epicutaneously as indicated by antigen-specific IgE responses [58–60]. Hsieh *et al.* have shown that Balb/c mice sensitized to OVA by application of OVA to the skin respond to oral challenge with systemic anaphylaxis (measured by symptom score and plasma histamine) and histological changes in intestine and lung [61]. In the same study, the authors show that this sensitization process is IL-4 dependent. In addition, Strid *et al.* have shown that Balb/c mice exposed to peanut proteins via the skin develop peanut-specific IgE, IgG1, and a Th2-dominated T-cell cytokine response [62]. Epicutaneous exposure to peanut was shown to not only abrogate oral tolerance responses, but also prime for Th2-skewed immunity. During oral challenge, the mice epicutaneously primed with peanut developed symptoms of anaphylaxis. The latter study [62] required mild abrasion of the skin (by stripping with tape) for sensitization, but exposure via the skin results in an allergenic immune response in the absence of exogenous adjuvants. It is not clear what factors in the skin predispose to this allergenic response, or if endotoxin in OVA preparations or endogenous adjuvant activity in peanut are critical in the development of sensitization.

The only study to examine the role of TLR4 in epicutaneous sensitization to OVA used CT as adjuvant, and did not show an influence of TLR4 on allergic sensitization to OVA [63]. These studies have not yet been done in the absence of adjuvant.

These studies clearly show that allergic sensitization resulting in food-allergic-type symptoms can be generated by cutaneous sensitization. The link between oral challenge and cutaneous symptoms as seen in patients with food allergy has not yet been clearly modeled. It has been shown that mice orally sensitized to a model food allergen (transgenic expression of α-AI) will develop immediate (mast-cell mediated) and delayed (T-cell mediated) cutaneous hypersensitivity reactions in response to intradermal injection in the footpads [5]. In addition, several murine models of food antigen-induced anaphylaxis report transient cutaneous symptoms, including itching and swelling around the eyes, ears, and mouth, in response to oral challenge [9,10]. Delayed cutaneous reactions in response to oral challenge have not yet been convincingly modeled, although it has been reported that mice sensitized to milk developed atopic dermatitis-like lesions in response to mouse chow contaminated with milk proteins [64].

Pathophysiology of immediate hypersensitivity reactions in the gut

Experimental models of food allergy have been used to elucidate the consequences of allergen challenge in the gastrointestinal tract. As outlined above, rats or mice systemically sensitized to OVA develop increased ion secretion, epithelial permeability, and intestinal motility in response to allergen challenge. Ussing chambers have been particularly instrumental in uncovering mechanisms of epithelial dysfunction. Intestinal segments are mounted in Ussing chambers that immobilize the tissue between oxygenated chambers bathing the luminal or serosal sides of the tissue. Tissues are voltage clamped so that the Short circuit current (Isc) is equal and opposite to the current generated by the tissue by active transport. Therefore, Isc is a measure of active transport of the tissue. The compartmentalization of buffers bathing the serosal and luminal sides of the tissue also allow for measurement of permeability to small and large molecular weight tracers. Tissues can also be "challenged" with allergen on the luminal or serosal side of the intestinal segment. As outlined in the section on models of systemic sensitization to food proteins, luminal allergen challenge of sensitized mice and rats produce a local immediate hypersensitivity response, mediated by mast cells [28,65], and characterized by increased chloride ion secretion and permeability to macromolecules. There is bi-directional communication between mast cells and enteric nerves within the gastrointestinal tract [66,67], and mast cell–nerve interactions are critical to the generation of secretory and motility changes in response to allergen challenge [65,68]. Different mast cell mediators appear to mediate effects on epithelial ion secretion and barrier function. Ion secretion is driven by mast-cell-derived histamine, serotonin, and prostaglandins [24]. In contrast, mast cell proteases, including tryptase acting on protease-activated-receptor 2 (PAR2), appear to be major mediators of epithelial permeability changes in the gastrointestinal tract [69,70].

Studies have demonstrated that in the gastrointestinal tract there is a mast-cell-dependent "late-phase" response generated after oral allergen challenge [71–73]. In the stomach this is mediated by mast-cell-derived TNF-α [72]. The late-phase response in the small intestine is characterized by a mononuclear cell infiltrate, disrupted epithelial barrier function, and ion secretion [73]. Immediate effects of mast cell degranulation on epithelial cells combined with a late-phase response are likely underlying mechanisms responsible for allergen-induced diarrhea *in vivo*, which has been confirmed to be mast cell dependent [29]. The central role of mast cells in allergen-induced pathophysiology of the gastrointestinal tract is shown schematically in Fig. 43.1.

Early studies using the Ussing chamber system to examine epithelial responses to allergen demonstrated that addition of OVA to the luminal or serosal side of intestinal segments from systemically sensitized rats resulted in a rapid ion secretion response (15 seconds when added serosally, 3 minutes when added luminally) [24]. The difference in the response time reflects the time required for antigen to cross the epithelial cell layer prior to triggering lamina propria mast cells that degranulate and cause epithelial ion secretion. Within the last 10 years, it has been shown that this rapid transepithelial antigen transport across intestinal epithelial cells is a feature of sensitized intestine [27,28,74,75]. Rapid transepithelial transport is antigen specific [27], and is mediated by IgE and CD23 on the epithelial cell surface [74,75]. This enhanced uptake is mast cell independent [28], and epithelial CD23 expression is regulated by IL-4 and IgE [74]. Recently these findings have been extended to human systems [76–80], and we have recently shown that CD23 and food-specific IgE are present within stool of food-allergic patients (post-food challenge), but not in controls [76]. It has not yet been shown if interference with this system can prevent anaphylaxis in murine models of food-induced anaphylaxis, although blocking antibodies against CD23 prevent the development of local hypersensitivity reactions in the gut [75]. Figure 43.2 illustrates the role of CD23 in the transepithelial transport of IgE. Improving barrier function through the use of glucagon-like peptide 2 (GLP-2) has also been shown to prevent local hypersensitivity reactions in the gut through a CD23-independent mechanism [81]. Clearly factors that prevent uptake of allergen from the gastrointestinal lumen are effective in prevention of allergen-induced gastrointestinal dysfunction. Probiotics have also been shown to enhance intestinal epithelial barrier function [82], which may be one mechanism by which they may have therapeutic effect.

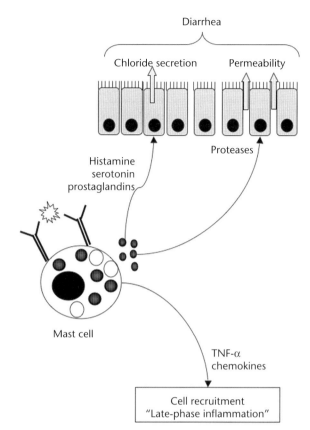

Figure 43.1 Mast cell mediators and the pathophysiology of gastrointestinal hypersensitivity reactions.
Mast cells are required for allergen-induced increases in epithelial chloride secretion and permeability, two driving forces for onset of diarrhea. Mast cells produce a vast array of bioactive mediators, and these have differing effects on pathophysiology. Rapidly released mediators such as histamine, serotonin, and prostaglandins have immediate (within minutes) effects on epithelial chloride secretion. Proteases impair epithelial barrier function within 30–60 minutes, whereas mast-cell-derived cytokines and chemokines can participate in late-phase inflammatory reactions occurring within hours to days after allergen challenge.

Harnessing host–microbial interactions for therapy

The ability of microbial products to downregulate allergic sensitization to food proteins has been of significant interest in the development of potential therapeutics. The use of CpG oligodeoxynucleotides (ODN), bacterial vectors and adjuvants, and probiotics have been tested in animal models for their ability to prevent or treat experimental food allergy. Bashir *et al.* have shown that administration of CpG ODN together with peanut and CT results in impairment of sensitization to peanut (reduced IgE, reduced IL-13, enhanced IFN-γ) and abolishment of peanut-induced anaphylaxis [54]. The same group has also shown that helminth infection inhibits development of allergic sensitization and anaphylaxis in response to peanut challenge,

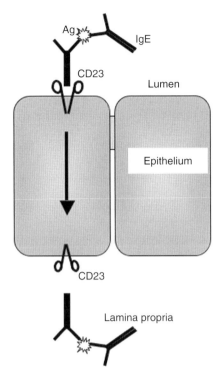

Figure 43.2 CD23 facilitates the entry of antigen from the gut lumen. CD23 is constitutively expressed in human intestinal epithelium, and is induced in rodent models of food allergy. CD23 facilitates the apical-to-basolateral transport of IgE–antigen complexes and delivers these complexes to immune cells in the lamina propria.

via an IL-10-dependent pathway [83], which supports the hypothesis that exposure to microbial products can promote the development of regulatory cells that suppress allergic sensitization. This is also supported by studies showing that helminth infections are protective against intestinal inflammation in murine colitis models through IL-10-dependent [84] and -independent [85,86] pathways. Although a helminth-based therapy has been developed for ulcerative colitis [87], this approach has not been studied as a therapeutic option in food-allergic disorders.

Of major interest in the development of therapeutics is a means of inhibiting pre-existing sensitization. Two studies have been published using HKL as an adjuvant to inhibit sensitization and reactivity to peanut. Li et al. showed that administration of HKL to peanut-sensitized mice inhibited peanut-specific IgE, peanut-induced anaphylaxis, and modified the peanut-specific Th2/Th1 cytokine balance [88]. Frick et al. used peanut- or milk-sensitized dogs to show that HKL plus specific antigen could significantly inhibit antigen-induced allergic responsiveness and skin test reactivity [35]. Other studies testing the effect of HKL on OVA-induced airway hyperresponsiveness have shown that HKL induces IFN-γ-producing "Th1 regulatory" cells that express the regulatory transcription factor Foxp3 and suppress allergic inflammation in an IL-10-dependent manner [89]. These Th1-like Tregs are generated by CD8+ DCs, and by

an IL-10- and IL-12-dependent mechanism. It is likely that the same mechanism is responsible for the suppression of peanut-specific IgE and peanut-induced anaphylaxis, but this has not been directly tested.

Another experimental approach to immunotherapy has been to administer modified (non-IgE binding) recombinant peanut allergens. These were administered to peanut-sensitized mice by intrarectal administration within a heat-killed E. coli vector [90]. Despite the heavy microbial load normally present within the large intestine, administration of the E. coli vector itself had some transient immunomodulatory effects, but maximal prolonged suppression of IgE- and peanut-induced anaphylaxis was observed with E. coli carrying modified peanut proteins. The mechanism by which this preparation has immunomodulatory effects, or if this suppression of anaphylaxis is mediated by regulatory cells that suppress peanut-specific T- and B-cells, is currently under investigation.

Probiotics have been shown to have clinical efficacy in patients with atopic dermatitis or food allergen-exacerbated eczema [91–95]; however, relatively little has been investigated in experimental animal models. Adel-Patient et al. generated Lactococcus lactis strains expressing the milk protein BLG and administered them orally to mice [96]. After administration, mice were sensitized to BLG by intraperitoneal injection in incomplete Freund's adjuvant. Only one of the test strains inhibited BLG-specific IgE in serum, but several of the strains induced a significant increase in BLG-specific IgG2a. Surprisingly both Th1 and Th2 cytokines were enhanced by administration of BLG-expressing L. lactis strains. Although a BLG-expressing Lactobacillus casei has also been developed [97], the effect of these strains on clinical reactivity to BLG in mice has not been reported to date. Kim et al. reported that administration of Bifidobacterium bifidum, Lactobacillus casei, or E. coli to mice in the mouse chow significantly reduced OVA-specific IgE and IgG1 in a murine model of oral sensitization to OVA [98]. Anaphylaxis symptoms were not assessed. Oral administration of probiotics (VSL-3) to mice with experimental colitis has been shown to inhibit inflammation (in both Th1-mediated and innate-immunity-mediated models of colitis) in a TLR9-dependent manner [99]. Given the fact that CpG has been shown to inhibit peanut-induced anaphylaxis in a murine model of food allergy [54], the use of oral probiotics may also potentially activate TLR9 and downregulate allergic sensitization in food allergy; however, this remains speculative at this point.

Reductionist models for food-allergy research

Animal models are not the only experimental approach to food allergy, and reductionist models have been used to examine specific aspects of the allergic response to food allergens. The use of Ussing chambers has been introduced in a previous section of the chapter. Ussing chambers can be used not only for the *in vitro* measurement of local hypersensitivity reactions of gastrointestinal tissue from animal models, but modified chambers have been developed for use with patient biopsies [100,101]. This technique has been reported as a potential diagnostic tool for food-allergic disorders [100], and has been used to study transepithelial antigen trafficking in inflammatory bowel disease [101]. In cases where endoscopy and biopsy are called for, this technique may be valuable for studying local responses to food allergens in humans.

Modeling of the human gastrointestinal epithelium can also be done using cell lines that polarize when grown on filter supports. T84 cells, Caco-2 cells, HT-29 subclones, and HCA-7 cells all polarize when grown on transwell filters. These cell lines form tight junctions and have well-differentiated apical and basolateral domains. Human intestinal cell monolayers have been used to address issues related to transepithelial allergen transport [102,103], antibody-mediated antigen uptake [76,77,79], and when co-cultured with immune cells can model epithelial pathophysiology in response to local immune activation [104].

Mast cells, like human epithelial cells, have also been modeled using cell line systems. The most common is the rat basophil leukemia cell line, or RBL. This cell line has been transfected with the human high-affinity IgE receptor, and through this method can be used to assess the reactivity of human serum samples to different allergens [105,106]. Bischoff and colleagues have also published protocols for the isolation of human intestinal mast cells [107], which allows for the study of tissue-specific characteristics of human mast cells.

Reductionist approaches may be most useful for modeling the interaction of cells and allergens within the gastrointestinal mucosa, as access to intestinal tissues from food-allergic patients is limited due to the invasive measures needed to acquire them. The development of co-culture systems will then begin to address cell–cell interactions in a well-controlled experimental environment, and can begin to move findings using rodent systems into a human tissue-based experimental system.

References

1 Knippels LM, Penninks AH, Spanhaak S, Houben GF. Oral sensitization to food proteins: a Brown Norway rat model. *Clin Exp Allergy* 1998;28:368–75.

2 Knippels LM, Penninks AH, Smit JJ, Houben GF. Immune-mediated effects upon oral challenge of ovalbumin-sensitized Brown Norway rats: further characterization of a rat food allergy model. *Toxicol Appl Pharmacol* 1999;156:161–9.

3 Akiyama H, Teshima R, Sakushima JI, *et al.* Examination of oral sensitization with ovalbumin in Brown Norway rats and three strains of mice. *Immunol Lett* 2001;78:1–5.

4 Prescott VE, Campbell PM, Moore A, *et al.* Transgenic expression of bean alpha-amylase inhibitor in peas results in altered structure and immunogenicity. *J Agric Food Chem* 2005;53:9023–30.

5 Prescott VE, Forbes E, Foster PS, *et al.* Mechanistic analysis of experimental food allergen-induced cutaneous reactions. *J Leukoc Biol* 2006;80:258–66.

6 Shreffler WG, Castro RR, Kucuk ZY, *et al.* The major glycoprotein allergen from *Arachis hypogaea*, Ara h 1, is a ligand of dendritic cell-specific ICAM-grabbing nonintegrin and acts as a Th2 adjuvant *in vitro. J Immunol* 2006;177:3677–85.

7 Charbonnier AS, Hammad H, Gosset P, *et al.* Der p 1-pulsed myeloid and plasmacytoid dendritic cells from house dust mite-sensitized allergic patients dysregulate the T cell response. *J Leukoc Biol* 2003;73:91–9.

8 Hammad H, Charbonnier AS, Duez C, *et al.* Th2 polarization by Der p 1–pulsed monocyte-derived dendritic cells is due to the allergic status of the donors. *Blood* 2001;98:1135–41.

9 Snider DP, Marshall JS, Perdue MH, Liang H. Production of IgE antibody and allergic sensitization of intestinal and peripheral tissues after oral immunization with protein Ag and cholera toxin. *J Immunol* 1994;153:647–57.

10 Li XM, Serebrisky D, Lee SY, *et al.* A murine model of peanut anaphylaxis: T- and B-cell responses to a major peanut allergen mimic human responses. *J Allergy Clin Immunol* 2000; 106:150–8.

11 Li XM, Schofield BH, Huang CK, *et al.* A murine model of IgE-mediated cow's milk hypersensitivity. *J Allergy Clin Immunol* 1999;103:206–14.

12 Adel-Patient K, Bernard H, Ah-Leung S, *et al.* Peanut- and cow's milk-specific IgE, Th2 cells and local anaphylactic reaction are induced in Balb/c mice orally sensitized with cholera toxin. *Allergy* 2005;60:658–64.

13 Morafo V, Srivastava K, Huang CK, *et al.* Genetic susceptibility to food allergy is linked to differential TH2–TH1 responses in C3H/HeJ and BALB/c mice. *J Allergy Clin Immunol* 2003;111:1122–8.

14 Pons L, Ponnappan U, Hall RA, *et al.* Soy immunotherapy for peanut-allergic mice: modulation of the peanut-allergic response. *J Allergy Clin Immunol* 2004;114:915–21.

15 Frossard CP, Hauser C, Eigenmann PA. Antigen-specific secretory IgA antibodies in the gut are decreased in a mouse model of food allergy. *J Allergy Clin Immunol* 2004;114:377–82.

16 Frossard CP, Tropia L, Hauser C, Eigenmann PA. Lymphocytes in Peyer patches regulate clinical tolerance in a murine model of food allergy. *J Allergy Clin Immunol.* 2004;113:958–64.

17 Byars NE, Ferraresi RW. Intestinal anaphylaxis in the rat as a model of food allergy. *Clin Exp Immunol* 1976;24:352–6.

18 Byars NE, Ferraresi RW. Inhibition of rat intestinal anaphylaxis by various anti-inflammatory agents. *Agents Actions* 1980;10:252–7.

19 Perdue MH, Chung M, Gall DG. Effect of intestinal anaphylaxis on gut function in the rat. *Gastroenterology* 1984;86:391–7.

20 Bloch KJ, Walker WA. Effect of locally induced intestinal anaphylaxis on the uptake of a bystander antigen. *J Allergy Clin Immunol* 1981;67:312–6.

21 Scott RB, Diamant SC, Gall DG. Motility effects of intestinal anaphylaxis in the rat. *Am J Physiol* 1988;255:G505–11.

22 Perdue MH, Gall DG. Transport abnormalities during intestinal anaphylaxis in the rat: effect of antiallergic agents. *J Allergy Clin Immunol* 1985;76:498–503.

23 Crowe SE, Soda K, Stanisz AM, Perdue MH. Intestinal permeability in allergic rats: nerve involvement in antigen-induced changes. *Am J Physiol* 1993;264:G617–23.

24 Crowe SE, Sestini P, Perdue MH. Allergic reactions of rat jejunal mucosa. Ion transport responses to luminal antigen and inflammatory mediators. *Gastroenterology* 1990;99:74–82.

25 Kosecka U, Marshall JS, Crowe SE, et al. Pertussis toxin stimulates hypersensitivity and enhances nerve-mediated antigen uptake in rat intestine. *Am J Physiol* 1994;267:G745–53.

26 Perdue MH, Gall DG. Intestinal anaphylaxis in the rat: jejunal response to *in vitro* antigen exposure. *Am J Physiol* 1986;250:G427–31.

27 Berin MC, Kiliaan AJ, Yang PC, et al. Rapid transepithelial antigen transport in rat jejunum: impact of sensitization and the hypersensitivity reaction. *Gastroenterology* 1997;113:856–64.

28 Berin MC, Kiliaan AJ, Yang PC, et al. The influence of mast cells on pathways of transepithelial antigen transport in rat intestine. *J Immunol* 1998;161:2561–6.

29 Brandt EB, Strait RT, Hershko D, et al. Mast cells are required for experimental oral allergen-induced diarrhea. *J Clin Invest* 2003;112:1666–77.

30 Alvarez D, Swirski FK, Yang TC, et al. Inhalation tolerance is induced selectively in thoracic lymph nodes but executed pervasively at distant mucosal and nonmucosal tissues. *J Immunol* 2006;176:2568–80.

31 Kweon MN, Yamamoto M, Kajiki M, et al. Systemically derived large intestinal CD4(+) Th2 cells play a central role in STAT6-mediated allergic diarrhea. *J Clin Invest*. 2000;106:199–206.

32 Chesney CJ. Food sensitivity in the dog: a quantitative study. *J Small Anim Pract* 2002;43:203–7.

33 Jackson HA, Jackson MW, Coblentz L, Hammerberg B. Evaluation of the clinical and allergen specific serum immunoglobulin E responses to oral challenge with cornstarch, corn, soy and a soy hydrolysate diet in dogs with spontaneous food allergy. *Vet Dermatol* 2003;14:181–7.

34 Jackson HA, Hammerberg B. Evaluation of a spontaneous canine model of immunoglobulin E-mediated food hypersensitivity: dynamic changes in serum and fecal allergen-specific immunoglobulin E values relative to dietary change. *Comp Med* 2002;52:316–21.

35 Frick OL, Teuber SS, Buchanan BB, et al. Allergen immunotherapy with heat-killed *Listeria monocytogenes* alleviates peanut and food-induced anaphylaxis in dogs. *Allergy* 2005;60:243–50.

36 Teuber SS, Del Val G, Morigasaki S, et al. The atopic dog as a model of peanut and tree nut food allergy. *J Allergy Clin Immunol* 2002;110:921–7.

37 Helm RM, Furuta GT, Stanley JS, et al. A neonatal swine model for peanut allergy. *J Allergy Clin Immunol* 2002;109:136–42.

38 Hogan SP, Mishra A, Brandt EB, et al. A pathological function for eotaxin and eosinophils in eosinophilic gastrointestinal inflammation. *Nat Immunol* 2001;2:353–60.

39 Hogan SP, Mishra A, Brandt EB, et al. A critical role for eotaxin in experimental oral antigen-induced eosinophilic gastrointestinal allergy. *Proc Natl Acad Sci USA* 2000;97:6681–6.

40 Untersmayr E, Scholl I, Swoboda I, et al. Antacid medication inhibits digestion of dietary proteins and causes food allergy: a fish allergy model in BALB/c mice. *J Allergy Clin Immunol* 2003;112:616–23.

41 Saunders PR, Santos J, Hanssen NP, et al. Physical and psychological stress in rats enhances colonic epithelial permeability via peripheral CRH. *Dig Dis Sci* 2002;47:208–15.

42 Santos J, Saunders PR, Hanssen NP, et al. Corticotropin-releasing hormone mimics stress-induced colonic epithelial pathophysiology in the rat. *Am J Physiol* 1999;277:G391–9.

43 Yang PC, Jury J, Soderholm JD, et al. Chronic psychological stress in rats induces intestinal sensitization to luminal antigens. *Am J Pathol* 2006;168:104–14; quiz 363.

44 Yamaguchi N, Sugita R, Miki A, et al. Gastrointestinal Candida colonisation promotes sensitisation against food antigens by affecting the mucosal barrier in mice. *Gut* 2006;55:954–60.

45 Fowler S, Powrie F. CTLA-4 expression on antigen-specific cells but not IL-10 secretion is required for oral tolerance. *Eur J Immunol* 2002;32:2997–3006.

46 van Wijk F, Hoeks S, Nierkens S, et al. CTLA-4 signaling regulates the intensity of hypersensitivity responses to food antigens, but is not decisive in the induction of sensitization. *J Immunol* 2005;174:174–9.

47 Watanabe T, Katsukura H, Shirai Y, et al. Helper CD4+ T cells for IgE response to a dietary antigen develop in the liver. *J Allergy Clin Immunol* 2003;111:1375–85.

48 Anjuere F, Luci C, Lebens M, et al. *In vivo* adjuvant-induced mobilization and maturation of gut dendritic cells after oral administration of cholera toxin. *J Immunol* 2004;173:5103–11.

49 Shreedhar VK, Kelsall BL, Neutra MR. Cholera toxin induces migration of dendritic cells from the subepithelial dome region to T- and B-cell areas of Peyer's patches. *Infect Immun* 2003;71:504–9.

50 Wannemuehler MJ, Kiyono H, Babb JL, et al. Lipopolysaccharide (LPS) regulation of the immune response: LPS converts germfree mice to sensitivity to oral tolerance induction. *J Immunol* 1982;129:959–65.

51 Moreau MC, Corthier G. Effect of the gastrointestinal microflora on induction and maintenance of oral tolerance to ovalbumin in C3H/HeJ mice. *Infect Immun* 1988;56:2766–8.

52 Gaboriau-Routhiau V, Moreau MC. Gut flora allows recovery of oral tolerance to ovalbumin in mice after transient breakdown mediated by cholera toxin or *Escherichia coli* heat-labile enterotoxin. *Pediatr Res* 1996;39:625–9.

53 Sudo N, Sawamura S, Tanaka K, et al. The requirement of intestinal bacterial flora for the development of an IgE production system fully susceptible to oral tolerance induction. *J Immunol* 1997;159:1739–45.

54 Bashir ME, Louie S, Shi HN, Nagler-Anderson C. Toll-like receptor 4 signaling by intestinal microbes influences susceptibility to food allergy. *J Immunol* 2004;172:6978–87.

55 Berin MC, Zheng Y, Domaradzki M, *et al.* Role of TLR4 in allergic sensitization to food proteins in mice. *Allergy* 2006;61:64–71.

56 Chambers SJ, Wickham MS, Regoli M, *et al.* Rapid *in vivo* transport of proteins from digested allergen across pre-sensitized gut. *Biochem Biophys Res Commun* 2004;325:1258–63.

57 Campbell DJ, Kim CH, Butcher EC. Chemokines in the systemic organization of immunity. *Immunol Rev* 2003;195:58–71.

58 Wang LF, Lin JY, Hsieh KH, Lin RH. Epicutaneous exposure of protein antigen induces a predominant Th2-like response with high IgE production in mice. *J Immunol* 1996;156:4077–82.

59 Spergel JM, Mizoguchi E, Brewer JP, *et al.* Epicutaneous sensitization with protein antigen induces localized allergic dermatitis and hyperresponsiveness to methacholine after single exposure to aerosolized antigen in mice. *J Clin Invest* 1998;101:1614–22.

60 Herrick CA, MacLeod H, Glusac E, *et al.* Th2 responses induced by epicutaneous or inhalational protein exposure are differentially dependent on IL-4. *J Clin Invest* 2000;105:765–75.

61 Hsieh KY, Tsai CC, Wu CH, Lin RH. Epicutaneous exposure to protein antigen and food allergy. *Clin Exp Allergy* 2003; 33:1067–75.

62 Strid J, Hourihane J, Kimber I, *et al.* Epicutaneous exposure to peanut protein prevents oral tolerance and enhances allergic sensitization. *Clin Exp Allergy* 2005;35:757–66.

63 Kahlon R, Dutz JP. Skin immune responses to peptide and protein antigen are TLR4 independent. *Cell Immunol* 2003;226:116–23.

64 Li XM, Kleiner G, Huang CK, *et al.* Murine model of atopic dermatitis associated with food hypersensitivity. *J Allergy Clin Immunol* 2001;107:693–702.

65 Perdue MH, Masson S, Wershil BK, Galli SJ. Role of mast cells in ion transport abnormalities associated with intestinal anaphylaxis. Correction of the diminished secretory response in genetically mast cell-deficient W/Wv mice by bone marrow transplantation. *J Clin Invest* 1991;87:687–93.

66 Stead RH, Dixon MF, Bramwell NH, *et al.* Mast cells are closely apposed to nerves in the human gastrointestinal mucosa. *Gastroenterology* 1989;97:575–85.

67 Stead RH, Tomioka M, Quinonez G, *et al.* Intestinal mucosal mast cells in normal and nematode-infected rat intestines are in intimate contact with peptidergic nerves. *Proc Natl Acad Sci USA* 1987;84:2975–9.

68 Oliver MR, Tan DT, Kirk DR, *et al.* Colonic and jejunal motor disturbances after colonic antigen challenge of sensitized rat. *Gastroenterology* 1997;112:1996–2005.

69 Jacob C, Yang PC, Darmoul D, *et al.* Mast cell tryptase controls paracellular permeability of the intestine. Role of protease-activated receptor 2 and beta-arrestins. *J Biol Chem* 2005; 280:31936–48.

70 Scudamore CL, Thornton EM, McMillan L, *et al.* Release of the mucosal mast cell granule chymase, rat mast cell protease-II, during anaphylaxis is associated with the rapid development

of paracellular permeability to macromolecules in rat jejunum. *J Exp Med* 1995;182:1871–81.

71 Wershil BK, Furuta GT, Wang ZS, Galli SJ. Mast cell-dependent neutrophil and mononuclear cell recruitment in immunoglobulin E-induced gastric reactions in mice. *Gastroenterology* 1996;110:1482–90.

72 Furuta GT, Schmidt-Choudhury A, Wang MY, *et al.* Mast cell-dependent tumor necrosis factor alpha production participates in allergic gastric inflammation in mice. *Gastroenterology* 1997;113:1560–9.

73 Yang PC, Berin MC, Yu L, Perdue MH. Mucosal pathophysiology and inflammatory changes in the late phase of the intestinal allergic reaction in the rat. *Am J Pathol* 2001;158:681–90.

74 Yu LC, Yang PC, Berin MC, *et al.* Enhanced transepithelial antigen transport in intestine of allergic mice is mediated by IgE/CD23 and regulated by interleukin-4. *Gastroenterology* 2001;121:370–81.

75 Yang PC, Berin MC, Yu LC, *et al.* Enhanced intestinal transepithelial antigen transport in allergic rats is mediated by IgE and CD23 (FcepsilonRII). *J Clin Invest* 2000;106:879–86.

76 Li H, Nowak-Wegrzyn A, Charlop-Powers Z, *et al.* Transcytosis of IgE–antigen complexes by CD23a in human intestinal epithelial cells and its role in food allergy. *Gastroenterology* 2006;131:47–58.

77 Tu Y, Perdue MH. CD23-mediated transport of IgE/immune complexes across human intestinal epithelium: role of p38 MAPK. *Am J Physiol Gastrointest Liver Physiol* 2006;291:G532–8.

78 Tu Y, Salim S, Bourgeois J, *et al.* CD23-mediated IgE transport across human intestinal epithelium: inhibition by blocking sites of translation or binding. *Gastroenterology* 2005;129:928–40.

79 Montagnac G, Molla-Herman A, Bouchet J, *et al.* Intracellular trafficking of CD23: differential regulation in humans and mice by both extracellular and intracellular exons. *J Immunol* 2005;174:5562–72.

80 Montagnac G, Yu LC, Bevilacqua C, *et al* Differential role for CD23 splice forms in apical to basolateral transcytosis of IgE/allergen complexes. *Traffic* 2005;6:230–42.

81 Cameron HL, Yang PC, Perdue MH. Glucagon-like peptide-2-enhanced barrier function reduces pathophysiology in a model of food allergy. *Am J Physiol Gastrointest Liver Physiol* 2003;284: G905–12.

82 Madsen K, Cornish A, Soper P, *et al.* Probiotic bacteria enhance murine and human intestinal epithelial barrier function. *Gastroenterology* 2001;121:580–91.

83 Bashir ME, Andersen P, Fuss IJ, *et al.* An enteric helminth infection protects against an allergic response to dietary antigen. *J Immunol* 2002;169:3284–92.

84 Hunter MM, Wang A, Hirota CL, McKay DM. Neutralizing anti-IL-10 antibody blocks the protective effect of tapeworm infection in a murine model of chemically induced colitis. *J Immunol* 2005;174:7368–75.

85 Metwali A, Setiawan T, Blum AM, *et al.* Induction of CD8+ regulatory T cells in the intestine by *Heligmosomoides polygyrus* infection. *Am J Physiol Gastrointest Liver Physiol* 2006;291: G253–9.

86 Elliott DE, Setiawan T, Metwali A, *et al. Heligmosomoides polygyrus* inhibits established colitis in IL-10-deficient mice. *Eur J Immunol* 2004;34:2690–8.

87 Summers RW, Elliott DE, Urban Jr JF, *et al.* Trichuris suis therapy for active ulcerative colitis: a randomized controlled trial. *Gastroenterology* 2005;128:825–32.

88 Li XM, Srivastava K, Huleatt JW, *et al.* Engineered recombinant peanut protein and heat-killed *Listeria monocytogenes* coadministration protects against peanut-induced anaphylaxis in a murine model. *J Immunol* 2003;170:3289–95.

89 Stock P, Akbari O, Berry G, *et al.* Induction of T helper type 1-like regulatory cells that express Foxp3 and protect against airway hyper-reactivity. *Nat Immunol* 2004;5:1149–56.

90 Li XM, Srivastava K, Grishin A, *et al.* Persistent protective effect of heat-killed *Escherichia coli* producing "engineered," recombinant peanut proteins in a murine model of peanut allergy. *J Allergy Clin Immunol* 2003;112:159–67.

91 Kalliomaki M, Salminen S, Poussa T, *et al.* Probiotics and prevention of atopic disease: 4-year follow-up of a randomised placebo-controlled trial. *Lancet* 2003;361:1869–71.

92 Kalliomaki M, Salminen S, Arvilommi H, *et al.* Probiotics in primary prevention of atopic disease: a randomised placebo-controlled trial. *Lancet* 2001;357:1076–9.

93 Sistek D, Kelly R, Wickens K, *et al.* Is the effect of probiotics on atopic dermatitis confined to food sensitized children? *Clin Exp Allergy* 2006;36:629–33.

94 Rosenfeldt V, Benfeldt E, Valerius NH, *et al.* Effect of probiotics on gastrointestinal symptoms and small intestinal permeability in children with atopic dermatitis. *J Pediatr* 2004;145:612–16.

95 Rosenfeldt V, Benfeldt E, Nielsen SD, *et al.* Effect of probiotic Lactobacillus strains in children with atopic dermatitis. *J Allergy Clin Immunol.* 2003;111:389–95.

96 Adel-Patient K, Ah-Leung S, Creminon C, *et al.* Oral administration of recombinant *Lactococcus lactis* expressing bovine beta-lactoglobulin partially prevents mice from sensitization. *Clin Exp Allergy* 2005;35:539–46.

97 Hazebrouck S, Oozeer R, Adel-Patient K, *et al.* Constitutive delivery of bovine {beta}-lactoglobulin to the digestive tract of gnotobiotic mice by engineered *Lactobacillus casei. Appl Environ Microbiol* 2006;72:7460–67.

98 Kim H, Kwack K, Kim DY, Ji GE. Oral probiotic bacterial administration suppressed allergic responses in an ovalbumin-induced allergy mouse model. *FEMS Immunol Med Microbiol* 2005;45:259–67.

99 Rachmilewitz D, Katakura K, Karmeli F, *et al.* Toll-like receptor 9 signaling mediates the anti-inflammatory effects of probiotics in murine experimental colitis. *Gastroenterology* 2004;126:520–8.

100 Bijlsma PB, Backhaus B, Weidenhiller M, *et al.* Food allergy diagnosis by detection of antigen-induced electrophysiological changes and histamine release in human intestinal biopsies during mucosa-oxygenation. *Inflamm Res* 2004;53:S29–30.

101 Wallon C, Braaf Y, Wolving M, *et al.* Endoscopic biopsies in using chambers evaluated for studies of macromolecular permeability in the human colon. *Scand J Gastroenterol* 2005;40:586–95.

102 Moreno FJ, Rubio LA, Olano A, Clemente A. Uptake of 2S albumin allergens, Ber e 1 and Ses i 1, across human intestinal epithelial Caco-2 cell monolayers. *J Agric Food Chem* 2006; 54:8631–9.

103 Bernasconi E, Fritsche R, Corthesy B. Specific effects of denaturation, hydrolysis and exposure to *Lactococcus lactis* on bovine beta-lactoglobulin transepithelial transport, antigenicity and allergenicity. *Clin Exp Allergy* 2006;36:803–14.

104 Heyman M, Darmon N, Dupont C, *et al.* Mononuclear cells from infants allergic to cow's milk secrete tumor necrosis factor alpha, altering intestinal function. *Gastroenterology* 1994;106:1514–23.

105 Dibbern Jr DA, Palmer GW, Williams PB, *et al.* RBL cells expressing human Fc epsilon RI are a sensitive tool for exploring functional IgE–allergen interactions: studies with sera from peanut-sensitive patients. *J Immunol Methods* 2003;274:37–45.

106 Vogel L, Luttkopf D, Hatahet L, *et al.* Development of a functional *in vitro* assay as a novel tool for the standardization of allergen extracts in the human system. *Allergy* 2005; 60:1021–8.

107 Sellge G, Bischoff SC. Isolation, culture, and characterization of intestinal mast cells. *Methods Mol Biol* 2006;315:123–38.

CHAPTER 44

Food Allergy: Psychological Considerations

Lourdes B. de Asis and Ronald A. Simon

KEY CONCEPTS

- Food allergic patients, particularly children and adolescents, are subject to increased stress and social disruption, which can lead to diminished quality of life and increased risk-taking behavior.

- The key features differentiating the person with food aversion or food sensitivity from the person with a true food allergy are: (i) the absence or inconsistent finding of recognized signs and symptoms, physical findings, and laboratory evaluation supportive of an allergic, toxic, enzymatic, or pharmacological reaction to a specific food and (ii) the inability to reproduce symptoms or physical changes under adequately controlled double-blind food challenge conditions.

- Single-blinded placebo-controlled (SBPC) challenges may be performed to confirm neuropsychological complaints associated with food ingestion.

- There are four elements necessary to accomplish this type of challenge: (i) a single substance (food/additive/substance etc.); (ii) that produces a consistent reaction (even totally subjective); (iii) with a known amount; and (iv) in a set time frame.

- The benefits of elemination diets on behavior and cognition in autistic children remain questionable.

- Depression, but not schizophrenia, has been shown to have a well established link with celiac disease.

- Patients with complaints of multiple food intolerance/sensitivities, as frequently seen in multiple chemical sensitivity (MCS)/idiopathic environmental intolerance (IEI) syndromes have frequently been shown to have underlying somatoform, depression, or panic disorders.

Introduction

Food is central to our physical and social development from our earliest memory as individuals and as a society. Since childhood, the sight, smell, and taste of food are inextricably linked to experiences that shape our personalities and how we relate to the world. It is therefore small wonder that food is involved in numerous psychological and somatic disorders with psychological overtones such as anorexia, bulimia, obesity, and many others [1]. Food-related behavior has not only been the means of expression of psychological disorder, but food itself has been implicated in the causation and exacerbation of emotional and psychological problems. In food-allergic patients, the anxiety and limitations imposed by their condition have been recognized to have significant impact on quality of life. There has also been increased interest in the psychological response to the restrictions on diet and lifestyle required of patients and their families.

Food Allergy: Adverse Reactions to Foods and Food Additives, 4th edition.
Edited by Dean D. Metcalfe, Hugh A. Sampson, and Ronald A. Simon.
© 2008 Blackwell Publishing. ISBN: 978-1-4501-5129-0.

This chapter addresses these issues and provides the practicing allergist with an approach to managing and counseling patients with documented food allergies as well as psychogenic food reactions. It also examines the current literature on the association between food sensitivity and psychological diseases, such as autism and schizophrenia. It is worth noting Pearson's observation [2] that effective communication between the patients, their families, and the medical practitioner, is a critical component in the management of these patients.

Psychological responses to food allergy

The most common abnormal psychological responses to physical illness include denial, anxiety, anger, depression, and dependency. These psychological states are a reaction to loss of health. The extent of psychopathology and impaired somatic functioning depends on the degree to which emotional issues related to the illness are resolved [3]. With this in mind, allergic patients have not been found to have significantly increased prevalence of psychological problems compared to non-allergic controls [4].

Food allergy carries with it the additional psychological burden of dietary restriction and vigilance and continuous anxiety regarding the consequences of accidental exposure. Primeau et al. [5] studied the impact of peanut allergy on quality of life and family relations in children and adults compared to patients of similar age group with a rheumatological disease. Peanut-allergic children, as reported by their parents, were found to have significantly more disruption in their daily activities and increased impairment of familial social interactions compared to the families of children with rheumatological disease. However, the families of peanut-allergic children scored better on mastery and coping mechanisms. The reverse was true of peanut-allergic adults who scored worse on mastery and coping mechanisms associated with their disease, but had less personal strain and familial disruption than adults with rheumatological disease. This difference was attributed not only to the greater vigilance parents practice over the management of their children's allergies, leading to better mastery and coping, but also to higher stress levels. Peanut-allergic adults were less compulsive regarding management of their own allergies, and thus had less stress and social disruption. This study also emphasized the significant psychological burden of a food allergy diagnosis on families and their need for educational and emotional support.

Other studies by Bollinger and colleagues [6] found that food allergy had significant effect on meal preparation, family social activities, stress levels, and school attendance. Avery [7] compared the quality of life scores of peanut-allergic children and children with insulin-dependent diabetes mellitus and found that peanut-allergic children had poorer quality life and had more fear of adverse events, anxiety about eating, and felt more restricted regarding physical activities, but felt safer when they ate in familiar places or when carrying epinephrine kits.

Adolescents and young adults are especially vulnerable and have been found to be particularly high risk for fatal food-allergic reactions. The risk-taking behaviors and coping mechanisms of this group of patients was examined by Sampson, Munoz-Furlong, and Sicherer [8] using anonymous questionnaires. Their findings revealed that a significant number engage in risk-taking behaviors such as ingesting potentially unsafe food and failure to "always" carry epinephrine. These behaviors may be related to the increased sense of "social isolation" [9] and reports of "feeling different" which have been found in this group as a result of their food allergies. Participants in this study thought that educating other students about food allergy, wider meal selection, and having pre-selected staff members with whom to discuss meal selection would help them cope better at school. This study further recommended increased education of teens, young adults, and their peers with emphasis on the symptoms of anaphylaxis, the importance of carrying and using injectable epinephrine, and avoidance of "unsafe" foods.

Food allergy and psychological disorders

It is recognized that the experience and expression of illness reflects the interaction between the physical and psychological states of an individual, such that an individual's mental state can influence physiological changes, including the reactivity of the immune system [10,11]. Moreover, the response to physical stimuli, such as the wheal and flare reaction to intradermal testing [12] and hyperreactivity of the bronchial airways [13] are reported to be influenced by mental events. Psychologically mediated allergic changes can be classified into a non-specific autonomic nervous system response to emotional arousal, such as an asthma attack due to fright or violent emotion, and changes due to suggestion or conditioning to specific stimuli [14]. It has been reported that nasal, eye, and airway symptoms as well as changes in eosinophil levels, nasal secretion, bronchoconstriction, and gastrointestinal (GI) and skin blood flow can be experimentally induced by suggestion alone [15,16]. These findings emphasize the importance of performing diagnostic tests, particularly challenge/provocation procedures, under-blinded, placebo-controlled conditions.

Definition of terms
In 1984, the Royal College of Physicians and the British Nutrition Program formed a joint committee to address the public's concern about food processing and food allergies. In their report [17], they defined two main disorders: food intolerance or adverse physical reaction to a specific food or food ingredient that is reproducible under-blinded challenge conditions; and food aversion or "pseudo-food allergy," as Pearson called it [14], which includes psychological avoidance of food and psychogenic physical reactions to food due to emotions associated with the food rather than a physical response to the food itself, that is not reproducible in a blinded challenge. Food allergy is classified under food intolerance or adverse reaction with characteristic clinical and immunological abnormalities that may be immediate IgE-mediated or non-IgE mediated.

The key features differentiating the person with food aversion or food sensitivity, as they are currently called, from the person with a true food allergy or adverse food reaction are: (i) the absence or inconsistent finding of recognized signs and symptoms, physical findings, and laboratory evaluation supportive of an allergic, toxic, enzymatic, or pharmacological reaction to a specific food and (ii) the inability to reproduce symptoms or physical changes under adequately controlled double-blind food challenge conditions. Double-blind placebo-controlled food challenge (DBPCFC) in an appropriate clinical setting is the gold standard in the diagnosis of food allergy [18] and is the best method to avoid patient and observer bias [19].

Autism

Childhood autism is characterized by significant abnormal or impaired development in social interaction and communication, and restricted repertoire of activity and interests [1]. Immunological abnormalities, gluten sensitivity, and food allergy have been proposed to play a role in the pathogenesis and management of autism [20–22]. However, evidence supporting the beneficial effects of dietary manipulation on behavior and cognition in children with autism spectrum disorder has consisted mainly of anecdotal reports and small trials.

Bidet and colleagues [23] reported increased basophil degranulation to food allergens in 10 autistic children and Lucarelli [24] reported improvement in behavioral disturbance in 36 autistic children placed on a cow's milk elimination diet. More recently, two small trials examined the benefit of gluten and casein-free diets in autistic children. One trial [25] reported reduction in autistic traits but equivocal results on cognitive skills, and on linguistic and motor ability. The trial by Knivsberg [26] studied 10 autistic children over 1 year and reported improvement in the children on the gluten and casein-free diets.

Other studies by Sponheim [27], Renzoni, [28], and Pavone [29] were unable to demonstrate improvement in behavior with a gluten-free diet, or any association between autism and food allergy or celiac disease. Studies by Walker-Smith [30] and McCarthy [31] failed to demonstrate an increased prevalence of celiac disease in autistic patients using anti-gliadin assays and jejunal biopsies.

Lymphocytic infiltration in the upper and lower GI tract [32], immune activation [33], and abnormal lymphocytic responses to dietary antigens [34] have also been recently reported in children with autism, but the relevance of these findings to cognitive function or to development of autism is still unclear.

These studies demonstrate the need for large-scale quality-controlled trials in this area. Given the lack of hard evidence supporting the benefits of dietary manipulation in preventing or treating autistic patients, implementation of rigorous elimination diets should be undertaken with great caution. Such unproven measures may divert the autistic patient's family from more useful treatments and contribute to poor nutrition and further social isolation in families already facing great difficulties.

Schizophrenia

In 1966, it was proposed by Dohan [35] that gluten played a significant role in aggravating the symptoms of schizophrenia and that a gluten-free diet was of therapeutic value to these patients. Studies of the rate of mental hospital admissions for schizophrenic women and change in wheat consumption during World War II in the United States, Canada, Norway, Sweden, and Finland reported a high correlation further supporting this hypothesis [36,37]. Eaton and colleagues [38] reported increased risk of schizophrenia in patients with celiac disease in their analysis of Danish national registers [39].

Dohan and other researchers [40–42] also reported improvement in schizophrenic patients when placed on a gluten-free diet with improvement seen as early as 1 month and others needing 6–12 months, and deterioration when given a gluten challenge. However, only some schizophrenics, those who were chronically ill, had a poor prognosis, and had nuclear schizophrenia, seemed to respond best. Reports that the incidence of anti-gliadin antibodies were elevated in schizophrenic patients, and that wheat gluten had endorphin-like and opioid antagonist polypeptides properties that can cross into the brain in experimental animals initially lent support to this hypothesis [43–45].

Subsequent studies of gliadin antibody levels in schizophrenics and follow-up intestinal biopsies in antibody-positive patients did not find an increased incidence of coeliac disease (CD) in schizophrenic patients [46–48]. Other studies have failed to find any improvement in schizophrenic patients with a gluten-free diet. Potkin [49] studied eight schizophrenic patients who were placed on a closely supervised gluten-, cereal grains-, and milk-free diet for at least 13 weeks. They then underwent DBPC gluten challenge for a period of 5–8 weeks. No deterioration in clinical status was observed using the Brief Psychiatric Rating Scale (BPRS). Other researchers [50,51] were also unable to demonstrate any improvement with a gluten-free diet for a period as long as 9 months. West and colleagues [52], using data from the UK General Practice Research Database, a database of approximately 3 million patients, found no increased risk of schizophrenia in patients with celiac disease compared with the general population.

Milk was reported in one case to be associated with psychotic symptoms in a 14-year-old female with a history of GI intolerance to milk who developed symptoms on double-blind challenge [53]. Elevated IgA antibodies to gliadin, β-lactoglobulin, and casein were reported in 25 schizophrenic patients compared to controls, but the clinical relevance of this finding is unclear [54]. Other researchers [55,48] have not found elevated food antibodies in schizophrenic patients.

Coeliac disease and psychiatric disorders

CD, or gluten-sensitive enteropathy, is a chronic disease of the small intestinal mucosa with intermittent diarrhea, abdominal pain, distension, and irritability induced by gliadin, the prolamin protein of wheat [56]. Aside from the resulting weight loss and malabsorption, neurological and psychiatric illnesses have also been reported in patients with CD [57,58].

A high prevalence of anxiety, depression, and disruptive behavioral disorders has been reported in adults and adolescents with CD [59–61]. The prevalence of these disorders has been attributed to the reduction in the quality of life due to chronic disease in these patients [59,60] and serotonergic dysfunction due to impaired availability of tryptophan related to either malabsorption or impaired transport [62]. Hallert and Sedvall [63] reported significant increases in monoamine metabolites and tryptophan in the cerebrospinal fluid in patients with CD after being on a gluten-free diet for 1 year. De Santis and colleagues [64] reported a case of a patient with undiagnosed and untreated CD with psychiatric disorder. The patient's psychiatric symptoms disappeared and frontal cortex abnormalities normalized as documented by single photon emission computed tomography (SPECT) after beginning a gluten-free diet. Addolorato [59] studied 35 patients with CD, anxiety, and depression for 1 year on a gluten-free diet. They reported a significant decrease in anxiety state to values similar to controls after 1 year on the gluten-free diet without significant reduction in depression. They attributed these findings to the fact that anxiety in CD patients is predominantly reactive, and related to poor quality of life due to chronic illness, whereas depression is a characteristic of CD. They recommend that patients with CD obtain psychological support to improve compliance to treatment and limit-related disease complications. Pynnonen [65] also reported significant improvement in depressive symptoms in adolescents with celiac disease after 3 months on a gluten-free diet.

Hallert [63] studied 12 patients with CD and depression and reported no improvement in depressive symptoms after 1 year on a gluten-free diet despite improvement in small intestinal biopsies. However, he reported significant reduction in depression as evaluated by the Minnesota Multiphasic Personality Inventory (MMPI) after 6 months on oral pyridoxine (vitamin B6) therapy (80mg/day). Their findings suggest that the metabolic effects of pyridoxine deficiency may influence central nervous mechanisms regulating mood in CD.

Somatoform disorders

In 1984, Rix and colleagues [66] studied the psychiatric characteristics of 19 patients who believed they had allergies to multiple foods but were subsequently found not to be allergic on skin testing and double-blind provocation. These patients attributed to food allergy a variety of symptoms such as lethargy, head pain or tightness, abdominal discomfort, nausea, depression and irritability among others. The authors found this group to be almost identical, in terms of psychiatric symptoms, with a group of new psychiatric patients who attended an outpatient clinic. The majority of these patients had depressive neurotic complaints, which under current classification criteria could be categorized under the somatoform disorders.

The characteristic feature of the somatoform disorders is the presence of multiple physical symptoms that cannot be explained by a medical condition or by another mental disorder, and that cause significant social or occupational dysfunction [1]. Somatization disorder, conversion disorder, pain disorder, hypochondriasis, and body dysmorphic disorder are included in this category.

Somatization disorder is of special interest because food intolerance is a common complaint in these patients. Patients with this disorder complain of numerous physical problems over several years with onset before age 30. These complaints cannot be fully explained by any known medical condition, or if they occur in the presence of a medical condition, the resulting functional impairment is in excess of what would be expected.

Criteria for diagnosis require that the patient report at least four pain symptoms, two GI symptoms (which may include multiple food intolerance), one sexual symptom, and one pseudoneurological symptom. Patients with this disorder have increased suggestibility and are more likely to complain of multiple problems [67]. Other studies [68–70] have also found increased frequency of somatoform disorders, depression, and anxiety in community samples of professionals and students reporting intolerance to foods that are not confirmed by allergy skin testing or oral challenge.

Patients with somatoform disorders are the most frequently encountered type of patient who present with an unconfirmed food allergy and non-specific symptoms. They present a special challenge to the physician and require extra effort and support in terms of time, education, and attempts to build a rapport, since most patients will reject a psychiatric referral if they do not have a good relationship with their physicians and if they feel that their emotional and physical problems are not taken seriously.

Panic disorder and environmental intolerance

Self-reported multiple food intolerances/sensitivities have been reported to be frequently associated with idiopathic environmental intolerance (IEI), formerly called multiple chemical sensitivities (MCS) [66,71,72]. In 1987, Cullen [73] introduced the term "MCS," which he defined as "An acquired disorder characterized by recurrent symptoms, referable to multiple organ systems, occurring in response to demonstrable exposure to many chemically unrelated compounds at doses far below those established in the general population to cause harmful effects. No single widely accepted test of physiological function can be shown to correlate with symptoms." Other terms for IEI are cerebral allergy, chemically induced immune dysregulation, total allergy syndrome, and ecological illness [74].

The most common complaints are fatigue, headache, nausea, malaise, pain, mucosal irritation, disorientation, and dizziness, which are mostly non-specific. No gross or microscopic evidence of inflammation or other objective signs of pathology have been associated with IEI. As in somatoform disorders, these patients have multiple chronic symptoms and have previously consulted with numerous physicians and other health-care professionals without satisfaction nor any finding of underlying immunological, autoimmune, or any physical

12 Fry L, Mason AA, Pearson RS. Effect of hypnosis on allergic skin responses in asthma and hay fever. *BMJ* 1964;51:1145–8.

13 Godfrey S, Silverman M. Demonstration of placebo response in asthma by means of exercise testing. *J Psychosom Res* 1973;17:293–7.

14 Pearson DJ. Pseudo food allergy. *BMJ* 1986;292:221–2.

15 Horton DJ, Sude WL, Kinsman RA, *et al*. Bronchoconstrictive suggestions in asthma: a role for airways hyperreactivity and emotions. *Am Rev Respir Dis* 1978;117:1029–38.

16 Graham DR, Wolf S, Wolff H. Changes in tissue sensitivity associated with varying life situations and emotions: their relevance to allergy. *J Allergy* 1950;21:478–86.

17 Food intolerance and food aversion. A Joint report of the Royal College of Physicians and the British Nutrition Foundation. *J R Coll Physicians Lond.* 1984 Apr;18(2):83-123.

18 Metcalfe DD, Sampson HA. Workshop on experimental methodology for clinical studies of adverse reactions to foods and food additives. *J Allergy Clin Immunol* 1990;86:421–42.

19 Atkins FM. A critical evaluation of clinical trials in adverse reactions to foods in adults. *J Allergy Clin Immunol* 1986; 78:174–81.

20 Coleman M. Autism: non-drug biologic treatments. In: Gilbert C (ed.) *Diagnosis and Treatment of Autism*. New York: Plenum Press, 1989:219–35.

21 Goodwin MS, Cowen MA, Goodwin TC. Malabsorption and cerebral dysfunction: a multicariate and comparative study of autistic children. *J Autism Child Schiz* 1971;1:48–62.

22 Tsaltas MO, Jefferson T. A pilot study on allergic responses. *J Autism Dev Disord* 1986;16:91–2.

23 Bidet B, Leboyer M, Descours B, *et al*. Allergic sensitization in infantile autism. *J Autism Dev Disord* 1993;23:419–20.

24 Lucarelli S, Frediani T, Zingoni AM, *et al*. Food allergy and infantile autism. *Panminerva Med* 1995;37:137–41.

25 Millward C, Ferriter M, Calver S, Connel-Jones G. Gluten- and casein-free diets for autistic spectrum disorder. *Cochrane Database Syst Rev* 2004;2:CD003498.

26 Knivsberg AM, Reichelt KL, Hoien T, Nodland M. A randomised, controlled study of dietary intervention in autistic syndromes. *Nutr Neurosci* 2002;5:251–61.

27 Sponheim E. Gluten-free diet in infantile autism. A therapeutic trial. *Tidsskr Nor Laegeforen* 1991;111:704–7.

28 Renzoni E, Beltrami V, Sestani P, *et al*. Brief report: allergological evaluation of children with autism. *J Autism Dev Disord* 1995;25:327–33.

29 Pavone L, Fiumara A, Bottaro G, *et al*. Autism and coeliac disease: failure to validate the hypothesis that a link might exist. *Biol Psyhciatr* 1997;42:72–5.

30 Walker-Smith J. Gastrointestinal disease and autism-the result of a survey. *Symposium on Autism*. Sidney, Australia: Abbott Laboratories, 1973.

31 McCarthy DM, Coleman M. Response of intestinal mucosa to gluten challenge in autistic subjects. *Lancet* 1979;2:877–8.

32 Ashwood P, Anthony A, Pellicer AA, *et al*. Intestinal lymphocyte populations in children with regressive autism: evidence for extensive mucosal immunopathology. *J Clin Immunol* 2003; 23:504–17.

33 Ashwood P, Anthony A, Torrente F, Wakefield AJ. Spontaneous mucosal lymphocyte cytokine profiles in children with autism and gastrointestinal symptoms: mucosal immune activation and reduced counter regulatory interleukin-10. *J Clin Immunol* 2004;24:664–73.

34 Jyonouchi H, Geng L, Ruby A, Zimmerman-Bier B. Dysregulated innate immune responses in young children with autism spectrum disorders: their relationship to gastrointestinal symptoms and dietary intervention. *Neuropsychobiology* 2005; 51:77–85.

35 Dohan FC. Cereals and schizophrenia-data and hypotheses. *Acta Psychiatr Scand* 1966;42:125–52.

36 Dohan FC. Coeliac disease and schizophrenia. *Lancet* 1970;1:897–8.

37 Dohan FC, Harper EH, Clark MH, *et al*. Is schizophrenia rare if grain is rare? *Biol Psychiatr* 1984;19:385–99.

38 Eaton W, Mortensen PB, Agerbo E, *et al*. Coeliac disease and schizophrenia: population based case control study with linkage of Danish national registers. *BMJ* 2004;328:1017.

39 Campbell EB, Foley S. celiac disease and schizophrenia: data do not support hypothesis. *BMJ* 2004;328:1017.

40 Dohan FC, Grasberger JC. Relapsed schizophrenics: earlier discharge from the hospital after cereal-free, milk-free diet. *Am J Psychiatr* 1973;130:685–8.

41 Singh MM, Kay SR. Wheat gluten as a pathogenic factor in schizophrenia. *Science* 1976;191:401–2.

42 Rice JR, Ham CH, Gore WE. Another look at gluten in schizophrenia. *Am J Psychiatr* 1978;135:1417–18.

43 Hemmings WA, Williams EW. Transport of large breakdown products of dietary protein through the gut wall. *Gut* 1978;8:715–23.

44 Zioudrou C, Streaty RA, Klee WA. Opioid peptides derived from food proteins. The exorphins. *J Biol Chem* 1979; 254:2446–9.

45 Klee WA, Zioudrou C, Streaty RA. Endorphins, peptides with opioid activity isolated from wheat gluten, and their possible role in the etiology of schixophrenia In: Usdin E (ed.) *Endorphins in Mental Health Research*. New York: Macmillan, 1978.

46 Stevens FM, Lloyd RS, Geraghty SMJ, *et al*. Schizophrenia and coeliac disease – the nature of the relationship. *Psychol Med* 1977;7:259–63.

47 Dean G, Hanniffy L, Steven F, *et al*. Schizophrenia and coeliac disease. *J Med Assoc* 1975;68:545–6.

48 Peleg R, Ben-Zion ZI, Peleg A, *et al*. "Bread madness" revisited: screening for specific celiac antibodies among schizophrenia patients. *Eur Psychiatr* 2004;19:311–14.

49 Potkin SG, Weinberger D, Kleinman J, *et al*. Wheat gluten challenge in schizophrenic patients. *Am J Psychiatr* 1981; 138:1208–11.

50 Storms LH, Clopton JM, Wright C. Effects of gluten on schizophrenia. *Arch Gen Psychiatr* 1982;39:323–7.

51 Osborne M, Crayton JW, Javaid J, Davis JM. Lack of effect of gluten-free diet on neuroleptic blood levels in schizophrenic patients. *Biol Psychiatr* 1982;17:627–9.

52 West J, Logan RF, Hubbard RB, Card TR. Risk of schizophrenia in people with celiac disease, ulcerative colitis and Crohn's disease: a general population-based study. *Alimen Pharmacol Ther* 2006;23:71–4.

53 Denman AM. The relevance of immunopathology to research into schizophrenia. In: Hemmings J (ed.) *Biochemistry of Schizophrenia and Addiction*. Lancaster: MTP Press, 1980.

54 Reichelt KL, Landmark J. Specific IgA antibody increases in schizophrenia. *Biol Psychiatr* 1995;37:410–13.

55 Kinnell HG, Kirkwood E, Lewis C. Food antibodies in schizophrenia. *Psychol Med* 1982;12:85.

56 Corrazza GR, Gasbarrini G. Coeliac disease in adults. *Bailiere Clin Gastroenterol* 1995;9:329–50.

57 Gobbi G, Bouquet F, Greco L, *et al*. Coeliac disease, epilepsy and cerebral calcifications. *Lancet* 1992;340:439–443.

58 Hallert C, Derefeldt T. Psychic disturbances in adult coeliac disease. I. Clinical observations. *Scand J Gastroenterol* 1982;17:17–19.

59 Addorato G, Stefanini GF, Capristo E, *et al*. Anxiety and depression in adult untreated celiac subjects and in patients affected by inflammatory bowel disease: a personality trait or a reactive illness? *Hepatogastroenterology* 1996;43:1153–7.

60 Hallert C, Astrom J, Sedvall G. Psychic disturbances in adult coeliac disease. III. Reduced central monoamine metabolism and signs of depression. *Scand J Gastroenterol* 1982; 17:25–28.

61 Pynnonen PA, Isometsa ET, Aronen ET, *et al*. Mental disorders in adolescents with celiac disease. *Psychosom* 2004; 45:325–35.

62 Hernanz A, Polanco I. Plasma precursor amino acids of central nervous system monoamines in children with coeliac disease. *Gut* 1991;32:1478–81.

63 Hallert C, Astrom J, Walan A. Reversal of psychopathology in adult celiac disease with the aid of pyridoxine (vitamin B6). *Scand J Gastroentrol* 1983;18:299–304.

64 De Santis A, Addorato G, Romito A, *et al*. Schizophrenic symptoms and SPECT abnormalities in a coeliac patient: regression after a gluten-free diet. *J Intern Med* 1997;242:421–3.

65 Pynnonen PA, Isometsa ET, Verkasalo MA, *et al*. Gluten-free diet may alleviate depressive and behavioural symptoms in adolescents with celiac disease: a follow-up case-series study. *BMC Psychiatr* 2005;5:14.

66 Rix KJB, Pearson DJ, Bentley SJ. A psychiatric study of patients with supposed food allergy. *Br J Psych* 1984;145:121–6.

67 Woodruff R, Clayton P, Guze S. Hysteria-studies of diagnosis, outcome, and prevalence. *JAMA* 1971;215:425–8.

68 Vatn MH, Grimstad IA, Thorsen L, *et al*. Adverse reactions to food: assessment by double blind placebo-controlled food challenge and clinical, psychosomatic and immunological analysis. *Digestion* 1995;56:419–26.

69 Knibb RC, Armstrong A, Booth DA, *et al*. Psychological characteristics of people with perceived food intolerance in a community sample. *J Psychosom Res* 1999;57:545–54.

70 Bell IR, Schartz GE, Peterson JM, Amend D. Symptom and personality profiles of young adults from a college student population with self-reported illness from foods and chemicals. *J Am Coll Nutr* 1993;12:693–702.

71 Bell IR, Schwartz GE, Amend D, *et al*. Sensitization to early life stress and response to chemical odors in older adults. *Biol Psychiatr* 1994;35:857–63.

72 Ross GH. Clinical characteristics of chemical sensitivity: an illustrative case history of asthma and MCS. *Environ Health Perspect* 1997;105:437–41.

73 Cullen MR. The worker with multiple chemical hypersensitivities: an overview. *State Art Rev Occup Med* 1987;2:655–61.

74 Green MA. "Allergic to everything": 20th century syndrome. *JAMA* 1985;253:842.

75 Brodsky CM. "Allergic to everything": a medical subculture. *Psychosomatics* 1983;24:731–42.

76 Terr AI. Clinical ecology in the workplace. *J Occup Med* 1989;31:257–61.

77 Stewart DE, Raskin J. Psychiatric assessment of patients with 20th century disease. *Can Med Assoc J* 1985;133:1001–6.

78 Bailer J, Witthoft M, Paul C, *et al*. Evidence for overlap between idiopathic environmental intolerance and somatoform disorders. *Psychosom Med* 2005;67:921–9.

79 Simon G, Daniell W, Stockbridge H, *et al*. Immonologic, psychological and neuropsychological factors in multiple chemical sensitivity: a controlled study. *Ann Intern Med* 1993: 119:97–103.

80 Black DW, Rathe A, Golstein RB. Environmental illness: a controlled study of 26 subjects with "20th century disease." *JAMA* 1990;264:3166–70.

81 Dietel A, Jordan L, Muhlinghaus T, *et al*. Psychiatric disorders of environmental outpatients- results of the standardized psychiatric interview (CIDI) from the German multi-center study on Multiple Chemical Sensitivity (MCS). *Psychother Psychosom Med Psychol* 2006;56:162–71.

82 Papo D, Eberlein- Konig B, Berresheim HW, *et al*. Chemosensory function and psychological profile in patients with multiple chemical sensitivity: comparison with odor-sensitive and asymptomatic controls. *J Psychosom Res* 2006; 60:199–209.

83 Binkley KE, Kutcher S. Panic response to sodium lactate infusion in patients with multiple chemical sensitivity syndrome. *J Allergy Clin Immunol* 1997;99:570–4.

84 Poonal N, Antony MM, Binkley KE, *et al*. Carbon dioxide inhalation challenges in idiopathcic environmental intolerance. *J Allergy Clin Immunol* 2000;105:358–63.

85 Leznoff A. Provocative challenges in patients with multiple chemical sensitivity. *J Allergy Clin Immunol* 1997; 99:438–42.

86 Binkley K, King N, Poonal N, *et al*. Idiopathic environmental intolerance: increased prevalence of panic disorder-associated

cholecystokinin B receptor allele 7. *J Allergy Clin Immunol* 2001;107:887–90.

87 Young E, Patel S, Stoneham M, *et al*. The prevalence of reaction to food additives in a survey population. *J Coll Phys* 1987;721:214–47.

88 Young E, Stoneham MD, Petruckevitch A, *et al*. A population study of food intolerance. *Lancet* 1994;343:1127–30.

89 Howard LM, Wessely S. Psychiatry in the allergy clinic: the nature and management of patients with non-allergic symptoms. *Clin Exp Allergy* 1995;25:503–14.

90 Bass C, Benjamin S. The management of chronic somatisation. *Br J Psychiatr* 1993;162:472–80.

91 Buchwald A, Rudick Davis D. The symptoms of major depression. *J Abn Psychol* 1993;102:197–205.

92 Munoz-Furlong A. Daily coping strategies for patients and their families. *Pediatrics* 2003;111:1654–61.

93 Cohen BL, Noone S, Munoz-Furlong A, Sicherer SH. Development of a questionnaire to measure quality of life in families with a child with food allergy. *J Allergy Clin Immunol* 2004;114:1159–63.

94 Coleman MT, Newton KS. Supporting self-management in patients with chronic illness. *Am Fam Phy* 2005;72:1503–10.

45

CHAPTER 45
Foods and Rheumatological Diseases

Lisa K. Stamp and Leslie G. Cleland

KEY CONCEPTS

- There is little convincing evidence for rheumatoid arthritis (RA) occurring as a result of food allergy.
- Patients with RA commonly associate certain foods with increased joint symptoms, although in many cases this is not confirmed by formal assessments.
- Individual patients with RA may have an improvement in disease control on elimination of certain foods from the diet.
- Prolonged periods of fasting or hypocaloric diets should be avoided due to potential adverse outcomes.
- In patients with RA, long-term dietary supplementation with n-3 fatty acids is associated with improvements in disease activity when combined with disease modifying anti-rheumatic drug therapy.

Introduction

Broadly speaking food has been linked to joint symptoms in three ways. Firstly, primary food allergy can be associated with self-limited arthralgia (joint pain) and/or arthritis (joint inflammation) in addition to the other manifestations of allergy such as urticaria [1]. Secondly, reactive arthritis or Reiter's syndrome may be associated with a preceding gastrointestinal infection such as *Campylobacter*, acquired from eating contaminated food products. Thirdly, patients with primary inflammatory arthritis often report a link between certain foods and joint symptoms in regard to both disease timing and severity of symptoms. The causal link between diet and inflammatory arthritis is strongest for gout [2,3]. However, patients with other forms of inflammatory arthritis such as rheumatoid arthritis (RA) sometimes report an association between their symptoms and food. The frequency with which RA occurs as a consequence of true food allergy is uncertain and perhaps not frequent. Notwithstanding, certain foods seem to have a significant impact on disease activity for some individuals with RA and elimination of particular foods may benefit some patients. However, there is currently no easy way to predict who will respond to dietary avoidance strategies. There is more robust evidence for the benefits of dietary supplementation with n-3 fatty acids in RA. The focus of this chapter is the relationship between foods and RA.

Food Allergy: Adverse Reactions to Foods and Food Additives, 4th edition.
Edited by Dean D. Metcalfe, Hugh A. Sampson, and Ronald A. Simon.
© 2008 Blackwell Publishing, ISBN: 978-1-4501-5129-0.

Rheumatoid arthritis

RA is a chronic condition which affects 1–2% of the general population. The hallmark of RA is inflammation of the synovial lining of the joints. Early in the course of the disease the inflammation results in joint pain, swelling, and stiffness. Over time, the joints become damaged by erosion of bone and cartilage by inflamed synovial tissue (pannus), which leads to joint deformities and functional impairment. Disease classification criteria for RA rest on the pattern of joint involvement (symmetrical polyarthritis involving the small joints of the hands and feet), presence of rheumatoid factor (RF) in serum, and radiographic evidence of peri-articular erosions. Further laboratory features which aid the diagnosis of RA include elevated C-reactive protein (CRP) and antibodies against cyclic citrullinated peptide (CCP).

The aims of management in RA are reduction of symptoms, prevention of joint damage, and preservation of joint function. Pharmacological therapies, which are the mainstay of treatment, can be broadly classified into three groups:

1 Non-steroidal anti-inflammatory drugs (NSAIDs) which act rapidly to reduce pain but have no beneficial effect on long-term disease progression.

2 Corticosteroids which rapidly control inflammation and may reduce joint erosion, but are associated with many non-trivial unwanted effects.

3 Disease modifying anti-rheumatic drugs (DMARDs) (e.g. methotrexate, salazopyrin, tumor necrosis factor (TNF) blockers) which in general are slow to act but prevent long-term joint destruction and improve functional outcomes.

In addition to these standard medical therapies, patients frequently request information regarding alternative and/or complementary therapies, including dietary therapies for management of their disease. Up to 75% of RA patients believe food influences their symptoms and it has been reported that as many as 50% try dietary manipulation in an attempt to control their symptoms [4,5]. By contrast, relatively few physicians would regard diet as contributing to the etiology of RA or as having a significant role in the management of RA.

Diet in the etiology of rheumatoid arthritis

A number of genetic factors have been shown to predispose to RA. As heritability is well short of 100%, it follows that environmental factors contribute substantially to etiology. A number of epidemiological studies have examined the role of diet in the etiology of RA. A decreased risk of developing RA has been reported with high consumption of fish, a rich source of n-3 fatty acids [6]. Consumption of β-cryptoxanthin (a carotenoid found in fruit and vegetables) has also been associated with reduced risk for RA [7,8]. Some but not all studies have reported an increased risk of developing RA with high red meat consumption [9–11] and caffeine intake [12–14].

Evidence for an RA-like illness as a result of food allergy is sparse. Panush described two patients who developed subjective and objective evidence of a non-erosive, RF negative, palindromic inflammatory arthritis after exposure to shrimp and nitrites [15].

Genetics in the etiology of rheumatoid arthritis: the potential interaction with food

Twin studies provide a means for assessing the relative extent of contributions by genetic and environmental factors to multi-factorial diseases. In RA, the concordance rate in monozygotic twins is reported to be 12% [16] to 15% [17]. Quantitative genetic analysis using the data from both of these cohorts has demonstrated that the "heritability" or extent to which liability to RA is explained by genetic variation in the population is about 60% [18].

Human leukocyte antigen (HLA) class II alleles are among the most important genetic contributors to RA. HLA antigens are surface membrane molecules that play a central role in specific immunity through their ability to present peptide fragments that have been processed by antigen-presenting cells (APCs). HLA-DR molecules are strongly expressed on APCs, especially dendritic cells. They present peptides derived from both endogenous and exogenous antigens to CD4+ve T-cells. The HLA genes within the major histocompatibility complex (MHC) comprise the class I loci (A, B, and C) and the class II loci (DQ, DR, and DP). The alleles at these respective loci occur in non-random associations known as haplotypes. The strongest allelic associations in RA are with subtypes of HLA-DR4 and HLA-DR1, in particular

HLA-DR*0401, HLA-DR*0404, and HLA-DR*0101. These HLA-DR specificities are determined by the HLA-DRβ1 locus and have a conserved amino acid sequence in the third hypervariable region of the DRβ chain, known as the "shared epitope." The "shared epitope" is situated within the region of the DRβ chain that forms part of the peptide-binding groove which presents the antigen. It is this "shared epitope" portion that is thought to confer the risk of RA [19]. The canonical feature of the shared epitope is a positively charged pocket lined by neutral and positively charged amino acids. This configuration is favorable for presentation of peptide fragments with appropriately located negative charge. The "shared epitope" provides a potential mechanism whereby an individual may inherit a susceptibility to RA. According to this scenario, when a predisposed person meets a potentially pathogenic antigen in an appropriate immunological context (with endogenous and exogenous co-stimulatory molecules signaling a "danger" context), a pathogenic immune response may occur directed against either exogenous and endogenous antigens or both. From the perspective of a possible allergic component to RA, it is notable that the HLA-DR4 alleles have been associated with atopy. While food is an abundant source of exogenous antigens, presentation of peptides within the specialized immunological tissues of the gut mucosa generally evokes immunological tolerance rather than responsiveness because "danger signals" that promote the latter are typically lacking.

Food allergy/intolerance in rheumatoid arthritis

A number of case reports link symptom severity with certain foods in RA (Table 45.1). In all of these reports patients responded with an improvement in arthritic symptoms on elimination of the offending food from the diet. Van der Laar et al. have also reported on two patients with RA who had raised serum IgE concentrations to several foods, which reduced after elimination of the foods from the diet. This was accompanied by an improvement in clinical symptoms and a reduction in mast cells in both the synovial membrane and proximal small intestine [20]. However, while a number of patients describe food-related aggravation of symptoms, this often is not substantiated by more formal assessment [15].

The concept of food allergy/intolerance in RA has led to studies examining the effects of dietary manipulation on disease activity in RA. Dietary manipulation can be divided into two categories: exclusion diets where foods thought to increase symptoms are removed from the diet and supplementation diets where foods that improve symptoms are added to the diet. In RA, exclusion diets have been shown to be of some value in individual patients only. In comparison, supplementation of the diet with n-3 fatty acids has been shown to benefit groups of patients in randomized controlled trials. In this section we review the evidence for exclusion diets in RA.

Table 45.1 Reports of food allergy/intolerance in RA

Case summary	Allergen	Effect of removal of putative food allergen from diet	Effect of re-introduction of putative food allergen from diet	Reference
RF−ve RA, extra-articular manifestations, ↑ESR, ↑IgE	Cereals (skin prick test positive)	Remission	Recurrence of symptoms	[21]
Erosive RF−ve RA, 11 years duration	Milk and cheese	Significant improvement with ↓ESR, able to stop prednisone	Recurrence of symptoms within 24 hours of re-introduction of dairy products IgE antibodies to milk and cheese became positive during re-challenge	[22]
Active RA, 35 years duration	Corn	Improved, ↓ESR, able to stop DMARDs	Recurrence of symptoms	[23]
RF−ve arthritis elbow and tenosynovitis	Milk (RAST+ve for cow's milk)	Improved	Recurrence of symptoms	[24]
Spondylitis	Milk and wheat (serum-specific IgE+ve for milk and wheat)	Marked improvement	Recurrence of symptoms	[24]
RF+ve inflammatory arthritis	Milk (↑IgG anti-milk antibodies)	Improved	Challenges with milk resulted in deterioration of symptoms	[25]
Juvenile RA, 6 years duration, RF−ve	Cow's milk (lactose intolerant; IgG and IgM anti-milk antibodies)	Marked improvement	Multiple challenges resulted in recurrence of symptoms	[26]
Monoarthritis form of juvenile chronic arthritis, ANA−ve	Milk	Improved but not resolution	Swelling of the affected joint after milk challenge After 2 years patient asymptomatic and tolerating milk	[27]

ANA, antinuclear antibody; ESR, erythrocyte sedimentation rate; RAST, radioallergosorbent tests.

Elemental diets

Elemental diets are designed to provide foods in their simplest forms, thus proteins are provided as amino acids, carbohydrates as glucose or small saccharides, and fats as medium chain triglycerides. Such diets are thought to be hypoallergenic and thereby provide a means for determining whether food allergy/intolerance has a role in RA. There have been several studies using such diets in RA. Haugen et al. conducted a prospective, double-blind, controlled study in 20 patients with active RA. For 3 weeks patients received either an elemental diet or a control diet consisting of well mixed and blended soup which contained milk, meat, corn, and wheat. In the fourth week of the study all patients returned to their normal diet. While 3/10 patients in the elemental group and 2/7 patients in the control group improved, overall there was no significant difference between the two groups [28]. In a larger study by Holst-Jensen et al., 4 weeks of an artificial elemental peptide diet was compared to normal diet in 30 patients. Patients were assessed at baseline, at the end of the 4 weeks on the study diet and then at 3 and 6 months. While there were improvements in pain and Health Assessment Questionnaire (HAQ) scores at 4 weeks these improvements were lost by 3 months. Only one patient in the elemental

diet group was classified as a "responder" according to their predetermined criteria (ACR20 improvement (see box)) [29]. Similar findings with individual patient improvement, particularly in the more subjective aspects of disease assessment, have been reported by Kavanagh et al. [30]. While individual patients may benefit from such elemental diets, there is insufficient evidence to support their routine use in the management of RA. Furthermore, the benefits appear to be short-lived once patients return to a normal diet and the long-term sustainability of such diets is questionable.

ACR20 response

20% improvement in 5 of 7 core set variables, first two required:
Tender joint count
Swollen joint count
Acute-phase reactant
Patients' pain
Patients' global assessment of disease activity
Physicians' global assessment of disease activity
Physical disability
Reproduced from Felson D et al. [31], with permission from John Wiley and Sons, Inc.

Elimination diets

Elimination diets remove foods that are thought to be allergenic or "arthritogenic" in the case of RA, from the diet. An elimination diet needs to be continued for at least 3 weeks and is usually followed by gradual re-introduction of potentially offending foods. Such a diet trial is considered to be positive if elimination of those potentially allergenic foods from the diet results in clinical improvement with a subsequent deterioration after re-introduction. However, such studies are usually single-blind as patients are aware of what they eat, and a double-blind, placebo-controlled food challenge is the only validated test for the diagnosis of food allergy/intolerance.

As with elemental diets, elimination diets have been reported to be of some benefit in individual patients with RA. One such elimination diet, the Dong diet, contains little meat except occasional fish and chicken, no herbs or spices, dairy products, additives or preservatives, and no alcohol. The Dong diet was created by Dr. Dong after his personal experience of remission of arthritis with such a diet and gained widespread popularity among patients [32]. However, a 10-week double-blind, controlled study of the Dong diet in 33 patients with RA showed no overall benefit, although 2/11 patients did improve while on the Dong diet with subsequent deterioration after return to normal diet [33].

To achieve an even more restrictive diet, van der Laar et al. used artificial foods in order to remove potential allergens from the diet. Ninety-four patients with RA consumed their normal diet for 4 weeks and were then assigned either to an "allergen-free" (free of all potentially allergenic foods, additives, and preservatives) or "allergen-restricted" diet (contained milk proteins and yellow azo colorings) for 4 weeks, followed by a return to normal diet for the final 4 weeks of the study. Seventy-eight of the 94 patients completed the study and while there were subjective improvements in both groups, there was no difference between the two diets [34].

The majority of patients with RA are treated with DMARDs in an attempt to provide long-term control of the disease. Withholding or stopping DMARD therapy for the purposes of studying the effects of dietary manipulation would no longer be considered ethical. In addition, therapy in the 21st century is far more intensive than even 10 years ago, thus there would be very few patients with RA on no DMARD therapy. However, in the early 1980s Darlington et al. examined the effects of an elimination diet in 53 patients with RA receiving no DMARD treatment [35]. Patients were allocated to 6 weeks of dietary therapy immediately or 6 weeks of placebo followed by 6 weeks of dietary therapy. During the first week of the diet therapy phase, patients were only allowed foods thought very unlikely to cause symptoms; during the ensuing 5 weeks other foods considered more likely to cause symptoms, such as cereals, were gradually re-introduced. During the diet therapy phase there were significant improvements in pain, swollen joint count, and erythrocyte sedimentation rate (ESR). Interestingly, 9/10 (90%) patients with a family history of atopy had a good response to the diet therapy as compared to 24/34 (70.6%) patients with no family history of atopy ($p < 0.05$) [35]. While these results are encouraging, patients who do not require DMARD therapy are likely to have milder disease and the results of dietary studies in these patients may not be generalizable to those with more active or severe disease.

Compliance with such restrictive diets may be problematic, especially in the long term. Beri et al. undertook a complex dietary study in 27 patients with RA, whereby an isocaloric diet consisting of fruit, vegetables, sugar, and refined oil was consumed for 2 weeks, followed by stepwise 2 weekly additions of wheat, rice, milk, and finally non-vegetarian foods. Of the 52% of patients who completed the study, 71% sustained clinical improvement. However, only 3/27 patients adhered to the diet for 10 months [36].

These studies demonstrate that individual patients may respond to dietary manipulation and that compliance with dietary therapy is a major limiting factor in many cases. Determining an appropriate diet for an individual might be expected to result in clinical improvements and increased compliance. Skin prick test (SPT) of potential allergens is one means of determining if an allergy exists. In an attempt to "individualize" dietary manipulation, Karatay et al. studied 20 patients with RA who had a positive SPT for at least one food and 20 RA patients with negative SPT. All patients had clinically inactive disease at study entry. Initially patients underwent an elimination diet for 12 days in which the most common allergenic foods were avoided. This was followed by a 12-day "challenge phase" during which SPT-positive foods were added and finally a 12-day "re-elimination" phase whereby the SPT-positive foods were removed. In the control SPT-negative group, corn, which is reported to be a common allergenic food in RA, and rice, which is not thought to be an allergenic food, were added in increasing amounts. At the end of the challenge phase, swollen and tender joint counts, pain, patient and physician global assessment, morning stiffness, ESR, and CRP all increased significantly in the SPT-positive group. In the SPT-negative group only pain and patient global assessment increased during the "challenge phase." This increase in disease activity was observed in 13/18 (72%) SPT-positive patients compared to 3/20 (17%) SPT-negative patients during the "challenge phase" and continued in all but one patient during the "re-elimination" phase [37]. The authors concluded that food allergy may be a triggering factor in RA and that an individualized avoidance diet may be helpful in some patients. SPT may not be practical for many patients; thus in patients who believe their arthritis is due to or worsened by a particular food, objective measures of disease activity should be undertaken before and after one or more cycles of removal of the putative "food allergen." The resulting evidence may then be used by both the patient and physician to determine whether long-term avoidance of the "food allergen" is warranted.

Vegetarian and vegan diets

Vegan and vegetarian diets have been the subject of a number of studies in patients with RA. In the largest study, 66 patients with active RA were randomized to either a gluten-free vegan diet or a well-balanced non-vegetarian diet for 12 months. Only 58% of the vegan diet group and 89% of the control group completed at least 9 months of the study. At the 12-month endpoint 41% of the vegan diet group and 4% of the control group achieved an ACR20 response. Radiographic progression was similar in both groups. In those patients on the study diet who achieved the ACR20 response, a significant reduction in serum IgG-anti-gliadin antibodies and IgG-β-lactoglobulin antibodies was observed. The authors suggest a diminished immune response to exogenous food antigens may have had a role in the observed clinical benefits [38].

Other studies of vegetarian/vegan diets have been preceded by a period of fasting. In a 13-month prospective, single-blind trial, 27 patients with active RA were randomized to a 7–10 day fast followed by gradual re-introduction of foods, which were eliminated if they resulted in symptom deterioration. During the first 3½ months a gluten-free vegan diet was allowed with subsequent introduction of milk-based products and gluten. Twenty-six matched control patients with active RA continued their normal diet. In the diet group, improvements were noted as early as 1 month after entry with significant reductions in tender and swollen joint counts, duration of morning stiffness, ESR, and CRP. The improvements persisted throughout the duration of the study [39]. Of note, 10/27 (37%) patients in the diet group and 9/26 (35%) in the control group withdrew during the study period. Disease flare was the cause for withdrawal in 4/10 patients in the diet group and 7/9 in the control group while one patient in the diet group was unable to tolerate the diet. Importantly some patients were consuming cod-liver oil prior to and during the study period, although the exact numbers and doses are not revealed. As discussed below, cod-liver oil is rich in n-3 fatty acids which have been shown to provide a benefit in patients with RA. In those patients taking the cod-liver oil supplement, it is possible that the change in diet produced a more significant alteration in the ratio of dietary n-3/n-6 fatty acids, in favor of the less inflammatory n-3 fats, thereby contributing to at least some of the observed benefits. Ten of the 27 patients in the diet group who identified foods that exacerbated their symptoms were studied further. Of these 10 patients, 8 were classified as responders and 2 as non-responders to the dietary

regimen. However, in 9/10 patients there was no associated antibody activity to the suspected foods. Only one patient who suspected meat aggravated his arthritis symptoms was found to have elevated concentrations of IgM anti-BSA antibody activity, which subsequently reduced dramatically during the study period in parallel with a reduction in disease activity [40].

Living food consists of an uncooked vegan diet, rich in lactobacilli, with no animal products or added salt. Such a diet has been reported to result in subjective improvement in arthritis symptoms but no change in objective measures of disease activity in patients with RA [41]. Furthermore, the diet was poorly tolerated with half of the patients withdrawing due to adverse events (in particular nausea and diarrhea).

It has been suggested that a vegan diet which is also low in all kinds of fats is more likely to provide benefit to RA patients. In an uncontrolled trial, 24 patients with active RA maintained such a diet for 4 weeks. Compliance was not a problem with this diet, and improvements were observed in tender and swollen joint counts as well as pain scores. However, there was no improvement in duration of morning stiffness, ESR, or CRP [42]. Further, longer-term, double-blind-controlled studies of this diet are required.

Overall like elimination and elemental diets, vegetarian/vegan diets may be of benefit in some RA patients. However, restrictive diets are problematic with regard to compliance and there currently is no way to predict which patients will respond.

Mediterranean diet

The Mediterranean diet (MD) is characterized by a high consumption of fruits, vegetables, cereals, legumes and fish, moderate amounts of wine and olive oil as the primary source of fat. Such a diet is thought to be healthy and appears to be helpful in the secondary prevention of coronary artery disease [43]. The MD has been compared to a typical Western diet in 56 patients with active RA. Patients in both groups were provided with lunch and dinner at a hospital cafeteria for the first 3 weeks. During these 3 weeks patients in the MD group were instructed on Mediterranean food and its preparation and were provided with written instructions and recipes to use during the ensuing 9 weeks of the study, during which period they prepared their food at home. At the end of the 12-week study period there was a significant reduction in the disease activity score (DAS28) (see box), HAQ, swollen joint count, and CRP in patients on the MD compared to baseline, while there were no significant changes in the control group [44]. At least some of the improvements may be due to the increased intake of olive oil which is rich in oleic acid, a precursor to eicosatrienoic acid, which like the n-3 fatty acids can inhibit arachidonic acid (AA) metabolism (see below).

Fasting

Total and sub-total fasting have preceded some studies of vegetarian/vegan diets. In most cases improvements were observed during the fasting period, but rapidly disappeared on re-introduction of food [39,46–48]. Patients with RA frequently lose weight during periods of active disease. However, even patients with well-controlled disease have a lower body cell mass compared to healthy controls [49,50]. Rheumatoid cachexia is a term used to describe the severe loss of body cell mass that may occur (for recent review see [51]). This reduction in body cell mass can occur despite adequate protein and calorie intake and is associated with increased resting energy expenditure and protein catabolism as well as reduced physical activity. Diets which restrict protein and calorie intake may further compound this loss of body cell mass and should be avoided. In this regard, fasting which can only be maintained for short periods may still be detrimental. Given that the benefits of fasting are modest and short-lived when compared with the chronic nature of RA, fasting is an impractical approach to the management of RA.

Potential mechanisms of food intolerance/allergy rheumatoid arthritis

A number of potential mechanisms have been postulated for the observed responses in those patients who respond to elimination of suspected food allergens.

Disease and psychological factors

Patients who are willing to undertake dietary manipulation studies, particularly diets that involve fasting or are severely restrictive, may differ from the general RA population. One study which examined the psychological characteristics of patients participating in a study of a fasting/vegetarian diet, reported that study participants believed more in "alternative" treatments and less in "standard" medical treatments, had a higher perceived ability to control their own health and a lower perception that chance affected their health and response to treatment than non-study participants. Furthermore, those study participants who responded to the diet believed less in ordinary medical treatment than the non-responders [52]. While these data suggest that psychological factors do indeed play a role, one would not usually expect

clinical improvements to last for such an extended period of time (12 months) if this was the sole explanation.

Patients who are prepared to take part in dietary studies may also differ with respect to the severity of disease. In the study by Kjeldsen-Kragh *et al.*, study participants had shorter disease duration and less steroid and DMARD therapy suggesting milder disease compared to a group of non-study participants [52].

Weight loss

In the majority of dietary studies in RA, weight loss has been observed despite the dietary protocols aiming to be isocaloric. In general, weight loss *per se* has not been associated with improved disease control in these studies [35,39]. However, significant associations between reduction in body mass index and reduction in swollen joint count [53] and between weight loss and improved grip strength [31] have been reported. More recently, analysis of data from three previous studies of lacto-vegetarian, vegan, or MD suggests that weight loss *per se* does contribute to the observed improvements in disease control in patients on these kinds of diets [54].

Alterations in pro-inflammatory cytokines

A number of pro-inflammatory cytokines including interleukin (IL)-1, IL-6, and TNF are important in the inflammation and tissue destruction observed in RA.

Serum and synovial fluid IL-6 concentrations are increased in patients with RA. IL-6 has a role in regulation of the acute phase response, activation of T-cells, and may have a role in bone destruction [55]. A significant reduction in IL-6, along with a decrease in ESR and CRP, has been observed after a 7-day fast in 10 patients with RA [56].

IL-1β and TNF are both implicated in the tissue destruction seen in RA [57–59]. Biological agent therapies that block TNF or IL-1β activities have been shown to reduce disease activity and prevent joint damage in RA [60,61]. Recently, a small study has examined the effect of allergenic foods on serum TNF and IL-1β concentrations in patients with RA. In patients challenged with foods, which had previously resulted in a positive SPT, serum TNF and IL-1β concentrations increased along with an increase in clinical disease activity [62]. The authors concluded that food allergy may be a "triggering" rather than a causative factor in RA and that such allergy may increase the concentration of TNF and IL-1β.

Alterations in dietary fatty acid composition

Dietary polyunsaturated fatty acids (PUFAs) are subject to remodeling and incorporated into cell membrane phospholipids. The C20 PUFAs are released from cell membranes by phospholipase A_2 and can then be metabolized to inflammatory lipid mediators known as eicosanoids (prostaglandins (PG) and leukotrienes (LT)). The n-6 fatty acid, linoleic acid (LA), is converted to AA, the precursor for the pro-inflammatory eicosanoids PGE_2, PGI_2, thromboxane (TX)A_2,

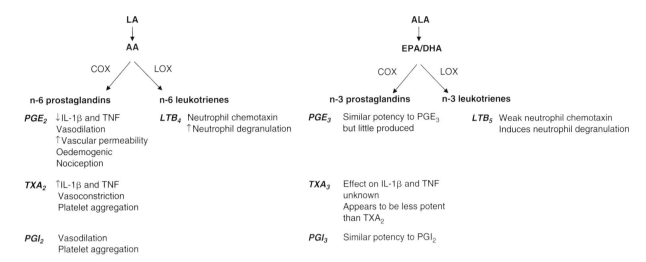

Figure 45.1 Metabolism of LA and ALA.

and LTB_4 (Fig. 45.1). In comparison, the n-3 fatty acid, α-linoleic acid (ALA), can be converted in a limited way to eicosapentaneoic acid (EPA). EPA is a substrate inhibitor of AA metabolism to eicosanoids and EPA itself can be converted to the three series eicosanoids (PGE_3, TXA_3, PGI_3, LTB_5), which are generally less inflammatory than the AA-derived eicosanoids (Fig. 45.1). The limited conversion of ALA to EPA within the context of a Western diet has led to the use of dietary supplements of EPA rich fish oils as a means of achieving anti-inflammatory effects. Alteration of dietary fatty acids may therefore modulate inflammatory disease expression (discussed further in section of n-3 fatty acids).

After a 1-week fast, the relative proportion of both AA and EPA has been shown to increase in serum and platelets. Although the increase in AA and EPA was small in neutrophils, there was a reduction in LTB_4 release from stimulated neutrophils *ex vivo* [38]. While plasma AA concentrations have been shown to decrease in patients on a vegan diet, concentrations returned to baseline values when the diet was changed to lacto-vegetarian. In comparison, EPA decreased with both the vegan and lacto-vegetarian diets [63]. However, fatty acid concentrations were no different between diet responders and non-responders, suggesting that other mechanisms must be responsible for the observed benefits of such diets [62].

Alterations in intestinal microbial flora

The intestine is a rich source of microbes and the balance of microbes present contributes to an individual's overall health. Changes in intestinal microbial flora are believed to contribute to many chronic diseases [64]. For example, patients with RA have a high carriage rate of *Clostridium perfringens* compared to healthy controls. Furthermore, those patients with active RA had significantly higher clostridia counts compared to those with inactive disease [65]. Genetic variations in the way individuals respond to normal gut

flora may also contribute. *Proteus mirabilis*, a normal bowel commensal, contains an amino acid sequence similar to that found in the "shared epitope" and patients with RA have higher titers of antibodies directed against this sequence compared to both patients with ankylosing spondylitis and healthy controls [66]. Furthermore, patients with active RA have higher concentrations of anti-*proteus* antibodies compared to patients with inactive RA, healthy controls and healthy HLA-identical same sexed siblings [67].

The diet can have a significant impact on fecal microbial flora and may thus provide a mechanism for alterations in disease activity. With respect to *Proteus mirabilis*, in RA patients who fasted for 7–10 days followed by 1-year vegetarian diet, there was a significant reduction in anti-*proteus* antibodies, which was greater in those patients who responded to the dietary therapy. Furthermore, a correlation was seen between reduced antibody levels and the extent of reduction in disease activity [68]. Alterations in fecal microbial flora, which correlate with improvements in disease activity, have also been observed in patients on a vegan diet, although individual organisms could not be identified with the method employed [69]. However, in a more recent study, neither fasting for 8 days nor a 2-week vegetarian MD altered fecal bacterial counts despite a significant reduction in the DAS28 score in the fasting group [70].

Altered intestinal permeability and gut antigen handling

The gastrointestinal epithelium is a complex structure which allows entry of essential nutrients while at the same time providing a critical barrier which prevents antigens in the lumen gaining access to the circulation. Abnormal intestinal permeability may have a role in the pathogenesis of autoimmune disorders [71]. In a small study of five patients with RA, fasting decreased intestinal permeability and was accompanied by improved disease control. Furthermore, when patients were started on a lacto-vegetarian diet, intestinal permeability and disease activity both increased [72]. Although limited, such data suggest that alterations in intestinal permeability, which allows increased entry of "arthritogenic" pathogens, may have a role in RA.

In addition to providing a physical barrier, the gut has a highly developed immune system (known as mucosa-associated lymphoid tissue (MALT)), that protects the host from potentially harmful pathogens, while simultaneously "tolerating" or allowing entry of "beneficial" antigens. MALT, which includes Peyers patches, has a preference for production of IgA, in particular secretory IgA, which is released into the gut lumen where it binds and prevents antigens from attaching to intestinal cells and gaining entry. In both patients with RA and healthy controls, short-term fasting has been reported to enhance mucosal antigen-specific B-cell responses but not systemic immune responses [73]. Thus activation of the mucosal immune system may not be reflected in the serum. A recent study has investigated this link among the mucosal immune system, food antibodies, and RA by examining jejunal fluid as well as serum [65]. In comparison to healthy controls, patients with RA had significantly increased concentrations of IgM in jejunal fluid. While there was an increase in IgA and IgG concentrations, this did not reach statistical significance. The activities of jejunal IgA, IgM, and IgG antibodies against a variety of different food antigens were also increased. The authors suggest that mucosal immune activation is important in the pathogenesis of RA, at least in some patients, and that apparent food intolerance may reflect the additive effect of hypersensitivity reactions [74].

Dietary n-3 supplementation and rheumatoid arthritis

n-3 fatty acids, which are abundant in fish and fish oils, have been shown to have a beneficial effect in patients with both early [75] and long-standing RA when combined with standard DMARD therapies (for review see [76]). For maximal benefits of n-3 supplementation to be achieved, the background diet should be low in competitor n-6 fatty acids [77]. Only one study has examined the effects of a diet containing hypoallergenic foods as well as being high in mono- and polyunsaturated fatty acids and low in saturated fatty acids. In this 24-week double-blind randomized, controlled study, 50 patients with RA were randomized to the experimental diet or a balanced control diet. In the experimental diet group, modest improvements were observed in all clinical variables although only ESR and tender joint count improved significantly [78]. The relative contributions of fatty acids and hypoallergenic foods to the outcomes could not be distinguished.

Like most of the DMARDs, there is a latent period of 6–12 weeks before benefits of n-3 supplements are observed and it is important that patients appreciate the lack of immediate effect when they commence n-3 supplements. The latent period can be shortened with use of higher doses [79–82].

Many patients with RA use NSAIDs on a regular or as required basis. Dietary supplementation with n-3 fatty acids has been shown to reduce NSAID requirements [83–86]. NSAIDs are associated with gastrointestinal toxicity and may contribute to an increase in risk of cardiovascular disease [87–88]. Furthermore, NSAIDs alter the ratio of TXA_2/PGE_2 in favor of TXA_2, which increases monocyte production of the pro-inflammatory cytokines IL-1β and TNF [89]. Thus the reduction in NSAID requirement associated with n-3 supplementation has a number of additional benefits including reduction in cardiovascular and gastrointestinal risk and potentially less joint damage.

The dose of n-3 fatty acids (EPA + DHA) required for the anti-inflammatory effect is 2.7 g/day, which equates to at least nine standard fish oil capsules daily. Perhaps a more efficient way of ingesting sufficient n-3 fatty acids is through bottled fish oil; 15 ml of fish oil, taken on fruit juice is for many patients easier to consume than large numbers of capsules and is significantly cheaper (~45 cents/day compared to ~$3.00/day for capsules).

Anti-inflammatory mechanisms of n-3 fatty acids

Fish and fish oils are rich in the n-3 long-chain fatty acids EPA (20:5 n-3) and docosahexaenoic acid (DHA; 22:5 n-3). EPA and DHA can be incorporated into cell membranes and tissues and may displace the n-6-derived AA (20:4 n-6). These n-3 and n-6 fatty acids are released from cell membranes and are metabolized by cyclo-oxygense (COX) or lipoxygenase (LOX) and the terminal synthases to the eicosanoids (PG and TX) and LT, respectively (Fig. 45.1). In general the n-6-derived eicosanoids (PGE_2, TXA_2, PGI_2, LTB_4) are more pro-inflammatory than their n-3-derived counterparts (PGE_3, TXA_3, PGI_3, LTB_5). In humans, dietary supplementation with n-3 fatty acids has been shown to reduce production of PGE_2 [90,91], TXA_2 [91], and LTB_4 [92], and increase production of TXA_3 [93] and LTB_5 [94]. DHA can be converted to C22 oxylipids, which also have anti-inflammatory properties.

In addition to their effects on eicosanoid production, n-3 fatty acids have been shown to decrease production of IL-1β and TNF, which are important mediators of tissues damage in RA, in both healthy subjects and patients with RA [81,90,91,95,96].

Matrix metalloproteinases (MMPs) have a pivotal role in cartilage degradation and bone erosion in RA. *In vitro* studies have demonstrated that n-3 fatty acids can suppress MMP expression and reduce proteoglycan degradation in IL-1-stimulated bovine chondrocytes [97,98]. Thus n-3 fatty acids may have the ability to reduce cartilage damage in inflamed joints.

As discussed above, class II MHC molecules (HLA-DR) are strongly expressed on APCs and present antigen to T-cells. *In vitro*, the n-3 fatty acids EPA and/or DHA reduce monocyte expression of HLA-DR and HLA-DP molecules [99], and reduce the ability of monocytes to present antigen to autologous lymphocytes [100]. In RA, one could speculate that n-3 fatty acids may inhibit APC function and suppress pathogenic T-cell activation, thereby reducing disease activity.

Cardiovascular risk in rheumatoid arthritis and the benefits of n-3 supplements

Patients with RA have an increased risk of death with a standardized mortality ratio of ~2 and most excess deaths are attributable to cardiovascular and cerebrovascular disease [101]. The risk of non-fatal myocardial infarction is also increased in patients with RA. In the Nurses' Health Study the adjusted relative risk (RR) of myocardial infarction in women with RA compared to women without RA was 2.0 (95% CI: 1.23–3.29). Furthermore, women with RA for >10 years had a RR of myocardial infarction of 3.1 (95% CI: 1.64–5.87) compared to women without RA [102]. There is no increase in traditional cardiovascular risk factors in patients to explain the observed increase [103]. The inflammatory process as well as use of NSAIDs may contribute to the increase risk [104]. In both primary and secondary prevention studies, n-3 fatty acid supplementation has been shown to reduce cardiovascular mortality [105]. To date there have been no studies examining whether n-3 fatty acid supplementation reduces cardiovascular morbidity and mortality in RA. However, a recent study has shown that patients with early RA taking n-3 fatty acid supplementation have lower triglycerides, increased "good" HDL cholesterol, lower CRP, less NSAID use, greater disease suppression, and reduced platelet synthesis of TXA_2 compared to patients not taking fish oil [58]. All of these factors would be expected to reduce cardiovascular risk.

Potential side effects of n-3 supplements

The most common adverse effects of n-3 fatty acid supplements are a fishy after-taste, gastrointestinal upset and nausea. In general these adverse effects are mild and can be controlled by taking the supplement with food. Fish can contain toxins, including methylmercury, polychlorinated biphenyls (PCBs), and dioxins which would accumulate in humans who consume contaminated fish on a regular basis. These toxins are in general reduced to acceptable limits in readily available commercial fish oils during processing.

Summary

Dietary restriction may prove useful in controlling RA in suitably motivated patients. Difficulties encountered in sustaining exclusion and other rigorous diets militate against a general application. By contrast dietary fish in appropriate doses is relatively easy to take as a dietary additive. The preferred method is to take bottled fish oil on juice with the two glass technique (quickly swallow 15 ml of fish oil layered on juice, then begin slowly sipping a juice chaser immediately, followed by food). This is the least expensive and most convenient way to achieve an anti-inflammatory dose of fish oil, since the equivalent dose of capsules is 14 × 1000 mg capsules. The symptomatic benefits of fish oil are delayed until the second or third month of treatment and include reduced reliance on NSAIDs, which carry risk for serious gastrointestinal and cardiovascular events. Fish oil in the long term also improves disease control and remission rates with DMARD therapy. There are thus two contrasting approaches, which are not mutually exclusive: elimination of candidate food allergens and arthritogens, while maintaining balance in the diet otherwise, and ingestion of increased amounts of the n-3 fatty acids EPA and DHA in essentially pharmacological, anti-inflammatory doses as a dietary supplement. The latter approach is generally applicable, while the former in practice may be best applied in those who are well disposed to dietary avoidance strategies.

References

1 Golding D. Is there an allergic synovitis? *J Roy Soc Med* 1990; 83:312–14.

2 Choi H, Liu S, Curhan G. Intake of purine-rich foods, protein, and dairy products and relationship to serum levels of uric acid. *Arthritis Rheum* 2005;52:283–9.

3 Choi H, Atkinson K, Karlson E, *et al.* Purine-rich foods, dairy and protein intake, and the risk of gout in men. *N Engl J Med* 2004;350:1093–103.

4 Martin RH. The role of nutrition and diet in rheumatoid arthritis. *Proc Nutr Soc* 1998;57:231–4.

5 Salminen E, Heikkila S, Poussa T, *et al.* Female patients tend to alter their diet following the diagnosis of rheumatoid arthritis and breast cancer. *Prev Med* 2002;34:529–35.

6 Shapiro JA, Koepsell TD, Voigt LF, *et al.* Diet and rheumatoid arthritis in women: a possible protective effect of fish consumption. *Epidemiology* 1996;7:256–63.

7 Cerhan J, Saag K, Merlino L, *et al.* Antioxidant micronutrients and risk of rheumatoid arthritis in a cohort of older women. *Am J Epidemiol* 2003;157:345–54.

8 Pattison D, Symmons D, Lunt M, *et al.* Dietary β-cryptoxanthin and inflammatory polyarthritis: results from a population-based prospective study. *Am J Clin Nutr* 2005;82:451–5.

9 Pattison D, Symmons D, Lunt M, *et al.* Dietary risk factors for the development of inflammatory polyarthritis. Evidence for a high level of red meat consumption. *Arthritis Rheum* 2004;50: 3804–12.

10 Grant W. The role of red meat in the expression of rheumatoid arthritis. *Br J Nutr* 2000;84:589–95.

11 Pedersen M, Stripp C, Klarlund M, *et al.* Diet and risk of rheumatoid arthritis in a prospective cohort. *J Rheumatol* 2005;32:1249–52.

12 Mikuls T, Cerhan J, Criswell L, *et al.* Coffee, tea, and caffeine consumption and risk of rheumatoid arthritis. *Arthritis Rheum* 2002;46:83–91.

13 Heliovaara M, Aho K, Knekt P, *et al.* Coffee consumption, rheumatoid factor, and the risk of rheumatoid arthritis. *Ann Rheum Dis* 2000;59:631–5.

14 Karlson E, Mandl L, Aweh G, *et al.* Coffee consumption and risk of rheumatoid arthritis. *Arthritis Rheum* 2003;48:3055–60.

15 Panush RS. Food induced (allergic) arthritis: clinical and serological studies. *J Rheumatol* 1990;17:291–4.

16 Aho K, Koskenvuo M, Tuominen J, *et al.* Occurrence of rheumatoid arthritis in a nationwide series of twins. *J Rheumatol* 1986;13:899–902.

17 Silman A, MacGregor A, Thomson W, *et al.* Twin concordance rates for rheumatoid arthritis: results from a nationwide study. *Br J Rheumatol* 1993;32:903–7.

18 MacGregor A, Snieder H, Rigby A, *et al.* Characterizing the quantitative genetic contribution to rheumatoid arthritis using data from twins. *Arthritis Rheum* 2000;43:30–7.

19 Gregersen P, Silver J, Winchester R. The shared epitope hypothesis: an approach to understanding the molecular genetics of susceptibility to rheumatoid arthritis. *Arthritis Rheum* 1987;30:1205–13.

20 van der Laar MA, Aalbers M, Bruins F, *et al.* Food intolerance in rheumatoid arthritis. II. Clinical and histologic aspects. *Ann Rheum Dis* 1992;51:303–6.

21 Lunardi C, Bambara L, Biasi D, *et al.* Food allergy and rheumatoid arthritis. *Clin Exp Rheumatol* 1988;6:423–5.

22 Parke AL, Hughes GRV. Rheumatoid arthritis and food: a case study. *BMJ* 1981;282:2027–9.

23 Williams R. Rheumatoid arthritis and food: a case study (letter). *BMJ* 1981;283:563.

24 Pacor M, Lunardi C, Di Lorenzo G, *et al.* Food allergy and seronegative arthritis: a report of two cases. *Clin Rheumatol* 2001;20:279–81.

25 Panush RS, Stroud RM, Webster EM. Food-induced (allergic) arthritis: inflammatory arthritis exacerbated by milk. *Arthritis Rheum* 1986;29:220–6.

26 Ratner D, Eshel E, Vigder K. Juvenile rheumatoid arthritis and milk allergy. *J Roy Soc Med* 1985;78:410–13.

27 Schrander J, Marcelis C, de Vries R, *et al.* Does food intolerance play a role in juvenile chronic arthritis? *Br J Rheumatol* 1997;36:905–8.

28 Haugen M, Kjeldsen-Kragh J, Forre O. A pilot study of the effect of an elemental diet in the management of rheumatoid arthritis. *Clin Exp Rheumatol* 1994;12:275–9.

29 Holst-Jensen SE, Pfeiffer-Jensen M, Monsrud M, *et al.* Treatment of rheumatoid arthritis with a peptide diet. A randomized, controlled trial. *Scand J Rheumatol* 1998;27:329–36.

30 Kavanagh R, Workman E, Nash P, *et al.* The effects of elemental diet and subsequent food reintroduction on rheumatoid arthritis. *Br J Rheumatol* 1995;34:270–3.

31 Felson D, Anderson J, Boers M, *et al.* The American College of Rheumatology preliminary definition of improvement in rheumatoid arthritis. *Arthritis Rheum* 1995;38:727–35.

32 Ziff M. Diet in the treatment of rheumatoid arthritis. *Arthritis Rheum* 1983;26:457–61.

33 Panush R, Carter R, Katz P, *et al.* Diet therapy for rheumatoid arthritis. *Arthritis Rheum* 1983;26:462–71.

34 van der Laar MA, van der Korst JK. Food intolerance in rheumatoid arthritis. I. A double blind, controlled trial of the clinical effects of elimination of milk allergens and azo dyes. *Ann Rheum Dis* 1992;51:298–302.

35 Darlington LG, Ramsey NW, Mansfield JR. Placebo-controlled, blind study of dietary manipulation therapy in rheumatoid arthritis. *Lancet* 1986:236–8.

36 Beri D, Malaviya AN, Shandilya R, *et al.* Effect of dietary restrictions on disease activity in rheumatoid arthritis. *Ann Rheum Dis* 1988;47:69–72.

37 Karatay S, Erdem T, Kiziltunc A, *et al.* General or personal diet: the individualized model for diet challenges in patients with rheumatoid arthritis. *Rheumatol Int* 2006;26:556–60.

38 Hafstrom I, Ringertz B, Spangberg A, *et al.* A vegan diet free of gluten improves the signs and symptoms of rheumatoid arthritis: the effects on arthritis correlate with a reduction in antibodies to food antigens. *Rheumatology* 2001;40:1175–9.

39 Kjeldsen-Kragh J, Borchgrevink C, Mowinkel P, *et al.* Controlled trial of fasting and one-year vegetarian diet in rheumatoid arthritis. *Lancet* 1991;338:899–902.

40 Kjeldsen-Kragh, Hvatum M, Haugen M, *et al.* Antibodies against dietary antigens in rheumatoid arthritis patients treated with fasting and one-year vegetarian diet. *Clin Exp Rheumatol* 1995;13:167–72.

41 Nenonen M, Helve T, Rauma A, *et al.* Uncooked, lactobacilli-rich, vegan food and rheumatoid arthritis. *Br J Rheumatol* 1998;37:274–81.

42 McDougall J, Bruce B, Spiller G, *et al.* Effects of a very low-fat vegan diet in subjects with rheumatoid arthritis. *J Altern Complement Med* 2002;8:71–5.

43 de Lorgeril M, Renaud S, Mamelle N, *et al.* Mediterranean alpha-linolenic acid-rich diet in secondary prevention of coronary heart disease. *Lancet* 1994;343:1454–9.

44 Skoldstam L, Hagfors L, Johansson G. An experimental study of a Mediterranean diet intervention for patients with rheumatoid arthritis. *Ann Rheum Dis* 2003;62:208–14.

45 Prevoo M, van't Hof M, van Leeuwen M, *et al.* Modified disease activity scores that include twenty-eight-joint counts. *Arthritis Rheum* 1995;38:44–8.

46 Skoldstam L, Larsson L, Lindstrom F. Effects of fasting and lactovegetarian diet on rheumatoid arthritis. *Scand J Rheumatol* 1979;8:249–55.

47 Hafstrom I, Ringertz B, Gyllenhammar H, *et al.* Effects of fasting on disease activity, neutrophil function, fatty acid composition, and leukotriene biosynthesis in patients with rheumatoid arthritis. *Arthritis Rheum* 1988;31:585–92.

48 Uden A-M, Trang L, Venizelos N, *et al.* Neutrophil functions and clinical performance after total fasting in patients with rheumatoid arthritis. *Ann Rheum Dis* 1983;42:45–51.

49 Roubenoff R, Cannon J, Kehayias JJ, *et al.* Rheumatoid cachexia: cytokine-driven hypermetabolism accompanying reduced body cell mass in chronic inflammation. *J Clin Invest* 1994;93:2379–86.

50 Walsmith J, Abad L, Kehayias J, *et al.* Tumor necrosis factor-α is associated with less body mass in women with rheumatoid arthritis. *J Rheumatol* 2004;31:23–9.

51 Rall L, Roubenoff R. Rheumatoid cachexia: metabolic abnormalities, mechanisms and interventions. *Rheumatology* 2004;43:1219–23.

52 Kjeldsen-Kragh J, Haugen M, Forre O, *et al.* Vegetarian diet for patients with rheumatoid arthritis: Can the clinical effects be explained by the psychological characteristics of the patients? *Br J Rheumatol* 1994;33:569–75.

53 Hansen GV, Nielsen L, Kluger E, *et al.* Nutritional status of Danish rheumatoid arthritis patients and effects of a diet adjusted in energy intake, fish-meal, and antioxidants. *Scand J Rheumatol* 1996;25:325–30.

54 Skoldstam L, Brudin L, Hagfors L, *et al.* Weight reduction is not a major reason for improvement in rheumatoid arthritis from lacto-vegetarian, vegan or Mediterranean diets. *Nutr J* 2005;4:15–21.

55 Wong P, Campbell I, Egan P, *et al.* The role of the interleukin-6 family of cytokines in inflammatory arthritis and bone turnover. *Arthritis Rheum* 2003;48:1177–89.

56 Fraser D, Thoen J, Djoseland O, *et al.* Serum levels of interleukin-6 and dehydroepiandrosterone sulphate in response to either fasting or a ketogenic diet in rheumatoid arthritis patients. *Clin Exp Rheumatol* 2000;18:357–62.

57 Arend WP, Dayer J-M. Inhibition of the production and effects of interleukin-1 and tumor necrosis factor-α in rheumatoid arthritis. *Arthritis Rheum* 1995;38:151–60.

58 Badolato R, Oppenheim J. Role of cytokines, acute-phase proteins and chemokines in the progression of rheumatoid arthritis. *Semin Arthritis Rheum* 1996;26:526–38.

59 Brennan FM, Maini RN, Feldmann M. TNF-α – a pivotal role in rheumatoid arthritis. *Br J Rheumatol* 1992;31:293–8.

60 Keystone EC, Kavanagh AF, Sharp J, *et al.* Radiographic, clinical, and functional outcomes of treatment with Adalimumab (a human anti-tumor necrosis factor monoclonal antibody) in patients with active rheumatoid arthritis receiving methotrexate therapy. *Arthritis Rheum* 2004;50:1400–11.

61 Dayer J-M, Feige U, Edwards C, Burger D. Anti-interleukin-1 therapy in rheumatic diseases. *Curr Opin Rheumatol* 2001;13:170–6.

62 Karatay S, Erdem T, Yildirim K, *et al.* The effect of individualized diet challenges consisting of allergenic foods on TNF-α and IL-1β levels in patients with rheumatoid arthritis. *Rheumatology* 2004;43:1429–33.

63 Haugen MA, Kjeldsen-Kragh J, Bjerve KS, *et al.* Changes in plasma phospholipid fatty acids and their relationship to disease activity in rheumatoid arthritis patients treated with a vegetarian diet. *Br J Nutr* 1994;72:555–66.

64 Hawrelak J, Meyers S. The causes of intestinal dysbiosis: a review. *Altern Med Rev* 2004;9:180–97.

65 Shinebaum R, Neumann VC, Cooke EM, *et al.* Comparison of faecal florae in patients with rheumatoid arthritis and controls. *Br J Rheumatol* 1987;26:329–33.

66 Wilson C, Ebringer A, Ahmadi K, *et al.* Shared amino acid sequences between major histocompatibility complex class II glycoproteins, type XI collagen and *Proteus mirabilis* in rheumatoid arthritis. *Ann Rheum Dis* 1995;54:216–20.

67 Deighton C, Gray J, Bint A, *et al.* Anti-*Proteus* antibodies in rheumatoid arthritis same-sexed sibships. *Br J Rheumatol* 1992;31:241–5.

68 Kjeldsen-Kragh J, Rashid T, Dybwad A, *et al.* Decrease in anti-*proteus mirabilis* but not anti-*Escherichia coli* antibody levels in rheumatoid arthritis patients treated with fasting and a one year vegetarian diet. *Ann Rheum Dis* 1995;54:221–4.

69 Peltonen R, Nenonen M, Helve T, *et al.* Faecal microbial flora and disease activity in rheumatoid arthritis during a vegan diet. *Br J Rheumatol* 1997;36:64–8.

70 Michalsen A, Riegert M, Ludtke R, *et al.* Mediterranean diet or extended fasting's influence on changing the intestinal microflora, immunoglobulin A secretion and clinical outcome in patients with rheumatoid arthritis and fibromyalgia: an observational study. *BMC Complement Altern Med* 2005;5:22–31.

71 Arrieta M, Bistritz L, Meddings J. Alterations in intestinal permeability. *Gut* 2006;55:1512–20.

72 Sundqvist T, Lindstrom F, Magnusson K, *et al.* Influence of fasting on intestinal permeability and disease activity in patients with rheumatoid arthritis. *Scand J Rheumatol* 1982;11:33–8.

73 Trollmo C, Verdrengh M, Tarkowski A. Fasting enhances mucosal antigen specific B cell responses in rheumatoid arthritis. *Ann Rheum Dis* 1997;56:130–4.

74 Hvatum M, Kanerud L, Hallgren R, *et al.* The gut–joint axis: cross reactive food antibodies in rheumatoid arthritis. *Gut* 2006;55:1240–7.

75 Cleland L, Caughey G, James M, *et al.* Reduction of cardiovascular risk factors with longterm fish oil treatment in early rheumatoid arthritis. *J Rheumatol* 2006;33:1973–9.

76 Stamp LK, James M, Cleland L. Diet and rheumatoid arthritis: a review of the literature. *Semin Arthritis Rheum* 2005;35:77–94.

77 Adam O, Beringer C, Kless T, *et al.* Anti-inflammatory effects of a low arachidonic acid diet and fish oil in patients with rheumatoid arthritis. *Rheumatol Int* 2003;23:27–36.

78 Sarzi-Puttini P, Comi D, Boccassini L, *et al.* Diet therapy for rheumatoid arthritis. A controlled double-blind study of two different dietary regimens. *Scand J Rheumatol* 2000;29:302–7.

79 Cleland LG, French JK, Betts WH, *et al.* Clinical and biochemical effects of dietary fish oil supplements in rheumatoid arthritis. *J Rheumatol* 1988;15:1471–5.

80 Volker D, Fitzgerald P, Major G, *et al.* Efficacy of fish oil concentrate in the treatment of rheumatoid arthritis. *J Rheumatol* 2000;27:2343–6.

81 Kremer JM, Lawrence DA, Jubiz W, *et al.* Dietary fish oil and olive oil supplementation in patients with rheumatoid arthritis. *Arthritis Rheum* 1990;33:810–19.

82 Leeb B, Sautner J, Andel I, Rintelen B. Intravenous application of omega-3 fatty acids in patients with active rheumatoid arthritis. The ORA-1 trial. An open pilot study. *Lipids* 2006;41:29–34.

83 Belch JJ, Ansell D, Madhok R, *et al.* Effects of altering dietary essential fatty acids on requirements for non-steroidal

anti-inflammatory drugs in patients with rheumatitis: a double blind placebo controlled study. *Ann Rheum Dis* 1988;47:96–104.

84 Lau CS, Morley KD, Belch JJF. Effects of fish oil supplementation on non-steroidal anti-inflammatory requirement in patients with mild rheumatoid arthritis – a double blind placebo controlled trial. *Br J Rheumatol* 1993;32:982–9.

85 Skoldstam L, Borjesson O, Kjallman A, *et al.* Effect of six months of fish oil supplementation in stable rheumatoid arthritis. A double-blind, controlled study. *Scand J Rheumatol* 1992; 21:178–85.

86 Kjeldsen-Kragh J, Lund JA, Riise T, *et al.* Dietary omega-3 fatty acid supplementation and naproxen treatment in patients with rheumatoid arthritis. *J Rheumatol* 1992;19:1531–6.

87 Johnsen S, Larsson H, Tarone R, *et al.* Risk of hospitalization for myocardial infarction among users of rofecoxib, celecoxib, and other NSAIDs. *Arch Int Med* 2005;165:978–84.

88 Hippisley-Cox J, Coupland C. Risk of myocardial infarction in patients taking cyclo-oxygenase-2 inhibitors or conventional non-steroidal anti-inflammatory drugs: population based nested case-control analysis. *BMJ* 2005;330:1366–73.

89 Penglis P, Cleland LG, Demasi M, *et al.* Differential regulation of prostaglandin E_2 and thromboxane A_2 production in human monocytes: implications for the use of cyclooxygenase inhibitors. *J Immunol* 2000;165:1605–11.

90 Endres S, Ghorbani R, Kelley V, *et al.* The effect of dietary supplementation with n-3 polyunsaturated fatty acids on the synthesis of interleukin-1 and tumor necrosis factor by mononuclear cells. *N Engl J Med* 1989;320:265–71.

91 Caughey GE, Mantzioris E, Gibson RA, *et al.* The effect on human tumor necrosis factor-α and interleukin-1β production of diets enriched in n-3 fatty acids from vegetable oil or fish oil. *Am J Clin Nutr* 1996;63:116–22.

92 Lee TH, Hoover RL, Williams JD, *et al.* Effect of dietary enrichment with eicosapentaenoic and docosahexaenoic acids on *in vitro* neutrophil and monocyte and leucocyte leukotriene generation and neutrophil function. *N Engl J Med* 1985;312: 1217–24.

93 Fischer S, Weber P. Thromboxane A_3 is formed in human platelets after dietary eicosapentaenoic acid. *Biochem Biophys Res Comm* 1983;116:1091–9.

94 Sperling RI, Benincaso A, Knoell C, *et al.* Dietary omega-3 polyunsaturated fatty acids inhibit phosphoinositide formation and chemotaxis in neutrophils. *J Clin Invest* 1993;91:651–60.

95 Molvig J, Pociot F, Worsaae H, *et al.* Dietary supplementation with omega-3 polyunsaturated fatty acids decreases mononuclear cell proliferation and interleukin-1β content but not monokine secretion in healthy and insulin-dependent diabetic individuals. *Scand J Immunol* 1991;34:399–410.

96 Meydani SN, Endres S, Woods M, *et al.* Oral (n-3) fatty acid supplementation suppresses cytokine production and lymphocyte proliferation: comparison between young and older women. *J Nutr* 1991;121:547–55.

97 Curtis C, Hughes C, Flannery C, *et al.* n-3 fatty acids specifically modulate catabolic factors involved in articular cartilage degradation. *J Biol Chem* 2000;275:721–4.

98 Curtis C, Rees S, Little C, *et al.* Pathological indicators of degradation and inflammation in human osteoarthritis cartilage are abrogated by exposure to n-3 fatty acids. *Arthritis Rheum* 2002;46:1544–53.

99 Hughes DA, Southon S, Pinder A. (n-3) Polyunsaturated fatty acids modulate the expression of functionally associated molecules on human monocytes *in vitro*. *J Nutr* 1996;126: 603–10.

100 Hughes DA, Pinder AC. n-3 polyunsaturated fatty acids inhibit the antigen-presenting function of human monocytes. *Am J Clin Nutr* 2000;71:357S–60S.

101 Wolfe F, Mitchell D, Sibley J, *et al.* The mortality of rheumatoid arthritis. *Arthritis Rheum* 1994;37:481–94.

102 Solomon D, Karlson E, Rimm E, *et al.* Cardiovascular morbidity and mortality in women diagnosed with rheumatoid arthritis. *Circulation* 2003;107:1303–7.

103 Solomon D, Curhan G, Rimm E, *et al.* Cardiovascular risk factors in women with and without rheumatoid arthritis. *Arthritis Rheum* 2004;50:3444–9.

104 van Doornum S, Jennings G, Wicks I. Reducing the cardiovascular disease burden in rheumatoid arthritis. *Med J Aust* 2006;184: 287–90.

105 Wang C, Harris WS, Chung M, *et al.* n-3 Fatty acids from fish or fish-oil supplements, but not α-linoleic acid, benefit cardiovascular disease outcomes in primary- and secondary-prevention studies: a systematic review. *Am J Clin Nutr* 2006;84:5–17.

46

CHAPTER 46

Therapeutic Approaches Under Development

Miae Oh, Hugh A. Sampson, and Xiu-Min Li

KEY CONCEPTS

- Food allergy-induced anaphylaxis continues to increase despite current treatment modalities.
- Improved food allergy immunotherapy is needed.
- In general, therapeutic measures provide a shift from a Th2 to a Th1 response.
- Immunotherapies may be allergen-specific or non-specific.
- Future therapies must be safe, applicable, and practical.

Introduction

Food allergy affects almost 4% of the American population [1]. The prevalence is higher than initially deemed. As with other atopic disorders, the incidence of food allergy is reportedly increasing [2]. Current treatment modalities include patient education, dietary restrictions, antihistamines, and self-administered injectable epinephrine. However, despite these measures, accidental ingestions and anaphylaxis continue to occur in sensitized patients. As a result, adverse reactions to foods are the leading single cause of anaphylaxis treated in emergency departments in the United States [3]. An estimated 30,000 episodes of food-induced anaphylaxis occur each year, resulting in an estimated 150 deaths, with peanuts and tree nuts accounting for the vast majority of fatalities [4]. Therefore, an improved modality of treatment is imperative.

In the past, immunotherapeutic approaches for food hypersensitivities had been translated from allergic rhinitis therapies. Although subcutaneous immunotherapy has been successful in treating allergic rhinitis, it has, unfortunately, resulted in increased adverse systemic reactions and has proven unacceptable for the treatment of food allergy [5,6]. However, in the advent of the "hygiene hypothesis," there have been various novel approaches to the treatment

of atopic disorders. The "hygiene hypothesis" postulates that increased hygiene and the lack of immunostimulatory pathogens early in childhood have resulted in a skewing of the Th1 and Th2 response [7]. Consequently, due to an increased persistent Th2 immune response, there is a growing prevalence of allergic disorders. Much of the research in future therapies aim at providing a lasting, clinical improvement by downregulating the Th2 immune response.

Several immunotherapeutic approaches are being investigated as treatments for food allergy. In reviewing these future therapies, we have divided the subject matter into allergen-specific and non-specific immunotherapies. As we discuss individual therapies, we hope to clarify the potential benefits of each approach.

Allergen-specific immunotherapy (Table 46.1)

DNA-based immunotherapy
Plasmid DNA-based immunotherapy

In plasmid DNA-based immunotherapy, a bacterial plasmid vector is manufactured which contains a specific allergen-encoding DNA insert. Immunization with the plasmid DNA (pDNA) theoretically results in uptake by antigen-presenting cells, which then transcribe and express the product. The allergen is then presented by major histocompatibility complex molecules to lymphocytes. These antigens, in turn, induce a Th1 response that is attributed to immunostimulatory sequences (ISS), consisting of unmethylated cytosine and guanine motifs (CpG motifs) in the pDNA backbone [8].

Food Allergy: Adverse Reactions to Foods and Food Additives, 4th edition.
Edited by Dean D. Metcalfe, Hugh A. Sampson, and Ronald A. Simon.
© 2008 Blackwell Publishing, ISBN: 978-1-4501-5129-0.

Previous data have shown the efficacy of a pDNA vaccine encoding house-dust mite allergen in a rat asthma model. The immunized rats had decreased IgE, histamine release, and airway hyperresponsiveness [9]. In order to investigate the effect of this therapy on peanut anaphylaxis, Li *et al.* immunized naïve AKR/J and C3H/HeJ mice with pDNA encoding Ara h2 (pAra h2) prior to peanut sensitization [10]. The vaccine provided some protective effect in AKR mice, but C3H-treated mice had anaphylactic reactions following peanut challenge. In addition, the pAra h2 vaccine did not effectively prevent the development of peanut-specific IgE levels in AKR or BALB/C mice, which indicated that this form of pDNA immunotherapy does not effectively protect against IgE-mediated peanut hypersensitivity. Furthermore, the variable effects in the different strains of mice likely reflect the genetically heterogeneous human population. Currently, this form of therapy remains experimental and cannot be viewed as safe or efficacious for treating food allergy.

Immunostimulatory-oligodeoxynucleotides immunotherapy

Another DNA-based immunotherapeutic approach consists of synthetic immunostimulatory-oligodeoxynucleotides containing CpG motifs (ISS-ODN). ISS-ODN has been shown to be highly immunogenic, promoting a Th1 response [11]. In addition, ISS-ODN/protein conjugates have been shown to promote a more robust Th1 response, than ISS-ODN alone or as a co-injection of ISS-ODN with allergen [12]. The postulated mechanism of action is believed to involve TLR9 that is expressed on plasmacytoid dendritic cells and upon stimulation induce secretion of IL-12, which induces Th1 development [13]. Previous studies indicate that immunotherapy with ISS-ODN conjugated to house-dust mite and

Table 46.1 Allergen-specific immunotherapies

Approach	Therapy	Effect	Comment
pDNA	Encoding wAra h2 (pAra h2, i.m.) [10]	Prophylactic protocol: no effect on IgE, increased IgG2a, prevented anaphylaxis in AKR mice, induced anaphylaxis in C3H/J mice.	Concerns regarding safety.
ISS-ODN	ISS-conjugated-Ara h2 (i.d.) [16]	Prophylactic protocol on C3H/J mice: partially prevented Ara h2 induced anaphylaxis in C3H/J mice; no significant reduction in IgE levels, increased Th1 cytokine levels.	Difficult to prepare material; no data on desensitization of established peanut allergy.
Peptides	20-mer Ara h2 peptide mixture (s.c.)	Therapeutic protocol in C3H/J mice: reduced Ara h2-specific IgE levels, reduced anaphylaxis scores, increased IFN-γ production by cultured splenocytes.	Very expensive to manufacture.
Engineered protein	mAra h2 (i.n. or s.c.) [20]	Therapeutic protocol in C3H/J mice: reduced IgE, IL-4, and anaphylaxis scores, did not increase IFN-γ in cultured splenocytes.	Frequent i.n. administration; s.c. immunotherapy provided little protection.
	mAra h123 + HKLM (s.c.) [22]	Therapeutic protocol in C3H/J mice: reduced peanut-specific IgE, partially protected from anaphylaxis, reduced IL-4, IL-5, IL-13 and increased IFN-γ production by splenocytes.	Safety remains to be determined. Long-lasting therapeutic effect has not been established.
	HKE-MP123 (p.r.) [23,24]	Therapeutic protocol in C3H/J mice: reduced peanut-specific IgE partially protected from anaphylaxis, reduced IL-4, IL-5, Il-13, and IL-10 production by splenocytes and increased IFN-γ and TGF-β production by splenocytes. Therapeutic effect lasted at least 10 weeks.	Less concern regarding activating mast cells, little concern about safety of vaccine administration, relatively long-lasting effect.
Oral desensitization	Cow's milk (p.o.) [27,28]	70–80% of patients were able to tolerate 40–200 ml of cow's milk/day.	Up to 44% of patients spontaneously outgrow cow's milk hypersensitivity on elimination diet; there was no placebo control group.
Sublingual desensitization	Hazelnut extract (p.o.) [31]	Patients tolerated 5 times more hazelnut than prior to desensitization; increased IL-10, IgG4.	Required a large amount of hazelnut to provoke a reaction prior to desensitization.

w, wild type; p, plasmid; m modified; i.m., intramuscular; i.n., intranasal; p.r., per rectum; i.d., intradermal; s.c., subcutaneous; p.o., per os; ISS-ODN, immunostimulatory-oligonucleotide; HKLM, heat-killed *Listeria monocytogenes*; HKE, heat-killed *Esherichia coli*.

common ragweed allergens improve symptom scores in sensitized patients as well as provide a lasting Th1 response [13–15]. Based on these promising results, this approach was applied to a murine peanut-allergy model. In preliminary studies, Li *et al.* utilized ISS/Ara h2 conjugates as prophylactic therapy in murine models of peanut-induced anaphylaxis [16]. When C3H/HeJ mice were immunized with ISS/Ara h2 and then sensitized to peanut, the treated mice did not exhibit obvious symptoms following an oral peanut challenge, whereas the control mice did. These findings suggest that ISS/Ara h2 immunization had a prophylactic effect on a peanut-induced allergic response in an antigen-specific manner. Further studies will be required to see if ISS/Ara h2 immunization can reverse a type I reaction in peanut-sensitized mice.

Peptide immunotherapy

Peptide immunotherapy is an approach which involves overlapping peptides, 10–20 amino acids in length, or short segments representing T-cell epitopes of known allergenic protein. These short sequences theoretically preclude IgE cross-linking on mast cell and basophil receptors, while stimulating antigen-presenting cells and T-cells [17]. Initial studies involved peptides representing T-cell epitopes on the major cat allergen Fel d1 in cat-allergic patients with asthma. One study showed a dose–response-related decrease in nasal and pulmonary symptoms in treated subjects compared to control groups [18]. In a murine peanut allergy model, Li *et al.* showed in a preliminary study that treatment with a 20-mer Ara h2 overlapping mixture of peptides reduced serum Ara h2-specific IgE, and reduced plasma histamine levels and symptom scores following oral peanut challenge, while increasing INF-γ production by spleen cells. Although seemingly promising, standardizing a large mixture of peptide fragments in a vaccine is technically challenging, and the preparation of such a vaccine is very costly.

Engineered protein immunotherapy

In engineered recombinant protein immunotherapy, the allergen is modified by altering one or two amino acids within an allergenic epitope to eliminate IgE binding, while retaining the T-cell epitopes largely intact to promote proliferation. In order to precisely modify the relevant protein, well-characterized allergens and IgE-binding epitopes are required. Using known sequences and IgE-binding epitopes of the three major peanut proteins Ara h1, Ara h2, Ara h3, all allergenic epitopes were modified to produce peanut proteins that bound little or no peanut-specific IgE [19]. Li *et al.* used the modified Ara h 1–3 (mAra h123) in murine model of peanut anaphylaxis and demonstrated beneficial effects [20]. The mice were treated with intranasal mAra h 1–3, which decreased peanut-specific IgE levels and anaphylactic symptoms following peanut challenge compared to control groups. However, to achieve this response, frequent

intranasal administrations were required. Interestingly, subcutaneous administrations of the modified protein, the standard route for immunotherapy, did not produce comparable protection.

In an attempt to improve the Th1 immunostimulatory response, heat-killed *Listeria monocytogenes* (HKLM) was administered as an adjuvant with the engineered peanut protein. Previous data supported the use of HKLM as an adjuvant and its ability to produce a Th1 response in a murine model [21]. Li *et al.* demonstrated that subcutaneous injections with HKLM and mAra h1–3 were able to desensitize a peanut-allergic murine models [22–25]. Compared to mAra h1–3 alone, the vaccine with the combination of HKLM and mAra h1–3 showed improved post-challenge clinical score, body temperature, airway response, and plasma histamine, when given rectally or subcutaneously. Subsequently, experiments utilizing a heat-killed bacterial adjuvant, heat-killed *Escherichia coli*, which is utilized to produce the mutated Ara h1, −2, and −3 (HKE-MP123), yielded similar effective results in the peanut-allergic murine model. Since the HKE-MP123 is administered into an environment replete with *Escherichia coli* and other bacteria, there is little concern about safety of administering such a vaccine. Therefore this approach appears to be superior to co-administration of HKL and purified, engineered peanut proteins. This investigation is currently pursuing commercial production for clinical study.

Oral immunotherapy

Food hypersensitivity is believed to be due to the failure in the induction of oral tolerance [26]. The rationale for utilizing gastrointestinal mucosa for immunotherapy depends on the normal immune system's capacity to induce immune tolerance via the gastrointestinal tract, despite the high exposure of numerous bacteria and dietary antigens. Although the exact mechanism of action is unknown, various factors seem to be involved in the immunologic mechanism of oral tolerance such as exposure to high or low doses of antigens, processing by dendritic cells, and activation of T-regulatory cells. High-dose antigens promote lymphocyte anergy or deletion, whereas low-dose tolerance is mediated by regulatory T-cells – Th3 (suppression via TGF-β), Tr1 (suppression via IL-10), or CD4+CD25+ (possibly via surface bound TGF-β). Dendritic cells process antigens and are activated to secrete cytokines that play a crucial role in determining the balance between tolerance and immunity. This balance is dependent on expression of specific co-stimulatory molecules and the cytokines released into the lymphocytes' milieu [26].

Although oral immunotherapy for food allergy has been received with skepticism in the past [27–29], recent studies have shown its potential as a future therapy [30–35]. Patriarca *et al.* have shown effects of oral immunotherapy on various foods. They reported that a majority of 59 subjects enrolled (83.3%) were "desensitized" and able to consume their respective IgE-mediated allergens after the completion of the protocol, in particular cow's milk (120 ml), egg (1 whole egg), and cod fish (160 mg) [31]. Increasing doses of the allergen were given over 60–84 days, depending on the food. In addition, skin prick test size had decreased, specific IgE levels had decreased, and specific IgG$_4$ levels had increased. However, subjects had to remain on almost daily oral immunotherapy in order to maintain the desensitized state. A control group of patients that were on an elimination diet failed the double-blind-placebo-controlled food challenges (DBPCFC) after a 6-month observation period. There was no placebo control group in this trial. Meglio *et al.* found that 15 of 21 children (71.4%) were able to consume 200 ml of cow's milk, while 3 of 21 (14.3%) were able to consume 40–80 ml/day after a 6-month oral desensitization protocol [36]. The subjects were approximately 6 years old or older and had positive DBPCFC on average 23 days prior to the initiation of therapy. Diluted cow's milk protein 0.06 mg was given initially, doubling every 7 days until day 70, after which the cow's milk protein was doubled every 16 days until 200 ml of undiluted cow's milk was achieved in a 6-month period. A DBPCFC was performed after completion of the therapy with 18 of the 21 children experiencing a negative DBPCFC. Skin prick test showed a significant decrease in wheal size in all 18 patients that passed the DBPCFC ($p < 0.001$). However, there was no significant change in serum-specific IgE levels before and after treatment. In addition, no placebo control group was utilized in this study.

Previous reports indicated that spontaneous resolution of food allergy may occur in 19–44% of patients that are on elimination diet [37]. Although this may be a confounding factor, these two studies show that a population of food-allergic patients could become desensitized with oral immunotherapy. However as reported by Rolinck-Werninghaus *et al.* [38] (Allergy 2005), patients must continue oral immunotherapy on a daily basis in order to maintain the desensitized state.

Sublingual immunotherapy

Similarly, sublingual immunotherapy (SLIT) has been a topic of interest due to its simple administration and effectiveness in other allergic disorders, particularly allergic rhinitis. A meta-analysis by Wilson *et al.* [39] encompassing 22 studies with 484 SLIT recipients and 475 placebo recipients with allergic rhinitis to dust mite, grass, *Parietaria*, olive, ragweed, *Cupressus*, and cat showed a decrease in symptom scores and medication usage. Although the exact mechanism for SLIT is unknown, there is a decrease in the IgE/IgG$_4$ ratio, as seen in subcutaneous immunotherapy for aeroallergens [40]. During SLIT, the allergen extract is held under the tongue for 1–2 minutes to allow the antigen to be captured by oral Langerhans-like dendritic cells (LLDCs). Due to the effectiveness noted in patients with allergic rhinitis, there is an increasing interest in attempting to desensitize patients with food hypersensitivity. A placebo-controlled

SLIT trial with standardized hazelnut extract, by Enrique *et al.*, showed that SLIT-treated subjects could be at least partially desensitized and were able to tolerate an increase in the amount of hazelnut that provoked objective symptoms compared to placebo-treated subjects [41]. Twenty-three patients with anaphylaxis, angioedema, or oral allergy syndrome without birch pollen sensitization, who had positive DBPCFC to hazelnut, participated in the study. The SLIT recipients underwent a 4-day build-up period to a maintenance dose of 188.15 µg of Cor a1 and 121.9 µg of Cor a8 for 2–3 months. The subjects were then assessed by a follow-up DBPCFC to hazelnut. The mean quantity of hazelnut that provoked objective symptoms increased from 2.29 to 11.56 g ($p = 0.02$) in the treated group compared to 3.49–4.14 g (no statistical significance) in the placebo group. There was an increase in IL-10 and IgG$_4$ in the treated group. A large quantity of hazelnut was often required to provoke objective symptoms in subjects even prior to desensitization. Therefore, further studies will be needed to assess the effectiveness, general applicability, and safety of this method.

Non-specific immunotherapy (Table 46.2)

Traditional Chinese medicine

Traditional Chinese medicine (TCM) has been used for centuries in Asia, and still plays a role in mainstream medicine in all Asian countries. Recently, there has been an increased interest in TCM as a source of future therapies in the field of allergy and asthma. Li *et al.* reported an herbal therapy for asthma called MSSM-002 that decreased airway hyper-reactivity, mucous production, Th2 cytokine profile, and airway remodeling, without suppressing IFN-γ in a murine asthma model [42]. A clinical trial completed in asthmatic subjects in China, using ASHMI (Anti-asthma Herbal Medicine Intervention), which is derived from MSSM-002, demonstrated results that were consistent with the findings reported in the murine asthma model [43]. Phase I clinical trials of ASHMI have now started in the United States.

The successful application of TCM to asthma led to the investigation of TCM as a possible treatment for food allergy. An herbal formulation for food allergy composed of nine herbs called Food Allergy Herbal Formula-2 (FAHF-2) has been studied in a well-characterized peanut-allergic murine model. FAHF-2 has been shown to successfully prevent anaphylactic reactions to peanut for up to 4 weeks post-therapy, when given at the induction of peanut hypersensitivity (3 weeks post-sensitization and boosting) [44]. Although it is known that immunotherapy that is initiated early in atopic disorders suppresses the disease, most studies suggest that the treatments started in established disease are often ineffective. In response to this, Qu *et al.* showed that FAHF-2 can block anaphylactic reactions in mice with established peanut allergy mice and that this protection lasts up to 6 months post-therapy, which is 25% of an

Table 46.2 Non-specific immunotherapies

Approach	Therapy	Effect	Comment
Chinese herbal medicine	FAHF2 (p.o.) [34]	Therapeutic protocol in peanut-allergic C3H/J mice: reduced peanut-specific IgE, IL-4, IL-5, and IL-13, completely blocked anaphylaxis in established peanut allergy, enhanced IFN-γ production.	Safe and well tolerated, most potent effect on peanut allergy, long-term protection, less costly.
Probiotics	LGG (p.o.) [38,39,42,43]	Therapeutic protocol in cow's milk-protein-allergic infants: increased fecal IgA, decreased fecal AT and TNF-α post-challenge.	May decrease intestinal inflammation in cow's milk-allergic patients.
	LGG (p.o.) [47]	Therapeutic protocol in peanut-allergic C3H/J mice: did not significantly reduce anaphylaxis to peanut, plasma histamine, or IgE levels, reduced IL-4 but not IL-13 levels, minimal increase in IFN-γ production.	Does not protect against IgE-mediated peanut reactions.
	ImmuSoy (p.o.) [46,47]	Therapeutic protocol in peanut-allergic C3H/J mice: protected against anaphylaxis, reduced histamine and peanut-specific IgE levels, reduced IL-4 and IL-13, increased IFN-γ production.	Safe and well tolerated, does not protect against peanut anaphylaxis as FAHF2, further studies are needed.
Humanized anti-IgE	TNX-901 (s.c.) [50]	Therapeutic protocol in peanut-allergic patients: patients that received the 450-mg dose increased their threshold sensitivity to peanut from 178 to 2805 mg.	Provides partial protection against accidental peanut ingestion, requires multiple injections, is expensive.
Cytokines	IL-12 (p.o.) [51]	Therapeutic and prophylactic protocol in peanut-allergic C3H/J mice: reduced anaphylaxis, decreased peanut-specific IgE levels, decreased IgG1/IgG2a ratio, increased IFN-γ/IL-4 and IFN-γ/IL-4 ratios.	Decreased anaphylaxis to peanut, is expensive.
	Anti-IL-5 (mepolizumab) (i.v.) [52]	Case report on AEE patient: decreased emesis and dysphagia, decreased esophageal eosinophils/hpf on biopsy.	Further studies are required.

p.o., per os; s.c., subcutaneous, i.v., intravenous; AT, α1-antitrypsin; AEE, allergic eosinophilic esophagitis; hpf, high-power field.

average mouse lifespan (ref). C3H/HeJ mice were sensitized and boosted for 8 weeks and subsequently received FAHF-2 treatment twice daily for 7 weeks. They were then challenged 1 day and 4 weeks post-therapy. Although all the sham-treated mice developed anaphylactic reactions, none of the FAHF-2-treated mice had anaphylactic reactions. Consistent with these results, FAHF-2 blocked histamine release. Peanut-specific-IgE levels were significantly lower, whereas IgG2a levels were increased in FAHF-2 treated mice, but not in sham-treated mice. Cell culture supernatants of peanut-stimulated splenocytes and mesenteric lymph node cells from FAHF-2-treated mice contained significantly lower levels of Th2 cytokines, IL-4, IL-5, and IL-13, and significantly higher levels of IFN-γ than cell cultures from sham-treated mice. FAHF-2 also showed beneficial immunomodulatory effects on Th1 and Th2 responses of peripheral mononuclear cells from children with peanut allergy and asthma [45].

In order to find the key components in FAHF-2, Kattan et al. studied the effects of the individual herbs in a peanut-allergic murine model at doses equivalent to those in FAHF-2 (submitted). Interestingly, none of the nine herbs individually suppressed plasma histamine, IgE, or anaphylactic symptoms as well as FAHF-2. Furthermore, a simplified form of FAHF-2 (sFAHF-2), composed of the individual herbs that appeared most effective in reducing anaphylaxis and/or Th2 cytokine profile, was investigated. Although sFAHF-2 administration produced a decrease in IgE, plasma histamine, and anaphylaxis scores, the degree of improvement was significantly less than the whole formula. This study showed that the components in the FAHF-2 herbal mixture have a synergistic or additive effect that no single herb was able to accomplish.

The exact mechanism of action of FAHF-2 is unknown. However, one of the herbs, Gui Zhi showed some protection against anaphylaxis but did not inhibit Th2 cytokines or IgE, suggesting that mast cells or basophils could be its target of action. In addition, Ling Zhi reduced IgE levels, but did not reduce IL-4 and IL-13 or protect from anaphylaxis, indicating that its effects could be directed at B-cells. Further studies to determine the mechanism of action are in progress. No immune suppression and no hepatic or renal toxicities were detected in these studies. FAHF-2 is a potential therapy for food allergy and has been approved for Phase I and II clinical trials. If efficacious in human trials, FAHF-2 has several advantages over other novel treatments: it is administered orally, provides long-lasting protection, and has an excellent safety profile that makes it one of the more favorable therapies for food allergy.

Probiotics

The commensal gut flora has been considered to have an important role in the maturation of the immune system. This belief has been reinforced by the advent of the "hygiene hypothesis." Animal studies have suggested that the lack of sufficient intestinal microbial stimuli may promote a persistent Th2 response [46,47]. As a result, there has been a growing interest in utilizing probiotics to establish healthy intestinal microbiota and subsequently, an interest in studying its effects on the immune system. The possible mechanism of action of probiotics involves promoting a potentially anti-allergic process involving Toll-like receptors (TLRs) and intracellular nucleotide oligomerization domains (NOD1 and NOD2). These domains recognize conserved pathogen-associated molecular patterns (PAMPs) [48]. As a result, there is an enhanced Th1 response, increased TGF-β, specific IgA production, and increased gut barrier function [49].

There are a number of studies regarding probiotics and atopic disease. In a randomized placebo-controlled study, Kalliomaki *et al.* showed that *Lactobacillus rhamnosus GG* (LGG) therapy given to pregnant women and infants postnatally for 6 months could possibly prevent atopic dermatitis for up to 4 years in high-risk families [49,50]. Another randomized placebo-controlled study by Brouwer *et al.* found that LGG was not an adequate therapy when initiated in patients with active atopic dermatitis under 5 months of age [51]. Although the effects of LGG are controversial for the treatment of atopic dermatitis, Kalliomaki's study suggests that it may provide some protection against atopic dermatitis in infants.

Few data are available regarding probiotic therapy and food allergy. Some studies show possible improvement in intestinal inflammation in patients with cow's milk-protein allergy following treatment with LGG [52,53]. One study found increased INF-γ secretion by the peripheral blood mononuclear cells of cow's milk-allergic patients treated with LGG [54]. Other studies on probiotics have suggested that koji mold fermentation may show some promise. Products that incorporate koji fermentation include miso (fermented soybean paste), shoyu (soy sauce), and sake (rice

wine) [55]. The beneficial effects of soy products were suggested in a cross-sectional study evaluating soy intake and the prevalence of allergic rhinitis in 1002 pregnant Japanese women. This study showed an inverse relationship between dietary soy intake, including miso, and allergic rhinitis [56]. A recent study by Zhang *et al.* showed that a fermented soy probiotic therapy called ImmuSoy, a proprietary koji fermentation product made by fermenting defatted soybeans with *Aspergillus oryzae* and lactic acid bacteria (*Pedicoccus parvalus* and *Enterococcus faecium*), prevented reactions in a well-characterized murine model of peanut anaphylaxis [57,58]. In this study, peanut-sensitized mice were divided into six treatment groups and received 4 weeks of either ImmuSoy (9×10^7 cfu/g of chow), ImmuSoy $2 \times$ (1.8×10^8 cfu/g of chow), irradiated-ImmuSoy $2 \times$ (irradiated 1.8×10^8 cfu/g of chow), LGG (9×10^7 cfu/g of chow), sham treatment or no treatment. Four weeks after treatment, the mice were challenged to peanut. At both doses, irradiated-ImmuSoy and ImmuSoy were able to protect the peanut-sensitized mice from developing anaphylactic symptoms. In addition, there were significant reductions in plasma histamine and peanut-specific IgE levels in the ImmuSoy-treated mice. Splenocyte cultures from ImmuSoy-treated mice showed decreased IL-4 and IL-13 production, increased IFN-γ production, and no change in TNF-α production. These results showed that ImmuSoy and irradiated-ImmuSoy have immunomodulatory properties that may be applicable to the treatment of peanut allergy.

Humanized, monoclonal anti-IgE antibody

In type I hypersensitivity reactions, an allergen binds and cross-links two IgE molecules that are bound to their receptors, FcϵRI and FcϵRII, found on mast cells and basophils. As a result, the mast cells and basophils degranulate, releasing histamine, tryptase, and other type I mediators. Engineered monoclonal anti-IgE antibodies bind to the Fc region of IgE molecules and prevent the binding of IgE to its receptors. This markedly decreases IgE bound to mast cells and basophils, which in turn increases their threshold of activation and improves asthma and allergic rhinitis symptoms [59,60]. With a potentially wide application for atopic diseases, there was a question as to whether this therapy would be useful for treating food allergy. Leung *et al.* showed promising results in a multi-center, randomized, placebo-controlled trial of anti-IgE therapy in peanut-allergic patients [61]. Eighty-four patients underwent DBPCFC to determine the amount of peanut necessary to provoke an allergic reaction (threshold dose). These patients were randomized to three treatment groups of anti-IgE therapy (150, 300, and 450 mg) and a placebo group. After weekly anti-IgE injections for 4 weeks, the patients underwent a second oral food challenge to peanut. Patients treated with 450 mg of anti-IgE were able to tolerate an increased amount of peanut, from a level equal to approximately half a peanut kernel (178 mg) to approximately nine peanut kernals (2805 mg), which would protect against most unintentional ingestions. In addition, since most food-allergic patients have other atopic symptoms, this therapy may also provide some benefit by decreasing asthma and allergic rhinitis symptoms. Currently, there is no similar ongoing clinical trial for peanut allergy.

Cytokine therapy

Atopic disorders are characterized by Th2 cytokines such as IL-4, IL-5, and IL-13, whereas non-allergic responses are typified by Th1 cytokines such as IL-12 and IFN-γ. Cytokine-based therapies typically consist of administering a specific cytokine or by inhibiting a cytokine with monoclonal antibodies in order to promote a Th1 response rather than a Th2 response. With respect to food allergy, there has been one study by Lee et al. that showed the prophylactic and therapeutic effects of administering oral IL-12 in a peanut-allergic murine model [62]. When IL-12 was given prophylactically during oral sensitization to peanut, or 3 weeks after sensitization was completed, it not only attenuated the allergic reaction to peanut but also decreased plasma histamine levels, peanut-specific IgE levels, and reduced IgG1/IgG2a levels. In addition, both treatment groups also had increased IFN-γ/IL-4 and IFN-γ /IL-5 ratios in splenocyte cultures. Although further studies are needed, oral IL-12 could possibly be used for food allergy therapy.

With the advent of humanized anti-IL-5, interest has increased in its effects on eosinophilic disorders. Case reports of anti-IL-5 treatment for hypereosinophilic syndromes showed potential benefit in treating these disorders [63]. Of particular interest is the report of an 18-year-old patient with eosinophilic esophagitis who received anti-IL-5 therapy. Prior to treatment he had dysphagia, emesis 3–4 times per week, marked esophageal strictures and persistent esophageal eosinophils >200 cells/high-power field. He failed dietary restrictions, topical fluticasone, and oral prednisone therapies. Following three doses of anti-IL-5 therapy, he had no emesis, decreased inflammation of his esophagus, and >10-fold decrease in the mean number of tissue eosinophils in his esophagus. These results suggest a possible therapeutic use for anti-IL-5 in patients with allergic eosinophilic esophagitis. Currently these patients are being treated with severely restrictive diets and amino-acid-based formulas that are unpalatable and have social and emotional repercussions.

Conclusion

Research into novel therapies for food allergy has reached that stage where it offers the possibility of effective treatment, and perhaps a cure for this often debilitating disorder. FAHF-2, because of its ability to completely suppress peanut-induced anaphylaxis in a model of established peanut allergy, is entering Phase I clinical trials and offers a novel approach to treat patients with a broad spectrum of food allergies. Novel immunotherapeutic strategies including engineered

recombinant proteins and ISS as adjuvants show promise in "curing" food-allergic responses.

References

1 Sampson HA. Update on food allergy. *J Allergy Clin Immunol* 2004;113:805–19; quiz 820.

2 Sicherer SH, Munoz-Furlong A, Sampson HA. Prevalence of peanut and tree nut allergy in the United States determined by means of a random digit dial telephone survey: a 5-year follow-up study. *J Allergy Clin Immunol* 2003;112:1203–7.

3 Sampson HA. Anaphylaxis and emergency treatment. *Pediatrics* 2003;111:1601–8.

4 Bock SA, Munoz-Furlong A, Sampson HA. Fatalities due to anaphylactic reactions to foods. *J Allergy Clin Immunol* 2001;107:191–3.

5 Oppenheimer JJ, Nelson HS, Bock SA, et al. Treatment of peanut allergy with rush immunotherapy. *J Allergy Clin Immunol* 1992 ;90:256–62.

6 Nelson HS, Lahr J, Rule R, et al. Treatment of anaphylactic sensitivity to peanuts by immunotherapy with injections of aqueous peanut extract. *J Allergy Clin Immunol* 1997;99:744–51.

7 Strachan DP. Hay fever, hygiene, and household size. *BMJ* 1989;299:1259–60.

8 Sato Y, Roman M, Tighe H, et al. Immunostimulatory DNA sequences necessary for effective intradermal gene immunization. *Science* 1996;273:352–4.

9 Hsu CH, Chua KY, Tao MH, et al. Immunoprophylaxis of allergen-induced immunoglobulin E synthesis and airway hyperresponsiveness *in vivo* by genetic immunization. *Nat Med* 1996;2:540–4.

10 Li X, Huang CK, Schofield BH, et al. Strain-dependent induction of allergic sensitization caused by peanut allergen DNA immunization in mice. *J Immunol* 1999;162:3045–52.

11 Roman M, Martin-Orozco E, Goodman JS, et al. Immunostimulatory DNA sequences function as T helper-1-promoting adjuvants. *Nat Med* 1997;3:849–54.

12 Tighe H, Takabayashi K, Schwartz D, et al. Conjugation of immunostimulatory DNA to the short ragweed allergen amb a 1 enhances its immunogenicity and reduces its allergenicity. *J Allergy Clin Immunol* 2000;106:124–34.

13 Creticos PS, Schroeder JT, Hamilton RG, et al. Immunotherapy with a ragweed-Toll-like receptor 9 agonist vaccine for allergic rhinitis. *N Engl J Med* 2006;355:1445–55.

14 Mo JH, Park SW, Rhee CS, et al. Suppression of allergic response by CpG motif oligodeoxynucleotide-house-dust mite conjugate in animal model of allergic rhinitis. *Am J Rhinol* 2006;20:212–18.

15 Simons FE, Shikishima Y, Van Nest G, et al. Selective immune redirection in humans with ragweed allergy by injecting Amb a 1 linked to immunostimulatory DNA. *J Allergy Clin Immunol* 2004;113:1144–51.

16 Srivastava K, Li XM, Bannon GA. Investigation of the use of ISS-linked Ara h2 for the treatment of peanut-induced allergy (abstract). *J Allergy Clin Immunol* 2001;107:S233.

17 Briner TJ, Kuo MC, Keating KM, et al. Peripheral T-cell tolerance induced in naive and primed mice by subcutaneous injection of

peptides from the major cat allergen Fel d I. *Proc Natl Acad Sci USA* 1993;90:7608–12.

18 Norman PS, Ohman Jr JL, Long AA, *et al*. Treatment of cat allergy with T-cell reactive peptides. *Am J Respir Crit Care Med* 1996;154:1623–8.

19 Stanley JS, King N, Burks AW, *et al*. Identification and mutational analysis of the immunodominant IgE binding epitopes of the major peanut allergen Ara h 2. *Arch Biochem Biophys* 1997;342:244–53.

20 Srivastava KD, Li X, King N, *et al*. Immunotherapy with modified peanut allergens in a murine model of peanut allergy. *J Allergy Clin Immunol* 2002;109:S287–S287.

21 Yeung VP, Gieni RS, Umetsu DT, DeKruyff RH. Heat-killed *Listeria monocytogenes* as an adjuvant converts established murine Th2-dominated immune responses into Th1-dominated responses. *J Immunol* 1998;161:4146–52.

22 Li J, Srivastava KD, Huleatt J, *et al*. Investigation of efficacy of co-administration of heat killed listeria with modified peanut protein for the treatment of peanut-induced hypersensitivity in a murine model. *J Allergy Clin Immunol* 2002;109:S93–S93.

23 Li X, Srivastava KD, Grishin A, *et al*. Persistent effect of immunotherapy with "Engineered" recombinant peanut protein and a bacterial adjuvant on peanut hypersensitivity. *J Allergy Clin Immunol* 2003;111:S195–S195.

24 Li X, Srivastava K, Grishin A, *et al*. Persistent protective effect of heat-killed *Escherichia coli* producing "engineered," recombinant peanut proteins in a murine model of peanut allergy. *J Allergy Clin Immunol* 2003;112:159–67.

25 Grishin A, Srivastava K, Sampson H, Li X. Generation of heat-killed *E. coli* expressing cow milk proteins for immunotherapy regiment for the milk allergic mice. *J Allergy Clin Immunol* 2004;113:S325–S325.

26 Chehade M, Mayer L. Oral tolerance and its relation to food hypersensitivities. *J Allergy Clin Immunol* 2005;115:3–12; quiz 13.

27 Bahna SL. Oral desensitization with cow's milk in IgE-mediated cow's milk allergy. *Contra! Monogr Allergy* 1996;32:233–5.

28 Goldstein GB, Heiner DC. Clinical and immunological perspectives in food sensitivity. a review. *J Allergy* 1970;46:270–91.

29 May CD, Remigio L, Feldman J, *et al*. A study of serum antibodies to isolated milk proteins and ovalbumin in infants and children. *Clin Allergy* 1977;7:583–95.

30 Patriarca C, Romano A, Venuti A, *et al*. Oral specific hyposensitization in the management of patients allergic to food. *Allergol Immunopathol (Madr)* 1984;12:275–81.

31 Patriarca G, Nucera E, Roncallo C, *et al*. Oral desensitizing treatment in food allergy: clinical and immunological results. *Aliment Pharmacol Ther* 2003;17:459–65.

32 Patriarca G, Schiavino D, Nucera E, *et al*. Food allergy in children: results of a standardized protocol for oral desensitization. *Hepatogastroenterology* 1998;45:52–8.

33 Nucera E, Schiavino D, D'Ambrosio C, *et al*. Immunological aspects of oral desensitization in food allergy. *Dig Dis Sci* 2000;45:637–41.

34 Wuthrich B. Oral desensitization with cow's milk in cow's milk allergy. *Pro! Monogr Allergy* 1996;32:236–40.

35 Bauer A, Ekanayake Mudiyanselage S, Wigger-Alberti W, Elsner P. Oral rush desensitization to milk. *Allergy* 1999;54:894–5.

36 Meglio P, Bartone E, Plantamura M, *et al*. A protocol for oral desensitization in children with IgE-mediated cow's milk allergy. *Allergy* 2004;59:980–7.

37 Bock SA. The natural history of food sensitivity. *J Allergy Clin Immunol* 1982;69:173–7.

38 Rolink-Werninghaus C, Staden U, Melhi A, Hamelmann E, Beyer K, Niggemann B. Specific oral tolerance induction with food in children: transient or persistent effect on food allergy? Allegry. 2005 Oct;60(10):1320–2.

39 Wilson DR, Lima MT, Durham SR. Sublingual immunotherapy for alleric rhinitis: systematic review and meta-analysis. Cochran Database Syst Rev. 2003;(2):CD002893.

40 Mascarell L, Van Overtvelt L, Moingeon P. Novel ways for immune intervention in immunotherapy: mucosal allergy vaccines. *Immunol Allergy Clin North Am* 2006;26:283–306, vii–viii.

41 Enrique E, Pineda F, Malek T, *et al*. Sublingual immunotherapy for hazelnut food allergy: a randomized, double-blind, placebo-controlled study with a standardized hazelnut extract. *J Allergy Clin Immunol* 2005;116:1073–9.

42 Li XM, Huang CK, Zhang TF, *et al*. The chinese herbal medicine formula MSSM-002 suppresses allergic airway hyperreactivity and modulates TH1/TH2 responses in a murine model of allergic asthma. *J Allergy Clin Immunol* 2000;106:660–8.

43 Wen MC, Wei CH, Hu ZQ, *et al*. Efficacy and tolerability of anti-asthma herbal medicine intervention in adult patients with moderate–severe allergic asthma. *J Allergy Clin Immunol* 2005;116:517–24.

44 Srivastava KD, Kattan JD, Zou ZM, *et al*. The Chinese herbal medicine formula FAHF-2 completely blocks anaphylactic reactions in a murine model of peanut allergy. *J Allergy Clin Immunol* 2005;115:171–8.

45 Ko J, Busse PJ, Shek L, *et al*. Effect of Chinese herbal formulas on T cell responses in patients with peanut allergy or asthma. *J Allergy Clin Immunol* 2005;115:S34.

46 Sudo N, Sawamura S, Tanaka K, *et al*. The requirement of intestinal bacterial flora for the development of an IgE production system fully susceptible to oral tolerance induction. *J Immunol* 1997;159:1739–45.

47 Oyama N, Sudo N, Sogawa H, Kubo C. Antibiotic use during infancy promotes a shift in the T(H)1/T(H)2 balance toward T(H)2-dominant immunity in mice. *J Allergy Clin Immunol* 2001;107:153–9.

48 Rautava S, Kalliomaki M, Isolauri E. New therapeutic strategy for combating the increasing burden of allergic disease: Probiotics-A Nutrition, Allergy, Mucosal Immunology and Intestinal Microbiota (NAMI) Research Group report. *J Allergy Clin Immunol* 2005;116:31–7.

49 Kalliomaki M, Salminen S, Arvilommi H, *et al*. Probiotics in primary prevention of atopic disease: a randomised placebo-controlled trial. *Lancet* 20017;357:1076–9.

50 Kalliomaki M, Salminen S, Poussa T, *et al*. Probiotics and prevention of atopic disease: 4-year follow-up of a randomised placebo-controlled trial. *Lancet* 2003;361:1869–71.

51 Brouwer ML, Wolt-Plompen SA, Dubois AE, *et al.* No effects of probiotics on atopic dermatitis in infancy: a randomized placebo-controlled trial. *Clin Exp Allergy* 2006;36:899–906.

52 Majamaa H, Isolauri E. Probiotics: a novel approach in the management of food allergy. *J Allergy Clin Immunol* 1997;99: 179–85.

53 Viljanen M, Kuitunen M, Haahtela T, *et al.* Probiotic effects on faecal inflammatory markers and on faecal IgA in food allergic atopiceczema/dermatitis syndrome infants. *Pediatr Allergy Immunol* 2005;16:65–71.

54 Pohjavuori E, Viljanen M, Korpela R, *et al.* Lactobacillus GG effect in increasing IFN-gamma production in infants with cow's milk allergy. *J Allergy Clin Immunol* 2004;114:131–6.

55 Yamane Y, Fujita J, Shimizu R, *et al.* Production of cellulose- and xylan-degrading enzymes by a koji mold, aspergillus oryzae, and their contribution to the maceration of rice endosperm cell wall. *J Biosci Bioeng* 2002;93:9–14.

56 Miyake Y, Sasaki S, Ohya Y, *et al.* Soy, isoflavones, and prevalence of allergic rhinitis in Japanese women: the Osaka Maternal and Child Health Study. *J Allergy Clin Immunol* 2005; 115:1176–83.

57 Zhang T, Pan W, Takebe M, *et al.* Effects of ImmuSoy as a food supplement for altering peanut allergic reactions. *J Allergy Clin Immunol* 2005;115:S35–S35.

58 Pan W, Zhang T, Takebe M, *et al.* Comparison of efficacy of a novel probiotic from koji fermentation(ImmuSoy) with LGG on peanut allergy. *J. Allergy Clin Immunol* 2006;117:S327–S327.

59 Casale TB, Bernstein IL, Busse WW, *et al.* Use of an anti-IgE humanized monoclonal antibody in ragweed-induced allergic rhinitis. *J Allergy Clin Immunol* 1997;100:110–21.

60 Milgrom H, Fick Jr RB, Su JQ, *et al.* Treatment of allergic asthma with monoclonal anti-IgE antibody. rhuMAb-E25 Study Group. *N Engl J Med* 1999;341:1966–73.

61 Leung DY, Sampson HA, Yunginger JW, *et al.* Effect of anti-IgE therapy in patients with peanut allergy. *N Engl J Med* 2003;348:986–93.

62 Lee SY, Huang CK, Zhang TF, *et al.* Oral administration of IL-12 suppresses anaphylactic reactions in a murine model of peanut hypersensitivity. *Clin Immunol* 2001;101:220–8.

63 Garrett JK, Jameson SC, Thomson B, *et al.* Anti-interleukin-5 (mepolizumab) therapy for hypereosinophilic syndromes. *J Allergy Clin Immunol* 2004;113:115–19.

CHAPTER 47

Food-Dependent Exercise- and Pressure-Induced Syndromes

Adam N. Williams and Ronald A. Simon

KEY CONCEPTS

- Food-dependent exercise-induced anaphylaxis (FDEIA) is a physical allergy syndrome that occurs only in response to exercise preceded by food ingestion.

- The importance of food in eliciting attacks of exercise-induced anaphylaxis (EIA) in some patients may be under-recognized, and many patients diagnosed with EIA may in fact have FDEIA.

- Food-specific FDEIA has been reported with many different types of food, and in some patients, attacks follow ingestion of any food (non-specific FDEIA).

- The main treatment for FDEIA is avoidance of ingestion of implicated foods at least 4 hours before exercise.

- Convincing evidence for a role of food allergy in other physical urticaria syndromes is currently lacking.

Introduction

The body of literature describing the association between physical allergy syndromes with the ingestion of food has grown significantly in the past decade. In these food-dependent physical allergy syndromes, it appears that two or more stimuli, which independently do not provoke an allergic response, do so when combined in sufficient temporal relationship. The clinical manifestations of the allergic response range in severity from itching and hives to anaphylactic shock. The two recognized physical allergy syndromes in which food ingestion contributes a "sub-threshold" precipitating factor are food-dependent exercise-induced anaphylaxis (FDEIA) and food-dependent delayed pressure urticaria (FDDPU).

Definitions

The clinical syndrome of exercise-induced anaphylaxis (EIA) has been described in several comprehensive reviews [1–11]. It is a physical allergy syndrome with onset generally during or within minutes of completion of exercise. Initial symptoms consist of a sensation of generalized

fatigue, warmth, pruritus, cutaneous erythema, and urticaria. Progression to other systemic symptoms including angioedema, dyspnea, cough, wheezing, nausea, vomiting, abdominal cramping, diarrhea, malaise, laryngeal edema, hypotension, vascular collapse, and loss of consciousness can follow. The attack can last from 30 minutes to 4 hours. Headache may persist following an attack for 24–72 hours. Various types and intensities of exercise may precipitate attacks. Jogging is the most commonly reported provoking exercise, but walking, bicycling, racquet sports, skiing, aerobics, dancing, soccer, and swimming have also been reported. Importantly, other reported provoking activities include horseback riding, raking leaves, and shoveling snow [10,11].

In one case series evaluating the frequency of various etiologies of anaphylaxis, exercise is considered the cause of anaphylaxis in 5–10% of patients (10–12% of patients with identifiable causes) referred to allergy and immunology clinics after presenting to acute care centers with anaphylaxis [12].

EIA appears to be associated with atopy in up to 50% of patients [1]. Women with EIA appear to be at least twice as likely as men to respond to epidemiologic surveys, but whether they in fact are more likely to experience EIA, as has been stated in other reviews on the subject, is unknown [13].

Little is known about the natural history of EIA, but lifestyle modification can certainly reduce the frequency and severity of attacks. Shadick *et al.* report on the 10-year

---

Food Allergy: Adverse Reactions to Foods and Food Additives, 4th edition.
Edited by Dean D. Metcalfe, Hugh A. Sampson, and Ronald A. Simon.
© 2008 Blackwell Publishing. ISBN: 978-1-4501-5129-0.

follow-up survey results of one cohort of 279 patients with EIA [13]. The response rate of women was twice that of men. The mean age at the time of first EIA attack was 26 years, with a range of 3–66 years. Forty-seven percent of respondents reported a decrease in the frequency of attacks, and 41% reported being completely free of attacks, in the preceding year. Subjects reported reducing attacks by avoiding exercise during extremely hot or cold weather (44%), restricting exercise during allergy season (36%) or humid weather (33%), and avoiding certain foods before exercise (37%).

Though considered by some to be another example of exercise-induced urticaria and anaphylaxis [9], there is rather convincing evidence that cholinergic urticaria (CU) is clinically distinct from EIA [14,15]. First, exercise, not heat, sweat, nor rise in body temperature has been identified to be the provoking factor for EIA. Second, the hives that occur in EIA are typically larger and distinct in appearance from the classic punctuate hives seen in CU. Third, CU can be associated with bronchospasm but vascular collapse occurs rarely. Laryngeal edema and stridor can occur in EIA, but no change in pulmonary function was observed in patients with EIA who underwent exercise challenge. Finally, studies have found elevated tryptase levels following attacks of EIA, but not CU [16,17].

FDEIA refers to a physical allergy syndrome in which attacks of EIA occur only when exercise is preceded by ingestion of a specific food (specific FDEIA) or any food (non-specific EIA).

A far less common type of exercise-induced urticaria and anaphylaxis, variant-type EIA, has been identified. These patients have attacks characterized by eruptions of punctuate urticaria, progression to vascular collapse, and are precipitated by exercise only and not passive warming [1,18].

Delayed pressure urticaria is a physical urticaria characterized by the development of hives and angioedema 30 minutes to 6 hours after the application of a sustained pressure stimulus on the skin. Underlying chronic idiopathic urticaria is usually present. A few reports have suggested that food may play a role in some cases of DPU.

Food-dependent, exercise-induced anaphylaxis

Epidemiology

In recent years, it has become clearer that a subset of patients with EIA can completely prevent exercise-induced attacks by avoiding either specific foods or non-specific food ingestion in the hours before exercise. In the survey results of their cohort of 279 patients with EIA, Shadick *et al.* reported that 37% of patients were able to reduce or eliminate attacks by avoiding certain foods [13]. A report of survey results obtained from another cohort of 199 EIA patients noted 54% of patients considered food ingestion or intake of specific foods to be a factor in the development of attacks [19].

In order to determine the prevalence of FDEIA in pre-adolescent school children in Japan, Aihara and colleagues conducted a survey of junior high school nurses representing 76,226 students in Yokohama [20]. Twenty-four cases of EIA (12 boys and 12 girls) and 13 cases of FDEIA (11 boys and 2 girls) were identified, with prevalences of 0.031% and 0.017%, respectively. Ten of 12 patients with FDEIA had other allergic disorders.

In a review of 167 cases of FDEIA in the Japanese literature since 1983, Harada and colleagues [21] described several characteristics of the disease, including a recent upward trend in the number of reports of FDEIA, male predominance, adolescents accounting for more than half of the cases, and a history of atopy in 40% of affected individuals.

Clinical features

The first case of EIA associated with food ingestion was reported by Maulitz *et al.* in 1979 [22]. This case involved a runner who developed anaphylactic reactions when he ran within 8–12 hours of ingestion of shellfish. The patient ran regularly, averaging 50–130 km per week. Over a 3-year period prior to diagnosis of the condition, the patient sustained approximately 10 bouts of transient facial flushing and edema, with diffuse urticaria and pruritus occurring during or immediately after exercise. Two of the reactions resulted in almost complete upper airway obstruction requiring emergency therapy with epinephrine and antihistamines. The patient had no initial suspicion of allergic sensitivity to, or clinical reactions following, shellfish ingestion, but eventually the association with exercise was made. During further evaluation, he had positive immediate reactions with epicutaneous skin testing to clams, oysters, shrimp, crab, peanuts, trees, grasses, and weeds. Once the diagnosis was made and causative foods identified, avoidance of ingestion of these foods for at least 12 hours prior to exercise resulted in almost complete elimination of any further reactions.

In all cases of FDEIA, ingestion of the implicated food or non-specific food ingestion followed by exercise provokes the attack, and neither food ingestion nor exercise alone is sufficient. The nature of the attacks in FDEIA is indistinguishable from those described in patients with EIA. In their report on the clinical characteristics of 54 patients with FDEIA, Romano *et al.* found the most common symptoms to be pruritus (94% of patients), urticaria (85%), and angioedema (83%). Other common symptoms included flushing (74%), dyspnea (70%), gastrointestinal disturbances (nausea, diarrhea, colic, vomiting: 35%), hypotension (33%), and upper respiratory disturbances (choking, throat constriction, and hoarseness: 30%) [23].

The most common implicated foods are wheat, shellfish, alcohol, and a variety of fruits and vegetables, though over 40 different foods have been reported (see Table 47.1). In Japan, wheat and shellfish are implicated in the majority of cases of FDEIA, whereas case series reports from the

Table 47.1 Foods reported to be associated with FDEIA

>10 cases reported	<10 cases reported	
Alcohol	Apple	Mushroom
Barley	Almonds	Mustard
Celery	Banana	Onion
Cheese	Beef	Orange
Milk	Cabbage	Peas
Oats	Chicken	Pear
Peach	Corn	Penicillium
Peanut	Egg	(contaminated food)
Rye	Fennel	Pistachio
Soybean	Fish	Poppy seed
Shellfish	Garlic	Pork
Strawberry	Grape	Potato
Tomato	Hazelnut	Rice
Wheat	Kiwi	Snail
	Lentil	Spinach
	Lettuce	Umeboshi
	Litchi	(combination w/wheat)
		Walnut

United States and Europe implicate a wider variety of foods [13,15,22–42].

In a subset of patients with EIA associated with food ingestion, a specific food cannot be identified. Among the 54 patients with FDEIA reported by Romano et al., a causative food could not be identified by history or specific IgE testing in six subjects [23]. Another case series of 11 Japanese patients with FDEIA, 4 were not sensitive to any specific food [25].

As with EIA, a variety of types and intensities of exercise can provoke attacks. Running, jogging, walking, soccer, dancing, and racquet sports are the most commonly reported provoking exercises for FDEIA [13,23,25]. The time between food ingestion and exercise generally ranges between 30 minutes and 4 hours, with the vast majority occurring within 2 hours [23]. The distance runner first described by Maulitz et al. in 1979 reported attacks 5, 20, and 24 hours after shellfish ingestion [22], but no cases of food-and-exercise challenge (FEC) confirmed cases with ingestion-to-exercise intervals greater than 6 hours have been reported. Whether the intensity of exertion correlates with the severity of the attack remains unclear, but the duration of exercise necessary to provoke an attack can range from 10 to 50 minutes. A single case of FDEIA has been reported in which the attack only occurred if the food (celery) was ingested within 2 hours after exercise [30].

It is unknown whether the amount of allergen ingested has an impact on the elicitation or severity of the attacks in FDEIA. Case series reporting FEC results do not specify the amount of food ingested prior to exercise. Hanakawa

and colleagues reported a case of FDEIA in which the systemic allergic reaction depended on the amount of allergen ingested [43]. A 24-year-old woman with EIA associated with wheat ingestion had a class 2 positive radioallergoabsorbent test (RAST) for wheat and gluten, class 3 positive RAST for rye, and positive skin prick tests (SPTs) for wheat, bread, gluten, and udon (Japanese wheat noodles). Challenge tests with bread were performed. Exercise following ingestion of 64g, but not 45g, of bread induced generalized urticaria. Challenge tests with udon also provoked urticaria in a dose-dependent manner: 200g, but not 100 or 150g, elicited symptoms. They concluded that a negative challenge in patients suspected to have FDEIA may result from an insufficient amount of ingested food allergen (or sub-threshold exercise).

In some cases, a combination of two different foods followed by exercise may be required to elicit a reaction. Aihara et al. [28] reported a case of a 14-year-old boy with FDEIA diagnosed by provocation testing with the simultaneous ingestion of wheat and umeboshi (unripe plums pickled in brine and other ingredients, used in Japanese cooking), followed by exercise. Provocation tests with wheat or umeboshi alone failed to produce the transient increase in plasma histamine levels and drop in forced expiratory volume in 1 second (FEV1) elicited by the combination of food allergens. Again, this could partly account for negative challenge tests in patients with a strong clinical history for FDEIA. More recently, a case of FDEIA was reported in a 48-year-old woman that could only be provoked by a combination of food additives, ethanol, wheat flour, and exercise, whereas exercise challenges with or without ingestion of food additives, ethanol or wheat individually were negative [39].

Cross-reactivity of allergenic food components may also play an important role in FDEIA. Palosuo et al. examined the sera of 23 adult patients with wheat-dependent EIA for cross-reactivity of wheat omega-5 gliadin with other cereal proteins. They found that gamma-70 and gamma-35 secalins in rye and gamma-3 in barley cross-react with omega-5 gliadin [44]. In addition, two patients in their cohort of wheat-specific FDEIA reported exercise-induced allergic symptoms after rye ingestion. This suggests that rye and barley may also elicit exercise-induced symptoms in patients with wheat-specific EIA. Romano et al. noted that in their cohort of patients with FDEIA, 9 of 14 patients with tomato-specific FDEIA had positive skin tests for grasses with structural cross-reactivity with tomato. IgE cross-reactivity has also been reported in patients with mustard-specific FDEIA to mugwort pollen, celery-dependent FDEIA to mugwort pollen, and snail-dependent FDEIA to dust mite allergen [34,35,45].

Aspirin, non-steroidal anti-inflammatory drugs (NSAIDs), and possibly other medications may have a key role in eliciting or enhancing food-dependent, exercise-induced reactions. Dohi et al. described two patients who recalled that aspirin taken 30 or 60 minutes before food intake provoked exercise-induced reactions that were more severe than without aspirin [25]. In another case series of three patients with FDEIA, Harada *et al.* found that aspirin added to FEC was required to provoke a systemic reaction in two patients, and was sufficient to provoke systemic symptoms when combined with food (without exercise) in one patient [46].

In order to investigate the effect of aspirin in provocation tests and in SPT of patients with FDEIA, Aihara *et al.* performed provocation challenges with combinations of food, exercise, and aspirin. Pre-treatment with aspirin was associated with enhanced SPT reactions to food, but not histamine, in five of eight (62.5%) patients. Of three patients who did not react to food and exercise, two reacted when challenged with the combination of food, exercise, and aspirin. In addition, two of three patients with positive challenges to food and exercise also had a positive challenge when food was combined with aspirin instead of exercise [47]. In another case series, Dohi *et al.* described three patients in whom aspirin ingestion followed by specific foods and exercise elicited more severe attacks with less exercise than when food and exercise were not preceded by aspirin ingestion [48]. Taken together, these data suggest aspirin may contribute to the severity of FDEIA reactions. Cross-reactivity of this aspirin effect on FDEIA severity with NSAIDs is supported by the finding by Romano *et al.* that three of five patients who reported taking aspirin shortly before FDEIA attacks had also taken NSAIDs before other FDEIA attacks [23].

Other factors that appear to be capable of contributing to the elicitation or severity of FDEIA attacks include psychological stress, abnormal response of the autonomic nervous system, menstruation, fatigue, lack of sleep, and seasonal variation [23,25].

Diagnostic considerations

Differentiating FDEIA from other clinical entities involving food, exercise, urticaria, respiratory symptoms, or collapse may be difficult (Table 47.2). Unless the association of exercise-induced attacks with specific or non-specific food ingestion can be identified historically, patients with FDEIA may be misdiagnosed as having EIA. Idiopathic anaphylaxis, food- and drug-induced anaphylaxis, and anaphylaxis associated with systemic mastocytosis lack a clear association with exertion.

CU should also be distinguished from FDEIA. As discussed above, CU is a physical urticaria syndrome characterized by small, punctate wheals that develop in response to elevation in body temperature such as through exercise, exposure to hot water, sweating, fever, or emotional stress. The symptoms are generally limited to the skin, can be associated with wheezing, but not stridor, laryngeal edema, or vascular collapse. The provocation of the other physical urticarias by

Table 47.2 Differential Diagnosis of FDEIA

Differential diagnosis of FDEIA
Anaphylaxis syndromes
Idiopathic
Food induced
Drug induced
Exercise-induced syndromes
Exercise-induced anaphylaxis
Physical urticarias
Cholinergic
Delayed pressure
Solar
Aquagenic
Exercise-induced bronchospasm
Cardiac arrythmias
Other
Other urticaria
Idiopathic/autoimmune urticaria
Systemic mastocytosis
Vasovagal syncope–presyncope
Carcinoid syndrome
Psychogenic
Shock
Septic
Cardiogenic
Hypovolemic

exposure to sunlight, water, vibration, and pressure should be readily distinguished from FDEIA on the basis of history.

The phenomenon of exercise-induced bronchospasm that can occur in patients with asthma presents with dyspnea, cough, and wheezing provoked by exercise but is rarely associated with pruritus, urticaria, upper respiratory obstruction, or vascular collapse. Non-allergic causes of vascular collapse such as neurocardiogenic syncope and cardiac arrhythmias that can be associated with exercise and/or food ingestion also lack these characteristic features of anaphylaxis.

Diagnosing underlying food sensitivity in patients with FDEIA may prove difficult. The history is the most important diagnostic tool. Special emphasis should be placed on obtaining a detailed account of the symptoms of the attack, timing in relation to food and exercise, specific foods and/or medications (as well as quantities) ingested prior to attack, and other allergic history. The best clue comes from the presence of intermittent or sporadic exercise-induced reactions superimposed on the baseline of consistent, uneventful exercise. Although a specific food is usually implicated as a co-precipitating factor (specific FDEIA), some patients suffer from EIA after any food ingestion (non-specific FDEIA) [23]. In many cases of FDEIA, the association with food ingestion may not have been made, thereby unnecessarily restricting affected patients' ability to exercise. Some cases may even be labeled idiopathic. A confounding factor that may complicate the process of making an accurate diagnosis may be the lag in time between ingestion and reaction. This may rarely extend to 12–24 hours, making the association with a specific food trigger extremely difficult. The association of EIA episodes with a specific food may also be missed in cases when the implicated food is a dietary staple such as wheat. Varjonen *et al.*, for example, reported a series of five patients who could only associate the attacks of anaphylaxis with exercise, but were found to have detectable IgE on SPT and were able to exercise safely be eliminating wheat from the diet [49]. The accurate diagnosis can further be obscured by the requirement, in at least a few cases, of other factors such as aspirin or NSAID ingestion, psychological stress, menstruation, and seasonal or temperature variation. Some patients considered to have exercise-induced or "idiopathic" anaphylaxis without apparent relationship to food may in fact be reacting to unidentified ingestants, a combination of allergenic ingestants, or a cross-reacting ingestant.

Specific IgE testing in the form of SPT or RAST can be quite useful, especially as an opportunity to minimize exercise restrictions for affected patients. The vast majority of cases of FDEIA with a specific food identified as a co-precipitating factor have positive SPTs to the implicated food. Based on their findings in 54 patients with FDEIA, Romano and colleagues stress the importance of both *in vivo* and *in vitro* testing to an extensive panel of foods [23]. After detailed histories, patients were subjected to SPT to 26 commercial food allergens, SPTs with 15 fresh foods, and RAST for 31 food allergens. Forty-eight patients had suspected a particular food in association with attacks; six could not recall a certain food. Fifty-two patients were positive to at least one food; two had no positive results at all. All suspect foods were positive and each of the three tests revealed varying degrees of sensitivity, with positive results not discovered by the other tests. Exercise challenges following meals lacking the foods that elicited positive results on SPT or RAST failed to elicit reactions.

In another study of 19 patients referred for evaluation for anaphylaxis that occurred during or immediately following exercise, screening SPT and/or RAST to foods ingested prior to the episode of EIA revealed sensitization in 17. Avoidance of the identified foods 5 hours prior to exercise successfully prevented recurrence in 15 of these patients during the follow-up period (median 2 years) [29].

Special consideration of the limitations of specific IgE testing in the evaluation of patients with possible wheat-dependent EIA should be noted. Omega-5 gliadin (the major allergen responsible for wheat-dependent EIA) exists in the insoluble gliadin fraction of wheat proteins, which is lacking from commercial testing reagents [44,50]. The clinical implication is that the detection of IgE sensitization to wheat with commercial test reagents is impaired and this may lead to the incorrect diagnosis of EIA or nonspecific FDEIA, rather than wheat-specific EIA. *In vitro* IgE testing to omega-5 gliadin is not currently commercially available.

Though considered to be the gold-standard for confirming the diagnosis of FDEIA, the role of food-and-exercise provocation challenges in the clinical setting is unclear. The decision to perform such provocation challenges should include consideration of the risk of patient harm resulting from positive challenges, the possibility of a false-negative challenge, and the ease of avoidance of the suspected food prior to exercise. One approach used by some authors [23,29] is performing observed exercise challenges following meals lacking the suspected food(s), thereby providing reassurance that patients can safely exercise as long as the implicated food is eliminated from the diet.

Pathophysiology

The mechanism whereby exercise and food ingestion elicit the allergic response resulting in urticaria and anaphylaxis is not entirely understood. Food and exercise appear to act as two sub-threshold stimuli that individually are inadequate to produce mediator release from mast cells or basophils, yet when combined in a temporal relationship can produce mast cell or basophil degranulation. Support for the concept that mast cell degranulation is involved comes from studies involving electron microscopy of biopsy specimens obtained from exercise-induced urticarial lesions in patients with EIA showing ultrastructural evidence of mast cell degranulation [17]. Furthermore, a number of endogenous peptides can release histamine from mast cells both *in vivo* and *in vitro* [51]. These peptides include substance P, vasoactive intestinal peptide (VIP), calcitonin gene-related peptide (CGRP), gastrin, pentagastrin, and endorphins [51–54]. Release of these peptides occurs via various stimuli, including exercise, digestion, anxiety, pain, and local irritation. Any of these factors could be involved in physical urticarias or other allergic syndromes, including chronic urticaria, asthma, allergic rhinitis, and anaphylaxis, but studies showing increases in any of these endogenous peptides in response to exercise in patients with FDEIA are lacking.

Increased levels of histamine and tryptase have been observed after exercise in patients with EIA [3,16]. Exercise alone was sufficient to produce a rise in histamine in 6 of 11 patients with FDEIA, and exercise preceded by provocative foods was necessary in one additional patient [25].

Kivity *et al.* studied the effect of compound 48/80, a mast cell degranulating agent, on SPT in five subjects with FDEIA who had previous skin reactivity to provocative foods and five normal controls. Intradermal injection of compound 48/80 was associated with a much larger wheal response in four subjects with FDEIA as compared to controls after FECs, but not after food- or exercise-only challenges. The histamine wheal response in these subjects was not significantly changed [55]. Similar increases in exercise-induced wheal responses have been found in other studies using compound 48/80 and codeine [56,57]. These findings suggest reactions in patients with FDEIA are produced by a direct effect of exercise and food allergen on mast cell releasability, rather than an increased sensitivity to histamine. This also implies that IgE and food antigens may interact with mast cells to lower the threshold to another stimulus, such as exercise, to produce the anaphylactic response.

The high prevalence of atopic diseases in patients with FDEIA and the finding that most patients with challenge-proven food-specific FDEIA have detectable IgE antibodies to implicated foods on SPT or RAST leave little doubt that IgE plays an important role in triggering attacks of FDEIA [20,21,23,25]. In addition to possible effects on mast cell releasability, exercise may also serve to facilitate increased small intestine allergen absorption. In one study of six patients with wheat-dependent EIA and four healthy controls, Matsuo et al. found that serum levels of gliadin, a major wheat allergen, rose in parallel with allergic responses following wheat ingestion and exercise [58]. An explanation for this observation comes from studies on the effects of exercise on intestinal function and hemodynamics showing that reduction of splanchnic blood flow from exercise causes epithelial barrier disruption and increases in intestinal permeability [59–61].

Other studies involving wheat-dependent FDEIA in Japan have provided further support for IgE-mediated food allergy in at least this subset of patients. Some of the IgE-binding epitopes for two important allergens in wheat-dependent FDEIA, omega-5 gliadin and a high-molecular-weight glutenin, have been identified [62,63]. In both cases, the epitope appears to be linear, rather than conformational. Interestingly, neither wheat-sensitive subjects with atopic dermatitis nor healthy controls demonstrated reactivity with epitope-specific IgE testing.

Of the additional cofactors that have been reported to possibly contribute to FDEIA attacks, the potential role of aspirin in enhancing FDEIA reactions has been most widely studied. Aspirin and other NSAIDs are capable of provoking or exacerbating hives in up to 30% of patients with chronic urticaria and angioedema through inhibition of cyclooxygenase-1 (COX-1) [64]. The observation that aspirin and other NSAIDs appear to provoke or exacerbate reactions in patients with FDEIA could, at least in part, also be attributable to COX-1 inhibition, but other mechanisms may also be involved. Aspirin, like exercise, appears to increase intestinal permeability through damage to gut epithelial tight junctions [65]. Matsuo et al. showed that co-ingestion of aspirin and wheat in patients with wheat-dependent EIA resulted in a rise in serum levels of gliadin and clinical allergic reactions [58]. Further studies are required to determine what potential role other cofactors such as medications, psychological stress, menstruation, fatigue, and lack of sleep may play in FDEIA responses.

Taken together, these observations provide some insight into the processes whereby food and exercise combine to produce anaphylactic reactions (see Fig. 47.1). In sensitized individuals, immunologically intact food antigen is absorbed, but in the absence of exercise, an immune response does not occur. When food ingestion is followed by exercise, the clinically observed reaction that follows is likely brought about by at least two key concomitant mechanisms: enhanced mast cell releasability and altered intestinal permeability. Serum levels of a number of the endogenous peptides known to induce mast cell degranulation including substance P, VIP, CGRP, gastrin, pentagastrin, and endorphins have been shown to increase in response to exercise [55–58]. In addition, intestinal epithelial barrier disruption associated with reduced splanchnic blood flow leads to altered intestinal permeability and the potential for enhanced absorption of immunologically intact food antigens [62–65]. Aspirin and

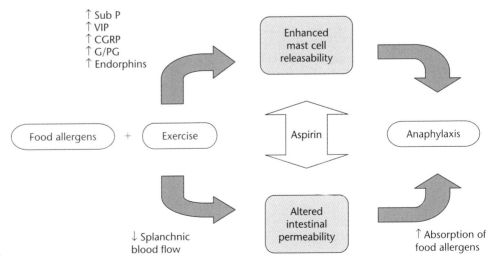

Figure 47.1 Schematic representation of role of exercise in food-specific EIA. Sub P, substance P; VIP, vasoactive intestinal peptide; CGRP, calcitonin gene-related peptide; G/PG, gastrin/pentagastrin.

NSAIDs can further potentiate these effects through COX-1 inhibition (and increased mast cell releasing factors, such as LTC4) and disruption of intestinal epithelial tight junctions. The result is the observed clinical allergic reaction.

Treatment

Avoidance of ingestion of any implicated foods in sufficient temporal proximity to exercise is the cornerstone of management of FDEIA. Prospective, controlled studies designed to evaluate the minimal time interval between provoking foods and exercise are lacking, but for patients with specific FDEIA, avoidance of implicated foods 4–6 hours prior to exercise usually prevents an urticarial or anaphylactic reaction following exercise. In cases of non-specific FDEIA, avoidance of all foods for at least 6–8 hours prior to exercise is recommended [66]. Of 43 patients with food-specific FDEIA advised to avoid implicated foods for 4 hours prior to exercise, none had experienced reactions after a mean of over 4 years of follow-up. In addition, none of the five patients with non-specific FDEIA advised to avoid exercise for at least 4 hours after any meal had experienced reactions [23]. Because lower levels of exertion such as walking and activities not considered to be exercise such as yard work and ironing clothes have been reported to provoke EIA, some patients might prefer complete avoidance of implicated foods [31]. Inquiring about and tailoring exercise regimes as indicated to avoid co-precipitating factors such as aspirin and NSAID ingestion, menstruation, seasonal variation, and extremes of weather should also be considered [13].

The utility of various medications taken prior to exercise in patients with FDEIA has not been established. Antihistamines taken either daily or one-half hour before exercise may help blunt the attack [67]. However, no data exist to suggest that this therapy can eliminate or prevent episodes. Oral cromolyn has also been reported to successfully prevent attacks [28,68]. The leukotriene antagonists, zafirlukast and montelukast, have been shown to attenuate exercise-induced bronchoconstriction, but no studies have evaluated this class of agents in FDEIA so far [69,70].

When attacks do occur, early intervention should help decrease their severity [1]. Patients should have a clear understanding of the early signs and symptoms of anaphylaxis, and immediate cessation of exercise when they occur is recommended. Self-injectable epinephrine should be prescribed for all patients along with the recommendation to carry it during exercise. Patients with a history of life-threatening reactions should also consider wearing a medical alert bracelet and avoid exercising alone. Emergency treatment at the time of the reaction may be lifesaving, although deaths attributed to FDEIA are rare [10,71].

The potential role of other treatment modalities such as anti-IgE therapy or other immunomodulatory agents requires investigation. Whether induction of tolerance to exercise following food ingestion can be achieved remains unknown. In their report on the results of a survey of patients with EIA, Wade *et al.* reported one patient who remained free from exercise-induced attacks while walking 5 miles per day, but EIA symptoms recurred following resumption of exercise after a several month period of inactivity. Other patients have described a "refractory period" following an attack of EIA, during which time they could exercise without risk of subsequent attack [19].

Delayed pressure urticaria

Clinical features

DPU is another syndrome in which the association has been made between the ingestion of food and the development of a physically induced cutaneous reaction [72–80]. This unusual disease, which is more prevalent than previously appreciated, is characterized by the delayed onset of deep cutaneous swellings in areas exposed to prolonged pressure of variable intensity. The appearance of the pressure-induced swelling of the hands and feet is indistinguishable from that of angioedema. The onset of lesions can occur within 30 minutes to 9 hours of application of pressure from a variety of stimuli (e.g. for the feet, prolonged walking on a hard surface; for the shoulder, carrying luggage; and for the hands, hammering nails). The lesions usually peak 6–9 hours after pressure and may last as long as 36 hours. There may be a refractory period for development of new lesions in locations with recent urticaria [81]. In 30–90% of patients, DPU can be associated with chronic idiopathic urticaria [75,77,79]. Some patients develop "flu-like" symptoms (malaise, arthralgias, and fever) in association with the skin lesions. Almost half patients with DPU have an elevated erythrocyte sedimentation rate (ESR) and mild leukocytosis with or without eosinophilia. Usually the delayed pressure symptoms and reactivity parallel the activity of the chronic urticaria and can persist up to 30 years. The condition often creates a significant functional disability, especially in individuals whose occupations require heavy physical labor, such as carpenters, constructions workers, and auto mechanics [75].

Diagnosis

DPU is best diagnosed by a thorough history. Many patients have been incorrectly diagnosed as having refractory angioedema in association with their chronic urticaria. The diagnosis can be confirmed using several tests [74–77,80,81]. The simplest and most reliable test utilizes 15 lb of weight split into two sandbags connected by a thin strap. This device is then suspended over the shoulder for a period of 15 minutes while the patient is walking [74]. The shoulder is examined 4–8 hours after challenge for the development of a deep, often painful, erythematous swelling. In most cases the test is positive initially. In patients with a good history and a negative initial test, a follow-up test at least 48 hours later may be positive. The test can be negative when the disease is quiescent or in remission.

Pathophysiology

The pathogenesis of DPU remains unclear. Lesions can be induced by injections of compound 48/80 into the skin, suggesting that release of mast cell mediators may be important in lesion induction [82]. Increased histamine levels have been shown in skin blisters above the lesions [77]. Biopsy specimens reveal mild mononuclear perivascular infiltrates with some eosinophils and a small number of polymorphonuclear leukocytes [83]. Fibrin deposition and edema among the collagen fibers at the pressure challenge site suggest a similarity between the lesions of DPU and those generated by the cutaneous late-phase reaction seen after allergen injection [84]. Barlow [85] proposes a lower threshold in DPU patients to form wheals compared to control subjects. Hermes and colleagues noted endothelial cell upregulation of tumor necrosis factor (TNF)-α and IL-3 in non-lesional skin of patients with DPU, and upregulation of TNF-α production in perivascular cells [86]. They suggest a role for these cytokines in the pathogenesis of DPU by an induction of sub-threshold inflammation in endothelial cells of uninvolved skin. Kallikrein generation [77], leukotriene production [77], and cytokine release in lesions [82] have been hypothesized but, to date, not confirmed. As with other causes of urticaria, aspirin appears to have a potentiating effect on the development of urticarial lesions in DPU [87,88].

Treatment

The pressure-induced lesions of most patients with DPU respond poorly to standard drugs used in the treatment of chronic urticaria and angioedema. The only medications that consistently relieve the delayed pressure symptoms are systemic corticosteroids [74–76,79]. Some patients require relatively high doses of these agents and prolonged therapy to remain functional and able to work. The delayed pressure component often does not respond to conventional H1 antihistamine alone or to a combination of H1 and H2 antihistamines [71–76,79]. Cetirizine reportedly has been effective in some patients [88,89]. Leukotriene antagonists have been shown effective in chronic idiopathic urticaria but are poorly studied in DPU [91–95]. Berkun and colleagues [94] reported the first case of a patient with steroid-dependent DPU responding to the leukotriene antagonist montelukast. One small randomized, double-blind study of 20 patients with DPU comparing loratadine to loratadine plus montelukast found the combination to be more effective at suppressing pressure-induced reactions than loratadine alone [95]. Another small study showed the addition of theophylline to cetirizine to be more effective than cetirizine monotherapy [96]. Sulfasalazine, at doses used in inflammatory bowel disease, was found to be an effective steroid-sparing

agent for angioedema in two patients with refractory DPU [97]. Some patients [75] respond partially to NSAIDs, but this has not been observed consistently [79]. Limited studies have demonstrated the effectiveness of higher potency topical corticosteroids [98,99]. High-dose intravenous immunoglobulin induced remission or improved symptoms in five of eight patients with DPU considered to be severe and refractory to other therapies or responding only to oral corticosteroids [100]. The role in DPU of other agents used with some success in chronic idiopathic urticaria such as antimalarials [101], hydroxychloroquine [102], cyclosporine [103], dapsone [104,105], pentoxifylline [105], methotrexate [106], stanozolol [107], and calcineurin inhibitors [108] remains to be seen.

Food-related delayed pressure urticaria

Specific causal factors for DPU are rarely identified; however, Davis and colleagues [109] identified specific food ingestion as an exacerbating factor. In this report, six selected patients with challenge-proven DPU and chronic idiopathic urticaria were studied, all of whom required daily prednisone for symptomatic control. The patients either fasted, receiving only water, or were given a diet of unflavored Vivonex for a minimum of 48 hours. In five of the six patients, both spontaneous urticarial lesions and pressure-induced symptoms cleared after 24–48 hours of fasting. A control group of patients with chronic urticaria was treated in the same way, but none responded to the fast. All patients who had resolution of urticaria with fasting had at least one positive delayed cutaneous reaction (measured at 6 hours) on SPT with food antigens. Ingestion of foods producing a positive delayed cutaneous reaction was followed within 2–24 hours by recurrence of spontaneous and pressure-induced urticaria. Interestingly, RAST to foods causing positive delayed cutaneous reactions and recurrence of urticaria were negative.

A subsequent report described two patients with DPU in whom lesions could be elicited when they had eaten typical foods but not when they had been on at least 5 days of an elimination diet [110]. Skin testing was not described, however. In another study by Czarnetzki *et al.* [111], 13 patients with DPU and positive cutaneous prick testing responses to foods failed to respond to elimination diets. All of the subjects underwent testing to a large battery of common allergens, including food extracts. Seven of these patients had positive early cutaneous reactions (15 minutes), and six developed positive late cutaneous reactions (after 6 hours). None of the patients, however, showed any improvement on diets that eliminated those food antigens to which they developed a late cutaneous reaction. It is not clear whether any of the patients fasted for any prolonged period of time to exclude other allergens that were not part of the skin test battery.

Although a role for food ingestion in the causation of DPU has been suggested, it has not been well documented or proved. In over 20 years since the report by Davis *et al.* [109]

summarized above, few studies convincingly implicating food ingestion as a possible cause of DPU have been published. Vidal *et al.* reported one additional case of delayed pressure urticaria that appeared to occur only in association with egg ingestion [112]. Whereas none of the patients reported in the case series by Davis *et al.* had detectable IgE to the suspected foods, this patient did have egg-specific IgE detected on RAST and SPT.

Thus, while efforts to exclude specific foods as contributing factors to cutaneous eruptions in patients with DPU appear unlikely to contribute significantly, given the high morbidity of DPU in some patients, including the potential requirement for long-term systemic corticosteroid therapy, it may be worthwhile to consider ingestants as aggravating factors in almost any patient with DPU.

Other food/physical syndromes

Strong evidence for the role of food in eliciting other physical allergy syndromes is lacking. Zuberbier and colleagues [113] describe the case of a 43-year-old woman with angioedema resulting from a combination of non-specific food intake and elevation of body temperature. Pseudoallergic reactions to hot, cold, or spicy foods may elicit CU responses, but true allergic responses involving food ingestion have not been reported to contribute to other physical urticaria syndromes including dermographism, solar urticaria, aquagenic urticaria, or vibratory angioedema.

Conclusions

Of the physical allergy syndromes, food allergy appears to play a role in a significant subset of patients with EIA and possibly DPU. In the case of FDEIA, the historical association of specific or non-specific food ingestion with the exercise-induced attacks may not be readily apparent but may not be uncommon. As a result, in patients with EIA in whom the possibility that food may be contributing to anaphylaxis attacks cannot be excluded historically, a thorough investigation including specific IgE testing to a variety of common foods should be considered. Because nearly all patients with specific FDEIA are able to prevent attacks of EIA by avoiding suspected foods 4 hours before exercise, this approach may contribute significantly to the quality of life in patients who may otherwise impose disabling restrictions on their physical activity in an effort to avoid attacks. Though the role of food allergy in DPU is less clear, the significant morbidity of pressure avoidance and lack of proven non-toxic therapies for this condition also warrant consideration of foods as potential co-precipitants. Future studies are clearly needed to help guide clinicians in the management and treatment of these chronic conditions.

References

1 Sheffer AL, Austen KR. Exercise induced anaphylaxis. *J Allergy Clin Immunol* 1980;66:106–11.

2 Lewis J, Lieberman P, Treadwell G, Erffmeyer J. Exercise induced urticaria, angioedema, and anaphylactoid episodes. *J Allergy Clin Immunol* 1981;68:432–7.

3 Sheffer AL, Soter NA, McFadden ER, Austen KR. Exercise induced anaphylaxis: a distinct form of physical allergy. *J Allergy Clin Immunol* 1983;7:311–16.

4 Kapla AP, Natbony SF, Tawil AP, *et al.* Exercise-induced anaphylaxis as a manifestation of cholinergic urticaria. *J Allergy Clin Immunol* 1981;68:319–24.

5 Songsiridej V, Busse WW. Exercise-induced anaphylaxis. *Clin Allergy* 1983;13:317–21.

6 Casale TB, Kehey TM, Kaliner M. Exercise-induced anaphylactic syndromes: insights into diagnostic and pathophysiologic features. *JAMA* 1986;255:2049–53.

7 Tilles S, Schocket A, Milgrom H. Exercise-induced anaphylaxis related to specific foods. *J Pediatrics* 1995;127:587–9.

8 Tilles SA, Schocket AL. Exercise-induced anaphylaxis. *Pact Allergy Immunol* 1994;9:64–7.

9 Volcheck GW, Li JT. Exercise-induced urticaria and anaphylaxis. *Mayo Clin Proc* 1997;72:140–7.

10 Lieberman P, Kemp SF, Oppenheimer J, *et al.* The diagnosis and management of anaphylaxis: an updated practice parameter. *J Allergy Clin Immunol* 2005;115:S483–523.

11 Castells MC, Horan RF, Sheffer AL. Exercise-induced anaphylaxis. *Curr Allergy Asthma Rep* 2003;3:15–21.

12 Webb LM, Lieberman P. Anaphylaxis: a review of 601 cases. *Ann Allergy Asthma Immunol* 2006;97:39–43.

13 Shadick NA, Liang MH, Partridge AJ, *et al.* The natural history of exercise-induced anaphylaxis: survey results from a 10-year follow-up study. *J Allergy Clin Immunol* 1999;104:123–7.

14 Kaplan A. Urticaria and angioedema. In: Adkinson NF, Yuninger JW, Busse WW, Bochner BS, Holgate ST, Simons FER (eds.) *Middleton's Allergy Principles and Practice*, 6th edn. Philadelphia, PA: Mosby, 2003:1537–58.

15 Perkins DN, Keith PK. Food- and exercise-induced anaphylaxis: importance of history in diagnosis. *Ann Allergy Asthma Clin Immunol* 2002;89:15–23.

16 Schwartz H. Elevated serum tryptase in exercise-induced anaphylaxis. *J Allergy Clin Immunol* 1995;95:917–19.

17 Sheffer AL, Tong AKF, Murphy GF, *et al.* Exercise-induced anaphylaxis: a serious form of physical allergy associated with mast cell degranulation. *J Allergy Clin Immunol* 1985;75:479–84.

18 Sheffer AL, Austen KF. Exercise-induced anaphylaxis. *J Allergy Clin Immunol* 1984;73:699–703.

19 Wade JP, Liang MH, Sheffer AL. Exercise-induced anaphylaxis: epidemiologic observations. *Prog Clin Biol Res* 1989;297: 175–82.

20 Aihara Y, Takahashi Y, Kotoyori T, *et al.* Frequency of food-dependent, exercise-induced anaphylaxis in Japanese junior-high-school students. *J Allergy Clin Immunol* 2001;108:1035–9.

21 Harada S, Horikawa T, Icihashi M. A study of food-dependent exercise-induced anaphylaxis by analyzing the Japanese cases reported in the literature. *Aerugi* 2000;49:1066–73.

22 Maulitz RM, Pratt DS, Schocket AL. Exercise-induced anaphylactic reaction to shellfish. *J Allergy Clin Immunol* 1979;63:433–4.

23 Romano A, Di Fonso M, Guiffreda F, *et al.* Food-dependent exercise-induced anaphylaxis: clinical and laboratory findings in 54 subjects. *Int Arch Allergy Immunol* 2001;125:264–72.

24 Silverstein SR, Frommer DA, Dobozin B, Rosen P. Celery dependent exercise-induced anaphylaxis. *J Emerg Med* 1986;4:195–9.

25 Dohi M, Suko M, Sugiyama H, *et al.* Food-dependent exercise induced anaphylaxis: a study on eleven Japanese cases. *J Allergy Clin Immunol* 1992;87:34–40.

26 Anibarro B, Domiguez C, Diaz JM, *et al.* Apple-dependent exercise-induced anaphylaxis. *Allergy* 1994;49:482.

27 Munoz MF, Lopez CJM, Villas F, *et al.* Exercise-induced anaphylactic reaction to hazel-nut. *Allergy* 1994;49:314–16.

28 Aihara Y, Kotoyori T, Takahashi Y, *et al.* The necessity for dual food intake to provoke food-dependent exercise-induced anaphylaxis (FEIAn): a case report of FEIAn with simultaneous intake of wheat and umeboshi. *J Allergy Clin Immunol* 2001;107:1100–5.

29 Guinnepain MT, Eliot C, Raffard M, *et al.* Exercise-induced anaphylaxis: useful screening of food sensitization. *Ann Allergy Asthma Immunol* 1996;77:491–6.

30 Kidd JM, Cohen SH, Sosman AL, Fink JN. Food-dependent exercise induced anaphylaxis. *J Allergy Clin Immunol* 1983;71:407–11.

31 Biederman T, Schopf P, Rueff F, Przybilla B. Exertion-induced anaphylaxis after eating pork and beef. *Dtsch Med Wochenschr* 1999;124:456–8.

32 Novey HS, Fairshter RD, Salness K, *et al.* Postprandial exercise-induced anaphylaxis. *J Allergy Clin Immunol* 1983;71:498–504.

33 Fiocchi A, Mirri GP, Santini I, *et al.* Exercise-induced anaphylaxis after food contaminant ingestion in double-blinded, placebo-controlled, food-exercise challenge. *J Allergy Clin Immunol* 1997;100:424–5.

34 Figueroa J, Blanco C, Dumpierrez AG, *et al.* Mustard allergy confirmed by double-blind placebo-controlled food challenges: clinical features and cross-reactivity with mugwort pollen and plant-derived foods. *Allergy* 2005;60:48–55.

35 Longo G, Barbi E, Puppin F. Exercise-induced anaphylaxis to snails. *Allergy* 2000;55:513–14.

36 Senna G, Mistrello G, Roncarlo D, *et al.* Exercise-induced anaphylaxis to grape. *Allergy* 2001;56:1235–6.

37 Garcia-Ara MC, Sanchez AV, Boyano Martinez MT, *et al.* Cow's milk-dependent, exercise-induced anaphylaxis: case report of a patient with previous allergy to cow's milk. *J Allergy Clin Immunol* 2003;111:647–8.

38 Pauls JD, Cross D. Food-dependent exercise-induced anaphylaxis to corn. *J Allergy Clin Immunol* 1998;101:853–4.

39 Fiedler EM, Zuberbier T, Worm M. A combination of wheat-flour, ethanol and food additives inducing FDEIA. *Allergy* 2002;57:1090–1.

40 Kutting B, Brehler R. Exercise-induced anaphylaxis. *Allergy* 2000;55:585–6.

41 Perez-Pimiento AJ, Moneo I, Santaolalla M, *et al.* Anaphylactic reaction to young garlic. *Allergy* 1999;54:626–9.

42 Porcel S, Sanchez AB, Rodriguez E, *et al.* Food-dependent exercise-induced anaphylaxis to pistachio. *J Investig Allergol Clin Immunol* 2006;16:71–3.

43 Hanakawa Y, Tohyama M, Shirakata Y, *et al.* Food-dependent exercise-induced anaphylaxis: a case related to the amount of food allergen ingested. *Br J Dermatol* 1998;138:898–900.

44 Palosuo K, Alenius H, Varjonen E, *et al.* Rye-gamma-70 and gamma-35 secalins and barley gamma-3 hordein cross-react with omega-5 gliadian, a major allergen in wheat-dependent exercise-induced anaphylaxis. *Clin Exp Allergy* 2001;31:466–73.

45 Dreborg S. Food allergy in pollen-sensitive patients. *Ann Allergy* 1988;61:41–6.

46 Harada S, Horikawa T, Ashida M, *et al.* Aspirin enhances the induction of type I allergic symptoms when combined with food and exercise in patients with food-dependent exercise-induced anaphylaxis. *Br J Dermatol* 2001;145:336–9.

47 Aihara M, Miyazawa, Osuna H, *et al.* Food-dependent exercise-induced anaphylaxis: influence of concurrent aspirin administration on skin testing and provocation. *Br J Dermatol* 2002; 146:466–72.

48 Dohi M, Suki M, Sugiyama H, *et al.* 3 cases of food-dependent exercise-induced anaphylaxis in which aspirin intake exacerbated anaphylactic symptoms. *Arerugi* 1990;39:1598–604.

49 Varjonen E, Vainio E, Kalimo K. Life-threatening, recurrent anaphylaxis caused by allergy to gliadin and exercise. *Clin Exp Allergy* 1997;27:162–6.

50 Paluoso K. Update on wheat hypersensitivity. *Curr Opin Allergy Clin Immunol* 2003;205–9.

51 Foreman JC, Piotrowski W. Peptides and histamine release. *J Allergy Clin Immunol* 1984;74:127–31.

52 Miadonna A, Tedeschi A, Leggieri E, *et al.* Activity of substance P on human skin and nasal airways. *Ann Allergy* 1988; 61:220–3.

53 Wallengren J, Moller H, Ekman R. Occurrence of substance PI vasoactive intestinal peptide, and calcitonin gene-related peptide in dermographism and cold urticaria. *Arch Dermatol Res* 1987;279:512–15.

54 Tharp MD, Thirlby R, Sullivan TJ. Gastrin induces histamine release from human cutaneous mast cells. *J Allergy Clin Immunol* 1984;74:159–65.

55 Kivity S, Ephraim S, Greif J, *et al.* The effect of food and exercise on the skin response to compound 48/80 in patients with food associated exercise induced urticaria angioedema. *J Allergy Clin Immunol* 1988;81:1155–8.

56 Errington G, Mekori Y, Silvers W, Schocket A. Altered mast cell threshold in exercise-induced anaphylaxis. *J Allergy Clin Immunol* 1985;75:193.

57 Lin RY, Barnard M. Skin testing with food, codeine, and histamine in exercise-induced anaphylaxis. *Ann Allergy* 1993;70:475–8.

58 Matsuo H, Morimoto K, Akaki T, *et al.* Exercise and aspirin increase levels of circulating gliadin peptides in patients with

wheat-dependent exercise-induced anaphylaxis. *Clin Exp Allergy* 2005;35:461–6.

59 Pals KL, Chang RT, Ryan AJ, *et al*. Effect of running intensity on intestinal permeability. *J Appl Physiol* 1997;82:571–6.

60 Ryan AJ, Chang RT, Gisolfi CV. Gastrointestinal permeability following aspirin intake and prolonged running. *Med Sci Sports Exerc* 1996;28:698–705.

61 Otte JA, Oostveen E, Geelkerken RH, *et al*. Exercise induces gastric ischemia in healthy volunteers: a tonometric study. *J Appl Physiol* 2001;91:866–71.

62 Matsuo H, Kohno K, Niihara H, *et al*. Specific IgE determination to epitope peptides of omega-5 gliadin and high molecular weight glutenin is a useful tool for diagnosis of wheat-dependent exercise-induced anaphylaxis. *J Immunol* 2005;175:8116–22.

63 Battais F, Mothes T, Moneret-Vautirn DA, *et al*. Identification of IgE binding epitopes on gliadins for patients with food allergy to wheat. *Allergy* 2005;60:815–21.

64 Mathison DA, Lumry WR, Stevenson DD, *et al*. Aspirin in chronic urticaria and/or angioedema: studies of sensitivity and desensitization. *J Allergy Clin Immunol* 1982;69:135.

65 Somasundaram S, Hayllar H, Rafi S, *et al*. The biochemical basis of non-steroidal anti-inflammatory drug-induced damage to the gastro-intestinal tract: a review and a hypothesis. *Scand J Gastroenterol* 1995;30:289–99.

66 Tilles S, Schocket A, Milgrom H. Exercise-induced anaphylaxis related to specific foods. *J Pediatr* 1995;127:587–9.

67 Fujimoto S, Kurihara N, Hirata K, *et al*. Successful prophylaxis of wheat-dependent exercise-induced anaphylaxis with terfenadine. *Intern Med* 1995;34:654–6.

68 Juji F, Suko M. Effectiveness of disodium cromoglycate in food-dependent, exercise-induced anaphylaxis: a case report. *Ann Allergy* 1994;72:452–4.

69 Dessanges J, Prefaut C, Taytard A, *et al*. The effect of zafirlukast on repetitive exercise-induced bronchoconstriction: the possible role of leukotrienes in exercise-induced refractoriness. *J Allergy Clin Immunol* 1999;104:1155–61.

70 Pearlman DS, van Adelsberg J, Philip G, *et al*. Onset and duration of protection against exercise-induced bronchoconstriction by a single oral dose of montelukast. *Ann Allergy Asthma Immunol* 2006;97:98–104.

71 Noma T, Yoshigawa I, Ogawa N, *et al*. Fatal buckwheat dependent exercise-induced anaphylaxis. *Asian Pac J Allergy Immunol* 2001;19:283–6.

72 Kalz M, Bower C, Prichard H. Delayed and persistent dermographia. *Arch Dermatol Syph* 1950;61:772–80.

73 Baughman RD, Jillson OE. Seven specific types of urticaria: with special reference to delayed persistent dermographism. *Ann Allergy* 1963;21:248–55.

74 Ryan TJ, Shim-Young N, Turk JL. Delayed pressure urticaria. *Br J Dermatol* 1968;80:485–90.

75 Warin R, Champion RH. *Urticaria*. London: WB Saunders, 1974.

76 Sussman GL, Harvey RP, Schocket AL. Delayed pressure urticaria. *J Allergy Clin Immunol* 1982;70:337–42.

77 Czarnetzki B. *Urticaria*. Berlin: Springer-Verlag, 1986.

78 Czarnetzki B, Meentken J, Rosenbach T, Pokropp A. Clinical, pharmacological and immunological aspects of delayed pressure urticaria. *Br J Dermatol* 1984;111:315–23.

79 Dover JS, Black AK, Ward AM, Greaves MW. Delayed pressure urticaria: clinical features, laboratory investigations, and response therapy of 44 patients. *J Am Acad Dermatol* 1988;18:1289–98.

80 Lawlor F, Kobza Black A. Delayed pressure urticaria. *Immunol Allergy Clin North Am* 2004;24:247–58.

81 Estes SA, Yung CW. Delayed pressure urticaria: an investigation of some parameters of lesion induction. *Am Acad Dermatol* 1981;5:25–31.

82 Davis K, Mekori Y, Kohler P, Schocket A. Late cutaneous reactions in patients with delayed pressure urticaria. *J Allergy Clin Immunol* 1984;73:810–12.

83 Czarnetzki B, Meentken J, Kolde G, Brocket E. Morphology of the cellular infiltrate in delayed pressure urticaria. *J Am Acad Dermatol* 1985;12:253–9.

84 Mekori Y, Dobozin B, Schocket A, *et al*. Delayed pressure urticaria histologically resembles cutaneous late-phase reactions. *Arch Dermatol* 1988;124:230–5.

85 Barlow RJ. Diagnosis and incidence of delayed pressure urticaria in patients with chronic urticaria. *J Am Acad Derm* 1999;29:954–8.

86 Hermes B, Prochazka AK, Haas N, *et al*. Upregulation of TNF-alpha and IL-3 expression in lesional and uninvolved skin in different types of urticaria. *J Allergy Clin Immunol* 1999;103:307–14.

87 Doeglas H. Reactions to asprin and food additives inpatients with chronic urticaria, including the physical urticarias. *Br J Dermatol* 1975;93:135–44.

88 Murdoch RD, Pollock L, Young E. Effects of food additives on leukocyte histamine release in normal and urticaria subjects. *J Roy Coll Phys Lond* 1987;21:251–6.

89 Kontou-Fili K, Maniatakou G, Paleologos G, Atom K. Cetrizine inhibits delayed pressure urticaria (part 2): skin biopsy findings. *Ann Allergy* 1990;65:520–2.

90 Kontou-Fili K, Maniatakou G, Demaka P, *et al*. Therapeutic effects of cetrizine in delayed pressure urticaria (part 1): effects on weight tests and skin window cytology. *Ann Allergy* 1990;65:517–19.

91 Chu TK, Warren MS. Zafirlukast (Accolate) in the treatment of chronic idiopathic urticaria – a case series. *J Allergy Clin Immunol* 1998;101:s155.

92 Spector S, Tan TA. Leukotrienes in chronic urticaria. *J Allergy Clin Immunol* 1998;101:572.

93 Ellis MH. Successful treatment of chronic urticaria with leukotriene antagonists. *J Allergy Clin Immunol* 1998;102:876–7.

94 Berkun Y, Shalit M. Successful treatment of delayed pressure urticaria with montelukast. *Allergy* 2000;55:203–4.

95 Nettis E, Pannofino A, Cavallo E. Efficacy of montelukast, in combination with loratadine, in the treatment of delayed pressure urticaria. *J Allergy and Clin Immunol* 2003;112:212–13.

96 Kalogeromitros D, Kempuraj D, Katsorou-Katsari A. Theophylline as "add-on" therapy in patients with delayed pressure urticaria: prospective self-controlled study. *Int J Immunopathol Pharmacol* 2005;18:595–602.

97 Engler RJ, Squire E, Benson P. Chronic sulfasalazine therapy in the treatment of delayed pressure urticaria and angioedema. *Ann Allergy Asthma Immunol* 1995;74:155–9.

98 Vena GA, Cassano N, D'Argento, *et al*. Clobetasol propionate 0.05% in a novel foam formulation is safe and effective in the short-term treatment of patients with delayed pressure urticaria: a randomized, double-blind, placebo-controlled trial. *Br J Dermatol* 2006;154:353–6.

99 Barlow R, Macdonald DM. The effects of topical corticosteroids on delayed pressure urticaria. *Arch Dermatol Res* 1995;287:285–8.

100 Dawn G, Urcelay M, Ah-Weng A, *et al*. Effect of high-dose intravenous immunoglobulin in delayed pressure urticaria. *Br J Dermatol* 2003;149:836–40.

101 Koranda FC. Antimalarials. *J Am Acad Dermatol* 1981;4:650–5.

102 Lopez LR, Davis KC, Kohler PF, Schocket AL. The hypocomplementemic urticarial-vasculitis syndrome: therapeutic response to hydroxychloroquine. *J Allergy Clin Immunol* 1984;73:600–3.

103 Loria MP, Dambra PP, D'Oronzio L, *et al*. Cyclosporin A in patients affected by chronic idiopathic urticaria: a therapeutic alternative. *Immunopharmacol Immunotoxicol* 2001;23:205–13.

104 Boehm I, Bauer R, Bieber T. Urticaria treated with dapsone. *Allergy* 1999;54:765–6.

105 Nurnberg W, Grabbe J, Czarnetzki BM. Urticarial vasculitis syndrome effectively treated with dapsone and pentoxifylline. *Acta Derm Venereol* 1995;75:54–6.

106 Gach JE, Sabroe RA, Greaves MW, Kobza-Black A. Methotrexate-responsive chronic idiopathic urticaria: a report of two cases. *Br J Dermatol* 2001;145:340–3.

107 Parsad D, Pandhi R, Juneja A. Stanozolol in chronic urticaria: a double-blinded placebo controlled trial. *J Dermatol* 2001;28:299–302.

108 Kessel A, Bamberger E, Toubi E. Tacrolimus in the treatment of severe chronic idiopathic urticaria: an open-label prospective study. *J Am Acad Dermatol* 2005;52:145–8.

109 Davis K, Mekori Y, Kohler P, Schocket A. Possible role of diet in delayed pressure urticaria – preliminary report. *J Allergy Clin Immunol* 1986;77:566–9.

110 Rajka P, Mork NJ. Clinical observations of the mechanisms of delayed pressure urticaria. In: Chamion RH, Greaves MW, Black AK, Pye RJ (eds.) *The Urticarias*. New York: Churchill Livingstone, 1985:191–3.

111 Czarnetzki B, Cap H, Forck G. Late cutaneous reactions to common allergens in patients with delayed pressure urticaria. *Br J Dermatol* 1987;117:695–701.

112 Vidal C, Moreno E, Rodriguez M, *et al*. Delayed pressure urticaria and egg allergy. *Int J Dermatol* 1991;30:674.

113 Zuberbier T, Bohm M, Czarnetzki B. Food intake in combination with a rise in body temperature: a newly identifiable cause of angioedema. *J Allergy Clin Immunol* 1993;91:1226–7.

APPENDIX

Allergen Avoidance Handouts

Wheat avoidance

All manufactured food products that contain wheat as an ingredient are required by US law to *list the word "Wheat" on the product label*. The law states that any species in the genus *Triticum* is considered wheat.

The following ingredients should be avoided when eliminating wheat from the diet:

Bread crumbs
Bulgur
Cereal extract
Couscous
Durum, durum flour, durum wheat
Emmer
Einkorn
Farina
Flour (all wheat types such as all purpose, cake, enriched, graham, high protein or high gluten, pastry)
Kamut
Semolina
Spelt
Sprouted wheat
Triticale
Vital wheat gluten
Wheat (bran, germ, gluten, grass, malt, starch)
Whole-wheat berries

• Wheat may be found in ale, baking mixes, baked products, batter-fried foods, beer, breaded foods, breakfast cereals, candy, crackers, frankfurters and processed meats, ice cream products, salad dressings, sauces, soups, soy sauce, and surimi. *Please read product labels carefully before purchasing or consuming any item.*
• The following flour substitutes are available and may be used by the wheat allergic child *if tolerated*: amaranth, arrowroot, buckwheat, corn, millet, oat, potato, rice, soybean, tapioca, and quinoa flour. *Please check with your doctor* before including these in your diet.

Source: Jaffe Food Allergy Institute, 2007.

Food Allergy: Adverse Reactions to Foods and Food Additives, 4th edition.
Edited by Dean D. Metcalfe, Hugh A. Sampson, and Ronald A. Simon.
© 2008 Blackwell Publishing, ISBN: 978-1-4501-5129-0.

Soy avoidance

All manufactured food products that contain soy as an ingredient are required by US law to *list the word "Soy" on the product label*.

The following ingredients indicate the presence of soy protein:

Edamame
Miso
Natto
Shoyu sauce
Soy (fiber, flour, grits, nuts, sprouts)
Soy (milk, yogurt, ice cream, cheese)
Soy protein (concentrate, hydrolyzed, isolate)
Soy sauce
Tamari
Tempeh
Textured vegetable protein
Tofu

• Soy protein may be found in numerous products such as breads, cookies, crackers, canned broth and soups, canned tuna and meat, breakfast cereals, high protein energy bars and snacks, low fat peanut butters, and processed meats. *Please read product labels carefully before purchasing or consuming any item.*
• Asian cuisines are considered high risk for individuals with soy allergy due to the common use of soy as an ingredient and the risk of cross-contamination even if a soy-free item is ordered.
• Studies show that most individuals with soy allergy may safely eat products containing soy oil and soy lecithin. Soy oil is exempt from US labeling laws.

Source: Jaffe Food Allergy Institute, 2007.

Peanut avoidance

All manufactured food products that contain peanut protein as an ingredient are required by US law to *list the word "Peanut" on the product label*.

The following ingredients indicate the presence of peanut protein:

Beer nuts
Ground nuts
Mixed nuts
Peanut (including peanut flour and peanut butter)

• Peanut protein is found in *Arachis* oil, cold pressed, expressed, expelled, and extruded peanut oils. Highly processed peanut oil has been shown to be safe for the vast majority of individuals allergic to peanut. As the degree of processing of commercial peanut oil may be difficult to determine, avoidance is prudent.

• Nu-Nuts® and other artificial flavored nuts contain peanut protein.

• Ethnic restaurants (such as Chinese, African, Indonesian, Thai, and Vietnamese), bakeries, and ice cream parlors are considered high risk for individuals with peanut allergy due to the common use of peanut and the risk of cross-contamination *even if a peanut-free item is ordered.*

• Peanut butter and/or peanut flour have been used in chili and spaghetti sauce as thickeners. Always ask if peanut was used in a recipe.

• Many candies and chocolates contain peanut or run the risk of cross-contact with peanut protein.

• Lupine or lupin is a legume that may cause an allergic reaction in those with peanut allergy. Lupine is used in this country in many gluten-free and high protein products. In many European countries (particularly Italy and France), lupine flour and or peanut flour may be mixed with wheat flour in baked goods.

• Many tree nuts are processed with peanuts and therefore may contain trace amounts of peanut protein. Extreme caution is advised.

• *Please read all product labels carefully before purchasing and consuming any item.*

Source: Jaffe Food Allergy Institute, 2007.

Egg avoidance

All manufactured food products that contain egg as an ingredient are required by US law to *list the word "Egg" on the product label.*

The following ingredients indicate the presence of egg protein:

Albumin
Egg (white, yolk, dried, powdered, solids)
Egg substitutes
Eggnog
Globulin
Lecithin
Lysozyme
Mayonnaise
Meringue
Ovalbumin
Ovovitellin

• Egg protein may be found in numerous products such as baked goods, breaded foods, cream fillings, custards, candies, canned soups, casseroles, frostings, ice creams, lollipops, marshmallows, marzipan, pastas, salad dressings, and meat-based dishes such as meatballs or meatloaf. *Please read product labels carefully before purchasing or consuming any item.*

• Egg whites and shells may also be used as a clarifying agent in soup stocks, consommés, wine, alcohol-based and coffee drinks.

• A shiny glazed or yellow colored baked good may indicate the presence of egg protein.

• For each egg, one of the following may be substituted in recipes:
  – 1 teaspoon baking powder, 1 tablespoon water and 1 tablespoon vinegar
  – 1 teaspoon yeast dissolved in ¼ cup warm water.
  – 1½ tablespoon water, 1½ tablespoon oil, and 1 teaspoon baking powder.
  – 1 packet gelatin and 2 tablespoon warm water (mix just prior to use).
  – 2 tablespoon fruit puree may be used for binding, but not leavening.

MMR vaccine

The American Academy of Pediatrics has stated that egg allergy is not a contraindication for the MMR vaccine. Several studies have indicated that the MMR vaccine can safely be administered to all patients with egg allergy.

Source: Jaffe Food Allergy Institute, 2007.

Tree nut avoidance

All manufactured food products that contain a tree nut as an ingredient are required by US law to *list the specific tree nut on the product label.*

The following common nuts are considered tree nuts under US law:

Almond
Brazil nut
Cashew
Chestnut
Filbert/hazelnut
Macadamia nut
Pecan
Pine nut (pignolia nut)
Pistachio
Walnut

The following are uncommon, additional tree nuts which require disclosure by US law; however, the risk of allergic reaction to these nuts is unknown:

Beech nut Butter nut Chinquapin Coconut Ginkgo Hickory Lychee nut Pili nut Shea nut

- Tree nut proteins may be found in cereals, crackers, cookies, candy, chocolates, energy bars, flavored coffee, frozen desserts, marinades, barbeque sauces, and some cold cuts, such as Mortadella. *Read product labels carefully before purchasing or consuming any item.*
- Tree nut protein will be found in foods such as gianduja (a creamy mixture of chocolate and chopped almonds and hazelnuts although other nuts may be used), marzipan (almond paste), nougat, Nu-Nuts® artificial nuts, pesto, and nut meal.
- Tree nut oils may contain nut protein and should be avoided.
- Ethnic restaurants (such as Chinese, African, Indian, Thai, and Vietnamese), ice cream parlors, and bakeries are considered high risk for individuals with tree nut allergy due to the common use of nuts and the risk of cross-contamination *even if a tree nut-free item is ordered.*
- Avoid natural extracts such as pure almond extract, and natural wintergreen extract (for the filbert/hazelnut allergy). Imitation or artificially flavored extracts are generally safe.
- The following are not considered nuts: nutmeg, water chestnuts, and butternut squash.
- Tree nut oils are sometimes used in lotions and soaps. Shea nut, not usually found in food products, is often used in lotions.
- Some alcoholic beverages may contain nut flavoring and should be avoided. These beverages are not currently regulated by the new labeling laws, therefore, it may be necessary to call the manufacturer to determine the safety of ingredients such as natural flavoring.

Source: Jaffe Food Allergy Institute, 2007.

Shellfish avoidance

All manufactured food products that contain crustacean shellfish as an ingredient are required by US law to *list the specific crustacean shellfish on the product label.*

Crustacean
Shrimp (prawns, crevette)
Lobster (langouste, langoustine, scampo, coral, tomalley)
Crab
Crawfish (crayfish, ecrevisse)

Mollusks are not considered major allergens under food labeling laws. They may not be fully disclosed on a product label.

Mollusks
Abalone
Clam
Cockle
Mussel
Oyster

Octopus
Scallop
Snail (escargot)
Squid (calamari)

The following ingredients may indicate the presence of shellfish protein:

Bouillabaisse
Fish stock
Flavoring
Seafood flavoring
Surimi

- Some sensitive individuals may react to aerosolized shellfish protein through cooking vapors.
- Fish and seafood restaurants are considered high risk due to the risk of cross-contamination even if a non-shellfish item is ordered.
- Carrageen is a marine algae, not a fish, and is considered safe for those avoiding fish and shellfish.

Please read all product labels carefully before purchasing and consuming any item.

Source: Jaffe Food Allergy Institute, 2007.

Milk avoidance

All manufactured food products that contain milk as an ingredient are required by US law to *list the word "Milk" on the product label.* Milk protein is found in all dairy products including milk, butter, cheese, cream, custard, yogurt, ice cream, and puddings.

The following ingredients indicate the presence of milk protein:

Artificial butter flavor, butter fat, and butter oil
Casein and caseinates (in all forms)
Cheese flavor
Curds
Ghee
Hydrolysates (casein, milk protein, protein, whey, whey protein)
Lactalbumin, lactalbumin phosphate, lactoglobulin, lactoferrin, lactulose
Nougat
Rennet, rennet casein
Recaldent™ (used in teeth-whitening chewing gums)
Simplesse®
Whey (in all forms)

- Milk protein may be found in numerous manufactured products such as many margarines, breads, cookies, cakes, chewing gum, cold cuts, crackers, cereals, non-dairy products, processed and canned meats, and frozen and refrigerated soy products. *Please read product labels carefully before purchasing or consuming any item.*

- Many frozen and refrigerated soy-based products are manufactured on dairy equipment and run the risk of cross-contact with milk protein.
- Sheep and goat's milk is not considered safe for those with cow's milk allergy as most cow's milk-allergic individuals are also allergic to goat's milk.
- Shellfish is occasionally dipped in milk as a preservative. Please ask if there is any risk of milk contact when purchasing shellfish.
- *Kosher dairy*: A "D" or the word "dairy" following the circled K or U on a product label indicates the presence of milk protein or a risk of milk protein contamination. These products should be avoided.
- *Kosher pareve*: A product labeled pareve is considered milk free under kosher dietary law. However, a food product may be considered pareve even if it contains a very small amount of milk protein – potentially enough to cause an allergic reaction in susceptible individuals. Do not assume pareve products are always safe.

Ingredients that *do not* contain milk are:
Cocoa butter, coconut milk, calcium lactate, calcium stearoyl lactylate, oleoresein, cream of tartar, sodium stearoyl lactylate, and lactic acid (although lactic acid starter culture may contain milk).

Nutrition
Milk is an important dietary source of protein, calcium, vitamin D, and vitamin B12. Please discuss a safe dietary alternative to cow's milk with your doctor or dietitian.
Source: Jaffe Food Allergy Institute, 2007.

Sesame avoidance

The following ingredients indicate the presence of sesame protein:

Sesame flour
Sesame oil
Sesame seeds
Sesame paste – tahini

Other foods that may contain the presence of sesame seed protein:

Bakery products such as breads, rolls, and bagels
Bread crumbs, breadings, and prepared breaded products
Breakfast cereals such as Granola, Muesli, and Kashi brand cereals
Snacks such as tortillas chips, pretzels, rice cakes, crackers, and Japanese snack mixes
High protein bars, energy bars, and low carbohydrate products
Salad dressings, spice mixes, and marinades

Exotic, ethnic, vegetarian and "natural" foods that commonly have sesame seed protein as an ingredient:

Baba Ghanoush
Falafel
Goma-dofu (Japanese custard)

Halvah
Hummus
Pasteli (Greek dessert)
Sushi
Vegetarian burgers
Japanese and Chinese dipping sauces and marinades

- Cross-contamination with sesame may occur in bakeries, bagel shops, and Chinese and Japanese restaurants.
- Some herbal drinks may contain sesame including Aqua Libra, a British herbal beverage.
- Sesame may also be used in soaps, cosmetics, creams, and massage oils where it may be listed as Sesamum Indicum.
Source: Jaffe Food Allergy Institute, 2007.

Index

Page numbers in *italics* represent figures; those in **bold** represent tables.